Review of Pathology

and Genetics

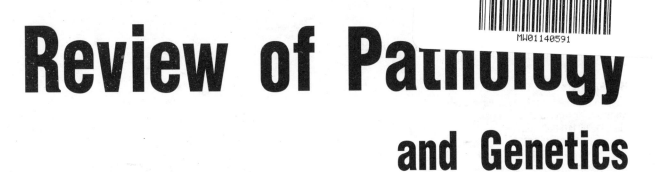

Seventh Edition

Free
Interactive DVD-ROM
(Contains Live Lecture
on Immunology)

Gobind Rai Garg MBBS MD
(Gold Medalist)
Ex-Assistant Professor (Pharmacology)
MAMC, Delhi, India
Director
Ayush Institute of Medical Sciences
Delhi, India

Sparsh Gupta MBBS MD
(Gold Medalist)
Assistant Professor (Pharmacology)
VMMC and Safdarjung Hospital, Delhi, India

JAYPEE *The Health Sciences Publisher*
New Delhi | London | Panama | Philadelphia

Jaypee Brothers Medical Publishers (P) Ltd

Headquarters

Jaypee Brothers Medical Publishers (P) Ltd
4838/24, Ansari Road, Daryaganj
New Delhi 110 002, India
Phone: +91-11-43574357
Fax: +91-11-43574314
Email: jaypee@jaypeebrothers.com

Overseas Offices

J.P. Medical Ltd
83, Victoria Street, London
SW1H 0HW (UK)
Phone: +44-20 3170 8910
Fax: +44 (0)20 3008 6180
Email: info@jpmedpub.com

Jaypee Medical Inc.
The Bourse
111, South Independence Mall East
Suite 835, Philadelphia, PA 19106, USA
Phone: +1 267-519-9789
Email: joe.rusko@jaypeebrothers.com

Jaypee Brothers Medical Publishers (P) Ltd
Bhotahity, Kathmandu, Nepal
Phone: +977-9741283608
Email: Kathmandu@jaypeebrothers.com

Jaypee-Highlights Medical Publishers Inc
City of Knowledge, Bld. 237, Clayton
Panama City, Panama
Phone: +1 507-301-0496
Fax: +1 507-301-0499
Email: cservice@jphmedical.com

Jaypee Brothers Medical Publishers (P) Ltd
17/1-B, Babar Road, Block-B, Shaymali
Mohammadpur, Dhaka-1207
Bangladesh
Mobile: +08801912003485
Email: jaypeedhaka@gmail.com

Website: www.jaypeebrothers.com
Website: www.jaypeedigital.com

Assistant Editors: **Mrs Praveen Kumari, Mrs Krishna Gupta**

Review of Pathology and Genetics

First Edition: 2009
Second Edition: 2010
Third Edition: 2011
Fourth Edition: 2012
Fifth Edition: 2013
Sixth Edition 2014
Seventh Edition **2015**

ISBN: 978-93-5152-867-8

Printed at: Sanat Printers

Dedicated to

My parents, wife Praveen,
son Ayush and other family members
— *Gobind Rai Garg*

My family members and
my teachers (Shri SK Suri and Mrs V Gopalan)

— *Sparsh Gupta*

Preface to the Seventh Edition

We acknowledge the support shown by each of our esteemed readers (present and past) for placing the book at the **numero uno position amongst the pathology books for PGMEE**. We are also highly grateful for the **wonderful response to the lecture DVD on immunology**. To meet the expectations of students, we have tried to further improve this seventh edition.

The book has been fully colored to increase its appeal to the esteemed readers. Along with this edition of the book, we are again providing a free lecture in the form of an **educational DVD**. We have intentionally chosen the topic of 'Immunology' because apart from being very important, it is considered as one of the most difficult chapters of Pathology. We hope that after viewing this DVD, immunology will no longer remain a difficult topic to comprehend.

Dear friends, the apprehension regarding the **National Eligibility Cum Entrance Test (NEET)** has now been taken care of as the examination pattern has not been modified drastically. Cracking the NEET exam and other important PG examinations require a thorough knowledge and understanding of the subject. Readers of this book have got an edge over others because of the strong theory and conceptual questions. This along with the key points given under the heading of various boxes in the chapters has helped many of you to get extremely good ranks in NEET 2013, 14 and 2015.

It is a humble request from our side that **all the chapters** (and not only general pathology) of this book has to be read by the student so as to maximise the benefit. This is because many additional concepts and questions asked frequently in the exam have been explained in systemic pathology chapters. This is one important point which came as a gist differentiating the people getting a good rank in NEET versus those who did not.

In our constant endeavour to improvise the book, there has been incorporation of important additions in almost all chapters along with the new section of **Most recent questions.** The question bank of the every chapter has been subdivided into smaller portions. It will help students to solve MCQs after reading the theory of a particular topic of a chapter.

For getting a grasp on the NEET questions in a better way, a new section in the end comprising of **Image Based Questions** has also been added.

In this seventh edition, we have added a **lot of diagrams** and **flow charts** to make learning interesting and easier. Another salient feature of this edition is the updating of **appropriate authentic references** from standard textbooks particularly in regard **to the controversial questions** so that reader gets all the relevant information under one roof. Other salient features of the current edition are:

- All references have been updated from **Robbins 9th edition**
- The *question bank has been expanded* and includes the most recent questions
- *More color plates* for image based questions have been added
- A summary of important information added in **Robbins 9th edition** has been mentioned separately at the end of each chapter.

We have fully revised the book and corrected the typographical and some other errors present in the previous editions. We have also added plenty of vital information under the heading of 'Concept', 'Info' and 'Subject Links' at multiple places in almost all the chapters in the book. Further, we have also expanded some of the old topics.

Questions from latest entrance examinations of AIIMS have been added. Several other questions have been incorporated from PGI, DNB and other state PG entrance examinations. In some topics, there are contradictions between different books. In such a situation, we have quoted the text from Harrison's Principles of Internal Medicine, 18th edition.

To help the students to understand the subject better, **Dr Gobind** has started **Ayush Institute of Medical Sciences**. Any query regarding the admission in the same maybe addressed to Dr Gobind at the under mentioned e-mail ID.

We must admit hereby that despite keeping an eagle's eye for any inaccuracy regarding factual information or typographical errors, some mistakes must have crept in inadvertently. You are requested to communicate these errors and send your valuable suggestions for the improvement of this book. Your suggestions, appreciation and criticism are most welcome.

April 2015

Gobind Rai Garg
Sparsh Gupta

E-mail: gobind_garg@yahoo.co.in
healing_sparsh@yahoo.co.in

Preface to the First Edition

Pathology is one of the most difficult and at the same time most important subject in various postgraduate entrance examinations.

As we experienced it ourselves, most of the students preparing for postgraduate entrance examinations are in a dilemma, whether to study antegrade or retrograde. Antegrade study takes a lot of time and due to bulky textbooks, some important questions are likely to be missed. In a retrograde study, the students are likely to answer the frequently asked MCQs but new questions are not covered. We have tried to overcome the shortcomings of both of the methods while keeping the advantages intact.

In this book, we have given a concise and enriched text in each chapter followed by MCQs from various postgraduate entrance examinations and other important questions likely to come. The text provides the advantage of antegrade study in a short span of time.

After going through the book, it will be easier for the student to solve the questions of most recent examinations, which are given at the end of the book.

Eighth edition of Robbins is just to strike the Indian market. We have arranged this edition directly from US and added the references from its text. Further, important differences between 7th and 8th edition of Robbins have been mentioned with the relevant questions.

It is very difficult and at times very confusing to remember large number of pathological features. To make learning easy, several easy to grasp MNEMONICS have been given throughout the text.

Despite our best efforts, some mistakes might have crept in, which we request all our readers to kindly bring to our notice. Your suggestions, appreciation and criticism are most welcome.

Gobind Rai Garg
Sparsh Gupta

E-mail: gobind_garg@yahoo.co.in
healing_sparsh@yahoo.co.in

Acknowledgments

When emotions are profound, words sometimes are not sufficient to express our thanks and gratitude. With these few words, we would like to thank our teachers at University College of Medical Sciences and Guru Teg Bahadur Hospital, Delhi, for the foundation they helped to lay in shaping our careers.

We are especially thankful to Dr KK Sharma, Ex-Professor and Head, Department of Pharmacology, UCMS, Delhi who has been a father-figure to whole of the department. Prof CD Tripathi, (Director-Professor and Head, VMMC and Safdarjung Hospital).

We would also like to acknowledge the encouragement and guidance of Prof CD Tripathi, (Director Professor and Head, Pharmacology, VMMC and Safdarjung Hospital), Dr SK Bhattacharya (Professor and Head, Hindu Rao Hospital), Dr Uma Tekur (Director Professor, MAMC), Col (Dr) AG Mathur (Professor, ACMS), Dr Vandana Roy (MAMC) and Dr Shalini Chawla (MAMC), all professors in the department of Pharmacology, in the completion of this book.

We feel immense pleasure in conveying our sincere thanks to all the residents of department of Pharmacology at VMMC, MAMC and ACMS for their indispensable help and support.

No words can describe the immense contribution of our parents, Ms Praveen Garg, Ms Ruhee, Mr Nitin Misra, Ms Dhwani Gupta, Mr Rohit Singla and Mrs Komal Singla, without whose support this book could not have seen the light of the day.

We want to extend our special thanks to Dr Sonal Aggarwal (ESI Hospital, Delhi) and Dr Raina SG (AIIMS, Delhi) for their unconditional support in the making of this edition.

We would also like to extend our special thanks to Dr Sonal Pruthi (UCMS, Delhi), Dr Smiley M Gupta (Kerala), Dr Saurabh Jain (TSMA, Tver, Russia), Dr Amrita Talwar (ACMS, Delhi), Dr Avinash A, Dr Nikita Mary Baby, Dr Mamta Nikhurpa, Dr Rihas Mohammed, Dr Anuradha Tiwari (ACMS, Delhi) and Dr Sandeep Goel (MD Radiodiagnosis, AIIMS).

Although it is impossible to acknowledge the contribution of all individually, we extend our heartfelt thanks to:

- Dr Bhupinder Singh Kalra, Assistant Professor (Pharmacology), MAMC, Delhi
- Lt Col (Dr) Dick BS Brashier, Associate Professor (Pharmacology), AFMC, Pune
- Lt Col (Dr) Sushil Sharma, Associate Professor (Pharmacology), AFMC, Pune
- Lt Col (Dr) Dahiya, Associate Professor (Pharmacology), AFMC, Pune
- Dr Nitin Jain, DCH, DNB (Pediatrics, Std), Delhi
- Dr Sushant Verma, MS (General Surgery), MAMC, Delhi
- Dr Kapil Dev Mehta, MD (Pharmacology), UCMS, Delhi
- Dr Saurabh Arya, MD (Pharmacology), UCMS, Delhi
- Dr Deepak Marwah, MD (Pediatrics), MAMC, Delhi
- Dr Shubh Vatsya, MD (Medicine), MAMC, Delhi
- Mr Rajesh Sharma, MBA
- Dr Puneet Dwivedi DA (Std), Hindu Rao Hospital, Delhi
- Dr Sandeep Agnihotri, DVD, Safdarjung Hospital, Delhi
- Dr Harsh Vardhan Gupta MD, Pediatrics (Std), Patiala
- Mr Tarsem Garg, LLB, DM, SBOP
- Dr Pardeep Bansal, MD (Radiodiagnosis), UCMS, Delhi
- Dr Pankaj Bansal, MS (Orthopedics), RML Hospital, Delhi
- Dr Pradeep Goyal, MD (Radiodiagnosis), LHMC, Delhi
- Dr Rakesh Mittal, MS (Surgery), Safdarjung Hospital, Delhi
- Dr Amit Miglani, DM (Gastroenterology), PGI, Chandigarh
- Dr Sachin Gupta DA, DMC (Ludhiana)
- Dr Reenu Gupta DGO BMC (Bangalore)
- Dr Shiv Narayan Goel, MCh (Urology), KEM, Mumbai

- Dr Kamal Jindal, Assistant Professor (Physiology), LHMC, Delhi
- Dr Gaurav Jindal, MD, Radiodiagnosis Resident, Boston, USA
- Dr Saket Kant, MD (Medicine UCMS), DM (Endocrinology, BHU)
- Dr Mukesh Kr Joon, DM (Cardiology), Udaipur, Rajasthan
- Dr Amit Garg, Assistant Professor (Psychiatry), IHBAS, Delhi
- Dr Garima Mahajan, MD (Pathology), UCMS, Delhi
- Dr Ravi Gupta, MD (Psychiatry), Jolly Grants Medical College, Dehradun, Uttarakhand
- Dr Shashank Mohanty, MD (Medicine), Udaipur, Rajasthan
- Dr Amit Shersia, MS (Orthopedics), MAMC, Delhi
- Dr Mohit Gupta, DCP, DNB (Pathology), Delhi
- Dr Mayank Dhamija, DCH, DNB (Pediatrics), DNB (Hemato-oncology), Delhi

Last but not the least, we would like to thank Shri Jitendar P Vij (Group Chairman), M/s Jaypee Brothers Medical Publishers (P) Ltd, New Delhi, India, publishers of this book and the entire PGMEE team, for their keen interest, innovative suggestions and hardwork in bringing out this edition.

April 2015

Gobind Rai Garg
Sparsh Gupta

From the Publisher's Desk
We request all the readers to provide us their
valuable suggestions/errors (if any)
at: *jppgmee@gmail.com*
so as to help us in further improvement of this book in the subsequent edition

References

- Robbin's Pathological Basis of Diseases, 9th edition
- Harsh Mohan's Textbook of Pathology, 7th edition
- Harrison's Principles of Internal Medicine, 18th edition
- Current Medical Diagnosis and Treatment 2015
- Wintrobe's Clinical Hematology, 12th edition
- Ackerman's Surgical Pathology, 10th edition
- Sternberg's Diagnostic Surgical Pathology, 5th edition

SYMBOLS USED IN BOXES ON 'HIGH YIELD POINTS'

- **Key points**
- **Definition**
- **Mnemonic**
- **Concept**

- **Questions asked in most recent exam**

Contents

CELL AS A UNIT OF HEALTH AND DISEASE

- **Virchow** coined the term 'cellular pathology'
- **The human genome** contains roughly **3.2 billion DNA base pairs** and only about 2% is used for coding of proteins.
- **80% of the human genome either binds proteins,** implying it is involved in regulating gene expression, or can be assigned some functional activity, mostly related to the regulation of gene expression, often in a cell-type specific fashion.
- The **two most common forms** of **DNA variation** in the **huxivxiiiman genome** are *single-nucleotide polymorphisms (SNPs) and copy number variations (CNVs).*
- **SNPs** are variants at single nucleotide positions and are almost always biallelic (i.e., only two choices exist at a given site within the population, such as A or T).
- **CNVs** are a more recently identified form of genetic variation consisting of different numbers of large contiguous stretches of DNA from 1000 base pairs to millions of base pairs.
- Epigenetics is defined as heritable changes in gene expression that are not caused by alterations in DNA sequence.
- Nuclear chromatin exists in two basic forms:

> 1. Cytochemically dense and transcriptionally inactive heterochromatin and
> 2. Cytochemically dispersed and transcriptionally active euchromatin

- Different histone modifications are generically called as *marks*. The modifications include methylation, acetylation, or phosphorylation of specific amino acid residues on the histones.

Gene regulation can also be done through noncoding RNAs which can be of the following subtypes:

a. *MicroRNAs* (miRNA): The miRNAs are small RNA molecules 22 nucleotides in length which do not encode proteins. They function primarily to modulate the translation of target mRNAs into their corresponding proteins.
b. *Long noncoding RNAs* (lncRNA): RNAs are >200 nucleotides in length. Its example includes **XIST**, which is transcribed from the X chromosome and plays an essential role in *physiologic X chromosome inactivation.*

MiRNA associated with cancers are called oncomiRs. They act by increasing the number of cancer causing genes and suppress the tumor suppressor genes.

The non coding RNAs fall into several classes:

- **Piwi-interacting RNAs** (piRNAs), the most common type of small noncoding RNA, which (like miRs) are believed to have a role in post-transcriptional gene silencing;
- **Sno RNAs**, which are important in maturation of rRNA and the assembly of ribosomes; and
- **Long intervening noncoding RNAs (lincRNAs)**, some of which regulate the activity of chromatin "writers," the factors that modify histones and thereby control gene expression

CELLULAR HOUSEKEEPING (as per 9th edition of Robbins)

Organelles	Key points
Mitochondria	Oxidative phosphorylation Intermediates for heme synthesis Intrinsic pathway of Apoptosis (programmed cell death)
Smooth endoplasmic reticulum (SER)	Abundant in gonads and liver Used for lipoprotein and steroid hormone synthesis, Required for converting the hydrophobic compounds like drugs into water-soluble molecules Sequestration of calcium
Proteasomes	Required for selectively chewing of denatured proteins using ubiquitin. Also needed for presentation of peptides in context of the class I major histocompatibility molecules
Peroxisomes	Breakdown of fatty acids

Contd...

Contd...

Organelles	Key points
Plasma membrane proteins	Phosphatidylinositol serves as scaffold for intracellular proteins as well as for the generation of intracellular second signals like diacylglycerol and inositol trisphosphate. Phosphatidylserine is required for apoptosis (programmed cell death) and on platelets, it serves as a cofactor in the clotting of blood. Glycolipids are important in cell-cell and cell-matrix interactions, including inflammatory cell recruitment and sperm-egg interactions.
Lysosomes	Most cytosolic enzymes prefer to work at pH 7.4 whereas lysosomal enzymes function best at pH 5 or less.
Golgi apparatus	Mannose 6 phosphateQ is the marker

- *Channel proteins* create hydrophilic pores, which, when open, permit *rapid movement* of solutes (usually restricted by size and charge)
- *Carrier proteins* bind their specific solute and undergo a series of conformational changes to transfer the ligand across the membrane; their transport is relatively *slow*.

- Exocytosis is the process by which large molecules are exported from cells. In this process, proteins synthesized and packaged within the RER and Golgi apparatus are concentrated in secretory vesicles, which then fuse with the plasma membrane and expel their contents.
- Transcytosis is the movement of endocytosed vesicles between the apical and basolateral compartments of cells. It is a mechanism for transferring large amounts of intact proteins across epithelial barriers.
- Potocytosis is literally "cellular sipping." whereas *pinocytosis* is "*cellular drinking*"
- Endocytosis is the uptake of fluids or macromolecules by the cell. It could be of the following types:
1. *Caveolae-mediated endocytosis:* **Caveolin**Q *is the major structural protein of caveole.* Internalization of caveolae with any bound molecules and associated extracellular fluid is sometimes called potocytosis—literally "cellular sipping."
2. *Pinocytosis and receptor mediated endocytosis: Pinocytosis* ("cellular drinking") describes a fluid-phase process during which the plasma membrane invaginates and is pinched off to form a cytoplasmic vesicle. *Receptor-mediated endocytosis* is the major uptake mechanism for certain macromolecules like **transferrin** and **low-density lipoprotein** (LDL).
- *Most cytosolic enzymes prefer to work at pH 7.4 whereas* **lysosomal enzymes** function best at **pH 5 or less.**

Cytoskeleton

The ability of cells to adopt a particular shape, maintain polarity, organize the relationship of intracellular organelles, and move about depends on the intracellular scaffolding of proteins called the cytoskeleton. The three major classes of cytoskeletal proteins are:
i. *Actin microfilaments* are 5- to 9-nm diameter fibrils formed from the **g**lobular protein actin (**G**-actin), the most abundant cytosolic protein in cells.
ii. *Intermediate filaments* are 10-nm diameter fibrils that impart tensile strength and allow cells to bear mechanical stress. The examples include:

- *Lamin A, B, and C:* nuclear lamina of all cells
- *Vimentin:* mesenchymal cells (fibroblasts, endothelium)
- *Desmin:* muscle cells, forming the scaffold on which actin and myosin contract
- *Neurofilaments:* axons of neurons, imparting strength and rigidity
- *Glial fibrillary acidic protein:* glial cells around neurons
- *Cytokeratins:* 30 different types are present, hence can be used as cell markers

Clinical significance!

Since they have characteristic tissue-specific patterns of expression, they are useful for assigning a cell of origin for poorly differentiated tumors.
iii. *Microtubules*: these are 25-nm-thick fibrils composed of non-covalently polymerized dimers of α- and β-tubulin arrayed in constantly elongating or shrinking hollow tubes with a defined polarity. Within cells, microtubules are required to move vesicles, organelles, or other molecules around cells along microtubules. There are two varieties of these motor proteins: kinesins (for anterograde transport) and dyneins (for retrograde transport).

Mitochondrial function: key points

- *Intermembrane space* in the mitochondria is the *chief site of ATP synthesis.*
- *Thermogenin* is an inner membrane protein which is used to generate heat by uncoupling electron transport chain with ATP generation. It is present in high concentration in brown fat and is useful to generate heat by *non-shivering thermogenesis*.
- **Warburg effect:** it is the phenomenon in which rapidly growing cells (both benign and malignant) upregulate **glucose and glutamine uptake** and decrease their production of ATP per glucose molecule. This is responsible for providing metabolic intermediates which are useful for cellular growth and maintenance.

Receptors

Cell-surface receptors are generally transmembrane proteins with extra cellular domains that bind soluble secreted ligands. They can be of the following types:
1. **Ion channels** (typically at the synapse between electrically excitable cells)
2. *G protein coupled receptors*: activate an associated GTP-binding regulatory protein
3. **Enzymatic receptors**: activate an associated enzyme usually tyrosine kinase
4. Receptors which trigger a proteolytic event or a change in protein binding or stability that activates a latent transcription factor. Examples include Notch, Wnt, and Hedgehog receptors which regulate normal development.

Transcription factors

- **MYC** and **JUN** are the transcription factors that regulate the expression of genes that are needed for **growth.**
- **p53** is a transcription factor that triggers the expression of genes that lead to **growth arrest.**

Summary of growth factors and the receptors

The major role of growth factors is to stimulate the activity of genes that are required for cell growth and cell division. They are also involved in the non-growth activities, including migration, differentiation, and synthetic capacity. Some important examples include:
a. **Epidermal Growth Factor and Transforming Growth Factor-α.**

The "EGF receptor family" includes four membrane receptors with intrinsic tyrosine kinase activity. The examples include *EGFR1 involved in lung cancer, head and neck, breast* etc. and the ERBB2 receptor (also known as HER2) *involved in breast cancer*

b. **Hepatocyte Growth Factor** (also known as **scatter factor**)

HGF acts as a morphogen in embryonic development, promotes cell migration and enhances hepatocyte survival. MET is the receptor for HGF, it has intrinsic tyrosine kinase activity and is frequently over-expressed or mutated in tumors, particularly *renal and thyroid papillary carcinomas*.

c. *Platelet-Derived Growth Factor*
   PDGF is stored in platelet granules and is released on platelet activation.
d. *Vascular Endothelial Growth Factor*

- *VEGF-A* is the **major** *angiogenic* **factor** (inducing blood vessel development) after injury and in tumors.
- VEGF-B and PlGF (placental growth factor) are involved in embryonic vessel development, and VEGF-C and -D stimulate both angiogenesis and lymphatic development (lymphangiogenesis).
- In adults, VEGFs are also involved in the maintenance of normal adult endothelium and not involved in angiogenesis.
- *Hypoxia is the most important inducer of VEGF production*.
- **VEGFR-2** is highly expressed in **endothelium** and is the **most important for angiogenesis.**
- Anti-VEGF antibodies are being used for a number of ophthalmic diseases including "wet" age-related macular degeneration, the angiogenesis associated with retinopathy of prematurity; and diabetic macular edema.

e. *Fibroblast Growth Factor* (FGF-7)
- *FGF-7* is also referred to as *keratinocyte growth factor* (KGF).
f. *Transforming Growth Factor-β*

TGF-β has multiple and often opposing effects depending on the tissue and concurrent signals. Agents with such multiplicity of effects are called pleiotropic.

- *TGF-β* is involved in *scar formation after injury*. It also drives fibrosis in lung, liver, and kidneys in conditions of chronic inflammation.
- *TGF-β* is an *anti-inflammatory cytokine* that serves to limit and terminate inflammatory responses.

Extracellular matrix

- *Laminin* is the most abundant glycoprotein in *basement membrane*
- The major constituents of basement membrane are amorphous **nonfibrillar type IV collagen** and **laminin.**
- **Collagens** are typically composed of three separate polypeptide chains braided into a ropelike **triple helixQ**.

CHAPTER 1

Cell Injury

Pathology is a science dealing with the study of diseases. Four important components of pathology are *etiology* (causative factors), *pathogenesis* (mechanism or process by which disease develops), *morphology* (appearance of cells, tissues or organs) and *clinical features*.

CELL INJURY

Disease occurs due to alteration of the functions of tissues or cells at the microscopic level. The various causes of cell injury include:

1. **Hypoxia:** It is the **most common cause of cell injury**. It results due to decrease in oxygen supply to the cells. Hypoxia may be caused by

    a. *Ischemia:* Results due to decrease in blood supply. It is the *most common cause of hypoxia*[Q]
    b. *Anemia:* Results due to decrease in oxygen carrying capacity of blood
    c. *Cardio-respiratory disease:* Results from decreased oxygenation of blood due to cardiac or respiratory disease.

2. **Physical Agents:** Cell injury may occur due to radiation exposure, pressure, burns, frost bite etc.
3. **Chemical Agents:** Many drugs, poisons and chemicals can result in cell injury.
4. **Infections:** Various infectious agents like bacteria, virus, fungus and parasites etc can cause cell injury.
5. **Immunological reactions:** These include hypersensitivity reactions and autoimmune diseases.
6. **Genetic causes:** Cell injury can also result due to derangement of the genes.
7. **Nutritional imbalance:** Cell injury can result due to deficiency of vitamins, minerals etc.

> **Hypoxia** is the most common cause of cell injury.

> **Ischemia** is the most common cause of hypoxia.

> **Neurons** are the **most sensitive** cells in the body. They are most commonly damaged due to global hypoxia.

Clinical Importance

At a the cellular level, the protective effect in mammalian cells against hypoxic injury is induction of a transcription factor called as hypoxia inducible factor 1 which promotes blood vessel formation, stimulates cell survival pathways and enhances anaerobic glycolysis. The only reliable clinical strategy to decrease ischemic brain and spinal cord injury is transient reduction of core body temperature to 92°F.

In response to injury, a cell/tissue can have following consequences:
- *Adaptation*: The cell changes its physiological functions in response to an injurious stimulus.
- *Reversible cell injury*
- *Irreversible cell injury.*

1. **REVERSIBLE CELL INJURY:** As already discussed, hypoxia is the most common cause of cell injury. Oxygen is an important requirement of mitochondria for the formation of ATP; therefore, hypoxia will result in **earliest involvement of mitochondria**[Q] resulting in decreased formation of ATP. All cellular processes requiring ATP for normal functioning will be affected. Important organelles affected are *cell membranes* (require ATP for functioning of Na⁺ - K⁺ pump), *endoplasmic reticulum* (require ATP for protein synthesis) *and nucleus.*

> *Concept*
>
> The only reliable clinical strategy to decrease ischemic brain and spinal cord injury is transient reduction of core body temperature to 92°F.

Cell Injury

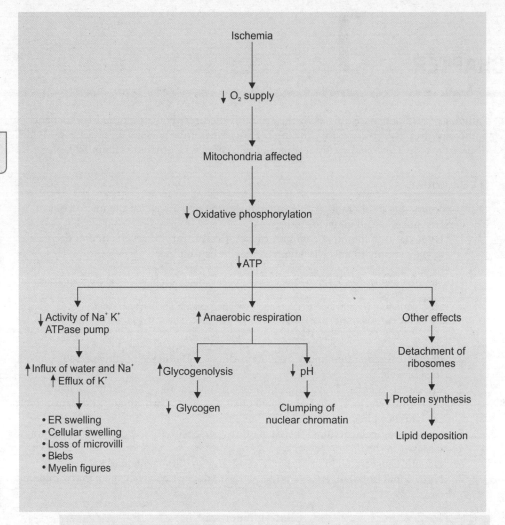

> **Mitochondria** is the *earliest organelle* affected in cell injury.

> **Hydropic change** or swelling of the cell due to increased water entry is the *earliest change* seen in reversible cell injury.

> **Pyknosis** is nuclear condensation
> **Karyorrhexis** is fragmentation of the nucleus.
> **Karyolysis** is nuclear dissolution

- *Swelling of organelles* like endoplasmic reticulum results in decreased protein synthesis
- *Bleb formation* results due to outpouching from the cell membrane to accommodate more water.
- *Loss of microvilli*
- Formation of *myelin figures* due to breakdown of membranes of cellular organelles like endoplasmic reticulum. These are composed of *phospholipids*[Q]. Myelin figures are intracellular whorls of laminated lipid material (resembling myelin of nerves). When these are present in membrane bound structures containing lysosomal enzymes, these are known as *myeloid bodies or myelinoid bodies.*

All the features discussed above are of reversible cell injury because if the injurious agent is removed at this point, cell can recover back to its normal state of functioning. However, if the stimulus continues, then irreversible cell injury ensues.

2. **IRREVERSIBLE CELL INJURY:** Features of irreversible cell injury include
   - **Damage to cell membrane:** It results due to continued influx of water, loss of membrane phospholipids and loss of protective amino acids (like glycine). Damage to cell membranes result in massive influx of calcium.
   - **Calcium influx:** Massive influx of Ca^{2+} results in the formation of *large flocculent mitochondrial densities* and activation of enzymes.
   - **Nuclear changes:** These are the most specific microscopic features of irreversible cell injury. These include: *Pyknosis, *Karyorrhexis and *Karyolysis.

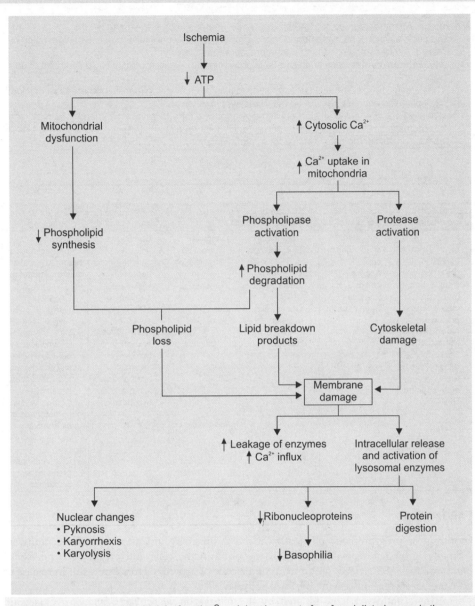

Inability to reverse mitochondrial dysfunction[Q] and development of profound disturbances in the membrane function characterize irreversibility[Q].

Irreversible cell injury may be necrosis or apoptosis (Programmed cell death)

Necrosis	Apoptosis
Always pathological	May be **physiological** or **pathological**
Associated with disruption of cellular homeostasis (e.g. ischemia, hypoxia & poisoning)	Important for development, homeostasis & elimination of pathogens & tumor cells
Affects contiguous (adjacent) group of cells	Affect single cells
Cell size is increased	Cell size is **shrunken**
Passive	**Active**
Causes inflammatory reaction	**No inflammatory** reaction
Plasma membrane is disrupted	Plasma membrane is **intact**
'Smear pattern' on electrophoresis	**Step ladder pattern** is seen

3

Mnemonic: Apoptosis can be considered as suicide whereas necrosis as murder. Like
- Murder is always done by someone else (i.e. pathological) whereas suicide can be committed by oneself (physiological) or due to undue pressure (pathological).
- A person can murder many people (affects group of cells) whereas suicide can be committed only by oneself (affect single cells).
- The person who is being killed doesn't need to plan or do anything (passive) whereas for suicide, lot of planning and effort has to be made (active process).
- When a person is being killed, he will make a lot of efforts to save himself and thus may lead to accumulation of other people or police (equivalent to inflammatory mediators coming there) whereas in suicide no help is called for (no-inflammation).

Concept

Liquefactive necrosis is seen in CNS specifically because there is **lack of extracellular architecture** in brain and the brain is **rich in liquefactive hydrolytic enzymes**.

Concept

Coagulative necrosis is associated with **'tomb stone'** appearance of affected tissue

Concept

Caseous necrosis is seen in **tuberculosis** and **systemic fungal infections** (like histoplasmosis) because of the presence of *high lipid content in the cell wall* in these organisms. So, there is cheese like appearance of the necrotic material.

Concept

In fibrinoid necrosis, there is no deposition of fibrin. Fibrinoid means the appearance of the necrotic material in this case is similar to fibrin. Due to inflammation seen in these conditions, there is increased vessel permeability which causes plasma proteins to be deposited in the vessel wall. The microscopic appearance is like fibrin but the actual composition is plasma proteins.

Type of neorosis

Coagulative necrosis	Liquefactive necrosis	Caseous necrosis	Fat necrosis	Fibrinoid necrosis	Gangrenous necrosis
– Most common^Q type of necrosis – Loss of nucleus with the cellular outline being preserved – Associated with ischemia – Seen in organs (heart, liver, kidney etc.) **except BRAIN^Q.**	– Enzymatic destruction of cells – Abscess formation – Pancreatitis – Seen in **brain**	– Combination of coagulative and liquefactive necrosis – Characteristic of **TB^Q** – Cheese like appearance of the necrotic material.	– Action of lipases on fatty tissue – Seen in breast, omentum and pancreatitis^Q	– Complexes of antigens and antibodies are deposited in vessel wall with leakage of fibrinogen out of vessels – Seen in PAN^Q Aschoff bodies^Q (in rheumatic heart disease) and malignant hypertension^Q.	(Surgically used term; necrosis of tissue with super-added putrefaction) – Dry gangrene is similar to coagulative necrosis – Wet gangrene is similar to liquefactive necrosis and is due to secondary infection – Noma is gangrenous lesion of vulva or mouth (cancrum oris) – Fournier's gangrene is seen in scrotum

APOPTOSIS

Apoptosis or programmed cell death can be induced by intrinsic or extrinsic pathway. Normally, growth factors bind to their receptors in the cells and prevent the release of *cytochrome C and SMAC*. So, withdrawal or absence of growth factors can result in release of these mediators and initiate the intrinsic pathway.

Intrinsic pathway: It is initiated by the release of *cytochrome C and SMAC* (second mitochondrial activator of caspases) from the *mitochondrial inter-membrane* space. Upon release into the cytoplasm, cytochrome C associates with dATP, procaspase-9 and APAF-1 (apoptosis activating factor -1) leading to sequential activation of caspase-9 and effector caspases {Caspases- 3 and -7}. On the other hand, upon release, SMAC binds and blocks the function of IAPs (Inhibitor of Apoptosis Proteins). Normally, IAPs are responsible for causing the blocking the activation of caspases and keep cells alive and so, neutralization of IAPs permits the initiation of a caspase cascade.

Extrinsic pathway: It is activated by *binding of Fas ligand to CD95 (Fas; member of TNF receptor family) or binding of TRAIL (TNF related apoptosis inducing ligand) to death receptors DR4 and DR5*. This induces the *association of FADD (Fas- associated death domain) and procaspase-8 to death domain motifs* of the receptors resulting in *activation of caspase 8 (in humans caspase 10)* which finally activates **caspases- 3 and 7** that **are final effector caspases.** Cellular proteins particularly a caspase antagonist called FLIP, binds to procaspase-8 but can not activate it. This is important because some viruses produce homologues of FLIP and protect themselves from Fas mediated apoptosis.

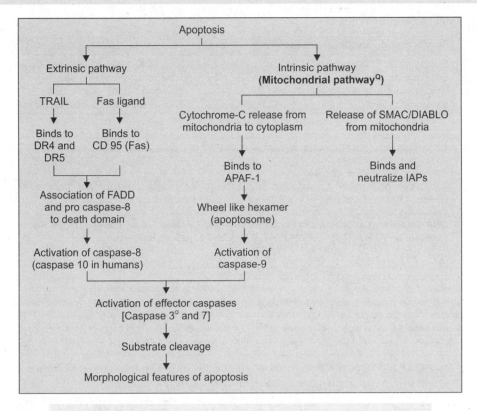

Mnemonic: Short Story to understand the pathogenesis of apoptosis.

Suppose, a person is working in some institution. If he leaves his job, this will be equivalent to apoptosis. There are two reasons due to which that person can leave the work. 1. This person is fired from work (equivalent to extrinsic pathway through death receptors). 2. Person is not given pay for long time, so that the person himself gives resignation (equivalent to intrinsic pathway, due to absence of growth factors). In latter case, before giving resignation, the person will talk to his colleagues, whether he should leave or not. Some of them will suggest him to leave (equivalent to pro-apoptotic gene products like bak, bid etc.) and some of them will stop him and suggest to wait (equivalent to anti-apoptotic factors like bcl-2, bcl-xL etc.) This regulation has been discussed below.

REGULATION OF APOPTOSIS

Regulation is primarily by **bcl-2 family** of genes *located on chromosome 18*. Some members of this family like bak, bid, bin, bcl-x**S** (to remember, S for **s**timulate apoptosis) stimulate apoptosis whereas others like bcl-2, bcl-xL (to remember, L for **l**ower apoptosis) etc inhibit apoptosis.

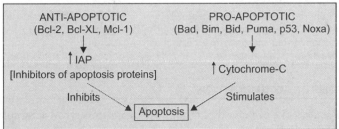

Normal cells have bcl-2 and bcl-xL present in the mitochondrial membrane. They inhibit apoptosis because their protein products prevent the leakage of mitochondrial cyt 'c' into the cytoplasm. When there is absence of growth factors or hormones, bcl-2 and bcl-xL are replaced by bax, bin etc. resulting in increased permeability of mitochondrial membrane. This result in stimulation of intrinsic pathway of apoptosis (described above in flowchart).

EXAMPLES OF APOPTOSIS

Physiological conditions	Pathological conditions
1. Endometrial cells (Menstruation) 2. Cell removal during embryogenesis 3. Virus infected cells and Neoplastic cells by cytotoxic T cells	1. Councilman bodies: Viral hepatitis 2. Gland atrophy following duct obliteration as in cystic fibrosis 3. Graft versus host disease (GVHD)

> Apoptotic cells express molecules facilitating their uptake by adjacent cells/macrophages. This leads to **absence of inflammatory response** in apoptosis.

Diagnosis of apoptosis
1. **Chromatin condensation** seen by hematoxylin, Feulgen and acridine orange staining.
2. Estimation of cytochrome 'c'
3. Estimation of activated caspase
4. **Estimation of Annexin V** (apoptotic cells express *phosphatidylserine* on the outer layer of plasma membrane because of which these cells are recognized by the dye *Annexin V*^{Q}. Some cells also express high concentration of *thrombospondin*).
5. **DNA breakdown at specific sites can be detected by 'step ladder pattern' on gel electrophoresis or TUNEL (TdT mediated d-UTP Nick End Labelling) technique.**

Clinical Significance of apoptosis in cancers

Mutated cells are cleared normally in the body by apoptosis but in cancers, apoptosis is decreased. Commonly it could be due to mutation in p53 gene or increased expression of genes like bcl-2. The bcl-2 over expression is seen with translocation (14;18) preventing the apoptosis of abnormal B lymphocytes which proliferate then and result in the development of B cell follicular lymphoma.

> On agarose gel electrophoresis, ladder pattern^Q is seen in apoptosis (in necrosis, smeared pattern is seen).

3. **ADAPTATION:** Cells may show adaptation to injury by various processes like atrophy, hypertrophy, hyperplasia, metaplasia, dysplasia etc.

Atrophy	Hypertrophy	Hyperplasia
• Reduced size of an organ or tissue resulting from a decrease in cell size and number. • Caused by ischemia, ageing, malnutrition etc. • May result due to chronic absence of stimulus (disuse atrophy).	• Increase in size and function of cells. • Results due to increase in growth factors or trophic stimuli. • Includes puberty, lactating breasts and skeletal muscle fibres (in body builders).	• Increase in number of cells in tissues/organ. • Results due to increase in growth factors, increased expression of growth promoting genes and increased DNA synthesis. • It persists so long as the stimulus is present. • e.g. breast development at puberty, endometrial hyperplasia, benign hyperplasia of prostate, hyperplasia of liver cells after partial hepatectomy.

Metaplasia	Dysplasia
• **Reversible change** in which one differentiated cell type (epithelial or mesenchymal) is replaced by another cell type. • Results from "reprogramming" of stem cells that are known to exist in normal tissues, or of undifferentiated mesenchymal cells in connective tissue.	• Abnormal multiplication of cells characterized by change in size, shape and loss of cellular organization • The basement membrane is intact^Q • Can progress to cancer

> **Epithelial metaplasia**: Barret's esophagus (squamous to intestinal columnar epithelium).
>
> **Connective tissue metaplasia**: myositis ossificans (bone formation in muscle after trauma)

INTRACELLULAR ACCUMULATIONS

Various substances like proteins, lipids, pigments, calcium etc. can accumulate in cells.

1. **Proteins:** Proteins are synthesized as polypeptides on ribosomes. These are then re-arranged into α-helix or β sheets and folded. **Chaperones** *help in protein folding* and transportation across endoplasmic reticulum and golgi apparatus. Chaperones thus can be induced by stress (like heat shock proteins; hsp 70 and hsp 90). They also prevent 'misfolding' of proteins. However, if misfolding occurs, chaperones facilitate degradation of damaged protein via ubiquitin-proteasome complex.

Disorders with protein defects

Defect in transport and secretion of proteins	Misfolded/unfolded proteins
Accumulation of proteins inside cells	Initially increase chaperone concentration, Later, these induce apoptosis by activating caspases
• α_1 – Antitrypsin deficiency [Q] • Cystic fibrosis [Q]	• Alzheimer's Disease[Q] • Huntington's Disease • Parkinson's Disease

2. **Lipids:**
   - *Triglycerides:* Fatty change in liver, heart and kidney (stained with Sudan IV or Oil Red O).
   - *Cholesterol:* Atherosclerosis, xanthoma
   - *Complex lipids:* Sphingolipidosis

3. **Endogenous Pigments:**

Lipofuscin (wear and tear pigment)	Melanin	Hemosiderin
- Perinuclear, brown coloured pigment - Responsible for *brown atrophy*[Q] of liver and heart - It is derived through lipid peroxidation of polyunsaturated lipids of subcellular membranes and is indicative of free radical injury[Q] to the cell - Seen in aging, protein energy malnutrition and cancer cachexia.	- Only naturally occurring endogenous black pigment derived from tyrosine[Q] - Responsible for pigmentation of skin and hair	- Golden yellow pigment - Seen at sites of hemorrhage or bruise[Q] - Also seen in hemochromatosis[Q] (Iron overload)

> **Lipofuscin** is an important indicator of *free radical injury*

4. **Hyaline change:** It is any intracellular or extracellular accumulation that has pink homogenous appearance.

Intracellular	Extracellular
- Mallory alcoholic hyaline - Russell bodies (seen in multiple myeloma) - Zenker's hyaline change	- Hyaline membrane in newborns - Hyaline arteriosclerosis - Corpora amylacea in prostate, brain, spinal cord in elderly, old lung infarct

INFO: The deposition of such hyaline like material and the associated sclerosis is important in diseases affecting the kidneys (glomerulopathies).

> *Concept*
> **Zenker's degeneration** is a true necrosis (**coagulative necrosis**) affecting skeletal muscles (more commonly) and cardiac muscles (less commonly) during acute infections like **typhoid**. Rectus and the diaphragm are the usual muscles affected.

5. **Calcification:** Pathologic calcification is the abnormal tissue deposition of calcium salts, together with smaller amounts of iron, magnesium, and other mineral salts. It can be of the following two types:

Dystrophic	Metastatic
- Seen in dead tissues[Q] - Serum calcium is normal[Q] - Seen at sites of necrosis[Q] - Often causes organ dysfunction - Examples include: 　**R** – **R**heumatic heart disease (in cardiac valves) 　**A** – **A**theromatous plaque 　**T** – **T**ubercular lymph node 　Tumors (**MOST** for **PG**) 　• **M** – **M**enigioma, **M**esothelioma 　• **O** – Papillary carcinoma of **O**vary (serous ovarian cystadenoma) 　• **S** – Papillary carcinoma of **S**alivary gland 　• **T** – Papillary carcinoma of **T**hyroid 　• **P**rolactinoma 　• **G**lucagonoma	- Seen in living tissues also - Association with elevated serum Ca^{2+} - Does not cause clinical dysfunction - Seen in 　• Hyperparathyroidism[Q] 　• Renal failure[Q] 　• Vitamin D intoxication[Q] 　• Sarcoidosis[Q] 　• Milk alkali syndrome[Q] 　• Multiple myeloma[Q] 　• Metastatic tumors to bone[Q] - Found in organs which loose acid and have alkaline environment inside them [like **lungs (most commonly)**, kidneys, stomach, systemic artery, pulmonary veins etc]

> *m*
> **D** for **Dead** and **D** for **Dystrophic**. So, at sites of necrosis or death of cells, we have dystrophic calcification

> **Calcification begins in mitochondria** of all organs *except* kidney (begin in basement membrane)

> **Lungs** are the **commonest site for metastatic calcification**

Note: *Hypercalemia normally is responsible for metastatic calcification but it also accentuates dystrophic calcification.

REPERFUSION INJURY

It is seen with cerebral or myocardial injury. On re-establishment of blood flow, there is increased recruitment of white blood cells which cause inflammation as well as generation of more free radicals.

> **Reperfusion injury** is characteristically seen in cardiac cells appearing as **contraction bands after myocardial infarction.**

CELLULAR AGEING

Features of ageing include decreased oxidative phosphorylation, decreased synthesis of nucleic acids and proteins, deposition of lipofuscin, accumulation of glycosylation products and abnormally folded proteins. The most effective way to prolong life is calories restriction because of a family of proteins called **SIRTUINS**. The latter have histone deacetylase activity and promote expression of genes whose products increase longevity.

> A defect in DNA helicase enzyme (required for DNA replication and repair) results in premature ageing (**WERNER SYNDROME**)

The best-studied mammalian sirtuin is Sirt-1[Q] which has been shown to improve glucose tolerance and enhance β cell insulin secretion. It is implicated in diabetes[Q].

- Ends of the chromosomes are known as telomeres. Enzyme *telomerase* helps in keeping the length of telomere constant. *Decreased activity* of this enzyme is *associated with ageing* whereas excessive activity is associated with cancers.

> Decreased activity of **telomerase** is associated with ageing whereas its **excessive activity** is associated with **cancers**.

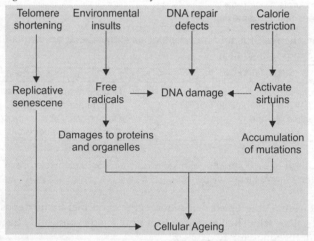

> **Fenton reaction:** $H_2O_2 + Fe^{2+} \rightarrow Fe^{2+} + OH^- + OH^-$

FREE RADICAL INJURY

Free radical injury is caused by the following mechanisms:
1. Oxidative stress/reactive oxygen species (O_2^-, H_2O_2, OH)
2. Radiation exposure
3. Drugs (carbon tetrachloride, paracetamol)
4. Metals (iron, copper):

> **Free radicals in reperfusion injury** are produced by **neutrophils**

Nitric oxide (NO), an important chemical mediator generated by endothelial cells, macrophages, neurons, and other cell types can act as a free radical and can also be converted to highly reactive peroxynitrite anion ($ONOO^-$) as well as NO_2 and NO_3.

Mechanism of Free Radical Injury

It can result in lipid peroxidation, DNA breaks and fragmentation of the proteins. This is associated with formation of more free radicals thereby making free radical induced injury as an autocatalytic reaction.

Antioxidants

Antioxidants may act by inhibiting the generation of free radials or scavenging the already present free radicals. These may be divided into enzymatic and non-enzymatic.

Enzymatic	Non-enzymatic
a. Superoxide dismutase	a. Vitamin E
b. Catalase	b. Sulfhydryl containing compounds: cysteine and glutathione
c. Glutathione peroxidase	c. Serum proteins: Albumin, Ceruloplasmin and Transferrin

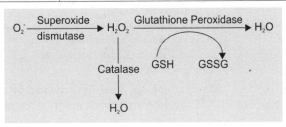

Concept

The intracellular ratio of oxidized glutathione (GSSG) to reduced glutathione (GSH) is a reflection of the oxidative state of the cell and is an important aspect of the cell's ability to detoxify reactive oxygen species.

- Catalase is present in peroxisomes and decomposes H_2O_2 into O_2 and H_2O. ($2 H_2O_2 \rightarrow O_2 + 2 H_2O$).
- Superoxide dismutase is found in many cell types and converts superoxide ions to H_2O_2. ($2 O_2^- + 2 H \rightarrow H_2O_2 + O_2$). This group includes both manganese-superoxide dismutase, which is localized in mitochondria, and copper-zinc-superoxide. dismutase, which is found in the cytosol.
- Glutathione peroxidase also protects against injury by catalyzing free radical breakdown. ($H_2O_2 + 2 GSH \rightarrow GSSG$ [glutathione homodimer] $+ 2 H_2O$, or $2 OH + 2 GSH \rightarrow GSSG + 2 H_2O$).

Clinical importance: Deficiency of SOD 1 gene may result in motor neuron disorder. This finding strengthens the view that SOD protects brain from free radial injury.

CHEMICAL FIXATIVES

- Chemical fixatives are used to preserve tissue from degradation, and to maintain the structure of the cell and of sub-cellular components such as cell organelles (e.g., nucleus, endoplasmic reticulum, mitochondria).
- The most common fixative for light microscopy is 10% neutral buffered formalin (4% formaldehyde in phosphate buffered saline).
- For electron microscopy, the most commonly used fixative is glutaraldehyde, usually as a 2.5% solution in phosphate buffered saline.
- These fixatives preserve tissues or cells mainly by irreversibly cross-linking proteins.
- Frozen section is a rapid way to fix and mount histology sections. It is used in surgical removal of tumors, and allow rapid determination of margin (that the tumor has been completely removed). It is done using a refrigeration device called a cryostat. The frozen tissue is sliced using a microtome, and the frozen slices are mounted on a glass slide and stained the same way as other methods.

The most common fixative for **light microscopy** is **10% neutral buffered formalin** (4% formaldehyde in phosphate buffered saline).

For **electron microscopy**, the most commonly used fixative is **glutaraldehyde**.

Commonly Used Stains

Substance	Stain
Glycogen	Carmine (best), PAS with diastase sensitivity
Lipids	Sudan black, Oil Red 'O'
Amyloid	Congo Red, Thioflavin T (for JG apparatus of kidney) and S
Calcium	Von Kossa, Alzarine Red
Hemosiderin	Perl's stain
Trichrome	Collagen^Q appears blue, while smooth muscle^Q appears red.

MULTIPLE CHOICE QUESTIONS

CELL INJURY, NECROSIS, APOPTOSIS

1. CD 95 is a marker of *(AIIMS Nov 2012)*
   (a) Intrinsic pathway of apoptosis
   (b) Extrinsic pathway of apoptosis
   (c) Necrosis of cell
   (d) Cellular adaption

2. Which of the following is the characteristic of irreversible injury on electron microscopy?
   (a) Disruption of ribosomes *(AIIMS May 2012)*
   (b) Amorphous densities in mitochondria
   (c) Swelling of endoplasmic reticulum
   (d) Cell swelling

3. Caspases are associated with which of the following?
   (a) Hydopic degeneration *(AIIMS May 2010)*
   (b) Collagen hyalinization
   (c) Embryogenesis
   (d) Fatty degeneration

4. Caspases are seen in which of the following?
   (a) Cell division *(AI 2010)*
   (b) Apoptosis
   (c) Necrosis
   (d) Inflammation

5. Light microscopic characteristic feature of apoptosis is:
   (a) Intact cell membrane *(AI 2010)*
   (b) Eosinophilic cytoplasm
   (c) Nuclear moulding
   (d) Condensation of the nucleus

6. Coagulative necrosis is found in which infection?
   (a) TB *(AI 2009, AIIMS May' 10)*
   (b) Sarcoidosis
   (c) Gangrene
   (d) Fungal infection

7. Organelle which plays a pivotal role in apoptosis is:
   (a) Cytoplasm *(AI 2011, 09, AIIMS May 2010)*
   (b) Golgi complex
   (c) Mitochondria
   (d) Nucleus

8. All of the following statements are true regarding reversible cell injury, except *(AI 2005)*
   (a) Formation of amorphous densities in the mitochondrial matrix
   (b) Diminished generation of adenosine triphosphate (ATP).
   (c) Formation of blebs in the plasma membrane.
   (d) Detachment of ribosomes from the granular endoplasmic reticulum.

9. Fibrinoid necrosis may be observed in all of the following, except: *(AI 2005)*
   (a) Malignant hypertension
   (b) Polyarteritis nodosa
   (c) Diabetic glomerulosclerosis
   (d) Aschoff's nodule

10. In apoptosis, Apaf-I is activated by release of which of the following substances from the mitochondria?
    (a) Bcl-2 *(AI 2005)*
    (b) Bax
    (c) Bcl-XL
    (d) Cytochrome C

11. Which of the following is an anti-apoptotic gene?
    (a) C-myc *(AI 2004)*
    (b) p 53
    (c) Bcl-2
    (d) Bax

12. Annexin V on non-permeable cell is indicative of:
    (a) Apoptosis *(AIIMS May 2009)*
    (b) Necrosis
    (c) Cell entering replication phase
    (d) Cell cycle arrest

13. Ultra-structural finding of irreversible injury
    (a) Ribosomal detachment from endoplasmic reticulum
    (b) Amorphous densities in mitochondria
    (c) Formation of phagolysosomes *(AIIMS Nov 2007)*
    (d) Cell swelling

14. Caspases are involved in *(AIIMS Nov 2007)*
    (a) Necrosis
    (b) Apoptosis
    (c) Atherosclerosis
    (d) Inflammation

15. True about Apoptosis are all except:
    (a) Inflammation is present *(AIIMS May 2007)*
    (b) Chromosomal breakage
    (c) Clumping of chromatin
    (d) Cell shrinkage

16. The following is an antiapoptotic gene
    (a) Bax *(AIIMS Nov 2006)*
    (b) Bad
    (c) Bcl-X
    (d) Bim

17. Cytosolic cytochrome C plays an important function in
    (a) Apoptosis *(AIIMS Nov 2006)*
    (b) Cell necrosis
    (c) Electron transport chain
    (d) Cell division

18. **Most pathognomic sign of irreversible cell injury**
    (a) Amorphous densities in mitochondria
    (b) Swelling of the cell membrane   *(AIIMS Nov 2006)*
    (c) Ribosomes detached from endoplasmic reticulum
    (d) Clumping of nuclear chromatin

19. **Internucleosomal cleavage of DNA is characteristic of**
    (a) Reversible cell injury   *(AIIMS Nov 2005)*
    (b) Irreversible cell injury
    (c) Necrosis
    (d) Apoptosis

20. **Programmed cell death is known as:**
    (a) Cytolysis   *(AIIMS Nov 2005)*
    (b) Apoptosis
    (c) Necrosis
    (d) Proptosis

21. **Ladder pattern of DNA electrophoresis in apoptosis is caused by the action of the following enzyme:**
    (a) Endonuclease   *(AIIMS Nov 2004)*
    (b) Transglutaminase
    (c) DNAse
    (d) Caspase

22. **Which finding on electron microscopy indicates irreversible cell injury?**   *(AIIMS Nov 2002)*
    (a) Dilatation of endoplasmic reticulum
    (b) Dissociation of ribosomes from rough endoplasmic reticulum
    (c) Flocculent densities in the mitochondria
    (d) Myelin figures

23. **True about apoptosis is all, except:**   *(AIIMS Nov 2001)*
    (a) Considerable apoptosis may occur in a tissue before it becomes apparent in histology
    (b) Apoptotic cells appear round mass of the intensely eosinophilic cytoplasm with dense nuclear chromatin fragments
    (c) Apoptosis of cells induce inflammatory reaction
    (d) Macrophages phagocytose the apoptotic cells and degrade them

24. **Morphological changes of apoptosis include**
    (a) Cytoplasmic blebs   *(PGI Dec 01)*
    (b) Inflammation
    (c) Nuclear fragmentation
    (d) Spindle formation
    (e) Cell swelling

25. **True about apoptosis**   *(PGI June 2003)*
    (a) Migration of Leukocytes
    (b) End products are phagocytosed by macrophage
    (c) Intranuclear fragmentation of DNA
    (d) Activation of caspases
    (e) Annexin V is a marker of apoptotic cell

26. **Which of the following is the hallmark of programmed cell death?**   *(Delhi PG 2009 RP)*
    (a) Apoptosis
    (b) Coagulation necrosis

    (c) Fibrinoid necrosis
    (d) Liquefaction necrosis

27. **Which of the following is an inhibitor of apoptosis?**
    (a) Bad   *(Delhi PG-2006)*
    (b) Bax
    (c) Bcl-2
    (d) All of the above

28. **Inhibitor of apoptosis is:**   *(Delhi PG-2005, DNB-2007)*
    (a) p53
    (b) Ras
    (c) Myc
    (d) Bcl-2

29. **Apoptosis is associated with all of the following features except:**   *(Karnataka 2009)*
    (a) Cell shrinkage
    (b) Intact cellular contents
    (c) Inflammation
    (d) Nucleosome size fragmentation of nucleus

30. **Liquefactive necrosis is typically seen in**
    (a) Ischemic necrosis of the heart   *(Karnataka 2006)*
    (b) Ischemic necrosis of the brain
    (c) Ischemic necrosis of the intestine
    (d) Tuberculosis

31. **All of the following are morphological features of apoptosis except**   *(Karnataka 2004)*
    (a) Cell shrinkage
    (b) Chromatin condensation
    (c) Inflammation
    (d) Apoptotic bodies

32. **Coagulative necrosis as a primary event is most often seen in all except:**   *(AP 2002)*
    (a) Kidneys
    (b) CNS
    (c) Spleen
    (d) Liver

33. **Liquefactive necrosis is seen in:**
    (a) Heart
    (b) Brain
    (c) Lung
    (d) Spleen

34. **Irreversible injury in cell is**   *(UP 2000)*
    (a) Deposition of Ca++ in mitochondria
    (b) Swelling
    (c) Mitotic figure
    (d) Ribosomal detachment

35. **Apoptosis is**   *(UP-98, 2004)*
    (a) Cell degeneration
    (b) Type of cell injury
    (c) Cell regeneration
    (d) Cell activation

36. **Pyogenic infection and brain infarction are associated with** *(UP 2008)*
    (a) Coagulative necrosis
    (b) Liquefactive necrosis
    (c) Caseous necrosis
    (d) Fat necrosis

37. **In apoptosis initiation:** *(UP 2008)*
    (a) The death receptors induce apoptosis when it engaged by *fas* ligand system
    (b) Cytochrome C binds to a protein Apoptosis Activating (Apaf-1) Factor – 1
    (c) Apoptosis may be initiated by caspase activation
    (d) Apoptosis mediated through DNA damage

38. **Apoptosis is alternatively called as** *(RJ 2005)*
    (a) Ischemic cell death
    (b) Programmed cell death
    (c) Post traumtic cell death
    (d) All

39. **First cellular change in hypoxia:** *(Kolkata 2003)*
    (a) Decreased oxidative phosphorylation in mitochondria
    (b) Cellular swelling
    (c) Alteration in cellular membrane permeability
    (d) Clumping of nuclear chromatin

40. **About apoptosis, true statement is:** *(Bihar 2003)*
    (a) Injury due to hypoxia
    (b) Inflammatory reaction is present
    (c) Councilman bodies is associated with apoptosis
    (d) Cell membrane is damaged

41. **Fournier's gangrene is seen in:**
    (a) Nose *(Jharkhand 2006)*
    (b) Scrotal skin
    (c) Oral cavity
    (d) All are true

42. **Coagulative necrosis is seen in:** *(Jharkhand 2006)*
    (a) Brain
    (b) Breast
    (c) Liver
    (d) All

43. A patient Fahim presents to the hospital with jaundice, right upper quadrant pain and fatigue. He tests positive for hepatitis B surface antigen. The serum bilirubin levels is 4.8mg/dl (direct is 0.8mg/dl and indirect bilirubin is 4.0mg/dl), AST levels is 300 U/L, ALT is 325 U/L and alkaline phosphatase is within normal limits. The elevation in AST and ALT can be explained by which of the following?
    (a) Bleb formation
    (b) Cell membrane rupture
    (c) Clumping of nuclear chromatin
    (d) Swelling of endoplasmic reticulum

44. A 23-year-old lady Sweety was driving her car when she had to apply brakes suddenly. She suffered from "steering wheel" injury in the right breast. After 5 days of pain and tenderness at the site of trauma, she noticed the presence "lump" which was persistent since the day of trauma. Dr. M. Spartan does an excision biopsy and observed the presence of an amorphous basophilic material within the mass. The amorphous material is an example of
    (a) Apocrine metaplasia.
    (b) Dystrophic fat necrosis
    (c) Enzymatic fat necrosis
    (d) Granulomatous inflammation

45. A patient Subbu is diagnosed with a cancer. It was observed that he shows a poor response to a commonly used anti-cancer drug which acts by increasing programmed cell death. Inactivation of which of the following molecules/genes is responsible for the resistance shown in the tumor cells?
    (a) Granzyme and perforin
    (b) Bcl-2
    (c) p53
    (d) Cytochrome P450

46. Dr Maalu Gupta is carrying out an experiment in which a genetic mutation decreased the cell survival of a cell culture line. These cells have clumping of the nuclear chromatin and reduced size as compared to normal cells. Which of the following is the most likely involved gene in the above described situation?
    (a) Fas
    (b) Bax
    (c) Bcl-2
    (d) Myc

47-49. ...Read the following statement for questions 49, 50 and 51 carefully and answer the associated questions.
A 50-year old male Braj Singh presented to the medicine emergency room with retrosternal chest pain of 15 minutes duration. He also had sweating and mild dyspnea. The physician immediately gave him a nitrate tablet to be kept sublingually following which his chest pain decreased significantly.

47. Which of the following best represents the biochemical change in the myocardial cells of this patient during the transient hypoxia?
    (a) Decreased hydrogen ion concentration
    (b) Increase in oxidative phosphorylation
    (c) Loss of intracellular Na^+ and water
    (d) Stimulation of anaerobic glycolysis and glycogenolysis

48. Which of the following if accumulated is suggestive of reversible cell injury due to hypoperfusion of different organs during this duration of myocardial ischemia?
    (a) Carbon dioxide
    (b) Creatinine
    (c) Lactic acid
    (d) Troponin I

49. If we presume that the patient has experienced several similar episodes of pain over the last 10 hours, which of the following ultra-structural changes would most likely indicate irreversible myocardial cell injury in this patient?
    (a) Myofibril relaxation
    (b) Disaggregation of polysomes
    (c) Mitochondrial vacuolization
    (d) Disaggregation of nuclear granules

50. A 55-year-old man, Vikas develops a thrombus in his left anterior descending coronary artery. The area of myocardium supplied by this vessel is irreversibly injured. The thrombus is destroyed by the infusion of streptokinase, which is a plasminogen activator, and the injured area is reperfused. The patient, however, develops an arrhythmia and dies. An electron microscopic (EM) picture taken of the irreversibly injured myocardium reveals the presence of large, dark, irregular amorphic densities within mitochondria. What are these abnormal structures?
    (a) Apoptotic bodies
    (b) Flocculent densities
    (c) Myelin figures
    (d) Psammoma bodies
    (e) Russell bodies

51. Which one of the listed statements best describes the mechanism through which Fas(CD95) initiates apoptosis?
    (a) BCL2 product blocks channels
    (b) Cytochrome activates Apaf-1
    (c) FADD stimulates caspase 8
    (d) TNF inhibits Ikb
    (e) TRADD stimulates FAD

Most Recent Questions

52.1. In apoptosis, cytochrome C acts through:
    (a) Apaf 1
    (b) Bcl-2
    (c) FADD
    (d) TNF

52.2. Cells most sensitive to hypoxia are:
    (a) Myocardial cells
    (b) Neurons
    (c) Hepatocytes
    (d) Renal tubular epithelial cells

52.3. In cell death, myelin figures are derived from:
    (a) Nucleus
    (b) Cell membrane
    (c) Cytoplasm
    (d) Mitochondria

52.4. Irreversible cell injury is characterised by which of the following?
    (a) Mitochondrial densities
    (b) Cellular swelling

(c) Blebs
(d) Myelin figures

52.5. Coagulative necrosis as a primary event is most often seen in all except:
    (a) Kidneys
    (b) CNS
    (c) Spleen
    (d) Liver

52.6. Liquefactive necrosis is seen in:
    (a) Heart
    (b) Brain
    (c) Lung
    (d) Spleen

52.7. Organelle that plays a pivotal role in apoptosis:
    (a) Endoplasmic reticulum
    (b) Golgi complex
    (c) Mitochondria
    (d) Nucleus

52.8. Intracellular calcification begins in which of the following organelles?
    (a) Mitochondria
    (b) Golgi body
    (c) Lysososme
    (d) Endoplasmic reticulum

52.9. Which of the following induces apoptosis in a cell?
    (a) Oleic acid   *(AIIMS Nov 2013)*
    (b) Isoprenoids
    (c) Myristic acid
    (d) Glucocorticoids

52.10. Which of the following is not seen is apoptosis?
    (a) Chromatin condensation   *(AIIMS Nov 2013)*
    (b) DNA fragmentation
    (c) Inflammation
    (d) Cell membrane shrinkage

52.11. Following gene when mutated protects tumor cells from Apoptosis
    (a) BCL – 2
    (b) BRCA
    (c) RB
    (d) TGF – β

52.12. Following is seen in both apoptosis and necrosis:
    (a) Both may be physiological
    (b) Both may be pathological
    (c) Inflammation
    (d) Intact cell membrane

CELLULAR ADAPTATION, INTRACELLULAR ACCUMULATION

53. Psammoma bodies are seen in all *except*:
    (a) Follicular carcinoma of thyroid   *(AI 2011,09)*
    (b) Papillary carcinoma of thyroid
    (c) Serous cystadenoma of ovary
    (d) Meningioma

54. **True about metastatic calcification is**
    (a) Calcium level is normal   *(AIIMS May 2009)*
    (b) Occur in dead and dying tissue
    (c) Occur in damaged heart valve
    (d) Mitochondria involved earliest

55. **Both hyperplasia and hypertrophy are seen in?**
    (a) Breast enlargement during lactation
    (b) Uterus during pregnancy   *(AIIMS May 2009)*
    (c) Skeletal muscle enlargement during exercise
    (d) Left ventricular hypertrophy during heart failure

56. **Which of the following is not a common site for metastatic calcification?**   *(AIIMS Nov 2005)*
    (a) Gastric mucosa
    (b) Kidney
    (c) Parathyroid
    (d) Lung

57. **Calcification of soft tissues without any disturbance of calcium metabolism is called**
    (a) Inotrophic calcification   *(AIIMS Nov 2004)*
    (b) Monotrophic calcification
    (c) Dystrophic calcification
    (d) Calcium induced calcification

58. **The light brown perinuclear pigment seen on H & E staining of the cardiac muscle fibres in the grossly normal appearing heart of an 83 year old man at autopsy is due to deposition as:**
    (a) Hemosiderin   *(AIIMS May 2003)*
    (b) Lipochrome
    (c) Cholesterol metabolite
    (d) Anthracotic pigment

59. **Dystrophic calcification is seen in:**
    (a) Rickets   *(AIIMS Nov 2002)*
    (b) Hyperparathyroidism
    (c) Atheromatous plaque
    (d) Vitamin A intoxication

60. **The Fenton reaction leads to free radical generation when:**   *(AIIMS Nov 2002)*
    (a) Radiant energy is absorbed by water
    (b) Hydrogen peroxide is formed by Myeloperoxidase
    (c) Ferrous ions are converted to ferric ions
    (d) Nitric oxide is converted to peroxynitrite anion

61. **Mallory hyaline is seen in:**   *(PGI Dec 2000)*
    (a) Alcoholic liver disease
    (b) Hepatocellular carcinoma
    (c) Wilson's disease
    (d) I.C.C. (Indian childhood cirrhosis)
    (e) Biliary cirrhosis

62. **Heterotopic calcification occurs in:**
    (a) Ankylosing spondylitis   *(PGI Dec 2000)*
    (b) Reiter's syndrome
    (c) Forrestier's disease
    (d) Rheumatoid arthritis
    (e) Gouty arthritis

63. **Pigmentation in the liver is caused by all except:**
    (a) Lipofuscin   *(PGI Dec 01)*
    (b) Pseudomelanin
    (c) Wilson's disease
    (d) Malarial pigment
    (e) Bile pigment

64. **Wear and tear pigment in the body refers to**
    (a) Lipochrome   *(Karnataka 2006)*
    (b) Melanin
    (c) Anthracotic pigment
    (d) Hemosiderin

65. **Mallory hyaline bodies are seen all Except:**
    (a) Indian childhood cirrhosis   *(AI 97) (UP 2004)*
    (b) Wilson's disease
    (c) Alcoholic hepatitis
    (d) Crigler-Najjar syndrome

66. **"Russell's body" are accumulations of:**   *(UP 2006)*
    (a) Cholesterol
    (b) Immunoglobulins
    (c) Lipoproteins
    (d) Phospholipids

67. **Dystrophic calcification is seen in:**   *(UP 2006)*
    (a) Atheroma
    (b) Paget's disease
    (c) Renal osteodystrophy
    (d) Milk-alkali syndrome

68. **Brown atrophy is due to**   *(AP 2000)*
    (a) Fatty necrosis
    (b) Hemosiderin
    (c) Lipofuscin
    (d) Ceruloplasmin

69. **Psammoma bodies are typically associated with all of the following neoplasms except**   *(AP 2001)*
    (a) Medulloblastoma
    (b) Meningioma
    (c) Papillary carcinoma of the thyroid
    (d) Papillary serous cystadenocarcinoma of the ovary

70. **Transformation of one epithelium to other epithelium is known as**   *(AP 2001)*
    (a) Dysplasia
    (b) Hyperplasia
    (c) Neoplasia
    (d) Metaplasia

71. **All are true about metaplasia except**   *(AP 2004)*
    (a) Slow growth   *(AIIMS 1996, UP 2002)*
    (b) Reverse back to normal with appropriate treatment
    (c) Irreversible
    (d) If persistent may induce cancer transformation

72. **About hyperplasia, which of the following statement is false?**   *(AP 2007)*
    (a) ↑ no of cells
    (b) ↑ size of the affected cell

(c) Endometrial response to estrogen is an example
(d) All

73. **Example of hypertrophy is:** *(Kolkata 2004)*
(a) Breast in puberty
(b) Uterus during pregnancy
(c) Ovary after menopause
(d) Liver after resection

74. **Metastatic calcification occurs in all except:**
(a) Kidney *(Bihar 2005)*
(b) Atheroma
(c) Fundus of stomach
(d) Pulmonary veins

75. **Dystrophic calcification is:** *(Jharkhand 2006)*
(a) Calcification in dead tissue
(b) Calcification in living tissue
(c) Calcification in dead man
(d) None

76. **An old man Muthoot has difficulty in urination associated with increased urge and frequency. He has to get up several times in night to relieve himself. There is no history of any burning micturition and lower back pain. On rectal examination, he has enlarged prostate. Which of the following represents the most likely change in the bladder of this patient?**
(a) Hyperplasia
(b) Atrophy
(c) Hypertrophy
(d) Metaplasia

77. **An increase in the size of a cell in response to stress is called as hypertrophy. Which of the following does not represent the example of smooth muscle hypertrophy as an adaptive response to the relevant situation?**
(a) Urinary bladder in urine outflow obstruction
(b) Small intestine in intestinal obstruction
(c) Triceps in body builders
(d) None of the above

78. **A patient Ramu Kaka presented with complaints of slow progressive breathlessness, redness in the eyes and skin lesions. His chest X ray had bilateral hilar lymphadenopathy. His serum ACE levels were elevated. On doing Kveim test, it came out to be positive. Final confirmation was done with a biopsy which demonstrated presence of non-caseous granuloma. A diagnosis of sarcoidosis was established. Which of the following statements regarding calcification and sarcoidosis is not true?**
(a) The calcification in sarcoidosis begins at a cellular level in mitochondria
(b) There is presence of dystrophic calcification
(c) The granulomatous lesions contain macrophages which cause activation of vitamin D precursors
(d) None of the above

79. **A 50-year-old male alcoholic, Rajesh presents with symptoms of liver disease and is found to have mildly elevated liver enzymes. A liver biopsy examined with a routine hematoxylin and eosin (H & E) stain reveals abnormal clear spaces in the cytoplasm of most of the hepatocytes. Which of the following materials is most likely forming cytoplasm spaces?**
(a) Calcium
(b) Cholesterol
(c) Hemosiderin
(d) Lipofuscin
(e) Triglyceride

80. **A 36-year-old woman, Geeta presents with intermittent pelvic pain. Physical examination reveals a 3-cm mass in the area of her right ovary. Histologic sections from this ovarian mass reveal a papillary tumor with multiple, scattered small, round, laminated calcifications. Which of the following is the basic defect producing these abnormal structures?**
(a) Bacterial infection
(b) Dystrophic calcification
(c) Enzymatic necrosis
(d) Metastatic calcification
(e) Viral infection

81. **A 28-year-old male executive presents to the doctor with complaints of "heartburn" non responsive to usual medicines undergoes endoscopy with biopsy of the distal esophagus is taken. What type of mucosa is normal for the distal esophagus?**
(a) Ciliated, columnar epithelium
(b) Keratinized, stratified, squamous epithelium
(c) Non-keratinized, simple, squamous epitheliu
(d) Non-keratinized, stratified, squamous epithelium

Most Recent Questions

82.1. **True about psammoma bodies are all except:**
(a) Seen in meningioma
(b) Concentric whorled appearance
(c) Contains calcium deposits
(d) Seen in teratoma

82.2. **Metastatic calcification is most often seen in:**
(a) Lymph nodes
(b) Lungs
(c) Kidney
(d) Liver

82.3. **Russell bodies are seen in:**
(a) Lymphocytes
(b) Neutrophils
(c) Macrophages
(d) Plasma cells

82.4. **Psammoma bodies show which type of calcification:**
(a) Metastatic
(b) Dystrophic
(c) Secondary
(d) Any of the above

82.5. Gamma Gandy bodies contain hemosiderin and:
(a) Na+
(b) Ca++
(c) Mg++
(d) K+

82.6. Oncocytes are modified form of which of the following:
(a) Lysososmes
(b) Endoplasmic reticulum
(c) Mitochondria
(d) None of the above

MISCELLANEOUS: FREE RADICAL INJURY: STAINS

83. Which of the following is the most common fixative used in electron microscopy? *(AIIMS Nov 2012)*
(a) Glutaraldehyde
(b) Formalin
(c) Picric acid
(d) Absolute Alcohol

84. The fixative used in histopathology: *(AIIMS May 2012)*
(a) 10% buffered neutral formalin
(b) Bouins fixative
(c) Glutaraldehyde
(d) Ethyl alcohol

85. Which is the most commonly used fixative in histopathological specimens? *(AI 2011)*
(a) Glutaraldehyde
(b) Formaldehyde
(c) Alcohol
(d) Picric acid

86. Lipid in the tissue is detected by: *(AIIMS Nov 2009)*
(a) PAS
(b) Myeloperoxidase
(c) Oil Red O
(d) Mucicarmine

87. The most abundant glycoprotein present in basement membrane is: *(AI 2004)*
(a) Laminin
(b) Fibronectin
(c) Collagen type 4
(d) Heparan sulphate

88. Enzyme that protects the brain from free radical injury is: *(AI 2001)*
(a) Myeloperoxidase
(b) Superoxide dismutase
(c) MAO
(d) Hydroxylase

89. Increased incidence of cancer in old age is due to
(a) Telomerase reactivation *(AIIMS May 2009)*
(b) Telomerase deactivation
(c) Inactivation of protooncogene
(d) Increase in apoptosis

90. Stain not used for lipid *(AIIMS Nov 2007)*
(a) Oil red O
(b) Congo red
(c) Sudan III
(d) Sudan black

91. Acridine orange is a fluorescent dye used to bind
(a) DNA and RNA *(AIIMS Nov 2007)*
(b) Protein
(c) Lipid
(d) Carbohydrates

92. PAS stains the following except *(AIIMS Nov 2007)*
(a) Glycogen
(b) Lipids
(c) Fungal cell wall
(d) Basement membrane of bacteria

93. All are components of basement membrane except
(a) Nidogen *(AIIMS Nov 2007)*
(b) Laminin
(c) Entactin
(d) Rhodopsin

94. Which of the following pigments are involved in free radical injury? *(AIIMS Nov 2006)*
(a) Lipofuscin
(b) Melanin
(c) Bilirubin
(d) Hematin

95. True about cell ageing: *(AIIMS Nov 2001)*
(a) Free radicals injury
(b) Mitochondria are increased
(c) Lipofuscin accumulation in the cell
(d) Size of cell increased

96. Neutrophil secretes: *(PGI Dec 2002)*
(a) Superoxide dismutase
(b) Myeloperoxidase
(c) Lysosomal enzyme
(d) Catalase
(e) Cathepsin G

97. Which of the following is a peroxisomal free radical scavenger? *(Delhi PG 2006)*
(a) Superoxide dismutase
(b) Glutathione peroxidase
(c) Catalase
(d) All of the above

98. Crooke's hyaline body is present in: *(Kolkata 2001)*
(a) Yellow fever
(b) Basophil cells of the pituitary gland in Cushing's syndrome
(c) Parkinsonism
(d) Huntington's disease

99. An autopsy is performed on a 65-year-old man, Suresh who died of congestive heart failure. Sections of the

liver reveal yellow-brown granules in the cytoplasm of most of the hepatocytes. Which of the following stains would be most useful to demonstrate with positive staining that these yellow-brown cytoplasmic granules are in fact composed of hemosiderin (iron)?
(a) Oil red O stain
(b) Oil red O stain
(c) Periodic acid- Schiff stain
(d) Prussian blue stain
(e) Sudan black B stain
(f) Trichrome stain

100. An AIDS patient Khalil develops symptoms of pneumonia, and Pneumocystis carinii is suspected as the causative organism. Bronchial lavage is performed. Which of the following stains would be most helpful in demonstrating the organism's cysts on slides made from the lavage fluid?
(a) Alcian blue
(b) Hematoxylin and eosin
(c) Methenamine silver
(d) Trichrome stain

101. Which process makes the bacteria 'tasty' to the macrophages: *(Kolkata 2008)*
(a) Margination
(b) Diapedesis
(c) Opsonisation
(d) Chemotaxis

102. In an evaluation of a 7-year-old boy, Ram who has had recurrent infections since the first year of life, findings include enlargement of the liver and spleen, lymph node inflammation, and a superficial dermatitis resembling eczema. Microscopic examination of a series of peripheral blood smears taken during the course of a staphylococcal infection indicates that the bactericidal capacity of the boy's neutrophils is impaired or absent. Which of the following is the most likely cause of this child's illness?
(a) Defect in the enzyme NADPH oxidase
(b) Defect in the enzyme adenosine deaminase (ADA)
(c) Defect in the IL-2 receptor
(d) Developmental defect at the pre-B stage
(e) Developmental failure of pharyngeal pouches 3 and 4

Most Recent Questions

102.1. Which of the following is a negative stain?
(a) Fontana
(b) ZN stain
(c) Nigrosin
(d) Albert stain

102.2. Stain used for melanin is:
(a) Oil red
(b) Gomori methamine silver stain
(c) Masson fontana stain
(d) PAS stain

102.3. Which of the following statements about Telomerase is true?
(a) Has RNA polymerase activity
(b) Causes carcinogenesis
(c) Present in somatic cells
(d) Absent in germ cells

EXPLANATIONS

1. **Ans. (b) Extrinsic pathway of apoptosis** *(Ref: Robbins 8/e p29-30, 9/e p56)*
   In the activation of Extrinsic pathway of apoptosis, *binding of Fas ligand* takes place to *CD95* (Fas; member of TNF receptor family) *or binding of TRAIL* (TNF related apoptosis inducing ligand) attaches *to* death receptors *DR4 and DR5.* This induces the *association of FADD* (Fas- associated death domain) *and procaspase-8 to death domain motifs* of the receptors resulting in *activation of caspase 8 (in humans caspase 10)* which finally activates **caspases- 3 and 7** that **are final effector caspases**

2. **Ans. (b) Amorphous densities in mitochondria** *(Ref: Robbins 8/e p14-19, 9/e p42,50)*
   Two phenomena consistently characterize irreversibility:
   1. *The first is the inability to reverse mitochondrial dysfunction* (lack of oxidative phosphorylation and ATP generation) even after resolution of the original injury.
   2. *The second is the development of profound disturbances in membrane function*
   So, the answer for the given question is 'Amorphous densities in mitochondria'.

   However, please remember friends that the Robbins in its 8th edition pg 14 mentions small amorphous densities to be present in reversible cell injury also. Therefore, the best answer for characterizing irreversibility of an injury is *'profound disturbances in membrane function'.*

3. **Ans. (c) Embryogenesis** *(Ref: Robbins 8/e p25, 9/e p52)*
   Caspases are cysteine proteases and are critical for the process of apoptosis. Physiologically, apoptosis is required to eliminate the cells no longer required and to maintain a steady number of various cell populations in tissues. The programmed cell death (apoptosis) is required at the time of different processes in embryogenesis like implantation, organogenesis, developmental involution and metamorphosis.

4. **Ans. (b) Apoptosis** *(Ref: Robbins 8/e p27, 9/e p53)*

5. **Ans. (d) Condensation of the nucleus** *(Ref: Robbins 8/e p14-15, 26-27, 9/e p53)*
   The morphologic features characteristic of apoptosis includes
   - **Cell shrinkage**: The cell is smaller in size having dense cytoplasm and the organelles are tightly packed.
   - **Chromatin condensation:** This is the *most characteristic feature* of apoptosis.
   - **Formation of cytoplasmic blebs and apoptotic bodies**
   Regarding option 'a'…'Plasma membranes are thought to remain intact till late stage of apoptosis, as well as is a normal cell.
   Regarding option "b", eosinophilic cytoplasm, it is a common feature of necrosis and apoptosis.

   > *Regarding option "c",* nuclear moulding is defined as the "The shape of one nucleus conforming around the shape of an adjacent nucleus". It is a *characteristic* of malignant cells.

6. **Ans. (a) TB > (c) Gangrene** *(Ref: Robbins 8/e p16, 9/e p43)*
   In the 7th edition of Robbins it was clearly stated that…"*Caseous necrosis, a distinctive form of coagulative necrosis, is encountered most often in foci of tuberculous infection. The term caseous is derived from the cheesy white gross appearance of the area of necrosis."*
   Regarding the option gangrene, it is not specified the type of gangrene and therefore, we go with the better option as tuberculosis in the given question. Moreover, according to Robbins, gangrenous necrosis is not a specific pattern of necrosis but is a term used in clinical practice.

   > Dry gangrene has coagulative necrosis whereas wet gangrene has liquefactive necrosis.

7. **Ans. (c) Mitochondria** *(Ref: Robbins 8/e p28, Harrison 18/e p681, 9/e p53)*

8. **Ans. (a) Formation of Amorphous densities in mitochondrial matrix** *(Ref: Robbins 7/e p19, 9/e p42)*
   Formation of amorphous densities in the mitochondrial matrix is a feature of irreversible injury and not reversible injury.
   - Decreased formation of ATP constitutes the critical mechanism of cell injury and occurs in both reversible as well as irreversible cell injury.

Features of Reversible cell injury	Features of irreversible cell injury

• Cellular swelling[Q]
• Loss of microvilli
• Formation of cytoplasmic blebs
• Endoplasmic reticulum swelling
• Detachment of ribosomes
• Myelin figures[Q]
• Clumping of nuclear chromatin[Q]
	• Large **flocculent, amorphous densities**[Q] in swollen mitochondria due to increased calcium influx.
	• Swelling and disruption of lysosomes and leakage of lysosomal enzymes in cytoplasm
	• **Decreased basophilia**[Q]
	• Severe damage to plasma membranes
	• Nuclear changes include
	  *Pyknosis (Nuclear condensation)
	  *Karyorrhexis (Nuclear fragmentation)
	  *Karyolysis (Nuclear dissolution)

9. **Ans. (c) Diabetic glomerulosclerosis** *(Ref: Robbins 7/e p214, 594, 1008, 9/e p44)*
   Fibrinoid necrosis is a distinctive morphological pattern of cell injury characterized by deposition of fibrin like proteinaceous material in walls of arteries. Areas of fibrinoid necrosis appear as smudgy eosinophilic regions with obscured underlying cellular details.
   Fibrinoid necrosis is seen in
   • *Malignant hypertension*
   • *Vasculitis like PAN*
   • *Acute Rheumatic Fever.*

10. **Ans. (d) Cytochrome C** *(Ref: Robbins 7/e p30; Harrison 17/e p506, 9/e p55)*
    Apoptosis or programmed cell death can be induced by intrinsic or extrinsic pathway. As can be seen in the intrinsic pathway; cyt c gets associated with APAF-1 which activates caspase and cause cell death.For detail see text.

11. **Ans. (c) bcl – 2** *(Ref: Robbins 7/e p29-30, Harrison 17/e p506)*

12. **Ans. (a) Apoptosis** *(Ref: Robbins 8/e p27, 9/e p56)*
    Apoptotic cells express phosphatidylserine in the outer layers of their plasma membranes. This phospholipid moves out from the inner layers where it is recognized by a number of receptors on the phagocytes. These lipids are also detected by binding of a protein called Annexin V. So, **Annexin V** staining is used to identify the apoptotic cells.

13. **Ans. (b) Amorphous densities in mitochondria** *(Ref: Robbins 7/e p12, 9/e p42)*
    See earlier explanation.

14. **Ans. (b) Apoptosis** *(Ref: Robbins 7/e p28, 9/e p53)*
    Caspases are present in *normal cells as inactive proenzymes* and when they are activated they *cleave proteins and induce apoptosis.* These are cysteine proteases.

15. **Ans. (a) Inflammation is present** *(Ref: Robbins 7/e p31, 27, 9/e p56)*
    In *Apoptosis* the dead cell is rapidly cleared, before its contents have leaked out, and therefore cell death by this pathway **does not elicit an inflammatory reaction**[Q] in the host.

16. **Ans. (c) Bcl-X** *(Ref: Robbins 7/e p29, 9/e p55)*

17. **Ans. (a) Apoptosis** *(Ref: Robbins 7/e p26, 9/e p55)*

   > • **Cytosolic cytochrome C** and **Apaf-1** are involved in **intrinsic pathway of apoptosis**[Q].
   > • **Mitochondrial cyt 'c'** and not cytosolic cyt'c' is involved in **aerobic respiration**[Q].

18. **Ans. (a) Amorphous densities in mitochondria** *(Ref: Robbin's 7/e p12, 9/e p50)*
    Two phenomenon's consistently characterize irreversible cell injury:
    • Large amorphous densities in the mitochondria (this indicates inability to reverse mitochondrial dysfunction)
    • Development of profound disturbance in membrane function

19. **Ans. (d) Apoptosis** *(Ref: Robbin's 7/e p27; Robbins 8/e p27, 9/e p52)*
    The inter-nucleosomal cleavage of DNA into oligonucleosomes (in multiples of 180-200 base pairs) is brought about by Ca^{2+} and Mg^{2+} dependent **endonucleases** and is characteristic of apoptosis.

20. **Ans. (b) Apoptosis** *(Ref: Robbins 7/e p26, 27, 9/e p52)*

21. **Ans. (a) Endonuclease** *(Ref: Robbins 7/e p26, 27, 28; 8/e pg28)*
    • **Endonucleases** are enzymes which cause **internucleosomal cleavage** of DNA into oligonucleosomes, the latter being visualized by *agarose gel electrophoresis* as **DNA ladders.**
    • **In necrosis, smeared pattern is commonly seen**

22. **Ans. (c) Flocculent densities in mitochondria** *(Ref: Robbins's 7/e p12, 9/e p50)*

23. **Ans. (c) Apoptosis of cells induce inflammatory reaction** *(Ref: Robbins 7/e p27, 9/e p56)*
    Remember important features of apoptosis

    - Formation of **cytoplasmic blebs and apoptotic bodies**[Q]
    - **Cell Shrinkage**[Q]: The cells are smaller in size and the cytoplasm is dense.
    - **Chromatin condensation**[Q]: This is the **most characteristic features of apoptosis**.
    - Absence of inflammation[Q]
    - **Gel Electrophoresis** of DNA shows **'Step ladder'**[Q] **Pattern**.

24. **Ans. (a) Cytoplasmic blebs; (c) Nuclear Fragmentation:** *(Ref: Robbins 7/e p26, 9/e p53)*
    Apoptosis is a programmed cell death.
    During apoptosis, cells destined to die activate enzymes that degrade the cell's own nuclear DNA and nuclear and cytoplasmic proteins. There is no inflammatory reaction elicited by host.
    - **Spindle formation** is found in cell division in **mitosis**.
    - During necrosis, cell swelling is seen.

Differences between apoptosis and necrosis		
Feature	Necrosis	Apoptosis
Cell size	Enlarged (swollen)	Reduced (shrink)
Nucleus	Pyknosis/Karyorrhexis/Karyolysis	Fragmentation into nucleosome-sized fragments
Plasma membrane	Disrupted	Intact; altered structure, especially orientation of lipids
Cellular contents	Enzymatic digestion; may leak out of cell	Intact; may be released in apoptotic bodies
Adjacent inflammation	Frequent	No
Role in body	Invariably pathologic (culmination of irreversible cell injury)	Often physiologic. May be pathologic after cell injury as DNA damage.
Proapoptotic		Bak; Bax; Bim; P53 gene; Caspases TNFRI; Fas [CD95]; FADD (Fas associated death domain)
Anti-apoptotic		Bcl-2/bcl-X; FLIP; Apaf-1 (Apoptosis activating factor-1) Cytochrome C

25. **Ans. (b) End products are phagocytosed by macrophage; (c) Intranuclear fragmentation of DNA; (d) Activation of caspases; (e) Annexin V is a marker of apoptotic cell** *(Ref: Harsh Mohan 5th/53, Robbins 7/e p25-3l, 9/e p53)*

26. **Ans. (a) Apoptosis** *(Ref: Robbins 8/e p25, 9/e p52)*

27. **Ans. (c) Bcl-2** *(Ref: Robbins 7/e p31, 32)*

Inhibitors of apoptosis:	Promoters of apoptosis:	Sensors of apoptosis:
Bcl-2	Bax	Bad
Bcl-XL	BAK	Bim
	P-53 activation	Bid
	Ischemic injury	Noxa
	Death of virus infected cells	PUMA
	Neurodegenerative diseases	

28. **Ans. (d) Bcl-2** *(Ref: Robbins 7/e p29, 31, 32, 9/e p55)*

29. **Ans. (c) Inflammation** *(Ref: Robbins 7/e p26, 9/e p53)*

30. **Ans. (b) Ischemic necrosis of the brain** *(Ref: Robbins 7/e p21-22, 9/e p43)*

31. **Ans. (c) Inflammation** *(Ref: Robbin 7/e p27, 9/e p56)*

32. **Ans. (b) CNS** *(Ref: Robbins 8/e p15, 7/e p22, 9/e p43)*

33. **Ans. (b) Brain** *(Ref: Robbins 8/e p15, 7/e p22, 9/e p43)*

34. **Ans. (a) Deposition of Ca^{++} in mitochondria** *(Ref: Robbins 8/e p13-14; 7/e p11, 9/e p47)*

35. **Ans. (b) Type of cell injury** *(Ref: Robbins 8/e p25; 7/e p26-28, 9/e p52)*

36. **Ans. (b) Liquefactive necrosis** *(Ref: Robbins 7/e p22, 8/e p1300, 9/e p43)*

37. **Ans. (a) The death receptors induce apoptosis when it engaged by *fas* ligand system** *(Ref: Robbins 8/e p29; 7/e p30, 9/e p56)*

38. **Ans. (b) Programmed cell death** *(Ref: Robbins 8/e p25, 9/e p52)*

39. **Ans. (a) Decreased oxidative phosphorylation in mitochondria** *(Ref: Robbins 8/e p18-19, 7/e p15, 9/e p45)*

40. **Ans. (c) Councilman bodies is a type of apoptosis** *(Ref: Robbins 8/e p25; 7/e 26, 9/e p823)*

41. **Ans. (b) Scrotal skin**

42. **Ans. (c) Liver** *(Ref: Robbins 7/e p21, 8/e p15; 9/e p43)*

43. **Ans. (b) Cell membrane rupture** *(Ref: Robbins 8/e p23, 9/e p49-50)*
    The symptoms and the medical reports of the patient are suggestive of liver cell injury. Out of the options provided, rupture of the cell membrane is the only cellular change suggestive of irreversible cell injury. All others may be seen in reversible cell injury as well.

    > Infact, the enzymes normally are stored inside the cells but in irreversible injury which is usually associated with cell membrane damage, these intracellular enzymes leak out and their serum levels are elevated. This is the basis of the commonly prescribed diagnostic tests.

44. **Ans. (b) Dystrophic fat necrosis** *(Ref: Robbins 8/e p16-17, 9/e p65)*
    The situation described above is a typical description of a traumatic fat necrosis. This condition needs to be distinguished from enzymatic fat necrosis. The hint is in the stem of the question which describes the presence of amorphous basophilic material. This is suggestive of calcification and such pattern of calcification of previous damaged tissue is termed dystrophic calcification.

    > Dystrophic calcification has normal serum calcium levels whereas metastatic classification is associated with increased calcium levels.

45. **Ans. (c) p53** *(Ref: Robbins 8/e p30,292, 9/e p53-55)*
    When anti-cancer drugs are administered, they induce the death of the tumor cells by activating p53 gene and increasing apoptosis. Tumor cells may show resistance to these drugs if there is a mutation in the p53 gene thereby preventing apoptosis. Bcl-2 promotes the cell growth by inhibiting apoptosis. Granzyme and perforin also increase apoptosis but in case of cytotoxic T cells. Cytochrome P450 is not associated with apoptosis.

46. **Ans. (c) Bcl-2** *(Ref: Robbins 8/e p28, 9/e p55)*
    The process being described in the stem of the question is apoptosis. Fas and Bax are genes which promote apoptosis. Bcl-2 is inhibitory for apoptosis. So, a Bcl-2 mutation is associated with an increase in apoptosis. Myc is involved in development of cancer and not directly associated with apoptosis.

47. **Ans. (d) Stimulation of anaerobic glycolysis and glycogenolysis** *(Ref: Robbins 8/e p18, 9/e p46)*
    The hypoxic cell damage results in decrease in oxidative phosphorylation followed by ATP depletion and increase in AMP and ADP. Increased phosphofructokinase and phosphorylase activities respectively stimulate anaerobic glycolysis and glycogenolysis. This results in decrease in intracellular pH and depletion of cellular glycogen stores. Decrease availability of ATP also results in failure of the Na^+ -K^+- ATPase pump, which then leads to increased cell Na^+ and water and decreased cell K^+.

    > Mitochondrion is the earliest organelle affected in cell injury.

48. **Ans. (c) Lactic acid** *(Ref: Robbins 8/e p18, 9/e p45)*
    Anaerobic glycolysis results in accumulation of cellular lactic acid in almost every organ having reduced perfusion. Lactate accumulation also causes reduced pH. Carbon dioxide and creatinine would increase in involvement of the lung and the kidneys respectively. But these are not common for every organ involvement.

    > Troponin I is increased in irreversible injury to the myocardium and is the best marker for diagnosing MI.

49. **Ans. (c) Mitochondrial vacuolization** *(Ref: Robbins 8/e p19, 9/e p46)*
    The appearance of vacuoles and phospholipid-containing amorphous densities within mitochondria generally signifies irreversible injury, and implies a permanent inability to generate further ATP via oxidative phosphorylation. When the mitochondria are injured irreversibly, the cell cannot recover.

    > - **Myofibril relaxation** is an early sign of **reversible injury** in cardiac myocytes. It is associated with intracellular ATP depletion and lactate accumulation due to anaerobic glycolysis during this period.
    > - **Disaggregation of polysomes** denotes the dissociation of rRNA from mRNA in reversible ischemic/hypoxic injury. ATP depletion promotes the dissolution of polysomes into monosomes as well as the detachment of ribosomes from the rough endoplasmic reticulum.
    > - **Disaggregation of granular and fibrillar elements of the nucleus** is associated with reversible cell injury. Another common nuclear change associated with reversible cell injury is clumping of nuclear chromatin due to a decrease in intracellular pH.

50. **Ans. (b) Flocculent densities** *(Ref: Robbins 7/e p15-16, 37-38, , 9/e p51)*
    - Irreversible cellular injury is characterized by severe damage to mitochondria (vacuole formation), extensive damage to plasma membranes and nuclei, and rupture of lysosomes.
    - Severe damage to mitochondria is characterized by the influx of calcium ions into the mitochondria and the subsequent formation of large, flocculent densities within the mitochondria. These **flocculent densities** are characteristically seen in **irreversibly injured** myocardial cells that undergo reperfusion soon after injury.

51. **Ans. (c) i.e. FADD stimulates caspase – 8** *(Ref: Robbins 7/e p26-32, , 9/e p56)*
    - Apoptosis has two basic phases: an initiation phase, during which caspases are activated, and an execution phase, during which cell death occurs.
    - The initiation phase has two distinct pathways: the extrinsic (receptor mediated) pathway and the intrinsic (or mitochondrial) pathway.
    - The extrinsic pathway is mediated by cell surface death receptors, two example of death receptors are type I TNF receptor (TNFR1) and Fas (CD95).
      Fas ligand (FasL), which is produced by immune cells, stimulates apoptosis by binding to Fas, which activates the cytoplasmic Fas-associated death domain protein (FADD), which in turn activates the caspase cascade via the activation of caspase 8.
    - In contrast to the extrinsic pathway, the intrinsic pathway does not involve death receptors and instead results from increased permeability of mitochondria.

52.1. **Ans. (a) Apaf 1** *(Ref: Robbins 8/e p29, 9/e p55)*
     On being released in the *cytosol*, **cytochrome *c* binds to a protein called Apaf-1** (apoptosis-activating factor-1 which is responsible for formation of a complex called *apoptosome*. This complex binds to caspase-9 which is a critical initiator caspase of the mitochondrial pathway of apoptosis.

NEET POINTS about APOPTOSIS

• **Mitochondrion** is the critical organelle required for apoptosis.
• **Chromatin condensation** is the most characteristic feature.
• Cell shrinkage is seen
• Gel electrophoresis demonstrates "**step ladder pattern**"
• **Annexin V** is the marker for apoptosis.
• **CD 95** is the molecular marker for apoptosis

52.2. **Ans. (b) Neurons** *(Ref: Robbins 8/e p11-2)*
     - The **neurons** are the **most sensitive cells** in the body to get injured because of hypoxia.
     - So, **Purkinje cells of the cerebellum** and **neurons of the hippocampus** are the most susceptible cells which get affected in hypoxic ischemic encephalopathy.

52.3. **Ans. (b) Cell membrane** *(Ref: Robbins 8/e p23, 9/e p50-51)*
     Dead cells may be replaced by large, whorled phospholipid masses called **myelin figures** that are derived from damaged cell membranes. These phospholipid precipitates are then either phagocytosed by other cells or further degraded into fatty acids.

52.4. **Ans. (a) Mitochondrial densities** *(Ref: Robbins 8/e p23-4, 9/e p50)*
     The two key features of irreversible injury are:
     - **Inability to reverse mitochondrial dysfunction**[Q] and
     - Development of **profound disturbances in the membrane function**[Q].

52.5. **Ans. (b) CNS** *(Ref: Robbins 8/e p15, 7/e p22, 9/e p43)*
     As discussed in text, central nervous system is characterized by the presence of *liquefactive necrosis*[Q] during ischemic injury.

52.6. **Ans. (b) Brain** *(Ref: Robbins 8/e p15, 7/e p22, 9/e p43)*
     As discussed earlier, CNS shows liquefactive necrosis.

52.7. **Ans. (c) Mitochondria** *(Ref: Robbins 8/e p28, 7/e p29, 9/e p15, 53)*
     Mitochondrion must be recognized not only as an organelle with vital roles in intermediary metabolism and oxidative phosphorylation, but also as a central regulatory structure of apoptosis.

52.8. **Ans. (a) Mitochondria** *(Ref: Robbins 8/e p19, 9/e p65-66)*
     Direct quote.. "Initiation of *intracellular calcification* occurs in the *mitochondria* of dead or dying cells that accumulate calcium".

52.9 Ans. (d) Glucocorticoids *(Ref: Underwood's Pathology 6/e p80)*

Glucocorticoids induce apoptosis while *sex steroids inhibit apoptosis*. ..Underwood Pathology

Inducers of apoptosis	Inhibitors of apoptosis
• Withdrawal of growth factor • Loss of matrix attachment • Glucocorticoids • Free radicals • Some viruses • Ionising radiation • DNA damage	• Growth factors • Extracellular matrix • **Sex steroids** • Some viral proteins

52.10. Ans. (c) Inflammation *(Ref: Robbin 8/e p26-7)*

Inflammation is **not** seen in apoptosis.

Chromatin condensation is the most characteristic feature of apoptosis. Other findings like cell membrane shrinkage and DNA fragmentation are also associated with apoptosis.

52.11. Ans (a) Bcl-2 *(Ref: Robbin 9th/ 8thed: pg606)*

We need to identify a gene which should be able to inhibit apoptosis. The answer therefore is bcl-2. It is seen to result in the development of follicular lymphoma.

52.12. Ans (b) Both may be pathological *(Ref: Robbin 9th/40)*

53. Ans. (a) Follicular carcinoma of Thyroid *(Ref: Robbins 8/e p38, 9/e p65)*

Tumors (MOST for PG)
• **M** – **M**eningioma
• **O** – Papillary carcinoma of **O**vary (serous ovarian cystadenoma)
• **S** – Papillary carcinoma of **S**alivary gland
• **T** – Papillary carcinoma of **T**hyroid
• **P**rolactinoma, **P**apillary type of renal cell carcinoma
• **G**lucagonoma

(Psammoma bodies are seen in papillary thyroid cancer and not follicular thyroid cancer)

54. Ans. (d) Mitochondria involved earliest *(Ref: Robbins 8/e p38, Robbins 7/e p41-42, 9/e p65)*

• When the calcium deposition occurs locally in dying tissues despite normal serum levels of calcium, it is known as *dystrophic calcification*. It is seen in atherosclerosis, tuberculous lymph node and aging or damaged heart valves.
• The deposition of calcium salts in otherwise normal tissues almost always results from hypercalcemia and is known as *metastatic calcification*.

Friends, Robbins 7th edn page 41-42 mentions that initiation of *intracellular calcification* occurs in the *mitochondria* of dead or dying cells that accumulate calcium. Nothing is mentioned regarding the involvement of mitochondria in metastatic calcification in either 8th or 7th edition of Robbins. However, we got an article on Medscape which states that "Within the cell it is the mitochondria that serves as the nidus for metastatic calcification".

55. Ans. (b) Uterus during pregnancy *(Ref: Robbins 8/e p6-8, 9/e p36)*

• *Hypertrophy refers to an increase in the size of cells, resulting in an increase in the size of the organ.* The increased size of the cells is due the synthesis of more structural components.
• The massive physiologic growth of the uterus during pregnancy is a good example of hormone-induced increase in the size of an organ that results from both hypertrophy and hyperplasia
• Regarding the 'a' choice, Breast enlargement during lactation; it is written in Robbins that prolactin and estrogen cause **hypertrophy of the breasts** during **lactation**. Hormonal *hyperplasia* is best exemplified by the proliferation of the glandular epithelium of the female *breast at puberty and during pregnancy*.

56. Ans. (c) Parathyroid *(Ref: Robbins 7/e p42, 9/e p65)*

• Metastatic calcification may occur widely throughout the body but principally affects:

> • *Interstitial tissues of gastric mucosa*[Q]
> • *Kidneys*[Q]
> • *Lungs*[Q]
> • *Systemic arteries*[Q] and
> • *Pulmonary veins*[Q]

• The common feature of all these sites, which makes them prone to calcification is that **can loose acid** and therefore they have an **internal alkaline component** favorable for metastatic calcification.

- Absence of derangement in calcium metabolism
- Often a cause of organ dysfunction.

57. **Ans. (c) Dystrophic calcification** *(Ref: Robbins 7/e p41, 8/e p38, 9/e p65)*

58. **Ans. (b) Lipochrome** *(Ref: Robbins 7/e p39, 9/e p64)*

    Regarding other options
    - Hemosiderin: It is a pigment deposited in conditions of excess iron.
    - Anthracotic pigment: It is pigment seen in the lung of coal

59. **Ans. (c) Atheromatous plaque** *(Ref: Robbins 7/e p41, 9/e p65)*
    - Atheromatous plaque would have dead cells, so, there is presence of dystrophic calcification.
    - **Mnemonic:** D for **D**ead and D for **D**ystrophic.

60. **Ans. (c) Ferrous ions are converted to ferric ions** *(Ref: Robbins' 7/e p16, 9/e p48)*
    - Free radicals are generated through **Fenton's reaction** which is $(H_2O_2 + Fe^{2+} \rightarrow Fe^{3+} + OH^+ + OH^-)$
    - In this reaction iron is converted from its ferrous to ferric form and a radical is generated.
    - The other options are also examples of free radical injury but the questions specifically about Fenton reaction.
    - The effects of these reactive species relevant to cell injury include: **Lipid peroxidation of membranes, oxidative modification of proteins and lesions in DNA.**

61. **Ans. (a) Alcoholic liver disease; (b) Hepatocellular carcinoma; (c) Wilson's disease; (d) I.C.C. (Indian childhood cirrhosis); (e) Biliary cirrhosis** *(Ref: Robbins' 7/e p905)*
    Mallory bodies: Scattered hepatocytes accumulate tangled skeins of cytokeratin intermediate filaments and other proteins, visible as eosinophilic cytoplasmic inclusions in degenerating hepatocytes. See details in chapter on 'Liver'.

62. **Ans. (a) Ankylosing spondylitis; (c) Forrestier's disease** *(Ref: Robbins' 7/e p41-2; Harrison17/e p1952)*
    Pathologic calcification (Heterotopic calcification) is the abnormal tissue deposition of calcium salts together with small amounts of iron, manganese and other mineral salts. It may be of **two types: Dystrophic calcification** or **Metastatic calcification**

    *In **ankylosing spondylitis** - There is calcification and ossification usually most prominent in anterior spinal ligament that gives "Flowing wax" appearance[Q] on the anterior bodies of vertebrae.

    *Diffuse idiopathic skeletal hyperostosis (Forrestier's disease[Q], ankylosing hyperostosis) affects spine and extra-spinal locations. It is an enthesopathy, causing bony overgrowths and ligamentous ossification and is characterized by flowing calcification over the anterolateral aspects of vertebrae.

63. **Ans. None** *(Ref: Harsh Mohan 5th/735; Robbins 7/e p39, 910, 914)*
    Pigmentation in liver is caused by:
    - **Lipofuscin:** It is an insoluble pigment known as lipochrome and 'wear and tear' pigment. It is seen in cells undergoing low, regressive changes and is particularly prominent in liver and heart of ageing patient or patients with severe malnutrition and cancer cachexia.
    - **Pseudomelanin:** After death, a dark greenish or blackish discoloration of the surface of the abdominal viscera results from the action of sulfated hydrogen upon the iron of disintegrated hemoglobin. Liver is also pigmented.
    - **Wilson's disease:** Copper is usually deposited in periportal hepatocytes in the form of reddish granules in cytoplasm or reddish cytoplasmic coloration stained by rubeanic acid or rhodamine stain for copper or orcein stain for copper associated protein. Copper also gets deposited in chronic obstructive cholestasis.
    - **Malarial pigment:** Liver colour varies from dark chocolate red to slate-grey even black depending upon the stage of congestion.
    - **In biliary cirrhosis** liver is enlarged and greenish-yellow in colour due to cholestasis. So liver is pigmented due to bile.

64. **Ans. (a) Lipochrome** *(Ref: Robbins 7/e p39, 9/e p64)*

65. **Ans. (d) Crigler-Najjar syndrome** *(Ref: Robbins 8/e p858; 7/e p905, Harsh Mohan 6/e p621-622)*

66. **Ans. (b) Immunoglobulins** *(Ref: Robbins 8/e p610; 7/e p680-681, 9/e p63)*

67. **Ans. (a) Atheroma** *(Ref: Robbins 8/e p38, 7/e p41-42, 9/e p65)*

68. **Ans. (c) Lipofuscin** *(Ref: Robbins 8/e p10,532; 7/e 10, 9/e p64)*

69. **Ans. (a) Medulloblastoma** *(Ref: Robbins 8/e p38, 1122; 7/e 41,1178,1407, 9/e p65)*

70. **Ans. (d) Metaplasia** *(Ref: Robbins 8/e p10,11; 7/e 10,11, 9/e p37)*

71. **Ans. (c) Irreversible** *(Ref: Robbins 8/e p265; 7/e 10), 9/e p37-38*

72. **Ans. (b) ↑ Size of affected cell** *(Ref: Robbins 8/e p8-9, 7/e p7 , 9/e p35)*

73. **Ans. (b) Uterus during pregnancy** *(Ref: Robbins 8/e p6, 7/e p7-8 , 9/e p34-36)*

Breast at Puberty	**Hyperplasia**
Breast during lactation	Hypertrophy
Uterus after resection	**Hyperplasia**
Uterus during pregnancy	Hyperplasia + Hypertrophy

74. **Ans. (b) Atheroma** *(Ref: Robbins 8/e p38; 7/e p41, 9/e p65)*

75. **Ans. (a) Calcification in dead tissue** *(Ref: Robbins 8/e p38, 7/e p41, 9/e p65)*

76. **Ans. (c) Hypertrophy** *(Ref: Robbins 8/e p6-7, 9/e p36)*
The patient is most likely suffering from benign hyperplasia of the prostate. The question however asks about the change in bladder which would be hypertrophy. This is secondary to the obstruction in the urine outflow following the smooth muscle in the bladder undergoes hypertrophy.

Benign prostatic hyperplasia is due to action of the hormone **dihydrotestosterone** and not testosterone.

77. **Ans. (c) Triceps in body builders** *(Ref: Robbins 8/e p6-7, 9/e p34)*
The enlargement of the triceps is an example of **skeletal muscle hypertrophy (not smooth muscle hypertrophy)**.

78. **Ans. (b) There is presence of dystrophic calcification** *(Ref: Robbins 8/e p38, 9/e p65)*
In sarcoidosis, there is presence of metastatic calcification because of the presence of increased concentration of calcitriol (most active form of vitamin D). Both the patterns of calcification begin in mitochondria.

79. **Ans. (e) Triglyceride** *(Ref: Robbins 7/e p35-37, 41-42; Chandrasoma, 3/8-10, 9/e p62)*
- Substance that can form clear spaces in the cytoplasm of cells as seen with a routine H&E stain include glycogen, lipid, and water. In the liver, clear spaces within hepatocytes are most likely to be lipid, this change being called fatty change or steatosis.
- Increased formation of triglycerides can result from alcohol use, as alcohol causes excess NADH formation (high NADH/NAD ratio), increases fatty acid synthesis, and decreases fatty acid oxidation.
- In contrast to lipid, **calcium** appears as a dark **blue-purple color** with routine H&E stains, while **hemosiderin**, which is formed from the breakdown of ferritin, appears as **yellow-brown granules**.
- **Lipofuscin** also appears as fine, granular, **golden –brown intracytoplasmic pigment**. It is an insoluble **"wear and tear" (ageing) pigment** found in **neurons, cardiac myocytes,** or **hepatocytes**.

80. **Ans. (b) Dystrophic calcification** *(Ref: Robbins 7/e p41-42; Henry/195-196, 9/e p65)*
- Dystrophic calcification is characterized by calcification in abnormal (dystrophic) tissue, while metastatic calcification is characterized by calcification in normal tissue.
- Examples of dystrophic calcification of damaged or abnormal heart valves, and calcification within tumors
- Small (microscopic) laminated calcifications within tumors are called Psammoma bodies and are due to single- cell necrosis. Psammoma bodies are characteristically found in papillary tumors, such as papillary carcinomas of the thyroid and papillary tumors of the ovary (especially papillary serous cystadenocarcinoma), but they can also be found in meningiomas or mesotheliomas.
- With dystrophic calcification the serum calcium levels are normal, while with metastatic calcification the serum calcium levels are elevated (hypercalcemia).

81. **Ans. (d) i.e. Non-keratinized, stratified, squamous epithelium** *(Ref: Robbins 8/e p770, 9/e p37)*
The esophagus is covered by non-keratinized, stratified, squamous epithelium for its entire length. Heartburn is usually a sign of gastric regurgitation of the acidic contents in the lower esophagus (acid reflux disease).

82.1. **Ans. (d) Seen in teratoma** *(Ref: Robbins 8/e p38, 9/e p65)*
The progressive acquisition of outer layers may create lamellated configurations, called **psammoma bodies** because of their resemblance to grains of sand. Some common cancers associated with psammoma bodies are:
- M – Meningioma, Mesothelioma
- O – Papillary carcinoma of Ovary (serous ovarian cystadenoma)
- S – Papillary carcinoma of Salivary gland
- T – Papillary carcinoma of Thyroid
- Prolactinoma
- Glucagonoma

82.2. Ans. (b) Lungs *(Ref: Dail and Hammar's Pulmonary Pathology: Non-neoplastic lung disease, Springer 3/e p777)*
Direct quote…'Lung are the most frequent involved of all organs.'
Ours is the only and the first book to give you an authentic reference for this one friends. This is in **sharp contrast to all our competitors** who give name and page number of books where this info is just not there. Try that yourself. You would find many such questions and answers in other chapters of this edition. Happy reading!

82.3. Ans. (d) Plasma cells *(Ref: Robbins 8/e p35, 7/e p37, 9/e p63)*
Russell bodies are homogenous eosinophilic inclusions that result from hugely distended endoplasmic reticulum.

82.4. Ans. (b) Dystrophic *(Ref: Robbins 8/e p38, 7/e p41 , 9/e p65)*
Direct quote… "On occasion single necrotic cells may constitute seed crystals that become encrusted by the mineral deposits. The progressive acquisition of outer layers may create lamellated configurations, called **psammoma bodies.**"

82.5. Ans. (b) Ca++ *(Ref: Harsh Mohan 6/e p106-107, Robbins 7/e p705)*
In chronic venous congestion of spleen, some of the hemorrhages overlying fibrous tissue get deposits of **hemosiderin and calcium**, these are called as **Gamma Gandy bodies** or **siderofibrotic nodules**.

82.6. Ans. (c) Mitochondria *(Ref: Robbins 8/e p35, 7/e p37 , 9/e p53)*
Oncocytes are epithelial cells stuffed with **mitochondria**, which impart the granular appearance to the cytoplasm.

83. Ans. (a) Glutaraldehyde *(Ref: Bancroft 6/e p53, Ackerman 9th/27)*

- Commonest fixative used for *light microscopic examination*: **10% buffered neutral formalin**
- Commonest fixative used for *electron microscopic examination*: Glutaraldehyde

84. Ans. (a) 10% buffered neutral formalin *(Ref: Bancroft 6/e p53, Ackerman 9th/27)*
- Commonest fixative used for *light microscopic examination*: **10% buffered neutral formalin**
- Commonest fixative used for *electron microscopic examination*: Glutaraldehyde

85. Ans. (b) Formaldehyde *(Ref: Bancroft 6/e p53)*
- Formaldehyde is the most commonly used fixative in histopathological specimens. See text for details.

86. Ans. (c) Oil Red O *(Ref: Bancroft histology 6/e p53)*

87. Ans. (a) Laminin *(Ref: Robbins 7/e p105, Harrison 17/e p2462 , 9/e p24)*
Laminin is the most abundant glycoprotein in basement membranes. Type IV collagen, laminin and nidogen are present in basement membranes.

Tendons and ligaments consist primarily of collagen type I whereas cartilage is mainly consisted of Type II collagen.

88. Ans. (b) Superoxide dismutase *(Ref: Robbins 7/e p17, Harrison's 17/e p2572 , 9/e p48)*
- Antioxidant enzymes include glutathione peroxidase, SOD and catalase.
- Deficiency of SOD 1 gene may result in motor neuron disorder. This finding strengthens the view that SOD protects brain from free radial injury.

89. Ans. (a) Telomerase reactivation *(Ref: Robbins 8/e p296-297 , 9/e p67)*

- After a fixed number of divisions, normal cells become arrested in a terminally non-dividing state known as **replicative senescence**. With each cell division there is some shortening of specialized structures, called telomeres, at the ends of chromosomes. Once the telomeres are shortened beyond a certain point, the loss of telomere function leads to activation of p53-dependent cell-cycle checkpoints, causing proliferative arrest or apoptosis. Thus, telomere shortening functions as a clock that counts cell divisions.
- In **germ cells**, telomere shortening is prevented by the sustained **function of the enzyme telomerase**, thus explaining the ability of these cells to **self-replicate extensively**. This enzyme is **absent in most somatic cells**, and hence they suffer progressive loss of telomeres.
- **Cancer cells** prevent telomere shortening by the reactivation of telomerase activity. Telomerase activity has been detected in more than 90% of human tumors. Telomerase activity and maintenance of telomere length are essential for the maintenance of replicative potential in cancer cells.

90. Ans. (b) Congo red *(Ref: Bancroft's histopathology 5th/204)*
Congo red is used for staining amyloid and not lipids

Stains for Lipids

• Oil red O	• Sudan black	• Sudan III and IV
• Filipin	• Schultz	• Nile blue sulfate

91. **Ans. (a) DNA and RNA** *(Ref: Bancroft 5th/236, 237, 238)*
    - **Acridine orange** is a nucleic acid selective fluorescent cationic dye useful for cell cycle determination.
    - It is cell-permeable, and interacts with DNA and RNA by intercalation or electrostatic attractions respectively and emits green and red right respectively.
    - **Acridine orange can be used in conjunction with ethidium bromide to differentiate between live and apoptotic cells.**

92. **Ans. (b) Lipids** *(Ref: Bancroft's histopathology 5th/204)*
    PAS (periodic acid-Schiff) stain is versatile and has been used to stain many structures including glycogen, mucin, mucoprotein, glycoprotein, as well as fungi. PAS is useful for outlining tissue structures, basement membranes, glomeruli, blood vessels and glycogen in the liver.

    > *Lipids are stained by oil red O and Sudan stains. (See explanation above)
    > *PAS can also stain glycolipids but here it is used for staining carbohydrate moiety of these compounds and not lipid portion.

93. **Ans. (d) Rhodopsin** *(Ref: Robbins 7/e p103, 9/e p24)*
    Basement membrane is Periodic Acid Schiff (PAS) positive amorphous structures that lie underneath epithelia of different organs and endothelial cells. It consists of

• **Laminin**	• *Fibronectin*	• *Tenascin*
• **Proteoglycans**	• **Entactin (Nidogen)**	• *Perlecan* (heparin sulphate)
• Collagen type IV		

94. **Ans. (a) Lipofuscin** *(Ref: Robbins 7/e p39 , 9/e p64)*
    Important points about Lipochrome or Lipofuscin.

    > *Also called '**wear and tear pigment**'[Q] or '**pigment of ageing**'[Q]
    > *Perinuclear in location
    > *Derived through **lipid peroxidation**[Q]
    > *Indicative of **free radical injury to the cell**
    > *Prominent in ageing[Q], severe malnutrition[Q] and cancer cachexia[Q]

95. **Ans. (c) Lipofuscin accumulation** *(Ref: Robbins 8/e p36, 39 – 41, 9/e p64)*

96. **Ans. (b) Myeloperoxidase; (e) Cathepsin G** *(Ref: Robbins 7/e p73)*

Granules of Neutrophils	
Specific granules	**Azurophil granules**
• Lactoferrin • Lysozyme • Type IV collagenase • Leucocyte adhesion molecules • Plasminogen activator • Phospholipase A$_2$	• Myeloperoxidase • Lysozyme • Cationic proteins • Acid hydrolase • Elastase • Non-specific collagenase • BPI • Defensin • Cathepsin G • Phospholipase A$_2$

97. **Ans. (d) All of the above** *(Ref: Robbins 7/e p17 , 9/e p48)*
    - Catalase is present in peroxisomes and decomposes H_2O_2 into O_2 and H_2O.
    - Superoxide dismutase is found in many cell types and converts superoxide ions to H2O2. This group includes both manganese-superoxide dismutase, which is localized in mitochondria, and copper-zinc-superoxide dismutase, which is found in the cytosol.
    - Glutathione peroxidase also protects against injury by catalyzing free radical breakdown.

98. **Ans. (b) Basophil cells of the pituitary gland in Cushing's syndrome** *(Ref: Robbins 8/e p1149)*

    > In Cushing syndrome, the normal granular, basophilic cytoplasm of the ACTH producing cells in the anterior pituitary becomes paler and homogenous. This is due to **accumulation** of intermediate **keratin filaments** [Q] in the cytoplasm.

99. **Ans. (c) Prussian blue stain** *(Ref: Robbins 7/e p39- 42, 9/e p64)*
    - Yellow-brown granules in hepatocytes as seen with routine hematoxylin and eosin (H&E) stain can be hemosiderin, bile, and Lipofuscin.

> - The special histologic stain for **hemosiderin**, which contains iron, is the **Prussian blue stain**[Q].
> - **Oil red O**[Q] and **Sudan black B**[Q] **stain** are both used to demonstrate **neutral lipids**[Q] in tissue sections.
> - **PAS (periodic acid –Schiff) stain**[Q] is used to demonstrate **carbohydrates**[Q].
> - **Trichrome stain**[Q] is used to demonstrate collagen or smooth muscle in tissue. With this stain **collagen**[Q] **appears blue,** while **smooth muscle**[Q] **appears red.**

100. Ans. (c) i.e. Methenamine silver *(Ref: Harsh Mohan 6/e p474)*

The appropriate stain is methenamine silver. The routine hematoxylin and eosin does not adequately demonstrate the organisms. The cysts, when stained with methenamine silver, have a characteristic cup or boat shape; the trophozoites are difficult to demonstrate without electron microscopy.

> - **Alcian blue** (choice A) is good for demonstrating **mucopolysaccharides**[Q].
> - **Hematoxylin and eosin** (choice B) is the **routine tissue stain**[Q] used in pathology laboratories.
> - **Trichrome stain** (choice D) is good for **distinguishing fibrous tissue from nerve and muscle**.

101. Ans. (c) Opsonisation *(Ref: Robbins 8/e p52-53, 7/e p59 , 9/e p78)*

102. Ans. (a) Defect in the enzyme NADPH oxidase *(Ref: Robbins 7/e p61-62, 243-244 , 9/e p79)*

Patients with chronic granulomatous disease have defective functioning of phagocytic neutrophils and monocytes.

- The most common cause of chronic granulomatous disease is defective NADPH oxidase, which is an enzyme on the membrane of lysosomes that converts O_2 to superoxide and stimulates oxygen burst. This deficiency results in recurrent infections with catalase-positive organisms, such as *S. aureus*. Key findings in chronic granulomatous disease include lymphadenitis, hepatosplenomegaly, eczematoid dermatitis, pulmonary infiltrates.

- A defect in the enzyme adenosine deaminase (ADA) is seen in the autosomal recessive (Swiss) form of severe combined immunodeficiency disease (SCID), while a defect in the IL-2 receptor is seen in the X-linked recessive form of SCID.

- A developmental defect at the pre-B stage is seen in X-linked agammaglobulinemia of Bruton, while developmental failure of pharyngeal pouches 3 and 4 is characteristic of DiGeorge's syndrome.

102.1. Ans. (c) Nigrosin

> - **Negative staining** is a technique in which the background is stained, leaving the actual specimen untouched, and thus visible. In contrast, with 'positive staining', the actual specimen is stained.
> - Examples of negative stains include **nigrosin** and **India Ink.**
> - **India ink** is used to make a diagnosis of **cryotococcal infection** by making its **capsule prominent.**

102.2. Ans. (c) Masson fontana stain *(Ref: Histopathology p150)*

Stain	Substance
Masson Fontana	Melanin
Oil red O	Neutral lipids and fatty acids
PAS	Glycogen, mucin, mucoprotein, glycoprotein and fungi
Gomori methamine silver stain	Fungi (like Cryptococcus, Coccidiodes and Pneumocystis jiroveci (carinii)

- Other stains for melanin are Schmorl's method and enzyme histochemical method called **DOPA-oxidase** (**most specific method**).

102.3. Ans. (b) Causes carcinogenesis *(Ref: Robbins 8/e p40, 9/e p67)*

- Telomerase is a specialized RNA-protein complex that uses its own RNA as a template for adding nucleotides to the ends of chromosomes.

- Regulatory protein sense the telomere length and they restrict the activity of telomerase to prevent unnecessary elongation.

- **Telomerase activity** is **highest** in **germ cells** and present at lower levels in stem cells, but it is usually undetectable in most somatic tissues

Decreased activity of **telomerase** is associated with ageing whereas its **excessive activity** is associated with **cancers**.

GOLDEN POINTS FOR QUICK REVISION
(CELL INJURY)

- *Hypoxia* is the most common cause of cell injury.
- *Neurons* are the most sensitive cell to hypoxic injury in the brain.
- *Coagulative necrosis* is associated with "*tombstone appearance*". It is seen with ischemic injury to all tissues *except central nervous system*.
- Best example of coexistence of hypertrophy and hyperplasia is *uterus during pregnancy* (gravid uterus).
- Most common metaplasia is squamous metaplasia in the lungs of smokers.
- **CD 95** plays a role in apoptosis.
- **Mitochondria** plays a pivotal role on apoptosis
- Marker for apoptosis *(programmed cell death)* is **annexin V**
- Most important **stimulatory gene for apoptosis is p53 gene** and most important *inhibitory gene* for apoptosis is *bcl family* (bcl-2) of genes.
- Key words associated with apoptosis: caspases, cytochrome C and embryogenesis
- '**Chromatin condensation**' is the **hallmark feature** of apoptosis.
- "*Step ladder pattern*" on gel electrophoresis is a feature of apoptosis. Stepladder fever is seen in typhoid/enteric fever.
- *Lipofuscin* is also known by several other names like '*lipochrome*', '*wear and tear*' *pigment*, *pigment of aging* and "*indicator of free radical injury*". It gets deposited mostly in heart and liver.
- The *endogenous brown-black pigments* include *melanin* (present in skin) and **homogentisic acid** (the black pigment in patients with *alkaptonuria*)
- *Dystrophic calcification:* **normal** serum calcium levels and in *dead tissues* (areas of necrosis).
- *Metastatic calcification:* **increased** serum calcium levels and in **living** tissues.
- "**Lungs**" are the commonest site for *metastatic calcification*. Other sites include stomach, pulmonary vein, systemic artery and kidneys.
- *Psammoma bodies:* meningioma, papillary thyroid carcinoma, prolactinoma, glucagonoma and serous cystadenoma of the ovary.
- **Gandy gamma body** is seen in **congestive splenomegaly.** It contains hemosiderin and calcium.
- *Oncocytes* are formed with modified *mitochondria.*
- Germ cells have the capacity for self renewal because of telomerase activation.
- **Cancer cells** have the phenomenon of '**telomerase reactivation**'.
- Germ cells have the maximum telomerase activity amongst all the cells of the body.
- *Cell cannibalization* required for self survival is called *autophagy*.
- **Necroptosis** is a *caspase independent process* which resembles necrosis morphologically and apoptosis mechanistically as a form of programmed cell death.
- **Pyroptosis** is a programmed cell death is accompanied by the release of fever inducing cytokine IL-1. It also involves **caspases 1 and 11**.
- Commonest *fixative used for light microscopic* examination: *10% buffered neutral formalin*
- Commonest fixative used for *electron microscopic* examination: **glutaraldehyde**

UPDATED INFORMATION FROM 9TH EDITION OF ROBBINS
Necroptosis and Pyroptosis

- Necroptosis resembles necrosis morphologically and apoptosis mechanistically as a form of programmed cell death. It is triggered by ligation of TNFR1, and viral proteins of RNA and DNA viruses.
- Necroptosis is caspase-independent but dependent on signaling by the RIP1 and RIP3 complex.
- RIP1-RIP3 signaling reduces mitochondrial ATP generation, causes production of ROS, and permeabilizes lysosomal membranes, thereby causing cellular swelling and membrane damage as occurs in necrosis.
- The release of cellular contents evokes an inflammatory reaction as in necrosis.

Pyroptosis occurs in cells infected by microbes. It involves activation of caspase-1 which cleaves the precursor form of IL-1 to generate biologically active IL-1. Caspase-1 along with closely related caspase-11 also lead to death of the infected cell.

Autophagy

- Autophagy is an adaptive response that is enhanced during nutrient deprivation, allowing the cell to cannibalize itself to survive. It involves sequestration of cellular organelles into cytoplasmic autophagic vacuoles (autophagosomes) that fuse with lysosomes and digest the enclosed material. The autophagosome formation is regulated by more than a dozen proteins that act in a coordinated and sequential manner.
- Dysregulation of autophagy occurs in many disease states including cancers, inflammatory bowel diseases, and neurodegenerative disorders. Autophagy plays a role in host defense against certain microbes.
- In *Alzheimer disease, formation of autophagosomes is accelerated* and in *Huntington disease, mutant huntingtin impairs autophagy.*

CHAPTER 2

Inflammation

Response of the blood vessels and cells to an injurious stimulus is called inflammation. It can be:

- *Acute inflammation:* It is of shorter duration (seconds, minutes, few hours)
- *Chronic inflammation:* It is of longer duration (weeks, months and years)

The changes seen in inflammation can be in the blood vessels (called vascular changes) and in the cells (called cellular changes).

I. **Vascular Changes**

1. *Vasoconstriction*: It is the *first*[Q] change in the blood vessels which is transient in nature. Clinically it is responsible for the blanching seen immediately after injury.

2. *Vasodilation*: Second change in the blood vessels lasting for a longer duration is vasodilation. It results in increased blood flow leading to redness (*rubor*) and the sensation of warmth (*color*).

3. *Increased permeability*: It is the *hallmark of acute inflammation*[Q] caused by separation of the endothelial cells resulting in movement of fluid, cells and proteins out of the blood vessels (collectively called as *exudate*). The *exudate* is a protein rich fluid which is responsible for the swelling (*tumor*) associated with an injury. It is *maximally seen in the venules*. The various mechanisms of increased vascular permeability are explained below:

> Increased vascular permeability is the **hallmark of acute inflammation**

MECHANISMS OF INCREASED VASCULAR PERMEABILITY			
Mechanism	**Caused by**	**Affected blood vessels**	**Properties of response**
1. Formation of endothelial gaps (***Immediate transient response***[Q])	Vasoactive mediators like histamine, leukotrienes, bradykinin and contraction of endothelial cell cytoskeleton	Venules	Rapid; Reversible; short lived (15 to 30 minutes)
2. Direct endothelial injury (***immediate sustained response***[Q])	Toxins, infections, burns, chemicals causing endothelial cell necrosis and detachment	Venules, capillaries and arterioles	Fast and may be long lived
3. Cytoskeletal reorganisation (**Endothelial cell retraction**[Q])	Due to cytokines and hypoxia	Mostly venules[Q]; capillaries may be also involved	***Reversible, delayed and prolonged***
4. Delayed prolonged leakage	Thermal and radiation injury induced endothelial cell damage	Venules and capillaries	Delayed and long lived
5. Leukocyte mediated endothelial injury	Activated leukocytes causing endothelial injury or detachment	Venules (mostly); pulmonary and glomerular capillaries	Late and long lived
6. Increased transcytosis	Formation of vesiculo-vacuolar organelles near inter cellular junctions by histamine and VEGF	Venules	
7. Leakage from new blood vessel	Mostly by vascular endothelial growth factor (VEGF) and less commonly by histamine and substance P	Sites of angiogenesis	

4. The loss of fluid results in concentration of red cells in small vessels and increased viscosity of the blood leading to slower blood flow and is called *stasis*.

> Formation of endothelial gaps (**Immediate transient response**) is the **commonest mechanism for increased permeability**.

> **Selectins** are responsible for **"rolling"** of neutrophils.

> Endothelial cell expression of E-selectin is a hallmark of acute cytokine mediated inflammation.

> β_2-Integrins are neutrophil adhesion molecules.

> **LAD1:** Integrin defects; recurrent infections and **delayed separation of umbilical cord stump**

> **LAD2:** Selectin defects; recurrent infections, **Bombay blood group** and mental retardation.

II. Cellular Changes

The sequence of events in the journey of leukocytes from the vessel lumen to the interstitial tissue, called *extravasation*, can be divided into the following steps:

1. *Margination*: Movement of the leukocytes which are normally moving in the centre of the blood vessel towards the periphery of the blood vessel is called as margination.

2. *Rolling*: It is the process of transient adhesion of leukocytes with the endothelial cells. *Selectins* are the most important molecules responsible for it. They interact with the complementary molecules resulting in transient adhesion. The selectins can be either.

   E selectin (CD 62E) – Present on cytokine-activated *endothelial cells* and interacts with sialyl lewis X receptor on the leukocyte.
   L selectin (CD 62L) – Present on *leukocytes* and interacts with glycoprotein adhesion molecules (GlyCAM-1), Mad CAM-1 and CD34 on endothelial cells.
   P selectin (CD 62P) – Present on *platelets and endothelial cells* and interacts with sialyl lewis X receptor on leukocytes.

3. *Adhesion*: It is firm attachment of the leukocytes to the endothelial cells. *Integrins* are the most important molecules promoting cell-cell or cell-matrix interactions by interacting with vascular cell adhesion molecule (VCAM) or intercellular adhesion molecule (ICAM). These can be of two types:

   β_1-**containing integrins**: These are also called VLA molecules and interact with VCAM-1 on endothelial cells.

   β_2-**containing integrins**: These are also called LFA-1 or Mac-1 and interact with ICAM-1 on endothelial cells.

Concept: Clinical importance of adhesion molecules (Harrison's 18th/478)

Leukocyte adhesion deficiency type 1 (LAD1) is caused *by a defect in the CD 18 molecule required for biosynthesis of the β_2 chain shared by the LFA-1 and Mac-1 integrins*. Poor adhesion is accompanied by defective aggregation and chemotaxis. So, these patients have **recurrent bacterial infections** involving skin, oral and genital mucosa, respiratory and intestinal tract; persistent leukocytosis because cells don't marginate and a history of **delayed separation of umbilical cord stump[Q]** is present.

Leukocyte adhesion deficiency type 2 (LAD2) is caused by the absence of *sialyl-Lewis X, the fucose-containing ligand for E-selectin, owing to a defect in the enzyme fucosyl transferase* responsible for binding fucose moieties to protein backbones. Patients have recurrent bacterial infections, platelet disfunction short stature, **Bombay blood group[Q]** and mental retardation. LAD 2 is also called as "congenital disorder of glycosylation IIc".

Leukocyte adhesion deficiency type 3 (LAD3) is caused by the *mutation in FERMT3 gene* resulting in impaired signaling for integrin activation. Patients have petechial hemorrhage, leucocytosis and recurrent infections.

*Both LAD1 and LAD2 are autosomal recessive conditions.

Endothelial Leukocyte adhesion molecules and their functions		
Endothelial molecule	*WBC receptor*	*Major role*
P-selectin	Sialyl- Lewis X	Rolling
E-selectin	Sialyl- Lewis X	Rolling, adhesion to activated endothelium
ICAM-1	CD 11/CD 18 (Integrins)	Adhesion, arrest, transmigration
VCAM-1	VLA 4, LPAM-1	Adhesion
Glycam-1	L-selectin	Lymphocytes homing to high endothelial venules
CD 31(PECAM)	CD 31	WBC migration through endothelium.

4. *Transmigration*: The step in the process of the migration of **the leukocytes[Q]** through the endothelium is called transmigration or *diapedesis*. The most important molecule responsible for diapedesis is called **PECAM-1** (platelet endothelial cell adhesion molecule) or **CD31**. Neutrophils predominate in the

inflammatory infiltrate during the first 6 to 24 hours, then are replaced by monocytes in 24 to 48 hours (*except in Pseudomonas infection in which neutrophils predominate over 2 to 4 days*).

5. *Chemotaxis*: It is **unidirectional movement**[Q] of the leukocytes towards antigens/bacteria in response to certain chemicals. These chemicals are called chemotactic stimuli. They can be:

   a. *Exogenous*: Bacterial products[Q]
   b. *Endogenous products*: C5a, LTB 4, IL-8

All the chemotactic agents mentioned above bind to G-protein coupled receptors (GPCRs) on the surface of leukocytes to cause actin polymerization and all movements. Other actin-regulating proteins like *filamin, gelsolin, profilin*, and *calmodulin* also interact with actin and myosin to produce contraction and cellular movement. The leukocytes degranulate to release lysosomal enzymes, cytokines and produce arachidonic acid metabolites. The leukocyte activation takes place due to GPCRs, cytokine receptors and Toll-like receptors (TLRs).

6. *Opsonisation*: Coating of the bacteria so that they are easily phagocytosed by the white blood cells is known as opsonisation.

   *Mnemonic corollary – friends I believe all of you have had waterballs or golgappe at some point of time in your life, u can have them both with and without water but in which condition do u think they are tastier? Well majority would answer the latter option i.e. 'with water'. The function of water is to make the golgappa tastier. Similarly, opsonins make the bacteria tastier for the leukocytes. Please remember that the WBCs can kill bacteria without opsonins also but opsonised bacteria are preferentially killed.

Chemicals causing opsonisation are called **opsonins**. These are:

   C3b[Q]
   Fc fragment of antibody or IgG[Q].
   Some serum proteins (like fibrinogen[Q], mannose binding lectin[Q] and C reactive protein[Q])

7. *Phagocytosis*: It is the process by which bacteria are killed/eaten up by the white blood cells. Lysosomes are important organelles required for phagocytosis.

Phagocytosis: It is characterized by 3 steps

a. **Recognition and attachment**: The particles to be ingested by leukocytes (microbes and dead cells) are recognized by receptors present on the surface of WBCs. These receptors are.
   i. *Scavenger receptors*: These bind microbes and oxidized or acetylated LDL particles.
   ii. *Mac-1 integrins*: These are present on the surface of macrophages.
   iii. *Mannose receptors*: These bind to mannose and fucose residues of glycoproteins in microbial cell wall. The presence of an additional terminal sialic acid or N-acetyl galactosamine in human cells prevents their destruction by WBCs.

b. **Engulfment**: There is formation of phagolysosome (due to fusion of the lysosomes and the phagosome containing the microbe) inside the leukocytes. This is followed by degranulation of leukocytes.

Concept

The clinical significance of phagolysosome formation is appreciated in an autosomal recessive disorder known as Chediak-Higashi syndrome. It is characterized by *reduced transfer of lysosomal enzymes to phagocytic vacuoles* in phagocytes, defective degranulation, and delayed microbial killing causing increased susceptibility to infections. The *polymorphs also exhibit defective random movements and have **defective chemotaxis***.

Clinical features: It includes neutropenia (decreased numbers of neutrophils), albinism (due to abnormalities in melanocytes), nerve defects, nystagmus and bleeding disorders (due to defect in neurons and platelets respectively). These patients also have reduced NK cell responsiveness.

The secretion of granule proteins by cytotoxic T cells is also affected which also contributes to the immunodeficiency. The gene for lysosomal trafficking is called LYST.

Leukocyte diapedesis, similar to increased vascular permeability, occurs predominantly in the **venules** (*except in the lungs, where it also occurs in capillaries*).

Example of **Opsonins** include **antibodies, complement proteins and lectins.**

Chemotaxis: It is unidirectional or *targeted movement* of the leukocytes towards antigens/bacteria.

Concept

IgG is produced by activated B cells called plasma cells. Bruton's disease is a defect in maturation of the B cells in which there is absence of immunoglobulin. So, *Bruton's disease* is characterized by *defective opsonisation*.

Phagocytosis (cell eating) requires **polymerization of actin** filaments whereas in contrast, *pinocytosis* (cell drinking) and *receptor mediated endocytosis* require *clathrin* coated pits.

The leukocytes in **Chediak-Higashi syndrome** have **giant granules** seen in peripheral blood smear which are due to aberrant organelle fusion.

O₂-dependent MPO system is most potent microbicidal system.

NADPH oxidase is also called by the name of respiratory burst oxidase.

Chronic granulomatous disease (CGD) is a disease caused due to a defect in NADPH oxidase activity and respiratory burst.

Concept

Chronic granulomatous disease is a disease caused due to a defect in NADPH oxidase activity characterised by repeated infections by catalase positive organisms; (bacterial infections mostly due to Staph. aureus and fungal due to Candida).

Nitroblue-tetrazolium test is the most widely known test for chronic granulomatous disease.

c. **Killing and degradation:** Final step in phagocytosis is the killing of infectious organism within the leukocytes. It can be accomplished by

i. **Oxygen dependent killing mechanism**

There is production of microbicidal reactive oxygen species within phagocytic vesicles by the following mechanism:

The final step in the microbial killing is due to reactive oxygen species called as 'respiratory burst'.

Phagocytes (i.e., neutrophils, monocytes, and macrophages) require an enzyme to produce reactive oxygen species to destroy bacteria after they ingest the bacteria in a process called phagocytosis. This enzyme is termed "phagocyte NADPH oxidase" (*PHOX*). The initial step in this process involves the one-electron reduction of molecular oxygen to produce superoxide free radical. Superoxide then undergoes a further series of reactions to produce products such as peroxide, hydroxyl radical and hypochlorite. The reactive oxygen species thus produced are toxic to bacteria and help the phagocyte kill them once they are ingested.

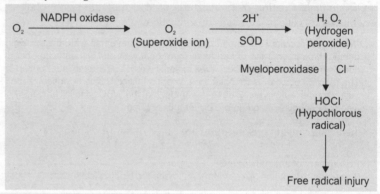

Chronic granulomatous disease (CGD) has a defective NADPH oxidase activity with recurrent infection and granuloma formation affecting gastrointestinal or genitourinary tract. CGD can be diagnosed with the following tests:

Nitroblue-tetrazolium (NBT) test: It is negative in chronic granulomatous disease and positive in normal individuals. This test depends upon the direct reduction of NBT by superoxide free radical to form an insoluble formazan. This test is simple to perform and gives rapid results, but only tells whether or not there is a problem with the PHOX enzymes, not how much they are affected.

Dihydrorhodamine (DHR) test: in this test, the whole blood is stained with DHR, incubated and stimulated produce superoxide radicals which reduce DHR to rhodamin in cells with normal function.

Cytochrome C reduction assay is an advanced test that tells physicians how much superoxide a patient's phagocytes can produce.

Difference between Myeloperoxidase deficiency and Chronic Granulomatous Disease (CGD)

In CGD, some phagocytosed organisms (catalase negative organisms like steptococci) can be killed because these organisms produce their own hydrogen peroxide which is used by neutrophilic myeloperoxidase to produce free radicals and kill them.

In myeloperoxidase deficiency, the enzyme myeloperoxidase is absent, so both catalase positive and catalase-negative organisms will survive within phagocytes and cause infections.

Enzymes involved in respiratory burst

- NADPH oxidase is chiefly responsible for the formation of hydrogen peroxide which plays the most important role in microbial killing.
- Catalase degrades hydrogen peroxide into water and oxygen.
- Superoxide dismutase (SOD) causes conversion of superoxide ion into hydrogen peroxide.

– Glutathione peroxidase causes conversion of reduced glutathione to its homodimer.

$$2OH^- + 2GSH \rightarrow 2H_2O + GSSG$$

Note: H_2O_2 – MPO – halide system is the most efficient way of killing the bacteria[Q].

ii. **Oxygen independent killing mechanism**
It can be done by various enzymes and proteins like
– *Lysozyme:* Cause hydrolysis of glycopeptide coat of bacteria.
– *Lactoferrin:* It is an iron binding protein.
– Bacterial permeability increasing protein.
– *Major basic protein*[Q] (MBP).
– *Defensins*: These are arginine rich peptides toxic to the microbes.
– *Cathelicidins*: These are antimicrobial proteins in the neutrophils and other cells They are highly effective against M. tuberculosis.

> **Major basic protein** is present in **Eosinophils** and is *toxic to parasites*.

IMPORTANT CHEMICAL MEDIATORS

Chemical mediators of inflammation may be present in cells (cellular) or in the plasma.

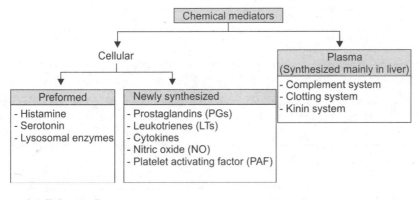

> *Concept*
> The synthesis of antimicrobial protein cathelicidin is stimulated by 1, 25 dihyroxyvitamin D. The importance of this non skeletal effect of vitamin D is that vitamin D deficiency can increase the chances of tubercular infections

Preformed Cellular Mediators

a. *Histamine*: It is formed from the amino acid 'histidine'. **Mast cells** are the richest source of histamine. It is also present in platelets and basophils. It causes **vasodilation (but vasoconstriction of large arteries)**, increased permeability (*immediate transient response*) and bronchoconstriction.

b. *Serotonin* (5-HT): Richest source of serotonin (5- hydroxytryptamine; 5- HT) is **platelets**. It has actions similar to histamine. It is also present in **enterochromaffin cells**.

c. *Lysosomal Enzymes*: These are present in the lysosomes of neutrophils and monocytes. Lysosomes contain two types of granules; Primary (azurophilic) and secondary (specific) granules.

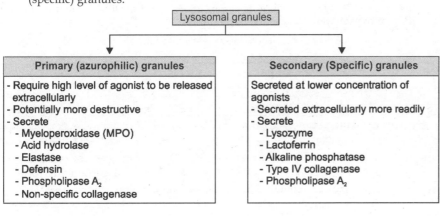

> Histamine is the most important chemical mediator of acute inflammation.

– Two major anti-proteases present in the body are α_1 antitrypsin and α_2 macroglobulin
– *Neutrophils also have **tertiary granules or C particles** which contain gelatinase and acid hydrolases.*

Newly Synthesized Cellular Mediators

a. *Nitric Oxide* (NO): It is formed from l-arginine with the help of enzyme nitric oxide synthase (NOS).

$$L\text{-Arginine} \xrightarrow[\text{NOS}]{\text{NADPH} + O_2} L\text{- Citrulline} + NO$$

Three isoforms of NOS are present in the body:

i. **e** NOS (Present in **e**ndothelium)
ii. **n** NOS (Present in **n**eurons)
iii. **i** NOS (**i**nducible form)

eNOS and nNOS are constitutively expressed whereas i NOS production is induced by cytokines like TNF α and IFN-γ.

Important actions of NO

Potent vasodilator
Reduction of platelet aggregation
Endogenous regulator of leucocyte recruitment
Also possess microbicidal action: NO acts as a free radical and can also be converted to highly reactive peroxynitrite anion ($ONOO^-$) as well as NO_2 and NO_3.

b. *Cytokines* : These are small proteinaceous molecules secreted by the inflammatory cells. These include interleukins, interferons and tumor necrosis factor- alpha (TNF-α). These can produce local and systemic effects. Most important cytokine responsible for systemic effects of inflammation are interleukin-1 (IL-1) and tumor necrosis factor- alpha (TNF-α).

IL-1, TNF-α		
Acute phase reaction	Endothelial and fibroblast effects	WBC effects
- Fever	• ↑ PGI_2 formation	• ↑ Secretion of IL-1 and IL-6
- Increased sleep	• ↑ Procoagulant	
- Decreased appetite	• ↑ Fibroblast	
- Neutrophilia	• ↑ Collagen	

Important info

Resolvins and protectins are anti inflammatory lipid mediators derived from polyunsaturated fatty acids which along with IL-10, TGF-β and lipoxins help in the termination of acute inflammatory response.

c. *Arachidonic acid metabolites* : Arachidonic acid (AA) is a 20-C fatty acid containing four double bonds. It must be released/mobilized from membrane phospholipids (PL) for oxygenation to various compounds.

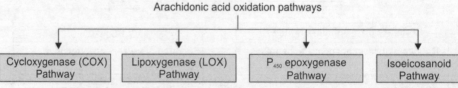

Arachidonic acid oxidation pathways

| Cycloxygenase (COX) Pathway | Lipoxygenase (LOX) Pathway | P_{450} epoxygenase Pathway | Isoeicosanoid Pathway |

i. **COX pathway:** Two type of COX-enzymes (also known as PGH synthase); COX-1 and COX-2 convert AA to PGG_2 first and then to PGH_2 [both are called cyclic endoperoxides]. Further fate of PGH_2 depend upon the enzyme present in a particular cell e.g. endothelium contain PGI_2 synthase and thus forms PGI_2 whereas platelets contain TXA_2 synthase and therefore synthesize TXA_2.

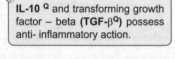

Nitric Oxide is synthesized from the amino acid l-arginine.

IL-1[Q] is the **most important cytokine** responsible for the **systemic effects** of inflammation

IL-10 [Q] and transforming growth factor – beta (**TGF-β**[Q]) possess anti- inflammatory action.

TGF-β is the **most important fibrogenic**[Q] agent

IL-1, IL-6, TNF-α and type I interferons contribute to acute phase response.

Pyrogenic cytokines
• Exogenous : LPS
• Endogenous : IL-1/TNFα
    ISNα/CNTF
    IL-6

Inflammation

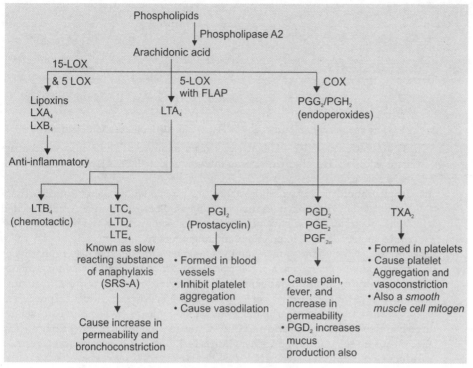

FLAP- **F**ive **L**ipoxygenase **A**ctivating **P**rotein

ii. **LOX-pathway:** AA can be acted upon different types of LOX enzymes.

    1. **5-LOX** (present in leukocytes, mast cells and dendritic cells) acts in the presence of FLAP [5-LOX activating protein] to convert AA to LTA_4. This product can be converted either to LTB_4 or to cysteinyl Leukotrienes (LTC_4, D_4 and E_4).

    2. **15-LOX** converts AA to 15-HETE which can be converted to Lipoxins (LXA_4 and LXB_4) with the action of 5-LOX. Lipoxins can also be synthesized by action of 12-LOX on LTA_4.

LTB_4 is a potent chemotactic molecule for T-lymphocytes, eosinophils, monocytes and mast cells whereas LTC_4, D_4 and F_4 are chemotactic for T-lymphocytes and eosinophils. Lipoxins[Q] cause activation of monocytes and macrophages and inhibition of neutrophils[Q]. These also inhibit NK cell cytotoxicity and are powerful coronary vasoconstrictors in vivo.

iii. **Epoxygenase pathway:** Cytochrome P450 may convert AA to 20-HETE or EET. Biological effects of EET are reduced by metabolism to less active DHET with the help of epoxide hydrolases.

    • EET may function as endothelium derived hyperpolarizing factor particularly in coronary circulation. It also possesses anti-inflammatory, anti-apoptotic and pro-angiogenic action.

    • 20-HETE cause vasoconstriction of renal arteries and has been implicated in the pathogenesis of hypertension. In contrast, EET possess antihypertensive properties via its vasodilating and natriuretic actions. Inhibitors of epoxide hydrolase [results in elevated levels of EET] are being developed as antihypertensive drugs.

COX-1 is mostly **constitutive** (house-keeping) whereas **COX-2** is **inducible**. However, in endothelium, kidney and CNS, even COX-2 is constitutively present.

$PGF_{2\alpha}$[Q] is a **vasoconstrictor** whereas PGD_2 and PGE_2 are vasodilators.

PGI_2 cause inhibition of platelet aggregation (**I** stands for **I**nhibition) and TXA_2 cause platelet aggregation (**A** for **a**ggregation)

LTC_4[Q] and LTC_4[Q] [primary components of **slow reacting substance of anaphylaxis; SRS-A**[Q]] are powerful bronchoconstrictors, increase permeability and mucus secretion in airways.

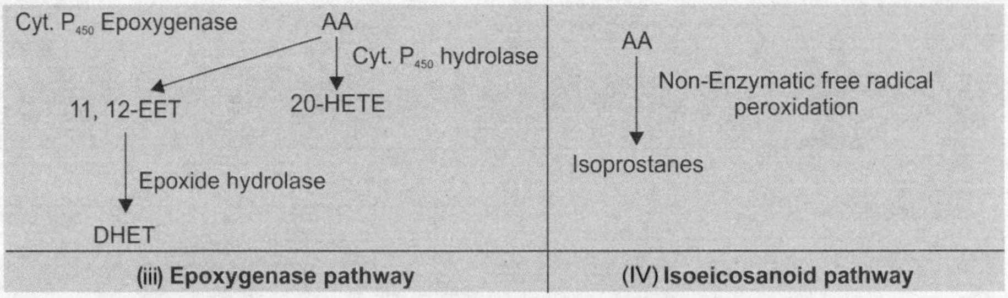

Abbreviations: DHET – Dihydroxyeicosatrienoic acid, EET – Epoxyeicosatrienoic acid, HETE – Hydroxyeicosatetraenoic acid, HPETE – Hydroxyperoxyeicosatetraenoic acid.

iv. **Isoeicosanoid pathway:** Isoprostanes are prostaglandin stereoisomers. These are formed by non-enzymatic free-radical based peroxidation of AA and related lipid substrates. These have potent vasoconstrictor activity and modulate WBC and platelet adhesive interactions and angiogenesis.

d. *Chemokines :* Chemokines are a family of ***small proteins*** that act primarily as ***chemoattractants*** *for specific types of leukocytes.* **They are classified into 4 major groups according to the arrangement of conserved cysteine residue in mature proteins.** Most the chemokines have four conserved cysteine residues (expressed as C). X means amino acid other than C. Thus, C-X-C means two conserved cysteines are separated by one amino acid and C-X3-C means separation by three amino acids. C-C means no separation and C-chemokines lack first and third conserved cysteine residues.

Chemokines

α-chemokines (C X C)	β-chemokines (C-C)	γ-chemokines (C chemokine)	CX_3C chemokine
• Primarily act on neutrophils • e.g. **IL-8**° • Cause activation and chemotaxis of neutrophils° • Induced by microbial products and other cytokines (mainly IL-1 and TNF)	• Attract all leukocytes except neutrophils° • **MCP-1** (Monocyte chemoattractant protein) • **RANTES** (regulated and normal T-cell expressed and secreted) • **Eotaxin** (selectively recruits eosinophils)	• Relatively selective for lymphocytes • attract T cell precursors to thymus • e.g. lymphotactin	• Chemotactic for monocytes and T cells • **Fractalkaline** is the only known member of this class

Note: Chemokines mediate their actions through chemokine receptors (CXCR or CCR). Certain receptors (CXCR4; CCR5) act as co-receptors for binding and entry of HIV into CD4 cells.

IL-8 is chemotactic for **neutrophils** whereas *Eotaxin selectively recruits eosinophils.*

Mediators Present in Plasma

a. **Complement system**

It consists of 20 complement proteins (and their breakdown products) present in the plasma. These are numbered C_1 to C_9. The complement system has the following four pathways:

- **Classic** activation pathway activated by antigen/antibody immune complexes,
- **Mannose binding lectin** activation pathway activated by microbes with terminal mannose groups
- **Alternativ**e activation pathway activated by microbes or tumor cells
- **Terminal** pathway that is common to the first three pathways and leads to the membrane attack complex that lyses cells.

Critical step in the functioning of the complement system is the **activation of C_3** (most abundant component).

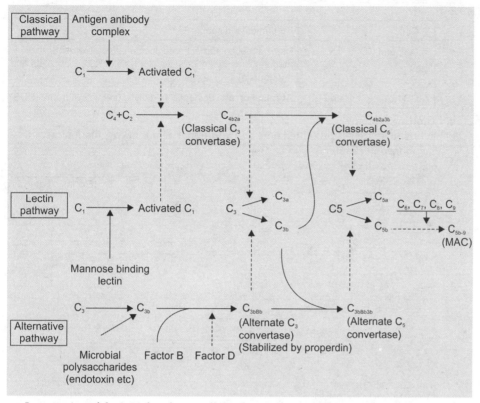

Classical Pathway activation: *decreased C_1, C_2, C_4, C_3;* with *normal factor B.*

Alternative pathway activation: *decreased factor B, C_3;* with *normal C_1, C_2 and C_4.*

Concept

C1 inhibitor (C1 INH) blocks binding of C1 to immune complex. So its deficiency causes excessive complement activation. This forms the basis of development of herediatary angioneurotic edema.

Irrespective of the initial pathway, all the three cause break down of activation of C_3 and result in the formation of membrane attack complex (MAC). This complex causes antigenic destruction.

FUNCTIONS OF IMPORTANT INDIVIDUAL COMPLEMENT PROTEINS

- C_{3a} and C_{5a} are also called **anaphylatoxins** which are chemicals causing release of histamine from mast cells. So, they cause vasodilation and increased vascular permeability.
- C_{3b} and inactive C_3 (C_{3i}) used for opsonisation.
- C_{5a} also has important role in chemotaxis.
- C_{5b-9} (Membrane Attack Complex; MAC) attacks and kills the antigen.

REGULATORY MOLECULES OF COMPLEMENT SYSTEM

- Decay accelerating factor (DAF) increases the dissociation of C_3 convertase.
- Factor I proteolytically cleaves C_{3b}.
- CD59 (Membrane inhibitor of reactive lysis) inhibits formation of MAC.
- Factor H, factor I and CD46 prevent exessive alternate pathway activation.

Deficiency of C2 is the most common complement deficiency and is associated with Streptococcal septicemia and lupus like syndrome in children.

Deficiency of complement component	Disease/Syndrome
1. C1 esterase Inhibitor	Hereditary angioneurotic edema (subcutaneous edema because of excessive complement activation)
2. Early complement proteins C_1, C_2, C_4	SLE and collagen vascular disorders
3. C_{3b} and C_{3b} inactivator	Recurrent pyogenic infections
4. C_5 to C_8	Bacterial infections with Neisseria and Toxoplasmosis

cont...

IgM and IgG (**IgM** > IgG) are responsible for activation of **classical pathway** whereas **IgA** is responsible for activation **alternate pathway**.

cont...

5. C_9	No particular disease
6. DAF and CD59	Paroxysmal nocturnal hemoglobinuria (complement mediated increased intravascular lysis of RBCs, platelets and neutrophils)
7. CD46, factors H and I	**Atypical** or 'non epidemic' hemolytic uremic syndrome (HUS)

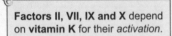

All the clotting factors are synthesized in the **liver** *except factor IV* (calcium) and a factor VIII carrier protein called *von Willebrand factor.*

Factors II, VII, IX and X depend on **vitamin K** for their *activation.*

Monitoring of **intrinsic pathway** is done using activated partial thromboplastin time **(aPTT)** and *extrinsic pathway* using prothrombin time *(PT)* or *International Sensitivity Index* (ISI)

Factor XII is the only protein in the coagulation cascade whose deficiency does not cause bleeding but rather results in a prothrombotic state.

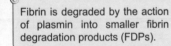

Fibrin is degraded by the action of plasmin into smaller fibrin degradation products (FDPs).

b. **Clotting system**

A brief overview is presented here and additional details of coagulation cascade are mentioned in **chapter 3.**

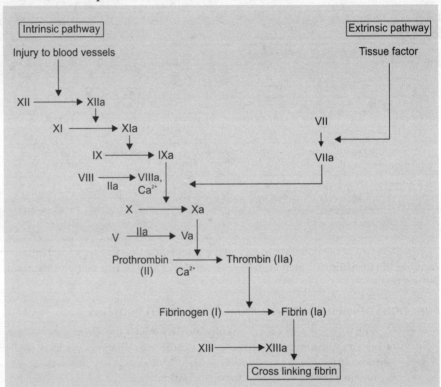

The most important function of clotting system activation is formation blood clot that helps to prevent excessive blood loss. Some of the components of the clotting system also play other roles e.g. fibrinogen is used for opsonisation and thrombin causes chemotaxis.

Clinical correlation: Deficiency of clotting factors VIII and IX resulting in hemophilia A and B respectively.

Why a patient of hemophilia would bleed inspite of a normal extrinsic pathway?

Answer: The main function of the extrinsic pathway in hemostasis is to produce initial limited thrombin activation upon tissue injury which is reinforced and amplified by a critical feedback loop whereby thrombin activates factors XI and IX of the intrinsic pathway. In addition, high levels of thrombin are required to activate TAFI (thrombin activatable fibrinolysis inhibitor) that augments fibrin deposition by inhibiting fibrinolysis. Thus, both inadequate coagulation (fibrinogenesis) and inappropriate clot removal (fibrinolysis) contribute to the bleeding manifestations in hemophilia.

c. **Kinin System**

It is initiated by activated factor XII (Hageman's factor)

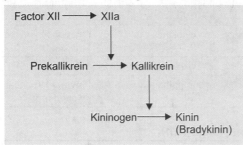

Kallikrein can also activate plasminogen into plasmin and cause activation of complement protein C5a

Functions of Bradykinin:

1. Contraction of smooth muscles
2. Pain
3. Dilation of the venules

The most important outcome of acute inflammation is clearance of the injurious stimuli and replacement of injured cells (resolution).

Morphological patterns of inflammation

Serous inflammation	Fibrinous inflammation	Catarrhal inflammation	Purulent inflammation
Presence of outpouring of thin fluid Effusion is fluid accumulation in cavities	Deposition of fibrin in extracellular space due to large vascular leaks Characteristic of inflammation in body cavity linings (meninges, pericardium)	Epithelial surface inflammation causes increased mucus secretion Seen in common cold	Purulent exudate is made of necrotic cells, neutrophils and edema fluid

CHRONIC INFLAMMATION

Chronic inflammation is characterized by infiltration with mononuclear cells (including macrophages, lymphocytes, and plasma cells), tissue destruction and healing by replacement of damaged tissue via angiogenesis and fibrosis. Macrophage is the dominant cell in chronic inflammation. It accumulates inside the tissue because of recruitment from circulation; local proliferation in tissue and immobilization at the site of inflammation. *Tissue destruction is the hallmark of chronic inflammation.*

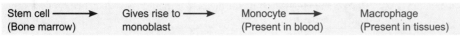

Macrophages have a life span ranging from months to years and they are given different names in different tissues e.g.

Liver	-	Kupffer cell
CNS	-	Microglia
Bone	-	Osteoclast
Lung	-	Alveolar macrophage or 'Dust cells'
Connective tissue	-	Histiocyte
Placenta	-	Hoffbauer cells
Spleen	-	Littoral cells
Kidney	-	Mesangial cells
Synovium	-	Type A lining cells

Inflammation

Monocytes and macrophages are the primary leukocytes in chronic inflammation.

Epithelioid cells are macrophages activated by interferon γ released from CD4 T cells

Warthin-Finkeldey giant cells are seen in **measles**.

Tumor giant cells like **Reed-Sternberg cells** are seen in **Hodgkin's lymphoma**

Amongst **IBD, Granuloma formation** is associated with **only Crohn's disease**; it is *not* seen in *ulcerative colitis*

Subsets of Activated Macrophages

Classically activated macrophages (M1)	Alternatively activated macrophages (M2)
Induced by microbial products and cytokines like IFN-γ[Q].	Induced by microbial products and cytokines like IL-4, IL-5[Q]
Release lysosomal enzymes, nitric oxide, IL-1and IL-12	Release IL-10[Q], TGF-β[Q]
Involved in microbicidal activities and pathogenic inflammation[Q]	Involved in anti-inflammatory actions and wound repair[Q]

GRANULOMATOUS INFLAMMATION

It is a type of chronic inflammation characterized by formation of granuloma. Granuloma is an *aggregation of macrophages surrounded by a collar of mononuclear cells* principally lymphocytes. Macrophages may get activated to form epithelioid cells (epithelium like cells). Some of the cells may fuse together to form a bigger cell called a **giant cell**. The giant cells can be primarily of the following types:

1. *Langerhans giant cell:* The nuclei in this giant cell are present in the periphery and in a horse shoe pattern. It is seen is **tuberculosis.**
2. *Foreign body giant cell:* The nuclei are arranged randomly or haphazardly here. It is seen in granuloma formed by *foreign bodies* like sutures, talc etc.
3. *Touton giant cells* are seen in *xanthomas, fat necrosis, xanthogranulomatous inflammtion and dermatofibroma.* They are formed by fusion of epithelioid cells and contain a ring of nuclei surrounded by foamy cytoplasm.
4. *Physiological giant cells* are seen in *osteoclasts, syncytiotrophoblasts and megakaryocytes.*

Common conditions resulting in granuloma formation with important features
- Tuberculosis
- Sarcoidosis (**Non caseating granuloma[Q]**)
- Brucellosis
- Cat scratch disease (**Stellate[Q]** shaped or **round granuloma**)
- Syphilis (**Gumma[Q]**)
- Lymphogranuloma inguinale
- Leprosy
- Inflammatory bowel disease (IBD)

The formation of a granuloma is discussed later in the chapter of 'immunity'.

Types of Cells

Depending on the regenerative capacity, cells can be divided into 3 categories.

1. Permanent cells	Cells of the body which **never divide** e.g. neurons, skeletal muscle fibres and cardiac myocytes.
2. Stable cells	They have a low rate of multiplication and are usually present is the G_0 **phase**. When given a stimulus, they enter the G1 phase and multiply e.g. Cells of proximal tubule of kidney, hepatocytes, pancreatic cells, fibroblasts etc.
3. Labile cells	These cells can regenerate throughout life e.g. hematopoietic cells, cells of skin, gastrointestinal mucosa etc.

WOUND HEALING

It is characterized by the process of regeneration of the damaged tissue by cells of the same type and replacement of the lost tissue with connective tissue. Regeneration refers to proliferation of cells and tissues to replace lost structures. It results in complete restitution of lost or damaged tissue.

Repair consists of a combination of regeneration and scar formation by the deposition of collagen. It may restore some original structures but can cause structural derangements.

Healing by Primary Intention

The healing of a clean uninfected wound is called healing by **first intention** or **primary union**. It involves the following changes.

Day	Features of wound
Day 0 (when the wound has formed)	Presence of blood clot in the incision
Day 1 (within 24 hours)	Neutrophilic infiltration + blood clot
Day 2 (24 to 48 hours)	Neutrophils + blood clot + continuous thin epithelial layer[Q]
Day 3	Macrophages replace neutrophils, Appearance of granulation tissue, type III collagen deposition begins but do not bridge the incision
Day 5	Abundant granulation tissue - Collagen fibrils bridge the incision - *Neovascularisation is maximum*[Q] - Full epithelial thickness with surface keratinization
End of 2nd week	Accumulation of collagen; fibroblast proliferation
1 month	Replacement of collagen type III with collagen type I (has greater tensile strength) due to action of collagenase enzyme

Vitamin C is required for the conversion of tropocollagen to collagen due to hydroxylation of lysine and proline residues providing stability to collagen molecules.

Healing by Secondary Intention

During healing by **secondary intention** or **secondary union**; inflammatory reaction being more intense, granulation tissue is abundant and a large scar is formed. The scar decreases in size after sometime; this is called as **scar contraction.**

Myofibroblasts are altered fibroblast having the presence of bundles of smooth muscle microfilaments α actin and vimentin immediately beneath the cell membrane and the cytoplasm which is responsible for the contractile properties of this cell. They arise from either tissue fibroblasts or fibrocytes in bone marrow or epithelial cells.

Wound strength is **10% after 1 week**[Q]; it increases rapidly during **next 4 weeks**[Q] and becomes **70% at the end of 3rd month**[Q]. The tensile strength of the wound keeps on increasing as time progresses.

The predominant collagen in adult skin is type I[Q] whereas in early granulation tissue, it is type III and I[Q].

The balance between extracellular matrix (ECM) synthesis and degradation results in *remodeling* of the connective tissue framework which is an important feature of chronic inflammation and wound repair. The collagen degradation is done by zinc dependent matrix metalloproteinases (MMP). Collagen degradation is important for tissue remodeling, angiogenesis and cancer metastasis. That is why *zinc deficiency is associated with impaired wound healing*. MMPs are synthesized by several cells like fibroblasts, macrophages, neutrophils, synovial cells, and some epithelial cells. Activated collagenases (a type of MMP) are rapidly inhibited by specific *tissue inhibitors of metalloproteinases (TIMPs)*, which are produced by most mesenchymal cells, thus preventing uncontrolled action of these proteases. The regulated activity is required for proper wound healing.

During wound healing, **complications** can arise from:

1. *Delayed wound healing*: Due to foreign body, ischemia, diabetes, malnutrition, hormones (glucocorticoids), infection or scurvy. Ascorbic acid deficiency causes reduced cross linking of tropocollagen to collagen and so, in this condition the patient has increased bleeding tendencies and poor wound healing.
2. *Deficient scar formation*: May lead to wound dehiscence and ulceration. Dehiscence or rupture of a wound is most common after abdominal surgery and is due to increased abdominal pressure.

Granulation tissue is fibroblasts + small blood vessel + chronic inflammatory cells (macrophage and lymphocytes)

Neo vascularisation is maximum on day 5.

Granulation tissue is the hallmark of the **fibrogenic repair.**

The chief cell responsible for **scar contraction** is **myofibroblast.**

Zinc is a cofactor in **collagenase**

Infections are the most common cause of impaired wound healing.

3. *Excessive formation of the repair components*: Certain conditions may arise because of increased granulation tissue or excessive collagen leading to keloid, hypertrophic scar and 'proud flesh'.

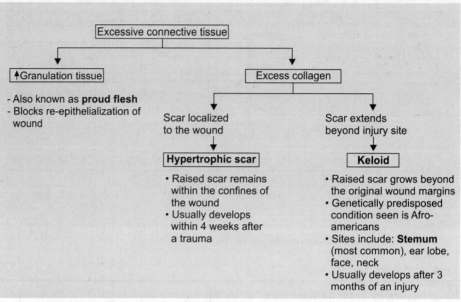

Sternum is commonest site for **keloid formation**

Intralesional steroids (triamcinolone) are the usual drugs for the managment of keloid.

Incisional scars or traumatic injuries may be followed by exuberant proliferation of fibroblasts and other connective tissue elements called *desmoids* or *aggressive fibromatoses*. These recur frequently after excision.

4. *Formation of contractures*: Contractures are particularly prone to develop on the palms, the soles, and the anterior aspect of the thorax. These are commonly seen after serious burns.

STEM CELLS

Definition: The most widely accepted stem cell definition is a cell with a unique capacity to produce unaltered daughter cells (*self-renewal*) and to generate specialized cell types (*potency*).

1. **Self-renewal** can be achieved in two ways:

Asymmetric cell division	Symmetric cell division
• Produces one daughter cell that is identical to the parental cell and one daughter cell that is different from the parental cell and is a progenitor or differentiated cell • Asymmetric cell division does not increase the number of stem cells.	• Produces two identical daughter cells

In human embryo in about 3rd week of development stem cells appear in yolk sac.

For stem cells to proliferate *in vitro*, they must divide symmetrically. Self-renewal alone cannot define stem cells, because any established cell line, e.g., HeLa cells proliferate by symmetric cell division.

2. **Potency** is used to indicate a cell's ability to differentiate into specialized cell types. This can be classified as:

In adults, most of the stem cells are found in the bone marrow, but a subset normally circulates in peripheral blood.

Totipotent cells	Multipotent cells	Oligopotent cells	Uni/Mono potent cells
Can form an entire organism autonomously.	Can form multiple cell lineages but cannot form all of the body's cell lineages.	Can form more than one cell lineage but are more restricted than multipotent cells.	Can form a single differentiated cell lineage.
Only zygote[Q] (fertilized egg) has this feature.	Hematopoietic[Q] stem cells	Neuron[Q] stem cells	Spermatogonial[Q] stem cells

Concept

Stem cells are used in bone marrow transplantation in treatment of various types of leukemia and lymphoma.

Terminally differentiated cells, such as fibroblast cells, also have a capacity to proliferate (which may be called self-renewal) but maintain the same cell type (e.g., no potency to form another cell type) and are not, therefore, considered unipotent cells.

Embryonic stem cells are pluripotent, that is, they are capable of forming all the tissues of the body

Adult stem cells are usually only able to differentiate into a particular tissue.

- Stem cells are located in special sites called **niches**.

Name of the cell	Location	Function
Oval cells[Q]	Canals of Herring of the liver	Forming hepatocytes and biliary cells
Satellite cells[Q]	Basal lamina of myotubules	Differentiate into myocytes after injury
Limbus cells[Q]	Canals of Schlemm[Q]	Stem cells for the cornea[Q]
Ito cells[Q]	Subendothelial space of Disse[Q]	Store vitamin A[Q]
Paneth cells	Bottom of crypts	Host defense against microorganisms

Other sites for stem cells are the base of the crypts of the colon and the dentate gyrus of the hippocampus.

Other Important Concepts in Stem Cell Biology

- Development naturally progresses from totipotent fertilized eggs to pluripotent epiblast cells, to multipotent cells, and finally to terminally differentiated cells.
- **Nuclear reprogramming:** The reversal of the terminally differentiated cells to totipotent or pluripotent cells (called *nuclear reprogramming*) has been achieved using *nuclear transplantation*, or *nuclear transfer* (NT), procedures (often called "cloning"), where the nucleus of a differentiated cell is transferred into an enucleated oocyte.
- **Stem cell plasticity or trans-differentiation:** The prevailing standard in developmental biology is that once cells are differentiated, their phenotypes are stable. However, a number of reports have shown that tissue stem cells, which are thought to be lineage-committed multipotent cells, possess the capacity to differentiate into cell types outside their lineage restrictions (called *trans-differentiation*). For example, hematopoietic stem cells may be converted into neurons as well as germ cells.

MULTIPLE CHOICE QUESTIONS

ACUTE INFLAMMATION, VASCULAR AND CELLULAR CHANGES

1. **In acute inflammation endothelial retraction leads to**
   (AIIMS Nov 2011)
   (a) Delayed transient increase in permeability
   (b) Immediate transient increase in permeability
   (c) Delayed prolonged increase in permeability
   (d) Immediate transient decrease in permeability

2. **After binding of complement and antibody on the surface of encapsulated bacteria, the process of phagocytosis by polymorphonuclear leukocytes involves which of the following?** *(AIIMS Nov 2011)*
   (a) Fc and C3b
   (b) Receptor-mediated endocytosis
   (c) Respiratory burst
   (d) Pseudopod extension

3. **Free radicals are generated by all except** *(AI 2011)*
   (a) Superoxide dismutase
   (b) NADPH Oxidase
   (c) Myeloperoxidase
   (d) NO synthase

4. **Which among the following is the hallmark of acute inflammation?** *(AI 2011, AIIMS May 2010)*
   (a) Vasoconstriction
   (b) Stasis
   (c) Vasodilation and increase in permeability
   (d) Leukocyte margination

5. **Main feature of chemotaxis is** *(AIIMS May 2010)*
   (a) Increased random movement of neutrophils
   (b) Increase adhesiveness to intima
   (c) Increased phagocytosis
   (d) Unidirectional locomotion of the neutrophils

6. **Characteristic of acute inflammation is:** *(AI 2009)*
   (a) Vasodilation and increased vascular permeability
   (b) Vasoconstriction
   (c) Platelet aggregation
   (d) Infiltration by neutrophils

7. **Which of the following helps in generating reactive O_2 intermediates in the neutrophils?**
   (a) NADPH oxidase *(AI '11, 08, AIIMS Nov 2008)*
   (b) SOD (superoxide dismutase)
   (c) Catalase
   (d) Glutathione peroxidase

8. **Basement membrane degeneration is mediated by:**
   (a) Metalloproteinases *(AI 2008)*
   (b) Oxidases
   (c) Elastases
   (d) Hydroxylases

9. **Delayed prolonged bleeding is caused by:**
   (a) Histamine *(AI 2008)*
   (b) Endothelial retraction
   (c) IL-1
   (d) Direct injury to endothelial cells

10. **Earliest transient change following tissue injury will be:** *(AI 2007)*
    (a) Neutropenia
    (b) Neutrophilia
    (c) Monocytosis
    (d) Lymphocytosis

11. **All of the following vascular changes are observed in acute inflammation, except:** *(AI 2005)*
    (a) Vasodilation
    (b) Stasis of blood
    (c) Increased vascular permeability
    (d) Decreased hydrostatic pressure

12. **The following host tissue responses can be seen in acute infection, except:** *(AI 2002)*
    (a) Exudation
    (b) Vasodilation
    (c) Margination
    (d) Granuloma formation

13. **Oxygen dependent killing is done through**
    (a) NADPH oxidase *(AI 2007)*
    (b) Superoxide dismutase
    (c) Catalase
    (d) Glutathione peroxidase

14. **Which of the following is not true?**
    (a) NADPH oxidase generate superoxide ion
    (b) MPO kills by OCl⁻ *(AIIMS May 2009)*
    (c) Chediak-Higashi syndrome is due to defective phagolysosome formation
    (d) In Bruton's disease there is normal opsonization

15. **Nitroblue tetrazolium test is used for?** *(AIIMS Nov 2008)*
    (a) Phagocytes
    (b) Complement
    (c) T cell
    (d) B cell

16. **In acute inflammation due to the contraction of endothelial cell cytoskeleton, which of the following results?** *(AIIMS Nov 2006)*
    (a) Delayed transient increase in permeability
    (b) Early transient increase
    (c) Delayed permanent increase
    (d) Early permanent increase

Inflammation

17. Diapedesis is: *(AIIMS Nov 2001)*
    (a) Immigration of leukocytes through the basement membrane
    (b) Immigration of the leukocytes through the vessel wall to the site of inflammation
    (c) Aggregation of platelets at the site of bleeding
    (d) Auto digestion of the cells

18. Endothelium leukocyte interaction during inflammation is mediated by/due to *(PGI, Dec 2003)*
    (a) Selectins
    (b) Integrins
    (c) Defensins
    (d) Endothelin

19. In genetic deficiency of MPO the increased susceptibility to infection is due to: *(Delhi PG 09 RP)*
    (a) Defective production of prostaglandins
    (b) Defective rolling of neutrophils
    (c) Inability to produce hydroxyl-halide radicals
    (d) Inability to produce hydrogen peroxide

20. After extravasation, leukocytes emigrate in the tissue towards the site of injury. It is called as
    (a) Margination *(UP 2005)*
    (b) Chemotaxis
    (c) Diapedesis
    (d) Pavementing

21. The complex process of leukocyte movements through the blood vessels are all except
    (a) Rolling *(UP 2008)*
    (b) Adhesion
    (c) Migration
    (d) Phagocytosis

22. All are true about exudate except *(RJ 2000)*
    (a) More protein
    (b) Less protein
    (c) More specific gravity
    (d) All

23. All of the following are signs of inflammation except
    (a) Pain *(AP 2001)*
    (b) Swelling
    (c) Redness
    (d) Absence of functional loss

24. Endogenous chemoattractant is: *(Bihar 2004)*
    (a) C5a
    (b) Bacterial products
    (c) Lipopolysaccharide A
    (d) C8

25. Which of the following statements in context of the enzyme 'E' shown in the diagram given below is correct?
    (a) It is a major mode of defense mechanism in eosinophils
    (b) Its deficiency results in Chediak Higashi syndrome
    (c) It causes formation of a more important bactericidal agent than defensins and lysozyme

(d) It is required for attracting the white blood cells near a targeted organism.

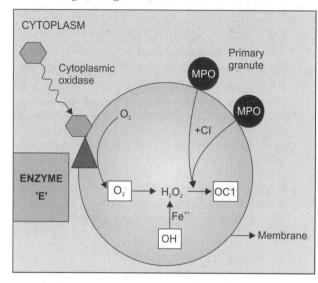

26. A middle aged scientist Sudarshan is working in the laboratory on the mechanisms involved in inflammation. He observes that the leucocytes leave the blood vessels and move towards the site of bacteria. Which of the following is likely to mediate this movement of the bacteria?
    (a) Histamine
    (b) C3b
    (c) C3a
    (d) C5a

27. Which of the following statements in context of endothelial cell contraction in inflammation is false?
    (a) Endothelial cell contraction is the commonest mechanism of increased permeability
    (b) Endothelial cell contraction is responsible for immediate transient response
    (c) It affects venules, capillaries and arterioles commonly.
    (d) It is associated with the release of histamine, substance P and bradykinin.

28. A 14 month old boy Chunnu is being evaluated for recurrent, indolent skin infections and gingivitis. On taking a detailed history from the mother, she tells very valuable point that he had delayed separation of the umbilical cord which occurred around 9-10 weeks after his birth. Which of the following proteins is most likely under-expressed in this boy?
    (a) Late complement components
    (b) Transcobalamin II
    (c) Integrins
    (d) α_2-globulins

29. A 5-year-old female Sukanya is hospitalized with fever and hemorrhagic skin lesions on her lower extremities. About five months ago she was successfully treated

with penicillin for bacterial meningitis. She likely to be suffering from which of the following immune system disorders?
(a) Pure T-cell dysfunction
(b) Ineffective intracellular killing
(c) Insufficient IgA production
(d) Inability to form the membrane-attack complex

30. A 3-year-old boy, Krish presents with recurrent bacterial and fungal infections primarily involving his skin and respiratory tract. Physical examination reveals the presence of oculocutan-eous albinism. Examination of a peripheral blood smear reveals large granules within neutrophils, lymphocytes, and monocytes. The total neutrophil count is found to be decreased. Further workup reveals ineffective bactericidal capabilities of neutrophils due to defective fusion of phagosomes with lysosomes. Which of the following is the most likely diagnosis?
(a) Ataxia-telangiectasia
(b) Chediak-Higashi syndrome
(c) Chronic granulomatous disease
(d) Ehlers-Danlos syndrome

Most Recent Questions

30.1. All of the following are a family of selectin except
(a) P selectin
(b) L selectin
(c) A selectin
(d) E selectin

30.2. Most important for diapedesis?
(a) PECAM
(b) Selectin
(c) Integrin
(d) Mucin like glycoprotein

30.3. In acute inflammation the tissue response consists of all except
(a) Vasodilatation
(b) Exudation
(c) Neutrophilic response
(d) Granuloma formation

30.4. The function common to neutrophils, monocytes, and macrophages is
(a) Immune response is reduced
(b) Phagocytosis
(c) Liberation of histamine
(d) Destruction of old erythrocytes

CHEMICAL MEDIATORS OF INFLAMMATION

31. The role of bradykinin in process of inflammation is:
(a) Vasoconstriction   *(AIIMS May 2012)*
(b) Bronchodilation
(c) Pain
(d) Increased vascular permeability

32. Which of the following is not a pyrogenic cytokine?
(a) IL - 1   *(AI 2012)*
(b) TNF
(c) IFN - α
(d) IL - 18

33. All of the following are true in respect of angioneurotic edema except?   *(AI 2012)*
(a) It is caused by deficiency of complement proteins
(b) It is more common in females
(c) It manifests as pitting edema
(d) It is an autosomal dominant disorder

34. Which of the following complement component can be activated is both common as well as alternative pathways?   *(AI 2011)*
(a) C1
(b) C2
(c) C3
(d) C4

35. Which of the following is not an inflammatory mediator?   *(AIIMS Nov 2010)*
(a) Tumor Necrosis Factor
(b) Myeloperoxidase
(c) Interferons
(d) Interleukin

36. Nephrocalcinosis in a systemic granulomatous disease is due to   *(AIIMS Nov 2010)*
(a) Over production of 1,25 dihydroxy vitamin D
(b) Dystrophic calcification
(c) Mutation in calcium sensing receptors
(d) Increased reabsorption of calcium

37. Bradykinin is for: *(AI 2010)*
(a) Pain
(b) Vasodilatation
(c) Vasoconstriction
(d) Increase vascular permeability

38. Most important bactericidal agent is: *(AI 2009)*
(a) Cationic basic protein
(b) Lactoferrin
(c) Lysozyme
(d) Reactive O_2 species

39. Bradykinin causes: *(AI 2008)*
(a) Vasoconstriction
(b) Pain at the site of inflammation
(c) Bronchodilation
(d) Decreased vascular permeability

40. Lewis triple response is caused due to:
(a) Histamine   *(AI 2008)*
(b) Axon reflex
(c) Injury to endothelium
(d) Increased permeability

41. Factor present in the final common terminal complement pathway is: *(AI 2007)*
(a) C4
(b) C3
(c) C5
(d) Protein B

42. To which of the following family of chemical mediators of inflammation, the Lipoxins belong?
    (a) Kinin system   (AI 2004)
    (b) Cytokines
    (c) Chemokines
    (d) Arachidonic acid metabolites

43. Both antibody dependent and independent complement pathway converge on which complement component?
    (a) C3   (AIIMS Nov 2008) (DNB 2008)
    (b) C5
    (c) C1q
    (d) C8

44. C-C beta chemokines includes   (AIIMS Nov 2006)
    (a) IL-8
    (b) Eotaxin
    (c) Lymphotactin
    (d) Fractalkine

45. All of the following are mediators of acute inflammation except   (AIIMS Nov 2005)
    (a) Angiotensin
    (b) Prostaglandin E2
    (c) Kallikrein
    (d) C3a

46. All of the following are mediators of inflammation except: (AIIMS May 2005)
    (a) Tumour necrosis factor-α (TNF-α)
    (b) Interleukin-1
    (c) Myeloperoxidase
    (d) Prostaglandins

47. Interleukin secreted by macrophages, stimulating lymphocytes is: (AIIMS May 2001)
    (a) IFN alpha
    (b) TNF alpha
    (c) IL-1
    (d) IL-6

48. Cytokines are secreted in sepsis and Systemic Inflammatory Response Syndrome (SIRS) by:
    (a) Neutrophils   (PGI Dec 01)
    (b) Adrenal
    (c) Platelets
    (d) Collecting duct
    (e) Renal cortex

49. Febrile response in CNS is mediated by (PGI Dec 2003)
    (a) Bacterial toxin.
    (b) IL-I
    (c) IL-6
    (d) Interferon
    (e) Tumor necrosis factor (TNF)

50. Cytokines: (PGI Dec 2005)
    (a) Includes interleukins
    (b) Produced only in sepsis
    (c) Are polypeptide (complex proteins)
    (d) Have highly specific action

51. Conversion of prothrombin to thrombin requires:
    (a) V only   (Delhi PG-2008)
    (b) V and Ca^{++}

(c) XII
(d) X and Ca^{++}

52. Which complement fragments are called 'anaphylatoxins'?
    (a) C3a and C3b   (Delhi PG-2006)
    (b) C3b and C5b
    (c) C5a and C3b
    (d) C3a and C5a

53. Cryoprecipitate is rich in which of the following clotting factors: (Delhi PG-2005)
    (a) Factor II
    (b) Factor V
    (c) Factor VII
    (d) Factor VIII

54. Most important mediator of chemotaxis is:
    (a) C3b   (Delhi PG-2005)
    (b) C5a
    (c) C5-7
    (d) C2

55. Histamine causes   (Delhi PG-2004)
    (a) Hypertension
    (b) Vasoconstriction
    (c) Vasodilation
    (d) Tachycardia

56. Which of the following is found in secondary granules of neutrophils?   (UP 2000)
    (a) Catalase
    (b) Gangliosidase
    (c) Proteolytic enzyme
    (d) Lactoferrin

57. All are mediators of neutrophils except:
    (a) Elastase   (UP 2004)
    (b) Cathepsin
    (c) Nitric oxide
    (d) Leukotrienes

58. Ultra-structurally, endothelial cells contain
    (a) Weibel Palade bodies   (UP 2004)
    (b) Langerhan's granules
    (c) Abundant glycogen
    (d) Kallikrein

59. Partial thromboplastin time correlates with:
    (a) Intrinsic and common pathway   (UP 2006)
    (b) Extrinsic and common pathway
    (c) Vessel wall integrity and intrinsic pathway
    (d) Platelet functions and common pathway

60. Bleeding time assesses: (UP 2006)
    (a) Extrinsic clotting pathway
    (b) Intrinsic clotting pathway
    (c) Fibrinogen level
    (d) Function of platelets

61. The estimation of the prothrombin level is useful in the following clotting factor deficiency, except: (UP 2006)
    (a) II
    (b) V
    (c) VII
    (d) IX

62. Which of the following is secondary mediator of the anaphylaxis is: *(UP 2006)*
(a) Histamine
(b) Proteases
(c) Eosinophilic chemotactic factor
(d) Leukotriene B$_4$

63. Birbeck's granules in the cytoplasm are seen in:
(a) Langerhans cells *(UP 2006)*
(b) Mast cells
(c) Myelocytes
(d) Thrombocytes

64. The Eosinophils secrete all except *(UP 2005)*
(a) Major basic protein *(UP 2007)*
(b) Hydrolytic enzyme
(c) Reactive form of O$_2$
(d) Eosinophilic chemotactic factor

65. In Lipooxygenase pathway of the arachidonic acid metabolism, which of the following products helps to promote the platelet aggregation and vasoconstriction?
(a) C5a *(UP 2008)*
(b) Thromboxane A2
(c) Leukotriene B4
(d) C1 activators

66. Chemotactic complement components are *(RJ 2001)*
(a) C3a
(b) C5a
(c) Both
(d) C3b

67. In inflammatory process, the prostaglandin E1and E2 cause *(AP 2000)*
(a) Vasodilatation
(b) Increased gastric output
(c) Decreased body temperature
(d) Vasoconstriction

68. Opsonins are *(AP 2006)*
(a) C3a
(b) IgM
(c) Carbohydrate binding proteins
(d) Selectins

69. Inflammatory mediator of generalized systemic inflammation is: *(Kolkata 2002)*
(a) IL-1
(b) IL-2
(c) Interferon alpha
(d) TNF

70. All are cytokines except: *(Kolkata 2002)*
(a) Monoclonal antibody
(b) Interleukin
(c) Chemokine
(d) TNF

71. An 8 year old girl Geetu presents to the physician with wheezing and difficulty in breathing. The breathlessness increases when she went to the fields to play with her friends. Her blood contains higher than normal concentration of IgE. The physician believes that the cell shown in the photograph below is implicated

in the pathogenesis of her condition. This cell is most similar to which of the following white blood cells?
(a) Neutrophil
(b) Monocyte
(c) Basophil
(d) Eosinophil

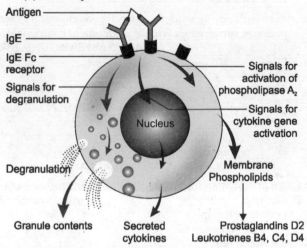

72. A 72 year-old man Kishori Lal presented to surgery OPD with a history of difficulty in micturition, increased frequency of urine and lower backache for the past 8 months. Digital rectal examination reveals an enlarged prostate with irregular surface. The surgeon orders for the serum PSA levels which are found to be increased and X ray spine shows osteoblastic lesions. A diagnosis of metastatic prostate cancer is made. Mr Lal also complaints of significant weight loss, loss of appetite and loss of energy over the past 45 days. His current complaints can be attributed to which of the following?
(a) Fibroblast growth factor
(b) Interleukin-2
(c) Tumor necrosis factor-α
(d) Vascular endothelial growth factor

73. A 14-year-old girl Radha has high grade fever. She goes to a physician Dr. Jeeva Roy who orders for some blood investigations. A complete blood count with differential implies the presence of a viral infection. Which of the following best describes the cells that indicate a viral etiology to her illness?
(a) They are basophilic with spherical dark-stained nuclei
(b) They are precursors of osteoclasts and liver Kupffer cells
(c) They contain a peripheral hyalomere and central granulomere
(d) They have azurophilic granules and multilobed nuclei

74. A 28-year-old woman, Vimla is being evaluated to find the cause of her urine turning a dark brown color after a recent upper respiratory tract infection. She has been otherwise symptomatic, and her blood pressure has been within normal limits. Urinalysis finds moderate blood present with red cells and red cell casts. Immunofluorescence examination of a renal biopsy reveals deposits of IgA within the mesangium. These clinical findings suggest that her disorder is associated with activation of the alternate complement system. Which of the following serum laboratory findings is the most suggestive of activation of the alternate complement system rather than the classic complement system?

	Serum C2	Serum C3	Serum C4
(a)	Decreased	Normal	Normal
(b)	Normal	Decreased	Normal
(c)	Normal	Normal	Decreased
(d)	Decreased	Normal	Decreased
(e)	Decreased	Decreased	Decreased

75. An 18-year-old woman, Sheila is being evaluated for recurrent facial edema, especially around her lips. She also has recurrent bouts of intense abdo-minal pain and cramps, sometimes associated with vomiting. Laboratory examination finds decreased C4, while levels of C3, decay-accelerating factor, and IgE are within normal limits. A deficiency of which one of the following substances is most likely to be associated with these clinical findings?
    (a) β2-integrins
    (b) C1 esterase inhibitor
    (c) Decay-accelerating factor
    (d) Complement components C3 and C5

Most Recent Questions

75.1. Fever occurs due to:
    (a) IL 1
    (b) Endorphin
    (c) Enkephalin
    (d) Histamine

75.2. E cadherin gene deficiency is seen in:
    (a) Gastric cancer
    (b) Intestinal cancer
    (c) Thyroid cancer
    (d) Pancreatic cancer

75.3. Cell-matrix adhesions are mediated by?
    (a) Cadherins
    (b) Integrins
    (c) Selectins
    (d) Calmodulin

75.4. Pro inflammatory Cytokines include all of the following except:
    (a) Interleukin 1
    (b) Interleukin-10
    (c) Interleukin 6
    (d) TNF- Alpha

75.5. The most important source of histamine:
    (a) Mast cells
    (b) Eosinophil
    (c) Neutrophil
    (d) Macrophages

75.6. Following injury to a blood vessel, immediate haemostasis is achieved by which of the following?
    (a) Fibrin deposition
    (b) Vasoconstriction
    (c) Platelet adhesion
    (d) Thrombosis

75.7. PAF causes all except
    (a) Bronchoconstriction
    (b) Vasoconstriction
    (c) Decreased vascular permeability
    (d) Vasodilation

75.8. Eosinophils are activated by:
    (a) IL1
    (b) IL5
    (c) IL4
    (d) IL6

75.9. Both antibody dependent and independent comple-ment pathway converge on which complement compo-nent?
    (a) C3
    (b) C5
    (c) C1q
    (d) C8

75.10. Cryoprecipitate is rich in which of the following clot-ting factors?
    (a) Factor II
    (b) Factor V
    (c) Factor VII
    (d) Factor VIII

75.11. Prostaglandins are synthesized from:
    (a) Linoleic acid
    (b) Linolenic acid
    (c) Arachidonic acid
    (d) Butyric acid

75.12. Which chemical mediator is an arachidonic acid metabolite produced by cyclo-oxygenase pathway?
    (a) LXA4
    (b) LXB4
    (c) 5HETE
    (d) PGH2

75.13. Procalcitonin is used as marker of
    (a) Cardiac dysfunction in acute coronary syndrome
    (b) Menstrual periodicity
    (c) Pituitary function
    (d) Sepsis

CHRONIC INFLAMMATION; GRANULOMATOUS INFLAMMATION

76. The epithelioid cell and multinucleated giant cells of Granulomatous inflammation are derived from:
    (a) Basophils   *(AI 2002)*
    (b) Eosinophils
    (c) CD4-T lymphocytes
    (d) Monocytes-Macrophages

77. Granuloma is pathological feature of all, except
    (a) Giant cell arteritis   *(AIIMS Nov 2001)*
    (b) Microscopic polyangiitis
    (c) Wegener's granulomatosis
    (d) Churg Strauss disease

78. Granulomatous inflammatory reaction is caused by all, except: *(AIIMS Nov 2001)*
    (a) M. tuberculosis
    (b) M. leprae
    (c) Yersinia pestis
    (d) Mycoplasma

79. Non-caseating granulomas are seen in all of the following except   *(AIIMS May 2001)*
    (a) Byssinosis
    (b) Hodgkin's lymphoma
    (c) Metastatic carcinoma of lung
    (d) Tuberculosis

80. Epithelioid granuloma is caused by:
    (a) Neutrophil   *(PGI Dec 2002)*
    (b) Cytotoxic T-cells
    (c) Helper T-cells
    (d) NK cells

81. Caseous necrosis in granuloma are not found in
    (a) Tuberculosis   *(PGI June 2006)*
    (b) Leprosy
    (c) Histoplasmosis
    (d) CMV
    (e) Wegener's granulomatosis

82. The most important function of epithelioid cells in tuberculosis is: *(Delhi PG 2010)*
    (a) Phagocytosis
    (b) Secretory
    (c) Antigenic
    (d) Healing

83. Necrotizing epithelioid cell granulomas are seen in all, except: *(Delhi PG 09 RP)*
    (a) Tuberculosis
    (b) Wegener's granulomatosis

    (c) Cat Scratch disease
    (d) Leprosy

84. Epithelioid granulomatous lesions are found in all of the following diseases, except:
    (a) Tuberculosis   *(Delhi PG-2005)*
    (b) Sarcoidosis
    (c) Berylliosis
    (d) Pneumocystis carinii

85. Caseous granuloma is seen in   *(UP 2004)*
    (a) Histoplasmosis
    (b) Silicosis
    (c) Sarcoidosis
    (d) Foreign body

86. Non-caseating granuloma is characteristically seen in
    (a) Syphilis   *(RJ 2003)*
    (b) Sarcoidosis
    (c) Tuberculosis
    (d) Histoplasmosis

87. All are granulomatous diseases except   *(RJ 2006)*
    (a) Syphilis
    (b) Sarcoidosis
    (c) Schistosomiasis
    (d) P. carinii

88. Which of the following is the most characteristic of granuloma: *(Kolkata 2003)*
    (a) Epithelioid cell
    (b) Giant cell
    (c) Fibroblasts
    (d) Endothelial cell

89. Caseating granuloma are seen in: *(Bihar 2003)*
    (a) Histoplasmosis
    (b) Sarcoidosis
    (c) Coccidiodomycosis
    (d) All

90. A 28 year old young man Alok Nath presents to the clinic with a maculopapular rash on the palms and soles, oral ulcers, malaise, lymphadenopathy and weight loss. He has a history of a painless genital lesion 2 months ago after an unprotected intercourse about 10 weeks back. Biopsy shows the presence of a granuloma. The figure shows a very important step in the pathogenesis of this condition. Identify the cell marked '?' in the figure.
    (a) CD8 T cell
    (b) T_H1
    (c) T_H2
    (d) Langhans cell

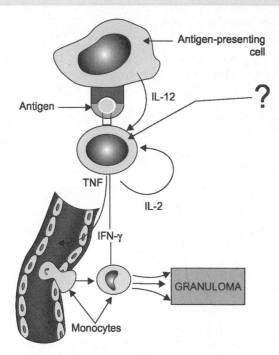

91. A 45-year-old poor man Teja has a chronic cough, a cavitary lesion of the lung, and is sputum positive for acid-fast bacilli. Which of the following is the principle form of defense by which the patient's body fights against this infection?
    (a) Antibody-mediated phagocytosis
    (b) Cell-mediated immunity
    (c) IgA-mediated hypersensitivity
    (d) Neutrophil ingestion of bacteria

92. A 36-year-old man, Avnish presents with a cough, fever, night sweats, and weight loss. A chest X-ray reveals irregular densities in the upper lobe of his right lung. Histologic sections from this area reveal groups of epithelioid cells with rare acid-fast bacilli and a few scattered giant cells. At the centre of these groups of epithelioid cells are granular areas of necrosis. What is the source of these epithelioid cells?
    (a) Bronchial cells
    (b) Pneumocytes
    (c) Lymphocytes
    (d) Monocytes

Most Recent Questions

92.1. In a granuloma, epithelioid cells and giant cells and derived from
    (a) T – lymphocytes
    (b) Monocyte – macrophages
    (c) B – lymphocytes
    (d) Mast cells

92.2. In a lymph node showing non necrotizing and non–caseating granuloma which of the following is suspected?
    (a) Toxoplaxmosis
    (b) Lymphogranuloma venereum
    (c) Cat scratch disease
    (d) Kikuchis lymphadenitis

92.3. Which of these is not a granulomatous disease
    (a) Leprosy
    (b) Tuberculosis
    (c) Sarcoidosis
    (d) Amebiasis

WOUND HEALING; STEM CELL BIOLOGY

93. Which one of the following statements is not correct regarding 'Stem cell'? *(DPG 2011)*
    (a) Developmental elasticity
    (b) Transdifferentiation
    (c) Can be harvested from embryo
    (d) "Knockout mice" made possible because of it

94. An adult old man gets burn injury to his hands. Over few weeks, the burned skin heals without the need for skin grafting. The most critical factor responsible for the rapid healing in this case is: *(AIIMS May 2003)*
    (a) Remnant skin appendages
    (b) Underlying connective tissues
    (c) Minimal edema and erythema
    (d) Granulation tissue

95. Absolute lymphocytosis is seen in
    (a) SLE
    (b) T.B.
    (c) CLL
    (d) Brucellosis

96. Which of the following is absolutely essential for wound healing? *(Karnataka 2009)*
    (a) Vitamin D
    (b) Carbohydrates
    (c) Vitamin C
    (d) Balanced diet

97. Chronic granulomatous disease is: *(Karnataka 2009)*
    (a) Associated with formation of multiple granulomas
    (b) A benign neoplastic process
    (c) A parasitic disease
    (d) Acquired leukocyte function defect

98. In regeneration *(UP 2002)*
    (a) Granulation tissue
    (b) Repairing by same type of tissue
    (c) Repairing by different type of tissue
    (d) Cellular proliferation is largely regulated by biochemical factors

99. Wound contraction is mediated by:
    (a) Epithelial cells *(Jharkhand 2005)*
    (b) Myofibroblasts
    (c) Collagen
    (d) Elastin

53

100. A 45-year-old man, Suveen presents with pain in the mid portion of his chest. The pain is associated with eating and swallowing food. Endoscopic examination reveals an ulcerated area in the lower portion of his esophagus. Histologic sections of tissue taken from this area reveal an ulceration of the esophageal mucosa that is filled with blood, fibrin, proliferating blood vessels, and proliferating fibroblasts. Mitosis is easily found, and most of the cells have prominent nucleoli. Which of the following statements best describes this ulcerated area?
(a) Caseating granulomatous inflammation
(b) Dysplastic epithelium
(c) Granulation tissue
(d) Squamous cell carcinoma
(e) Noncaseating granulomatous inflammation

Most Recent Questions

100.1. Which of the following adhesion molecules is involved in morphogenesis?
(a) Osteopontin
(b) Osteonectin SPARC
(c) Tenascin
(d) Thrombospondins

100.2. When a cell transforms itself into different lineage the ability us know as:
(a) De-differentiation
(b) Re-differentiation
(c) Trans-differentiation
(d) Sub-differentiation

100.3. Prion disease is caused by:
(a) Misfolding of protein
(b) Denaturation of proteins
(c) Reduced formation of proteins
(d) Exces formation of proteins

100.4. Maximum collagen in wound healing is seen at which stage of healing?
(a) End of first week
(b) End of second week
(c) End of third week
(d) End of 2 months

100.5. "Oval cells" are seen in the stem cells of which of the following tissues?
(a) Skin
(b) Cornea
(c) Liver
(d) Bone

100.6. First sign of wound injury is:
(a) Epithelialization
(b) Dilatation of capillaries
(c) Leukocytic infiltration
(d) Localized edema

100.7. Which of the following is the source of hepatic stem cells?
(a) Limbus cells
(b) Ito cell
(c) Oval cell
(d) Paneth cell

100.8. Vitamin used for post translational modification of glutamic acid to gamma carboxy glutamate is
(a) A
(b) D
(c) E
(d) K

100.9. Tensile strength of wound after laparoscopic cholecystectomy in a 30 year old woman depends upon:
(a) Replacement of type 3 collagen   *(AIIMS Nov 2013)*
(b) Extensive cross-linking of tropocollagen
(c) Macrophage activity
(d) Granulation tissue

100.10. One of the following statements about hematopoietic stem cell is false?
(a) Stem cells have self renewal property
(b) Subset of stem cells normally circulate in peripheral blood
(c) Marrow derived stem cells can seed other tissues and develop into non hematopoietic cells as well
(d) Stem cells resemble lymphoblasts morphologically

Inflammation

EXPLANATIONS

1. **Ans. (c) Delayed prolonged increase in permeability** *(Ref: Robbins 8th/45, 9/e p74)*

2. **Ans. (d) Pseudopod extension** *(Ref: Robbins 9/e p78)*
   Typically the phagocytosis of microbes and dead cells is initiated by recognition of the particles by receptors expressed on the leukocyte surface. ***Mannose receptors and scavenger receptors*** are two important receptors that function to bind and ingest microbes. The efficiency of phagocytosis is greatly enhanced when microbes are opsonized by specific proteins (opsonins) for which the phagocytes express high-affinity receptors. Binding of a particle to phagocytic leukocyte receptors initiates the process of active phagocytosis of the particle. During engulfment, **extensions of the cytoplasm (pseudopods) flow around the particle to be engulfed**, eventually resulting in complete enclosure of the particle within a phagosome created by the plasma membrane of the cell
   Direct concept quote from Robbins to clarify the answer;
   How is phagocytosis different from pinocytosis and receptor mediated endocytosis

   > **In contrast to phagocytosis**, fluid phase pinocytosis and receptor-mediated endocytosis of small particles involve internalization into clathrin[Q] coated pits and vesicles and are **not dependent on the actin cytoskeleton**.

   - Option 'a' Both Fc fragment of IgG and C3b are required in opsonisation. It takes place before phagocytosis.
   - Option 'c' respiratory burst occurs after the formation of the phagolysosome.

3. **Ans. (a) Superoxide dismutase** *(Ref: Robbins 8th/21 9/e p48)*
   Superoxide dismutase (SOD) is an anti oxidant enzyme
   Some clarification regarding option 'd'.... 'Nitric oxide (NO), an important chemical mediator generated by endothelial cells, macrophages, neurons, and other cell types can act as a free radical and can also be converted to highly reactive peroxynitrite anion (ONOO-) as well as NO_2 and NO^{3-}.

4. **Ans. (c) Vasodilation and increase in permeability** *(Ref: Robbins 8th/46-47 9/e p74)*
   Direct quote "a hallmark of acute inflammation is increased vascular permeability leading to the escape of protein-rich exudate into the extravascular tissue, causing edema".

5. **Ans. (d) Unidirectional locomotion of the neutrophils** *(Ref: Robbins 8th/50 9/e p77)*
   Chemotaxis is defined as locomotion oriented along a chemical gradient.

6. **Ans. (a) Vasodilation and increased vascular permeability** *(Ref: Robbins 8th/45 9/e p74)*

7. **Ans. (a) NADPH oxidase** *(Ref: Robbins 8th/53, 7th/42-3 9/e p79)*
   Within the phagocytes, the following reaction takes place:
   The initiating enzyme for this process is NADPH oxidase (also called **respiratory burst oxidase**).
   Glutathione peroxidase, glutathione reductase and superoxide dismutase are examples of anti-oxidants. They reduce free radical formation.

8. **Ans. (a) Metalloproteinases** *(Ref: Robbins, 7th/103, 110, 312 9/e p105)*
   - Extracellular Matrix (ECM) comprises of interstitial matrix and basement membrane. The degradation of collagen and other ECM proteins is achieved by a family of matrix metalloproteinases (MMPs) which are dependent on zinc ions for their activity.
   - MMP8 and MMP2 are collagenases which cleave type IV collagen of basement membranes.
   - MMPs also have a role in tumour cell invasion.

9. **Ans. (d) Direct injury to endothelial cells**... *For details see text (Ref: Robbins 7th/35, 36 9/e p74)*

10. **Ans. (b) Neutrophilia** *(Ref: Robbins 7th/56; Chandrasoma Taylor 3rd/41 9/e p77)*
    - Neutrophils predominate during the first 6 to 24 hours (Neutrophilia). These are replaced by monocytes/macrophages in 24 to 48 hours.

11. **Ans. (d) Decreased hydrostatic pressure** *(Ref: Robbins 7th/50-51 9/e p73-74)*
    With acute inflammation, *hydrostatic pressure is increased* (due to increased blood flow from vasodilation) and at the same time *osmotic pressure is reduced* because of protein leakage (due to increased permeability)

12. **Ans. (d) Granuloma formation** *(Ref: Robbins 7th/56, 517 9/e p97)*
    - **Granuloma formation is characteristic of chronic granulomatous inflammation** and is not seen in acute inflammation.
    - *Vasodilation, increase in permeability, exudation, margination, rolling etc. are seen in acute inflammation.*

13. **Ans. (a) NADPH oxidase** *(Ref: Robbins 7th/60, 16, Robbins 8th/53 9/e p48)*
    - *The generation of reactive oxygen intermediates is due to the rapid activation of an enzyme; NADPH oxidase which is involved in oxygen dependent killing.*
    - *Catalase, superoxide dismutase and glutathione peroxidase are free radical scavengers that prevent oxygen mediated injury.*

14. **Ans. (d) In Bruton's disease there is normal opsonization** *(Ref: Robbins 8th/231-232,55 9/e p240-241)*

    > **Bruton's agammaglobulinemia** is an X-linked immunodeficiency disorder *characterized by the failure of B-cell precursors (pro-B cells and pre-B cells) to mature into B cells* due to *mutation of B-cell tyrosine kinase (Btk)*. Btk is required for the maturation of pre-B cell to mature B cell. So, plasma cells derived from B cells are absent and therefore, production of immunoglobulins is impaired. The disease is **seen almost entirely in males**. It *usually does not become apparent until about 6 months, when maternal immunoglobulins are depleted.*
    > Opsonisation is a process by which preferential phagocytsosis of the opsonised bacteria is done by neutrophils and macrophages. This process also requires antibodies. In **Bruton's disease** therefore, the **opsonisation is defective**. Other options have been explained in the review of chapter 2 in detail.

15. **Ans. (a) Phagocytes** *(Ref: Harrison 17th/384, Robbins 8/e 55 9/e p79)*
    The **nitroblue-tetrazolium (NBT) test** is the original and most widely known **test for chronic granulomatous disease**. It is negative in chronic granulomatous disease and positive in normal individuals. It is used for detecting the production of reactive oxygen species in the phagocytes. The basis of the test has been discussed in the text.

16. **Ans. (b) Early transient increase** *(Ref: Robbin's 7/e 51-52 9/e p74)*
    The hallmark of acute inflammation is increased vascular permeability.

Name of Mechanism	Involved Mechanism
Early transient increase	Endothelial cell contraction
Delayed transient increase in permeability	Direct endothelial injury
Delayed permanent increase	Endothelial cell retraction, endothelial cell damage

17. **Ans. (b) Immigration of the leukocytes through the vessel wall to the site of inflammation** *(Ref: Robbins 7/e 54, 8/e50, 9/e p76)*
    Diapedesis or Transmigration

    > Definition: Migration of the leukocytes through the endothelium.
    > Most important molecule for diapedesis is **CD31or PECAM-1[Q]** (platelet endothelial cell adhesion molecule).
    > **Occurs predominantly in the venules** (except in the lungs, where it also occurs in capillaries).

18. **Ans. (a) Selectins; (b) Integrins** *(Ref: Robbins 7th/54, 8th/49-50 9/e p76)*
    - Endothelium and WBC interact through the molecules like Immunoglobulins (family molecules e.g. ICAM-I, VCAM-I), Integrins, Mucin-like glycoprotein and selectins.

Molecule	Function	Deficiency disease
Integrin	Firm adhesion	LAD I
Selectin	Rolling and loose adhesion	LAD II

    - **Defensins** are cationic arginine rich peptides having broad antimicrobial activity found in **Azurophil granules** of neutrophils.
    - **Endothelin** is a potent endothelial derived **vasoconstrictor**

19. **Ans. (c) Inability to produce hydroxyl-halide radicals** *(Ref: Robbins 8th/53, 56, 9/e p79)*

20. **Ans. (b) Chemotaxis** *(Ref: Robbins 8th/51-52; 7th/53-57,9/e p77)*

21. **Ans. (d) Phagocytosis** *(Ref: Robbins 8th/48-49, 7th/53-54, 9/e p75)*

22. **Ans. (b) Less protein** *(Ref: Robbins 8th/46, 7th/49, 9/e p73)*

23. **Ans. (d) Absence of functional loss** *(Ref: Robbins 8th/44; 7th/79, 9/e p71)*

24. **Ans. (a) C5a** *(Ref: Robbins 8th/66; 7th/56, 9/e p77)*

25. **Ans. (c) It causes formation of a more important bactericidal agent than defensins and lysozyme** *(Ref: Robbins 8th/53, 9/e p79-80)*
    The enzyme 'E' in the figure is NADPH oxidase. It is more important bactericidal agent than defensins and lysozyme. Its deficiency is associated with chronic granulomatous disease.

Inflammation

Major basic protein is the defense mechanism present in **eosinophils**. It is highly effective against parasites. So, parasitic infection is associated with eosinophilia.

Chediak Higashi syndrome is due to **defective LYST protein** and is associated with defective phagolysosome formation. Patients also have albinism, recurrent infections, neurological diseases and increased bleeding tendency.

Chemotaxis is required for attracting the white blood cells near a targeted organism.

26. **Ans. (d) C5a** *(Ref: Robbins 8th/50, 9/e p77)*

The movement of the leucocytes described in the question is known as chemotaxis. It is a unidirectional movement of the cells along a chemical gradient. The chemotactic molecules include:

Exogenous chemotactic molecules	Endogenous chemotactic molecules
• Bacterial products[Q]	• C5a[Q] • LTB4[Q] • IL-8[Q]

27. **Ans. (c) It affects venules, capillaries and arterioles commonly.** *(Ref: Robbins 8th/47, 9/e p74)*

Direct quote from Robbins.....'*Endothelial cell contraction is classically seen in the venules 20 to 60 μm in diameter leaving the capillaries and the arterioles unaffected*'.

For more details, see text.

28. **Ans. (c) Integrins** *(Ref: Robbins 8th/49-50, 9/e p76)*

Explanation:

The clinical features and history described in the stem of the question are consistent with a diagnosis of leukocyte adhesion deficiency. Clinical findings associated with this syndrome include late separation of the umbilical cord, poor wound healing, recurrent skin infections (**without formation of pus),** gingivitis and periodontitis.

In immune deficiencies, late separation of the umbilical cord alone should raise the question of **L**eukocyte **A**dhesion **D**eficiency type **I (LAD I)**.

LAD I is an autosomal recessive condition caused by absence of the CD18 antigen that is necessary for the formation of integrins **(Choice c)**. Integrins are essential for the migration of leukocytes from the blood vessels to the tissues to exert their effect. A leukocyte circulating in the blood vessel undergoes a well-characterized multistep process of reaching the site of infection.

* One of the initial steps is **rolling** mediated by selectins.
* The subsequent step is firm **adhesion** which is mediated by integrins.
* Then **transmigration** takes place followed by **chemotaxis**.

Wound healing, umbilical cord detachment, and the fighting against cutaneous infections all depend on the ability of neutrophils to exit the intravascular space and initiate inflammation in the skin.

* (Choice a) Deficiency of late complement components (i.e. C5b-9) results in an inability to form the complement membrane attack complex and a greater risk of severe infections caused by *Neisseria* organism.
* (Choice b) **Transcobalamin II** is a **carrier protein for vitamin B12** after it is absorbed in the ileum. Its deficiency is not associated with immunodeficiency.
* (Choice d) α_2-globulins are normal serum proteins (like haptoglobin, ceruloplasmin and α_2-macroglobulin) produced by the liver and kidneys.

29. **Ans. (d) Inability to form the membrane-attack complex.** *(Ref: Robbins 8th/64, also read explanation below)*

Patients having deficiency of the complement factors that form the membrane attack complex (MAC i.e. C5b-9 complex) experience recurrent infections by Neisseria species (Choice d). The Neisseria disease in these patients is mild because the remainder of the immune system is intact. MAC is the final end-product of complement activation and it forms a pore in the bacterial cell membrane leading to cell lysis.

(Choice A) Pure T-cell dysfunction is thymic hypoplasia seen in Di George syndrome. In this condition, there is congenital absence of the thymus and parathyroid glands caused by maldevelopment of the 3rd and 4th pharyngeal pouches. So, patients have pure T-cell lymphopenia (causing recurrent viral and fungal infections) and hypocalcemia. (Choice B) Chronic granulomatous disease (CGD) is an example of deficient intracellular killing due to absent NADPH oxidase.

(Choice C) Young adults infected with Neisseria meningitidis may be at increased risk for disseminated infection if they produce too much serum IgA antibody. In these patients IgA attaches to the bacteria and blocks attachment of the IgM and IgG antibodies that induce complement-mediated bacterial lysis. Normally, IgM and IgG activity helps protect against bacterial dissemination.

30. **Ans. (b) Chediak-Higashi syndrome** *(Ref: Robbins 7th/61-62, 155-156)*

Chediak-Higashi syndrome is an autosomal recessive disorder characterized by the abnormal fusion of phagosomes with lysosomes, which results in ineffective bactericidal capabilities of neutrophils and monocytes. These abnormal leukocytes develop giant intracytoplasmic lysosomes. Abnormal formation of melanosomes in these individuals results in oculocutaneous albinism. Most of these patients eventually develop an "accelerated phase" in which an aggressive lymphoproliferative disease, possibly the result of an Epstein-Barr viral infection, results in pancytopenia and death.

30.1. Ans. (c) A selectin *(Ref: Robbins 8/e p49, 9/e p76)*

Selectins are a family of proteins that are involved in the cellular process of rolling interactions. The following are the three types of selectins:

- E selectin (CD 62E) – Present on cytokine-activated *endothelial cells* and interacts with sialyl lewis X receptor on the leukocyte.
- L selectin (CD 62L) – Present on *leukocytes* and interacts with glycoprotein adhesion molecules (GlyCAM-1), Mad CAM-1 and CD34 on endothelial cells.
- P selectin (CD 62P) – Present on *platelets and endothelial cells* and interacts with sialyl lewis X receptor on leukocytes.

30.2. Ans. (a) PECAM *(Ref: Robbins 8/e p50, 9/e p77)*

- The process of leukocyte recruitment is *migration of the leukocytes through the endothelium,* called transmigration or *diapedesis.*
- Transmigration of leukocytes occurs mainly in **post-capillary venules**.
- Several adhesion molecules present in the intercellular junctions between endothelial cells are involved in the migration of leukocytes. These molecules include a member of the immunoglobulin superfamily called **PECAM-1** (platelet endothelial cell adhesion molecule) or **CD31** and several junctional adhesion molecules.

30.3. Ans. (d) Granuloma formation *(Ref: Robbins 9/e p97)*

- Granuloma formation is associated with chronic inflammation and **not** with acute inflammation.

30.4. Ans. (b) Phagocytosis

Friends, the first option actually confused lot of people when the question was asked because of the word 'immune'. Read the complete option carefully before answering the questions in the exam.

31. Ans. (d) Increased vascular permeability > (c) Pain *(Ref: Robbins 8th/65-6, 9/e p89)*

Functions of Bradykinin:

1. Increases vascular permeability
2. Contraction of smooth muscles
3. Dilation of the blood vessels
4. Pain when injected into the skin

- Out of these actions of bradykinin, the increase in vessel permeability is a better answer as it is the hallmark of acute inflammation.

32. Ans. (d) IL - 18 *(Ref: Robbins 8th/74, Harrison 18th/144 , 9/e p99)*

Pyrogens are substances which cause fever. These can be either exogenous or endogenous. The **endogenous pyrogens** (also called as the **pyrogenic cytokines**) include:

- IL-1[Q]
- IL-6 [Q]
- Tumor necrosis factor [Q] (TNF)
- Ciliary neurotopic factor [Q] (CNTF)
- IFN-α[Q] (alpha)

Harrison clearly mentions that the **IL-18**[Q] which is a *member of IL-1 family* **does not** appear to be a pyrogenic cytokine.

Important points about regulation of body temperature

PGE$_2$[Q] is the final mediator responsible for causing elevation of the thermoregulatory set point by increasing the concentration of cAMP. **Exogenous pyrogens** include microbial products and toxins; classical example is **endotoxin**[Q] produced by gram negative bacteria. Body temperature is regulated at the level of the hypothalamus. Most individuals with **hypothalamic damage** have **subnormal** and not supranormal body temperature.

33. Ans. (c) It manifests as pitting edema *(Ref: Harrison 17th/2066, 18th/2711-3)*

- Angioneurotic edema is a localised **non pitting edema**[Q] involving deeper layers of the skin and subcutaneous tissue. It is an **autosomal dominant**[Q] clinical condition caused by deficiency of C1 inhibitor protein (a complement regulatory protein) and associated with elevated levels of bradykinin. It is more common in **females**[Q].
- Diagnosis of hereditary angioedema is suggested by the presence of *lack of pruritus and urticarial lesions,* prominence of *recurrent gastrointestinal attacks of colic* and *episodes of laryngeal edema*. The levels of complement proteins **C1is normal** but levels of **C2 and C4 are depleted**.
- **Danazol**[Q] is the drug which can be used for hereditary angioedema.

34. Ans. (c) C3 *(Ref: Robbins 8th/63-64 , 9/e p88)*

The complement proteins can be activated by 3 pathways; classical, lectin and alternate pathways. Terminal pathway is common to the first three pathways and is present at the level of post activation stage of C3. It eventually leads to the membrane attack complex that lyses cells.

As can be seen in the text, C3 is the first common complement protein to be activated in both classical and alternate pathway.

35. Ans. (b) Myeloperoxidase *(Ref: Robbins 8th/57, 63 , 9/e p83)*

Myeloperoxidase (MPO) is an enzyme present in primary (or azurophilic) granules of the neutrophils. In the presence of a halide such as Cl-, MPO converts H_2O_2 to HOCl• (hypochlorous radical) during the process of respiratory burst.

36. Ans. (a) Over production of 1, 25 dihydroxy vitamin D *(Ref: Robbins 8th/433-6, Heptinstall's pathology of the kidney, LWW, Volume 1; 6th/1051, Interstitial Lung Disease by Schwarz 5th/458-9)*

Nephrocalcinosis is defined as calcification of the renal interstitium and tubules. It is associated with hypercalcemia. In chronic granulomatous inflammation, the important cells involved are macrophages and lymphocytes.

Direct quote Heptinstall's … **'Sarcoidosis and other granulomatous diseases can be cause of hypercalcemia and hypercalciuria owing to exces vitamin D from extra renal conversion of 1,25 (OH)2D3.** Nephrocalcinosis was found to be associated with 22% patients with chronic sarcoidosis'.

In other granulomatous conditions (like **Sarcoidosis**), there is presence of **metastatic calcification due to activation** of **vitamin D precursor by macrophages**…….Robbins

Interstitial Lung Disease 5th .. 'Hypercalciuria is seen in almost a third of patients with sarcoidosis. Serum calcium levels in sarcoidosis rise with serum vitamin D levels. This dysregulation of calcium metabolism appears to be modulated through abnormal synthesis of vitamin D by **activated pulmonary macrophages and granulomatous tissue that leads to excessive hydroxylation of 25- monohydroxylated vitamin D precursors**. This could be an adaptive response to the antigen in sarcoidosis.'

37. Ans. (a, b, d) *(Ref: Robbins 8th/65, 7th/45, 9/e p89)*

Friends, in our opinion the question should have been asked with an "except" because bradykinin **has the following effects**:

- Increases vascular permeability
- Arteriolar dilation
- Bronchial smooth muscle contraction
- Pain at the site of injections/inflammation

Since *increased vascular permeability* is the most *characteristic feature of acute inflammation,* some people were of the opinion that this could be single best option to be marked presuming the stem of question was correct.

38. Ans. (d) Reactive oxygen species *(Ref: Robbins 8th/53, 9/e p79)*

H_2O_2- MPO- halide system is the most efficient bactericidal system of neutrophils.

39. Ans. (b) Pain at the site of inflammation *(Ref: Robbin 7th/e 45, 9/e p89)*

40. Ans. (a) Histamine *(Ref: Goodman & Gilman 10th/650)*

Histamine is a vasoactive amine that is located in most body tissues but is highly concentrated in the lungs, skin, and gastrointestinal tract. It is stored in mast cells and basophils.

When it is injected intradermally it causes the triple response consisting of:

- Red spot: Due to capillary dilatation
- Wheal: Due to exudation of fluid from capillaries and venules
- Flare: Redness in the surrounding area due to arteriolar dilation mediated by axon reflex.

41. Ans. (c) C5 *(Ref: Harrison 17th/2030-2032, Robbins 8th/63-64, 9/e p88)*

- The terminal pathway that is common to all pathways of the complement system leads to the membrane attack complex and consists of factors C5, C6, C7, C8 and C9 (C_{5b6789}).

42. Ans. (d) Arachidonic acid metabolites *(Ref: Robbins 7th/69; Katzung 11th/314-323, 9/e p85)*

Lipoxins are a recent addition to the family of bioactive products generated from arachidonic acid. They have anti-inflammatory activity (explained in text).

43. Ans. (a) C3 *(Ref: Harrison 17th/2030, 9/e p88)*

44. Ans. (b) Eotaxin *(Ref: Robbins 8th/62-63; 7th/71, 9/e p87)*

45. Ans. (a) Angiotensin *(Ref: Robbin's 7th/g 63, 74, 75, 9/e p83)*

Kallikreins like bradykinin, PGs and complement components are mediators of acute inflammation.

46. Ans. (c) Myeloperoxidase *(Ref: Robbins 7th/74, 75, 9/e p83)*

47. Ans. (c) IL – 1 > (d) IL-6 *(Ref: Javetz, 22nd/1291, Walter Israel 7th/227)*
- Macrophages release IL – 1 which stimulates the T – helper cells.
- The T – cells in response proliferate and release IL – 2 which in turn further stimulates T – cell proliferation and B cell proliferation and differentiation into plasma cells.
- Please note that even IL-6 (produced by macrophages) acts on late stages of B cell differentiation enhancing antibody formation. Still, IL-1 being the most important cytokine having systemic effects of inflammation has been chosen as the answer here in preference to IL-6.

48. Ans. (a) Neutrophils; (c) Platelets *(Ref: Harrison' 18th/2223-5, Robbins 7th/202)*
Cytokines are peptide mediators or intercellular messengers which regulate immunological, inflammatory and reparative host responses. They are produced by widely distributed cells like macrophage, monocytes, lymphocytes, platelets, fibroblast, endothelium, stromal cells etc.

Criteria for SIRS (2 or more of the following conditions)
• **Fever**[Q] (oral temperature >38°C) or **hypothermia**[Q] (<36°C) • **Tachypnea**[Q] (>24 breaths/minute) • **Tachycardia** [Q] (>90 beats/minute) • **Leukocytosis**[Q] (>12,000/μl), **leucopenia**[Q] (<4,000/μl), or **>10%**[Q] **bands**

49. Ans. (a) Bacterial toxin; (b) IL-1; (d) Interferon; (e) TNF *(Ref: Harrison 18th/143-5)*
Fever is produced in response to substances called pyrogens that act by stimulating prostaglandin synthesis in the vascular and perivascular cells of hypothalamus. They can be classified as:
- **Exogenous pyrogens** - endotoxin of gram '-' bacteria, superantigens (gram '+' bacteria)
- **Endogenous pyrogens** - IL-1, TNF-α, IL-6, Ciliary neurotropic factor and IFN-α.

PGE$_2$ is the most important chemical responsible for **elevation of hypothalamic set point** in the body. So, NSAIDs reduce fever by inhibiting cyclooxygenase and reducing prostaglandin concentration.

50. Ans. (a) Includes interleukins; (c) Are polypeptide (complex protein): *(Ref: Ananthanarayan 7th/143; Harrison 16th/1915, Robbins 7th/202)*
Cytokines are peptide mediators or intracellular messengers produced by wide variety of haemopoietic and non- haemopoietic type of cells in response to immuno, inflammatory or infectious disease states. Most of the lymphokines exhibit multiple biological effects and same effect may be caused by different lymphokines.

Classification of cytokines

1.	Cytokines that mediate innate immunity - IL-1, TNF, IFN, IL-6. IL-12
	• Are involved in both innate and adaptive immunity.
2.	Cytokines regulating lymphocyte growth, activation and differentiation (IL-2, IL-4, IL-12, IL-15, TGF-β)
	• IL-2 is a growth factor for T-cells.
	• IL-4 stimulates differentiation to TH2 pathway.
	• IL-12 stimulates differentiation to T H1 pathway.
	• IL-15 stimulates the growth and activity of NK cells.
	• IL-10 and TGF-β down regulate immune responses.
3.	Cytokines that activate inflammatory cells:
	• IL-5 activates eosinophils.
	• TNF induces acute inflammation by acting on neutrophils and endothelial cells.
4.	Cytokines that affect movement of WBCs (chemotaxis).
5.	Cytokines that stimulate hematopoiesis e.g. GM-CSF, G-CSF, stem cell factor.

- Same cytokine can be produced by different cells
- Same cytokine can have multiple actions (pleiotropic in nature).

51. Ans. (d) X; Ca^{++} *(Ref: Robbins 7th/128, 8th/119, 9/e p118)*

52. Ans. (d) C3a and C5a *(Ref: Robbins 7th/64, 8th/64, 9/e p89)*
- Anaphylatoxins are chemicals which increase vascular permeability and cause vasodilation mainly by releasing histamine from mast cells.

Inflammation

- C3a, C5a and to a small extent C4a are called anaphylatoxins.

> **C5a** is also a powerful **chemotactic agent** for neutrophils, monocytes, eosinophils and basophils.
> **C3b** and C3bi are required for **opsonisation** and favor phagocytosis by neutrophils and macrophages.

53. **Ans. (d) VIII** *(Ref: Robbins 7th/664, T. Singh 1st/258)*
    - Cryoprecipitate is a source of **Fibrinogen (factor I), Factor VIII and Von-Willebrand factor**[Q]
    - Treatment of choice for **Hemophilia A**[Q], **von Willebrand disease**[Q] and **hypofibrinogenemic states**[Q].
    - If factor VIII is unavailable, cryoprecipitate may be an alternative, since each unit contains about 80 IU of factor VIII.

54. **Ans. (b) C5a** *(Ref: Robbins 7th/56, 9/e p77)*

Role of different mediators in Inflammation

Increased vascular permeability	Chemotaxis, leukocyte recruitment and activation
(a) C3a and C5a	(a) C5a
(b) Vasoactive amines	(b) Leukotriene B_4
(c) Leukotriene C_4, D_4, E_4	(c) Chemokines
(d) PAF	(d) IL-8
(e) Substance P	(e) Bacterial products
(f) Bradykinin	(f) TNF
Fever	**Vasodilatation**
(a) IL-1	(a) NO
(b) TNF	(b) Histamine
(c) Prostaglandins	(c) Prostaglandins
Tissue damage	**Pain**
(a) Neutrophil/macrophage lysosomal enzymes	(a) Prostaglandin
(b) NO and reactive oxygen species	(b) Bradykinin

55. **Ans. (c) Vasodilation** *(Ref: Robbins 7th/64, 9/e p73)*

56. **Ans. (d) Lactoferrin** *(Ref: Robbins 8th/54; 7th/61, 9/e p80)*

57. **Ans. None** *(Ref: Robbins 8th/53-54; 7th/69, 9/e p80)*
    Cathepsin G is a serine protease secreted by activated neutrophils that play a role in the inflammatory response.

58. **Ans. (a) Weibel-Palade bodies** *(Ref: Robbins 8th/490; 7th/54,513, 9/e p76)*

59. **Ans. (a) Intrinsic and common pathway** *(Ref: Robbins 8th/120,666; 7th/469, 9/e p118)*

60. **Ans. (d) Function of platelets** *(Ref: Robbins 8th/666; 7th/469)*

61. **Ans. (d) IX** *(Ref: Harsh Mohan 6th/330, Robbins 8th/119, 7th/128, 9/e p119)*

62. **Ans. (d) Leukotriene B_4** *(Ref: Robbins 8th/200; 7th/208, 9/e p203)*

63. **Ans. (a) Langerhans cells** *(Ref: Robbins 8th/1166; 7th/701, 9/e p622)*

> *Birbeck granules* are rod shaped/*Tennis-racket shaped* cytoplasmic organelles with a central linear density and a striated appearance. They are diagnostic microscopic feature in *Langerhans cell histiocytosis (Histiocytosis X)*

64. **Ans. (b) Hydrolytic enzyme** *(Ref: Robbins 8th/54; 7th/82,209)*

65. **Ans. (b) Thromboxane A_2** *(Ref: Robbins 8th/58, 7th/125-127, 9/e p84)*

66. **Ans. (b) C5a** *(Ref: Robbins 8th/64, 7th/56, 9/e p77)*

67. **Ans. (a) Vasodilatation** *(Ref: Robbins 8th/66; 7th/69, 9/e p85)*

68. **Ans. (c) Carbohydrate binding proteins** *(Ref: Robbins 8th/51-53; 7th/59, 9/e p78)*

69. **Ans. (a) IL-1** *(Ref: Robbins 8th/57, 61, 7th/71, 9/e p86)*

70. **Ans. (a) Monoclonal antibody** *(Ref: Robbins 8th/61-63, 7th/71, 9/e p86)*

71. **Ans. (c) Basophil** *(Ref: Robbins 8th/200, 9/e p203)*
    The girl is most likely suffering from an acute attack of bronchial asthma. The figure shows the presence of an activated mast cell. These cells are similar to the basophils.

72. **Ans. (c) Tumor necrosis factor-α** *(Ref: Robbins 8th/61,320, 9/e p330)*

Cachexia, or wasting due to cancer, manifests with weakness, weight loss, anorexia, anemia, and infection. The principal cytokine responsible for such manifestations is tumor necrosis-α (TNF-α). Fibroblast growth factor is involved in wound healing. Interleukin-2 (IL-2) is an immune-stimulant produced by activated T cells. Vascular endothelial growth factor is important in the proliferation of blood vessels in a growing tumor.

73. **Ans. (a) They are basophilic with spherical dark-stained nuclei** *(Ref: Robbins 8th/72, 9/e p96)*
Lymphocytosis is associated with viral infection. These cells are **generally small and are basophilic with spherical dark-stained nuclei normally** constituting nearly 30% of leukocytes. There are two types of lymphocytes: T cells (involved in cell-mediated immunity) and B cells (involved in humoral immunity).

> Monocytes are precursors of osteoclasts and liver Kupffer cells (option b) and also give rise to tissue macrophages and alveolar macrophages.
> Platelets contain a peripheral hyalomere and central granulomere (option c).
> Neutrophils have azurophilic granules and multilobed nuclei (option d). They increase in number in response to bacterial infection.

74. **Ans. (b) Serum C2 normal, C3 decreased, C4 normal** *(Ref: Robbins 7th/64-67, 9/e p88)*
   - Activation of the complement cascade can produce local deposition of C3, which can be seen with special histologic techniques. If a patient has widespread activation of the complement system, then serum assays of C3 levels might be decreased.
   - In particular, activation of the classic complement pathway decreases levels of the early complement components, namely, C1, C4, and C2. In contrast, activation of the alternate complement pathway, decreases levels of C3, but the levels of the early factors (C2 and C4) are normal.
   - An example of a disorder associated with the activation of the alternate complement system is IgA nephropathy (Berger's disease), which is characterized by the deposition of IgA in the mesangium of the glomeruli.

75. **Ans. (b) C1 esterase inhibitor** *(Ref: Robbins 7th/66-67, 9/e p89)*
   - **Deficiencies of C1 esterase inhibitor** result in recurrent angioedema, which refers to **episodic non-pitting edema** of soft tissue, such as the face. Severe abdominal pain and cramps, occasionally accompanied by vomiting, may be caused by edema of the gastrointestinal tract (GI). C1 inhibitor not only inactivates C1, but also inhibits other pathways, such as the conversion of prekallikrein to kallikrein. It also leads to excess production of C2, and bradykinin. It is the uncontrolled activation of bradykinin that produces the angioedema,
   - A deficiency of **decay accelerating factor** (DAF), which breaks down the C3 convertase complex, is seen in **paroxysmal nocturnal hemoglobinuria** (PNH).

75.1. **Ans. (a) IL 1** *(Ref: Robbins 8/e p61,66 , 9/e p83, 90)*

Role in Inflammation	Mediators
Vasodilation	Prostaglandins
	Nitric oxide
	Histamine
Increased vascular permeability	Histamine and serotonin
	C3a and C5a (by liberating vasoactive amines from mast cells, other cells)
	Bradykinin
	Leukotrienes C_4, D_4, E_4
	PAF
	Substance P
Chemotaxis, leukocyte recruitment and activation	TNF, IL-1
	Chemokines
	C3a, C5a
	Leukotriene B_4
	(Bacterial products, e.g., N-formyl methyl peptides)
Fever	**IL-1**, TNF
	Prostaglandins
Pain	Prostaglandins
	Bradykinin
Tissue damage	Lysosomal enzymes of leukocytes
	Reactive oxygen species
	Nitric oxide

75.2. Ans. (a) Gastric cancer *(Ref: Robbins 8/e p96, 9/e p297)*

Cadherin is derived from the "calcium-dependent adherence protein." It participates in interactions between cells of the same type. The linkage of cadherins with the cytoskeleton occurs through the catenins. The cell -to-cell interactions mediated by cadherin and catenins play a major role in regulating cell motility, proliferation, and differentiation and account for the inhibition of cell proliferation that occurs when cultured normal cells contact each other ("**contact inhibition**").

- Reduced function of **E-cadherin** is associated with certain types of **breast and gastric cancer.**
- Mutation and altered expression of the *Wnt/β-catenin* pathway is implicated in in *gastrointestinal and liver cancer* development.

75.3. Ans. (b) Integrins *(Ref: Robbins 8/e p96, 9/e p24)*

The cell adhesion molecules (CAMs) are classified into four main families:
- Immunoglobulin family CAMs
- *Cadherins*
- *Integrins:* bind to extracellular matrix (ECM) proteins such as fibronectin, laminin, and osteopontin providing a connection between cells and extracellular matrix (ECM)
- *Selectins*
  - *Cadherins and integrins link the cell surface with the cytoskeleton through binding to actin and intermediate filaments.*
  - *Laminin* is the most abundant glycoprotein in the basement membrane and has binding domains for both ECM and cell surface receptors.

75.4. Ans. (b) Interleukin-10 *(Ref: Robbins 8/e p56;Cytokines and Pain/pg 3, 9/e p86)*

The following are the anti inflammatory cytokines:
- IL-10
- TGF-β
- IL-4
- IL-13

75.5. Ans. (a) Mast cells *(Ref: Robbins 8/e p57, 9/e p83)*

The richest sources of *histamine* are the **mast cells** that are normally present in the connective tissue adjacent to blood vessels. It is also found in blood basophils and platelets.

75.6. Ans. (b) Vasoconstriction *(Ref: Robbins 8/e p115 .... Not given in 8/9 edition of Robbins)*

After initial injury there is a brief period of arteriolar vasoconstriction mediated by reflex neurogenic mechanisms and augmented by the local secretion of factors such as endothelin(a potent endothelium-derived vasoconstrictor.

75.7. Ans. (c) Decreased vascular permeability *(Ref: Robbins 8/e p60, 9/e p73)*

PAF is another phospholipid-derived mediator having the following inflammatory effects:
- Platelet aggregation
- Vasoconstriction
- Bronchoconstriction
- ***At extremely low concentration, it may cause vasodilation and increased venular permeability***
- Increases leukocyte adhesion to endothelium (by enhancing integrin-mediated leukocyte binding), chemotaxis, degranulation, and the oxidative burst.
- Stimulates the synthesis of other mediators, particularly eicosanoids, by leukocytes and other cells.

75.8. Ans. (b) IL-5 *(Ref: Robbins 8/e p200)*

IL-5 is required for the development and maturation of the eosinophil.

75.9. Ans. (a) C3 ....already discussed earlier in text and AIIMS question *(Ref: Robbins 9/e p88, Harison 17/e 2030)*

75.10. Ans. (d) Factor VIII *(Ref: Robbins 7/e p664)*

Cryoprecipitate is a **rich source of Factor VIII.** Have a glance at the flowchart given below.

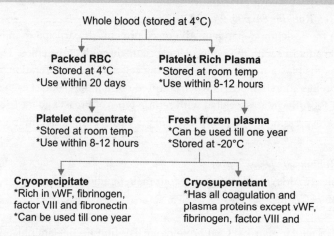

Whole blood (stored at 4°C)

Packed RBC
*Stored at 4°C
*Use within 20 days

Platelet Rich Plasma
*Stored at room temp
*Use within 8-12 hours

Platelet concentrate
*Stored at room temp
*Use within 8-12 hours

Fresh frozen plasma
*Can be used till one year
*Stored at -20°C

Cryoprecipitate
*Rich in vWF, fibrinogen, factor VIII and fibronectin
*Can be used till one year

Cryosupernetant
*Has all coagulation and plasma proteins except vWF, fibrinogen, factor VIII and

75.11. Ans. (c) Arachidonic acid *(Ref: Robbins 9/e p84)*

Arachidonic acid is an essential fatty acid which is acted on by the enzyme **cyclo-oxygenase**[Q] (COX) leading to the formation of the prostaglandins.

Also know:

- **Linoleic, linolenic and arachidonic acid** are examples of polyunsaturated **essential fatty acids**[Q] (PUFA) which means they cannot be synthesized in the human body.
- **Docosahexaenoic acid**[Q] is an *essential fatty acid* present in **breast milk** which is required for **myelination of nerves**[Q].
- **Richest source** of PUFA is **safflower oil**[Q]
- **Coconut oil**[Q] is the **poorest source** of PUFA

75.12. Ans. (d) PGH2 *(Ref: Robbins 9/e p84)*

75.13. Ans. (d) Procalcitonin *(Ref: Harrison 18th/3419)*

Procalcitonin is an acute phase reactant which is now useful for being a marker of sepsis. It is in fact utilized for differentiating the bacterial and aseptic meningitis.

76. Ans. (d) Monocyte macrophages *(Ref: Robbins 7th/82 – 83, 9/e p97)*

Delayed type hypersensitivity (as seen in TB) results from accumulation of mononuclear cells around small veins and venules, producing a perivascular cuffing. Monocytes transform into macrophages which undergo morphological changes to produce epithelioid cells.

77. Ans. (b) Microscopic polyangiitis *(Ref: Robbins Illustrated 7th/540)*

- **Microscopic polyangiitis** is a small vessel vasculitis showing the presence of necrotizing inflammation of the affected vessels without the presence of granuloma.

Systemic vasculitis causing granulomas	Systemic vasculitis causing necrotizing inflammation
• Giant cell arteritis	• Polyarteritis nodosa (PAN)
• Takayasu's disease	• Microscopic polyangiitis
• Wegener's granulomatosis	• Wegener's granulomatosis
• Churg-Strauss syndrome	• Churg-Strauss syndrome

78. Ans. (d) Mycoplasma *(Ref: Robbins 8th/802 9/e p97)*

- **Granulomatous inflammation** is a distinctive pattern of chronic inflammatory reaction characterized by focal accumulations of activated macrophages, which often develop an epithelial-like (epithelioid) appearance.
- **Tuberculosis** is the prototype of the granulomatous diseases, but **sarcoidosis, Crohn's disease, cat-scratch disease, lymphogranuloma inguinale, leprosy, brucellosis, syphilis, some mycotic infections, berylliosis, and reactions of irritant lipids** are also included.
- In Robbins (8th ed, page 802), *Yersinia* has also been mentioned to be associated with granulomatous inflammation. So, the answer of exclusion is Mycoplasma.

79. Ans. (c) Metastatic carcinoma of the lung *(see below)*

Friends, remember that fungal and mycobacterial granulomas are usually associated with central necrosis but all large caseating granulomas come from small non-caseating granulomas. Granuloma can be seen in both Byssinosis and Hodgkin's lymphomas.

- Granulomas are also seen in Hodgkin's disease (Dorland's, 28/p 716)
- So, metastatic carcinoma of lung is the answer of exclusion.

Inflammation

80. **Ans. (c) Helper T-cell** *(Ref: Robbins 7th/83, Anderson's pathology 10th/583 9/e p97-98)*
Granuloma is a focus of chronic inflammation consisting of a microscopic aggregation of macrophages that are transformed into epithelium–like cells surrounded by a collar of mononuclear WBC, principally lymphocytes and occasionally plasma cells.
CD 4 Helper T-cells are involved in granuloma formation as it secretes IFN-γ, IL-2 and IL-12.

81. **Ans. (b) Leprosy; (d) CMV; (e) Wegener's granulomatosis** *(Ref: Robbins 7th/83,8th/73, 9/e p98)*
Caseous necrosis is characteristic of tubercular granuloma, rare in others type of granulomatous disease. TB granuloma is a prototype of immune granuloma. These are caused by insoluble particles; typically microbes that are capable of inducing a cell mediated immune response.
Granulomatous lesions may develop in liver in CMV infection.

82. **Ans. (a) Phagocytosis** *(Ref: Robbins 7th/381, Harsh Mohan 6th/153, 9/e p97)*
Epithelioid cells and giant cells are apposed to the surface and encompass the foreign body.

83. **Ans. (d) Leprosy** *(Ref: Robbins 8th/73, 9/e p98)*
Examples of Diseases with Granulomatous Inflammation

Disease	Cause	Tissue Reaction
Tuberculosis	**Mycobacterium tuberculosis**	**Noncaseating tubercle (granuloma prototype):** focus of epithelioid cells, rimmed by fibroblasts, lymphocytes, histiocytes and **Langhans giant cell.** Caseating tubercle: central amorphous granular debris, loss of all cellular detail; acid-fast bacilli
Leprosy	**Mycobacterium leprae**	**Acid-fast bacilli** in macrophages; **non-caseating** granulomas
Syphilis	**Treponema pallidum**	**Gumma:** lesion enclosing wall of histiocytes; plasma cell infiltrate; central cells are necrotic without loss of cellular outline
Cat-scratch disease	Gram-negative bacillus	**Rounded or stellate granuloma** containing central granular debris and recognizable neutrophils; giant cells uncommon

84. **Ans. (d) Pneumocystis carinii** *(Ref: Robbins 7th/216, 756, 9/e p98)*

85. **Ans. (a) Histoplasmosis** *(Ref: Robbins 8th/718; 7th/754-755, 739)*

86. **Ans. (b) Sarcoidosis** *(Ref: Robbins 8th/701, 7th/738, 9/e p98)*

87. **Ans. (d) P. carinii** *(Ref: Robbins 8th/246, 7th/82-83, 9/e p98)*

88. **Ans. (a) Epithelioid cell** *(Ref: Robbins 8th/73-74, 7th/82, 9/e p97-98)*

89. **Ans. (a) Histoplasmosis** *(Ref: Robbins 8th/717-718; 7th/676)*

90. **Ans. (b) T_H1** *(Ref: Robbins 8th/208, 9/e p210)*
The history is highly suggestive of a sexually transmitted disease, **syphilis** that is characterized by the formation of granuloma in the affected lesions. The formation of a granuloma is associated with activation of a T_H1 cell which causes release of cytokines like IFN-γ causing macrophage activation and IL-2 having an autocrine stimulatory effect.

91. **Ans. (b) Cell-mediated immunity** *(Ref: Robbins 8th/73-4, 9/e p97-98)*
The principle host defense in mycobacterial infections is cell-mediated immunity, which causes formation of granulomas. In many infectious diseases characterized by granuloma formation, the organisms may persist intracellularly for years in the granulomas to be a source of activation of the infection later.
While antibody-mediated phagocytosis and neutrophil ingestion of bacteria (options a and d) are a major source of host defense against many bacteria but they are not active against Mycobacteria.
IgA-mediated hypersensitivity (option c) is not involved in the body's defense against Mycobacteria.

92. **Ans. (d) Monocytes** *(Ref: Robbins 7th/79-83, 381-386, 9/e p97)*
Granulomatous inflammation is characterized by the presence of granulomas, which by definition are aggregates of activated macrophages (**epithelioid cells, not epithelial cells**). These cells may be surrounded by mononuclear cells. The source of macrophages (histiocytes) is monocytes from the peripheral blood.

92.1. **Ans. (b) Monocyte – macrophages** *(Ref: Robbins 9/e p97)*
Monocytes and macrophages fuse together resulting in the formation of epithelioid cells giant cells.

- **Langhans giant**[Q] cell is seen in **tuberculosis**. They have *horse shoe shaped nucleus.*
- *Reed Sternberg cells* are seen in *Hodgkin's lymphoma*[Q].
- *Touton giant* cells are seen **xanthoma**[Q].

92.2. Ans. (a) Toxoplaxmosis

This is a characteristic feature of toxoplasmosis.

Also know

- Toxoplasmosis is transmitted by *cat*[Q] *(definitive host). Man is the intermediate host*[Q].
- It is diagnosed by **Sabin Feldman dye test**[Q].
- **Chorioretinitis**[Q] is the commonest manifestation of this disease when **transmitted congenitally**. In the *acquired disease, there is usually absence of symptoms.*
- *Drug of choice* for toxoplasmosis is **combination of pyrimethamine and sulfadiazine**[Q].
- **Drug of choice** for toxoplasmosis in **pregnancy** is **spiramycin**[Q].

92.3. Ans. (d) Amebiasis *(Ref: Robbins 9/e p98)*

93. Ans. (a) Developmental elasticity *(Ref: Robbins 8th/82-5; Harrison 17th/426... Not in 9/ Edition of Robbins)*

Stem cells show the property of developmental plasticity (Not developmental elasticity) which is also known as transdifferentiation.

A change in stem cell differentiation from one cell type to another is called transdifferentiation, and the multiplicity of stem cell differentiation options is known as developmental plasticity. ...Robbins 8th/85.

94. Ans. (a) Remnant skin appendages *(Ref: Love & Bailey 23rd/189)*

- Skin consists of two layers. Epidermis which is the most superficial layer of the skin constantly replaced from the basal layer and the dermis which is thicker than epidermis and contains adnexal structures. The importance of these adnexal structures is that they contain epithelial cells can proliferate and can heal a partial thickness wound by epithelialization.

95. Ans. (b) TB; (c) CLL; (d) Brucellosis *(Ref: P.J. Mehta 14th – 374)*

Absolute lymphocytosis	Relative lymphocytosis
1. Bacterial infections like tuberculosis, brucellosis, syphilis, pertussis, and toxoplasmosis. 2. Viral infections like mumps, rubella, and infectious mononucleosis. 3. Leukemia (chronic lymphocytic). 4. Thyrotoxicosis	1. All causes of neutropenia. 2. Infective hepatitis 3. Convalescence from acute injection. 4. Infant with infections, malnutrition and avitaminosis.

96. Ans. (c) Vitamin C *(Ref: Robbins 7th/114, 9/e p106)*

Healing is modified by a number of influences (including both *systemic and local host factors*) frequently impairing the quality and adequacy of both inflammation and repair.

Ascorbic acid deficiency causes **reduced cross linking of tropocollagen to collagen**[Q]
So, the patient has increased bleeding tendencies and poor wound healing.

97. Ans. (a) Associated with formation of multiple granulomas *(Ref: Robbins 7th/62, 8th/56, 9/e p79, Harrison 18th/387)*

It is a congenital and not acquired leucocyte function defect.

98. Ans. (b) Repairing by same type of tissue *(Ref: Robbins 8th/92-94, 7th/88, 9/e p101)*

99. Ans. (b) Myofibroblasts *(Ref: Robbins 8th/104, 7th/113 , 9/e p105)*

100. Ans. (c) Granulation tissue *(Ref: Robbins 7th/107, 110, 112-113 , 9/e p103)*

Tissue repair involves the formation of granulation tissue, which histologically is characterized by a combination of proliferating fibroblasts and proliferating blood vessels. Proliferating cells are cells that are rapidly dividing and usually have prominent nucleoli.

100.1. Ans. (c) Tenascin *(Ref: Robbins 8/e p96)*

Name of adhesion molecule	Function
Osteonectin (SPARC)	Tissue remodeling in response to injury , Angiogenesis inhibitor
Thrombospondins	Inhibit angiogenesis
Osteopontin	Regulates calcification Mediator of leukocyte migration in inflammation, Vascular remodeling Fibrosis in various organs
Tenascin **family**	Morphogenesis Cell adhesion

Inflammation

SPARC is **s**ecreted **p**rotein **a**cidic and **r**ich in **c**ysteine.

100.2. Ans. (c) Trans-differentiation *(Ref: Robbins 8/e p85, 9/e p26-27)*

Tissue stem cells which are thought to be lineage-committed multipotent cells, possess the capacity to differentiate into cell types outside their lineage restrictions (called *trans-differentiation*). For example, hematopoietic stem cells may be converted into neurons as well as germ cells.

100.3. Ans. (a) Misfolding of protein *(Ref: Robbins 8/e p1308-9 , 9/e p1281)*

Prions are abnormal forms of a cellular protein that cause transmissible neurodegenerative disorders. This group of disorders includes:

- Creutzfeldt-Jakob disease[Q] (CJD),
- Gerstmann-Sträussler-Scheinker syndrome[Q] (GSS),
- Fatal familial insomnia[Q], and
- Kuru[Q] in humans;
- Scrapie in sheep and goats; mink-transmissible encephalopathy; chronic wasting disease of deer and elk; and *bovine spongiform encephalopathy*[Q]
- The *prion protein* (PrP) is both **infectious**[Q] and **transmissible**[Q].
- These disorders are predominantly characterized by **"spongiform change"** caused by intracellular vacuoles in neurons and glia.
- In pathogenesis, the disease occurs when the PrP undergoes a conformational change from its normal α-helix-containing isoform (PrP^c) to an abnormal β-pleated sheet isoform, usually termed PrP^{sc} (for scrapie). It is associated with resistance to the digestive action of proteases.

100.4. Ans. (c) End of third week *(Ref: Robbins 8/e p102-3, 9/e p106-108)* **Measurements in Wound Healing: Science and Practice Springer 2012 pg 112-3**

Measurements in Wound Healing… *"maximum collagen production occurs at **20 days**".* The remodeling of the collagen continues beyond this duration.

Also know for future NEET questions

- *TGF-β is the most important fibrogenic agent*
- Wound strength is **10% after 1 week**[Q]; it increases rapidly during **next 4 weeks**[Q] and becomes **70% at the end of 3rd month**[Q].
- The tensile strength of the wound keeps on increasing as time progresses.
- Collagen is the most abundant protein in the body
- *Type I collagen* is the *major component* of extracellular matrix in skin.
- **Type III collagen** which is also normally present in skin, becomes **more prominent and important during the repair process.**

100.5. Ans. (c) Liver *(Ref: Robbins 8/e p85-6, 9/e p28)*

Name of the cell	Location	Function
Oval cells[Q]	**Canals of Herring** of the **liver**	Forming hepatocytes and biliary cells
Satellite cells[Q]	Basal lamina of myotubules	Differentiate into myocytes after injury
Limbus cells[Q]	Canals of Schlemm[Q]	Stem cells for the cornea[Q]
Ito cells[Q]	Subendothelial space of Disse[Q]	Store vitamin A[Q]
Paneth cells	Bottom of crypts	Host defense against microorganisms

100.6. Ans. (b) Dilatation of capillaries….(Ref: Robbins 8/e p46, 102, 7/e p107, 9/e p106)

Direct quote.. "the cutaneous wound healing is divided into the three phases: inflammation proliferation and maturation." One of the earliest manifestations of inflammation is dilation of the capillaries.

100.7. Ans. (c) Oval cell….discussed in detail in a different question *(Ref: Robbins 8/e p83, 7/e p91, 9/e p28)*

100.8. Ans. (d) K *(Ref: Robbins 9/e p442, 119)*

All previous exam questions

- Vitamin K is required for the activation of **factors 2,7,9,10**[Q]
- The reason why vitamin K is required for these factors is the *gamma carboxylation of glutamate*[Q].
- Vitamin K is the other vitamin apart from vitamin D whose deficiency can cause **osteoporosis**[Q].
- Vitamin K deficiency can cause **Hemorrhagic disease of newborn**[Q].

- **Earliest indicator** for **vitamin K deficiency** is **increased PT^Q** value.
- **Diet^Q** and **intestinal bacteria^Q** are the chief source of vitamin K in the human body.
- **Liver^Q** is the main organ for **storage of vitamin K^Q**.

100.9. Ans. (b) Extensive cross linking of tropocollagen *(Ref: Robbin 8/e p 105-6)*

Fibrillar collagens (mostly type I collagen) form a major portion of the connective tissue in repair sites and are essential for the development of strength in healing wounds.

Net collagen accumulation, however, depends not only on increased collagen synthesis but also on decreased degradation.

The *recovery of tensile strength* results from the excess of collagen synthesis over collagen degradation during the first 2 months of healing, and, at later times, from *structural modifications of collagen fibers* (**cross-linking, increased fiber size**) after collagen synthesis ceases.

100.10. Ans. (b) Subset of stem cells normally circulate in peripheral blood *(Ref: Robbin 9/e p 581)*

Hematopoietic stem cells have two essential properties that are required for the maintenance of hematopoiesis: pluripotency and the capacity for self-renewal. Pluripotency refers to the ability of a single HSC to generate all mature blood cells. When an HSC divides, at least one daughter cell must self renew to avoid stem cell depletion. Self-renewing divisions occur within a specialized marrow niche, in which stromal cells and secreted factors nurture and protect the HSCs. During stress, HSCs are mobilized from the bone marrow and appear in the peripheral blood.

Remember HSC resemble blasts morphologically.

GOLDEN POINTS FOR QUICK REVISION

(INFLAMMATION)

- **Celsus** was the frost person to describe the **four cardinal signs of inflammation**: *rubor* (redness), *tumor* (swelling), *calor* (heat), and *dolor* (pain). These signs are hallmarks of acute inflammation.
- **Rudolf Virchow** added the fifth clinical sign '**loss of function**' *(function laesa)*
- **Elie Metchnikoff** discovered the process of *phagocytosis* by observing the ingestion of rose thorns by amebocytes of starfish larvae and of bacteria by mammalian leukocytes.
- **Sir Thomas Lewis** established the concept that *chemical substances, such as* **histamine** *(produced locally in response to injury), mediate the vascular changes of inflammation.*

- **Increased vascular permeability** is the hallmark feature of acute inflammation.
- **Endothelial cell contraction** is the most common mechanism of increased vascular permeability.
- "**Selectins**" are responsible for '**rolling**' whereas "*integrins*" are required for "*adhesion*".
- Transmigration (also called **diapedesis**) requires PECAM molecule or **CD31**.
- Chemotaxis: single direction targeted movement of WBCs like neutrophils caused by exogenous molecule (bacterial products) or endogenous molecules (C5a, LTB4 or IL-8)
- Opsonisation requires special chemicals called opsonins (complement proteins like C3b, lectins and antibodies)
- *Phagocytic receptors* include **mannose receptors, scavenger receptors and receptors for various opsonins.**
- *Scavenger receptors* were originally defined as molecules that bind and mediate endocytosis of oxidized or acetylated low-density lipoprotein (LDL) particles that can **no longer** interact with the conventional LDL receptor.
- The **H$_2$O$_2$-MPO-halide system** is the most efficient bactericidal system of **neutrophils**.
- **Nitroblue tetrazolium** test is used for monitoring the functioning of phagocytes and is useful in patients suffering from *chronic granulomatous disease*.
- In the *absence of effective TH17 responses*, individuals are susceptible to fungal and bacterial infections, and the skin abscesses that develop are "**cold abscesses**," lacking the classic features of acute inflammation, such as warmth and redness.
- *Arachidonic acid is derived from* the conversion of essential fatty acid **linoleic acid**.
- The **prostaglandins** are involved in the pathogenesis of *pain* and *fever* in inflammation. Also know that PGE2 is hyperalgesic
- *Lipoxins* are also generated from AA by the **lipoxygenase pathway.** They **suppress inflammation** by inhibiting the recruitment of leukocytes. Formation of lipoxins requires two cell populations (**leucocytes and platelets**) for the transcellular biosynthesis. Leukocytes, particularly neutrophils, produce intermediates in lipoxin synthesis, and these are converted to lipoxins by platelets interacting with the leukocytes.
- Stable tissues have a limited capacity to regenerate after injury the *only exception* being **liver**.

Inflammation

- Neutrophil extracellular traps **(NETs)** are **extracellular fibrillar networks** which provide a high concentration of antimicrobial substances at sites of infection. They are produced **by neutrophils** in response to chemicals mainly **interferons**. NET formation is dependent on platelet activation and it is associated with the pathogenesis of autoimmune conditions like **SLE.**
- **Eculizumab** prevents the conversion of C5 to C5a. This inhibitor not only reduces the hemolysis and attendant transfusion requirements in patients of **paroxysmal nocturnal hemoglobinuria** (PNH), but also lowers the risk of thrombosis by up to 90%.

UPDATED INFORMATION FROM 9TH EDITION OF ROBBINS

Neutrophil Extracellular Traps

- Neutrophil extracellular traps **(NETs)** are **extracellular fibrillar networks** that provide a high concentration of antimicrobial substances at sites of infection and prevent the spread of the microbes by trapping them in the fibrils.
- They are produced by **neutrophils** in response to infectious pathogens (mainly bacteria and fungi) and inflammatory mediators (e.g., chemokines, cytokines [*mainly interferons*], complement proteins, and ROS).
- The extracellular traps consist of a viscous meshwork of nuclear chromatin that binds and concentrates granule proteins such as antimicrobial peptides and enzymes.
- In the process of NET formation, the nuclei of the neutrophils are lost, leading to death of the cells.
- The formation of NETs is dependent on *platelet activation.*
- The nuclear chromatin in the NETs, which includes histones and associated DNA, has been postulated to be a source of nuclear antigens in systemic autoimmune diseases especially **systemic lupus erythematosus (SLE)**.

Tertiary lymphoid organs......... Robbins 9th/96

The accumulated lymphocytes, antigen-presenting cells, and plasma cells cluster together to form lymphoid tissues resembling lymph nodes. These are called tertiary lymphoid organs; this type of *lymphoid organogenesis* is often seen in the synovium of patients with long-standing rheumatoid arthritis and in the thyroid in Hashimoto thyroiditis.

NOTES

3

Hemodynamics

HEMODYNAMICS

In a normal blood vessel like capillary, there are two forces (Starling forces) acting on the fluid in the circulation. The **hydrostatic pressure** causes fluid movement from inside the vessel to outside and the **colloid osmotic pressure** (mostly due to proteins) is responsible for the reverse movement of fluid from outside the vessel to the inside. The capillary hydrostatic and osmotic forces are normally balanced so that there is no *net* loss or gain of fluid across the capillary bed. However, *increased* hydrostatic pressure or *diminished* plasma osmotic pressure leads to a net accumulation of extravascular fluid *(edema)*.

In edema, the excessive interstitial fluid can be either an exudate or a transudate.

A transudate is a fluid with low protein content (most of which is albumin) and a specific gravity of less than 1.012. It is essentially an ultrafiltrate of blood plasma that results from osmotic or hydrostatic imbalance across the vessel wall without an increase in vascular permeability.

An exudate is an inflammatory extravascular fluid that has a high protein concentration, cellular debris, and a specific gravity above 1.020. It is formed mainly due to alteration in the normal permeability of small blood vessels in the area of injury.

Causes and conditions associated with edema

↑ Hydrostatic pressure	↓ Plasma osmotic pressure	Lymphatic obstruction (Lymphedema)	Sodium retention	Inflammation
• CHF • Ascites (Cirrhosis) • Venous obstruction due to thrombosis of physical inactivity • Arteriolar dilation	• Liver cirrhosis • Malnutrition • Protein-losing gastroenteropathy	• After surgery or irratiation • Neoplasia • Inflammatory	• ↑ Salt intake • ↓ Renal perfusion • ↑ RAAS activity	• Acute and chronic inflammation

When edema is influenced by gravity, it is called *dependent edema* and it is a characteristic feature of congestive heart failure (particularly the right ventricle).
• Edema due to a renal cause (as in Nephrotic syndrome) is more severe and affects all parts of body equally. However, it is initially appreciated in tissue with loose tissue matrix such as around eyes and is called periorbital edema.

Hyperemia	Congestion
• **Active** process due to arteriolar dilation	• **Passive** process due to impaired venous outflow
• **Edema** is **absent**	• Edema is present
• **Red color** of the tissues	• **Blue red color** of the tissue (due to deoxyhemoglobin)
• Seen in **Inflammation**	• Seen in *Right heart failure*, portal venous obstruction in *cirrhosis*.

In chronic passive congestion, there is chronic hypoxia and capillary rupture leading to hemorrhage foci. Phagocytosis of red cells results in hemosiderin-laden macrophages.

Pulmonary Congestion

In acute pulmonary congestion there is presence of engorged alveolar capillaries and focal intra-alveolar hemorrhage.

In chronic pulmonary congestion there is presence of thickened and fibrotic septa and alveoli contain hemosiderin laden macrophages (heart failure cells).

Transudate is **protein-poor** and cell-poor fluid.

Exudate is **protein-rich** and **cell-rich fluid**.

Concept

Breast lymphedema (inflammatory carcinoma) is due to blockage of subcutaneous lymphatics by malignant cells.

Severe generalized edema is called **anasarca**.

Heart failure cells are present in the **lungs** and *NOT* in the heart. These are **hemosiderin laden macrophages**.

Fibrosis associated with Chronic passive congestion of the liver (in heart failure) is called as **cardiac cirrhosis**.

Hepatic Congestion

Acute hepatic congestion manifest as central vein and sinusoidal distension with degeneration of central hepatocytes.

In chronic hepatic congestion, central region of lobule shows loss of cells and have red brown color which is accentuated against surrounding normal liver (called **nutmeg liver**). Initially there is centrilobular necrosis and presence of hemosiderin laden macrophages. In long standing congestion (as in heart failure), there is presence of hepatic fibrosis called **cardiac cirrhosis**.

HEMOSTASIS

It is defined as a sequence of events leading to cessation of bleeding by the formation of a stable fibrin-platelet hemostatic plug. The process involves the vascular endothelium, platelets and the coagulation system.

1. **Vascular Endothelium**

   After an injury, there is *transient vasoconstriction* of the vessel *due to endothelin*. This is followed by the activation of thrombogenic factors which include:

   a. *Alteration in the blood flow* resulting in turbulence and stasis favoring the clot formation.

   b. There is release of tissue factor from the injured cells activating the factor VII (extrinsic pathway) and exposure to subendothelial collagen causing activating of factor XII (intrinsic pathway). The endothelial cells also release von Willebrand factor (vWF) which binds to exposed collagen and facilitates platelet adhesion.

   c. There is also release of inhibitors of plasminogen activator (PAIs) which inhibit fibrinolysis. Reduction in the endothelial formation of antithrombotic factors (like nitric oxide, prostacyclin and thrombomodulin) also occurs.

2. **Platelets**

   Initially vWF binds with the collagen followed by the binding of the platelets with vWF through the glycoprotein Ib factor. The platelets then undergo a shape change and their degranulation occurs. The granules in the platelets can be

   a. *Alpha granules* having P-selectin, fibrinogen, fibronectin, factors V and VIII, platelet factor 4, platelet-derived growth factor, and transforming growth factor-β.

   b. *Delta granules* or *delta bodies* having ADP, ATP, ionized calcium, histamine, serotonin, and epinephrine.

   The release of granule mediators result in release of calcium (required in the coagulation cascade), ADP (potent mediator of platelet aggregation) and the surface expression of *phospholipid complexes*, which provide the platform for the coagulation cascade. The platelets also synthesize thromboxane A_2 (TXA_2) which is a potent vasoconstrictor and is also responsible for platelet aggregation. The platelets bind to each other by binding to fibrinogen using Gp IIb-IIIa.

3. **The Coagulation System**

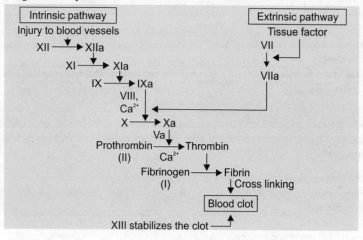

Concept

A defect in the glycoprotein **Ib** factor results in defective platelet adhesion known as **Bernard Soulier syndrome** whereas deficiency of *Gp IIb/IIIa* lead to *Glanzmann thrombasthenia*, a disorder having defective platelet aggregation.

The clotting system can be activated by intrinsic or the extrinsic pathway. The intrinsic pathway is activated by exposing factor XII to thrombogenic surfaces (like glass and other negatively charged surfaces) whereas extrinsic pathway requires exogenous trigger (provided originally by tissue extracts). The division is artifact because extrinsic pathway is physiologically relevant for after vascular damage whereas intrinsic pathway is of relevance in vitro.

> **PT** is prolonged by **deficiency** of VII, X, V, prothrombin **(II)** and fibrinogen **(I)** and oral anticoagulants like **warfarin**.

Prothrombin Time (PT)
- It is used to monitor the functioning of the **extrinsic and the common** coagulation pathways.
- Normal PT is **12-16 seconds**.

Activated partial thromboplastin time (aPTT)
- It is used to monitor the functioning of the intrinsic and the common coagulation pathways.
- Normal aPTT is 26-34 seconds.
- A relatively rare cause of prolonged aPTT is presence of antibodies against coagulation plasma proteins called inhibitors. It can be seen due to the following reasons:
Hemophilia A and B patients receiving clotting factors to control their bleeding episodes, Pregnancy, Autoimmune diseases, Malignancies (lymphoma, prostate cancer) and Dermatologic conditions This has been dealt extensively in chapter-8 of this book.

Thrombin time (TT)
- It is used for testing the conversion of fibrinogen into fibrin and depends on adequate fibrinogen levels.

Bleeding time (BT)
- It is the time taken for a standardized skin puncture to stop bleeding
- It tests the ability of blood vessels to constrict and platelets to form a hemostatic plug.

Fibrin degradation products (FDPs)
- They are used to assess the fibrinolytic activity and they are increased in disseminated intravascular coagulation (DIC).

> **aPTT** is prolonged by **deficiency** of factors XII, XI, IX, III, X, V, **prothrombin and fibrinogen** and drugs like **heparin**.

> Thrombin time is elevated in afibrinogenemia, dysfibrinogen-emia, heparin like inhibitors and DIC.

> **BT** is elevated in **quantitative** *(thrombocytopenia)* and **qualitative** *(thrombasthenia)* platelet defects.

Important anticoagulant substances are:
1. *Antithrombin III* – It inhibits activity of thrombin and other factors like XIIa, XIa, Xa and IXa. It is activated by binding to heparin- Like molecules.
2. *Proteins C and S* – Vitamin K dependent proteins which inactivate Va and VIIIa.
3. Endothelial prostacyclin (*PGI₂*) and nitric oxide (*NO*) are potent vasodilators and inhibitors of platelet aggregation.
4. *Tissue factor pathway inhibitor* – Derived from endothelium and inhibits tissue factor VIIa and Xa molecules.
5. *Thrombomodulin* is produced by all endothelial cells **except those in the cerebral microcirculation**^{Q}. It binds to thrombin and this complex activates protein C (in the presence protein S), which finally inactivates factor V and VIII. This action result in anticoagulant effect.

> *Thrombin is a procoagulant* but the **thrombin-thrombomodulin complex is an anticoagulant.**

> The binding of clotting factors II, VII, IX and X to calcium depends on the addition of γ **carboxylation of glutamic acid**^{Q} residues on these proteins using vitamin K as a cofactor. These clotting proteins are prothrombotic. *Proteins C and S* are two other vitamin K-dependent proteins which can inactivate factors Va and VIIIa. These are anticlotting factors.

THROMBOSIS

It is defined as the pathologic formation of intravascular fibrin-platelet thrombus.
Virchow's triad is required for thrombus formation. Its components are:
1. *Endothelial injury:* It can be due to the factors like vasculitis, hypertension, turbulent flow, bacterial endotoxins, homocystinuria, hypercholesterolemia, radiation etc. It is particularly important for thrombus formation occurring in the heart or in the arterial circulation.
2. *Alterations in the normal blood flow:* Both turbulence and stasis contribute to the development of thrombosis. Turbulence causes arterial whereas stasis causes venous thrombosis. It can also be seen with hyperviscosity syndromes like polycythemia and with deformed red cells as in sickle cell anemia.

> **Virchow's triad** = Endothelial injury + Alterations in the normal blood flow + Blood hypercoagulability

3. *Blood hypercoagulability:* It can be either primary or secondary hypercoagulable state.

Hypercoagulable states

Primary (Genetics)	Secondary (Acquired)
• Mutations in factor V (Most common) • Antithrombin III deficiency • Protein C or S deficiency • Fibrinolysis defects • Homocysteinemia • Allelic variations in prothrombin levels • Mutations in the methyl tetra hydro folate (MTHF) gene	• Prolonged bed rest or immobilization • Homocysteinemia • Tissue damage (Surgery, fracture, burns) • Cancer • MI, Prosthetic cardiac valves • DIC (Disseminated intravascular coagulation) • Heparin induced thrombocytopenia • Antiphospholipid antibody syndrome

Relationship between coagulation defect and site of thrombosis *(updated from Harrison18th/462)*

- *Factor V mutation (also called Leiden mutation) is the most common inherited cause of hypercoagulability* in which normal arginine is replaced by glutamine at position 506 making it resistant to degradation by protein C. This causes unchecked coagulation and it manifest with recurrent deep venous thrombosis.
- Antithrombin III, Protein C or Protein S deficiency are other genetic causes of hypercoagulability manifesting typically as venous thrombosis and recurrent thromboembolism in adolescence or early adult life.
- All conditions mentioned above would have presence of venous thrombosis except for the following:

Conditions with both arterial and venous thrombi

• Homocysteinuria[Q] • Antiphospholipid antibody[Q] • Hyperhomocysteinemia[Q] • Disseminated intravascular coagulation[Q] • Heparin induced thrombocytopenia[Q]	• Essential thrombocythemia[Q] • Cancer[Q] • PNH[Q] • Polycythemia vera[Q] • Dysfibrinogenemia[Q]

Arterial and Venous Thrombi

- An area of attachment to the underlying vessel or heart wall, frequently firmest at the point of origin, is characteristic of all thromboses. **Venous thrombi are called as stasis thrombi because they are formed in the sluggish venous circulation. These are also known as red thrombi as they contain more enmeshed red cells and relatively few platelets. Arterial thrombus contains more platelets and relatively less fibrin.**

Feature	Arterial thrombus	Venous thrombus
Pathogenesis	Endothelial injury or site of turbulence	Stasis of blood
Blood flow	Associated with **active** blood flow	Associated with sluggish blood flow
Sites	Coronary, cerebral and femoral arteries	Superficial and deep leg veins, ovarian/periuterine veins
Propagation	Grows in a **retrograde manner** from point of attachment	Grows in an antegrade manner from point of attachment
Gross	Lines of Zahn **present**	Lines of Zahn absent
Microscopic	Pale platelet layer alternating with dark red cell layer so also called as **white thrombi**	Red cells mixed with relatively less platelets, so also called as red thrombi
Occlusion	**Incomplete** lumen occlusion	Complete vessel occlusion
Complications	Ischemia and infarction of organs	Embolism, edema and ulceration

Factor V mutation (also called **Leiden mutation**) is the most common inherited cause of hypercoagulability

Hyperhomocystenemia is the only mixed disorder (**inherited as well as acquired**) which can cause **both venous and arterial thrombosis**

Lines of Zahn which are produced by the alternating pale layers of platelets mixed with some fibrin and darker layers containing more red cells.

Arterial thrombi arising in heart chambers or in the aortic lumen usually adhere to the wall of the underlying structure and are termed **mural thrombi.**

Hemodynamics

Postmortem clots are gelatinous with a dark red dependent portion where red cells have settled by gravity and a yellow *chicken fat* supernatant resembling melted and clotted chicken fat. These are usually not attached to the underlying wall whereas as discussed above, an area of attachment is characteristic of all thrombosis. Thrombi may form on heart valves as seen in **infective endocarditis; nonbacterial thrombotic endocarditis and verrucous (Libman-Sacks) endocarditis**.

EMBOLISM

An embolus is a detached intravascular solid, liquid, or gaseous mass that is carried downstream from its site of origin. It is most commonly composed of thromboembolism. The emboli may also be composed of other types like atheroemboli, fat emboli (most commonly with skeletal injuries), air emboli, amniotic fluid emboli and tumor emboli.

Pulmonary Emboli

Most of the pulmonary emboli arise in the ***deep leg veins above the level of the knee***. *Paradoxical embolus* is a rare embolus that can pass through an inter-atrial or inter-ventricular defect, thereby entering the systemic circulation. Most ***pulmonary emboli (60% to 80%) are clinically silent*** because they are small. They ***rarely may cause pulmonary infarction*** (because lungs have dual blood supply from pulmonary and bronchial vessels) manifesting clinically as breathlessness, pleuritic pain, hemoptysis and pleural effusion. Sudden death may occur if >60% of the pulmonary circulation is obstructed. Recurrent pulmonary emboli may also cause pulmonary hypertension which may lead to cor pulmonale.

Systemic Thromboembolism

Most of them arise in the heart and *the major sites of arterial embolization are the lower extremities* (75%), the brain (10%) and less commonly, the intestines, kidneys, spleen, and upper extremities.

Fat embolism

Fat embolism syndrome is characterized by ***pulmonary insufficiency, neurologic symptoms*** (irritability, restlessness and even coma), ***anemia, and thrombocytopenia*** (manifesting as diffuse petechial rash). It is seen after fractures of long bones (which contain fatty marrow) or after soft-tissue trauma. It is ***fatal only in 10%*** of cases. The pathogenesis involves both mechanical obstruction and free fatty acids causing local toxic injury to endothelium.

Infarct

It is an area of necrosis caused by occlusion of either the arterial supply or the venous drainage in a particular tissue. Nearly 99% of all infarcts result from thrombotic or embolic events, and almost all result from arterial occlusion. Venous thrombosis usually causes venous obstruction and congestion but can cause infarction (more in organs with a single venous outflow like testis and ovary). The infarcts may be either red (hemorrhagic) or white (anemic) and may be either septic or bland.

Feature	Red infarcts	White infarcts
Cause	• **Arterial occlusion** in **loose tissues** or organs having dual **blood supply** • **Venous occlusion** (in ovarian torsion)	• Arterial occlusions in solid organs with end arterial circulation
Affected organs	Lung and small intestine	Solid organs (heart, spleen, kidney)
Properties	**Ill define hemorrhagic margins** which change in color to brown	Well defined margins and progressively paler with time
Edema	Usually present	Usually absent

Disseminated Intravascular Coagulation (DIC)/Consumption Coagulopathy

DIC is an acute, subacute, or chronic thrombohemorrhagic disorder occurring as a secondary complication in a variety of diseases. It is characterized by activation of the coagulation sequence that leads to the formation of microthrombi throughout the microcirculation of the body. *As a consequence of the thrombotic diathesis, there is consumption of platelets, fibrin, and coagulation factors and, secondarily, activation of fibrinolytic mechanisms.*

Most common site for **venous thrombosis** is the deep leg veins in **below** the knee.

Most of the **pulmonary emboli** arise in the deep leg veins **above (femoral veins)** the level of the knee.

Fat embolism is seen after fractures of long bones and is **fatal only in 10%** of cases.

Concept

All **infarcts** tend to be **wedge shaped** with the occluded vessel at the apex and the periphery of the organ forming the base. The infarct microscopically has features of **ischemic coagulative necrosis**.

Hemodynamics

75

Causes of DIC				
Obstetrics complications	Infections	Neoplasm	Massive tissue injury	Miscellaneous
- Abruptio placenta - Retained dead fetus - Septic abortion - Amniotic fluid embolism - Toxemia	- Gram negative sepsis - Meningococcemia - Histoplasmosis - Aspergillosis - Malaria - Toxemia	- Ca pancreas - Ca prostate - Ca lung - Ca stomach - Acute promyelocytic leukemia	- Traumatic - Burns - Extensive surgery	- Acute intravascular hemolysis - Snake bite - Shock - Heat stroke - Vasculitis - Aortic aneurysm - Liver disease

Laboratory investigations in DIC reveal that
- Platelet count is decreased
- Prolonged PT/TT
- Decreased fibrinogen
- Elevated fibrin split products (D-dimers)

The management is to treat the underlying disorder.

SHOCK

It is defined as *systemic hypoperfusion* caused by reduction either in cardiac output or in the effective circulating blood volume.

Causes of Shock

- *Cardiogenic shock*: Presence of cardiac pump failure as seen with myocardial infarction, cardiac arrhythmia, cardiac tamponade and pulmonary embolism.
- *Hypovolemic shock*: Caused by reduction of blood volume due to hemorrhage, severe burns and severe dehydration.
- *Neurogenic shock*: Presence of generalized vasodilation due to anesthesia and CNS injury.
- *Anaphylactic shock*: Presence of generalized vasodilation due to type I hypersensitivity reaction
- *Septic shock*: It is due to release of endotoxins or bacterial cell wall lipopolysaccharides (gram negative infections) resulting in production of cytokines like TNF-alpha, IL-1and IL-6, vasodilation and hypotension, acute respiratory distress syndrome and multiple organ dysfunction syndrome. Pathogenesis of septic shock is explained in the flowchart below:

Concept

Most common cause of septic shock is gram positive bacteria now; so, the earlier term of endotoxic shock is not used now.

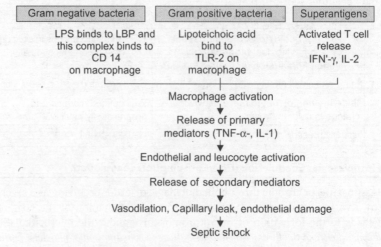

LPS: Lipopolysaccharide **LBP:** LPS Binding Protein **TLR:** Toll Like Receptor

Hemodynamics

STAGES OF SHOCK

Stage I: *Stage of compensation* in which perfusion to the vital organs is maintained by mechanisms like increased sympathetic tone, catecholamine release and activation of renin-angiotensin system.

Stage II: *Stage of decompensation* in which there is tissue hypoperfusion and other features like development of metabolic acidosis, electrolyte disturbances and renal insufficiency.

Stage III: *Irreversible stage* having irreversible tissue injury and multiple organ failure which is not even corrected by the removal of the underlying cause or correction of the hemodynamic disturbance.

FEATURES OF SHOCK

Brain	Ischemic encephalopathy
Heart	Coagulative necrosis or contraction band necrosis
Liver	Fatty change with hemorrhagic central necrosis; 'shock liver'
Kidneys	Extensive tubular ischemic injury (Acute tubular necrosis) leading to oliguria and electrolyte disturbances.
Adrenal	Cortical cell lipid depletion.
GIT	Hemorrhagic enteropathy.
Lungs are uncommonly affected but may show features of diffuse alveolar damage or shock lung.	

Clinical Features

In hypovolemic and cardiogenic shock, the patient presents with hypotension; a weak, rapid pulse; tachypnea; and cool, clammy, cyanotic skin. In septic shock, however, the skin may initially be warm and flushed because of peripheral vasodilation. Then, patients develop a second phase dominated by renal insufficiency and marked by a progressive fall in urine output as well as severe fluid and electrolyte imbalances.

MULTIPLE CHOICE QUESTIONS

HEMODYNAMICS AND HEMOSTASIS

1. **All are true about blood coagulation except?** *(AI 2011)*
   (a) Factor X is a part of both intrinsic and extrinsic pathway.
   (b) Extrinsic pathway is activated by contact of plasma with negatively charged surfaces.
   (c) Calcium is very important for coagulation.
   (d) Intrinsic pathway can be activated in vitro.

2. **Vitamin K is responsible for the carboxylation of which amino acid in the clotting factors?** *(AI 2011)*
   (a) Aspartate
   (b) Glutamate
   (c) Proline
   (d) Lysine

3. **Edema in nephrotic syndrome occurs due to**
   (a) Na+ and water restriction *(AIIMS Nov. 2010)*
   (b) Increased venous pressure
   (c) Decreased serum albumin
   (d) Decreased fibrinogen

4. **Thrombomodulin thrombin complex prevents clotting because:** *(DPG 2011)*
   (a) Thrombomodulin inhibits prothrombin activator
   (b) The complex activates antithrombin III
   (c) Thrombomodulin-thrombin complex activates heparin
   (d) The complex removes thrombin and also activates protein C which inactivates the activated factors V and VIII

5. **Vitamin K associated clotting factors are:**
   (a) IX, X *(AI 2010)*
   (b) I, V
   (c) VII, VIII
   (d) I, VIII

6. **All endothelial cells produce thrombomodulin except those found in:** *(AI 2005)*
   (a) Hepatic circulation
   (b) Cutaneous circulation
   (c) Cerebral microcirculation
   (d) Renal circulation

7. **Which of the following is a procoagulation protein?**
   (a) Thrombomodulin *(AI 2004)*
   (b) Protein C
   (c) Protein S
   (d) Thrombin

8. **All of the following are correct about Thromboxane A2 except:** *(AI 2001)*
   (a) Low dose aspirin inhibits its synthesis
   (b) Causes vasoconstriction in blood vessels
   (c) Causes bronchoconstriction
   (d) Secreted by WBC

9. **Coagulation defects associated with increased coagulation are seen in:** *(PGI Dec 2006)*
   (a) Increased Protein C
   (b) Increased Protein S
   (c) Increased Anti-thrombin III
   (d) Protein C resistance
   (e) Dysfibrinogenemia

10. **All of the following are anticoagulant substances except** *(Karnataka 2006)*
    (a) Antithrombin III
    (b) Protein S
    (c) vWF
    (d) Nitric oxide

11. **Cause of edema is** *(UP 2002)*
    (a) Decreased plasma protein concentration
    (b) Increased lymph flow
    (c) Increased ECF volume
    (d) Increased plasma protein concentration

12. **Endothelium derived relaxing factor (EDRF) is associated with:** *(UP 2004)*
    (a) Ras   (b) C-myc
    (c) Bcl   (d) N NOS

13. **Which is not involved in local hemostasis?**
    (a) Fibrinogen *(RJ 2004)*
    (b) Calcium
    (c) Vitamin K
    (d) Collagen

14. **Which is the following not synthesized in the liver?**
    (a) Factor II *(Jharkhand 2005)*
    (b) Factor VII
    (c) Factor IX
    (d) Factor VIII

15. **A 54 year old chronic alcoholic Adhiya Kumar is brought by his son as he has developed progressively increasing abdominal distension from past 3 months. The physician aspirates the abdominal fluid which is straw-colored and clear and is found to have protein content (mainly albumin) of 2.3 g/dl. Which of the following is a major contributor to the fluid accumulation in this patient?**
    (a) Blockage of lymphatics
    (b) Decreased oncotic pressure

(c) Decreased capillary permeability

(d) Inflammatory exudation

Most Recent Questions

15.1. Tissue thromboplastin activates:
- (a) Factor VII
- (b) Factor IV
- (c) Factor VI
- (d) Factor XII

15.2. Platelet adhesion to collagen is mediated by which of the following?
- (a) Factor VIII
- (b) Factor IX
- (c) Von willebrand factor
- (d) Fibronectin

15.3. Gandy gamma body is typically seen in chronic venous congestion of which of the following?
- (a) Lung
- (b) Kidney
- (c) Spleen
- (d) Liver

15.4. Extrinsic pathway of clotting factors is measured by?
- (a) Prothromin time
- (b) Activated partial thromboplastin time
- (c) Bleeding time
- (d) Clotting time

THROMBOSIS: EMBOLISM: INFARCT

16. Histologic sections of lung tissue from 66-year-old woman, Sheena with congestive heart failure and progressive breathing problems reveal numerous hemosiderin-laden cells within the alveoli. Which of the following is the cell of origin of these "heart failure cells"?
- (a) Endothelial cells
- (b) Pneumocytes
- (c) Lymphocytes
- (d) Macrophages

17. At autopsy, the spleen of a patient is noted to have a thickened capsule and many small, scarred areas. Microscopic examination of the scarred areas reveals fibrosis with hemosiderin and calcium deposition. This type of spleen is usually seen in conjunction with which of the following disorders?
- (a) Hepatic cirrhosis
- (b) Hodgkin's disease
- (c) Rheumatoid arthritis
- (d) Sickle cell anemia

18. Antiphospholipid syndrome is associated with all except: *(AI 2012)*
- (a) Recurrent abortion
- (b) Venous thrombosis
- (c) Pancytopenia
- (d) Antibody to lupus

19. Pale infarct is seen in all except: *(AIIMS Nov. 2010)*
- (a) Lungs
- (b) Spleen
- (c) Kidney
- (d) Heart

20. Congenital hypercoagulability states are all of the followings except
- (a) Protein C deficiency *(AIIMS Nov. 2010)*
- (b) Protein S deficiency
- (c) Anti-phospholipid antibody syndrome
- (d) MTHFR gene mutation

21. Fat embolism is commonly seen in: *(DPG 2011)*
- (a) Head injuries
- (b) Long bone fractures
- (c) Drowning
- (d) Hanging

22. Virchow's triad includes all except
- (a) Injury to vein
- (b) Venous thrombosis
- (c) Venous stasis
- (d) Hypercoagulability of blood

23. Hypercoagulability due to defective factor V gene is called: *(AIIMS Nov 2003)*
- (a) Lisbon mutation
- (b) Leiden mutation
- (c) Antiphospholipid syndrome
- (d) Inducible thrombocytopenia syndrome

24. Arterial thrombosis is seen in *(PGI June 2003)*
- (a) Homocysteinemia
- (b) Anti-phospholipid syndrome
- (c) Protein S deficiency
- (d) Protein C deficiency
- (e) Antithrombin III deficiency

25. Hemorrhagic infarction is seen in: *(PGI Dec 2002)*
- (a) Venous thrombosis
- (b) Thrombosis
- (c) Septicemia
- (d) Embolism
- (e) Central venous thrombosis

26. Hyperviscosity is seen in *(PGI Dec 2003, 04)*
- (a) Cryoglobulinemia.
- (b) Multiple myeloma.
- (c) MGUS.
- (d) Lymphoma.
- (e) Macroglobulinemia.

27. Predisposing factor for venous thrombosis:
- (a) AT III deficiency
- (b) Protein S deficiency
- (c) Protein C deficiency
- (d) Dysfibrinogenemia

28. Inherited coagulation disorders are:
- (a) Protein C deficiency *(PGI Dec 2005)*
- (b) Protein S deficiency
- (c) Leiden factor mutation
- (d) Lupus anticoagulant
- (e) Anti-cardiolipin

Hemodynamics

29. Which of the following statements about pulmonary emboli is not correct? *(Delhi PG 2009 RP)*
    (a) 60-80% pulmonary emboli are clinically silent
    (b) In more than 95% cases venous emboli originate from deep leg veins
    (c) Embolic obstruction of pulmonary vessels almost always cause pulmonary infarction
    (d) Embolic obstruction of medium sized arteries may result in pulmonary infarction

30. Which one of the following inherited disorders produces arterial thrombosis?
    (a) Factor V Leiden mutation *(Karnataka 2006)*
    (b) Antithrombin deficiency
    (c) Homocysteinemia
    (d) Protein S deficiency

31. Heart failure cells are seen in *(AP 2007)*
    (a) Chronic venous congestion of liver
    (b) Chronic venous congestion of lung
    (c) Acute venous congestion of lung
    (d) Acute venous congestion of liver

32. Necrosis with putrefaction is called as: *(Bihar 2005)*
    (a) Desiccation
    (b) Gangrene
    (c) Liquefaction
    (d) Coagulative necrosis

33. Lines of Zahn are found in: *(Jharkhand 2006)*
    (a) Thrombus
    (b) Infarct tissue
    (c) Postmortem clot
    (d) All

34. Chicken fat clot is: *(Jharkhand 2006)*
    (a) Postmortem clot
    (b) Thrombus
    (c) Infarct
    (d) All

35. The five stages of hemostasis are given below in random order. Put them into their correct order.

    (a) Clot dissolution
    (b) Blood coagulation
    (c) Vessel spasm
    (d) Clot retraction
    (e) Formation of platelet plug

    (a) cabed
    (b) acbde
    (c) cebda
    (d) ecdba

36. A 64 year old man Ojas Alok Nath resides in a city. He is a known case of hypertension and is a smoker too. One day, while watching tv, he developed severe pain in the chest. He is rushed to the medical emergency of the city hospital where this episode is diagnosed as unstable angina. The emergency medical officer Dr. Smiley Gupta immediately administers him an intravenous preparation of a glycoprotein IIb/IIIa inhibitor. The mechanism of action of this agent is the ability to
    (a) Dilate coronary arteries.
    (b) Inhibit platelet adhesion.
    (c) Inhibit platelet aggregation.
    (d) Lyses thrombi

37. A 62 year old man Ram Srinath is brought by his wife Shanti Devi after sustaining a fall in the washroom while taking bath. He has severe pain in his right leg. Dr. Amit Shersia, the orthopedic surgeon diagnoses it as fracture femur. He is discharged after administration of proper treatment. After about 12 days, Shanti observes that her husband has developed a swollen right leg below the knee. Ram is unable to move his limb properly and there is presence of tenderness too. Which of the following is the most likely complication in him?
    (a) Hematoma of the right thigh
    (b) Fat embolism
    (c) Gangrene in the right foot
    (d) Pulmonary thromboembolism

38. A 27-year-old woman, Shama presents with a history of losing pregnancies in the past 5 years. She also has a history of recurrent pains in her legs secondary to recurrent thrombosis. Her symptoms are most likely due to a deficiency of which one of the following substances?
    (a) PA inhibitors   (b) Protein C
    (c) Plasmin   (d) Thrombin

39. A 20-year-old male, Akash fractured his right femur. He was admitted to the hospital and over the next several days developed progressive respiratory problems. Despite extensive medical intervention, he died 3 days later. At the time of autopsy oil red O-positive material was seen in the small blood vessels of the lungs and brain. Which of the following was the most likely diagnosis?
    (a) Air emboli   (b) Amniotic fluid emboli
    (c) Fat emboli   (d) Paradoxical emboli

40. A pregnant woman develops deep, boring pain of her left thigh muscles associated with swelling and enhanced warmth of the same leg. The pain is worsened by extending the foot. The superficial veins of the leg are engorged. Her condition puts her at risk for which of the following?
    (a) Acute renal failure
    (b) Cerebral hemorrhage
    (c) Hepatic infarction
    (d) Pulmonary embolus

Most Recent Questions

40.1. White infarct is seen in:
    (a) Lung   (b) Intestine
    (c) Heart   (d) Ovary

40.2. Lines of Zahn occur in which of the following?
- (a) Postmortem clot
- (b) Infarct
- (c) Embolus
- (d) Coralline thrombus

40.3. White infarcts are seen in the following *except*:
- (a) Liver
- (b) Kidney
- (c) Spleen
- (d) Heart

SHOCK, DIC AND MISCELLANEOUS

41. All of the following are true about DIC except? *(AI 2012)*
- (a) Increased fibrinogen
- (b) Increased activated partial thromboplastin time
- (c) Decreased prothrombin time
- (d) Increased fibrin degradation products

42. The initiating mechanism in endotoxic shock is
- (a) Peripheral vasodilatation *(AIIMS Nov. 2010)*
- (b) Endothelial injury
- (c) Increased vascular permeability
- (d) Reduced cardiac output

43. The initiating mechanism in endotoxic shock is
- (a) Peripheral vasodilatation *(AIIMS Nov. 2010)*
- (b) Endothelial injury
- (c) Increased vascular permeability
- (d) Cytokine release

44. D-Dimer is the most sensitive diagnostic test for:
- (a) Pulmonary embolism *(DPG 2011)*
- (b) Acute pulmonary oedema
- (c) Cardiac tamponade
- (d) Acute myocardial infarction

45. Shock lung is characterized by
- (a) Alveolar proteinosis *(AIIMS May 2008; Nov 2007)*
- (b) Bronchiolitis obliterans
- (c) Diffuse pulmonary hemorrhage
- (d) Diffuse alveolar damage

46. The histological features of shock includes:
- (a) ATN
- (b) Pulmonary congestion
- (c) Depletion of lipids in adrenal cortex
- (d) Hepatic necrosis
- (e) Depletion of lymphocytes

47. Conditions associated with incoagulable state are:
- (a) Abruption placentae *(PGI Dec 2003, 2004)*
- (b) Acute promyelocytic leukemia
- (c) Severe falciparum malaria
- (d) Snake envenomation
- (e) Heparin overdose

48. Which of the following is a feature of Disseminated Intravascular Coagulation (DIC)?
- (a) Normal prothrombin time *(Karnataka 2006)*
- (b) Reduced plasma fibrinogen
- (c) Normal platelet count
- (d) Normal clotting time

49. A 29 year old woman Ruma is in labour but unfortunately during parturition, the placental membranes tear and amniotic fluid expressed into a lacerated cervical vein. Which of the following is the woman most likely to experience immediately following this event?
- (a) Placental abruption
- (b) Renal failure
- (c) Respiratory distress
- (d) Splinter hemorrhages

50. Irshaan has been diagnosed with acute promyelocytic leukemia recently. He presents suddenly in the medical emergency because of a dangerous complication of his malignancy called disseminated intravascular coagulation (DIC). In DIC, micro emboli form leading to obstruction of blood vessels and tissue hypoxia. The common clinical signs observed in patient may be due to which of the following?
- (a) Immunologic failure
- (b) Renal failure
- (c) Right ventricular failure
- (d) Hepatic failure

51. A primiparous woman Ritu at term experiences placental abruption and is rushed to the operating room for emergency Cesarean section. She develops shortness of breath, cyanosis, and copious bleeding from her surgical wounds. Levels of which of the following blood components is expected to rise in this setting?
- (a) Factor V
- (b) Fibrin degradation products
- (c) Fibrinogen
- (d) Plasminogen

52. A 24-year-old pregnant Heena sustains a placental abruption, and is admitted to the ICU where she begins bleeding from multiple sites, including oral mucous membranes. Which of the following studies would be most valuable in assessing this patient's condition?
- (a) Partial thromboplastin time, kininogen, and factor VIII levels
- (b) Platelet count, fibrinogen levels, and fibrin degradation products
- (c) Platelet count, thrombin time, and prekallikrein levels
- (d) Prothrombin time and factor VIII levels

EXPLANATIONS

1. **Ans. (b) Extrinsic pathway is activated by contact of plasma with negatively charged surfaces** *(Ref: Robbins 8th/119, 9/e 118)*
   Contact of plasma with negative charged surface activates intrinsic and not extrinsic pathways.

2. **Ans. (b) Glutamate** *(Ref: Robbins 8th/119, 9/e p119)*
   The binding of clotting factors II, VII, IX and X to calcium depends on the addition of γ carboxylation of glutamic acid residues on these proteins. This step requires vitamin K as a cofactor.

   ### Vitamin K dependent factors

Increasing clotting	Inhibiting clotting
• Clotting factors **II, VII, IX and X**	• Protein **C** and protein **S**

   Proteins C and S are two other vitamin K-dependent proteins which can inactivate factors Va and VIIIa. These are anticlotting factors.

3. **Ans. (c) Decreased serum albumin** *(Ref: Robbins 8th/922, 9/e p115)*
   Na+ and water retention is now the more important cause of edema in nephrotic syndrome. For details see the Chapter on Kidney.

   > Receptor Na+ and water retention is not to be confused with option (a) Na+ and water restriction.

4. **Ans. (d) The complex removes thrombin and also activates protein C which inactivates the activated factors V and VIII** *(Ref: Harrison 17th/364-5, Robbins 8th/116, 9/e p121)*

5. **Ans. (a) IX, X** *(Ref:Robbins 8th/118-119 9/e p119)*

6. **Ans. (c) Cerebral microcirculation** *(Ref: Ganong 21st/546, Robbins 7th/85, Robbins 8th/116, Harrison 17th/365, 9/e p121)*
   *'All endothelial cells **except** those in the **cerebral microcirculation** produce thrombomodulin, a thrombin protein, and express it on their surface'.*

7. **Ans. (d) Thrombin** *(Ref: Robbins 7th/127, Harrison 17th/364, 9/e p120-121)*
   • Thrombin is clotting factor IIa which participates in coagulation cascade by converting factor I [soluble protein fibrinogen] to factor Ia [insoluble fibrin].
   • Protein C and protein S are vitamin K dependent anticlotting proteins (remember factor II, VII, IX and X are vitamin-K dependent clotting factors). These act by inactivating factor Va and VIIIa.

   > • Thrombomodulin-thrombin complex activates protein C and thus the complex acts as an anticoagulant.

8. **Ans. (d) Secreted by WBC** *(Ref: Robbins 7th/68-70, 9/e p118)*
   Thromboxane A2 (TXA2) is synthesized and released from activated platelets (Not WBCs)
   • TXA$_2$ is also a powerful vasoconstrictor and bronchoconstrictor.
   • Low does aspirin (50-325 mg) is used as antiplatelet drug because it inhibits COX irreversibly and decreases formation of TXA$_2$ by platelets.

9. **Ans. (d) Protein C resistance; (e) Dysfibrinogenemia** *(Ref: Harrison 16th/1491, 9/e p123)*

10. **Ans. (c) Von Willebrand factor** *(Ref: Robbins 7th/125-126/129-130, 9/e p121,118)*

    > VWF (von Willebrand Factor) is produced by endothelial cells and it is required for platelet binding to collagen and other substances. So, it is a procoagulant factor.

11. **Ans. (a) Decreased plasma protein concentration** *(Ref: Robbins 8th/112; 7th/120-121, 9/e p114)*

12. **Ans. (d) nNOS** *(Ref: Robbins 8th/60, 7th/72-73, 9/e p80)*

13. **Ans. (c) Vitamin K** *(Ref: Robbins 8th/115-120, 7th/128, 9/e p118-119)*

14. **Ans. (d) Factor VIII** *(Ref: Robbins 8th/835; 7th/655, 9/e p47-118)*

Hemodynamics

15. **Ans. (b) Decreased oncotic pressure** *(Ref: Robbins 8th/112, 9/e p114)*

The patient in the stem of the question is most likely having liver cirrhosis secondary to chronic alcoholism. An important manifestation of this disease is reduced hepatic synthesis of albumin which is the most important contributor to plasma oncotic pressure. Also, ascites is associated with increased sodium and water retention because of stimulation of the renin-angiotensin aldosterone system (RAAS). A minor contribution is also because of hydrostatic forces (due to intra-hepatic scarring and partial obstruction of the portal venous return) resulting in fluid transudation and increased secretion of hepatic lymph.

15.1. **Ans. (a) Factor VII** *(Ref: Robbins 8/e p119, 7/e p128, 9/e p118)*

The extrinsic pathway is activated by tissue factor (thromboplastin) causing activation of factor VIIa. For details, refer to text.

15.2 **Ans. (c) Von willebrand factor** *(Ref: Robbin 8/e p116-8)*

Direct lines.. *"Von Willebrand factor functions as an adhesion bridge between subendothelial collagen and the glycoprotein Ib (Gp Ib) platelet receptor. Aggregation is accomplished by fibrinogen bridging GpIIb-IIIa receptors on different platelets."*

15.3 **Ans. (c) Spleen** *(Ref: Harsh Mohan 6th/52)*

Gamna-Gandy bodies in chronic venous congestion (CVC) of the spleen is characterized by calcific deposits admixed with haemosiderin on fibrous tissue.

15.4 **Ans. (a) Prothromin time** *(Ref: Robbin 9/e p119)*

Prothrombin time	Extrinsic pathway	Factor 5/7
Activated partial thromboplastin time	Intrinsic pathway	Factor 8
Bleeding time	Platelet function and platelet count	Platelet function and count

16. **Ans. (d) Macrophages** *(Ref: Robbins 7th/79-82, 122, 562, 9/e p116)*
    - Example of tissue macrophages are Kupffer cells (liver), alveolar macrophages (lung), osteoclasts (bone), Langerhan's cells (skin), microglial cells (central nervous system)
    - In the lung, alveolar macrophages can phagocytose the red blood cells that accumulate in alveoli in individuals with congestive heart failure. These cells contain hemosiderin and are referred to as "heart failure cells."

17. **Ans. (a) Hepatic cirrhosis** *(Ref: Robbins 8th/634, 9/e p530)*

The spleen shows the changes of chronic congestive splenomegaly, typically associated with hepatic cirrhosis. The described small scars are called Gandy-Gamma nodules which are due to the result of organization of old hemorrhages.

- *Hodgkin's disease* (choice B) produces large *splenic nodules* in which *Reed-Sternberg cells* can be found surrounded by mature lymphocytes, eosinophils, and neutrophils.
- *Rheumatoid arthritis* (choice C) and many other chronic inflammatory disorders induce reactive hyperplasia of the spleen with formation of many *large germinal centers in the splenic follicles*.
- *Sickle cell anemia* (choice D) produces many *small (often triangularly shaped) infarctions* in the spleen.

18. **Ans. (c) Pancytopenia** *(Ref: Harrison 17th/1795, Robbins 8th/123,215, 7th/133, 229, 9/e p124-125)*

Antiphospholipid antibody syndrome is characterized by antibodies against plasma proteins in complex with phospholipid. In **primary antiphospholipd antibody syndrome** there is hypercoagulable state without evidence of autoimmune disorders. In association with SLE or lupus, the name given is **secondary antiphospholipd antibody syndrome.** There is formation of antibody against **phospholipid beta– 2-glycoprotein 1 complex^Q.** It also binds to cardiolipin antigen and lead to **false positive test for syphilis^Q.** It also interferes with in vitro clotting time and so, called as lupus anticoagulant. In vivo, these patients have hypercoagulable state resulting in **arterial and venous thrombosis** resulting **spontaneous recurrent miscarriage** and focal or cerebral ischemia.

19. **Ans. (a) Lungs** *(Ref: Robbins 8th/128, 9/e p129)*

The Lungs have dual blood supply and so, they exhibit red infarct. The infarcts may be either red (hemorrhagic) or white (anemic) and may be either septic or bland.

All infarcts tend to be wedge shaped with the occluded vessel at the apex and the periphery of the organ forming the base. The infarct microscopically has features of **ischemic coagulative necrosis.**

20. **Ans. (c) Anti-phospholipid antibody syndrome** *(Ref: Robbins 8th/123, 9/e p123)*

Anti-phospholipid antibody syndrome is an acquired causes of hypercoagulability

Hypercoagulable states

Primary (Genetics)	Secondary (Acquired)
• Mutations in factor V (Most common) • Antithrombin III deficiency • Protein C or S deficiency • Fibrinolysis defects • Homocysteinemia • Allelic variations in prothrombin levels • Mutations in the methyl tetra hydro folate (MTHF) gene	• Prolonged bed rest or immobilization • Homocysteinemia • Tissue damage (Surgery, fracture, burns) • Cancer • MI, Prosthetic cardiac valves • DIC (Disseminated intravascular coagulation) • Heparin induced thrombocytopenia • Antiphospholipid antibody syndrome

21. **Ans. (b) Long bone fractures** *(Ref: Robbins 8th/126, 9/e p128)*

22. **Ans. (b) Venous thrombosis** *(Ref: Anderson 10th/387, Robbin's 7th/130, 9/e p122)*
    The factors that predispose to venous thrombosis were initially described by Virchow in 1856 and are known as **Virchow's triad**. These include
    • Stasis^Q • Vascular damage^Q • Hypercoagulability^Q

23. **Ans. (b) Leiden mutation** *(Ref: Robbins 7th/p131, Robbins 8th/122, 9/e p123)*
    • Mutation in factor V gene is caused by the substitution of glutamine for the normal arginine residue at position 506. It is known as **Leiden mutation and it is the most common inherited cause of hypercoagulability.**

    Note: **Lisbon mutation** is associated with a mutation in **thyroid peroxidase gene^Q**.

24. **Ans. (a) Homocysteinemia; (b) Antiphospholipid syndrome** *(Ref: Harrison 18th/462, 9/e p123)*

25. **Ans. (a) Venous thrombosis; (b) Thrombosis; (d) Embolism** *(Ref: Anderson's10th/2707)*
    Hemorrhagic infarction is seen in:
    • Hypercoagulable states (OCP use, pregnancy, polycythemia vera, malignancy etc.)
    • Embolism - Infarct is attributed to lysis of clot exposing infarct tissue and its permeable capillary bed to recirculating blood.
    • Venous thrombosis.

26. **Ans. (a) Cryoglobulinemia; (b). Multiple myeloma; (d) Lymphoma; (e) macroglobulinemia** *(Ref: William's Hematology 6/1268)*
    Hyperviscosity is seen in
    • Multiple myeloma
    • Lymphoplasmacytic lymphoma (Waldenstrom's macroglobulinemia)
    • Cryoglobulinemia
    • Myeloproliferative disorders
    MGUS (Monoclonal Gammopathy of uncertain significance): Here, M Protein can be identified in the serum of 1% of healthy individual >50 years of age and 3% in older than 70 yrs. It is the most common form of monoclonal gammopathy. In MGUS less than 3g/dL of monoclonal protein is present in serum and there is no Bence Jones proteinuria.

    Normal viscosity of blood is 1.8

27. **Ans. All.** *(Ref: Harrison 16th- 686, Robbin's 7th/132)*
    Dysfibrinogenemia produces hypercoagulable state and leads to thrombus formation in some patients. Other causes have already been discussed.

28. **Ans. (a) Protein C deficiency; (b) Protein S deficiency; (c) Leiden factor mutation** *(Ref: Harrison 16th/685; de Gruchy's 5th/420, Robbins 9/e p123)*
    Congenital coagulation disorders

• Hemophilia A and B • von Willebrand's disease • Fibrinogen absence or deficiency. • Prothrombin absence or deficiency. • Factor V deficiency.	• Factor VII deficiency. • Factor X (Stuart) deficiency. • Factor XII, XI deficiency. • Factor XIII deficiency. • Fitzgerald factor (HMWK) deficiency.

Hemodynamics

29. **Ans. (c) Embolic obstruction of pulmonary vessels almost always cause pulmonary infarction** *(Ref: Robbins 8th/126)*
As discussed is text, most pulmonary emboli (60% to 80%) are clinically silent because they are small. With time, they undergo organization and are incorporated into the vascular wall. Embolic obstruction of medium-sized arteries may result in pulmonary hemorrhage but usually does not cause pulmonary infarction because of the dual blood flow into the area from the bronchial circulation.

30. **Ans. (c) Homocysteinemia** *(Ref: Robbins 7th/131, 8th/122, Harrison 18th/462, 9/e p123)*

> Hyperhomocystenemia[Q] is a mixed disorder (inherited as well as acquired[Q]) which can cause both venous and arterial thrombosis[Q].

31. **Ans. (b) Chronic venous congestion of lung** *(Ref: Robbins 8th/535, 7th/122, 9/e p116)*

32. **Ans. (b) Gangrene** *(Ref: Robbins 8th/15; 7th/22, 9/e p43, 129)*

33. **Ans. (a) Thrombus** *(Ref: Robbins 8th/124; 7th/133, 9/e p125)*

34. **Ans. (a) Postmortem clot** *(Ref: Robbins 8th/124; 7th/133, 9/e p125)*

35. **Ans. (c) cebda** *(Ref: Robbins 8th/117-8, Harrison 18th/457-9, 9/e p116-119)*
Hemostasis is divided into five stages:
- Vessel spasm.
- Formation of the platelet plug.
- Blood coagulation or development of an insoluble fibrin clot.
- Clot retraction.
- Clot dissolution.

36. **Ans. (c) Inhibit platelet aggregation** *(Ref: Robbins 8th/118, 9/e p117-118)*
Glycoprotein IIb/IIIa inhibitors (tirofiban, eptifibatide and abciximab) prevent the action of the corresponding platelet surface receptor glycoprotein complex, which is required for formation of fibrinogen bridges between adjacent platelets (**platelet aggregation**).

37. **Ans. (d) Pulmonary thromboembolism** *(Ref: Robbins 8th/126-127, 9/e p127)*
The patient has prolonged immobilization of the limb resulting in venous stasis contributing to superficial and deep venous thrombosis. The most feared complication of the venous thrombi is their embolization to the lungs.
- Gangrene may occur as a complication of arterial and not venous obstruction.
- Hematomas usually appear immediately after a trauma and would have reduced in size after 12 days as has been mentioned in the stem of the question.
- Fat embolism occurs after fractures but symptoms appear 1-3 days after the trauma.

38. **Ans. (b) Protein C** *(Ref: Robbins 7th/129-130, 9/e p124)*
- Differential diagnosis of recurrent spontaneous abortions in women includes deficiencies of protein C and protein S, and the presence of the lupus anticoagulant, which is part of the anti-phospholipid syndrome.

39. **Ans. (c) Fat emboli** *(Ref: Robbins 7th/135-137, 9/e p128)*
- An embolus is a detached intravascular mass that has been carried by the blood to a site other than where it was formed. Most emboli originate from thrombi (thrombotic emboli), but they can also originate from material other than thrombi (non- thrombotic emboli). Types of non-thrombotic emboli include fat emboli, air emboli, and amniotic fluid emboli.
- Fat emboli, which result from severe trauma and fractures of long bones, will stain positively with an oil red O stain or Sudan black stain. They can be fatal as they can damage the endothelial cells and pneumocytes within the lungs.

40. **Ans. (d) Pulmonary embolus** *(Ref: Robbins 8th/126, 9/e p127)*

40.1. **Ans. (c) Heart** *(Ref: Robbins 8/e p128, 9/e p129-130)*

Feature	Red infarcts	White infarcts
Cause	• **Arterial occlusion** in **loose tissues** or organs having dual **blood supply** • **Venous occlusion** (in ovarian torsion)	• Arterial occlusions in solid organs with end arterial circulation
Affected organs	Lung and small intestine	Solid organs (heart, spleen, kidney)
Properties	**Ill define hemorrhagic margins** which change in color to brown	Well defined margins and progressively paler with time
Edema	Usually present	Usually absent

40.2. Ans. (d) Coralline thrombus *(Ref: Robbins 8/e p124, 9/e p125)*

Thrombi often have grossly and microscopically apparent laminations called **lines of Zahn**; these represent pale platelet and fibrin deposits alternating with darker red cell–rich layers. Such laminations signify that a thrombus has formed in flowing blood; their presence can therefore distinguish antemortem thrombosis from the bland non laminated clots occurring in postmortem clots.

In veins thrombi form coral-like system with framework of platelets, fibrin and trapped white blood cells; this is a coralline thrombus

40.3. Ans. (a) Liver.....see explanation of earlier question.... *(Ref: Robbins 8/e p128, 7/e p138)*

41. Ans. (c) Decreased prothrombin time *(Ref: Robbins 8th/674, 9/e p134, 664-665)*
Laboratory investigations in DIC the following:
- Platelet count is decreased
- Prolonged aPTT/PT/TT
- Decreased fibrinogen
- Elevated fibrin split products (D-dimers)

42. Ans. (b) Endothelial injury *(Ref: Robbins 8th/page 130,131, 9/e p131-132)*
The principle mechanisms for septic shock include:
- Peripheral vasodilation and pooling of blood
- Endothelial activation/injury
- Leukocyte-induced damage
- Disseminated intravascular coagulation
- Activation of cytokine cascades

If the question talks about the initiating mechanism, it should be preferably answered as cytokin release. If this option is not given then endothelial injury is the next best answer.
1. Thrombosis
2. Increase in vascular permeability
3. Vasodilation

The other three options are following this primary event of endothelial injury due to cytokine release.

43. Ans. (d) Release of cytokines *(Ref: Robbins 8th/130,131, 9/e p132-133)*

44. Ans. (a) Pulmonary Embolism *(Ref: Robbins 8th/126, 9/e p127)*
D-dimer is a fibrin degradation product, a small protein fragment present in the blood after a blood clot is degraded by fibrinolysis. It is so named because it contains two crosslinked D fragments of the fibrinogen protein. D-dimer concentration may be determined by a blood test to help diagnose thrombosis. D-dimer testing is of clinical use when there is a suspicion of deep venous thrombosis (DVT) or pulmonary embolism (PE). In patients suspected of disseminated intravascular coagulation (DIC), D-dimers may aid in the diagnosis.

45. Ans. (d) Diffuse alveolar damage *(Ref: Harrison 17th/1680-1681; Robbin's 7th/715, 9/e p134)*
Shock lung is also known as acute respiratory distress syndrome, diffuse alveolar damage, acute alveolar injury and acute lung injury.

46. Ans. (a) ATN; (b) Pulmonary congestion; (c) Depletion of lipid in adrenal cortex and (d) Hepatic necrosis *(Ref: Robbins 7th/141, 142, 9/e p134)*
Shock is characterized by failure of multiple organ systems due to systemic hypoperfusion caused by reduction either in cardiac output or in effective circulating blood volume.

Liver → Fatty changes with hemorrhagic central necrosis.
Kidneys → Extensive tubular ischemic injury (Acute tubular necrosis).
Lungs → Pulmonary congestion with diffuse alveolar damage.
Adrenal → Cortical cell lipid depletion.
Brain → Ischemic encephalopathy.
Heart → Coagulation necrosis or contraction band necrosis.
GIT → Hemorrhagic enteropathy.

47. Ans. (a) Abruptio placentae; (b) Acute pro-myelocytic leukemia; (c) Severe falciparum malaria (d) 'Snake envenomation; (e) Heparin overdose. *(Ref: Robbins 7th/657, KDT 5th/562, 9/e p664-665)*

48. Ans. (b) Reduced plasma fibrinogen level *(Ref: Robbins 7th/656-658, 9/e p664-665)*

Hemodynamics

49. **Ans. (c) Respiratory distress** *(Ref: Robbins 8th/127)*

    Respiratory distress immediately follows amniotic fluid embolism as the emboli consisting of squamous cells, lanugo, and mucus deposit in the pulmonary microcirculation, producing numerous tiny pulmonary infarcts. The dramatic respiratory distress may also reflect the action of prostaglandins and other bioactive compounds present in high concentrations in the amniotic fluid embolus.

    - Placental abruption (option a) is not a result of an amniotic fluid embolism.
    - Renal failure (option b) is most likely caused in peri-partum interval by eclampsia, hypovolemic shock, and ascending infections. Amniotic fluid embolism may produce shock and renal failure as well.
    - Splinter hemorrhages (option d) are small hemorrhages seen on toes and fingers due to **micro emboli arising in the arterial circulation**. *Amniotic fluid emboli arise in the veins* and deposit in the lungs.

50. **Ans. (b) Renal failure** *(Ref: Robbins 8th/125, 673-4, 9/e p664-665)*

    In DIC, micro-emboli may obstruct blood vessels and cause tissue hypoxia and necrotic damage to organ structures, such as the kidneys, heart, lungs, and brain. As a result, common clinical signs may be due to renal, circulatory, or respiratory failure, acute bleeding ulcers or convulsions and coma. A form of hemolytic anemia may develop as red cells are damaged as they pass through vessels partially blocked by thrombus.

51. **Ans. (b) Fibrin degradation products** *(Ref: Robbins 8th/673-674 , 9/e p664-665)*

    DIC or consumptive coagulopathy represents pathological activation of the coagulation system by another underlying disease, with consequent consumption and depletion of the cellular and humoral components of the coagulation cascade. The fibrinolytic mechanisms are also activated, and an uncontrolled cycle of bleeding and clotting develops. As a consequence, levels of all clotting proteins (options A and C) become depleted, platelet counts drop, and the fibrinolytic proteins are depleted as well (option D).

Fibrin degradation products (option B), which are normally low in the serum, rise markedly in this disease.

52. **Ans. (b) Platelet count, fibrinogen levels, and fibrin degradation products** *(Ref: Robbins 8th/673-674 , 9/e p664-665)*

    Disseminated intravascular coagulation (DIC) is characterized by consumption of both platelets and clotting factors.
    The best tests to order are platelet count (which will be markedly decreased), serum fibrinogen level (which will be low), and fibrin degradation products (which will be high).
    Prothrombin time (PT) and Partial thromboplastin time (PTT) are relatively non-specific. Thrombin time (TT) is a more specific measure of fibrinogen and would potentially be a useful test in this setting. However, specific measurement of factor VIII, kininogen, or prekallikrein levels would not be rational in evaluating DIC.

    ## GOLDEN POINTS FOR QUICK REVISION
    ### (HEMODYNAMICS)

    - Vitamin K dependent clotting factors are *factors 2,7,9,10* as well as anti clotting factors like *protein C* and *protein S*.
    - Thrombin is a procoagulant but *thrombin-thrombomodulin complex is an anticoagulant*.
    - **SLE** is most commonly associated with secondary anti phospholipid antibody syndrome and formation of **anti beta 2 glycoprotein antibody**.
    - **Leiden mutation** is the most common *inheritable cause* of hypercoagulability.
    - **White infarct** occurs with arterial occlusions in solid organs with end-arterial circulation (e.g., heart, spleen, and kidney).
    - **Red infarcts** occur in venous occlusions (e.g., testis), in loose tissues (e.g., lung), in organs with dual circulations (e.g., lung and small intestine).
    - **Lines of Zahn** are seen in antemortem clots.
    - **"Chicken fat"** appearance is seen in *post mortem* clots.

    ## UPDATED INFORMATION FROM 9TH EDITION OF ROBBINS

    - ADP is a component of dense body granules; thus, platelet activation and ADP release begets additional rounds of platelet activation, a phenomenon referred to as *recruitment*.

    - *Disseminated intravascular coagulation, hypotensive shock,* and metabolic disturbances (including insulin resistance and hyperglycemia) are referred to as the *clinical triad of septic shock.*

NOTES

4

Genetics

Genetics is the study of the genes. Genes are a part of chromosome and they code for a trait or character. The position of gene on a chromosome is called as a **locus**. Out of a total number of 46 chromosome, 22 pairs of chromosomes are homologous and are called *autosomes*. The 23rd pair is alike only in the females (have 2 similar X chromosomes) whereas in a male there is one X chromosome and one Y chromosome. The X and Y are therefore referred to as *sex chromosomes*.

The genetic makeup of an individual is called genotype whereas the manifested physical feature is called as phenotype.

The Gene are made up of nucleic acids like ribonucleic acid; RNA or deoxyribonucleic acid; DNA. RNA is present only in the nucleus whereas DNA is present in both the nucleus and mitochondria of a cell. These nucleic acids are made up of nucleotides whose composition includes nitrogenous base, a sugar (deoxyribose in DNA and ribose in RNA) and a phosphate group. The nitrogenous base can be either a purine (adenine, guanine) or pyrimidine (thymine, cytosine, uracil). The purines bind with the pyrimidines complementarily.

Alternate form of gene coding for different forms of a character is called allele. A normal gene has 2 alleles. When these code for same trait, it is known as homozygous state whereas if the alleles code for different traits, it is called heterozygous state.

If an allele manifests itself in a heterozygous state, it is called as dominant. The alternate allele which is unable to manifest itself in the heterozygous state is called as a recessive allele.

> The amount of the purine is equal with the corresponding pyrimidine which is called **Chargaff's rule.**

> The part of the DNA which is **ex**pressed is called **ex**on and the **int**ervening region is called **int**ron.

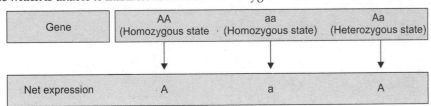

(So, 'A' is Dominant and 'a' is Recessive)

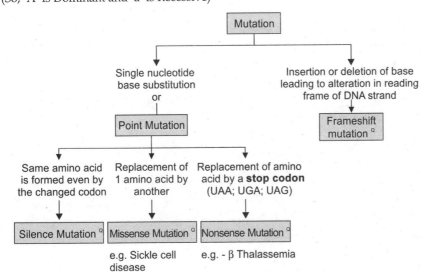

> **Mutation** is a *permanent* change in the DNA. The types of the mutations are given alongside.

> **Blood group** and histocompatibity antigens **(HLA)** are examples of *co-dominant* antigens.

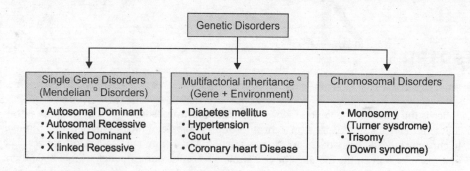

> In AD inheritance, heterozgotes with dominant mutant gene express disease.

> Homozygous individual for the dominant mutant gene usually die prenatally.

SINGLE GENE DISORDERS WITH MENDELIAN/CLASSICAL INHERITANCE

a. **Autosomal Dominant (AD) Inheritance Diseases**
   - Mutated genes can express themselves in *heterozygous state*.
   - Usually cause defect in the synthesis of *structural*[Q] or **non-enzyme** proteins.
   - These have *variable onset* (so, onset may be into adulthood).
   - These are characterized by **reduced penetrance**[Q] (individuals inherit the gene but can be phenotypically normal) and **variable expressibility**[Q] (the trait is seen in the individuals carrying the mutant gene but is expressed differently among individuals, e.g. patients of neurofibromatosis have variant from brownish skin spots to multiple skin tumors in different patients).

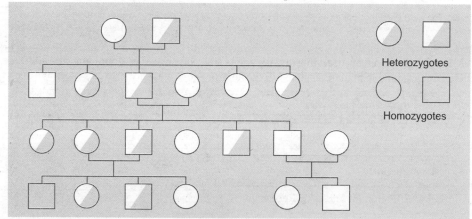

Heterozygotes

Homozygotes

Examples of autosomal dominant disorders
(Mnemonic: Vo Familial Hypercholesterolemia Autosomal DOMINANT Hai)

Vo	**V**on Willebrand Disease[Q]
Familial	**F**amilial Adenomatous Polyposis[Q]
Hypercholesterolemia	Hypercholesterolemia (Familial)
Autosomal	**A**dult polycystic kidney[Q]
D	**D**ystrophia myotonica[Q]
O	**O**steogenesis imperfecta[Q]
M	**M**arfan syndrome[Q]
I	Intermittent porphyria[Q]
N	**N**eurofibromatosis-1[Q]
A	**A**chondroplasia[Q]
N	**N**eurofibromatosis – 2[Q]
T	**T**uberous sclerosis[Q]
Hai	**H**untington's disease[Q]; *H*ereditary spherocytosis[Q]

There are the following types of autosomal dominant gene mutations:

Autosomal dominant disease mutations

Gain of Function	Loss of Function
Protein product of the mutant allele has properties not normally associated with the natural/wild-type protein	Leads to the reduced production of a gene product or give rise to an inactive protein
Less common	More common
Affects normal proteins with toxic properties	Affects regulatory proteins & subunits of multimeric proteins
e.g. *Huntington's disease*	e.g. *Osteogenesis imperfecta*

Concept

Dominant negative mutant allele is associated with the more common **"loss of function"** mutation. This type of mutation leads to not only reduced production of a gene product but the inactive polypeptide interferes with the functioning of a normall allele in a heterozygote. This usually affects structural proteins. At times, the inactive protein is a part of multiunit protein complex and it interferes with the normal functioning of other units of the same complex.

Example: **Osteogenesis imperfecta**

The collagen molecule is made up of triple helical molecule made up of three collagen chains arranged in a helical configuration. Each collagen chains in the helix must be normal for the normal assembly and stability of the collagen molecule. If there is a single mutant collagen chain, normal collagen trimers cannot be formed, and hence there is a marked deficiency of collagen.

SOME IMPORTANT AUTOSOMAL DOMINANT DISEASES

Marfan Syndrome

It is an autosomal dominant disease having mutation in the *fibrillin gene*[Q] on the chromosome 15q21. Fibrillin behaves as a scaffolding protein for the alignment of elastic fibers. So, any defect affects the following systems:

Skeletal Defects	CVS changes	Ocular changes
• Tall and thin built[Q] • Long and slender fingers and hands **(Archnodactyly)**[Q] • **Hyperextensible joints** (especially thumb[Q]) • Inward depressed sternum **(Pigeon breast deformity**[Q]**)**	• Mitral valve prolapse causing **mitral regurgitaiton**[Q] • **Medial** degeneration causing dissecting aortic aneurysm and **aortic regurgltation**[Q].	• Bilateral dislocation or subluxation of the lens (know as **Ectopia lentis**[Q])

Neurofibromatosis

Neurofibromatosis

NF-1 (von Recklinghausen Disease[Q])	NF-2 (Bilateral Acoustic Neurofibromatosis[Q])
• More common, seen in 90% patients[Q] • Presence of neural tumors of neurofibromas in the body which can be cutaneous, subcutaneous or plexiform • 6 or more pigmented skin lesions called 'cafe au lait' spots • Pigmented iris hamartoma called **Lisch Nodules**[Q]. • Associated skeletal muscle defects like scoliosis, bone cysts or tibial pseudoarthrosis • Risk of development of meningioma, pheochromocytomas and Wilm's tumor[Q].	• Less common, seen in 10% patients • **Bilateral acoustic neuromas**[Q] • **Multiple meningioma**[Q] • Cafe au lait spot are present but **Lisch nodules are absent**[Q].

Dominant negative mutant allele is associated with the more common **"loss of function"** mutation. Its clinical examples includes *Osteogenesis imperfecta, Ehler Danlos syndrome* and *Marfan's syndrome*.

Concept

In **Huntington's disease**, the protein formed *huntingtin* is different from normal protein by the fact that it is toxic to the neurons. So, **"gain of function"** mutation increases the amount of the toxic protein and hence, neurological features in the affected patients

Features of Marfan Syndrome
M - Mitral Valve Prolapse
A - Aortic Aneurysm
R - Retinal Detachment
F - Freely movable joints (hyperextensible joints), Fibrillin protein defect.
A - Arachnodactyly
N - Nine feet height (very tall person)
Disease - Dislocation of lens (Ectopia lentis)

Cause of death in **Marfan syndrome** is **Aortic dissection**. So, hypertension should be treated at the earliest in these patients.

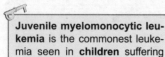

Juvenile myelomonocytic leukemia is the commonest leukemia seen in **children** suffering from **neurofibromatosis-1**

Note:
- *NF1 gene* is present on *chromosome 17*[Q] and its product called **neurofibromin** is a tumor suppressor gene which normally causes decreased activity of p21 ras oncoprotein.
- *NF2 gene* is present on *chromosome 22*[Q] and it normally produces **merlin** which is a protein causing contact inhibition of proliferation of Schwann cells.
- So, any mutation in NF1 or NF2 causes increased chances of tumor formation.

Ehler Danlos Syndrome (EDS)

It is an inherited tissue disease due to defect in collagen structure or synthesis. The clinical features include presence of hyperextensible skin (*cigarette paper skin*[Q]) which can be easily injured as it is fragile. There is also presence of *hyperextensible joints*. There are different variants of EDS having different modes of inheritance.

EDS type 3 (Hypermobility type)	AD inheritance; presence of joint hypermobility; pain and dislocation
EDS type 4 (Vascular type)	AD inheritance; defect in collagen type III; presence of thin skin; easy bruising; arterial and uterine rupture, small joint hyperextensibility
EDS type 6 (Kyphoscoliosis type)	AR inheritance, mutation in the enzyme lysyl hydroxylase resulting in formation of unstable collagen; there is presence of hypotonia, joint laxity, congenital scoliosis and ocular fragility.

m

Mnemonics: Count the number of letters in 'neurofibromatosis'. It is 17, so, NF1 is due to mutation in gene on chromosome 17. NF2 gene can be remembered as two letters (N and F) followed by 2 (of NF2) i.e. chromosome 22.

b. **Autosomal Recessive (AR) Inheritance Diseases**
   – Mutant genes express themselves *only in Homozygous state.*[Q]
   – Usually cause defect in the synthesis of an *enzyme protein*.[Q]
   – These have an *early* uniform *onset*[Q] (usually in childhood).
   – There is *complete penetrance*[Q] (persons having defective gene in homozygous state will have disease as well).
   – "*Inborn errors of metabolism*"are usually inherited as autosomal recessive disorders.[Q]
   – *If one parent is carrier and the other one is normal,* autosomal recessive disorders usually donot manifest but if an *affected baby* is born to such a couple, **Uniparental disomy (UPD)** should be suspected. UPD occurs when a person receives two copies of a chromosome, or part of a chromosome, from one parent and no copies from the other parent.

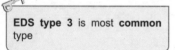

EDS type 3 is most **common** type

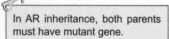

EDS type 4 is most **dangerous** type

Autosomal Recessive is the *most common* **Mendelian** mode of inheritance.

In AR inheritance, both parents must have mutant gene.

Pedigree in Autosomal Recessive Disorders

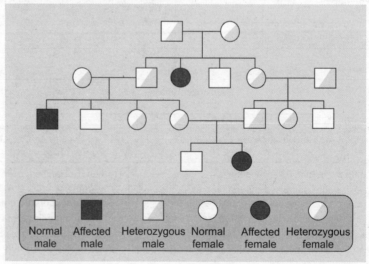

Examples of Autosomal Recessive Diseases
(Mnemonic: Fried Poori aur Garam **CHAWAL MAST** Hai**)**

Fried	Friedrich's ataxia[Q]
Poori aur	Phenylketonuria[Q]
Garam	Galactosemia[Q]
C	Cystic fibrosis[Q]
H	Hemochromatosis[Q]
A	α_1 – Antitrypsin deficiency[Q]
W	Wilson's disease[Q]
A	Alkaptonuria[Q]
L	Lysosomal and glycogen storage diseases[Q]
M	Muscular atrophy (both spinal as well as neurogenic)
A	Adrenal hyperplasia[Q] (congenital)
S	Sickle cell disease[Q]
T	Thalassemia[Q]
Hai	Homocystinuria[Q]

Uniparental disomy UPD should be suspected in an individual manifesting a recessive disorder, where only one parent is a carrier.

Some Important Autosomal Recessive Diseases

1. **Phenylketonuria (PKU):** It is caused by the deficiency of *enzyme phenylanine hydroxylase* resulting in inability to convert phenylalanine to tyrosine and resultant hyperphenylalaninemia. The clinical presentation is a child normal at birth but developing profound mental retardation by 6 months of age. The absence of tyrosine results in light-colored skin and hair. There is also presence of a *mousy or musty odor* to the sweat and urine *due to* secondary accumulation of a metabolite called *phenylacetate*.

   The management is done by the dietary restriction of phenylalanine.

2. **Alkaptonuria (Ochronosis):** It is caused by the *deficiency of homogentistic acid oxidase* resulting in the accumulation of homogentistic acid. The latter has an affinity for connective tissues (especially cartilage), resulting in a black discoloration **(ochronosis)**. The clinical features include the passage of normal coloured urine (which turn black on exposure to air), black cartilage, discoloration of the nose and ears and early onset of degenerative arthritis.

3. **Glycogen Storage Diseases:** These are a group of rare diseases that have in common a deficiency in an enzyme necessary for the metabolism of glycogen, which results in the accumulation of glycogen in the liver, heart, and skeletal muscle. Some salient types include:

Most AR disorders involve enzyme deficiencies.

Type	Name of disorder	Enzyme deficiency
Type I	**V**on Gierke's disease	Glucose-6-phosphatase
Type II	**P**ompe's disease	Acid maltase
Type III	**C**ori's disease	Debranching enzyme
Type IV	**A**nderson's disease	Branching enzyme
Type V	**M**cArdle's disease	Muscle phosphorylase
Type VI	**H**er's disease	Hepatic phosphorylase
Type VII	**T**arui's disease	Phosphofructokinase 1(PFK-1)

Tyrosine becomes an *essential* amino acid in *Phenylketonuria*

4. **Lysosomal Storage Diseases**

Disease	Enzyme Deficiency	Accumulating Substance
Tay-Sachs disease	Hexosaminidase A	GM2 ganglioside
Niemann-Pick disease	Sphingomyelinase	Sphingomyelin
Gaucher disease	Glucocerebrosidase	Glucocerebroside
Fabry disease	α-Galactosidase A	Ceramide trihexoside

Vitamin C/ascorbic acid provide partial relief in alkaptonuria

Metachromatic leukodystrophy	Aryl sulfatase A	Sulfatide
Hurler syndrome	α-1-Iduronidase	Dermatan sulfate Heparan sulfate
Hunter syndrome	L-Iduronosulfate sulfatase	Dermatan sulfate Heparan sulfate

Vo Physics Chemistry Aur Maths mein Hoshiyaar Tha is for different types of glycogen storage diseases in the exact order;
For the enzymes see the first letter and remember the alphabets A→B (Anderson with Branching) and C→D (Cori with Debranching)

Mnemonic

[Tarun Has Nine Shirts; Most Are Saffron, Few Are Green]

Disease		Deficiency	
Tarun – Tay Sachs	**Has**	–	**H**exosaminidase
Nine – Neimann Pick	**Shirts**	–	**S**phingomyelinase
Most – Metachromatic leukodystrophy	**Are Saffron**	–	**A**ryl **S**ulfatase
Few – Fabry	**Are Green**	–	**A**lpha **G**alactosidase

Tarun Has Nine Shirts; Most Are Saffron, Few Are Green

T Tay Sachs Disease
A Autosomal recessive
Y Young Deaths (< 4 years)
S Spot in the macula (Cherry red spot)
A Ashkenazi Jews (more commonly affected)
C Cytoplasmic vacuoles in dilated neurons in CNS
H Hexosaminidase A deficiency
S Storage disease (Lysosomal)

a. **Tay-Sachs Disease:** It is caused by the deficiency of the enzyme *hexosaminidase A* leading to *accumulation of GM2 ganglioside* in the lysosomes of the CNS and retina. It is common in *Ashkenazi Jews. Cherry red spot* is seen in the retina whereas dilated neurons with cytoplasmic vacuoles are seen in the CNS. The clinical presentation includes normal child at birth with onset of symptoms by 6 months. It is associated with progressive mental deterioration and motor incoordination and death by the age of 2-3 years. Electron microscopy shows the presence of distended lysosomes with whorled membranes.

b. **Niemann-Pick Disease:** It is caused by the deficiency of the enzyme *sphingomyelinase* leading to the accumulation of sphingomyelin within the lysosomes of the CNS and reticuloendothelial system. It is also commoner in Ashkenazi Jews. There is presence of a retinal *cherry-red spot* and CNS having distended neurons with a foamy cytoplasmic vacuolization. The clinical presentation includes normal child at birth with onset of symptoms by 6 months. It is associated with progressive *massive splenomegaly, lymphadenopathy, mental deterioration and motor manifestations* resulting in death by the age of 2 years.

c. **Gaucher Disease:** It is the **most common lysosomal storage disorder** caused by the *deficiency of glucocerebrosidase* leading to the accumulation of glucocerebroside predominantly in the lysosomes of the reticuloendothelial system. It is characterized by the presence of *hepatosplenomegaly, hypersplenism* leading to thrombocytopenia/pancytopenia, *lymphadenopathy and bone marrow involvement* leading to bone pain, deformities, and fractures. A subgroup of patients may also have CNS manifestations.

d. **Mucopolysaccharidosis (MPS):** These are a group of lysosomal storage disorders characterized by deficiencies of the lysosomal enzymes required for the degradation of mucopolysaccharides (glycosaminoglycans). The clinical features of the patients include *mental retardation, cloudy cornea, hepatosplenomegaly, skeletal deformities and coarse facial features, joint abnormalities and cardiac lesions.*

(**Mnemonic:** Remember the hunter has an ax**e/X**.)

Most of the metabolic disorders have autosomal recessive inheritance *except:*	
Her	– Hunter syndrome (X-linked recessive)
Left	– Lesch Nyhan syndrome (X-linked recessive)
Eye	– Ocular albinism (X-linked recessive)
Has	– Hypercholesterolemia (familial) (Autosomal Dominant)
Five	– Fabry's disease (X-linked recessive)
Pimples	– Porphyria [Acute intermittent] (Autosomal Dominant)

Electron microscopy in **Niemann-Pick's disease** shows the presence of distended lysosomes containing lamellated figures (**"zebra bodies"**).

X-LINKED RECESSIVE DISORDER

Males have an X and a Y chromosome. There is no corresponding locus for a mutant allele of the X chromosome on the Y chromosome. The mutant recessive gene on the X chromosome expresses itself in a male child because it is not suppressed by a normal allele whereas in the

Microscopically cells show the presence of **Gaucher's cells** which are enlarged macrophages with a fibrillary (**crumpled tissue-paper-like) cytoplasm.**

Genetics

female, the presence of a normal allele on other X-chromosome prevents the expression of the disease So, *females only act as carriers.*[Q]

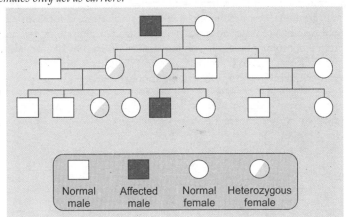

Normal male	Affected male
Normal female	Heterozygous female

Examples of X-linked recessive disorders

Less	Lesch Nyhan syndrome[Q]
H	**H**emophilia A and B[Q]; **H**unter syndrome[Q]
C	**C**hronic granulomatous disease[Q]
G is	**G**6PD deficiency[Q]
Detected	**D**uchhene muscular dystrophy[Q], **D**iabetes insipidus[Q]
Clinically in	**C**olor blindness[Q]
A	**A**gammaglobulinemia[Q] (*Bruton's disease*)
Fragile	**F**ragile X syndrome[Q], **F**abry Disease[Q]
Woman	**W**iskott Aldrich syndrome[Q]

X-LINKED DOMINANT DISORDERS

These are the conditions in which both heterozygous males and females are affected. All the sons of the affected male are normal and all the daughters are affected. The affected female transmits the disease to half of the sons and daughters.

Examples: *Hypophosphatemic type of vitamin D resistant rickets; Incontinentia pigmenti, Alport Syndrome and oro-facio-digital syndrome.*

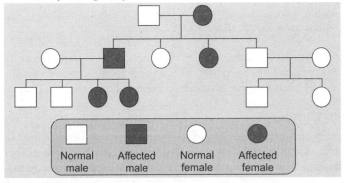

Normal male	Affected male
Normal female	Affected female

SINGLE GENE DISORDERS WITH NON-MENDELIAN INHERITANCE

Non-Mendelian Inheritance can be classified into the following categories:
- Mitochondrial inheritance
- Genomic Imprinting
- Triple Repeat Mutations
- Germline Mosaicism

MITOCHONDRIAL INHERITANCE

Mutation in the mitochondrial DNA has the characteristic feature of **maternal inheritance**[Q] because the ovum contains the mitochondria with their abundant cytoplasm whereas sperms contains minimal number of mitochondria. The fertilized oocyte degrades mtDNA carried from the sperm in a complex process involving the ubiquitin proteasome system. So, while mothers transmit their mtDNA to both their sons and daughters, only the daughters are able to transmit the inherited mtDNA to future generations.

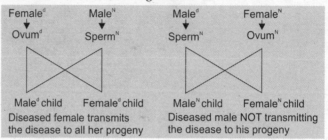

- d denotes diseased whereas N denotes normal individuals.

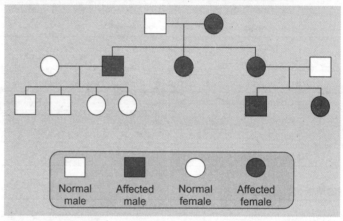

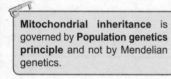

All offspring of an affected female will be having the disease and all daughters transmits the disease further to their progeny.

Affected sons **do not** transmit the disease to progeny

Mitochondrial inheritance is governed by **Population genetics principle** and not by Mendelian genetics.

Salient features of these diseases

- The **organs most commonly affected** in these diseases are the ones having large number of mitochondria inside them. Such organs include **CNS, skeletal muscle, cardiac muscle, liver and kidneys**.
- Tissues may have both normal/wild and mutant mitochondrial DNA.
- *Sons do not transmit the disease to progeny*[Q]
- *Examples* of mitochondrial inheritance *are Leber's optic neuropathy, Leigh's disease, MELAS (mitochondrial encephalopathy, lactic acidosis and stroke like syndrome) NARP syndrome (Neuropathy, ataxia, and retinitis pigmentosa.), Kearns-Sayre syndrome, Chronic progressive external ophthalmoplegia and Pearson syndrome.*

GENOMIC IMPRINTING

A person gets two alleles for a character; one from mother and second from father. Normally these two alleles are similar. But, in some cases these alleles are differentially expressed. i.e. either maternal gene become silent (only paternal gene express) or paternal gene become silent (only maternal express). In such a condition, if the chromosome containing the gene which is expressed undergoes deletion, there will be disease, whereas if homologous undergoes deletion, nothing will happen.

Imprinting selectively inactivates either the maternal or paternal allele. Thus maternal imprinting refers to transcriptional silencing of the maternal allele whereas paternal imprinting implies that the paternal allele is inactivated.

Example of genomic imprinting disorder is microdeletion of chromosome 15q11-13. If microdeletion occurs in maternal chromosome; Angelman syndrome results whereas paternal chromosomal microdeletion may cause Prader-Willi syndrome.

It is also seen in *Beckwith Wiedmann syndrome* and *Albright's hereditary osteodystrophy*.

The presence of mixutre of more than one type of an organellar genome within a tissue is called as **heteroplasmy**.

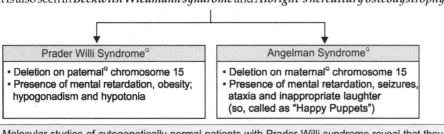

Prader Willi Syndrome[Q]	Angelman Syndrome[Q]
• Deletion on paternal[Q] chromosome 15 • Presence of mental retardation, obesity; hypogonadism and hypotonia	• Deletion on maternal[Q] chromosome 15 • Presence of mental retardation, seizures, ataxia and inappropriate laughter (so, called as "Happy Puppets")

- Molecular studies of cytogenetically normal patients with Prader Willi syndrome reveal that they have two maternal copies of chromosome 15.
- Inheritance of both chromosomes of a pair from one parent is called uniparental disomy. So, Prader Willi Syndrome may be due to UPD of maternal chromosome 15.
- Similarly Angelman syndrome patients might have uniparental disomy of paternal chromosome 15.

Genomic imprinting is defined as differential expression of a gene based on chromosomal inheritance from maternal or paternal origin

TRIPLE REPEAT MUTATIONS

The mutation in this disease group is characterized by a long repeating sequence of three nucleotides. It is characteristically different from other types of mutations because it is **dynamic** in nature. Dynamicity means that the **degree of amplification** of a sequence of three nucleotides **increases during gametogenesis**.

Chromosome 15 has its own **MAP**, so diseases associated with this chromosome are **M**arfan syndrome, **A**ngelman syndrome and **P**rader-Willi syndrome.

Trinucleotide repeat disorders

Expansions in non-coding regions	Expansions in coding regions
"Loss of function" type mutation	*"Gain of function"* type mutation
Mutant proteins aggregate as intranuclear inclusions	Mutant proteins interfere with other proteins
Examples: • Fragile X syndrome[Q] • Friedrich's ataxia[Q] • Myotonic dystrophy[Q]	*Examples:* • Huntington's disease[Q] • Spinobulbar muscular atrophy[Q] (Kennedy's disease) • Spinocerebellar ataxia types 1, 2, 3, 6, 7[Q]

The *trinucleotide repeat expansions* in the *non-coding regions* involve different repeats as *Fragile X syndrome (CGG[Q])*, *Friedrich's ataxia (GAA[Q])* and *Myotonic dystrophy (CTG[Q])*.

P for **p**aternal and **P**rader Willi whereas **m** for **m**aternal and **m** is present in Angel**m**an

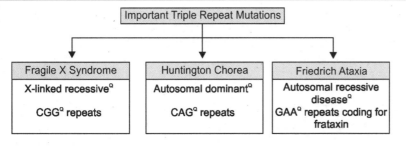

Fragile X Syndrome	Huntington Chorea	Friedrich Ataxia
X-linked recessive[Q]	Autosomal dominant[Q]	Autosomal recessive disease[Q]
CGG[Q] repeats	CAG[Q] repeats	GAA[Q] repeats coding for frataxin

Mom wears **SARI** – it stands for **S**eizures, **A**taxia, **R**etardation and **I**nappropriate laughter

Fragile X Syndrome

There is presence of triplet repeat mutations of **CGG** nucleotides. The mutation affects the *FMR-1 gene* (Familial Mental Retardation – 1 gene) present on the X chromosome. On karyotyping, the chromosome appears as broken (so, called fragile site). It is the *second most common* cause of mental retardation (*Down syndrome is the commonest cause*). The clinical features of patient include *long face with a large mandible, large everted ears and large testicles (macro-orchidism)*.[Q]

In the normal people, the number of CGG repeats is from 10 to 55. There is amplification of CGG repeat in carrier females to 55-200 CGG repeats which is called *premutation*. In diseased

The trinucleotide repeat expansions in the **coding regions** have all the presence of **CAG** repeat sequences.

individuals, the CGG repeats range from 200-4000 repeats called *full mutations*. During the process of oogenesis (*Not spermatogenesis*), amplification causes conversion of premutations to full mutations. This is responsible for **Sherman's Paradox**[Q] (the risk of mental retardation is much higher in grandsons than the brothers of transmitting males as the grandsons acquire a premutation from their grandfather which gets amplified to a mutation in their mother ova).

- Southern blot is useful for genetic counseling (it can differentiate between premutation and mutation prenatally and postnatally).

Huntington's Chorea

There is presence of **CAG** repeats associated with chromosome 4 that are responsible for the production of an abnormal neurotoxic protein called **Huntington**[Q]. It is associated with *caudate nucleus atrophy*. Clinical features include early onset of *progressive dementia* and presence of *choreiform movements* (due to inhibition of GABAergic neurons).

In Anticipation, additional trinucleotide repeats cause worsening of clinical features with each successive generation.

CONCEPT OF PLEIOTROPY

It describes the **genetic effect of a single gene on multiple phenotypic traits**. The underlying mechanism is that the gene codes for a product that is used by various cells, or has a signaling function on various targets. A classic example of pleiotropy is the human disease **phenylketonuria**.
Antagonistic pleiotropy refers to the expression of a gene resulting in multiple competing effects, some beneficial but others detrimental to the organism. An example is the p53 gene, which suppresses cancer, but also suppresses stem cells, which replenish worn-out tissue.

GONADAL/GERMLINE MOSAICISM

PCR is the method of choice for diagnosis of fragile X syndrome

Normally autosomal dominant disorders have affected parents but in some patients with autosomal dominant disorders, the parents are not affected. In such patients, the disorder results from a new mutation in the egg or the sperm from which they were derived; as such, their siblings are neither affected nor at increased risk of developing the disease.

However, in certain autosomal dominant disorders, exemplified by osteogenesis imperfecta[Q] and tuberous sclerosis[Q], phenotypically normal parents have more than one affected child. This may appear to clearly violate the laws of Mendelian inheritance but is explained by gonadal mosaicism.

A Hunter puts an animal in a **CAG** that has **FOUR** sides, four for association with **chromosome 4.**

Gonadal mosaicism results from a mutation that occurs postzygotically during early (embryonic) development. If the mutation affects only cells destined to form the gonads, the gametes carry the mutation, but the somatic cells of the individual are completely normal. Such an individual is said to exhibit *germ line* or *gonadal mosaicism*. A phenotypically normal parent who has germ line mosaicism can transmit the disease-causing mutation to the offspring through the mutant gamete. Since the progenitor cells of the gametes carry the mutation, there is a definite possibility that more than one child of such a parent would be affected. **Gonadal mosaicism should not be confused with mosaicism (explained below).**

MOSAICISM

Note: Presence of two or more populations of cell in the same individual is called mosaicism. This can be seen physiologically also as in case of normal females.

After fertilization of ovum

During mitotic division

One cell gets 1 extra chromosome / Other cell gets 1 less chromosome

(47,XXX) / (45, X)

Both the types of cells present in the same individual so, this is MOSAICISM

Gonadal/Germline Mosaicism is seen in *osteogenesis imperfecta and tuberous sclerosis.*

CHROMOSOMAL DISORDERS

Study of chromosomes is called **karyotyping.** It is done in cells like skin fibroblasts, peripheral blood lymphocytes and amniotic cells. The normal number of chromosomes in a somatic cell is diploid and is expressed as 46, XX or 46, XY.

A **karyotype** is a standard arrangement of a photographed or image stained chromosome pairs in **metaphase** stage in *order of decreasing length*.

- Mitosis is arrested in dividing cells in **metaphase stage** by use of colchicine. In this stage, individual chromosomes take the form of two chromatids connected at the centromere. The Short arm of chromosome is called "p" (petite) and long arm is reffered to as "q".

Banding technique and selected features				
	Q banding	**G banding**	**R (Reverse) banding**	**C banding**
Dye used	Quinacrine mustard	Trypsin followed by Giemsa	Alkaline solution followed by Giemsa	Chemical followed by Giemsa
Microscope used	Fluorescence microscopy	Light microscopy	Light microscopy	Light microscopy
Special features	*Temporary So, not used[Q] for routine cytogenetic analysis	*Permanent *MC technique[Q] for routine cytogenetic analysis	*Used for analyzing rearrangements involving the terminal ends[Q] of chromosomes *Gives pattern opposite to G banding	*Used for studying chromosomal translocations involving centromeric regions[Q]
Appearance of chromosomes	Bright fluorescent bands upon exposure to ultraviolet light; same as darkly stained G bands.	Darkly Stained G bands.	Darkly stained R bands correspond to light bands in G-banded chromosomes. Pattern is the reverse of G-banding.	Darkly stained C band centromeric region of the chromosome corresponds to region of constitutive heterochromatin.

Note: Q, G and R banding produce bands along entire length of chromosomes whereas for specific chromosomal structures, other types of banding may be used. Some of these include **T- banding** (for **T**elomeres), **C banding** (for **C**onstitutive heterochromatin) and **NOR-banding** (for **n**ucleolus-**o**rganizing **r**egions).

Sometimes, fluorodeoxyuridine (FUdR)[Q] banding is also done. It is a direct inhibitor of thymidylate synthetase and it can induce folate-sensitive fragile sites in chromosomes. Chromosomal fragile sites can induce mental retardation as is seen in fragile X syndrome[Q].

TYPES OF CHROMOSOMES

Metacentric	Centromere is in the center of the chromosome (the chromosome has two equal arms).
Submetacentric	Centromere is away from the center so that the arms are unequal in size (one arm shorter than the other). X chromosome is large submetacentric[Q] chromosome.
Acrocentric	Centromere is almost at the tip (one end) of the chromosome (one arm is much longer than the other). Y chromosome is small acrocentric[Q] chromosome
Telocentric	Centromere is at the extreme end of the replicating chromosome (chromosome has only one arm). Not seen in humans[Q].

CYTOGENETIC ABNORMALITIES

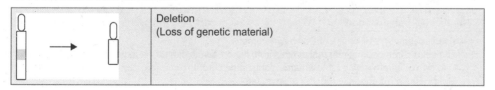

	Deletion (Loss of genetic material)

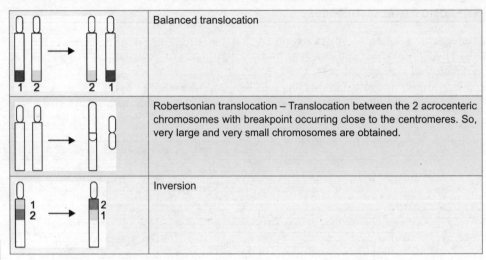

	Balanced translocation
	Robertsonian translocation – Translocation between the 2 acrocenteric chromosomes with breakpoint occurring close to the centromeres. So, very large and very small chromosomes are obtained.
	Inversion

> **Insertion, Deletion and Robertsonian translocation are associated with change in genetic material**

- The gametes contain half the number of chromosomes (haploid) and are represented as (23, X) or (23, Y).
- An exact multiple of haploid chromosomes is called **Euploidy** (2n, 3n, 4n … etc).
- When exact multiple of haploid chromosomes is not present, it is called **Aneuploidy**.

Genome mutations involve loss or gain of whole chromosomes, giving rise to monosomy or trisomy.

> **Unlike the above mentioned, inversion is NOT associated with change in genetic materials**

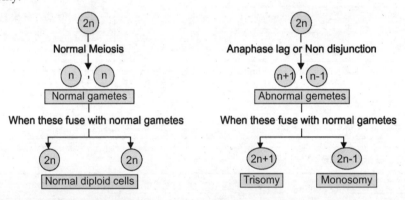

DOWN SYNDROME (TRISOMY 21)[Q]

- It is the most common of the chromosomal disorders[Q] and a major cause of mental retardation.[Q]

> **Note:** *Mitotic non-disjunction is responsible for development of mosaicism.*

- Genetics of Down syndrome.

> **Both monosomy and trisomy are types of genome mutations having aneuploidy.**

Meiotic nondisjunction of chromosome 21 occuring in the ovum
<ul><li>Seen in **95% cases** with trisomy 21. So, it is the **commonest cause** of Down syndrome</li><li>The extra chromosome is of **maternal origin**.</li><li>**Strong relation with maternal age**</li></ul>
Robertsonian translocation
<ul><li>Seen in about **4% of cases** of Down syndrome.</li><li>The extra chromosomal material derives from the presence of a robertsonian translocation of the long arm of chromosome 21 to another acrocentric chromosome (e.g., 22 or 14).</li><li>Most cases are frequently (but not always) familial.</li><li>**No relation with maternal age**</li></ul>

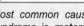

Mosaicism
• Seen in ~1% of Down syndrome patients
• Results from **mitotic nondisjunction of chromosome 21** during an early stage of embryogenesis.
• Patients have a mixture of cells with 46 and 47 chromosomes (mosaicism).
• **No relation with maternal age**.

*Most common cause of Down syndrome is **maternal meiotic non-disjunction**.*

- **Important signs of the disease include:**
  - Flat facial profile
  - Mental retardation
  - Microgenia (abnormally small chin)
  - Oblique palpebral fissures with epicanthic skin folds (**mongoloid slant)**
  - Muscle **hypotonia** (poor muscle tone)
  - Flat nasal bridge
  - Single palmar fold (**Simian crease**)
  - Curvature of little finger towards other four fingers (**Clinodactyly**)
  - Protruding tongue or macroglossia
  - White spots on the iris known as **Brushfield spots**
  - Excessive joint laxity including atlanto-axial instability
  - Excessive space between large toe and second toe (**Sandle toe**)
  - A single flexion furrow of the fifth finger
  - Higher number of ulnar loop dermatoglyphs

Advance maternal age has a strong influence on the incidence of trisomy 21 whereas it is not related to advanced paternal age.

Complications of Down syndrome are:
- Congenital cardiac defects (Most common is VSD)
- Increased risk of leukemia particularly **ALL (more commonly)** and specifically the **megakaryoblastic form** of AML (M7-AML)
- Hypothyroidism
- Reduced fertility in females (Males are totally infertile)
- Increased risk of respiratory tract infections

Down syndrome associated with **Robertsonian translocation** and **Mosaicism** has *no relation with maternal age.*

Screening for Down Syndrome

Many standard prenatal screens can discover Down syndrome. Amniocentesis and CVS are considered invasive procedures, in that they involve inserting instruments into the uterus, and therefore carry a small risk of causing fetal injury or miscarriage. The risks of miscarriage for CVS and amniocentesis are often quoted as 1% and 0.5% respectively. There are several common non-invasive screens that can indicate a fetus with Down syndrome. These are normally performed in the late first trimester or early second trimester. Due to the nature of screens, each has a significant chance of a false positive, suggesting a fetus with Down syndrome when, in fact, the fetus does not have this genetic abnormality. Screen positives must be verified before a Down syndrome diagnosis is made. Common screening procedures for Down syndrome are given in the Table below.

Down syndrome patients are having predisposition for **Hirschprung's disease, duodenal atresia, annular pancreas** and **Alzheimer's disease**

First and second trimester Down syndrome screens				
Screen	When performed (weeks gestation)	Detection rate	False positive rate	Description
Triple test	15-20	70%	5%	Maternal serum α-feto protein (Low) + Estriol (Low) + hCG (High) Triple test + inhibin-Alpha (High)
Quad screen	15–20	81%	5%	

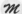

Features of Down Syndrome

My	Mental Retardation/ Micrognathia
C	Congenital heart disease/ Cataracts
H	Hypotonia/Hypothyroidism
I	Increased gap between 1st and 2nd toe (Sandle toe)
L	Leukemia risk/Lung problem (Increased risk of Respiratory Tract Infections)
D	Duodenal atresia
H	Hirshsprung's disease/Hearing loss
A	Alzheimer's disease/Atlanto-axial instability
S	Simian Crease
P	Protruding tongue
R	Round face/Rolling eye (nystagmus)
O	Occipit flat/Oblique palpabrel fissure
B	Brushfield spot/Brachycephaly
L	Low nasal bridge/Language problem
E	Epicanthic fold/Ear folded
M	Mongolian slant/Myoclonus

First Trimester Combined Test	10–13	85%	5%	Ultrasound to measure: *Nuchal Translucency (Increased) *Ductus venosus flow (reversed) *Nasal bone (hypoplasia) + hCG + Pregnancy associated plasma protein A; PAPPA (Low)
Integrated Test	10-13 and 15–20	95%	5%	Measurements from both the 1st Trimester Combined test and the 2nd trimester Quad test to yield a more accurate screening result.

2. Other Autosomal Trisomies

Trisomy 13 (Patau syndrome)	**Trisomy 18 (Edward syndrome)**
• Cleft lip or palate [Q] • Polydactyly[Q] • Microcephaly • Holoprosencephaly • Eye defects (Microphthalmia, Coloboma of iris, retinal dysplasia, cataract) • Capillary hemangiomata	• Prominent (extra) occiput • Micrognathia or small jaw[Q] • Hypertonia • Simple dermal arches on all digits • Very short fourth digit with single crease • Overlapping flexed fingers[Q]

Common features of both are *mental retardation, rocker bottom feet and congenital heart defects (VSD and PDA).*

Note: Ectodermal scalp defects, cleft lip and cleft palate points towards diagnosis of trisomy 13 whereas elongated skull and simple arches on all digits suggest trisomy 18.
(Mnemonic: p for **P**atau and **p**olydactyly as well as **p**alate defects and **e** for **E**dward and **e**xtra occciput).

TRISOMY 22

Cat Eye Syndrome is a rare condition caused by the **partial trisomy of chromosome 22** (The short arm (p) and a small section of the long arm (q) of Chromosome 22 is present three instead of the usual two times. The term "Cat Eye" syndrome was coined due to the particular appearance of the **vertical colobomas** in the eyes of some patients.

Klinefelter Syndrome

- *It is the most common chromosomal disorder of males associated with hypogonadism and infertility.*
- It is due to extra-X-chromosome. Classically, it is **47, XXY**. Other variants can have 48 XXXY, rarely 49 XXXY or mosaics can be there with some cells containing normal 46, XY and others 47, XXY.
- Classically, it results from **meiotic non- disjunction** of sex chromosomes [40% during spermatogenesis and 60% during **oogenesis**]. Mostly, non-disjunction occur during **1st meiotic division**.
- Extra X- chromosomes increase the **female like features,** i.e. feminization [as shown by atrophic testes, lack of secondary sexual characteristics, gynecomastia]. Further, Extra inactive X-chromosome appear as **Barr body**
- Presence of single Y- chromosome is enough for male phenotype. Thus XY, XXY, XXXY all are males.

Clinical Features of Klinefelter Syndrome

- Male sex
- Hypogonadism

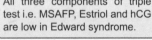

All three components of triple test i.e. MSAFP, Estriol and hCG are low in Edward syndrome.

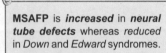

MSAFP is *increased* in *neural tube defects* whereas *reduced* in *Down* and *Edward* syndromes.

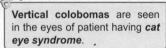

Vertical colobomas are seen in the eyes of patient having *cat eye syndrome.*

In Klinefelter's syndrome, there is ↓ testosterone and inhibin but ↑ LH and FSH, respectively

- Loss of secondary sexual characteristics
- Subnormal I^Q
- Disproportionately long arms and legs
- Gynecomastia
- There is increased risk of breast carcinoma, germ cell tumors (like embryonal cell carcinoma, teratoma and mediastinal germ cell tumors) and autoimmune diseases like SLE.
- Patients can develop cardiovascular problems. **Most commonly associated is mitral valve prolapse** followed by varicose veins.
- Due to less testosterone (hypogonadism), feedback inhibition is less and pituitary produces more LH and FSH.

Turner Syndrome

- *Most common cause of sex chromosomal abnormality in the females.*^{Q}
- Usually results from complete or partial monosomy of X chromosome and associated with hypogonadism in phenotypic females.^{Q} Patients have the (45X) karyotype or may be mosaics.

  - *Clinical features in infancy* include **edema of dorsum of hands and feet,**^{Q} neck webbing or edema of nape of neck (also produces **cystic hygroma**^{Q}) and **congenital cardiac defect** (particularly **preductal coarctation of the aorta**^{Q} and **bicuspid aortic valve**^{Q}).
  - *Clinical features in adolescence and adulthood* include short stature, low posterior hairline, webbing of neck, **cubitus valgus** (increased carrying angle),^{Q} **streak ovaries**^{Q} (contributing to infertility and amenorrhea), **coarctation of the aorta, broad chest and widely spaced nipples, short 4th metacarpal.**

> Autoimmune thyroiditis is not associated with Marfan syndrome. It is seen with *Down syndrome, Turner syndrome* and *Congenital rubella syndrome*

Noonan Syndrome

It is a relatively common autosomal dominant congenital disorder considered to be a type of dwarfism, that affects both males and females equally. It used to be referred to as the male version of Turner's syndrome; however, the genetic causes of Noonan syndrome and Turner syndrome are distinct. Genetics of Turner syndrome shows monosomy of X chromosome (XO) whereas **in Noonan syndrome, mostly mutation in genes on chromosome 12 is noted**. The principal features include congenital heart defect, short stature, learning problems, pectus excavatum, impaired blood clotting, and a characteristic configuration of facial features which is quite similar to Turner syndrome.

> **Turner's syndrome** is the most important cause of **primary amenorrhea**.
> *Pregnancy* is *overall* the commonest as well as the most important cause of *secondary amenorrhea*

Other Important Points

- Autosomal monosomies (loss of one chromosome) are incompatible with fetal development and are not found in live births. Only monosomy compatible with live birth is XO (Turner syndrome).
- Most of the trisomies occur due to meiotic non- disjunction whereas **Trisomy 7, mostly occur due to mitotic non- disjunction.**
- **Most of the meiotic non- disjunctions occur during 1st meiotic division. In Trisomy 18, it is more commonly seen in 2nd meiotic division.**

LYON'S HYPOTHESIS

- **Only one** of the X chromosome is **genetically active**.
- Other X of the paternal or maternal origin undergoes pyknosis and is rendered inactive.
- Inactivation of either maternal or paternal X occurs at random among all the cells of the blastocyst by **about 16th day of embryonic life.**^{Q}
- Inactivation of the same X chromosome persists in all the cells derived from each precursor cell. Inactivation of X is because of a gene called **Xist** which is causing gene silencing DNA methylation. So, all normal females are actually mosaics.

Note: *Number of drumsticks are equal to the number of Y-chromosomes*. Thus, these are one in a normal male (XY), zero in normal female (XX) and Turner's syndrome (XO).

The inactive X can be seen in the interphase nucleus as a small mass near the nuclear membrane called as the **Barr Body or X chromatin.**

Number of Barr bodies = Number of X chromosomes - 1.
So, they are **absent in normal males and Turner syndrome** whereas a *normal female has 1 barr body*

PEDIGREE ANALYSIS

Symbols Used

Male is represented as a square and female is represented as a circle. Affected individuals are represented by filling the circle or square by shading.

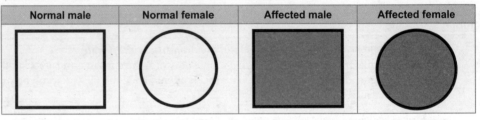

Normal male	Normal female	Affected male	Affected female

Two parents are joined by horizontal line and progeny is indicated by a vertical line.

Analysis

Step 1: First of all see whether there is mitochondrial inheritance or not. If female is transmitting the disease to all offsprings (both males and females) and male is not transmitting the disease to any child, it is **mitochondrial** inheritance.

Step 2: If mitochondrial inheritance is not present, now see whether the disease is inherited as dominant or recessive trait. In dominant inheritance, at least one member in all generations will have disease whereas in recessive inheritance, there will be some generations without disease also. Means, if offsprings of both unaffected parents carry the disease/character, it is recessive whereas if both affected parents produce normal offspring, it is dominantly inherited.

Step 3: Now see, whether it is sex-linked or autosomal by looking at the sex-predilection as
- If male is transmitting the disease only to daughters (all daughters) and not to the sons whereas female transmit the disease to half daughters and half of sons, it is **X-linked dominant**.
- If only males are affected in a pedigree, it is likely to be **X-linked recessive** disease (females act as carriers; only transmit the disease and themselves remain unaffected).
- If there is no sex-predilection and affected individuals transmit the disease to half of the offsprings, it is **autosomal dominant** disorder.
- If there is no sex-predilection and affected individuals transmit the disease to one fourth of the offsprings, it is likely to be **autosomal recessive** disorder.

LOCATION OF IMPORTANT GENES ON CHROMOSOMES

Gene	Chromosome	Gene	Chromosome
p73	1p	RET	10
Folate transporter	21q	WT-1	11p
Neuroblastoma	1p	vWF	12
Rhodopsin	3	Retinoblastoma	13q

Genetics

VHL	3p	BRCA-1	17q
ADPKD-2	4q	Fibrillin-1	15
ADC	5p	Fibrillin-2	5
MHC	6p	BRCA-2	13q
ARPKD	6	NF-1	17q
Cystic fibrosis	7q	p53	17p
MET	7	NF-2	22q

MULTIPLE CHOICE QUESTIONS

SINGLE GENE DISORDERS WITH CLASSICAL INHERITANCE

1. Which of the following is an autosomal recessive condition? *(AI 2012)*
   (a) Ataxia telangectasia
   (b) Peutz Jeghers syndrome
   (c) Neurofibromatosis
   (d) Tuberous sclerosis

2. Which of the following is an autosomal dominant metabolic disorder? *(AI 2004)*
   (a) Cystic fibrosis
   (b) Phenylketonuria
   (c) α-1 antitrypsin deficiency
   (d) Familial hypercholesterolemia

3. The approximate number of genes contained in the human genome is: *(AIIMS Nov 2002)*
   (a) 40,000
   (b) 30,000
   (c) 80,000
   (d) 1,00,000

4. True statements about α-1 anti-trypsin deficiency is
   (a) Autosomal dominant disease *(PGI June 2003)*
   (b) Emphysema
   (c) Fibrosis of portal tract
   (d) Diastase resistant positive hepatocytes
   (e) Orcein positive granules

5a. Autosomal recessive diseases are *(PGI June 2003)*
   (a) Hereditary spherocytosis
   (b) Thalassemia
   (c) Sickle cell anemia
   (d) Cystic fibrosis
   (e) Hemophilia A

5b. Autosomal dominant disorders are all except
   (a) Hereditary spherocytosis *(PGI Dec 2003)*
   (b) Thalassemia
   (c) Sickle cell anemia
   (d) Cystic fibrosis
   (e) Hemophilia

6. Which of the following disorders has been shown to be genetically transmitted by single autosomal dominant genes? *(Delhi PG 2010)*
   (a) Catatonic schizophrenia
   (b) Phenylketonuria
   (c) Creutzfeldt-Jakob's disease
   (d) Huntington's disease

7. Duchenne dystrophy is a: *(Delhi PG-2006)*
   (a) Autosomal dominant disorder
   (b) X-linked dominant disease
   (c) Autosomal recessive disease
   (d) X-linked recessive disease

8. Catastrophic variant of Ehler Danlos syndrome is
   (a) I
   (b) II
   (c) III
   (d) IV

9. Sickle cell disease is due to *(UP 2005)*
   (a) Point mutation
   (b) Frame shift mutation
   (c) Nucleotide receptor blockage
   (d) Non sequence mutation

10. All are autosomal dominant disorders except
   (a) Albinism *(UP 2007)*
   (b) Marfan's syndrome
   (c) Familial adenomatous polyposis
   (d) Von-Hippel Lindau syndrome

11. In Marfan's syndrome there is defect in protein
   (a) Collagen *(RJ 2000)*
   (b) Elastin
   (c) Fibrillin
   (d) All

12. Neurofibromatosis is *(RJ 2001)*
   (a) Autosomal dominant
   (b) AR
   (c) X-linked recessive
   (d) All

13. Blue black pigmentation in alkaptonuria is due to
   (a) Homogentisic acid *(RJ 2002)*
   (b) Oxalic acid
   (c) Glucouronic acid
   (d) All

14. A 26-year-old woman presents because of trouble with her vision. Physical examination reveals a very tall, thin woman with long, thin fingers. Examining her eyes reveals the lens of her left eye to be in the anterior chamber. Her blood levels of methionine and cystathionine are within normal levels. Which of the following is the most likely cause of this patient's signs and symptoms?
   (a) Abnormal copper metabolism
   (b) Decreased levels of vitamin D
   (c) Decreased lysyl hydroxylation of collagen
   (d) Defective synthesis of fibrillin
   (e) Defective synthesis of type I collagen

Genetics

Most Recent Questions

14.1. **Duchenne muscular dystrophy is inherited as:**
   (a) X linked
   (b) Autosomal dominant
   (c) Autosomal recessive
   (d) Codominant

14.2. **Inheritance of Gardner syndrome is:**
   (a) Autosomal recessive
   (b) Autosomal dominant
   (c) X linkeddominant
   (d) X linked recessive

14.3. **Which one of the following is an autosomal dominant disorder:**
   (a) Duchenn's muscular dystrophy
   (b) Fragile X syndrome
   (c) Fanconi's anemia
   (d) Huntington's chorea

14.4. **Adult polycystic kidney disease is inherited by:**
   (a) Autosomal dominant
   (b) Autosomal recessive
   (c) X-linked
   (d) Mitochondrial

14.5. **Neurofibroma is having which of the following inheritance?**
   (a) Autosomal dominant
   (b) Autosomal recessive
   (c) X-linked recessive
   (d) X-linked dominat

14.6. **Which of the following is the inheritance of Huntington's chorea?**
   (a) Autosomal dominant
   (b) Autosomal recessive
   (c) X-linked
   (d) Mitochondrial

14.7. **Hemophilia is associated with:**
   (a) X chromosome   (b) Y Chromosome
   (c) Chromosome 3   (d) Chromosome 16

14.8. **Which of the following is not X linked condition:**
   (a) Duchenne muscular dystrophy
   (b) Emery-Dreifuss muscular dystrophy
   (c) Facioscapulohumeral muscular dystrophy
   (d) Becker muscular dystrophy

14.9. **Which one is not a feature of cystic fibrosis?**
   (a) Autososmal recessive disease
   (b) Abonormal chloride transport
   (c) Affects intestine only
   (d) Increased risk of pulmonary infections

14.10. **Which of the following is an X-linked dominant disorder?**
   (a) Vitamin D resistant rickets
   (b) Familial hypercholesterolemia
   (c) Red green color blindness
   (d) Achondroplasia

SINGLE GENE DISORDERS WITH NON CLASSICAL INHERITANCE

15. **In Prader Willi syndrome, which of the following is increased?** *(AI 2012)*
   (a) LH
   (b) FSH
   (c) TSH
   (d) Ghrelin

16. **NARP syndrome is seen in:** *(AI 2011)*
   (a) Mitochondrial diseases
   (b) Glycogen storage diseases
   (c) Lysosomal storage diseases
   (d) Lipid storage diseases

17. **Maternal disomy of chromosome 15 is seen in:**
   (a) Prader-Willi syndrome *(AIIMS Nov 2010)*
   (b) Klinefelter's syndrome
   (c) Angelman syndrome
   (d) Turner's syndrome

18. **Two siblings with osteogenesis imperfecta have normal parents. The mode of inheritance is explained by which of the following?**
   (a) Anticipation *(AIIMS May 2010)*
   (b) Genomic imprinting
   (c) Germline mosaicism
   (d) New mutation

19. **Mitochondrial DNA (mt-DNA) is known for all except:**
   (a) Maternal inheritance *(DPG 2011)*
   (b) Heteroplasmy
   (c) Leber hereditary optic neuropathy is the prototype
   (d) Nemaline myopathy results due to mutations in mt-DNA

20. **Preferential expression of the gene depending upon the parent of origin is called:** *(AI 2009)*
   (a) Genomic imprinting
   (b) Mosaicism
   (c) Alleles
   (d) Chimerism

21. **Preferential expression of the gene depending upon the parent of origin is called:**
   (a) Anticipation *(AI 2008)*
   (b) Germ line mosaicism
   (c) Genomic imprinting
   (d) Aneuploidy

22. **Differential expression of same gene depending on parent of origin is referred to as:** *(AI 2005)*
   (a) Genomic imprinting
   (b) Mosaicism
   (c) Anticipation
   (d) Non-penetrance

23. A couple has two children affected with tuberous sclerosis. On detailed clinical and laboratory evaluation (including molecular studies) both parents are normal. Which one of the following explains the two affected children in this family?
    (a) Non penetrance   *(AIIMS May 2006)*
    (b) Uniparental disomy
    (c) Genomic imprinting
    (d) Germline mosaicism

24. Genomic imprinting is associated with:
    (a) Silencing of paternal chromosome   *(PGI Dec 01)*
    (b) Silencing of maternal chromosome
    (c) Angelman syndrome
    (d) Prader Willi syndrome
    (e) Gonadal mosaicism

25. Dominant negative inheritance is seen in:
    (a) Ehler Danlos syndrome   *(PGI Dec 2002)*
    (b) Marfan's syndrome
    (c) Hunter syndrome
    (d) Osteogenesis imperfecta
    (e) Hereditary retinoblastoma

26. True statements regarding the mitochondrial genes are: *(PGI Dec 2002)*
    (a) Paternal transmission
    (b) Maternal transmission
    (c) Mendelian inheritance
    (d) Mitochondrial myopathy
    (e) Horizontal inheritance

27. Mitochondrial DNA is   *(PGI June 2003)*
    (a) Paternally inherited
    (b) Maternally inherited
    (c) Horizontal inheritance
    (d) Vertical inheritance
    (e) Mendelian inheritance

28. Which of the following is/are an example/examples of non-Mendelian inheritance?
    (a) Genomic imprinting   *(Delhi PG 2009)*
    (b) Uniparental disomy
    (c) Mitochondrial inheritance
    (d) All of the above

29. Increasing severity of mental retardation in male members over generations is a result of:
    (a) Mitochondrial DNA mutation
    (b) Frameshift mutation   *(Delhi PG 2009 RP)*
    (c) Y linked disorder
    (d) Trinucleotide repeat mutation

30. All of the following are chromosomal breakage syndromes except   *(Karnataka 2004)*
    (a) Fanconi's anemia
    (b) Ehler-Danlos syndrome
    (c) Bloom's syndrome
    (d) Ataxia telangiectasia

31. All of the following are characterized by 'trinucleotide repeats' affecting the non-coding regions except
    (a) Friedrich's ataxia
    (b) Fragile X syndrome
    (c) Huntington's disease
    (d) Myotonic dystrophy

32. An 18 month old child Nonu is brought to a pediatrician. His mother noticed passage of altered color urine by him for past 2-3 days. Laboratory examination revealed it to be hematuria. Examination also reveals hypertension and an abdominal mass. A tumor is localized to the right kidney and biopsy reveals a stroma containing smooth and striated muscle, bone, cartilage, and fat, with areas of necrosis. The gene for this disorder has been localized to which of the following chromosomes?
    (a) 5
    (b) 11
    (c) 13
    (d) 17

33. Majority of the human characteristics are determined by multiple pairs of genes, many with alternate codes, accounting for some dissimilar forms that occur with certain genetic disorders. What type of inheritance involves multiple genes at different loci, with each gene exerting a small additive effect in determining a trait?
    (a) Polygenic inheritance
    (b) Multifactorial inheritance
    (c) Monofactorial inheritance
    (d) Collaborative inheritance

34. A 45-year-old male Arvind who was previously diagnosed with depression is now experiencing involuntary grimacing and strange movements of his arms and legs. Neurological examination shows normal strength and normal deep tendon reflexes. No sensory deficits are noted. The patient's grandfather died of a neurological disease at 65 years old, and the patient's father died of a similar disease at 58. This patient has an earlier onset of disease than either his father or grandfather is most likely explained by which of the following?
    (a) Increased penetrance
    (b) Pleiotropy
    (c) Anticipation
    (d) Mosaicism

35. A young boy, Rinku is being evaluated for developmental delay, mild autism, and mental retardation. Physical examination reveals the boy to have large, reverted ears and a long face with a large mandible. He is also found to have macroorchidism (large testes), and extensive workup reveals multiple tandem repeats of the nucleotide sequence CGG in his DNA Which of the following is the most likely diagnosis?

Genetics

(a) Fragile X syndrome
(b) Huntington's chorea
(c) Myotonic dystrophy
(d) Spinal-bulbar muscular atrophy
(e) Ataxia-telangiectasia

36. **A young man Ramkishore presents for an employment physical. He is very tall, has long fingers, and hyperflexible joints. He states that he has always been called "double jointed". Which of the following disorders is associated with this syndrome?**
 (a) Dissecting aortic aneurysm
 (b) Hepatosplenomegaly
 (c) Polycystic kidneys
 (d) Progressive neurologic dysfunction

Most Recent Questions

36.1. **Genomic imprinting is seen in –**
 (a) Klinefelter's syndrome
 (b) Down's syndrome
 (c) Angelman syndrome
 (d) Hydatidi form mole

36:2. **Mitochondrial chromosomal abnormality leads to:**
 (a) Leber's hereditary optic neuropathy
 (b) Angelman syndrome
 (c) Prader villi syndrome
 (d) Myotonic dystrophy

36.3. **One of the following disorders is due to maternal disomy**
 (a) Prader Willi syndrome
 (b) Angelman syndrome
 (c) Hydatidiform mole
 (d) Klinefelter's syndrome

36.4. **In Huntington chorea the causative mutation in the protein huntingtin is a**
 (a) Point mutation
 (b) Gene deletion
 (c) Frameshift mutation
 (d) Trinucleotide repeat expansion

CHROMOSOMAL DISORDERS AND KARYOTYPING

37. **No change of genetic material occurs in which of the following cytogenetic abnormalities?** *(AIIMS Nov 2012)*
 (a) Deletion   (b) Insertion
 (c) Translocation   (d) Inversion

38. **Patient present with skin bullae on sun exposure. There is a defect in which of the following?**
 (a) Thymidine dimers   *(AIIMS Nov 2012)*
 (b) Trinucleotide repeats
 (c) Sugar changes
 (d) DNA methylation

39. **Which of the following tests is used to differentiate the chromosome of normal and cancer cells?**
 (a) PCR   *(AIIMS Nov 2012)*

(b) Comparative genomic hybridization
(c) Western blotting
(d) Karyotyping

40. **Down's syndrome is associated with the clinical manifestation of mental retardation. Which of the following is not associated with Down's syndrome?**
 (a) Trisomy 21   *(AIIMS Nov 2011)*
 (b) Mosaic 21
 (c) Translocation t (14,21), t (21,21)
 (d) Deletion of 21

41. **The genetics involved in Down syndrome is:**
 (a) Maternal non-disjunction   *(AI 2010)*
 (b) Paternal non-disjunction
 (c) Mosaicism
 (d) Monosomy

42. **Karyotyping is done for:**   *(AI 2009)*
 (a) Chromosomal disorders
 (b) Autosomal recessive disorders
 (c) Autosomal dominant disorders
 (d) Linkage disorders

43. **Males who are sexually underdeveloped with rudimentary testes and prostate glands, sparse pubic and facial hair, long arms and legs and large hands and feet are likely to have the chromosome complement of:**
 (a) 45, XYY   *(AI 2004)*
 (b) 46, XY
 (c) 46, XXY
 (d) 46, X

44. **Which of the following procedures as routine technique for karyotyping using light microscopy?**
 (a) C-banding   *(AI 2003)*
 (b) G-banding
 (c) Q-banding
 (d) Brd V-staining

45. **A married middle aged female gives history of repeated abortions for the past 5 years. The prenatal karyogram of the conceptus is given below**

This karyogram suggests the following: *(AI 2003)*
 (a) Klinefelter's syndrome
 (b) Turner's syndrome
 (c) Down's syndrome
 (d) Patau's syndrome

46. **A nineteen year old female with short stature, wide spread nipples and primary amenorrhea most likely has a karyotype of:** *(AI 2003)*
    (a) 47, XX + 18
    (b) 46, XXY
    (c) 47, XXY
    (d) 45 X

47. **Karyotyping most commonly done under light microscopy:** *(AIIMS Nov 2009)*
    (a) G-banding
    (b) Q banding
    (c) C banding
    (d) R banding

48. **Effective polymerase reaction was repeated for 3 cycles on a DNA molecule. What will be the resulting formation of the copies?** *(AIIMS Nov 2001)*
    (a) Double number of copies
    (b) Three times the number of DNA molecule
    (c) Four times the number of DNA molecule
    (d) 8 times

49. **Y-chromosome is** *(AIIMS May 2007)*
    (a) Telocentric
    (b) Metacentric
    (c) Submetacentric
    (d) Acrocentric

50. **Which of the following is true of Klinefelter's syndrome:** *(PGI Dec 01)*
    (a) Chromosome pattern in 47 XXY
    (b) Mental retardation is present
    (c) Hypogonadism occurs
    (d) Increased FSH level
    (e) Eunuchoid proportions

51. **The classic karyotype of Klinefelter's syndrome is:**
    (a) 47 XXY *(Karnataka 2009)*
    (b) 45 XO
    (c) 48 XXXY
    (d) 46 XY/47 XXY

52. **Chromosomal abnormality in Mongolism is**
    (a) Trisomy 21 *(Karnataka 2005)*
    (b) Trisomy 22
    (c) Trisomy 17
    (d) Trisomy 5

53. **Trisomy 13 is identified as** *(Karnataka 2005)*
    (a) Edward's syndrome
    (b) Patau's syndrome
    (c) Down's syndrome
    (d) Klinefelter's syndrome

54. **In Down syndrome, there is non disjunction of chromosome** *(RJ 2000,2002)*
    (a) 13
    (b) 15
    (c) 18
    (d) 21

55. **Barr body is not seen in:** *(Kolkata 2008)*
    (a) Klinefelter syndrome
    (b) Turner syndrome
    (c) Normal female
    (d) XXX syndrome

56. **Karyotype is:** *(Jharkhand 2003)*
    (a) Size, shape and number of chromosome
    (b) Gene packing
    (c) DNA assay
    (d) None

57. **A 36-year-old retarded man with a strong history of mental retardation among male relatives undergoes genetic testing. His lymphocytes on metaphase arrest show a breakpoint at q27.3 on the X chromosome. This man is at increased risk for which of the following cardiovascular disorders?**
    (a) Aortic stenosis
    (b) Atrial septal defect
    (c) Mitral valve prolapse
    (d) Tricuspid atresia

58. **A 16-year-old female Bholi presents to Dr. Sindhu, a gynecologist because she has never had menstrual bleeding. She is 132 cm tall, weighs 44 kg, has swelling around the neck, increased carrying angle at the elbow and poorly developed secondary sexual characteristics. On performing a pelvic ultrasound, the physician observes her ovaries are small and elongated. Which of the following is the most likely cause of this patient's condition?**
    (a) Mitotic error in early development
    (b) Trinucleotide repeat expansion
    (c) Uniparental disomy
    (d) Balanced reciprocal translocation

59. **A 8-year-old boy Gullu with the Down's syndrome has an intelligence quotient (IQ) in the mid-normal range. Which of the following genetic mechanisms would most likely account for the discrepancy between the child's IQ and his appearance?**
    (a) Balanced translocation
    (b) Chiasma
    (c) Mosaicism
    (d) Spermiogenesis

60. **A tall man with gynecomastia and testicular atrophy has a testicular biopsy that shows sparse, completely hyalinized seminiferous tubules with a complete absence of germ cells and only rare Sertoli cells. Leydig cells are present in large clumps between the hyalinized tubules. Which of the following genetic disorders should be suspected?**
    (a) Testicular feminization syndrome
    (b) Trisomy 18
    (c) Trisomy 21
    (d) 47, XXY

Most Recent Questions

60.1. Patau syndrome is due to which of the following?
- (a) Trisomy 21
- (b) Trisomy 18
- (c) Trisomy 21
- (d) Trisomy 13

60.2. Osteogenesis imperfecta defect in:
- (a) Collagen type I
- (b) Elastin
- (c) Collagen type IV
- (d) Fibrillin 2

60.3. In marfan syndrome, the defect is in:
- (a) Fibrillin I
- (b) Fibrillin II
- (c) Collagen
- (d) Elastin

60.4. Karyotyping is done in which phase of cell cycle?
- (a) Anaphase
- (b) Metaphase
- (c) Telophase
- (d) S phase

60.5. The number of chromosomes in Turner syndrome is:
- (a) 47
- (b) 46
- (c) 45
- (a) 44

60.6. The number of chromosomes in Klinefelter syndrome is:
- (a) 47
- (b) 46
- (c) 45
- (d) 44

60.7. Chromosomes are visualized through light microscope with resolution of:
- (a) 5 Kb
- (b) 50 mb
- (c) 5
- (d) 500 Kb

60.8. Which of the following techniques can be used to detect exact localisation of a genetic locus? *(AIIMS May, Nov 2013)*
- (a) Chromosome painting
- (b) FISH
- (c) Comparative genomic hybridization
- (d) Western blot

60.9. If a chromosome divides in an axis perpendicular to usual axis of division it is going to form:
- (a) Ring chromosome
- (b) Isochromosome
- (c) Acrocentric chromosome
- (d) Subtelocentric chromosome

PEDIGREE ANALYSIS, GENE LOCATION, LYON HYPOTHESIS

61. BRCA 1 gene is located on? *(AIIMS May 2011)*
- (a) Chromosome 13
- (b) Chromosome 11
- (c) Chromosome 17
- (d) Chromosome 22

62. Males are more commonly affected than females in which of the following genetic disorders?
- (a) Autosomal Recessive Disorder *(AI 2010)*
- (b) Autosomal Dominant Disorder
- (c) X-linked Recessive Disorder
- (d) X-linked Dominant Disorder

63. In-situ DNA nick end labeling can quantitate:
- (a) Fraction of cells in apoptotic pathways
- (b) Fraction of cells in S phase *(AI 2005)*
- (c) p53 gene product
- (d) bcr/abl gene

64. The chances of having an unaffected baby, when both parents have achondroplasia, are: *(AI 2005)*
- (a) 0%
- (b) 25%
- (c) 50%
- (d) 100%

65. Study the following carefully: *(AI 2005)*

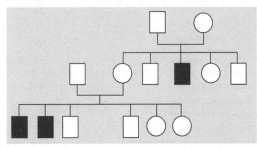

Read the pedigree. Inheritance pattern of the disease in the family is:
- (a) Autosomal recessive type
- (b) Autosomal dominant type
- (c) X-linked dominant type
- (d) X-linked recessive type

66. Kinky hair disease is a disorder where an affected child has peculiar white stubby hair, does not grow, brain degeneration is seen and dies by age of two years. Mrs. A is hesitant about having children because her two sisters had sons who had died from kinky hair disease. Her mother's brother also died of the same condition. Which of the following is the possible mode of inheritance in her family? *(AI 2004)*
- (a) X-linked recessive
- (b) X-linked dominant
- (c) Autosomal recessive
- (d) Autosomal dominant

67. An albino girl gets married to a normal boy, what are the chances of their having an affected child and what are the chances of their children being carriers?
- (a) None affected, all carriers *(AI 2003)*
- (b) All normal
- (c) 50% carriers
- (d) 50% affected, 50% carriers

68. The mother has sickle cell disease; Father is normal; Chances of children having sickle cell disease and sickle cell trait respectively are: *(AI 2001)*
- (a) 0 and 100%
- (b) 25 and 25%
- (c) 50 and 50%
- (d) 10 and 50%

69. **Father has a blood group B; Mother has AB; Children are not likely to have the following blood group:**
    (a) O   *(AI 2001)*
    (b) A
    (c) B
    (d) AB

70. **Gene therapy is used for:**   *(AIIMS May 2009)*
    (a) Cystic fibrosis
    (b) Sickle cell anemia
    (c) Thalassemia
    (d) All of the above

71. **Gene for major histocompatibility complex is located on which chromosome?**   *(AIIMS Nov 2008)*
    (a) Chromosome 10
    (b) Chromosome 6
    (c) X chromosome
    (d) Chromosome 13

72. **Gene for folate carrier protein is located on chromosome?**   *(AIIMS Nov 2008, May 2008)*
    (a) Chromosome 10
    (b) Chromosome 5
    (c) Chromosome 21
    (d) Chromosome 9

73. **Ability of stem cells to cross barrier of differentiation to transform into a cell of another lineage expressing the molecular characteristics of different cell type with the ability to perform the function of the new cell type is referred as:**   *(AIIMS Nov 2007)*
    (a) De differentiation
    (b) Re differentiation
    (c) Trans-differentiation
    (d) Sub differentiation

74. **If both husband and wife are suffering with achondroplasia, what are their chances of having a normal child**   *(AIIMS May 2004)*
    (a) 0%
    (b) 25%
    (c) 50%
    (d) 100%

75. **A one year old boy presented with hepatosplenomegaly and delayed milestones. The liver biopsy and bone marrow biopsy revealed presence of histiocytes with PAS-positive Diastase-resistant material in the cytoplasm. Electron-microscopic examination of these histiocytes is most likely to reveal the presence of:**   *(AIIMS Nov 2003)*
    (a) Birbeck's granules in the cytoplasm
    (b) Myelin figures in the cytoplasm
    (c) Parallel rays of tubular structures in lysosomes
    (d) Electron dense deposit in the mitochondria

76. **The gene that regulates normal morphogenesis during development is:**   *(AIIMS Nov 2002)*
    (a) FMR-1 gene
    (b) Homeobox gene
    (c) P-16
    (d) PTEN

77. **A baby's blood group was determined as O Rh negative. Select the blood group the baby's mother or father will not have**   *(AIIMS Nov 2002)*
    (a) A, Rh positive
    (b) B, Rh positive
    (c) AB, Rh negative
    (d) O, Rh positive

78. **Thalassemia occurs due to which mutation?**
    (a) Missense   *(PGI Dec 2000)*
    (b) Splicing
    (c) Transition
    (d) Frame-shift
    (e) Truncation

79. **Congenital syndrome associated with lympho-proliferative malignancy is:**   *(PGI June 2005)*
    (a) Bloom syndrome.
    (b) Fanconi's anemia
    (c) Turner syndrome.
    (d) Chediak Higashi syndrome.
    (e) Ataxia telangiectasia

80. **Loss of heterozygosity means:**   *(PGI Dec 2005)*
    (a) Loss of single arm of chromosome.
    (b) Loss of mutant allele in mutant gene
    (c) Loss of normal allele in mutant gene
    (d) Loss of normal allele in normal gene

81. **Long and short arm of chromosome are called respectively**   *(Delhi PG-2008)*
    (a) p and q
    (b) q and p
    (c) m and n
    (d) r and s

82. **Cystic fibrosis transmembrane conductance regulator gene is located on chromosome**   *(UP 2005)*
    (a) 5
    (b) 6
    (c) 7
    (d) 8

83. **Which one of the following is not a germ cell tumor?**
    (a) Dermoid   *(Nimhans 1991, AP 2000)*
    (b) Granulosa cell tumor
    (c) Choriocarcinoma
    (d) Gynandroblastoma

84. **A relatively recent advancement is the use of a technique called DNA fingerprinting. It is based in part on recombinant DNA technology and in part on those techniques originally used in medical genetics to detect slight variations in the genomes of different individuals. These techniques are used in forensic medicine to compare specimens from the suspect with those of the forensic specimen. What is being compared when DNA fingerprinting is used in forensics?**
    (a) The banding pattern
    (b) The triplet code
    (c) The haplotypes
    (d) The chromosomes

Genetics

85. Individual II-2 in the associated pedigree was diagnosed with hemophilia A. Which one of the following individuals would be most at risk for developing also hemophilia A?

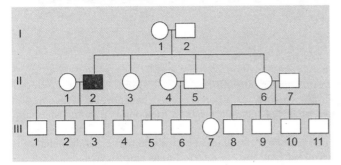

(a) II-3
(b) II-6
(c) III-3
(d) III-5
(e) III-8

86. A 22-year-old woman, Sheena presents with progressive bilateral loss of central vision. You obtain a detailed family history from this patient and produce the associated pedigree (dark circles or squares indicate affected individuals). Which of the following transmission patterns is most consistent with this patient's family history?

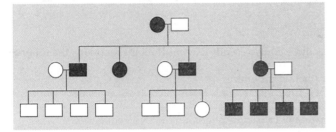

(a) Autosomal recessive
(b) Autosomal dominant
(c) X-linked recessive
(d) X-linked dominant
(e) Mitochondrial

87. A pathologist Dr. Gobind is examining four placentas from four different births. He notes the following characteristics in the four placentas:

Patient A: fused dichorionic diamnionic

Patient B: dichorionic diamnionic

Patient C: circumvallate placenta

Patient D: monochorionic diamnionic.

Which of the patients unquestionably gave birth to identical twins?

(a) Patient A
(b) Patient B
(c) Patient C
(d) Patient D

Most Recent Questions

87.1. True statement about inheritance of an X linked recessive trait is:
(a) 50% of boys of carrier mother are affected
(b) 50% of girls of diseased father are carrier
(c) Father transmits disease to the son
(d) Mother transmits the disease to the daughter

87.2. Gene for Wilm's tumor is located on:
(a) Chromosome 1
(b) Chromosome 10
(c) Chromosome 11
(d) Chromosome 12

87.3. Male to male transmission is not seen in:
(a) Autosomal dominant diseases
(b) Autosomal recessive disease
(c) X-linked dominant disease
(d) Genomic imprinting

87.4. Microarray is best characterised by:
(a) Study of multiple genes
(b) Study of disease
(c) Study of organisms
(d) Study of blood group

87.5. The technique used for separation and detection of RNA is which one of the following
(a) Northern blot
(b) Southern blot
(c) Eastern blot
(d) Western blot

87.6. Which of the following potentially represents the most dangerous situation?
(a) Rh+ve mother with 2nd Rh-ve child
(b) Rh-ve mother with 2nd Rh+ve child
(c) Rh+ve mother with 1st Rh-ve child
(d) Rh-ve mother with 1st Rh+ve child

87.7. The CFTR gene associated what cystic fibrosis is located on chromosome
(a) 5
(b) 12
(c) 4
(d) 7

87.8. In cystic fibrosis the most frequent pulmonary pathogen is
(a) Pseudomonas
(b) Enterococci
(c) Staphylococci
(d) Klebsiella

Genetics

EXPLANATIONS

1. **Ans. (a) Ataxia telangectasia** *(Ref: Robbins 8th/302-3, 1323-4, 9/e p242-243)*
   - **Ataxia** telangiectasiais an **autosomal recesive condition.**
   - Patients have increased *sensitivity to x-ray-induced chromosome abnormalities*.
   - Characterized by an ataxic-dyskinetic syndrome beginning in early childhood, caused by neuronal degeneration predominantly in the cerebellum, the subsequent development of telangiectasias in the conjunctiva and skin, and immunodeficiency.
   - The nuclei of cells in many organs (e.g., Schwann cells in dorsal root ganglia and peripheral nerves, endothelial cells as well as pituicytes) show a bizarre enlargement of the cell nucleus and are referred to as **amphicytes**.
   - The *lymph nodes, thymus,* and *gonads* are **hypoplastic**.
   - Clinical features include **recurrent sinopulmonary infections** and **unsteadiness in walking**.
   - Increased risk of development of lymphoid malignant disease (T-cell leukemia and lymphoma

   All other options are autosomal dominant conditions.

2. **Ans. (d) Familial hypercholesterolemia** *(Ref: Robbins 7th/152, 9/e p141)*
   Most of the metabolic disorders have **autosomal recessive inheritance except**:

Her	–	Her's disease [Liver phosphorylase deficiency]
Left	–	Lesch Nyhan syndrome
Eye	–	Ocular albinism
Has	–	Hunter syndrome and Hypercholesterolemia (familial)
Five	–	Fabry's disease
Pimples	–	Porphyria [Acute intermittent]

   Note: All these exceptions have X linked recessive inheritance **except** acute intermittent porphyria and familial hypercholesterolemia which are autosomal dominant disorders.

3. **Ans. (b) 30,000 genes** *(Ref: Robbins's 7th/1219, 8th/136)*
   Humans have a mere 30,000 genes rather than the 100,000 predicted only recently. Recent Robbins mentions the number of genes to 20,000 to 25,000.
   - **Genetics** is the study of **single or a few genes** and their phenotypic effects.
   - **Genomics** is the study of **all the genes** in the genome and their interactions. DNA microarray analysis of tumors is an excellent example of genomics in current clinical use.
   - **Epigenetics** is heritable changes in gene expression that are not caused by alteration in DNA sequences.

4. **Ans. (b) Emphysema; (c) Fibrosis of portal tact; (d) Diastase resistance positive hepatocytes;** *(Ref: Robbins 7th - 911, 912 , 9/e p850-851)*
   - This is an autosomal recessive disease characterized by deficiency of α_1 - antitrypsin (important protease inhibitor).
   - There is portal tract fibrosis in neonatal hepatitis. About 10 - 20% of newborn with α_1 – antitrypsin deficiency develop neonatal hepatitis and cholestasis.
   - Hepatocellular carcinoma develops in 2-3 % α_1 - antitrypsin deficiency in adults.
   - The treatment and cure, for severe hepatic disease is *orthotropic liver transplantation*.

5a. **Ans. (b) Thalassemia; (c) Sickle cell anemia; (d) Cystic fibrosis** *(Ref: Robbins 7th/151, 8th/141-2, 9/e p141)*
   - Hereditary spherocytosis is an autosomal dominant disorder
   - Hemophilia is an X-linked recessive disease.

   A broad generalization is that the physiologic metabolic enzyme deficiencies are all autosomal recessive whereas Structural defects are autosomal dominant.

5b. **Ans. (b) Thalassemia, (c) sickle cell disease, (d) cystic fibrosis, (e) hemophilia** *(Ref: Robbins 8th/652 , 9/e p141)*

6. **Ans. is d i.e. Huntington's disease** *(Ref: Harrison 17th/401 Robbins 7th/1393, 8th/141,168 , 9/e p141)*

7. **Ans. (d) X-linked recessive disease** *(Ref: Robbins 7th/1336 , 9/e p142)*

8. **Ans. (d) IV** *(Ref: Robbins 8th/145-146, 7th/155-156 , 9/e p146)*

9. **Ans. (a) Point mutation** *(Ref: Robbins 8th/645; 7th/628 , 9/e p138)*

10. **Ans. (a) Albinism** *(Ref: Robbins 8th/141-142, 7th/151 , 9/e p141-142)*

11. **Ans. (c) Fibrillin** *(Ref: Robbins 8th/144, 7th/154 , 9/e p144)*

12. **Ans. (a) Autosomal dominant** *(Ref: Robbins 8th/140, 7th/151 , 9/e p140)*

13. **Ans. (a) Homogentisic acid** *(Ref: Robbins 8th/155-156, 7th/167-168 , 9/e p64)*

14. **Ans. (d) Defective synthesis of fibrillin** *(Ref: Robbins 7th/104, 154-155 , 9/e p144)*
    The stem describes a patient of Marfan syndrome which is an autosomal dominant disorder that results from defective synthesis of fibrillin.

14.1. **Ans. (a) X linked** *(Ref: Robbins 8/e p142 , 9/e p142)*
    X-linked recessive disorder can be remembered by the following line:
    Less hCG is Detected Clinically in A Fragile Woman

Less	Lesch Nyhan syndrome[Q]
H	Hemophilia A and B[Q]; Hunter syndrome[Q]
C	Chronic granulomatous disease[Q]
G is	G6PD deficiency[Q]
Detected	Duchhene muscular dystrophy[Q], Diabetes insipidus[Q]
Clinically in	Color blindness[Q]
A	Agammaglobulinemia[Q] (*Bruton's disease*)
Fragile	Fragile X syndrome[Q], Fabry Disease[Q]
Woman	Wiskott Aldrich syndrome[Q]

14.2. **Ans. (b) Autosomal dominant** *(Ref: Robbins 8/e p816 , 9/e p806,809)*
    It is a subtype of familial adenomatous polyposis inherited as an **autososmal dominant disorder**.
    Gardener syndrome [Q] Intestinal polyps + epidermal cysts + fibromatosis + osteomas (of the mandible, long bones and skull).

14.3. **Ans. (d) Huntington's chorea** *(Ref: Robbins 8/e p141)*

Autosomal dominant disorders

Vo	Von Willebrand Disease[Q]
Familial	Familial Adenomatous Polyposis[Q]
Hypercholesterolemia	Hypercholesterolemia (Familial)
Autosomal	Adult polycystic kidney[Q]
D	Dystrophia myotonica[Q]
O	Osteogenesis imperfecta[Q]
M	Marfan syndrome[Q]
I	Intermittent porphyria[Q]
N	Neurofibromatosis-1[Q]
A	Achondroplasia[Q]
N	Neurofibromatosis–2[Q]
T	Tuberous sclerosis[Q]
Hai	Huntington's disease[Q]; Hereditary spherocytosis[Q]

14.4. **Ans. (a) Autosomal dominant...see earlier explanation** *(Ref: Robbins 9/e p141)*

14.5. **Ans. (a) Autosomal dominant...see earlier explanation** *(Ref: Robbins 9/e p141)*

14.6. **Ans. (a) Autosomal dominant...see earlier explanation** *(Ref: Robbins 9/e p141)*

14.7. **Ans. (a) X chromosome...explained earlier** *(Ref: Robbins 8/e p142, 9/e p142)*

14.8. Ans. (c)Facioscapulohumeral muscular dystrophy *(Ref: Robbins 8/e p142, 1270)*
- Facioscapulohumeral muscular dystrophy is an **autosomal dominant** disorder characterised by *facial weakness* (difficulty with eye closure and impaired smile) and *scapular winging*.

Progressive Muscular Dystrophies

Type	Inheritance	Clinical Features
Duchenne's	XR	Progressive weakness of girdle muscles Unable to walk after age 12 Progressive kyphoscoliosis Respiratory failure in 2d or 3d decade
Becker's	XR	Progressive weakness of girdle muscles Able to walk after age 15 Respiratory failure may develop by 4th decade
Limb-girdle	AD/AR	Slow progressive weakness of shoulder and hip girdle muscles
Emery-Dreifuss	XR/AD	Elbow contractures, humeral and peroneal weakness
Congenital	AR	Hypotonia, contractures, delayed milestones Progression to respiratory failure in some; static course in others
Myotonica (DM1, DM2)	AD	Slowly progressive weakness of face, shoulder girdle, and foot dorsiflexion Preferential proximal weakness in DM2
Facioscapulohumeral	AD[Q]	Slowly progressive weakness of face, shoulder girdle, and foot dorsiflexion
Oculopharyngeal	AD	Slowly progressive weakness of extraocular, pharyngeal, and limb muscles

14.9. Ans. (c) Affects intestine only *(Ref: Robbins 9/e 466-471)*
- **Cystic fibrosis** is also known as **salty baby syndrome[Q]** or **mucoviscidosis[Q]**. It is an **autosomal recessive[Q] genetic disorder** that affects most critically the lungs, and also the pancreas, liver, and intestine.
- It is characterized by abnormal transport of chloride and sodium across epithelium, leading to thick, viscous secretions
- Affected patients are prone to *Pseudomonas infections[Q]* for which a **combination of 3rd generation cepahalosporins and aminoglycoside[Q]** is used.
- The most commonly used form of testing is the sweat test using the drug that stimulates sweating (*pilocarpine iontophoresis[Q]*).
- Patients require repeated use of antibiotics and lung transplantation (in later stages) to survive.

14.10.Ans. (d) Vitamin D resistant rickets *(See Below)*

Vitamin D resistant rickets	X linked dominant due to PHEX gene
Familial hypercholesterolemia	Autosomal recessive
Red green colour blindness	X linked recessive
Achondroplasia	Autosomal dominant

15. Ans. (d) Ghrelin *(Ref: Robbins 8th/441-2, and 9/e 444, Pediatric endocrinology: mechanisms, manifestations, management 1st/26-8)*
- **Ghrelin** is a **growth hormone secretagogue** and the *only gut hormone with orexigenic* (means increasing food intake) property.
- It is primarily **produced in the stomach**. In children, its value is inversely related with body mass index and insulin values. It is postulated to play an important role in hyperphagia.

Direct quote from Pediatric endocrinology… *'fasting ghrelin levels were obtained in children with Prader Willi syndrome and found to be elevated 3-4 times when compared to children who are obese'*.

Pancreatic polypeptide Y (PYY) is normally secreted from endocrine cells of the **ileum and colon**. It reduces energy intake and its reduced levels in the patients of *Prader Willi syndrome* may contribute to hyperphagia and obesity.

16. Ans. (a) Mitochondrial Disorder *(Ref: Harrison 17th/316-317, Robbins 8th/1328)*

NARP syndrome (Neuropathy, ataxia, and retinitis pigmentosa), is a condition related to changes in mitochondrial DNA. For details, see text.

Genetics

17. Ans. (a) Prader-Willi syndrome *(Ref: Robbins 8th/172)*
Prader Willi syndrome could be present because of the following:
a.   Deletion of paternal chromosome 15 or
b.   Uniparental disomy of maternal chromosome 15.
For details, see text

18. Ans. (c) Germline mosaicism *(Ref: Robbins 8th/173)*
Gonadal mosaicism results from a mutation that occurs postzygotically during early (embryonic) development. If the mutation affects only cells destined to form the gonads, the gametes carry the mutation, but the somatic cells of the individual are **completely normal**. Such an individual is said to exhibit germ line or gonadal mosaicism. A phenotypically normal parent who has germ line mosaicism can transmit the disease-causing mutation to the offspring through the mutant gamete. Since the progenitor cells of the gametes carry the mutation, there is a definite possibility that more than one child of such a parent would be affected. It is seen with tuberous sclerosis and osteogenests imperfecta.

19. Ans. (d) Nemaline myopathy results due to mutations in mt-DNA *(Ref: Harrison 17th/2688, Robbins 8th/171)*
Nemaline myopathy is not a mitochondrial disease

Nemaline Myopathy

> Nemaline myopathy is a clinically heterogeneous condition and not a mitochondrial disease. Five genes have been associated with this myopathy. All code for thin filament–associated proteins, suggesting disturbed assembly or interplay of these structures as a pivotal mechanism. Mutations of the nebulin (NEB) gene account for most cases, including both severe neonatal and early childhood forms, inherited as autosomal recessive disorders.

20. Ans. (a) Genomic imprinting *(Ref: Robbins 8th/171-173, 9/e 173)*

21. Ans. (c) Genomic imprinting *(Ref: Robbin 7th/186 , 9/e 173)*

22. Ans. (a) Genomic imprinting *(Ref: Harrison's 17th/413, 18th/518; Robbins 7th/186. 8th/171-2 , 9/e 173)*
Genomic imprinting is the phenomenon that leads to preferential expression of an allele depending on its, parental origin. It is also seen in (**updated from HARRISON 18th**):

- *Wiedmann syndrome* (have two paternal but no maternal copies of *chromosome 11*).
- *Albright's hereditary* osteodystrophy (short stature, brachydactyly and PTH resistance). There is *mutation in the Gs α subunit*; individuals express the disease only when the mutation is inherited from the mother).

23. Ans. (d) Germline mosaicism *(Ref: Robbins 8th/173, 7th/187, Harrison 17th/1800, 9/e 174)*
Germline mosaicism is seen with osteogenesis imperfecta and tuberous sclerosis. For details, see text.

24. Ans. (a) Silencing of paternal chromosome; (b) Silencing of maternal chromosome; (c) Angelman syndrome; (d) Prader Willi syndrome: *(Ref: Robbins' 7th-1856, 8th/171-3 , 9/e 173)*

25. Ans. (a) Ehler Danlos syndrome; (b) Marfan's syndrome; (d) Osteogenesis imperfecta *(Ref: Robbins 7th/151 , 9/e 144-146)*
Dominant negative effects occurs when a **mutant polypeptide not only loses its own function but also interferes with the product of normal allele in a heterozygote,** thus causing more severe effects than deletion or non-sense mutations in the same gene. Structural proteins that contribute to multimeric structures are vulnerable to dominant negative effects, e.g. collagen.

> **Seen in: Osteogenesis imperfecta, Ehler Danlos syndrome, Marfan's syndrome.**

26. Ans. (b) Maternal transmission; (d) Mitochondrial myopathy: *(Ref: Harrison 18th/501, Robbins 8th/171)*
Human mitochondrial DNA (mt DNA)
- Examples include
  - Leber's Hereditary Optic Neuropathy,
  - Myoclonic Epilepsy with Ragged Red Fibers syndrome (MERRF),
  - Mitochondrial myopahty with Encephalopathy, Lactic Acidosis and Stroke (MELAS),
  - Autosomal dominant inherited mitochondrial myopathy with mitochondrial deletion (ADMIMY),
  - Kearns-Sayre syndrome,
  - Chronic progressive external ophthalmoplegia,
  - Pearson syndrome and
  - Neurogenic muscular weakness with ataxia and retinitis pigmentosa (NARP).

27. Ans. (b) Maternally transmitted. *(Ref: Robbins 7th/185 , 9/e 171)*

28. Ans. (d) All of the above *(Ref: Robbins 8th/167 , 9/e 168)*

Non- Mendelian inheritance can be classified into following four categories:

Trinucleotide repeat mutation disorders	Mitochondrial gene mutations	Genomic imprinting	Gonadal Mosaicism
• Fragile- X syndrome • Friedreich's Ataxia • Myotonic dystrophy • Huntington disease • Spinobulbar muscular atrophy (Kennedy disease) • Spinocerebellar ataxias	• Leber Hereditary Optic Neuropathy • Kearns-Sayre syndrome • Chronic progressive external ophthalmoplegia • Pearson syndrome • Neurogenic muscular weakness with ataxia and retinitis pigmentosa (NARP)	• Prader-Willi syndrome (Paternal deletion) • Angelman syndrome (maternal deletion)	• Tuberous sclerosis • Osteogenesis imperfecta

29. **Ans. (d) Trinucleotide repeat mutation** *(Ref:Robbins 8th/169-171 , 9/e 169)*

30. **Ans. (b) Ehlers-Danlos syndrome** *(Ref: Robbins 7th/155-6, Table 5.5 174 , 9/e 145-146)*
Chromosome breakage syndromes are associated with high level of chromosomal instability. Such conditions include. Fanconi anemia, Bloom syndrome and Ataxia telangiectasia.
Ehlers-Danlos syndrome (EDS)
• Genetic disorder resulting from defective synthesis of fibrillar collagen
• Skin is extraordinary stretchable, extremely fragile and vulnerable to trauma, joints are hypermobile
• Internal complications: rupture of colon, large arteries

31. **Ans. (c) Huntington's disease** *(Ref: Robbins 8th/168 , 9/e 168)*
Huntington's disease is characterized by trinucleotide repeats affecting the coding region. Rest all conditions mentioned in the options affects the non-coding regions.

32. **Ans. (b) 11** *(Ref: Robbins 8th/480-1 , 9/e 479)*
The diagnosis of this patient is **Wilms' tumor**. It occurs in children and typically presents with an abdominal mass as well as with hypertension, hematuria, nausea and intestinal obstruction. Since it is derived from mesonephric mesoderm, it can include mesodermal derivatives such as bone, cartilage, and muscle. The Wilms' tumor suppressor gene (WT-1) has been localized to chromosome 11 (11p).
Other options
• **Chromosome 5** (option a) is the site of the **tumor suppressor gene APC**, which is involved in the pathogenesis of colon cancer and familial adenomatous polyposis.
• **Chromosome 13** (option c) is the site of the tumor suppressor gene for **retinoblastoma and osteosarcoma** (Rb) as well as the BRCA-2 gene for breast cancer.
• **Chromosome 17** (option d) is the site of **p53** (involved in most human cancers), **NF-1** (neurofibromatosis type I), and **BRCA-1 (breast and ovarian cancer)**.

33. **Ans. (a) Polygenic inheritance** *(Ref: Robbins 8th/138 , 9/e 138)*
Polygenic inheritance involves multiple genes at different loci, with each gene exerting a small additive effect in determining a trait. Multifactorial inheritance is similar to polygenic inheritance in that multiple alleles at different loci affect the outcome; the difference is that multifactorial inheritance includes environmental effects on the genes.

34. **Ans. (c) Anticipation** *(Ref: Robbins 8th/168-170 , 9/e 169; 1297)*
Huntington disease manifests with the triad of movement disorder (chorea), behavioral abnormalities aggressiveness, apathy or depression), and dementia. Huntington disease is transmitted as an autosomal dominant trait with 100% penetrance, meaning that if a child inherits the abnormal gene, that child will inevitably develop Huntington disease. Most patients develop symptoms in their 40s or 50s. An earlier age of onset is associated with a larger number of trinucleotide repeats. During spermatogenesis, CAG repeats in the abnormal HD gene rapidly increase. Thus, patients who receive an abnormal gene from their fathers tend to develop the disease earlier in life. **(The number of trinucleotide repeats on HD gene remains the same during maternal transmission.)** The tendency for clinical symptoms to worsen and/or occur earlier in subsequent generations is called **anticipation**.

Anticipation is common in disorders associated with trinucleotide repeats as in **Fragile X syndrome, myotonic dystrophy** and **Friedreich ataxia**.

• (Choice A) The transmission of an abnormal gene from a parent to a child does not always cause disease. The likelihood that the properties of a gene will be expressed is called penetrance. Huntington disease is a disorder with 100% penetrance means all individuals who have an abnormal HD gene will develop Huntington disease.
• (Choice B) Sometimes, one gene mutation leads to multiple phenotypic abnormalities, a genetic phenomenon named "pleiotropy." In Huntington disease, pleiotropy is present because the mutation of one gene (HD) causes dysfunction of behavior, movement and cognition.
• (Choice D)The presence of two populations of cells with different genotypes in one patient is called mosaicism. Examples include milder forms of Turner (genotype 46XX/45X0), Klinefelter (46XY/47XXY), and Down syndromes.

35. Ans. (a) Fragile – X syndrome *(Ref: Robbins 7th/149, 181-183 , 9/e 169-171)*
The presentation in the stem of the question is characteristic of Fragile X syndrome.

36. Ans. is (a) i.e. Dissecting aortic aneurysm *(Ref: Robbins 8th/145 , 9/e 145)*

The patient has Marfan syndrome, an autosomal dominant disorder caused by a defect in the gene on chromosome 15 encoding fibrillin, a 350 kD glycoprotein. Fibrillin is a major component of elastin associated microfibrils, which are common in large blood vessels and the suspensory ligaments of the lens. Abnormal fibrillin predisposes for cystic medial necrosis of the aorta, which may be complicated by aortic dissection. Other features of the syndrome are subluxated lens of the eye, mitral valve prolapse, and a shortened life span (often due to aortic rupture).

36.1. Ans. (c) Angelman syndrome *(Ref: Robbins 8/e p171-2 , 9/e 172)*
Imprinting is a process associated with selective inactivation of either the maternal or paternal allele. Thus, *maternal imprinting* refers to transcriptional silencing of the maternal allele, whereas *paternal imprinting* implies that the paternal allele is inactivated. Imprinting occurs in the ovum or the sperm, before fertilization, and then is stably transmitted to all somatic cells through mitosis. The genomic imprinting is best illustrated by the following disorders: **Prader-Willi syndrome and Angelman syndrome.**

36.2. Ans. (a) Leber's hereditary optic neuropathy *(Ref: Robbins 8/e p171 , 9/e 172)*
Examples of mitochondrial inheritance are *Leber's optic neuropathy, Leigh's disease, MELAS* (*m*itochondrial *e*ncephalopathy, *l*actic *a*cidosis and *s*troke like syndrome) NARP syndrome (Neuropathy, ataxia, and retinitis pigmentosa), Kearns-Sayre syndrome, Chronic progressive external ophthalmoplegia and Pearson syndrome.

36.3. Ans. (d) Klinefelter's syndrome *(Ref: Robbins 8/e p165 , 9/e 173)*
Maternal disomy is associated with disorders like Prader-Willi syndrome and Angelman syndrome. It is also seen in other conditions like molar pregnancy and Beckwith-Wiedemann syndrome.

36.4. Ans. (d) Trinucleotide repeat expansion *(Ref: Robbins 9/e p168)*
Expansion of trinucleotide repeats is an important genetic cause of human disease, particularly neurodegenerative disorders. There are three key mechanisms by which unstable repeats cause diseases:
- Loss of function of the affected gene occurs in fragile X syndrome. In such cases the repeats are generally in non-coding part of the gene.
- A toxic gain of function by alterations of protein structure as in Huntington disease and spinocerebellar ataxias. In such cases the expansions occur in the coding regions of the genes.
- A toxic gain of function mediated by mRNA as is seen in fragile X tremor-ataxia syndrome. In this condition, the non coding parts of the gene are affected.

37. Ans. (d) Inversion *(Ref: Robbins 8th/138, 160)*

Inversion refers to a rearrangement that involves two breaks within a single chromosome with reincorporation of the inverted, intervening segment. It can be of the following two types:
a. An inversion involving only one arm of the chromosome is known as paracentric.
b. If the breaks are on opposite sides of the centromere, it is known as pericentric.
Inversions are often fully compatible with normal development. It is *not associated with change in genetic material.*

- *Deletion* refers to loss of a portion of a chromosome. Similarly, insertion would lead to increase (and not loss) in the genetic material.
- In a *translocation*, a segment of one chromosome is transferred to another. It can be of the following types:
  – In **balanced reciprocal translocation,** *there are single breaks in each of two chromosomes, with exchange of material. There is* **no loss of genetic material** *and so, the* **affected individual is likely to be phenotypically normal.** A balanced translocation carrier, however, is at increased risk for producing abnormal gametes.
  – *In **robertsonian translocation** (or centric fusion), a translocation between two acrocentric chromosomes. Typically the breaks occur close to the centromeres of each chromosome. Transfer of the segments then leads to one very large chromosome and one extremely small one. **Usually the small product is lost.** This loss is compatible with a normal phenotype because it carries only highly redundant genes.

Therefore, deletion, insertion and Robertsonian translocation would lead to change in genetic material.

38. Ans. (a) Thymidine dimers *(Ref: Robbins 8th/275, 302)*

Xeroderma pigmentosum

- **Autosomal recessive**[Q] inherited disorder of *defective DNA repair*[Q].
- Affected individuals are at increased risk for the development of skin cancers particularly following *exposure to the UV light* contained in sun rays.
- UV radiation causes *cross-linking of pyrimidine residues*, preventing normal DNA replication. Such DNA damage is repaired by the **nucleotide excision repair system**[Q].
- Deficiency of enzymes like *UV specific endonuclease (commonest), DNA polymerase and DNA ligase* is implicated

39. **Ans. (b)** Comparative genomic hybridization *(Ref: Robbins 8th/179, Harrison 18th/512)*
    - *Comparative genomic hybridization (CGH) differentiates between cancer and normal cells.*

Fluorescence in situ hybridization (FISH)

- The majority of FISH applications involve hybridization of one or two probes of interest as an adjunctive procedure to conventional chromosomal banding techniques. So, FISH can be utilized to identify specific chromosomes, characterize de novo duplications or deletions, and clarify subtle chromosomal rearrangements. Its *greatest utilization* in constitutional analysis is in *the detection of microdeletions*[Q].
- *In cancer cytogenetics, it is used extensively in the analysis of structural rearrangements*[Q].
- The usually performed FISH is metaphase FISH. However, **interphase analysis** can be used to make a rapid diagnosis in instances *when metaphase chromosome preparations are not yet available.* Interphase analysis also **increases the number of cells available for examination**, allows for investigation of nuclear organization, and provides results when cells do not progress to metaphase.
- The use of interphase FISH has increased recently, especially for analyses of **amniocentesis samples and cancer cytogenetics**[Q].
- FISH comparative genomic hybridization (CGH) is a method that can be used only when DNA is available from a specimen of interest. The **entire DNA specimen** from the **sample of interest** is **labeled in one color** (e.g., green), and the normal control DNA specimen is indicated by another color (e.g., red). These are mixed in equal amounts and hybridized to normal metaphase chromosomes. The **red-to-green ratio is analyzed** by a computer program that determines where the DNA of interest may have gains or losses of material.

40. **Ans. (d)** Deletion of 21 *(Ref: Robbins 8th/161-162)*
    Down syndrome is characterized by trisomy 21 (**NOT deletion of chromosome 21**). *For details see text.*

41. **Ans. (a) Maternal non-disjunction** *(Ref: Robbins 8th/161)*

Genetics of Down syndrome

- **Meiotic nondisjunction of chromosome 21 occuring in the ovum is** seen in *95% cases* with trisomy 21 and is the so, *commonest cause* of Down syndrome. The extra chromosome is of *maternal origin*.
- *There is a Strong relation* with maternal age
- It may also be seen with Robertsonian translocation and mosaicism.

42. **Ans. (a) Chromosomal disorders** *(Ref: Robbins 8th/158)*

- **Karyotyping** is the study of chromosomes
- Chromosomes are arrested in **metaphase** by **Colchicine**
- These are then stained by many stains. **Most commonly** used stain is **Giemsa stain**, so called **G-banding**
- The chromosomes are **arranged in order of decreasing length**
- Any alteration in number or structure of chromosomes can be easily detected by karyotyping

43. **Ans. (c) 46, XXY** *(Ref: Harrison's 17th/2340 – 2341, 411, Robbins 7th/179)*
    It is a typical case of Klinefelter syndrome. The features pointing towards this diagnosis are:
    - Male phenotype
    - Hypogonadism [rudimentary testes]
    - Decreased secondary sexual characteristics [sparse pubic and facial hairs]
    - Disproportionately long arms and legs.

    > Patients with Klinefelter syndrome have extra X chromosome, so they may be 47,XXY or 46XY/47 XXY mosaics.

    None of the options appear correct as an extra X chromosome in the male should increase the total number of chromosomes to 47 and hence 47 XXY should be the most appropriate answer. However an extra X – chromosome is the most essential aspect and hence, within the available options, the best answer is 46 XXY.

44. **Ans. (b) G-Banding** *(Ref: Harsh Mohan 6th/17, Robbins 8th/159, Cancer cytogenetics3rd/2010)*
G banding is the most widely used technique for routine cytogenetic analysis.' So, **G** banding is chosen as the answer of choice. For details of different banding techniques, please see text.

45. **Ans. (c) Down's syndrome** *(Ref: Robbins 7/175)*
- The given karyogram shows three chromosomes at 21 instead of a pair. It is called **Trisomy 21.**
- Trisomy 21 is synonymous with **Down's syndrome** and is the most common of the chromosomal disorders. It is a major cause of mental retardation.
- **Other trisomies** are Edward syndrome (Trisomy 18) and Patau syndrome (Trisomy 13)

46. **Ans. (d) 45X** *(Ref: Robbins 7/179-180)*
Given features (*Female, primary amenorrhea, short stature, widely spaced nipples*) suggests the diagnosis of **Turner's syndrome**.

Turner's Syndrome
Turner's syndrome is the *most common sex chromosomal disorder in phenotypic females.*
Turner's syndrome results from complete or partial loss of one X chromosome (45, XO) and is characterized by **hypogonadism in phenotypic females**

47. **Ans. (a) G-banding** *(Ref: Harsh Mohan 6th/17, Robbins 8th/159, Cancer cytogenetics 2010/3rd edition)*
Refer to the text for detail.

Q banding is easily ruled out because it does not require light microscopy. *Cancer cytogenetics* clearly mentions that 'sequence specific techniques like **T** banding; **C** banding and **NOR** banding have been replaced by in situ hybridization techniques. G banding is the most widely used technique for routine cytogenetic analysis.' So, **G** banding is chosen as the answer of choice.

48. **Ans. (d) Eight times** *(Ref: Harrison 17th/391)*
Friends, the number of copies of the particle after 'n' cycles of polymerase chain reaction is given by the formula 2^n times the original copies. So, the number of copies after 3 cycles would be $2^3 = 8$ times the original copies.
PCR is used to amplify DNA but RT – PCR (reverse transcriptase PCR) can be used for studying mRNA.

49. **Ans. (d) Acrocentric** *(Ref: Nelson 17th/382)*
X chromosome is Submetacentric and Y chromosome is Telocentric.

50. **Ans. (a) Chromosome pattern is 47 XXY; (b) Mental retardation is present; (c) Hypogonadism occurs; (d) Increased FSH level; (e) Eunuchoid proportions:** *(Ref: Harrison' 16th-2215, 2216, Robbins 7th/179, 8th/165)*
Klinefelter's syndrome is defined as male hypogonadism that occurs when there are two or more X chromosomes or one or more Y chromosomes. Characteristic changes are

- Hypogonadism comprising small, firm testes
- Hyalinized seminiferous tubules
- Failure of development of secondary sexual characters
- Chromosomal analysis reveals 47XXY chromosomal pattern (classic form) or 47XY/47XXY mosaicism.
- *Mental retardation* is seen.
- Plasma FSH, and LH level elevated.
- Plasma testosterone level averages half normal, plasma estradiol level elevated.
- Eunuchoid proportions is seen.

51. **Ans. (a) 47XXY** *(Ref:Robbins 7th/179, 8th/161-2)*
52. **Ans. (a) Trisomy 21** *(Ref: Robbins 7th/179, 8th/165)*
53. **Ans. (b) Patau syndrome** *(Ref: Robbins 7th/177)*
54. **Ans. (d) 21** *(Ref: Robbins 8th/161, 7th/175-176)*
55. **Ans. (b) Turner syndrome** *(Ref: Robbins 8th/165-167, 7th/179)*
56. **Ans. (a) Size, shape and number of chromosome** *(Ref: Robbins 8th/158-159; 7 th/170)*
57. **Ans. (c). Mitral valve prolapse** *(Ref: Robbins 8th/169)*
The patient in question is suffering from **Fragile X Syndrome** which is a familial form of mental retardation with features like lax skin and joints, flat feet, large ears, long narrow face with prominent jaw and nasal bridge and macro-orchidism. *Mitral valve prolapse and aortic root dilatation are the serious complications of this disorder.*

- Aortic regurgitation related to aortic root dilatation and not stenosis (option a) is seen.
- Common congenital cardiac malformations such as atrial septal defect (option b) or ventricular septal defect (option d) may be seen with Down's syndrome and not Fragile X syndrome.

58. **Ans. (a) Mitotic error in early development** *(Ref: Robbins 8th/165-6)*
The patient described in the stem of the question appears to have **Turner syndrome**. The clinical manifestations of this condition are as follows:

Phenotypic features	Urogenital anomalies	Cardiac anomalies	Lymphatic anomalies
*Short stature *Webbed neck *High palate *Low posterior hair line *"Shield" chest *Widely spaced nipples *Short fourth metacarpal	*Primary amenorrhea *"Streak" ovaries *Decreased estrogen and ↑ gonadotropins *Absent secondary sexual characteristics *Horseshoe kidney	*Coarctation of the aorta *Bicuspid aortic valve	*Cystic hygromas *Edema of extremities in neonates

Turner syndrome is genetically heterogeneous. The classic variant of complete monosomy (45, XO) occurs in a minority of patients, with most having **mosaicism**. In the mosaic population, one genetic line contains cells with a normal number of chromosomes (46, XX), while the other genetic line contains cells that are monosomic (45, XO). Both lines originate from a single zygote. While trisomies and non-mosaic monosomies typically result from meiotic non-disjunction, mosaicism arises secondary to mitotic errors after fertilization has taken place.

Sometimes, Turner syndrome individuals have normal karyotype (46 XX) with partial deletion of one or more arms of the X chromosome. This defect is termed "**partial monosomy**".

Other options

- **Trinucleotide repeat expansion** is responsible for diseases like **fragile X syndrome** (CGG repeats), **myotonic dystrophy** (CTG repeats), and **Huntington disease** (CAG repeats).
- **Uniparental disomy** occurs in **Prader-Willi syndrome** (maternal uniparental disomy) and **Angelman syndrome** (paternal uniparental disomy). Uniparental disomy is not associated with Turner syndrome.
- In **balanced form**, a reciprocal (Robertsonian) translocation is **clinically silent** because there is no excess or shortage of genetic material. An **unbalanced trisomy 21** (in which one chromosome 14 contains the long arms of both chromosomes 14 and 21) is responsible for **Down syndrome.**

59. **Ans. is (c) i.e. Mosaicism** *(Ref: Robbins 8th/161)*

Mosaicism is the term used when cells with more than one type of genetic constitution are present in the same organism. The situation in the question uncommonly occurs when nondisjunction of chromosome 21 occurs during mitosis (rather than meiosis) in one of the early cell divisions. The degree to which the individual expresses the characteristics of the syndrome depends on the number of cells involved and their distribution.

Balanced translocation (choice A) does not produce features of any syndrome, because critical genetic material is not lost, although progeny may be affected when the translocated chromosome is added to a complement of otherwise normal chromosomes.

Chiasma (choice B) refers to the "X"-shape of chromosomes undergoing exchange of genetic material in crossover.

Spermiogenesis (choice D) refers to the development of sperm precursors into mature sperm.

60. **Ans. is (d) i.e. 47, XXY** *(Ref: Robbins 8th/165)*

- The testicular changes described are those observed in Klinefelter's syndrome, most often due to 47, XXY genetics.
- Testicular feminization syndrome (choice A) is due to a genetically determined unresponsiveness to testosterone that produces a phenotypic female in an individual with 46, XY chromosomes.
- Trisomy 18 (choice B) is Edwards' syndrome, characterized by facial features that are small and delicate.
- Trisomy 21 (choice C) is the most common trisomy, Down syndrome.

60.1. **Ans. (d) Trisomy 13** *(Ref: Robbins 8/e p162)*

Trisomy 13 is known as **Patau syndrome** characterized by:

- *Mentalretardation, rocker bottom feet and congenital heart defects (VSD and PDA)*
- *Cleft lip/palate*
- *Polydactyly*
- *Microcephaly*
- *Eye defects* (microphthalmia, iris coloboma, cataract, retinal dysplasia)
- *Capillary hemangiomata*

Mnemonic: useful for AIIMS and NEET questions!

- **p** for **P**atau and **p**olydactyly as well as **p**alate defects: Patau syndrome (trisomy 13)
- **Edward syndrome (trisomy 18): e** for **E**dward and **E**xtra occiput (prominent occiput)

60.2. **Ans. (a) Collagen type I** *(Ref: Robbins 8/e p1211-2)*

- *Osteogenesis imperfecta* (or *brittle bone disease*[Q]) is a phenotypically diverse disorder caused by deficiencies in the synthesis of **type 1 collagen**[Q].
- It is the most common inherited disorder of connective tissue.
- It principally affects bone, but also impacts other tissues rich in type 1 collagen (joints, eyes, ears, skin, and teeth). It

is characterized by **bone fragility, hearing loss, blue sclera**^{Q} **and dentinogenesis imperfect**.

- Osteogenesis imperfecta usually results from autosomal dominant mutations in the genes that encode the α1 and α2 chains of collagen.

60.3. Ans. (a) Fibrillin I *(Ref: Robbins 8/e p144)*

- Fibrillin occurs in two homologous forms, fibrillin-1 and fibrillin-2, encoded by two separate genes, *FBN1* and *FBN2* mapped on chromosomes 15q21.1 and 5q23.31, respectively.
- Mutations of *FBN1* (affecting *fibrillin-1*^{Q}) underlie Marfan syndrome
- Mutations of the related *FBN2* gene (*fibrillin-2*^{Q}) are less common, and are associated with *congenital contractural arachnodactyly*, an autosomal dominant disorder characterized by skeletal abnormalities.

60.4. Ans. (b)Metaphase *(Ref: Robbins 8/e p158)*

Revise NEET info!

- Karyotyping is the study of chromosomes
- Chromosomes are arrested in metaphase by Colchicine^Q
- These are then stained by many stains. Most commonly used stain is Giemsa stain^Q, so called G-banding^Q
- The chromosomes are arranged in order of decreasing length^Q. Any alteration in number or structure of chromosomes can be easily detected by karyotyping

60.5. Ans. (c) 45 *(Ref: Robbins 8/e p165)*

Turner syndrome is the *most common cause of sex chromosomal abnormality in the females*. It usually results from complete or partial monosomy of X chromosome and associated with hypogonadism in phenotypic females.^{Q} Patients have the **(45X)** karyotype or may be mosaics.

60.6. Ans. (a) 47 *(Ref: Robbins 8/e p165)*

Klinefelter syndrome is *the most common chromosomal disorder of males associated with hypogonadism and infertility*. It is due to extra-X-chromosome. Classically, it is **47, XXY**. Other variants can have 48 XXXY, rarely 49 XXXY or mosaics can be there with some cells containing normal 46, XY and others 47, XXY.

60.7. Ans. (c) 5mb *(Ref: Encyclopedia of Genetics 3/e p29)*

Karyotype analysis detects both numerical and structural chromosomal aberrations (overall resolution is **5 Mega bases (Mb)**; breakpoint resolution is 5 to 15 Mb).

Table 1: Resolution provided by the various FISH techniques.

FISH technique	Resolution
Metaphase spreads	2-3 Mb
Prometaphase spreads	1 Mb
Mechanically stretched chromosomes	200-3000 kb
Interphase nuclei	50-1000 kb
Fiber FISH	1-300 kb
Mb, megabase = 1000000 base pairs	

60.8. Ans. (b) FISH *(Ref: Robbin 8/e p 179)*

FISH uses DNA probes that *recognize sequences specific to particular chromosomal regions.. (Ref: Robbind 8/e p179* Bacterial artificial chromosomes that span the entire human genome were created. These DNA clones are labeled with fluorescent dyes and applied to metaphase spreads or interphase nuclei. The *probe hybridizes to its homologous genomic sequence and thus labels a specific chromosomal region* that can be visualized under a fluorescent microscope.

Uses and advantages of FISH

- FISH can be performed on prenatal samples (e.g., cells obtained by amniocentesis, chorionic villus biopsy, or umbilical cord blood), peripheral blood lymphocytes, touch preparations from cancer biopsies, and even archival tissue sections.
- FISH has been used for detection of
  - Numeric abnormalities of chromosomes (aneuploidy);
  - For the demonstration of subtle microdeletions or complex translocations not detectable by routine karyotyping;
  - For analysis of gene amplification (e.g., *HER2/NEU* in breast cancer or *N-MYC* amplification in neuroblastomas);
  - For mapping newly isolated genes of interest to their chromosomal loci.
- The ability of FISH to *circumvent the need for dividing cells* is invaluable when a rapid diagnosis is warranted

Genetics

Chromosome painting

It is an extension of FISH, whereby probes are prepared for entire chromosomes.

Limitation of this technique: the number of chromosomes that can be *detected simultaneously* by chromosome painting is limited due to the availability of fluorescent dyes that emit different wavelengths of visible light.

This is overcome by the introduction of **spectral karyotyping** (also called **multicolor FISH**).

Comparative genomic hybridization

It is a method that can be used *only when DNA is available from a specimen of interest*. The entire DNA specimen from the sample of interest is labeled in one color (e.g., green), and the normal control DNA specimen is indicated by another color (e.g., red). These are mixed in equal amounts and hybridized to **normal metaphase** chromosomes.

The red-to-green ratio is analyzed by a computer program that determines where the DNA of interest may have gains or losses of material.

Currently used for detection of **cancer, mutations in mental retardation and the detection of microdeletions.**

60.9. Ans. (b) Isochromosome (*Ref: Robbin 8/e p160, The Principles of Clinical Cytogenetics 3/e p157-8*)

Isochromosome formation results when one arm of a chromosome is lost and the remaining arm is duplicated, resulting in a chromosome consisting of two short arms only or of two long arms.

- An isochromosome has morphologically identical genetic information in both arms.
- **The most common isochromosome** present in live births involves the **long arm of the X.**
- The Xq isochromosome is associated with monosomy for genes on the short arm of X and with trisomy for genes on the long arm of X.
- The reason for the formation of an isochrome is the centromere misdivision. Instead of *dividing longitudinally to separate the two sister chromatids, the centromere undergoes a transverse split that separated the two arms from one another... Principles of clinical cytogenetics*

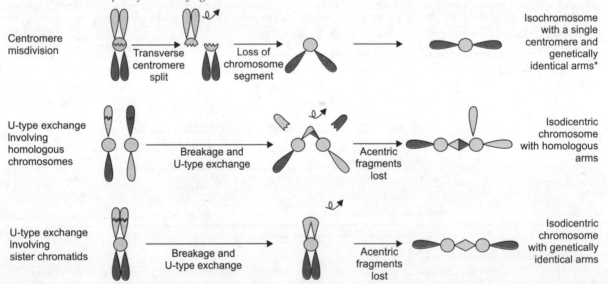

Figure: Some of the mechanism proposed for isochromosome formation. *Because recombination occurs during normal meionic cell division the arms of isochromromosome formed during meiosis would be identical only for markers close to the centromene

Previously asked questions on isochromosome

- **The most common isochromosome** present in live births involves the **long arm of the X** is seen in patient s affected with Turner syndrome.
- Testicular germ cell carcinoma has the presence of **gain of 12p** through **isochromosome formation** or amplification.

61. Ans. (c) Chromosome 17 (*Ref: Robbins 8th/1078, Harrison 17th/563*)

Features	BRCA1	BRCA2
Chromosome	17q21	13q12.3
Function	Tumor suppressor, Transcriptional regulation, Role in DNA repair	Tumor suppressor, Transcriptional regulation, Role in DNA repair

Genetics

Features	BRCA1	BRCA2
Age at onset	Younger age (40s to 50s)	50 years
% Single gene hereditary disorders	52%	32%
Risk of other tumors (varies with specific mutation)	Ovarian, Male breast cancer (lower than BRCA2), Prostate, colon, pancreas	Ovarian, Male breast cancer Prostate, pancreas, stomach, melanoma, colon
Pathology of breast cancers	Greater incidence of medullary carcinomas , poorly differentiated carcinomas, ER-, PR-, and *Her2/neu*-negative carcinomas, carcinomas with *p53* mutations	Similar to sporadic breast cancers

62. **Ans. (c) X-linked Recessive Disorder** *(Ref: Robbins 8th/142)*

Analysis of X linked recessive disorders

Males have an X and a Y chromosome. There is no corresponding locus for a mutant allele of the X chromosome on the Y chromosome. The mutant recessive gene on the X chromosome expresses itself in a *male child* because it is *not suppressed by a normal allele* whereas in the female, the presence of a normal allele on other X-chromosome prevents the expression of the disease so, *females only act as carriers.*[Q]

63. **Ans. (a) Fraction of cells in apoptotic pathways** *(Ref: The journal of Histochemistry & Cytochemistry:Volume 47 (5): 711-717, 1996: Wikipedia)*

In situ DNA nick end – labeling is an in-situ method for detecting areas of DNA which are nicked during apoptosis.

Terminal deoxynucleotidyl transferase mediated dUTP–biotin nick end labeling (TUNEL) is a method for detecting apoptotic cells that exhibit DNA fragmentation.

64. **Ans. (b) 25%** *(Ref: Harrison's 17th/385)*

Achondroplasia is an **autosomal dominant** condition.

Only one mutant allele is enough to cause disease. Thus, AA and Aa will be affected whereas aa will be unaffected. ['A' is mutant allele whereas 'a' is normal].

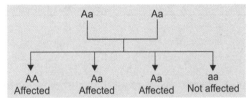

As is clear from the diagram, 3 out of 4, i.e. 75% of children will be affected and 1 out of 4, i.e. 25% children will be unaffected. However, please note that clinically the baby with AA genotype usually donot survive.

65. **Ans. (d) X linked Recessive** *(Ref: Robbins 8th/142)*

Presentation of disease only amongst males identifies the disorder as sex (X) linked. Because carrier mothers are not manifesting the disease, yet their sons do, the disorder can only be recessive. The disorder is thus X– linked recessive.

66. **Ans. (a) X – linked Recessive** *(Ref: Robbins 7th/172, 8th/142)*

The given disease is manifesting only in males, therefore it is sex-linked disease. Females are not affected, so they must be carriers. This is a classical inheritance feature of X-linked recessive disorder.

Remember:

- Male is having XY, i.e. only X-chromosome. So, *even if one mutant allele is present on X-chromosome, it will manifest* (whether recessive or dominant).
- Females are XX, so if one gene is mutated in X-chromosome, female will be phenotypically normal and genotypically carrier, *if inheritance is recessive but female will suffer from disease*, if it is X-linked dominant.
- There is *no sex predilection in autosomal dominant or recessive disorders*.

67. **Ans. (a) None affected, all carriers** *(Ref: Harrison 17/2332)*

Albinism is an autosomal recessive (AR) disorder

- AR disorders express only in homozygous state, i.e. if both alleles are mutant
- If 'A' is normal allele and 'a' is mutant, then the given cross in the question can be made as

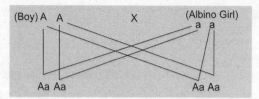

- Thus genotypically all offsprings are carriers and Phenotypically, all of then will be normal.

68. Ans. (a) 0 and 100% *(Ref: Harrison 17th/637)*

Sickle cell anemia is an autosomal recessive disorder.
- Sickle cell disease is the homozygous state of HbS (SS) where S stands for gene coding HbS.
- Sickle cell trait is the heterozygous state of HbS (SA) where A stands for absent gene.
- Normal individual has no gene for HbS (AA)

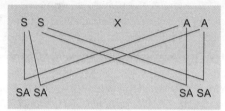

If the mother has sickle cell disease 'SS' and father is normal 'AA' all the offsprings will be 'SA'. Thus % of sickle cell disease (SS) will be zero and that of sickle cell trait (SA) will be 100%.

69. Ans. (a) Blood group O *(Ref: Harrison 17th/708)*
Major blood group system is ABO system. These are based on the presence of antigen on surface of RBCs Four blood groups according to this system are.

Blood Group	Antigen	Anti body (Isoagglutinins)
A	A	Anti – B
B	B	Anti – A
AB	A and B	None
O	None	Anti – A and Anti – B

- The genes that determine A and B phenotypes are found on chromosome 9p and are expressed in a Mendelian co-dominant manner.
- AB group is universal recipient (No antibody) and Blood group O is universal donor (No antigen)
- Blood group according to alleles can be

A	AA or Ai
B	BB or Bi
AB	AB
O	ii

[i means allele containing gene for no antigen]
- In the given question, father is blood group B [i.e. BB or Bi] and mother is AB. The cross can be

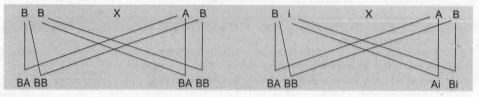

- Thus, phenotypically blood group can be A (Ai), B (Bi, BB) or AB (AB). Thus, none of the children can have O blood group.

70. Ans. (d) All of the above *(Ref: Harrison 17th/420, 18th/547-551)*
Gene transfer is a novel area of therapeutics in which the active agent is a nucleic acid sequence rather than a protein or small molecule. Most gene transfers are carried out using a vector or gene delivery vehicle because delivery of naked DNA

Genetics

or RNA to a cell is an inefficient process. More clear-cut success has been achieved in a gene therapy trial for another form of SCID, adenosine deaminase (ADA) deficiency. Other diseases likely to be amenable to transduction of hemaopietic stem cells (HSCs) include
- Wiskott-Aldrich syndrome
- Chronic granulomatous disease
- Sickle cell disease
- Thalassemia.

Clinical trials using recombinant adeno-associated vectors are now ongoing for muscular dystrophies, alpha-1 antitrypsin deficiency, lipoprotein lipase deficiency, hemophilia B, and a form of congenital blindness called Leber's congenital amaurosis.

71. Ans. (b) Chromosome 6 *(Ref: Harrison 17th/2045)*
- The human major histocompatibility complex (MHC), commonly called the human leukocyte antigen (HLA) complex, is a 4-megabase (Mb) region on chromosome 6 (6p21.3)[Q] that is densely packed with expressed genes.

72. Ans. (c) 21 *(Ref: Harrison 17th/644)*
Folate cofactors are one-carbon donors essential for the biosynthesis of purines and thymidylate. Mammalian cells are devoid of folate biosynthesis and are therefore folate auxotrophs that take up folate vitamins primarily via the reduced folate carrier (RFC). The gene for RFC is located on chromosome 21.

73. Ans. (c) Trans differentiation *(Ref: Robbins 7th/92 & Harrison 17th/426)*
Stem cell is defined as a cell with a unique capacity to produce unaltered daughter cells (*self-renewal*) and to generate specialized cell types (*potency*).
The prevailing paradigm in developmental biology is that once cells are differentiated, their phenotypes are stable. However, tissue stem cells, which are thought to be lineage-committed multipotent cells, possess the capacity to differentiate into cell types outside their lineage restrictions (called **trans-differentiation** or **stem cell plasticity**). For example, hematopoietic stem cells may be converted into neurons as well as germ cells.

74. Ans. (b) 25% *(Ref: Robbins 8th/141, 7th/151)*
Achondroplasia is an autosomal dominant disease.

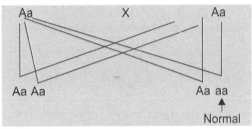

So, only 1 out of 4 children will be unaffected, i.e. 25% of children will be normal.

75. Ans. (c) Parallel rays of tubular structure in lysosomes *(Ref: Robbin 8th/152-153)*
- **PAS stain** is a widely used stain which gives positive reaction with glycogen (primarily) and non glycogen substances like glycoprotein, glycolipids, proteoglycans and neutral mucins.
- Whether the PAS positivity of a particular cell is due to presence of glycogen or due to latter can be differentiated with diastase (glycogen digesting enzyme).
- If the cell is PAS positive due to glycogen, the pretreatment with diastase will make it PAS negative. But if the cell is PAS positive due to non glycogen substances, the cell will retain its PAS positivity even after pretreatment with diastase. So, in the given question, the presence of PAS positive and diastase resistant material indicates presence of non glycogen substances.
- The clinical feature of delayed milestones and hepatosplenomegaly in 1 year old boy is suggestive of some lysosomal storage disorder (like Niemann Picks disease).
- This disease is characterized by the presence of large foam cells in bone marrow, liver and spleen. There is presence of pleomorphic inclusion of lipids in lysosomes enclosed in concentric or parallel lamellae.

76. Ans. (b) Homeobox gene *(Ref: Robbins 8th/452-3, 7th/305, 475)*
Classes of genes known to be important in normal morphogenesis during development include

- **Homeobox genes (HOX):** *The HOX genes have been implicated in the patterning of limbs, vertebrae, and craniofacial structures. HOX genes possess retinoic acid response elements (RAREs), and that the latter are required for mediating both physiologic and pathologic effects of retinoids during development.* Mutations of *HOXD13* cause *synpolydactyly* (extra digits) in heterozygous individuals and mutations of *HOXA13* cause *hand-foot-genital syndrome*, characterized by distal limb and distal urinary tract malformations.

- **PAX genes:** *PAX* genes are characterized by a 384 base pair sequence — the *paired box*. They code for DNA-binding proteins that are believed to function as transcription factors. In contrast to *HOX* genes, however, their expression patterns suggest that they act singly, rather than in a temporal or spatial combination.

- Mutation in **PAX3** causes **Waardenburg syndrome** (congenital pigment abnormalities and deafness).
- Mutation in **PAX6** causes **Aniridia** (congenital absence of the iris)
- **PAX2** mutations cause the "**renal-coloboma**" syndrome (developmental defects of the kidneys, eyes, ears, and brain).
- Translocations involving **PAX3** and **PAX7** are seen in **alveolar rhabdomyosarcomas**.
- Translocations involving **PAX5** are seen in subsets of **lymphomas**
- Translocations involving **PAX8** are seen in **thyroid cancers**.

Other options
FMR gene: It is involved in fragile X-syndrome.
PTEN gene: located on chromosome 10q is associated with endometrial cancers and glioblastoma.(phosphatase and tensin homologue)
p16 blocks cell cycle and is a tumor suppressor gene.

77. **Ans. (c) AB, Rh negative (Too obvious to explain friends)**

78. **Ans. (b) Splicing; (d) Frame-shift:** *(Ref: Harper' 27th/415, Robbins 8th/648-9)*
Important causes of thalassemia are:

β-**thalassemia:** A wide variety of mutations in β-globin gene may cause this including
• Promoter region mutations
• Chain terminator mutations include frameshift mutations.
• Splicing mutations
β^0-thalassemia, associated with total absence of β-globin chains in the homozygous state. Its commonest cause is chain termination.
β$^+$-**thalassemia**, characterized by reduced (but detectable) β-globin synthesis in the homozygous state. Its commonest cause is **splicing mutation**.
α-thalassemia: Mutations in α-globin gene are mainly unequal crossing over and large deletions and less commonly nonsense and Frame-shift mutations.

79. **Ans. (a) Bloom syndrome; (b) Fanconi's anemia; (d) Chediak Higashi syndrome; (e) Ataxia telangiectasia** *(Ref: Harrison 16th/643, 631, Robbins 7th/307)*
Bloom's syndrome, Fanconi anemia, Klinefelter syndrome, Ataxia telangiectasia and Kostman syndrome are associated with myeloid leukemia.

80. **Ans. (c) Loss of normal allele in mutant gene** *(Ref: Robbins 7th/299)*

"A child with inherited mutant RB allele in somatic cells is perfectly normal. Because such a child is a heterozygous at the Rb locus, it implies that heterozygosity for the Rb gene does not affect cell behavior. Cancer develops when the cell becomes homozygous for the mutant allele or in other words when the cell loses heterozygosity for the normal Rb gene (a condition known as LOH loss of heterozygosity)"

Thus, from these lines we interpret that loss of heterozygosity means loss of normal allele in mutant gene.

81. **Ans. (b) q and p** *(Ref: Robbins 6th/166, 7th/171)*
- Short arm of a chromosome is designated 'p' (for petit) and long arm is referred to as 'q'
- In a banded karyotype, each arm of the chromosome is divided into two or more regions by prominent bands.

- The regions are numbered (e.g. 1, 2, 3) from centromere outwards.
- Each region is further subdivided into bands and sub bands and these are ordered numerically as well.
- Thus, the notation Xp 21.2 refers to a chromosomal segment located on the short arm of the 'x' chromosome, in region 2, band 1 and sub band 2.

82. **Ans. (c) 7** *(Ref: Robbins 8th/465; 7th/490)*

Genetics

83. **Ans. (b) Granulosa cell tumor** *(Ref: Robbins 8th/1338; 7 th/1099)*

84. **Ans. (a) The banding pattern** *(Ref: Harrison 18th/521)*
   Banding patterns are analyzed in DNA fingerprinting to see if they match with the control specimen. Four bases i.e. guanine, adenine, cytosine, and thymine (uracil is substituted for thymine in RNA) are responsible for making the genetic code. A sequence of three of these bases forms the **triplet code** used in transmitting the genetic information needed for protein synthesis. The small variation in gene sequence (called as a **haplotype**) is thought to account for the individual differences in physical traits, behaviors, and disease susceptibility. Chromosomes contain all the genetic content of the genome.

85. **Ans. (e) III – 8** *(Ref: Robbins 7th/151- 152)*
   - Hemophilia. A is X-linked recessive disorder. It will be manifested in female having both the mutant alleles ($X^h X^h$) whereas X^hX will be carrier. On the other hand, in males, even one mutant gene will express, i.e. X^hY will be affected male
   - In the given pedigree, I-1 and I-2, both are unaffected, therefore male should be normal (xy) and female should be carrier (X^hX)
   - Now, if we see the inheritance, it will be

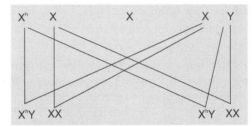

   - Therefore, half of the daughters are carrier and half are normal whereas half of males are normal whereas other half are affected.
   - In the given pedigree, II -5 (male) should be normal whereas II-2 (male) is affected. Females (II-3 and II-6) can be normal or carriers.
   - The affected male (X^hY), transmits the mutant genes to females only and not to males. Therefore, in the given pedigree, III-1, 2 will be normal. Females should be homozygous (X^hX^h) to manifest the disease, therefore III-3 and III-4 should be carriers.
   - As II-5 is a normal male, its progeny should be normal, if it is married to normal female (II-4). Thus, III-5, 6 and 7 should be normal
   - II-6 is a carrier female and therefore it will transmit the disease to sons. Thus, III-8 and III-9 have maximum risk of being affected by Hemophilia A.

86. **Ans. (e) Mitochondrial** *(Ref: Robbins 7th/33, 185, 1341-1342)*
   - In mitochondrial inheritance, mothers transmit the entire mitochondrial DNA to both male and female offspring, but only the daughters transmit it further. No transmission occurs through males.

87. **Ans. is (d) i.e. Patient D** *Read explanation below*
   Patient D is the mother of identical (monozygotic) twins. The chorion forms before the amnion, so the possible combinations are
   - Monoamnionic and monochorionic;
   - **Diamnionic and monochorionic; and**
   - **Diamnionic and dichorionic (either fused or separated).**
   The first two of these possibilities are seen only in identical twins. However, the latter can be seen either in fraternal or identical twins. Very early separation produces completely separate membranes with duplication of both chorion and amnion; somewhat later separation produces one chorion and two amnions; and very late separation produces one chorion and one amnion. A dichorionic, diamnionic placenta develops if splitting occurs early after fertilization, before the chorion forms. This type of placenta may occur with either monozygotic or dizygotic twins. Thus, we are unable to determine whether Patient A (choice A) or Patient B (choice B) had identical twins from the examination of the placentas. Patient C (choice C) did not have a twin pregnancy.

87.1. Ans. (a) 50% of boys of carrier mother are affected *(Ref: Robbins 8/e p142)*

Looking at the statements one by one:

- Carrier mother contributes to the transfer of one of the two boys getting the affected chromosome. So, 50% of boys of carrier mother are affected.
- Option "**b**"...All girls having diseased father are affected as carriers because they get the affected 'X' sperm from their fathers. However, these girls are not going to manifest the disease.
- Option "**c**"...fathers cannot transmit the disease to their sons as they transmit just the "Y" chromosome to them whereas the disease is "X" linked.
- Option "**d**"... mothers contribute to just one "X" chromosome and so, 50% of the daughters would become carriers if t other was a carrier.

87.2 Ans. (c) Chromosome 11 *(Ref: Robbins 8/e p479-80)*

Easiest way to remember that info..... count the number of letters in Wilms tumour..yea it is exactly 11...the location of both genes associated with Wilms tumour ☺

So, the two genes associated with Wilms tumour **WT1** gene (located on **chr 11p13**)and WT2 gene (located on **chr 11p15**).

87.3. Ans. (c) X-linked dominant disease *(Ref: Robbins 8/e p142)*

Since a male transmits only the 'Y' chromosome to his son, so obviously he cannot transmit any X linked disease.

87.4. Ans. (a) Study of multiple genes *(Ref: Robbins 8/e p174)*

Microarrays are gene chips used to **sequence genes or portions of genes.**In this technique, short sequences of DNA (oligonucleotides) that are complementary to the wild-type sequence and to known mutations are "tiled" adjacent to each other on the gene chip, and the DNA sample to be tested is hybridized to the array. Before hybridization the sample is labeled with fluorescent dyes. The hybridization (and consequently, the fluorescent signal emitted) will be strongest at the oligonucleotide that is complementary to wild-type sequence if no mutations are present, while the presence of a mutation will cause hybridization to occur at the complementary mutant oligonucleotide.

87.5. Ans. (a) Northern blot

•	Northern Blot	: **RNA** → North :	Roti
•	Southern Blot	: **DNA** → South :	Dosa
•	Western Blot	: **Proteins** → West :	Poha/Pizaa

87.6. Ans. (b) Rh-ve mother with 2nd Rh+ve child

- Rh-ve mother with 2nd Rh+ve child can result in the development of **hemolytic disease of newborn** or **erythroblastosis fetalis**. So, it is a dangerous condition.
- This condition is a **type II hypersensitivity** reaction.
- *This is Not to be confused with Hemorrhagic disease of the newborn* which is a coagulation disturbance in the newborns due to vitamin K deficiency. As a consequence of vitamin K deficiency there is an impaired production of coagulation factors II, VII, IX, X, C and S by the liver.

87.7. Ans. (d) 7 *(Ref: Robbins 9/e p466)*

87.8. Ans. (d) Pseudomonas *(Ref: Robbins 9/e p469)*

Pseudomonas aeruginosa species, in particular, colonize the lower respiratory tract, first intermittently and then chronically.

GOLDEN POINTS FOR QUICK REVISION / UPDATED INFORMATION FROM 9TH EDITION OF ROBBINS

(GENETICS)

- **Autosomal dominant disorders** are characterized by expression in heterozygous state; they affect males and females equally, and both sexes can transmit the disorder. It affects receptors and structural proteins.
- **Autosomal recessive diseases** occur when both copies of a gene are mutated; enzyme proteins are frequently involved. Males and females are affected equally.
- **X-linked disorders** are transmitted by heterozygous females to their sons, who manifest the disease. Female carriers usually are protected because of random inactivation of one X chromosome.
- **DiGeorge syndrome** (thymic hypoplasia with diminished T-cell immunity and parathyroid hypoplasia with hypocalcemia) and **Velocardiofacial** syndrome (congenital heart disease involving outflow tracts, facial dysmorphism, and developmental delay)

Genetics

- **Genomic Imprinting:** Imprinting involves transcriptional silencing of the paternal or maternal copies of certain genes during gametogenesis. For such genes, only one functional copy exists in the individual. Loss of the functional (not imprinted) allele by deletion gives rise to diseases. These disorders are also called as the *parent-of-origin* effects on gene function.
- In **Prader- Willi syndrome,** deletion of band q12 on long arm of paternal chromosome 15 occurs. Genes in this region of maternal chromosome 15 are imprinted so there is complete loss of their functions. Patients have mental retardation, short stature, hypotonia, hyperphagia, small hands and feet, and hypogonadism.
- In **Angelman syndrome** there is deletion of the same region from the maternal chromosome. Since genes on the corresponding region of paternal chromosome 15 are imprinted, these patients have mental retardation, ataxia, seizures, and inappropriate laughter.
- Inheritance of both chromosomes of a pair from one parent is called *uniparental disomy*. Angelman syndrome can also result from uniparental disomy of paternal chromosome 15.

NOTES

CHAPTER 5

Neoplasia

NEOPLASIA

Neoplasia refers to the process of new growth. The important feature of the growth associated with neoplasms is the fact that it is an uncoordinated growth of the tissue persisting even after the cessation of the stimulus which evoked the change. Oncology is the study of tumors or neoplasms. The tumors are usually composed of the:
1. Parenchyma – Made up of proliferating neoplastic cells
2. Stroma – Made up of connective tissue and blood vessels.

Benign Tumors

These are usually denoted by adding a suffix "- oma" to the cell of origin, so, these may be arising from fibroblastic cells (fibroma); cartilage cells (chondroma) or osteoblasts (osteoma). Adenoma and Papilloma are examples of benign tumors.

MALIGNANT TUMORS

Cancer is a generalized term used for all malignant tumors. These tumors can be of the following types:
1. **Sarcoma** - Arising from mesenchymal tissue.
2. **Carcinoma** – Tumor of epithelial cell origin derived from any germ layer. If this tumor is having a glandular pattern, it is called adenocarcinoma.

The divergent differentiation of parenchymal cells produces mixed tumors or pleomorphic tumors.

In teratoma, parenchymal cells are made up from more than one germ layer e.g. Dermoid cyst.

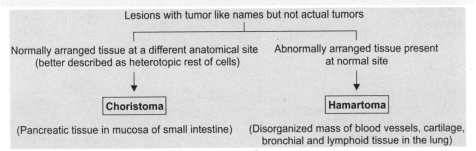

Lesions with tumor like names but not actual tumors

Normally arranged tissue at a different anatomical site (better described as heterotopic rest of cells) → **Choristoma** (Pancreatic tissue in mucosa of small intestine)

Abnormally arranged tissue present at normal site → **Hamartoma** (Disorganized mass of blood vessels, cartilage, bronchial and lymphoid tissue in the lung)

Characteristics of Neoplasia

I. **Anaplasia**: This is the hallmark of malignant transformation. The extent to which neoplastic cells resemble normal cells both morphologically and functionally is called differentiation. An *absence of differentiation* is called anaplasia.
The features of anaplasia are:
1. *Pleomorphism* – It is the variation in the size and shape of the cells.
2. *Hyperchromasia* – Increased nuclear material or DNA is responsible for dark staining of the cells called hyperchromasia. In normal cells, the nuclear cytoplasmic (or N: C) ratio is 1:4 whereas it becomes 1: 1 in anaplastic cells.
3. *Increased mitosis* gives rise to atypical bizarre mitotic figures.
4. *Loss of polarity* due to disturbed orientation of anaplastic cells.
5. Presence of tumor giant cells having big hyperchromatic nuclei.

Concept

Desmoplasia is a term used for stimulation of abundant collagenous stroma by the parenchymal cells.

Adenoma – Benign epithelial tumor arising from glands or forming a *glandular pattern*
Papilloma – Benign tumor with *finger–like projections*
Polyp – Tumor producing a visible projection above a mucosal surface protruding in the lumen.

Teratoma is derived from *ectoderm, endoderm* and *mesoderm*.

Choristoma - lesion with **normal differentiation** but **abnormal site**.

Hamartoma - lesion with **abnormal differentiation** but **normal site**.

Anaplasia is the hallmark of malignant transformation.

Concept of dysplasia

- Dysplasia is characterized by the abnormal proliferation of the cells which also exhibit pleomorphism. It is not cancer but can give rise to cancer as it is a preneoplastic lesion.
- When dysplastic changes involve entire thickness of the epithelium but the lesion remains confined to the normal tissue, it is called *carcinoma in situ*. When the cancer cells move beyond the normal tissue, it is said to be invasive.

Dysplasia is a *partially reversible* condition having **intact basement membrane**.

Key differentiating features between Metaplasia, Dysplasia and Anaplasia

Feature	Metaplasia	Dysplasia	Anaplasia
Definition	Reversible change in which one differentiated cell type (epithelial or mesenchymal) is replaced by another cell type	A change having loss in the uniformity of the individual cells and loss of architectural orientation	An *absence of differentiation* (extent to which neoplastic cells resemble normal cells both morphologically and functionally)
Pleomorphism (variation in the size and shape of cells/nuclei)	Absent	**Present**[Q] in low grade	**Present**[Q] in high grade
Reversibility	Reversible[Q]	**Reversible in early stages** (irreversible if whole epithelium is involved)	Irreversible[Q]
N:C ratio	Normal (1:4)	Increased (↑)	Increased (↑↑↑)
Hyperchromatism	Absent	Present (small degree)	Present (high degree)
Mitotic figures	Absent/minimal at normal places	**Typical mitotic figures**[Q] present at abnormal places	**Atypical mitotic figures**[Q] (multipolar spindles) present at abnormal places
Other features (Tumor giant cells[Q], hemorrhage, necrosis)	Absent	Absent	Present[Q]
Example	Barret's esophagus, myositis ossificans	Cervical dysplasia of squamous cells	Carcinoma of the cervix, carcinoma esophagus

Concept

When dysplastic changes involve entire thickness of the epithelium but the lesion remains confined to the normal tissue, it is called **carcinoma in situ**.

Malignant tumors have *upregulation of telomerase activity*.

Usually, **10⁹ cells** produce a clinically detectable tumor.

Almost all cancers can metastasize *except* **glioma** (malignancy of central nervous system) and the **rodent ulcer** (or **basal cell cancer** of the skin).

II. **Rate of growth:** The growth of a tumor correlates with the level of differentiation. Well-differentiated tumors have a slow proliferation rate. Recently, cancer stem cells or tumor-initiating cells (*T-ICs*) have been identified in breast cancer, glioblastoma multiforme (a brain tumor), and acute myeloid leukemia. These T-ICs are cells that allow a human tumor to grow and maintain itself definitely when transplanted into an immunodeficient mouse.

III. **Local invasion:** It is the second most reliable feature that differentiates malignant from benign tumors. The benign tumors are slow growing, cohesive, expansile masses that are usually capsulated. The malignant tumors show invasion, infiltration and destruction of the surrounding tissue.

IV. **Metastasis:** It is the *most reliable feature* of a malignant tumor, characterized by the spread of the tumor to other parts because of penetration into blood vessels, lymphatics and the body cavities.

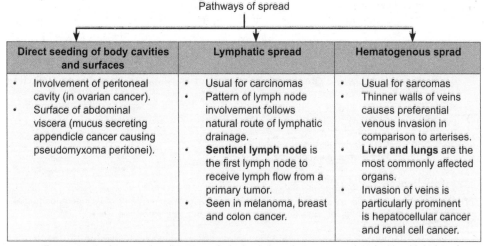

Pathways of spread

Direct seeding of body cavities and surfaces	Lymphatic spread	Hematogenous sprad
• Involvement of peritoneal cavity (in ovarian cancer). • Surface of abdominal viscera (mucus secreting appendicle cancer causing pseudomyxoma peritonei).	• Usual for carcinomas • Pattern of lymph node involvement follows natural route of lymphatic drainage. • **Sentinel lymph node** is the first lymph node to receive lymph flow from a primary tumor. • Seen in melanoma, breast and colon cancer.	• Usual for sarcomas • Thinner walls of veins causes preferential venous invasion in comparison to arterises. • **Liver and lungs** are the most commonly affected organs. • Invasion of veins is particularly prominent is hepatocellular cancer and renal cell cancer.

Sentinel lymph node is useful for **breast cancer, malignant melanoma** and **vulval cancer**.

Precursor lesions are localized morphologic change that are associated with a high risk of cancer. They can be of the following subtypes:

Precursor Lesions

With inflammation	Without inflammation	Benign tumors with malignant transformation
• Barret Esophagus due to chronic reflux disease • Squamous metaplasia of bronchus due to smoking • Colonic metaplasia in stomach due to pernicious anemia	• Endometrial hyperplasia • Leukoplakia of the oral cavity/penis/vulva	• Colonic villous adenoma

Concept

Monoclonality of tumors is assesed by ithe analysis of methylation patterns adjacent to the highly polymorphic locus of the human androgen receptor gene (**HUMARA**)and enzymes like glucose-6-phosphate dehydrogenase (**G6PD**), *iduronate-2-sulfatase* and *phosphoglycerate kinase*.

MONOCLONALITY OF TUMORS

- Most of the cancers arise from single clone of the cells (monoclonal in nature) by genetic transformation or mutation whereas non neoplastic proliferations are coming from multiple cells (polyclonal in nature). *Clonality of tumors can be assessed in women who are heterozygous for polymorphic X-linked markers because random X inactivation results in all females being mosaics with two cell populations.* **So, normally all females will be having both isoforms of the enzymes whereas malignant transformation results in a single marker being expressed**.
- For tumors with a specific translocation, such as in myeloid leukemias, the presence of the translocation can be used to assess clonality. **Immunoglobulin receptor** and *T-cell receptor* gene rearrangements serve as markers of clonality in **B**- and *T-cell lymphomas*, respectively.

m

For Autosomal dominant cancer syndrome, just remember the line:
Very Rich, Cute and Nice Men Hereditarily Like Familiar Females

GENETIC PREDISPOSITION TO CANCER/INHERITED CANCER SYNDROMES

I. **Autosomal dominant cancer syndrome**
   - Inheritance of a single mutant gene increases the risk of development of cancer.
   - Can be remembered as

Very	- Von Hippel Lindau (VHL) syndrome causing renal cell cancer
Rich	- Retinoblastoma
Cute and	- Cowden syndrome (PTEN gene)
Nice	- Neurofibromatosis 1, 2; Nevoid basal cell cancer syndrome
Men	- Melanoma: MEN (Multiple Endocrine Neoplasia) 1 and 2
Hereditarily	- Hereditary nonpolyposis colon cancer
Like	- Li-Fraumeni syndrome, LKB1 gene in Peutz Jeghers syndrome
Familiar	- Familial adenomatous polyposis
Females	- ovarian and breast tumor (will occur is **females** obviously)

Concept

Hereditary non polyposis colon cancer (**HNPCC**) is an **autosomal dominant** condition caused by *defective DNA repair* genes. All others are conditions associated with defective DNA repair genes are autosomal recessive.

Neoplasia

135

II. **Familial cancers**
   – These are cancers occurring at high frequency in families *without a clear defined pattern of transmission.* These usually show early age of onset and are present is 2 or more close relatives of the index case.
   – Include cancer of colon, ovary, breast, pancreas, etc.
III. **Autosomal recessive cancer syndrome (all of these are caused due to Defective DNA Repair)**

Big	-	**B**loom syndrome
F	-	**F**anconi anemia
A	-	**A**taxia telangiectasia
X	-	**X**eroderma pigmentosum

(mnemonic: - Big FAX)

Precancerous conditions are non- neoplastic conditions associated with cancer include endometrial hyperplasia, chronic gastritis, leukoplakia, ulcerative colitis and solar keratosis, etc.

> PET scanning requires the injection of **18 fluoro-deoxy-glucose** (18-FDG)

The seven fundamental changes in cell physiology that together determine the malignant phenotype are:
1. Self-sufficiency in growth signals: Due to oncogene activation
2. Insensitivity to growth-inhibitory signals
3. Evasion of apoptosis: Presence of resistance to apoptosis
4. Limitless replicative potential: Presence of unrestricted proliferative capacity due to telomerase activity
5. Development of sustained angiogenesis
6. Ability to invade and metastasize
7. Genomic instability resulting from defects in DNA repair

> *S phase* is characterized by doubling of the nuclear material. It is a *point of no return* in the cell cycle

The *eighth hallmark effect* is called **Warburg effect** or *aerobic glycolysis.* It is the shifting of glucose metabolism by *the cancer cells from the efficient mitochondria to glycolysis. This increases the glucose requirement of the tumor cells and is used for PET scanning in which we inject 18F-fluorodeoxyglucose which is preferentially taken by actively dividing tumor cells and hence, we make a diagnosis.*

CELL CYCLE AND CONTROL MECHANISMS

> Cyclin D is the **first cyclin** to increase in the cell cycle.

- Cell cycle consists of five phases. These include:

G_1	:	Pre-synthetic phase
S	:	Synthetic phase (DNA synthesis)
G_2	:	Post-synthetic pre-mitotic phase
M	:	Mitotic phase: Cells divide and produce new cells, which either directly re-enter next cycle or pass into non- proliferative G_0 phase
G_0	:	Quiescent state: Cells in this state remain quiescent for variable periods, but can be recruited in cell cycle if stimulated later.

- Resting (non-dividing) cells are in the G_0 stage of the cell cycle and must enter G_1 stage for replication. *The orderly progression of cells through the various phases of cell cycle is controlled by cyclins and cyclin-dependent kinases (CDKs), and by their inhibitors.*

> The **phosphorylation of** RB is a **molecular ON-OFF switch** for the cell cycle.

- CDKs are expressed constitutively during the cell cycle but in an inactive form whereas cyclins are synthesized during specific phases of the cell cycle, and their function is to activate the CDKs.
- Cyclins D, E, A, and B appear sequentially during the cell cycle and bind to one or more CDKs.

> The **initiation of DNA replication** involve the formation of an active complex between **cyclin E** and **CDK2**.

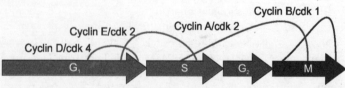

- During the G_1 phase of the cell cycle, cyclin D binds to and activates CDK4, forming a *cyclin D-CDK4 complex*. This complex has a critical role in the cell cycle by

Neoplasia

phosphorylating the retinoblastoma susceptibility protein (RB). *The phosphorylation of RB is a molecular ON-OFF switch for the cell cycle.* In its hypophosphorylated state, RB prevents cells from replicating by forming a tight, inactive complex with the transcription factor E2F. Phosphorylation of RB dissociates the complex and results in activation of E2F. *Thus, phosphorylation of RB eliminates the main barrier to cell-cycle progression and promotes cell replication.* Activated E2F results in transcription of target genes essential for progression through the S phase. These include cyclin E, DNA polymerases, thymidine kinase, dihydrofolate reductase, and several others.

- *Further progression through the S phase and the initiation of DNA replication involve the formation of an active complex between cyclin E and CDK2.* The next decision point in the cell cycle is the G_2/M transition. This transition is initiated by the E2F-mediated transcription of cyclin A, which forms the cyclin A-CDK2 complex that regulates events at the mitotic prophase. The main mediator that propels the cell beyond prophase is the cyclin B-CDK1 complex, which is activated by a *protein phosphatase (Cdc 25)*. Cyclin B-CDK1 activation causes the breakdown of the nuclear envelope and initiates mitosis.

> The main mediator that propels the cell **beyond prophase** is the **cyclin B-CDK1 complex**.

- Complexes of CDKs with cyclins A and B regulate some critical events at the G_2/M transition, such as the decrease in microtubule stability, the separation of centrosomes, and chromosome condensation. Exit from mitosis requires the inactivation of cyclin B-CDK1.

Cell-Cycle Inhibitors

The activity of cyclin-CDK complexes is tightly regulated by inhibitors, called CDK inhibitors. There are two main classes of CDK inhibitors: *the Cip/Kip and the INK4/ARF families.*

- *The Cip/Kip family* has three components, p21, p27, and p57, which bind to and inactivate the complexes formed between cyclins and CDKs. Transcriptional activation of p21 is under the control of *p53*

> G_1/S check-point is controlled by **p53** whereas G_2/M check-point has both p53 dependent as well independent mechanisms.

- The *human INK4a/ARF locus* (a notation for "*in*hibitor of *k*inase *4/a*lternative *r*eading *f*rame") encodes two proteins, p16INK4a and p14ARF, which block the cell cycle and act as tumor suppressors. p16INK4a competes with cyclin D for binding to CDK4 and inhibits the ability of the cyclin D-CDK4 complex to phosphorylate RB, thus causing cell-cycle arrest at late G_1 whereas p14ARF prevents p53 degradation.

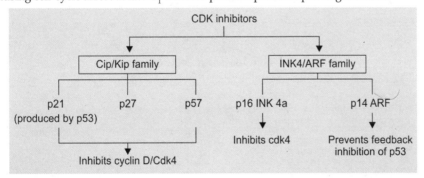

Cell-Cycle Checkpoints

The cell cycle has its own internal controls, called *checkpoints*. There are two main checkpoints, one at the G_1/S transition and another at G_2/M.

- The S phase is the point of no return in the cell cycle, and before a cell makes the final commitment to replicate, the **G1/S checkpoint** checks for DNA damage. If DNA damage is present, the DNA repair machinery and mechanisms that arrest the cell cycle are put in motion. The delay in cell-cycle progression provides the time needed for DNA repair; if the damage is not repairable, apoptotic pathways are activated to kill the cell. Thus, the G_1/S checkpoint prevents the replication of cells that have defects in DNA, which would be perpetuated as mutations or chromosomal breaks in the progeny of the cell.

Cells damaged by **ionizing radiation** activate the **G$_2$/M checkpoint** and arrest in G$_2$; defects in this checkpoint give rise to chromosomal abnormalities.

Proteins of the **RAD** and ataxia telangiectasia mutated **(ATM)** families act as **sensors**. Proteins of the **CHK kinase** families act as *transducers*.

p53 is called as "**guardian of the genome.**"

Prophase: The **chromatin is condensing** into chromosomes.

Metaphase: chromosomes **align at the metaphase plate**.

Anaphase: The **chromosomes split** and the kinetochore microtubules shorten.

Telophase: the **decondensing chromosomes** are surrounded by nuclear membranes.

- DNA damaged after its replication can still be repaired as long as the chromatids have not separated. The **G$_2$/M checkpoint** monitors the completion of DNA replication and checks whether the cell can safely initiate mitosis and separate sister chromatids. This checkpoint is particularly important in cells exposed to ionizing radiation.
- To function properly, cell-cycle checkpoints require sensors of DNA damage, signal transducers, and effector molecules. The sensors and transducers of DNA damage appear to be similar for the G$_1$/S and G$_2$/M checkpoints. The checkpoint effector molecules differ, depending on the cell-cycle stage at which they act. In the G$_1$/S checkpoint, cell-cycle arrest is mostly mediated through p53, which induces the cell-cycle inhibitor p21. Arrest of the cell cycle by the G$_2$/M checkpoint involves both p53-dependent (via cyclin A/cdK-2) and independent (via cdc 25) mechanisms.
- *p53 links cell damage with DNA repair, cell-cycle arrest, and apoptosis. In response to DNA damage, it is phosphorylated by genes that sense the damage and are involved in DNA repair. p53 assists in DNA repair by causing G1 arrest and inducing DNA repair genes. A cell with damaged DNA that cannot be repaired is directed by p53 to undergo apoptosis. With homozygous loss of p53, DNA damage goes unrepaired and mutations increase the chances of malignant transformation.*

Regulation of Cell Cycle

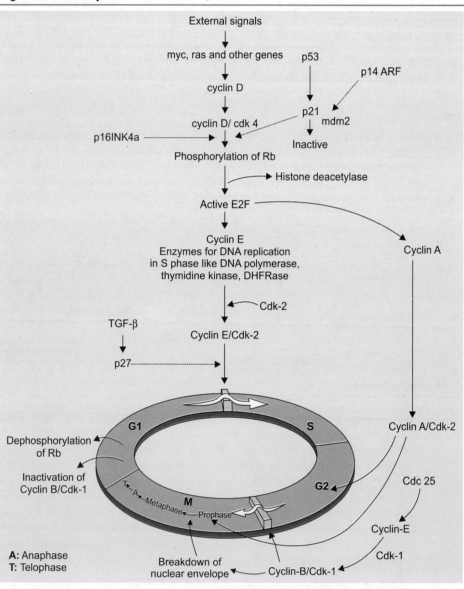

A: Anaphase
T: Telophase

CARCINOGENESIS

It is a multi-step process which requires accumulation of multiple genetic changes either as germline or somatic mutations. The following four are the principal targets of genetic damage:

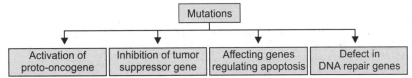

I. **Proto-Oncogenes**

Proto-oncogenes (Normal genes required for cell proliferation and differentiation)

Oncogenes (Genes promoting autonomous cell growth in cancer cells)

Oncoproteins (Proteins lacking regulatory control and responsible for promoting cell growth)

> **Proto-oncogenes** were discovered by **Harold Varmus** and **Michael Bishop**.

> The non receptor excessive tyrosine kinase activity associated with **CML** is countered by a *specific tyosine kinase inhibitor* drug called **imatinib**. This is an example of targeted drug therapy

Selected Oncogenes, their mode of activation and associated human tumors			
Category	**Proto-oncogenes**	**Mode of activation**	**Associated human tumor**
Growth factors			
PDGF-β chain	SIS	Overexpression	Astrocytoma Osteosarcoma
Fibroblast growth factors	HST-1 INT-2	Overexpression Amplification	Stomach cancer Bladder cancer Breast cancer Melanoma
TGF-α	TGFA	Overexpression	Astrocytomas Hepatocellular carcinomas
HGF	HGF	Overexpression	Thyroid cancer
Growth factor: Receptors			
EGF-receptor family	ERB-B1 (EGFR) ERB-B2	Overexpression Amplification	Squamous cell carcinomas of lung, gliomas Breast and ovarian cancers
CSF-1 receptor	FMS	Point mutation	Leukemia
Receptor for neurotrophic factors	RET	Point mutation	Multiple endocrine neoplasia 2A and B, familial medullary thyroid carcinomas
PDGF receptors	PDGF-R	Overexpression	Gliomas
Receptor for stem cell (steel factor)	KIT	Point mutation	Gastrointestinal stromal tumors and other soft tissue tumors
Proteins involved in signal transduction			
GTP-binding	K-RAS H-RAS N-RAS	Point mutation Point mutation Point mutation	Colon, lung and pancreatic tumors Bladder and kidney tumors Melanomas, hematologic malignancies
Non-receptor tyrosine kinase	ABL	Translocation	Chronic myeloid leukemia Acute lymphoblastic leukemia
RAS signal transduction	BRAF	Point mutation	Melanomas

Contd...

Contd...

WNT signal transduction	b-catenin	Point mutation Overexpression	Hepatoblastomas, hepatocellular carcinoma
Nuclear regulatory proteins			
Transcriptional activators	C-MYC N-MYC L-MYC	Translocation Amplification Amplification	Burkitt lymphoma Neuroblastoma, small cell carcinoma of lung Small cell carcinoma of lung
Cell-cycle regulators			
Cyclins	CYCLIN D CYCLIN E	Translocation Amplification Overexpression	Mantle cell lymphoma Breast and esophageal cancers Breast cancer
Cyclin dependent kinase	CDK4	Amplification or point mutation	Glioblastoma, melanoma, sarcoma

The **point mutation of the RAS family** gene is the single most common abnormality of dominant oncogenes in human tumors.

Neurofibromin (protein affected in neurofibromatosis 1) is an example of GAP whose mutation results in neurofibromatosis 1.

MYC is the most common nuclear transcription regulator affected in the human tumors.

MYC gene is associated with **"Conflict model"** in carcinogenesis

The Important Oncogenes Include

1. **RAS** – It is an example of signal transducing protein. Normally, inactive RAS binds to GDP and the presence of growth factor causes GDP to be exchanged by GTP causing RAS activation. The activated RAS binds to its farnesyl transferase receptor causing increased activation of MAP kinase and promoting mitogenesis. The activated RAS comes back to its normal inactive state due to the intrinsic GTPase activity which gets augmented due to a group of proteins called GTPase Activating Proteins (or *GAP*). Mutated RAS proteins bind to GAP without augmentation of GTPase activity resulting is uncontrolled mitogenesis and tumor formation.

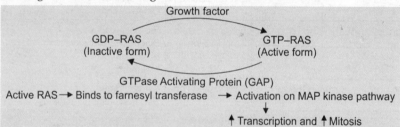

The different types of RAS affected in different tumors are:

K – RAS	Colon, lung and pancreatic tumors
N – RAS	Melanoma, blood tumors (AML)
H – RAS	Bladder and kidney tumors

2. **ABL** – It possess *non-receptor associated tyrosine kinase activity*. C-ABL present on chromosome 9 fuses with BCR gene on chromosome 22 and result in Philadelphia chromosome (t 9;22). The fusion gene possesses uncontrolled tyrosine kinase activity responsible for causing cancer development.

3. **MYC** – Normally in the presence of growth factors, increased levels of MYC along with another protein, MAX form a heterodimer and cause activation of transcription. Uncontrolled nuclear transcription gives rise to development of cancer. In the absence of growth factor, MYC can cause apoptosis. The types of MYC and the tumors associated with their mutation include:
   a. *C – MYC* - Burkitt's lymphoma
   b. *L- MYC* - Small cell lung cancer [**L**- for lung]
   c. *N- MYC* - Neuroblastoma [**N** for Neuroblastoma]

- ***Loss of function*** mutations in RET oncogene result in intestinal aganglionosis and Hirschsprung disease
- Gain of function mutations in RET oncogene result in Multiple Endocrine Neoplasia (MEN 2A/2B) syndromes.

Neoplasia

II. Tumor Suppressor Genes

These genes normally regulate cell growth (they do not prevent tumor formation, so the name is actually a misnomer). Any failure of growth regulation causes development of cancer.

Selected Tumor Suppressor Genes involved in Human Neoplasms				
Subcellular Location	Gene	Function	Tumors associated with Somatic Mutations	Tumors associated with Inherited Mutations
Cell surface	TGF-β receptor E-cadherin	Growth inhibition Cell adhesion	Carcinoma of colon Carcinoma of stomach	Unknown Familial gastric cancer
Inner aspect of plasma membrane	NF-1	Inhibition of RAS signal transduction and of p21 cell-cycle inhibitor	Neuroblastoma	Neurofibromatosis type 1 and sarcomas
Cytoskeleton	NF-2	Cytoskeleton stability	Schwannomas and meningiomas	Neurofibromatosis type 2, acoustic schwannomas and meningiomas
Cytosol	APC/β-catenin	Inhibition of signal transduction	Carcinomas of stomach, colon, pancreas; melanoma	Familial adenomatous polyposis coli/colon cancer
	PTEN	PI-3 kinase signal transduction	Endometrial and prostate cancers	Unknown
	SMAD 2 and SMAD 4	TGF-β signal transduction	Colon, pancreas tumors	Unknown
Nucleus	RB	Regulation of cell cycle	Retinoblastoma; osteosarcoma, carcinomas of breast, colon, lung	Retinoblastomas, osteosarcoma
	P53	Cell-cycle arrest and apoptosis in response to DNA damage	Most human cancers	Li-Fraumeni syndrome; multiple carcinomas and sarcomas
	WT-1	Nuclear transcription	Wilms tumor	Wilms tumor
	P16 (INK4a)	Regulation of cell cycle by inhibition of cyclin-dependent kinase	Pancreatic, breast and esophageal cancers	Malignant melanoma
	BRCA-1 and BRCA-2	DNA repair	Unknown	Carcinoma of female breast and ovary; carcinomas of male breast
	KLF-6	Transcription factor	Prostate	Unknown

Breast carcinoma is most common malignancy in females in India.
It is associated with mutations in BRCA1 and BRCA2 genes.

Some important tumor suppressor genes include:

1. **RB gene**
   - In the active or hypophosphorylated state, it is present in the non- multiplying cells. The oncogenic viruses cause phosphorylation of RB resulting in its inactivation. The RB inactivation results in cell multiplication by activation of the transcription factor E2F (as discussed earilar under control mechanism of cell cycle).

RB gene was the first tumor suppressor gene to be discovered.

Neoplasia

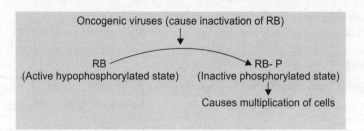

Concept of Loss of Heterozygosity (LOH)

- Retinoblastoma is a prime example of a tumor which is associated with loss of heterozygosity. This term is mostly used in the context of oncogenesis.
- Retinoblastoma develops when both the normal alleles of the Rb gene are inactivated or altered.
- In familial case of retinoblastoma, children are born with *one normal and one defective copy of the Rb gene.*
- Such a child is said to be heterozygous at the Rb locus (*one allele of the gene is normal while the other is a mutant*). So, till the time there is heterozygosity for the Rb gene, the cell behavior is not affected (no chances of cancer development).
- When there is a mutation affecting the second allele, the chances of cancer increases. It means that the cell *loses heterozygosity for the normal Rb gene (called as loss of heterozygosity)*.
- Loss of heterozygosity is the basis of two hit hypothesis of cancers (Knudson's hypothesis).

Knudson's Two Hit Hypothesis

According to this hypothesis, both the normal alleles should be inactivated for the development of retinoblastoma. Retinoblastoma can be of the following types:

a. **Inherited/Familial Retinoblastoma (40%)**

In hereditary cases of Retinoblastoma one genetic change (first hit) is inherited from the affected parent therefore it is present in all the somatic cells of the body. But one genetic change is not sufficient to produce cancer. The second mutation (second hit) is required to produce cancer. It occurs in the retinal cells (which are carrying the first mutation).

b. **Sporadic Retinoblastoma (60%)**

In sporadic cases both mutations (hits) occur somatically within a single retinal cell whose progeny then form the tumor.

2. **p 53 gene**

It is also known as '*molecular policeman*' and '*guardian of the genome*'. The gene is present on chromosome *17p*. The non-mutated p53 gene is also called as the 'wild type' of p53 gene and is associated with reduced risk of development of cancers. Any inactivation of p53 prevents successful DNA repair in a cell leading to the development of a tumor. The p53 gene codes for 53 KDa nuclear phophoprotein.

- In most of the cases, the inactivating mutations in both the alleles of p53 are acquired in somatic cells. However, sometimes individual may inherit one mutant p53 allele and the second acquired 'hit' may inactivate the normal p53 allele. This later condition is called **Li-Fraumeni syndrome** associated with development of *sarcoma, breast cancer, leukemia and brain tumors.*
- Human papilloma virus (HPV) causes inactivation of p53 through its E6 protein and so, is responsible for development of cancer of anal and genital region.

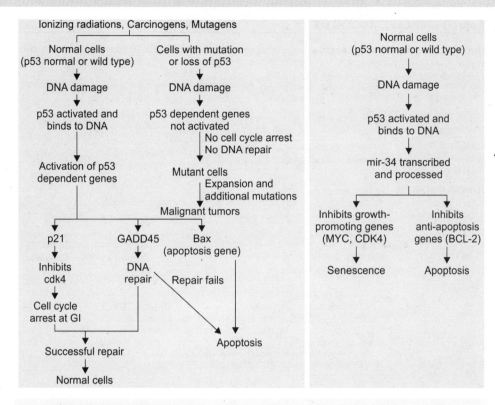

Note: p73 (big brother of p53) and p63 are other members of the family of p53 gene. p63 is esential for the differentiation of stratified squamous epithelia. p73 has pro-apoptotic effects after DNA damage induced by the chemotherapeutic agents.

3. **NF-1 and NF2 gene**

   NF- 1 gene gives rise to **neurofibromin** which is a GTPase activating protein (GAP). NF2 gives rise to neurofibromin 2 or **merlin** protein which inhibits the proliferation of Schwann cells. So, any mutation affecting any of these genes increases the chances of development of cancer.

III. **Genes Regulating Apoptosis**

   Apoptosis (or programmed cell death) is *promoted* by the genes *bax, bad, bcl- Xs and p53* whereas it is inhibited by bcl-2. Understandably, any increase in bcl-2 would cause inhibition of apoptosis and development of cancer. Normally chromosome 14 has immunoglobulin heavy chain gene whereas chromosome 18 has bcl-2 gene. In **follicular lymphoma**, there is presence of translocation **t (14:18)**[Q] which causes increased expression of bcl-2 thereby preventing apoptosis and inducing the development of cancer.

IV. **Genes Inhibiting DNA Repair**

   Defective DNA repair increases DNA instability increasing the chances of development of a cancer. This can be of the following three types:

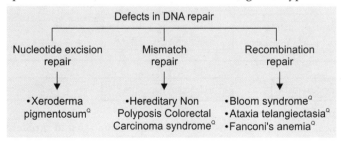

The **non-mutated p53 gene** is also called as the **'wild type'** of p53 gene and is associated with **reduced risk** of development of **cancers**.

Cancers carrying p53 mutations are relatively resistant to chemotherapy and radiotherapy.

Concept

MicroRNAs (miRNAs) are small RNA molecules which inhibit gene expression. They *DONOT encode proteins*. miRNAs get incorporated into a multiprotein complex called RISC (RNA-induced silencing complex). Then it can either cause target mRNA cleavage or repress its translation.

Mir34 family of miRNAs is **activated by p53 gene.** The targets of mir34 include pro-proliferative genes like cyclins and anti-apoptotic genes like bcl2. This is an important mechanism by which p53 gene is able to repress the function of other genes.

Small interfering RNAs (siRNAs) are similar to miRNA except that siRNA precursors are introduced by investigators into the cell. So, they are now used for **studying gene function.**

Additional features of diseases with defects in DNA repair by homologous recombination include *bone marrow depression (Fanconi's anemia)*, **developmental defects (Bloom syndrome)** and *neural symptoms (Ataxia telangiectasia).*

Neoplasia

MULTI-STEP CARCINOGENESIS

The normal epithelium undergoes sequential mutations in different genes eventually leading to development of carcinoma.

> **Multistep carcinogenesis** is best seen in cancers like **colon cancer**

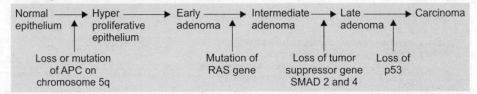

TUMOR GROWTH

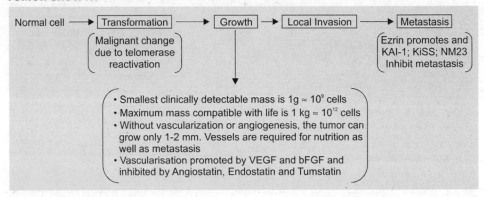

- Smallest clinically detectable mass is $1g \approx 10^9$ cells
- Maximum mass compatible with life is $1 \text{ kg} \approx 10^{12}$ cells
- Without vascularization or angiogenesis, the tumor can grow only 1-2 mm. Vessels are required for nutrition as well as metastasis
- Vascularisation promoted by VEGF and bFGF and inhibited by Angiostatin, Endostatin and Tumstatin

SPREAD OF TUMORS

> Genes **promoting** metastasis include **ezrin** (in rhabdomyosarcoma and osteosarcoma)
>
> Genes **inhibiting** metastasis include **NM23, KAI-1** (prostate cancer) and **Ki55** [malignant melanoma]

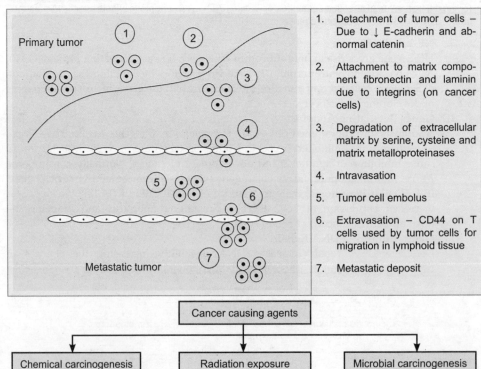

1. Detachment of tumor cells – Due to ↓ E-cadherin and abnormal catenin

2. Attachment to matrix component fibronectin and laminin due to integrins (on cancer cells)

3. Degradation of extracellular matrix by serine, cysteine and matrix metalloproteinases

4. Intravasation

5. Tumor cell embolus

6. Extravasation – CD44 on T cells used by tumor cells for migration in lymphoid tissue

7. Metastatic deposit

> **Sir Percival Pott** demonstrated the increased incidence of **scrotal skin cancer** in **chimney workers** exposed to chemical soot.

I. **Chemical Carcinogens**
   Chemical carcinogenesis has two steps called initiation and proliferation. Initiation can be by two types of agents

a. *Direct acting agents* – These are mutagens causing cancer by direct damage or modification of DNA.
b. *Indirect acting agents (also called as procarcinogens)* – These require metabolic conversion to form active carcinogens.

Initiators cause irreversible DNA damage. The proliferation of the tumor cells is done by promoters (chemicals causing multiplication of already mutated cells). The **promoters cause reversible DNA damage.** The *carcinogenic potential* of a chemical is tested by *Ames test*

Chemical Carcinogens

Alkylating agents	Acute myeloid leukemia, bladder cancer
Androgens	Prostate cancer
Aromatic amines (dyes)	Bladder cancer
Arsenic	Cancer of the lung, skin
Asbestos	Cancer of the lung, pleura, peritoneum
Benzene	Acute myelocytic leukemia
Chromium	Lung cancer
Diethylstilbestrol (prenatal)	Vaginal cancer (clear cell)
Epstein-Barr virus	Burkitt's lymphoma, nasal T cell lymphoma
Estrogens	Cancer of the endometrium, liver, breast
Ethyl alcohol	Cancer of the liver, esophagus, head and neck
Immunosuppressive agents (azathioprine, cyclosporine, glucocorticoids)	Non-Hodgkin's lymphoma
Nitrogen mustard gas	Cancer of the lung, head and neck, nasal sinuses
Nickel dust	Cancer of the lung, nasal sinuses
Oral contraceptives	Bladder and cervical cancer
Phenacetin	Cancer of the renal pelvis and bladder
Polycyclic hydrocarbons	Cancer of the lung, skin (especially squamous cell carcinoma of scrotal skin)
Schistosomiasis	Bladder cancer (squamous cell)
Sunlight (ultraviolet)	Skin cancer (squamous cell and melanoma)
Tobacco (including smokeless)	Cancer of the upper aerodigestive tract, bladder
Vinyl chloride	Liver cancer (angiosarcoma)

Radiation Exposure

UV Radiation
- It has three subtypes
  UV-A is 320 - 400 nm
  UV-B is 280 - 320 nm
  UV-C is 200 - 280 nm

UVC gets filtered by ozone layer, whereas UV-B^Q is the most carcinogenic UV ray to reach the earth

Exposure to UV rays
↓
Pyrimidine dimers in DNA
↓
Mutation in oncogenes and tumor suppressor genes
↓
↑Incidence of skin cancer

Ionizing Radiation
- It includes X-rays, γ rays α and β particles
- Maximum sensitivity is at G2 stage
- Exposure to ionizing radiation
  ↓
Cross-linking and chain break in nucleic acids
  ↓
↑cancer
- Most common are papillary thyroid cancer and leukemias **(except CLL)**
  Lung cancer is seen in uranium miners,
- The cells of skin, bone and GI tract are relatively to radiation induced neoplasms

Concept

Initiators cause **irreversible DNA damage**. The proliferation of the tumor cells is done by promoters (chemicals causing multiplication of already mutated cells). The **promoters** cause **reversible DNA damage**.

Concept

In **Ames test,** a modified bacterium *Salmonella typhimurium* is used, which is unable to produce histidine due to absence of histidine synthetase enzyme in it.

The modified bacteria are first put on a histidine free medium where it cannot grow.

Then it is put on the same medium but now having additionally the presence of the suspected mutagen. In the second case, the bacteria grow if the chemical has mutagenic potential.

The in *vitro mutagenic potential correlates well with the carcinogenic potential in vivo.*

CLL is the only leukemia **NOT** associated with **ionizing radiation** exposure

Basal cell carcinoma is the most common cancer due to **excessive UV light** exposure.

Squamous cell carinoma may develop in third degree **burn scars** and orifices of **chronically draining sinuses** (as in chronic ostemyelitis)

Neoplasia

Infectious Organisms

BACTERIA (H. PYLORI)

H. pylori is the first bacterium classified as a carcinogen. *H. pylori* infection is implicated in the genesis of both gastric adenocarcinomas and gastric lymphomas. The gastric lymphomas are of **B-cell origin**[Q] and are called MALT lymphomas (marginal zone-associated lymphomas) because the transformed B cells normally reside in the marginal zones of lymphoid follicles. *H. pylori* infection results in the formation of *H. pylori*-reactive T cells, which cause polyclonal B-cell proliferations. The MALT lymphoma is associated with **t(11;18)**[Q] translocation.

VIRUSES

Carcinogenic Viruses

RNA viruses	DNA viruses
• Human T cell leukemia virus-1 (HTLV-1) • Hepatitis C virus (HCV)	• Hepatitis B virus (HBV) • Human herpes virus 8 (HHV8) • Human papilloma virus (HPV) • Epstein-Barr virus (EBV)

Pathogenesis

HTLV-1

It is a RNA oncogenic virus which is transmitted by blood products, sexual intercourse or breast feeding. It has attraction for CD4 T cells (similar to HIV). HTLV-1 has a gene TAX. The **TAX protein**[Q] causes

1. Transcription of host genes involved in proliferation and differentiation of T-cells (e-FOS, IL-2 genes)
2. Genomic instability by inhibiting DNA repair function and by inhibiting cell cycle checkpoints activated by DNA damage

These contribute to increased chances of cancer by HTLV-1.

HCV

Hepatitis C virus (HCV) is also strongly associated with the development of hepatocellular carcinoma. This is associated with its ability to cause chronic liver cell injury and inflammation that is accompanied by liver regeneration. Mitotically active hepatocytes, surrounded by an altered environment, are presumably prone to genetic instability and cancer development.

EBV

It is a DNA oncogenic virus. It causes infection of epithelial cells of oropharynx and B- cells because of the presence of **CD21 molecule**[Q] on the surface of these cells. **LMP-1 gene**[Q] present in the EBV causes activation of NF-κβ and JAK/STAT signaling pathways thereby promoting B-cell survival and proliferation. (This increases the chances of B- cell lymphoma). Another EBV-encoded gene, *EBNA-2*, transactivates several host genes like cyclin D and the *src* family genes. The EBV genome also contains a viral cytokine, vIL-10 which prevents macrophages and monocytes from activating T cells and is required for EBV-dependent transformation of B cells. EBV acts a polyclonal B-cell mitogen followed by acquisition of **t(8;14)**[Q] translocation which ultimately results in development of Burkitt's lymphoma.

*EBV belongs to the herpes family and can cause the following cancers:
* African form of Burkitt's lymphoma
* B- cell lymphoma in immunosuppressed individuals
* Hodgkin's lymphoma
* Nasopharyngeal cancer

HHV8 is associated with **Primary effusion lymphoma** and **Multicentric Castleman's disease**

HCV is associated with **Lymphoplasmacytic lymphoma**

HTLV1 can cause **T-cell leukemia**/lymphoma and demyelinating disorder called **Tropical spastic paraparesis**.

EBV is associated with **'mixed cellularity' variant** of Hodgkin's lymphoma

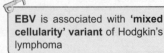

Nasopharyngeal cancer is the **only T cell malignancy** amongst the cancers caused by EBV

HBV

It encodes for **HBx protein**Q which disrupts the normal growth control of infected liver cells by activation of several growth promoting genes. HBx also causes inactivation of the tumor suppressor gene p53. This results in HBV causing hepatocellular cancer.

HPV

It is responsible for development of squamous cell carcinoma of cervix and anogenital lesion and in some cases, oral and laryngeal cancers. The virus gets integrated in the genome of host cells which is essential for the malignant transformation of the affected cells HPV 16 (more commonly) and HPV 18 (less commonly) are particularly important in carcinogenesis as they have viral genes **E6 and E7 which causes Rb and p53 gene inactivation respectively.** Since both p53 and Rb are tumor suppressor genes, so, their inactivation increases the chances of cancer development.

> **E6 gene** product **inhibits P53** suppressor gene
> **E7 gene** product **inhibits RB** suppressor gene

PARANEOPLASTIC SYNDROMES

Clinical syndromes	Major forms of underlying cancer	Causal mechanism
Endocrinopathies		
Cushing syndrome	Small cell carcinoma of lung Pancreatic carcinoma Neural tumors	ACTH or ACTH-like substance
Syndrome of inappropriate antidiuretic hormone secretion	Small cell carcinoma of lung; Intracranial neoplasms	Antidiuretic hormone or atrial natriuretic hormones
Hypercalcemia	Squamous cell carcinoma of lung Breast carcinoma Renal carcinoma Adult T-cell leukemia/lymphoma Ovarian carcinoma	Parathyroid hormone-related protein (PTHRP), TGF-α, TNF, IL-1
Hypoglycemia	Fibrosarcoma Other mesenchymal sarcomas Hepatocellular carcinoma	Insulin or insulin-like substance
Carcinoid syndrome	Bronchial adenoma (carcinoid) Pancreatic carcinoma Gastric carcinoma	Serotonin, bradykinin
Polycythemia	Renal carcinoma Cerebellar hemangioma Hepatocellular carcinoma	Erythropoietin
Nerve and Muscle Syndromes		
Myasthenia	Bronchogenic carcinoma	Immunologic
Disorders of the central and peripheral nervous systems	Breast carcinoma	
Dermatologic Disorders		
Acanthosis nigricans	Gastric carcinoma Lung carcinoma Uterine carcinoma	Immunologic; secretion of epidermal growth factor
Dermatomyositis	Bronchogenic, breast carcinoma	Immunologic
Osseous, Articular, and Soft Tissue Changes		
Hypertrophic osteoarthropathy and clubbing of the fingers	Bronchogenic carcinoma	Unknown

contd...

> **Cushing syndrome** is the most common **endocrinopathy**.

> **Hypercalcemia** is probably the most common paraneoplastic syndrome.

> **Trousseau phenomenon (Migratory thrombophlebitis)** is seen with **pancreatic** and **bronchogenic carcinoma**

contd...

Vascular and Hematologic Changes		
Venous thrombosis (Trousseau phenomenon)	Pancreatic carcinoma Bronchogenic carcinoma Other cancers	Tumor products (mucins that activate clotting)
Nonbacterial thrombotic endocarditis	Advanced cancers	Hypercoagulability
Anemia	Thymic neoplasms	Unknown
Others		
Nephrotic syndrome	Various cancers	Tumor antigens, immune complexes
ACTH, adrenocorticotropic hormone; TGF, transforming growth factor; TNF, tumor necrosis factor; IL, interleukin.		

Concept

Grading of a cancer is based on the **degree of differentiation** of the tumor cells and the number of mitoses within the tumor as presumed *correlates of the neoplasm's aggressiveness.*

Concept

The **staging** of cancers is based on the **size of the primary lesion, its extent of spread** to regional lymph nodes, and the presence or absence of **distant metastases.**

■ IMMUNOHISTOCHEMISTERY

It is a method for diagnosis of cancer.

1. **Categorization of undifferentiated malignant tumor:** Sometimes, many tumors like anaplastic carcinoma, lymphoma, melanoma and sarcoma are difficult to distinguish with routine H and E staining because of poor differentiation. So, immunohistochemical stains can help in diagnosis e.g.
   - Presence of cytokeratin points to epithelial origin (carcinoma).
   - Presence of desmin is specific for muscle cell origin.
   - Presence of Leucocyte Common Antigen (LCA) points to lymphoma.
2. **Determination of site of origin of metastatic tumor:** There are markers that point to the origin of tumor (primary) in a biopsy specimen of metastasis. Examples include *PSA (for prostate cancer) and thyroglobulin (for thyroid cancer).*
3. **Prognostic or therapeutic significance:** Estrogen/progesterone receptor detection has therapeutic value in breast carcinomas. Receptor positive breast cancers are susceptible to anti-estrogen therapy. Similarly, over-expression of erb-B2 protein suggests a poor prognosis.

■ TUMOR MARKERS

Tumor markers are biochemical substances (include cell-surface antigens, cytoplasmic proteins, enzymes, and hormones) which indicate the presence of a tumor.

Markers	Associated Cancers
Hormones	
Human chorionic gonadotropin (hCG)	Trophoblastic tumors, non-seminomatous testicular tumors
Calcitonin	Medullary carcinoma of thyroid
Catecholamine and metabolites	Pheochromocytoma and related tumors
Ectopic hormones	See above
Oncofetal Antigens	
α-Fetoprotein	Liver cell cancer, non-seminomatous germ cell tumors of testis
Carcinoembryonic antigen	Carcinomas of the colon, pancreas, lung, stomach, and heart
Isoenzymes	
Prostatic acid phosphatase	Prostate cancer
Neuron-specific enolase	Small cell cancer of lung, neuroblastoma

Concept

hCG is a **placental glycoprotein hormone** composed by α and β subunits. ***Alpha hCG is not used as tumor marker because it is similar to the FSH, LH and TSH.*** The beta subunit of hCG is typically measured as a tumor marker because it has unique sequence that are not shared with other human glycoprotein hormones. So, it is quite specific and there is no cross reactivity between beta subunits of these hormones.

contd...

Neoplasia

contd...

Specific Proteins	
Immunoglobulins	Multiple myeloma and other gammopathies
Prostate-specific antigen and prostate-specific membrane antigen	Prostate cancer
Mucins and Other Glycoproteins	
CA-125	Ovarian cancer
CA-19-9	Colon cancer, pancreatic cancer
CA-15-3	Breast cancer
New Molecular Markers	
p53, APC, RAS mutations in stool and serum	Colon cancer
p53 and RAS mutations in stool and serum	Pancreatic cancer
p53 and RAS mutations in sputum and serum	Lung cancer
p53 mutations in urine	Bladder cancer

The important antigens for the determination of specific tumor cell origin are:

Epithelial Tumors
- Breast: Alpha lactalbumin, GCDP-15, estrogen/progesterone
- Thyroid: Thyroglobulin, calcitonin
- Liver: AFP (α fetoprotein), HBsAg, keratin
- Prostate: Prostatic acid phosphatase, prostate specific antigen
- Mesothelioma: Keratin, Calretinin, mesothelin

Germ Cell Tumors
- Human chorionic gonadotropin, AFP (α-fetoprotein)

Mesenchymal Tumors
- Endothelial tumors: Factor VIII, CD 34,
- Melanoma: HMB 45, S 100
- Fibrohistiocytic tumors: Lysozyme, HAM 56
- Myogenic tumors: Desmin, smooth muscle specific antigen, myoglobin

Neuroendocrine Tumors
- Neuron specific enolase (NSE), chromogranin, synaptophysin
  - Malignant melanoma expresses HMB 45, S-100 and vimentin. **HMB 45** is present in melanosomes and is **more specific**. S-100 is more sensitive but is non-specific (also present in Langerhans' cell histiocytosis, neural tumors, and sarcomas like liposarcoma and chondrosarcoma)
  - Neurofibroma (a neural tumor) shows the presence of S100 and GFAP (Glial Fibrillary Acid Protein). Malignant tumors often lose expression of S-100 antigen.
  - Neuroblastoma expresses NSE, chromogranin and synaptophysin. NSE is more specific whereas chromogranin and synaptophysin are more sensitive tumor markers.
- Angiosarcoma expresses factor VIII, vimentin and CD34 antigen

Type of tumors associated with intermediate filaments:

Intermediate Filament	Normal Tissue Expression	Tumor
Cytokeratin	All epithelial cells	Carcinoma
Vimentin	Mesenchymal cells	Sarcomas
Desmin	Muscle cells	Leiomyoma Rhabdomyosarcoma
Glial Fibrillary Acidic Protein (GFAP)	Glial cells	Astrocytoma Ependymoma
Neurofilament	Neurons and Neural crest derivatives	Pheochromocytoma Neuroblastoma

Valproate embyopathy is due to mutation in **HOX gene**.

Vitamin A induced embryopathy is due to mutation in **TGF-β signaling pathway**.

t(12;15) (p13;q25) is associated with congenital infantile fibrosarcoma

In **malignant melanoma**, **HMB 45** is **more specific** whereas *S-100 is more sensitive.*

In **neuroblastoma**, **NSE is more specific** whereas *chromogranin and synaptophysin are more sensitive* tumor markers.

Tumor lysis syndrome is associated with **Burkitt lymphoma,** acute lymphoblastic leukemia **(ALL)**, chronic tumors **(CLL)** and uncommonly solid tumors.

It is associated with **hypocalce-mia** and *NOT* hypercalcemia.

CONCEPT OF TUMOR LYSIS SYNDROME

Tumor lysis syndrome is caused by destruction of large number of rapidly proliferating neoplastic cells. It is characterized by

- **Hyperuricemia** (due to increased turnover of nucleic acids)
- **Hyperkalemia** (due to release of the most abundant intracellular cation potassium)
- **Hyperphosphatemia** (due to release of intracellular phosphate)
- **Hypocalcemia** (due to complexing of calcium with the elevated phosphate)
- **Lactic acidosis**
- **Hyperuricemia** can cause uric acid precipitation in the kidney causing acute renal failure.

MULTIPLE CHOICE QUESTIONS

NEOPLASIA: General Aspects

1. Which of the following helps in differentiation of follicular carcinoma from follicular adenoma of thyroid gland? *(AI 2011, AIIMS May 2010)*
   - (a) Hurthle cell change
   - (b) Lining of tall columnar and cuboidal cells
   - (c) Vascular invasion
   - (d) Increased mitoses

2. All are malignant tumors, except: *(AI 2008)*
   - (a) Chloroma
   - (b) Fibromatosis
   - (c) Askin's tumor
   - (d) Liposarcoma

3. The following is not a feature of malignant transformation by cultured cells: *(AI 2005)*
   - (a) Increased cell density
   - (b) Increased requirement for growth factors
   - (c) Alterations of cytoskeletal structures
   - (d) Loss of anchorage

4. Which of the following carcinoma most frequently metastasizes to brain? *(AIIMS Nov 2005)*
   - (a) Small cell carcinoma lung
   - (b) Prostate cancer
   - (c) Rectal carcinoma
   - (d) Endometrial cancer

5. Chemotherapeutic drugs can cause:
   - (a) Only necrosis *(AIIMS May 2005)*
   - (b) Only apoptosis
   - (c) Both necrosis and apoptosis
   - (d) Anoikis

6. Reversible loss of polarity with abnormality in size and shape of cells is known as: *(AIIMS Nov 2001)*
   - (a) Metaplasia
   - (b) Dysplasia
   - (c) Hyperplasia
   - (d) Anaplasia

7. Predisposing factors for skin cancer are:
   - (a) Smoking *(PGI Dec 2000)*
   - (b) U-V-light
   - (c) Chronic ulcer
   - (d) Infrared light

8. Increased risk of cancer is seen in:
   - (a) Fibroadenoma of breast *(Delhi PG 2009 RP)*
   - (b) Bronchial asthma
   - (c) Chronic ulcerative colitis
   - (d) Leiomyoma of the uterus

9. A strong propensity for vascular invasion is seen in:
   - (a) Prostatic carcinoma *(Karnataka 2008)*
   - (b) Hepatocellular carcinoma
   - (c) Bronchogenic carcinoma
   - (d) Gastric carcinoma

10. Earliest changes of neoplastic transformation as seen at a microscopic level is called: *(Karnataka 2004)*
    - (a) Hyperplasia
    - (b) Metaplasia
    - (c) Dysplasia
    - (d) Carcinoma in situ

11. Squamous cell carcinoma spreads by: *(RJ 2000)*
    - (a) Hematogenous route
    - (b) Lymphatic route
    - (c) Direct invasion
    - (d) All

12. Which one of the following tumors does not cause bony metastasis? *(AP 2000)*
    - (a) Renal cell carcinoma
    - (b) Gastric carcinoma
    - (c) Thyroid carcinoma
    - (d) Breast carcinoma

13. Hamartoma is: *(AP 2003)*
    - (a) Proliferation of cells in foreign site
    - (b) Proliferation of native cells in tissue
    - (c) Malignant condition
    - (d) Acquired condition

14. Sure sign of malignancy is: *(AP 2005)*
    - (a) Mitoses
    - (b) Polychromasia
    - (c) Nuclear pleomorphism
    - (d) Metastasis

15. A lesion 3 cm away from gastroesophageal junction contain columnar epithelium, such a type of lesion is:
    - (a) Metaplasia *(Bihar 2004)*
    - (b) Hyperplasia
    - (c) Dysplasia
    - (d) Anaplasia

16. Malignancy is typically associated with disordered differentiation and maturation. Which of the following mentioned options best describes anaplasia?
    - (a) Hepatic tumor cells synthesizing bile
    - (b) Skin tumor cells producing keratin pearls

(c) Bronchial epithelial cells producing keratin pearls
(d) Muscle tumor cells forming giant cells

17. A 42 year-old woman Himanshi has an abnormal bloody discharge from her left nipple. She underwent the investigations and was diagnosed with an early stage breast cancer. Lumpectomy was performed and a slide was sent to the laboratory. The pathologist comments that there is significant desmoplasia in the surrounding tissue. The term 'desmoplasia' is best descriptive of which of the following?
(a) An irregular accumulation of blood vessels.
(b) Metastatic involvement of surrounding tissue.
(c) Normal tissue misplaced within another organ.
(d) Proliferation of non- neoplastic fibrous connective tissue.

18. All of the following are true of familial cancers except
(a) Early age of onset
(b) Arises in 2 or more relatives of index case
(c) Sometimes multiple tumors are present
(d) Present with specific marker phenotype

19. A 58 year old smoker Babu Bhai presents with long standing epigastric pain, occasional vomiting and significant weight loss. He did not respond to antacid and antibiotic therapy. A biopsy and other studies confirmed that he has gastric cancer at a stage that is associated with a very poor prognosis. Staging is based on which of the following?
(a) Degree of anaplasia
(b) Degree of differentiation of tumor cells
(c) Distribution and extent of disease
(d) Number of mitotic figures

20. Which of the following criteria can be used to determine if a pheochromocytoma lesion is benign or malignant?
(a) Blood vessel invasion
(b) Cannot be determined by microscopic examination
(c) Hemorrhage and necrosis
(d) Nuclear pleomorphism

Most Recent Questions

20.1. Which of the following is most reliable feature of malignant transformation of pheochromocytoma?
(a) Presence of mitotic figures
(b) Presence of metastasis to other organs
(c) Vascular/ capsular invasion
(d) All of the above

20.2. Overgrowth of a skin structure at a localised region is:
(a) Hamartoma
(b) Malignant tumor
(c) Choristoma
(d) Polyp

20.3. Cell-matrix adhesions are mediated by?
(a) Cadherins
(b) Integrins

(c) Selectins
(d) Calmodulin

20.4. Which of the following is not a labile cell?
(a) Bone marrow
(b) Epidermal cells
(c) Small intestine mucosa
(d) Hepatocytes

20.5. Which one is not the pre cancerous condition?
(a) Crohn's disease
(b) Ulcerative colitis
(c) Leukoplakia
(d) Xeroderma pigmentosum

20.6. Which of the following features differentiates invasive carcinoma from carcinoma in situ?
(a) Anaplasia
(b) Number of mitosis
(c) Basement membrane invasion
(d) Pleomorphism

20.7. Sure sign of malignancy is:
(a) Mitoses
(b) Polychromasia
(c) Nuclear pleomorphism
(d) Metastasis

20.8. Bimodality of incidence occurs in all, except
(a) Cancer penis in male
(b) Hodgkin's diseases
(c) Breast cancer in females
(d) Leukemia

CELLCYCLE AND ITS REGULATION

21. Ionizing radiation affects which stage of cell cycle
(a) G2 S
(b) G1 G2
(c) G2 M
(d) G0 G1

22. The correct sequence of cell cycle is: *(AI 2003)*
(a) G0-G1-S-G2-M
(b) G0-G1-G2-S-M
(c) G0-M-G2-S-G1
(d) G0-G1-S-M-G2

23. During which phase of the cell cycle the cellular content of DNA is doubled: *(AIIMS Nov 2005)*
(a) Mitotic phase
(b) G1 phase
(c) G2 phase
(d) S phase

24. The tumor suppressor gene p 53 induces cell cycle arrest at: *(AIIMS Nov 2005)*
(a) G_2-M phase
(b) S-G_2 phase
(c) G_1-S phase
(d) G_0 phase

Neoplasia

25. **Transition from G2 to M phase of the cell cycle is controlled by:** *(AIIMS Nov 2003)*
    (a) Retinoblastoma gene product
    (b) p53 protein
    (c) Cyclin E
    (d) Cyclin B

26. **Fixed time is required for which steps of cell cycle:**
    (a) S *(PGI Dec 2000)*
    (b) M
    (c) G_1
    (d) G_2
    (e) Go

27. **Regarding oncogenesis:** *(PGI June 2002)*
    (a) Topoisomerase II causes breaks in strands
    (b) p53 is the most common oncogene mutation causing malignancy in humans
    (c) At G2-M phase there is loss of inhibitors controlling cell-cycle
    (d) Decrease in telomerase activity causes anti-tumor effects

28. **Regarding oncogenesis:** *(PGI Dec 2002)*
    (a) Proto-oncogenes are activated by chromosomal translocation
    (b) Malignant transformations involves accumulation of mutations in proto-oncogenes and tumor suppressor genes
    (c) Point mutation of somatic cells
    (d) Increase in telomerase activity causes anti-tumor effects
    (e) At G2-M phase there is loss of inhibitors controlling cell cycle

29. **The tumor suppressor gene P53 induces cell arrest at:**
    (a) G_2- M phase *(AIIMS-Nov-05) (UP 2008)*
    (b) S- G_2 phase
    (c) G_1- S phase
    (d) G_0- phase

30. **Not a premalignant condition:** *(AP 2002)*
    (a) Fragile X syndrome
    (b) Down's syndrome
    (c) Blount's syndrome
    (d) Fanconi's syndrome

31. **Which is associated with G2M transition in cell cycle:**
    (a) Cyclin A *(Kolkata 2008)*
    (b) Cyclin B
    (c) Cyclin E
    (d) Cyclin D

Most Recent Questions

31.1. **E cadherin gene deficiency is seen in:**
    (a) Gastric cancer
    (b) Intestinal cancer
    (c) Thyroid cancer
    (d) Pancreatic cancer

31.2. **Li Fraumeni syndrome is due to mutation of which gene?**
    (a) p21
    (b) p53
    (c) p41
    (d) p43

31.3. **Which of the following is not a cyclin dependent kinase (CDK) inhibitor?**
    (a) p21
    (b) p27
    (c) p53
    (d) p57

31.4. **Cells are most radiosensitive in:**
    (a) S - phase
    (b) M -phase
    (c) Gl - phase
    (d) G0 - phase

GENETIC MECHANISMS OF CARCINOGENESIS: PROTO-ONCOGENE, TUMOUR SUPPRESSOR GENE, DEFECTIVE DNA REPAIR

32. **All are true about Fanconi anemia, except:** *(Bihar 2006)*
    (a) Defect in DNA repair
    (b) Bone marrow hyper function
    (c) Congenital anomaly present
    (d) Increased chances of cancer

33. **HER2/neu receptor plays a role in** *(AIIMS Nov. 2010)*
    (a) Predicting therapeutic response
    (b) Diagnosis of breast cancer
    (c) Screening of breast cancer
    (d) Recurrence of tumor

34. **The most common secondary malignancy in a patient having retinoblastoma is:** *(AI 2010)*
    (a) Osteosarcoma
    (b) Renal cell carcinoma
    (c) Pineoblastoma
    (d) Osteoblastoma

35. **Regarding Fanconi anemia, the wrong statement is:**
    (a) Autosomal dominant *(AI 2010)*
    (b) Bone marrow show pancytopenia
    (c) Usually aplastic anemia
    (d) It is due to defective DNA repair

36. **True statements about p53 gene are all except:** *(AI 2008)*
    (a) Arrests cell cycle at G_1 phase
    (b) Product is 53 kD protein
    (c) Located on chromosome 17
    (d) Wild/non-mutated form is associated with increased risk of childhood tumors

37. **Growth factor oncogene is:** *(AI 2008)*
    (a) Myc
    (b) Fos
    (c) Sis
    (d) Jun

38. **Rosettes are characteristically seen in:** *(AI 2008)*
    (a) Retinoblastoma
    (b) Melanoma
    (c) Dysgerminoma
    (d) Lymphoma

39. **The normal cellular counterparts of oncogenes are important for the following functions, except:** *(AI 2006)*
    (a) Promotion of cell cycle progression
    (b) Inhibition of apoptosis
    (c) Promotion of DNA repair
    (d) Promotion of nuclear transcription

40. **An example of a tumor suppressor gene is:** *(AI 2005)*
    (a) myc
    (b) fos
    (c) ras
    (d) Rb

41. **Lynch syndrome is associated with cancers of the:**
    (a) Breast, colon, ovary *(AIIMS Nov 2009)*
    (b) Breast, endometrium, ovary
    (c) Breast, colon, endometrium
    (d) Colon, endometrium, ovary

42. **Loss of heterozygosity associated with:**
    (a) Acute myeloid leukemia *(AIIMS May 2008)*
    (b) ALL
    (c) Retinoblastoma
    (d) Promyelocytic leukemia

43. **Which is not a tumor suppressor gene?**
    (a) WT-1 *(AIIMS May 2008)*
    (b) Rb
    (c) p53
    (d) ras

44. **The inheritance pattern of familial Retinoblastoma is:**
    (a) Autosomal recessive *(AIIMS Nov 2005)*
    (b) Autosomal dominant
    (c) X-linked dominant
    (d) X-linked recessive

45. **Which of the following is known as the "guardian of the genome"?** *(AIIMS May 2005)*
    (a) p53
    (b) Mdm2
    (c) p14
    (d) ATM

46. **The following statements are true about Tumor Suppressor Gene p53, except:** *(AIIMS Nov 2004)*
    (a) It regulates certain genes involved in cell cycle regulation
    (b) Its increased levels can induce apoptosis
    (c) Its activity in the cells decreases following UV irradiation and stimulates cell cycle
    (d) Mutations of the p53 gene are most common genetic alteration seen in human cancer

47. **In the mitogen activated protein kinase pathway, the activation of RAS is counteracted by:** *(AIIMS May 2004)*
    (a) Protein kinase C
    (b) GTPase activating protein
    (c) Phosphatidyl inositol
    (d) Inositol triphosphate

48. **Which of the following mutations in a tumor suppressor agent causes breast carcinoma?** *(AIIMS May 2002)*
    (a) p43   (b) p53
    (c) p73   (d) p83

49. **True about proto-oncogenes is:** *(PGI June' 06)*
    (a) Important for normal cell growth
    (b) May get converted into oncogenes
    (c) C-myc over-expression causes lymphoma
    (d) Their mutation causes retinoblastoma
    (e) Deletion cause Sickle cell disease

50. **True about oncogene is:** *(PGI Dec 2002)*
    (a) Present in normal cell
    (b) They are of viral origin
    (c) They are transduced from virus infected cells
    (d) P53 is most common oncogene mutation causing malignancy
    (e) Viral oncogenes are identical with humans cellular oncogenes

51. **Cancer cell survival is enhanced by:**
    (a) Suppression of p53 protein *(PGI June 2003)*
    (b) Over expression of p53 gene
    (c) bcl-2
    (d) bax
    (e) bad

52. **Following are required for normal growth:**
    (a) Proto-oncogenes *(PGI Dec 2003)*
    (b) Tumor suppressor genes
    (c) Oncogenes
    (d) DNA repair genes

53. **Xeroderma pigmentosum is caused due to a group of closely related abnormalities in:**
    (a) Mismatch repair *(Delhi PG 2010)*
    (b) Base excision repair
    (c) Nucleotide excision repair
    (d) SOS repair

54. **Increased expression of which of the following causes oncogenesis** *(Delhi PG-2004)*
    (a) IGF receptor
    (b) EGF receptor
    (c) GH receptor
    (d) Aldosterone receptor

55. **Tumor suppressor genes are all, except** *(Delhi PG-2004)*
    (a) APC
    (b) p53
    (c) Rb
    (d) C-myc

56. **Angiogenesis is:** *(UP 2007)*
    (a) Formation of the new blood vessels
    (b) Repair by connective tissues
    (c) Formation of the blood clot
    (d) All of the above

57. **Medullary carcinoma of thyroid is associated with mutation in:** *(AP 2003)*
    (a) RET
    (b) RAS
    (c) NF
    (d) Rb

58. **APC gene is located on which chromosome:**
    (a) Chromosome 5 *(AP 2008)*
    (b) Chromosome 6
    (c) Chromosome 9
    (d) Chromosome 11

59. **Proto-oncogene erb-B is not related to:** *(Kolkata 2003)*
    (a) Breast carcinoma
    (b) Small cell lung carcinoma
    (c) Non-small cell lung carcinoma
    (d) Ovarian carcinoma

60. **Most common genetic mutation in carcinogenesis involves:** *(Kolkata 2008)*
    (a) p53
    (b) Rb
    (c) HPC
    (d) PTEN

61 to 63. Read the following paragraph and answer questions 61-63.

It is now evident that most cases of sporadic colon cancer develop through the stepwise accumulation of various mutations. This transformation process is given in the diagram on next page.

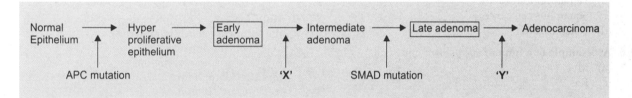

61. **Which of the following genes is most likely marked in the flowchart depiction as 'X'?**
    (a) N-myc
    (b) K-ras
    (c) Cyclin D
    (d) p53

62. **Which of the following is a true statement regarding the above gene?**
    (a) It is associated with the 'conflict model' of oncogenes
    (b) It is called as 'guardian of the genome'
    (c) It is active in hypopohosphorylated form
    (d) It is active in hyperphosphorylated form

63. **Which of the following genes is most likely marked in the flowchart as 'Y'?**
    (a) Cyclin D
    (b) K-ras
    (c) Wt-1 gene
    (d) p53

64. **Aisha, a 51 year old woman discovers a lump in her left breast on a weekly self-examination. Mammography is performed which confirms the presence of a suspicious "mass", and needle core biopsy is performed to determine whether the mass is malignant. Dr. Devesh, the pathologist confirmed the mass to be malignant and said that the tissue demonstrates amplification of *her-2/neu* oncogene. What kind of protein is the gene product of *Her-2/neu*?**
    (a) GTPase
    (b) GTPase-activating protein
    (c) Receptor tyrosine kinase
    (d) Retinoic acid receptor protein

65. **A patient Madhu undergoes total thyroidectomy for a mass lesion of the thyroid. During the surgery it is found that the parathyroid glands appeared enlarged. The thyroid lesion shows neuroendocrine-type cells and amyloid deposition. This patient's thyroid and parathyroid lesions may be related to which of the following oncogenes?**
    (a) bcl-2
    (b) C-myc
    (c) Ret
    (d) L-myc

66. **Dr. Marwah, a pediatrician, performing an ophthalmoscopic examination on a four-year-old boy, notices several small pigmented nodules in his irises. He also notices six light brown macules on the trunk of the child of variable sizes. This boy may have a propensity to develop tumors in which of the following structures?**
    (a) Bladder
    (b) Colon
    (c) Peripheral nerve
    (d) Skin

Most Recent Questions

66.1. **RET gene mutation is associated with which malignancy?**
    (a) Pheochromocytoma
    (b) Medullary carcinoma thyroid
    (c) Lymphoma
    (d) Renal cell carcinoma

66.2. Endometrial carcinoma is associated with which of the following tumor suppression gene mutation?
(a) P53
(b) Rb
(c) PTEN
(d) APC

66.3. The tumor suppressor gene p 53 induces cell cycle arrest at:
(a) G2 – M phase
(b) S – G2 phase
(c) G1 – S phase
(d) G0 phase

66.4. MYC gene is:
(a) Protein kinase inhibitor
(b) Growth factor inhibitor
(c) GTPase
(d) Transcription activator

66.5. Retinoblastoma is associated with which of the following tumours?
(a) Osteoclastoma
(b) Hepatocellular cancer
(c) Squamous cell cancer
(d) Osteosarcoma

66.6. An example of a tumour suppressor gene is:
(a) Myc
(b) Fos
(c) Ras
(d) RB

66.7. Which of the following is DNA repair defect?
(a) Retinoblastoma
(b) Neurofibromatosis
(c) Xeroderma pigmentosum
(d) MEN-I

66.8. Which of the following gene defect is associated with development of medullary carcinoma of thyroid:
(a) RET Proto Oncogene
(b) Fap gene
(c) Rb gene
(d) BRCA 1 gene

66.9. All of the following are tumor markers, except:
(a) Beta-2 macroglobulin
(b) HCG
(c) Alpha-fetoprotein
(d) CEA

66.10. An example of a tumor suppressor gene is:
(a) Myc
(b) Fos
(c) Ras
(d) Rb

66.11. Knudson two hit hypothesis is seen with
(a) Melanoma
(b) Retinoblastoma
(c) Ulcerative colitis
(d) Crohn disease

66.12. Retinoblastomas arising in the context of germ-line mutations not only may be bilateral, but also may be associated with _____ (so called "trilateral" retinoblastoma)

(a) Medulloblastoma
(b) Pinealoblastoma
(c) Neuroblastoma
(d) Hemangioblastoma

ETIOLOGICAL AGENTS FOR CANCER: CHEMICAL, RADIATION, MICROBES, MULTISTEP CARCINOGENESIS

67. Post transplant lymphoma is caused by which of the following? *(AIIMS May 2012)*
(a) CMV
(b) EBV
(c) Herpes simplex
(d) HHV-6

68. *H. pylori* infection is associated with development of which malignancy: *(DPG 2011)*
(a) MALTomas
(b) Atherosclerosis
(c) Sarcoma
(d) Gastrointestinal stromal tumor (GIST)

69. Helicobacter pylori infection is associated with all of the following conditions, except: *(DPG 2011)*
(a) Peptic ulcer disease
(b) Gastric adenocarcinoma
(c) B cell lymphoma
(d) Burkitt's lymphoma

70. Tumors associated with organisms are all except:
(a) Hepatocellular cancer *(AIIMS Nov 2009)*
(b) Non-small Cell Carcinoma of Lung
(c) Gastric cancer
(d) Nasopharyngeal cancer

71. Which of the following is essential for tumor metastasis?
(a) Angiogenesis *(AIIMS Nov 2008, DNB 2009)*
(b) Tumorogenesis
(c) Apoptosis
(d) Inhibition of tyrosine kinase activity

72. Which of the following statements about carcinogenesis is *false*? *(AIIMS May 2006)*
(a) Asbestos exposure increases the incidence of lung cancer
(b) Papilloma viruses produce tumors in animals but not in humans
(c) Exposure to aniline dyes predisposes to cancer of the urinary bladder
(d) Hepatitis B virus has been implicated in hepatocellular carcinoma

73. Which of the following is an oncogenic RNA virus?
(a) Hepatitis B virus *(Delhi PG 2009 RP)*
(b) Human papilloma virus
(c) Epstein Barr virus
(d) Hepatitis C virus

74. LMP-1 gene plays a role in oncogenesis induced by: *(Karnataka 2008)*
(a) Human T cell leukemia virus type I
(b) Hepatitis B virus

(c) Epstein-Barr virus
(d) Human papilloma virus

75. **Skin cancers develop due to sunlight exposure induced by:** *(Karnataka 2006)*
   (a) UVA rays   (b) UVB rays
   (c) UVC rays   (d) UVD rays

76. **Most radiosensitive tumor is:** *(RJ 2003)*
   (a) Renal cell carcinoma
   (b) Carcinoma colon
   (c) Hepatocellular carcinoma
   (d) Testicular seminoma

77. **Smoking is a risk factor for all carcinomas, except:**
   (a) Oral   *(RJ 2006)*
   (b) Bronchial
   (c) Bladder
   (d) Thyroid

78. **Workers exposed to polyvinyl chloride may develop following liver malignancy:** *(AP 2002)*
   (a) Cholangiocarcinoma
   (b) Fibrolamellar carcinoma
   (c) Angiosarcoma
   (d) All of the above

79. **Which among the following is not a neoplastic virus:**
   (a) Cytomegalovirus   *(Bihar 2006)*
   (b) Hepatitis B virus
   (c) Human papilloma virus
   (d) All of these

80. **A 37-year-old man, Gagan presents with increasing abdominal pain and jaundice. He gives a history of intake of groundnuts which did not taste appropriate. Physical examination reveals a large mass involving the right side of his liver, and a biopsy specimen from this mass confirms the diagnosis of liver cancer (hepatocellular carcinoma). Which of the following substances is most closely associated with the pathogenesis of this tumor?**
   (a) Aflaxotin B1
   (b) Direct-acting alkylating agents
   (c) Vinyl chloride
   (d) Azo dyes
   (e) Beta-Naphthylamine

81. **Biopsy of an ulcerated gastric lesion of a 26-year-old smoker Akki demonstrates glands containing cells with enlarged, hyperchromatic nuclei below the muscularis mucosa. Two tripolar mitotic figures are noted. With which of the following infectious agents has this type of lesion been most strongly associated?**
   (a) Epstein-Barr virus
   (b) Helicobacter pylori
   (c) Human papilloma virus
   (d) Molluscum contagiosum virus

82. **A man Alok Nath contracts HTLV-1 infection through sexual contact. Twenty-one years later he develops generalized lymphadenopathy with** hepatosplenomegaly, a skin rash, hypercalcemia, and an elevated white blood count. This man has most likely developed which of the following?
   (a) AIDS
   (b) Autoimmunity
   (c) Delayed hypersensitivity reaction
   (d) Leukemia
   (e) Recurrent infection

Most Recent Questions

82.1. **Thorium induced tumor is which of the following?**
   (a) Renal cell carcinoma
   (b) Lymphoma
   (c) Angiosarcoma of liver
   (d) Astrocytoma

82.2. **Radiation exposure during infancy has been linked to which one of the following carcinoma?**
   (a) Breast   (b) Melanoma
   (c) Thyroid   (d) Lung

82.3. **The following parasitic infections predispose to malignancies?**
   (a) Paragonimus westermani
   (b) Guinea worm infection
   (c) Clonorchiasis
   (d) Schistosomiasis

82.4. **Kaposi's sarcoma is seen with:**
   (a) HCV   (b) HPV
   (c) HSV   (d) HHV

82.5. **UV radiation has which of the following effects on the cells?**
   (a) Prevents formation of pyrimidine dimers
   (b) Stimulates formation of pyrimidine dimers
   (c) Prevents formation of purine dimers
   (d) All of the above

82.6. **The most radiosensitive cells are:**
   (a) Neutrophils   (b) Lymphocytes
   (c) Erythrocytes   (d) Megakaryocytes

82.7 **The SI unit of radiation absorbed dose is**
   (a) Rad   (b) Becquerel
   (c) Gray   (d) Sievert

82.8. **One of the following leukemia almost never develops after radiation?**
   (a) Acute myeloblastic leukemia
   (b) Chronic myeloid leukemia
   (c) Acute lumphoblastic leukemia
   (d) Chronic lymphocytic leukemia

PARANEOPLASTIC SYNDROMES, TUMOUR MARKERS, TUMOUR LYSIS SYNDROME

83. **A 20 year old female was diagnosed with granulose cell tumor of the ovary. Which of the following bio markers would be most useful for follow-up of patient?**

(a) CA 19-9 *(AIIMS Nov 2011)*
(b) CA50
(c) Inhibin
(d) Neuron – specific enolase

84. **Alpha fetoprotein is a marker of:** *(AI 2010)*
(a) Hepatoblastoma
(b) Seminoma
(c) Renal cell carcinoma
(d) Choriocarcinoma

85. **Hyperglycemia associated with:** *(AI 2010)*
(a) Multiple myeloma
(b) Ewing sarcoma
(c) Osteosarcoma
(d) Chondroblastoma

86. **Which of the following is Not associated with thymoma?** *(AI 2010)*
(a) SIADH
(b) Myasthenia gravis
(c) Polymyositis
(d) Hypogammaglobinemia

87. **Which of the following is not true about Neuroblastoma?** *(AI 2009)*
(a) Most common extracranial solid tumor in childhood
(b) >50% patients present with metastasis at time of diagnosis
(c) Lung metastases are common
(d) Involve aorta and its branches early

88. **Migratory thrombophlebitis is associated with all of the following malignancies, except:** *(AI 2008)*
(a) Prostate
(b) Lung
(c) GIT
(d) Pancreas

89. **HMB 45 is a tumor marker for:** *(AI 2008, DNB 2008)*
(a) Neuroblastoma
(b) Neurofibroma
(c) Malignant melanoma
(d) Angiosarcoma

90. **AFP is a marker of:** *(AIIMS Nov 2009)*
(a) Hepatoblastoma
(b) Seminoma
(c) Sertoli-Leydig cell tumor
(d) Choriocarcinoma

91. **An undifferentiated malignant tumor on immunohistochemical stain shows cytoplasmic positivity of most of the tumor cells for cytokeratin. The most probable diagnosis of the tumor is:**
(a) Sarcoma *(AIIMS May 2006)*
(b) Lymphoma
(c) Carcinoma
(d) Malignant melanoma

92. **For which one of the following tumors Gastrin is a biochemical marker?** *(AIIMS May 2005)*
(a) Medullary carcinoma of thyroid
(b) Pancreatic neuroendocrine tumor
(c) Pheochromocytoma
(d) Gastrointestinal stromal tumor

93. **All of the following are examples of tumor markers, except:**
(a) Alpha-HCG (α-HCG) *(AIIMS Nov 2004)*
(b) Alpha-Feto protein
(c) Thyroglobulin
(d) Beta 2-microglobulin

94. **Which of the following tumors have an increased elevation of placental alkaline phosphatase in the serum as well as a positive immunohistochemical staining for placental alkaline phosphatase?**
(a) Seminoma *(AIIMS May 2004)*
(b) Hepatoblastoma
(c) Hepatocellular carcinoma
(d) Peripheral neuroectodermal tumor

95. **In tumor lysis syndrome, all of the following are seen, except:** *(AIIMS May 2002)*
(a) Hypernatremia (b) Hypercalcemia
(c) Hyperkalemia (d) Hyperphosphatemia

96. **Uses of tumor marker are:** *(PGI Dec 2000)*
(a) Screening of a cancer
(b) Follow up of a cancer patient, esp. for knowing about recurrence
(c) Confirmation of a diagnosed cancer
(d) For monitoring the treatment of a cancer

97. **True about Carcinoembryonic antigen (CEA):**
(a) Useful for screening of carcinoma colon
(b) Gives confirmative evidence of Ca. colon
(c) Helpful for follow-up after resection *(PGI June 01)*
(d) Levels decrease immediately after resection of tumor
(e) Tumor size correlates with CEA level

98. **CA 125 is associated with:** *(PGI June 2002)*
(a) Colon ca (b) Breast ca
(c) Ovarian ca (d) Bronchogenic ca
(e) Pancreatic ca

99. **Secondaries are common in all, except:**
(a) Skull *(PGI June 01)*
(b) Hand and feet bones
(c) Proximal limb bones
(d) Pelvic
(e) Vertebrae

100. **Hybridoma refers to** *(Delhi PG 2009 RP)*
(a) Collision tumor
(b) A tumor of brown fat
(c) A hamartoma
(d) A technique for raising monoclonal antibodies

Neoplasia

101. **BCL2 is a marker for:** *(Delhi PG-2007)*
    (a) Follicular lymphoma
    (b) Mycosis fungoides
    (c) B-cell lymphoma
    (d) Mantle cell lymphoma

102. **Alpha-fetoproteins are a marker of:**
    (a) Secondaries in liver *(Karnataka 2005)*
    (b) Cholangiocarcinoma
    (c) Hepatoma
    (d) None of the above

103. **Increased level of alpha fetoprotein is found in**
    (a) Yolk sac tumor *(UP 2001)*
    (b) Seminoma
    (c) Teratoma
    (d) Choriocarcinoma

104. **Migratory thrombophlebitis is seen in:** *(UP 2007)*
    (a) Disseminated cancer
    (b) Rheumatic heart disease
    (c) Libman-Sachs endocarditis
    (d) All of the above

105. **A 65 years old male diagnosed by biopsy a case of lung carcinoma, with paraneoplastic syndrome and increased calcium. Probable cause is** *(UP 2008)*
    (a) Parathyroid hormone
    (b) Parathyroid hormone related peptide
    (c) Calcitonin
    (d) Calcitonin related peptide

106. **Which is associated with polycythemia:** *(RJ 2001)*
    (a) Gastric carcinoma
    (b) Fibrosarcoma
    (c) Cerebellar hemangioblastoma
    (d) All

107. **Serum AFP is increased in all, except:** *(RJ 2003)*
    (a) Acute hepatitis
    (b) Hepatocellular carcinoma
    (c) Hepatoma
    (d) Bladder carcinoma

108. **Carcinoembryonic antigen is elevated in all, except:**
    (a) Alcoholic cirrhosis *(RJ 2004)*
    (b) Ca colon
    (c) Ulcerative colitis
    (d) Emphysema

109. **Desmoid tumor arises from:**
    (a) Wall of the intestine *(TN 1991)(AP 2000)*
    (b) Anterior abdominal wall
    (c) Submucosa
    (d) Appendix

110. **Alpha-fetoprotein is a tumor marker of:**
    (a) Carcinoma ovary *(AP 2001)*
    (b) Liver malignancies
    (c) Endodermal sinus tumor of testis
    (d) Both (b) and (c)

111. **α-fetoprotein is seen in all except:** *(AP 2002)*
    (a) Hepatocellular carcinoma *(AI 1997)*
    (b) Carcinoma colon *(UP 1996)*
    (c) Pancreatic carcinoma
    (d) Germ cells of testes

112. **The diagnostic tumor marker of liver carcinoma is:**
    (a) CEA *(AP 2007)*
    (b) AFP
    (c) CA - 125
    (d) All of the above

113. **Spontaneous regression of tumor is seen in:**
    (a) Wilm's tumor *(Kolkata 2002)*
    (b) Neuroblastoma
    (c) Acute monocytic leukemia
    (d) Hepatoblastoma

114. **All of the following about tumor markers are properly matched, except:** *(Kolkata 2003)*
    (a) Prostate cancer - PSA
    (b) Colon cancer - CEA
    (c) Ovarian cancer – CA 125
    (d) Cholangiocarcinoma - AFP

115. **Popcorn calcification is seen in:** *(Kolkata 2005)*
    (a) Chondrosarcoma (b) Fibrous dysplasia
    (c) Osteoblastoma (d) Wilms' tumor

116. **Which one of the following is a frequent cause of serum alpha- fetoprotein level greater than 10 times the normal upper limit?** *(Bihar 2004)*
    (a) Seminoma
    (b) Hepatocellular carcinoma of liver
    (c) Cirrhosis of liver
    (d) Oat cell tumor of lung

117. **Rise of AFP is noted in all except:** *(Jharkhand 2004)*
    (a) Hepatocellular carcinoma
    (b) Cirrhosis
    (c) Germ cell tumor
    (d) Kidney tumor

118. **Catecholamines are increased in:** *(Jharkhand 2004)*
    (a) Neuroblastoma
    (b) Retinoblastoma
    (c) Medulloblastoma
    (d) Nephroblastoma

119. **A 60-year-old man, Shibu is found to have a 3.5-cm mass in the right upper lobe of his lung. A biopsy of this mass is diagnosed as a moderately differentiated squamous cell carcinoma. Workup reveals that no bone metastases are present, but laboratory examination reveals that the man's serum calcium levels are 11.5 mg/dL. This patient's paraneoplastic syndrome is most likely the result of the ectopic production of which of the following substances?**
    (a) Parathyroid hormone
    (b) Parathyroid hormone-related peptide
    (c) Calcitonin
    (d) Calcitonin-related peptide

120. During a routine physical examination, a 45-year-old woman Nusheen is noted to have a ruddy complexion. Her hematocrit is 52%. Her lungs are clear and she does not smoke. Serum erythropoietin levels are elevated. Cancer of which of the following organs is the most likely cause of her increased hematocrit?
    (a) Breast   (b) Colon
    (c) Kidney   (d) Stomach

121. A 62 year-old woman Omvati with advanced, metastatic lung cancer develops profound fatigue and weakness and alternating diarrhea and constipation. Physical examination demonstrates hyperpigmentation of skin, even in areas protected from the sun. Tumor involvement of which endocrine organ is most strongly suggested by this patient's presentation?
    (a) Adrenal gland   (b) Endocrine pancreas
    (c) Ovaries   (d) Pituitary gland

122. An old man Velu presents with complaints of abdominal and back pain, malaise, nausea, 8 kg weight loss and weakness, which have been present for 3 or 4 months. His history also reveals several episodes of unilateral leg swelling, which have involved both legs at different times. These findings are most consistent with which of the following diagnoses?
    (a) Pancreatic cancer
    (b) Primary sclerosing cholangitis
    (c) Splenic infarction
    (d) Reflux esophagitis

123. A 65-year-old woman Ramkali presents to the emergency room with a pathologic fracture of the shaft of her humerus. X-ray studies demonstrate multiple lytic and blastic bone lesions. Biopsy of one of these lesions shows adenocarcinoma. Which of the following is the most likely source of the primary tumor?
    (a) Breast   (b) Colon
    (c) Kidney   (d) Lung

Most Recent Questions

123.1. Tumor that follows rule of 10 is:
    (a) Pheochromocytoma
    (b) Oncocytoma
    (c) Lymphoma
    (d) Renal cell carcinoma

123.2. Which of the followingis a squamous cell carcinoma marker?
    (a) Vimentin   (b) Desmin
    (c) Cytokeratin   (d) Glial fibrillary acid protein

123.3. Marker for ovarian carcinoma in serum is:
    (a) CA-125
    (b) Fibronectin
    (c) Acid Phosphatase
    (d) PSA

123.4. Which of the following is a marker for carcinoma of lung and breast?
    (a) CEA   (b) AEP
    (c) HCG   (d) CA-15-3

123.5. Secondaries of all the following cause osteolytic lesions except:
    (a) Prostate   (b) Kidney
    (c) Bronchus   (d) Thyroid

123.6. Sacrococcygeal teratoma, marker is:
    (a) CEA   (b) β- HCG
    (c) S100   (d) CA-125

123.7. Which of the following mutation is seen in malignant melanoma?
    (a) N-myc   (b) CDKN2A
    (c) RET   (d) Rb

123.8. Marker of small cell cancer of lung is:
    (a) Chromogranin   (b) Cytokeratin
    (c) Desmin   (d) Vimentin

123.9. Which of the following is tumor marker of seminoma?
    (a) AFP   (b) LDH
    (c) PLAP   (d) HCG

123.10. Which of the following is a special stain for rhabdomyosarcoma?
    (a) Cytokeratin   (b) Synaptophysin
    (c) Desmin   (d) Myeloperoxidase

123.11. The most common cause of malignant adrenal mass is
    (a) Adrenocortical carcinoma
    (b) Malignant Phaeochromocytoma
    (c) Lymphoma
    (d) Metastasis from another solid tissue tumor

123.12. Commonest cancer in which metastasis is seen in brain in
    (a) Breast   (b) Lung
    (c) Kidney   (d) Intestines

123.13. Which of the following is incorrect about neuro-blastoma ?
    (a) Most common abdominal tumor in infants
    (b) X-ray abdomen shows calcification
    (c) Can show spontaneous regression
    (d) Urine contains 5H.I.A.A

EXPLANATIONS

1. Ans. (c) Vascular invasion (*Ref: Robbins 8th/1123, 9/e p1094*)

Robbins clearly write…. '*Microscopically, most follicular carcinomas are composed of fairly uniform cells forming small follicles. Follicular carcinomas may be grossly infiltrative or minimally invasive. The latter are sharply demarcated lesions that may be impossible to distinguish from follicular adenomas on gross examination.* **This distinction requires extensive histologic sampling of the tumor-capsule-thyroid interface, to exclude capsular and/or vascular invasion.** *Extensive invasion of adjacent thyroid parenchyma makes the diagnosis of carcinoma obvious in some cases*'.

- Ideal answer for a question for diagnosis of follicular cancer is **capsular invasion**[Q] (better than even vascular invasion) but in the given options, vascular invasion is the answer of choice.

Follicular Carcinoma: brushing up key points

- It is the 2nd most common form of thyroid cancer
- Seen in women of older age (40-50 yrs.)
- **Vascular invasion** is common (less lymphatic spread) to bone, lung, liver etc.
- **Microscopically**, there is presence of cells forming small follicles having colloid with NO Psammoma bodies. Uncommonly, cells have abundant, eosinophilic cytoplasm called as **Hurthle cells**[Q]
- Differentiation from follicular adenoma is based on the **presence of capsular invasion preferably** and **not** on vascular invasion[Q].

2. Ans. (b) Fibromatosis: (*Ref: Robbins 7th/770, 783-4, Harrison 16th/633, 9/e p1221-1222*)

- Fibromatosis are a group of **fibroblastic proliferations**. Though they are **locally aggressive**, they do not metastasize.

Fibromatosis

Superficial Fibromatosis	Deep Fibromatosis
*Palmar fibromatosis **(Dupuytren contracture)*** *Plantar fibromatosis *Penile fibromatosis **(Peyronie's disease)**	*Also called **desmoids tumors** *Greater tendency to recur *Grow in a locally aggressive manner *Arise isolated or as component of Gardner syndrome

3. Ans. (b) Increased requirement of growth factors (*Ref: Biology of the cell (2003) 357-364*)

Both normal cells and cancer cells can be cultured in-vitro. However, they behave quite differently

Normal cell	Cancer cell
Show **replicative senescence** i.e. cells pass through limited number of cell divisions before they decline in vigor and die. It may caused by **inability to synthesize telomerase**	They are immortal i.e. proliferate indefinitely in culture. Cancer cells in culture produce telomerase
Normal cells show the phenomenon of **contact inhibition** i.e. they proliferate until the surface of culture dish is covered by single layer of cells just touching each other	Show no contact inhibition. Even after the surface of dish is covered, the cells continue to divide
Nutrients and growth factors must be supplied to them in their tissue culture medium	**Do not require growth factors**
Normal karyotype is present	Mostly show abnormal karyotype

4. Ans. (a) Small cell carcinoma of lung (*Ref: Harrison 17th/2458; Robbins 8th/1339, 7th/1410 , 9/e p1315*)

Small cell carcinoma of lung most commonly metastasize to the brain. It accounts for about 40% of brain metastases.

Other Tumors Metastasizing to Brain are carcinomas of • Breast, • Melanoma, • Kidney, • GIT

5. Ans. (c) Both necrosis and apoptosis (*Ref: Harrison 17th/519 , 9/e p303, 315*)

- Chemotherapeutic drugs can cause both necrosis and apoptosis, but *it is apoptosis which is the basis of action of chemotherapeutic drugs.*
- **Anoikis** *refers to death of epithelial cells after removal from the normal milieu of substrate, particularly from cell to cell contact.*

6. Ans. (b) Dysplasia discussed in details in text. (*Ref: Robbins 7th/273-274 , 9/e p271*)

7. **Ans. (a) Smoking; (b) U-V-light; (c) Chronic ulcer:** *(Ref: Harrison' 16th/497, Robbins 9/e p1155)*

Risk factors

Melanoma	Basal cell and squamous cell carcinoma
• Family history of melanoma • Persistently changing mole • Presence of clinically atypical mole • Immunosuppression • Sun exposure	• Exposure to UV light principally UV-B • Male sex and Older age • Exposure to sun, arsenic, smoking, cyclic aromatic hydrocarbons in tar, soot or shale • HIV, HPV infection, immunosuppression. • Ionizing radiations, thermal burns • Certain scars and chronic ulcerations • Heritable conditions like albinism, Xeroderma pigmentosum, genetic mutations (PATCHED gene) • Premalignant conditions like Actinic keratosis, Bowen's disease, Erythroplasia of Queyrat.

8. **Ans. (c) Chronic ulcerative colitis** *(Ref: Robbins 8th/276 , 9/e p279)*
Certain non-neoplastic disorders—*the chronic atrophic gastritis of pernicious anemia, solar keratosis of the skin, chronic ulcerative colitis, and leukoplakia of the oral cavity, vulva, and penis*—have such a well-defined association with cancer that they have been termed *precancerous conditions.*

9. **Ans. (b) Hepatocellular carcinoma** *(Ref: Robbins 7th/925 , 9/e p274)*
Renal cell cancer and hepatocellular cancer have high tendency invasion of vascular channels.

10. **Ans. (c) Dysplasia** *(Ref: Robbins 7th/275, 276, 5 , 9/e p271-272)*
   - **Dysplasia** is the loss of uniformity of individual cells as well as their architectural orientation.
   - **Carcinoma *in situ*** (dysplastic changes are marked but lesion remains confined to normal tissue: pre-invasive neoplasm). ***Basement membrane is intact***.
   - **Anaplasia** is Complete lack of differentiation of cells both morphologically and functionally (Invasive Ca)

11. **Ans. (b) Lymphatic route** *(Ref: Robbins 8th/269, 7th/279-280 , 9/e p273)*

12. **Ans. (b) Gastric carcinoma** *(Ref: Robbins 8th/986; 7th/824 , 9/e p1207)*

13. **Ans. (b) Proliferation of native cells in tissue** *(Ref: Robbins 8th/262; 7th/272 , 9/e p267)*

14. **Ans. (d) Metastasis** *(Ref: Robbins 8th/269; 7th/268,279, 9/e p272)*

15. **Ans. (a) Metaplasia** *(Ref: Robbins 8th/10,265; 7th/10 , 9/e p271)*

16. **Ans (d) Muscle tumor cells forming giant cells** *(Ref: Robbins 8th/262-5, 9/e p270)*
Neoplastic cells may be similar to normal cells found in the tissue of origin, which defines the malignancy as "well differentiated" or "low grade." Alternatively, the neoplastic cells may lack most of the characteristic features of normal cells found in the tissue of origin, which defines the malignancy as "poorly differentiated" or "high grade." Tumors that contain neoplastic cells in the midst of this spectrum are termed "moderately differentiated" or "medium grade." If the neoplastic cells are described as anaplastic, they demonstrate a complete lack of differentiation.

Features of Anaplastic tumors
   - **Loss of cell polarity and normal tissue architecture**[Q]
   - Significant variation in shape and size of cells **(cellular pleomorphism)**[Q]
   - Deep staining of nuclei (**hyperchromatism**[Q]) and nuclear pleomorphism
   - Larger nuclei than those found in normal cells of the same tissue (**high nucleus-to-cytoplasm ratio**[Q])
   - Numerous often **abnormal mitoses**[Q]
   - **Giant multinucleated tumor cells**[Q]

The appearance of giant multinucleated cells in a muscle tumor would therefore suggest anaplasia.

(Choice A) Cells in hepatic tissue would be expected to synthesize bile. Therefore a hepatic tumor that synthesizes bile is described as being well-differentiated not anaplastic.
(Choice B and C) Cells in the epithelium would be expected to produce keratin pearls. Therefore an epithelial tumor that produces keratin pearls would be described as well-differentiated not anaplastic.

17. **Ans. (d) Proliferation of non- neoplastic fibrous connective tissue** *(Ref: Robbins 8th/260, 9/e p266)*
Desmoplasia refers to proliferation of non-neoplasitc fibrous connective tissue within a tumor and is common in breast cancer. An irregular accumulation of blood vessels is known as a hemangioma. An area of tissue misplaced within another organ is known as a choristoma.

18. **Ans. (d) Present with specific marker phenotypes.** *(Ref: Robbins 8th/275)*
The familial cancers are associated with the cancer occurring at a higher frequency in certain families without a clearly defined pattern of transmission[Q]. Features that characterize familial cancers include

- Early age at onset[Q]
- Tumors arising in two or more close relatives of the index case[Q]
- Sometimes multiple or bilateral tumors[Q]

Familial cancers are not associated with specific marker phenotypes[Q].

19. Ans. (c) Distribution and extent of disease *(Ref: Robbins 8th/323 , 9/e p332)*

Staging is based on clinical evaluation of the distribution and extent of the disease process and is contrasted with grading (based on histopathologic evaluation of a malignant neoplasm).

> **Mnemonic: S**taging includes **S**ize (extent of disease) and **S**pread (distribution) of the tumor.

20. Ans. (b) Cannot be determined by microscopic examination *(Ref: Robbins 8th/1159-1161, 9/e p1135)*

Pheochromocytomas, and their related counterparts in extra-adrenal sites called paragangliomas, are notorious because the only reliable indicator of metastatic potential is the presence of distant metastases. Very malignant-appearing tumors may not metastasize and benign-appearing tumors may produce metastases. These tumors should all be considered "potentially malignant."

20.1. Ans. (b) Presence of metastasis to other organs *(Ref: Robbins 8/e p1159-1161, 9/e p1135)*

Friends read these lines form Robbins to get a concept.. **"There is no histologic feature that reliably predicts clinical behavior**. Several histologic features, such as *numbers of mitoses, confluent tumor necrosis, and spindle cell morphology*, have been associated with an aggressive behavior and increased risk of metastasis, but these are not entirely reliable. Tumors with "benign" histologic features may metastasize, while bizarrely pleomorphic tumors may remain confined to the adrenal gland. In fact, *cellular and nuclear pleomorphism, including the presence of giant cells, and mitotic figures are often seen in benign pheochromocytomas*, while cellular monotony is paradoxically associated with an aggressive behavior. *Even capsular and vascular invasion may be encountered in benign lesions.* Therefore, the **definitive diagnosis of malignancy in pheochromocytomas** is based **exclusively on the presence of metastases.**

20.2. Ans (a) Hamartoma *(Ref: Robbins 8/e p262, 9/e p13)*

An overgrowth of a skin structure at a *localized region* is likely to be indigenous as well as benign; this is more likely to be a hamartoma.

- When a neoplasm, benign or malignant, produces a macroscopically visible projection above a mucosal surface and projects, for example, into the gastric or colonic lumen, it is termed a *polyp*
- *Hamartomas* present as disorganized but benign-appearing masses composed of cells indigenous to the particular site.
- *Choristoma* is a congenital anomaly which is described as a *heterotopic rest* of cells.

20.3. Ans (b) Integrins *(Ref: Robbins 8/e p49, 9/e p24)*

The cell adhesion molecules (CAMs) are classified into four main families:
- Immunoglobulin family CAMs
- *Cadherins*
- *Integrins:* bind to extracellular matrix (ECM) proteins such as fibronectin, laminin, and osteopontin **providing a connection between cells and extracellular matrix** (ECM)
- *Selectins*

20.4. Ans. (d) Hepatocytes *(Ref: Robbins 8/e p81-4, 7/e p90-91, 9/e p101)*

Permanent cells	Quiescent cells	Labile cells
• Cannot divide in postnatal life	• Low level of replication which increases only on stimulation	• Rapid rate of replication
• Neurons, skeletal muscles	• Liver cells, kidney cells	• Skin, GIT, oral cavity

20.5. Ans. (a) Crohn disease *(Ref: Robbins 9/e p279)*

- Ideal answer to this question is none but in the given situation, the answer of choice is Crohn disease because in the comparison of the two types of inflammatory bowel disease, Crohn disease is less likely to be associated with progression to cancer of the bowel.

20.6. Ans. (c) Basement membrane invasion *(Ref: Robbins 9/e p271)*

- **Basement membrane invasion**[Q] is the most important differentiating feature between **invasive carcinoma from carcinoma in situ.**

20.7. Ans. (d) Metastasis *(Ref: Robbins 9/e p272)*

Metastasis is the *most reliable feature* of a malignant tumor, characterized by the spread of the tumor to other parts because of penetration into blood vessels, lymphatics and the body cavities.

20.8 Ans. (a) Cancer penis in male *(Ref: Various books, internet)*
Diseases showing bimodality of age presentation (Mnemonic: **ABCDEGH**)
1. **A**ortic stenosis/acute leukemia – A.L.L > A.M.L
2. **B**reast cancer (Before advent of mammography
3. **C**rohn's disease
4. **D**ermatomyositis
5. **E**nthesioneurobalstoma
6. Thyroglossal cyst
7. **H**odgkin's lymphoma
8. Vulvar carcinoma *but NOT penile cancer*

21. **Ans. (c) G2M** *(Ref: Robbins 8th/286; Harrison 17th/516, 9/e p289)*
Direct quote from Robbins…. 'The G2/M checkpoint monitors the completion of the DNA replication and checks whether the cell can safely initiate the mitosis and separate sister chromatids. This checkpoint is particularly important in cells exposed to ionizing radiation. *Cells damaged by ionizing radiation activate G2/M checkpoint* and arrest in G2'.

22. **Ans. (a) G0-G1-S-G2-M** *(Ref: Robbins 7th/90, 9/e p25)*
- G_1/S check-point is controlled by **p53** whereas G_2/M check-point has both p53 dependent as well independent mechanisms.

23. **Ans. (d) S phase** *(Ref: Robbins 8th/86, 7th/90, 9/e p25)*

24. **Ans. (c) G1-S Phase** *(Ref: Robbins 7th/292, 9/e p295)*
- G_1/S check-point is controlled by p53 whereas G_2/M check-point has both p53 dependent as well as independent mechanisms.
- p53 induces the synthesis of p21 which inhibits cyclin D/Cdk4. This results in stoppage of activation of Rb and cell cycle is arrested in G_1/S phase.

25. **Ans. (d) Cyclin B** *(Ref: Robbins 7th/290-291, Robbins 8th/285-286 , 9/e p25-26)*
Examples of cyclin/CDK complexes controlling the cell cycle.

Cyclin B/CDK$_1$	Regulates the transition from G_2 to M phase
Cyclin D/CDK$_4$ Cyclin D/CDK$_6$ Cyclin E/CDK$_2$	Regulates the transition from G_1-S
Cyclin A/CDK$_2$ and cyclin B/CDK$_1$	Active in S phase

26. **Ans. (a) S; (b) M; (d) G_2:** *(Ref: Gray's anatomy 38th/55)*
- The time taken for S, G_2 and M phases are *similar* for most cell types, occupying about 6, 4 and 2 hours respectively.
- The *duration of G_1 shows considerable variation. It can be* as short as 2 hours in rapidly dividing cells like embryonic tissues or as long as 12 hours in some adult tissues.
- G_1 phase is most variable because, in this phase cells are not committed to DNA replication. They can either enter resting state or progress to next cell division.

27. **Ans. (a) Topoisomerase II causes break in strands; (c) At G2 M phase there is loss of inhibitors controlling cell cycle and (d) Decrease in telomerase activity causes anti-tumor effects.** *(Ref: Harrison 16th/453, 454, Robbins 7th/43, 292)*

- Topoisomerase I nicks DNA, relieving torsional tension of the replicating helix.
- Topoisomerase II introduces the double strand break to avoid DNA tangle.
- p53 it is a tumor supresser gene.
- With each cell division, there is some shortening of specialized structures called telomeres (present at ends of chromosomes). In germ cells, telomere shortening is prevented by the enzyme telomerase. This enzyme is absent from most somatic cells, and hence they suffer progressive loss of telomeres. Introduction of telomerase into normal human cells causes considerable extension of their life span, thus supporting that **telomerase loss is causally associated with loss of replication activity.** So, decrease telomerase activity causes anti tumor effect.
- Loss of inhibitors controlling cell cycle occurs at G_1-S phase/G_2-M phase.

28. **Ans. (a) Proto-oncogenes are activated by chromosomal translocation; (b) Malignant transformation involves accumulation of mutations in the proto-oncogenes and tumor suppressor gene in stepwise fashion; (c) point mutations of somatic cells; (e) At G2 M phase there is loss of inhibitors controlling cell cycle** *(Ref: Robbins' 7th/290, 314, 315, 9/e p284-286)*
Activation of proto-oncogene results in cancer causing oncogenes by following mechanisms:

Neoplasia

1. Single point mutation e.g. ras oncogene.
2. Gene amplification e.g. n-myc amplification in neuroblastoma.
3. Chromosomal translocation e.g. t (8:14) in Burkitt lymphoma results in c-myc over-expression and hence the tumor.
4. Promoter insertion.
5. Enhancer insertion.

The cell cycle has its own internal controls called checkpoints. There are two main checkpoints:

1. G_1-S transition- The S-phase is the point of no return in cell cycle. G_1-S checkpoint checks for DNA damage and prevents replication of defective cells.
2. At G_2M transition- The G_2M checkpoint monitors the completion of DNA replication and checks whether the cell can safely initiate cell division. Loss of inhibitors at this stage can lead to division of faulty cells and can lead to carcinogenesis.

- Defect in cell-cycle checkpoint components is a major cause of genetic instability in cancer cells.

29. Ans. (c) G_1- S phase *(Ref: Robbins 8th/290-292, 7th/302-303 , 9/e p294-295)*

30. Ans. (a) Fragile X syndrome *(Ref: Robbins 8th/169-170; 7th/181-183, 9/e p169)*

31. Ans. (b) Cyclin B *(Ref: Robbins 8th/286, 7th/290, 9/e p26)*

31.1. Ans. (a) Gastric cancer *(Ref: Robbins 8/e p96, 785, 9/e p291)*
Cadherin is derived from the "calcium-dependent adherence protein." It participates in interactions between cells of the same type. The linkage of cadherins with the cytoskeleton occurs through the catenins. The cell -to-cell interactions mediated by cadherin and catenins play a major role in regulating cell motility, proliferation, and differentiation and account for the inhibition of cell proliferation that occurs when cultured normal cells contact each other ("**contact inhibition**").
- Reduced function of **E-cadherin** is associated with certain types of **breast and gastric cancer.**
- Mutation and altered expression of the *Wnt/β-catenin* pathway is implicated in in *gastrointestinal and liver cancer* development.

31.2. Ans. (b) p53 *(Ref: Robbins 8/e p274, 290, 9/e p293-294)*
- The *p53* gene is located on chromosome **17p13.1**[Q], and it is the **most common target**[Q] for genetic alteration in human tumors.
- *A little over 50% of human tumors contain mutations in this gene.*
- In most cases, the inactivating mutations affect both *p53* alleles and are acquired in somatic cells (not inherited in the germ line).
- Less commonly, some individuals inherit one mutant *p53* allele. The **inheritance of one mutant allele predisposes individuals to develop malignant tumors** because only one additional "hit" is needed to inactivate the second, normal allele. Such individuals, said to have the *Li-Fraumeni syndrome* and have a greater chance of developing a malignant tumor at a younger age. These people tend to develop multiple primary tumors.
- Themost common types of tumors are sarcomas, breast cancer, leukemia, brain tumors, and carcinomas of the adrenal cortex.

31.3. Ans. (c) p53 *(Ref: (Ref: Robbins Illustrated 7/e p p 292, (Ref: Robbins 8/e p286, 9/e p25-26)*
Cyclins form complex with cyclin dependent kinases and regulate the transition of cell cycle from one stage to the other. These CDK complexes in turn are regulated by CDK inhibitor. The inhibitors control the cell cycle by balancing the activity of CDKs. The signals from these inhibitors determine whether a cell progresses through the cell cycle.
Changes in the level of these inhibitors may occur in some tumors, or possibly in aging cells.
- The cyclin dependent kinase inhibitors are

- p21 - p27 - p57 - p15 - p16 - p18 - p19

31.4. Ans. (b) M –phase
- Cells are most radiosensitive in **G_2M interphase**
- Cells are least radiosensitive in **S phase**

32. Ans. (b) Bone marrow hyper function *(Ref: Robbins 8th/663; 7th/647, 9/e p630)*

33. Ans. (a) Predicting therapeutic response *(Ref: Ackerman 's surgical pathology 9th/1818, Robbins 8th/1090, 9/e p1062)*

Friends, direct quote from Robbins....'*HER2/neu overexpression* is associated with *poorer survival* but its *main importance is as a predictor of response to agents that target this transmembrane protein (examples* trastuzumab or lapatinib)*.'
- The overexpression is due to *amplification* of the gene *HER2/neu* located on 17q21.
Ackerman writes.... HER2/new encodes a transmembrane glycoprotein with tyrosine kinase activity and its overexpression is a *good predictor of response to herceptin* (trastuzumab) but not a good predictor of response to chemotherapy or overall survival.

34. Ans. (a) Osteosarcoma *(Ref: Robbins 8th/287,1338, 1365, 9/e p293)*
- *Retinoblastoma is the most common primary intraocular malignancy of children.* Involvement of both eyes with pineal gland is called as trilateral retinoblastoma.
- The pinealoblastoma in association with retinoblastoma is a *primary tumor*.
- In approximately 40% of cases, retinoblastoma occurs in individuals who inherit a germ-line mutation of one RB allele. This variant of retinoblastoma (familial retinoblastoma) is inherited as an autosomal dominant trait and is associated with osteosarcoma. *Osteosarcoma* is therefore the commonest *secondary malignancy* associated with retinoblastoma.

35. Ans. (a) Austosomal dominant *(Ref: Robbins 8th/302, Harrison 665, 9/e p314-315)*
- Fanconi's anemia is an **autosomal recessive**[Q] disease characterized by progressive **pancytopenia**[Q], increased risk of malignancy **(solid tumors and AML**[Q]**)** and congenital developmental anomalies like short stature, café au lait spots, abnormalities affecting thumb, radius and genitourinary tract.
- Fanconi's anemia is associated with **BRCA gene**. The Fanconi anemia proteins and BRCA proteins form a **DNA-damage repair proteins** to correct intrastrand and interstrand DNA cross links induced by chemical cross-linking agents.

36. Ans. (d) Wild/non-mutated form is associated with increased risk of childhood tumors *(Ref: Robbin 7th/302-303, Harrison 17th/499-500, 8th/290-2, 9/e p294)*
- p53 gene is a tumor suppressor gene also known as **"guardian of the genome"**[Q] located on **short arm of chromosome 17**[Q] (17p). Its wild/non mutated form is associated with reduced risk of tumors.

37. Ans. (c) sis *(Ref: Robbins 7th/182)*
- A number of **nuclear transcription factors** are the products of oncogenes like **myc, fos, jun, myb and rel**. Out of these *myc is most commonly involved in tumors*[Q].
- **SIS oncogene** is the only example of a growth factor oncogene in the given options. Its over expression is seen in cancers like astrocytoma and osteosarcoma. The other growth factor are described is text.

38. Ans. (a) Retinoblastoma *(Ref: Robbins 7th/1442; Neuropathology for the Neuroradiologist: Rosettes and Pseudorosettes by F.J. Wippold and A. Perry)*
Rosettes consist of a halo or spoke-wheel arrangement of cells surrounding a central core or hub.

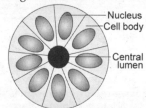

Rosettes may be considered primary or secondary manifestations of tumor architecture. Primary rosettes form as a characteristic growth pattern of a given tumor type, whereas secondary rosettes result from the influence of external factors on tumor growth.

Types of rosette	Flexner-Wintersteiner rosettes	Homer-Wright rosettes	True Ependymal Rosette	Perivascular Pseudorosette	Neurocytic rosette
Diagram					
Feature	*A halo of cells surrounds a largely empty central hub. Small cytoplasmic extensions from the cells project into the lumen	*A halo of cells surrounds a central hub that contains a meshwork of fibers	*The halo-like cluster of cells in each rosette surrounds an empty central lumen	*A halo of cells surrounds a blood vessel *Called 'pseudo' because the central structure is not actually formed by the tumor itself, but instead represents a native, non-neoplastic element	*Rosette is similar to the Homer Wright rosette, but the central fiber-rich neuropil island is larger and more irregular

Contd...

Contd...

Types of rosette	Flexner-Wintersteiner rosettes	Homer-Wright rosettes	True Ependymal Rosette	Perivascular Pseudorosette	Neurocytic rosette
Related tumors	Retinoblastoma[Q], Pineoblastomas, Medulloepitheliomas	Supratentorial PNETs, Retinoblastoma[Q], Pineoblastomas	Ependymoblastoma (rare form of PNET)	Medulloblastomas, PNETs, Central neurocytomas, Glioblastomas, Pilomyxoid astrocytomas	Central neurocytoma

> *Neuropil-rich rosettes are referred to as *pineocytomatous rosettes* in pineocytomas and *neurocytic rosettes* in central neurocytoma. These are similar to the Homer Wright rosette, but they are generally larger and more irregular in contour.

39. **Ans. (c) Promotion of DNA repair** *(Ref: Robbins 7th/293, 295), http://www.nature.com/scitable/topicpage/proto-onco-genes-to-oncogenes-to-cancer-883 by Heidi Chial, 9/e p284)*

The normal cellular counterpart of oncogene is known as proto-oncogene. Proto-oncogenes are important for cellular function related to growth and proliferation. Proteins encoded by these genes may function as growth factor ligands and receptors, signal transducers, transcription factors and cell cycle components.

Chial writes that 'proto-oncogenes encode proteins that function to *stimulate cell division, inhibit cell differentiation, and halt cell death*. All of these processes are important for normal human development and for the maintenance of tissues and organs. Oncogenes, however, typically exhibit increased production of these proteins, thus leading to increased cell division, decreased cell differentiation, and inhibition of cell death'. So, we can say that '**These genes may also inhibit apoptosis**'.

Promotion of DNA repair is the function of **tumor suppressor genes**. Promotion of DNA repair is protective from oncogenesis and is not the function of proto-oncogenes.

40. **Ans. (d) Rb** *(Ref: Robbins 7th/300, Harrison 17th/499, 496, 9/e p290)*
   - Tumor suppressor genes are the genes whose products down regulate the cell cycle, and thus apply brakes to cellular proliferation.
   - Rb gene is a tumor suppressor gene whereas Myc, fos and ras are all examples of proto-oncogenes.

41. **Ans. (d) Colon, endometrium, ovary** *(Ref: Harrison 17/page 575, Robbins 8th/821-822, 9/e p810)*
   - Lynch syndrome is an **autosomal dominant**[Q] disorder
   - It is also called as *Hereditary Non-polyposis Colon Cancer (HNPCC) syndrome*[Q]
   - It is caused because of **defective DNA repair genes**[Q] *leading to microsatellite instability.*
   - There is increased chance of multiple cancers (*colorectal area, endometrium, ovary, stomach, ureter, brain, small intestine, hepatobiliary tract and skin*)

42. **Ans. (c) Retinoblastoma** *(Ref: Robbins 7th/299, 9/e p292-293)*
   - Retinoblastoma is a prime example of a tumor which is associated with loss of heterozygosity.
   - Rb gene is a **tumor suppressor** gene located on **chromosome 13 q14**[Q].
   - Retinoblastoma develops when *both the normal alleles of the Rb gene are inactivated or altered*

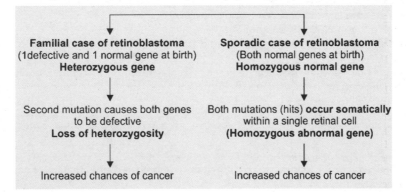

43. **Ans. (d) ras** *(Ref: Robbins 7th/295, 9/e p286)*

44. **Ans. (b) Autosomal dominant** *(Ref: Robbins 7th/1442, 299-300, 9/e p292-293)*
   - Retinoblastoma is a prime example of a tumor which is associated with loss of heterozygosity.
   - Rb gene is a **tumor suppressor** gene located on **chromosome 13 q14**[Q].

- Retinoblastoma develops when *both the normal alleles of the Rb gene are inactivated or altered.*
- **Familial retinoblastoma** is associated with **autosomal dominant inheritance**[Q] whereas the **Rb gene** is having **autosomal recessive** inheritance.

Hereditary/Familial retinoblastoma	Non-Hereditary/Sporadic retinoblastoma
• Seen in 40% cases • Usually bilateral and multifocal • Can also develop extraocular tumors (osteosarcoma and pinealoblastoma)	• Seen in 60% cases • Usually unilateral and unifocal

45. **Ans. (a) p53** *(Ref: Robbins 7th/302, 303, 304, 9/e p293)*

46. **Ans. (c) Its activity in the cells decreases following UV irradiation and stimulates cell cycle** *(Ref: Robbins 7th/302, 303, 8th/290-291, 9/e p293-294)*
    - p53 is a **tumor suppressor gene,** located on chromosome 17. It is also called as *"Guardian of the genome".*
    - At the time of DNA injury following irradiation, its **level increases and it acts to cause cell cycle arrest (G_1/S)**
    - The cell cycle arrest is to allow time for DNA repair. If repair is unsuccessful, p53 causes apoptosis of the cell by activating bax (apoptosis inducing gene). So, any exposure to UV irradiation would cause increased activity of p53 gene resulting in apoptosis and cell death.

47. **Ans. (b) GTPase activating protein** *(Ref: Robbins 8th/282, 7th/296-297, 9/e 286)*
    Activated ras is present in association with GTP. Enzyme GTPase will degrade GTP to GDP and result in inactivation of ras. Thus, GTPase activating protein will counteract the activation of ras.

48. **Ans. (b) p 53** *(Ref: Robbins Illustrated, 7th/1134, 9/e 294)*
    - Mutation in p53 tumor suppressor gene is strongly associated with breast cancer, as well as many other sarcomas and carcinomas. This condition is called as **Li-Fraumeni syndrome.**

49. **Ans. (a) Important for normal cell growth; (b) Oncogenesis; (c) C-myc over-expression causes lymphoma** *(Ref: Robbins 7th/292, 293, 295, 9/e 284)*
    - Genes that promote autonomous cell growth in cancer cells are called oncogenes and their **normal cellular counterparts** are called proto-oncogenes.
    - Proto-oncogenes are important for cellular function related to growth and proliferation.
    - Proto-oncogenes may be converted into cellular oncogenes that are involved in oncogenesis.
    - *c-myc* proto-oncogenes is expressed in virtually all eukaryotic cells and its persistent expression or over-expression is commonly found in tumors. Dysregulation of c-myc expression resulting from translocation of gene occurs in Burkitt's lymphoma.

50. **Ans. (c) They are transduced from virus infected cells** *(Ref: Ananthnarayan 7/580-1, Robbins' 7th/293, 302)*
    - **Viral oncogenes** (V-onc) commonly known as **'cancer genes'** which encode proteins triggering transformation of normal cells into cancer cells.
    - Proto-oncogenes are the **normal cellular genes** that promote normal growth and differentiation.
    - Oncogenes isolated from cancer cells are called cellular oncogenes (C-onc).
    - Proto-oncogenes are converted to oncogenes and cause cancer by:
      - Transduction into retrovirus (V-oncs) or
      - Changes in situ that affect their expression and function thereby converting them into cellular oncogene (C-oncs).
    - The transduction of oncogenes by the virus (e.g. retrovirus) is through recombination with DNA of a (normal) host cell that had been infected by the virus. Thus, they are of host cell origin. The virus act as transducing agent, carrying oncogenes from one cell to another.

    Viral oncogenes do not contain introns and that's how they are different from human oncogenes.

51. **Ans. (a) Suppression of P 53; (c) bcl-2** *(Ref: Robin's 7th/306, 274, 9/e 302)*
    - Cell survival would be seen when they are prevented from apoptosis. Genes that favor cell survival and protect from apoptosis are: - bcl-2 , bcl-xL
    - Genes that favor programmed cell death are: bax, bad, bcl-xL and p53.

52. **Ans. (a) Proto-oncogenes; (b) Tumor suppressor genes; (d) DNA repair genes** *(Ref: Robbins 7th/290, 298, 9/e 280)*

53. **Ans. is (c) i.e. Nucleotide excision repair** *(Ref: Harrison 17th/d/387 Robbins 7th/d 287, 9/e 314)*

54. Ans. (b) EGF Receptor *(Ref: Robbins 7th/295, 9/e 285)*

55. Ans. (d) C-Myc *(Ref: Robbins 7th/295, 300, 9/e 288)*
- C-myc is a proto-oncogene of transcriptional activator category and is associated with Burkitt's lymphoma.

Important points about p53

- Located on **chromosome 17** (17p 13.1).
- **Single most common** target for genetic alteration in human tumors.
- Also known as *Guardian of the Genome or molecular policeman*.
- p53 is not a cyclin-dependent inhibitor, rather it **elicits p21** which in turn is a CDK inhibitor and mediates
- G1/S arrest. So, it also called *Guardian of G1 checkpoint*. It induces DNA repair of genes (via GADD45). In case repair fails it induces apoptosis via BAX (the pro-apoptotic gene).
- Inheritance of mutated p53 gene increases the chances of multiple malignancies and is called **Li-Fraumeni syndrome**.
- **Mutation** in p53 gene causes the **resistance in tumors to radiation and chemotherapy**.

56. Ans. (a) Formation of the new blood vessels *(Ref: Robbins 8th/297; 7th/71-72, 9/e 305)*

57. Ans. (a) RET *(Ref: Robbins 8th/1124-1126, 7th/295, 9/e 284)*

58. Ans. (a) Chromosome 5 *(Ref: Robbins 8th/823, 7th/862, 9/e 296)*

59. Ans. (b) Small cell lung cancer *(Ref: Robbins 8th/722-723, 9/e 285)*

60. Ans. (a) p53 *(Ref: Robbins 8th/290-292, 7th/302-303, 9/e 294)*

61. Ans. (b) K-RAS *(Ref: Robbins 8th/308, 9/e 811)*
Read explanation below
Mostly colon adenocarcinoma develops from pre-existing adenomatous polyps (adenomas). Colon adenomas usually occur in patients in 50-60 years old and are considered premalignant. Early detection and excision of adenomatous polyps is therefore, an effective prophylaxis for colon adenocarcinoma.
The malignant potential of adenomatous polyps is determined by the following:

- **Size of the polyp:**
    - < 1cm - Unlikely to undergo malignant transformation
    - > 4cm- 40% risk of malignancy
- **Microscopic/Histologic appearance:** Villous adenomas are more prone to be malignant than tubular adenomas.
- **Degree of dysplasia.**

The transformation of normal mucosal cells into malignant ones is caused by a series of gene mutations called the "adenoma-to-carcinoma sequence." This sequence includes the *following steps*:
- Progression from normal mucosa to a small adenomatous polyp: Due to mutation of APC tumor   suppressor gene.
- Increase in the size of the polyps: It is due to mutation of K-ras proto-oncogene.
- Malignant transformation of adenoma into carcinoma requires mutation of two genes: p53 and DCC.
Increase in the size of adenomatous polyps (and, therefore, increase in their malignant potential) is attributed to K-ras protooncogene mutation which results in unregulated cell proliferation.

62. Ans. (d) It is active in hyperphosphorylated form *(Ref: Robbins 8th/282-3, 9/e 286)*
K-Ras is the proto-oncogene which is active in its phosphorylated form.

- Rb gene is active in its hypophosphorylated form.
- P53 gene is called as guardian of the genome.
- Myc gene promotes the cell growth in the presence of growth factors but it causes apoptosis in the absence of growth factors. So, it is said to be in a state of conflict because its activity is dependent on the absence or presence of growth factors.

63. Ans. (d) p53 *(Ref: Robbins 8th/308, 9/e 294)*
Read explanation of the above question and then read the text below

1. Colon cancer is one of the common malignancy whose incidence increases with age, and it affects males and females equally. The risk factors are discussed in detail in the chapter on GIT.
2. P53 gene also called as the "molecular policeman" triggers apoptosis of cells with damaged DNA. Mutation of p53 allows cells with genomic errors to enter the cell cycle. This mutation is considered the last "hit" in the adenoma-to-carcinoma sequence. Malignant transformation of adenoma into carcinoma requires mutation of two genes: p53 and DCC.

Evaluating the other options,
- (Choice A): Cyclin D is a protein that regulates cell cycle. Its overexpression is seen in breast, lung, and esophageal cancers, and certain types of lymphomas.

- (Choice B): K-ras protooncogene mutation is responsible for increase in the size of adenomatous polyps. Its mutation leads to uncontrolled cell proliferation.
- (Choice C) The mutation of WT-1, an anti-oncogene, leads to the development of Wilms tumor.

64. **Ans. (c) Receptor tyrosine kinase** (*Ref: Robbins 8th/281, 9/e 1062*)

Her-2/neu (also known as c-erb B2) is a receptor tyrosine kinase related to epidermal growth factor receptor. It is amplified at the DNA level and over-expressed at the protein level in some breast cancers. Trastuzumab is a monoclonal antibody targeted against her-2/neu.

Ras is a proto-oncogene mutated in a number of cancers. NF-1 is a GTPase-activating protein (GAP) aberrantly expressed in neurofibromatosis. A mutated variant of a retinoic acid receptor is expressed in M3 AML (acute promyelocytic leukemia).

65. **Ans. (c) Ret** (*Ref: Robbins 8th/1123-1124, 9/e 284*)

The thyroid lesion is medullary carcinoma of the thyroid. The coexistence of parathyroid hyperplasia suggests Sipple's syndrome (MEN II). These patients also tend to develop pheochromocytoma. Both MEN II and MEN III are associated with the ret oncogene. Please revise:

- Associate bcl-2 (option A) with follicular and undifferentiated lymphomas.
- Associate C-myc (option B) with Burkitt's lymphoma.
- Associate L-myc (option D) with small cell carcinoma of the lung.

66. **Ans. (c) Peripheral nerve** (*Ref: Robbins 8th/1341, 9/e 298*)

The disease is neurofibromatosis (von Recklinghausen's disease), which is characterized by café-au-lait spots (the light brown macules), Lisch nodules (pigmented iris hamartomas), and multiple peripheral nerve tumors (neurofibromas). The neurofibromas are initially benign, but may undergo malignant transformation. Café-au-lait spots are not considered to be premalignant lesions of skin (option D).

66.1. **Ans. (b) Medullary carcinoma thyroid** (*Ref: Robbins 8/e p280, 9/e 284*)

The RET protein is a receptor for the glial cell line–derived neurotrophic factor and structurally related proteins that promote cell survival during neural development. RET is normally expressed in neuroendocrine cells, such as parafollicular C cells of the thyroid, adrenal medulla, and parathyroid cell precursors. **Point mutations in the *RET* proto-oncogene** are associated with dominantly inherited **MEN types 2A[Q] and 2B[Q]** and **familial medullary thyroid carcinoma[Q]**.

RET gene mutation is more commonly associated with **medullary thyroid cancer than pheochromocytoma.**

Clinical significance of RET...(*Ref: Robbins 8/e p*

All individuals carrying **germline RET mutations** *are advised to undergo* **prophylactic thyroidectomy** *to prevent the inevitable development of medullary carcinomas.*

66.2. **Ans. (c) PTEN** (*Ref: Robbins 8/e p294, 9/e 298*)

Direct quote from Robbins… "*PTEN* (**P**hosphatase and *ten*sin homologue) is a membrane-associated phosphatase encoded by a gene on chromosome 10q23 that is mutated in **Cowden syndrome**, an autosomal dominant disorder marked by frequent benign growths, such as tumors of the skin appendages, and an increased incidence of epithelial cancers, particularly of **the breast, endometrium**, and **thyroid**.

66.3. **Ans. (c) G_1 – S phase** (*Ref: Robbins 8/e p290-1, 9/e 294*)

- The cell cycle has its own internal controls, called *checkpoints*. There are two main checkpoints, one at the **G1/S transition** and another at **G2/M.**
- In the **G1/S checkpoint, cell-cycle arrest is mostly mediated through p53**, which induces the cell-cycle inhibitor p21.
- Arrest of the cell cycle by the **G2/M checkpoint** involves **both p53-dependent (via cyclin A/cdK-2) and independent (via cdc 25)** mechanisms.

As can be deduced from above mentioned information that the p53 is associated with both the types of checkpoints. However, **G2/M checkpoint**can take place even without p53. Hence, option "c" is the preferred answer.

66.4. **Ans. (d) Transcription activator** (*Ref: Robbins 8/e p288*)

- A host of oncoproteins, including products of the *MYC, MYB, JUN, FOS*, and *REL* oncogenes, are transcription factors that regulate the expression of growth-promoting genes, such as cyclins.
- Out of all these,*MYC is most commonly involved in human tumors*[Q]
- MYC gene is associated with **"Conflict model"** in carcinogenesis

Tumors associated with different subtypes of MYC

C-*MYC*	Translocation	Burkitt lymphoma
N-*MYC*	Amplification	**N**euroblastoma, small-cell carcinoma of lung
L-*MYC*	Amplification	Small-cell carcinoma of **L**ung

66.5. Ans. (d) Osteosarcoma *(Ref: Robbins 8/e p293)*
- Rb gene is a **tumor suppressor** gene located on **chromosome 13 q14**[Q].
- Retinoblastoma develops when *both the normal alleles of the Rb gene are inactivated or altered.*
- **Familial retinoblastoma** is associated with **autosomal dominant inheritance**[Q] whereas the **Rb gene** is having **autosomal recessive** inheritance.

Hereditary/Familial retinoblastoma	Non-Hereditary/Sporadic retinoblastoma
• Seen in 40% cases • Usually **bilateral** and multifocal • Can also develop extraocular tumors **(osteosarcoma and pinealoblastoma)**	• Seen in **60% cases** (more common) • Usually **unilateral** and unifocal

66.6. Ans. (d) RB...explained earlier *(Ref: Robbins 9/e p291)*

66.7. Ans. (c) Xeroderma pigmentosum *(Ref: Robbins 8/e p275, 9/e 314)*

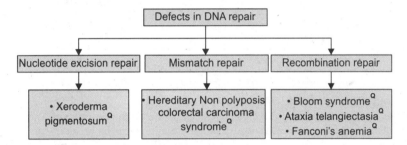

66.8. Ans. (a) RET Proto Oncogene *(Ref: Robbins 8/e p280, 9/e 284)*

66.9. Ans. (a) Beta-2 macroglobulin *(Ref: Robbins 8/e p327)*
Beta-2 **microglobulin** and not beta macroglobulin may be used as a tumor marker (as in multiple myeloma).

66.10. Ans. (d) Rb *(Ref: Robbins 8/e p286, 7/e p299-300, 9/e 291)*

66.11. Ans. (b) Retinoblastoma *(Ref: Robbins 9/e p 290)*

66.12. Ans. (b) Pinealoblastoma *(Ref: Robbins 9/e p 1339)*

Retinoblastoma is the most common primary intraocular malignancy of children. In the sporadic cases, both RB alleles are lost by somatic mutations. Retinoblastomas arising in the context of germline mutations are often bilateral. In addition, they may be associated with pinealoblastoma ("trilateral" retinoblastoma).

67. Ans. (b) EBV *(Ref: Robbins 8th/230, Harrison 18th/921, 1124, 9/e 327)*

Infectious Agent	Lymphoid Malignancy
Epstein-Barr virus	• Burkitt's lymphoma • Post–organ transplant lymphoma • Primary CNS diffuse large B cell lymphoma • Hodgkin's disease • Extranodal NK/T cell lymphoma, nasal type
HIV	• Diffuse large B cell lymphoma • Burkitt's lymphoma
Hepatitis C virus	• Lymphoplasmacytic lymphoma
Helicobacter pylori	• Gastric MALT lymphoma
Human herpesvirus 8	• Primary effusion lymphoma • Multicentric Castleman's disease
HTLV-I	• Adult T cell leukemia/lymphoma

68. Ans. (a) MALToma *(Ref: Harrison 17th/1858, Robbins 8th/316, 9/e 329)*

69. Ans. (d) Burkitt's lymphoma *(Ref: Robbins 7th/814, Robbins 8th/315-6, 9/e 329)*

70. Ans. (b) Non-small Cell Carcinoma of Lung *(Ref: Robbins 8th/277, 878, 9/e 325-329)*

CANCERS ASSOCIATED WITH INFECTIOUS AGENTS		
Opisthorchis, cholangitis	**Cholangiosarcoma, colon carcinoma**	**Liver flukes** (*Opisthorchis viverrini*)
		Bile acids
Chronic cholecystitis	Gallbladder cancer	Bacteria, gallbladder stones
Gastritis/ulcers	Gastric adenocarcinoma, MALT	Helicobacter pylori
Hepatitis	Hepatocellular carcinoma	Hepatitis B and/or C virus
Mononucleosis	B-cell non-Hodgkin lymphoma and Hodgkin lymphoma, nasopharyngeal cancer	Epstein-Barr virus
AIDS	Non-Hodgkin lymphoma, squamous cell carcinoma, Kaposi's sarcoma	Human immunodeficiency virus, human herpesvirus type 8
Osteomyelitis	Carcinoma in draining sinuses	Bacterial infection
Pelvic inflammatory disease, chronic cervicitis	Ovarian carcinoma, cervical/anal carcinoma	Gonorrhea, chlamydia, human papillomavirus
Chronic cystitis	Bladder, liver, rectal carcinoma	Schistosomiasis

Non small cell lung cancer is not reported to be associated with any infectious organism.

71. **Ans. (a) Angiogenesis** *(Ref: Harrison 17th/. 509, Robbins 9/e 305-306)*
Metastasis is a complex series of steps in which cancer cells leave the original tumor site and migrate to other parts of the body via the bloodstream or the lymphatic system. To do so, malignant cells break away from the primary tumor and degrade **proteins** of the **extracellular matrix** (ECM). One of the **critical events** required for metastasis is the growth of a new network of blood vessels, called tumor **angiogenesis**.
- Without vascularization or angiogenesis, the tumor can **grow only 1-2 mm**^{Q}. Vessels are also required for nutrition.
- Vascularisation *promoted by VEGF and bFGF* and **inhibited by Angiostatin, Endostatin and Tumstatin**^{Q}.
- It has been found that **angiogenesis inhibitors** would therefore prevent the growth of metastases.

72. **Ans. (b) Papilloma viruses produce tumors in animals but not in humans** *(Ref: Harrison 17th/487)*
All the options mention about the carcinogens. "Human papilloma virus is the most common etiological factor for cervical cancer"

73. **Ans. (d) Hepatitis C virus** *(Ref: Robbins 8th/315, 9/e 328)*
Hepatitis C virus (HCV) is only oncogenis RNA virus in the options. Others mentioned are oncogenic DNA viruses.

74. **Ans. (c) Epstein-Barr Virus** *(Ref: Robbins 7th/325-327, 9/e 328)*
LMP-1 gene plays a role in oncogenesis induced by EBV. For details, see text.

75. **Ans. (b) UV-B rays** *(Ref: Robbins 7th/323 , 9/e 324)*
Ultraviolet radiation is of 3 types; UV-A, UV-B and UV-C.
- **UVA** causes melanin oxidation with transient immediate darkening. Repeated exposure to UV radiation cause degenerative changes in elastin and collagen leading to wrinkling increased laxity and a leathery appearance. It is however used therapeutically in **PUVA therapy for the management of vitiligo, psoriasis and cutaneous T cell lymphoma**^{Q}.
- **UVB** can cause skin damage by formation of reactive oxygen species and formation of pyrimidine dimmers between adjacent pyrimidines on the same DNA strand. The latter can cause double base substitutions in the p53 resulting in the development of skin cancers. So, it is the **most dangerous for humans**. Exposure to UV rays also induces DNA repair, apoptosis or cell cycle arrest. The absence of this protective mechanism is seen in patients of **Xeroderma pigmentosum** causing high incidence of skin cancers.
- **UVC** is **not reaching** earth because it **gets filtered** by the protective **ozone layer**.

76. **Ans. (d) Testicular seminoma** *(Ref: Robbins 8th/989, 7th/1041)*

77. **Ans. (d) Thyroid** *(Ref: Robbins 8th/273-274, 7th/419 , 9/e 415)*

78. **Ans. (c) Angiosarcoma** *(Ref: Robbins 8th/274; 7th/550, 923 , 9/e 519)*

79. **Ans. (a) Cytomegalovirus** *(Ref: Robbins 8th/317-318; 7th/325 , 9/e 325-326)*

80. **Ans. (a) Aflatoxin – B1** *(Ref: Robbins 7th/319-323, 924 , 9/e 323)*
- Vinyl chloride is associated with angiosarcoma of the liver, not hepatocellular carcinoma.
- Azo dyes, such as butter yellow and scarlet red, have induced hepatocellular cancer in rats, but no human cases have

Neoplasia

been reported.
- There has been an increase in bladder cancer in workers in the aniline dye and rubber industries
- Aflatoxin B1, a natural product of the fungus Aspergillus flavus, is associated with the high incidence of hepatocellular carcinoma
- Hepatitis B virus is also highly associated with liver cancer.

81. Ans. (b) Helicobacter pylori *(Ref: Robbins 8th/785, 9/e 329)*
The patient has **gastric carcinoma**, which has been linked to prior gastric infection with **Helicobacter pylori**.

> - Epstein-Barr virus (option A) has been linked to African Burkitt's lymphoma and nasopharyngeal carcinoma.
> - Human papilloma virus (option C) has been linked to a variety of warts, condyloma, and genital cancers.
> - Molluscum contagiosum virus (option D) is a poxvirus that causes small tumor-like papules of the skin.

82. Ans. (d) Leukemia *(Ref: Robbins 8th/312, 9/e 325)*
HTLV-1, or human T-cell lymphotrophic virus 1, is an enveloped, single-stranded, RNA retrovirus whose infection can lead to T-cell leukemia 20-30 years after the infection. The HTLV-associated T-cell leukemia generally presents as described in the stem of the question and is very aggressive, progressing to death in less than 1 year.

82.1. Ans. (c) Angiosarcoma of liver *(Ref: Robbins 8/e p877 , 9/e 519)*
Angiosarcoma of the liver is a highly aggressive tumor which is associated with exposure to:
- **Vinyl chloride^Q,**
- **Arsenic^Q,** or
- **Thorotrast^Q.**

Thorotrast is a suspension containing particles of the radioactive compound thorium dioxide. It emits **alpha particles** due to which it has been found to be extremely carcinogenic.

82.2. Ans. (c) Thyroid *(Ref: Robbins 8/e p312, 425 and internet, 9/e p 325)*
The most radiosensitive organ sites in children in order of sensitivity are the thyroid gland, breasts, bone marrow (leukemia), brain and skin.

82.3. Ans. (c) Clonorchiasis *(Ref: Robbins 8/e p880, 9/e p 874)*
The following two parasites have definitive etiological association with malignancies:
- *Clonorchis sinensis*: cholangiocarcinoma^Q
- *Opisthorchis viverrini*: cholangiocarcinoma^Q
- *Schistosoma haematobium* : squamous cell cancer of urinary bladder^Q
- *Schistosoma* japonicum: colorectal cancer^Q

82.4. Ans. (d) HHV *(Ref: Robbins 8/e p313, 9/e p 254)*
- Kaposi sarcoma is caused by **HHV-8^Q** (Human Herpes Virus-8)or *KS-associated herpesvirus (KSHV)*
- It is a **vascular** tumor
- Most primary KSHV infections are asymptomatic.
- It can be treated by administration of **interferon-α**, adjunct chemotherapy or radiation therapy
- Classic KS is largely restricted to the surface of the body, and surgical resection is usually adequate for an excellent prognosis.

82.5. Ans. (b) Stimulates formation of pyrimidine dimers *(Ref: Robbins 8/e p312, 9/e p314)*
*Direct quote from Robbins.. **"The carcinogenicity of UV-B light is attributed to its formation of pyrimidine dimers in DNA"**. This type of DNA damage is repaired by the nucleotide excision repair pathway. The importance of the nucleotide excision repair pathway of DNA repair is illustrated by the high frequency of cancers in individuals with the hereditary disorder *xeroderma pigmentosum..*

82.6. Ans. (b) Lymphocytes *(Ref: Robbins, 9/e p430)*
- The **most radiosensitive** cell in the *blood* is the **lymphocytes^Q**.
- The **least radiosensitive** cell in the *blood* is the **platelets^Q**.
- **DNA^Q** is the most sensitive intracellular organelle to radiation.

82.7. Ans. (c) Gray *(Ref: Robbins 9/e p428)*
Gray (Gy) is a unit that expresses the energy absorbed by the target tissue per unit mass.

82.8. Ans. (d) Chronic lymphocytic leukemia *(Ref: Robbins 9/e p 431)*
The main sources of ionizing radiation are x-rays and gamma rays (electromagnetic waves of very high frequencies), high-energy neutrons, alpha particles (composed of two protons and two neutrons), and beta particles, which are essentially electrons.
Diagnostics is the most common source of radiation exposure in human beings.

Cancers associated with radiation	Cancers not associated with radiation
• ALL, AML and CML	• CLL
• Cancer of thyroid, breast and lung.	• Hodgkins lymphoma
• Cancer of CNS, bladder, ovary	• Cancer prostate/testis/cervix

83. Ans. (c) Inhibin *(Ref: Robbins 8th/1050, 9/e p1032)*
Granulosa cell tumor

- The most common type of ovarian tumor that is composed of cells that **stain positively with inhibin**^Q.
- Histologically, the cells may form **Call-Exner bodies**^Q
- The tumor cells may *secrete estrogens* and cause *precocious sexual development in girls* or increase the risk for *endometrial hyperplasia and carcinoma in women*.
- *Less commonly* granulosa cell tumors can *secrete androgens* and produce *masculinization*.

Concept: for future exam

- Tumor cells in **Sertoli-Leydig tumors (Androblastomas)** may *stain positively with inhibin, but Call-Exner bodies are not present*. Sertoli-Leydig tumors also may **secrete androgens and produce virilization in women**.
- The granulosa cell tumors vary in their clinical behavior, but they are considered to be potentially malignant.

84. Ans. (a) Hepatoblastoma *(Ref: Robbins 8th/327, 7th/339, 9/e p869-870, Harsh Mohan 6th/637)*
- AFP is glycoprotein synthesized in fetal life by yolk sac, fetal liver and fetal gastrointestinal tract. It is a **marker of hepatocellular cancer and non-seminomatous germ cell tumors of testes**. Elevated plasma AFP is also found less regularly in carcinomas of the colon, lung, and pancreas.

Important points about hepatoblastoma

- Arising from hepatic parenchymal cells
- The **most common tumor of young childhood**
- More commonly seen in *boys*
- The concentration of AFP is very high
- A *characteristic feature* of hepatoblastomas is the frequent *activation of the Wnt/β-catenin signaling pathway* by stabilizing mutations of β-catenin, contributing to the process of carcinogenesis.

85. Ans. (c) Osteosarcoma > (a) Multiple myeloma *(Ref: Journal....Cancer 42:603-610, 1978)*
The journal writes that............. "The clinical manifestations, resulting from the production of metabolically active substances by neoplastic tissue, have been labeled paraneoplastic syndromes. Adolescent patients with primary osteosarcoma demonstrate abnormal glucose, insulin and growth hormone responses to oral glucose loading in *78% of the study population*. No statistical association exists between any two of the three factors and, therefore, no primary abnormality can be identified. High somatomedin levels were noted in 72% of the group studied accompanied by simultaneous elevations of growth hormones. Studies of adrenal, gonadal and gonadotropic hormones were essentially normal, thereby ruling these out as associated endocrine abnormalities".
- Hyperglycemia is also associated with chondrosarcoma and fibrosarcoma.
- Some reports associate hyperglycemia with multiple myeloma too but we would prefer osteosarcoma as the answer here because the chances of hyperglycemia is more with osteosarcoma than multiple myeloma.

86. Ans. (a) SIADH *(Ref: Robbins 8th/636-637, 9/e p626-627)*
Thymoma is the commenest anterior mediastinal tumor which causes symptoms due to compression on the mediastinal structures. It is associated with the following paraneoplastic syndromes:
- Myasthenia gravis (most common)^Q
- *Acquired hypogammaglobulinemia*^Q
- *Pure red cell aplasia*^Q
- Graves disease
- Pernicious anemia
- Dermatomyositis-polymyositis
- Cushing syndrome.

Epstein-Barr virus may be associated with thymomas.
Thymoma is the commonest anterior mediastinal tumor.

Neoplasia

87. **Ans. (d) Involves aorta and its branches early** *(Ref: Robbins 8th/475-479, 9/e p476-479)*
See text in chapter-18

88. **Ans. (a) Prostate** *(Ref: Robbin 7th/354, 9/e p332)*
   - Migratory thrombophlebitis (**Trousseau sign**[Q]) is particularly associated with **adenocarcinomas of the pancreas, colon and lung**[Q] because of associated paraneoplastic syndrome resulting in hypercoagulability.

89. **Ans. (c) Malignant melanoma:** *(Ref Anderson pathology 144-152, 9/e p1149)*
   - Malignant melanoma expresses HMB 45, S-100 and vimentin.
   - **HMB 45** is present in melanosomes and is **more specific**[Q].
   - **S-100** is **more sensitive**[Q] but is non-specific (also present in Langerhans' cell histiocytosis, neural tumors, and sarcomas like liposarcoma and chondrosarcoma)

90. **Ans. (a) Hepatoblastoma** *(Ref: Robbins 8th/327, 7th/339, , 9/e p869-870, Harsh Mohan 6th/637)*

91. **Ans. (c) Carcinoma** *(Ref: Robbins 8th/324, 7th/336-337, 9/e p334)*
Immunohistochemistry is used for making categorization of undifferentiated tumors. The important examples include: Cytokeratin (carcinoma), Desmin (Leiomyoma and Rhabdomyosarcoma) and vimentin (Sarcomas).

92. **Ans. (b) Pancreatic neuroendocrine tumor** *(Ref: Harrison 17th/2354, Robbins 9/e 1121)*
   - Gastrin is secreted by *Gastrinomas,* which are neuroendocrine tumors most commonly found in duodenum.
   - Marker of medullary carcinoma of thyroid is calcitonin and GIST is CD117 (c-kit).

93. **Ans. (a) Alpha-hCG (α-hCG)** *(Ref: Robbins 7th/1045, 1046, 9/e 337-338, C.S.D.T. 11th/1071)*
Human chorionic gonadotropin (hCG)
The beta subunit of hCG is typically measured as a tumor marker because it has unique sequence that are not shared with other human glycoprotein hormones. So, it is quite specific.
Alpha hCG is not used as tumor marker because it is similar to the FSH, LH and TSH. So there can be cross reactivity between beta subunits of these hormones.

94. **Ans. (a) Seminoma** *(Ref: Harrison 17th/1925 & Robbins 8th//988-989)*
   - The normal serum alkaline phosphate consists of *4 isoenzymes* secreted from the following sites:
   a. Liver,   b. Bone,   c. Intestine,   d. Placenta
They are best differentiated by electrophoresis. Another approach is based on the differentiation between the different isoenzymes on the basis of heat susceptibility.

> - Alkaline phosphatase from individual tissues differ in susceptibility to inactivation by heat. The finding of an elevated serum alkaline phosphatase level in a patient with a **heat-stable fraction** strongly suggests that the **placenta or a tumor** is the source of the elevated enzyme in serum. *Susceptibility to inactivation by heat* increases, respectively, for the intestinal, liver, and *bone* alkaline phosphatase, bone being by far the *most sensitive* and the **liver** being **most resistant.**
> **Mnemonic**: bone burns but liver lasts

   - The conditions having *elevated placental alkaline phosphatase* include:
     - *Seminoma*
     - *Choriocarcinoma*
     - *Third trimester of pregnancy*

95. **Ans. (b) Hypercalcemia** *(Ref: Harrison, 17th/1736)*
Tumor lysis syndrome is associated with hyperphosphatemia due to release of intracellular phosphate by the destroyed cancer cells. This is followed by a decrease in serum calcium levels.

96. **Ans. (a) Screening of a cancer; (b) Follow up of a cancer patient, esp. for knowing about recurrence; (d) For monitoring the treatment of a cancer** *(Ref: Robbins' 7th/338, 9/e p338)*
   - **Uses of Tumor Markers**
     - Screening of Cancer e.g. in prostate carcinoma (PSA), ovarian carcinoma (CA-125).
     - Follow-up a cancer patient especially for knowing recurrence e.g. AFP in hepatocellular carcinoma, CEA in colon carcinoma.
     - For monitoring of a cancer e.g. AFP + HCG in testicular · malignancy, AFP in hepatocellular carcinoma.
     - Prognosis of a cancer e.g. HCG; AFP in testicular malignancy, CEA in colon Ca.

> Tumor markers are not specific, so, **cannot** be used for confirmation of diagnosis. *Confirmation is done by biopsy*

97. **Ans. (a) Useful for screening of Ca. colon; (c) Helpful for follow up after resection; (d) Levels decrease immediately after resection of tumor** *(Ref: Harrison' l6th/530, 531, Robbin 9/e p338)*

- • **Carcino embryonic antigen is used in Colon carcinoma as follows;**
  - – For screening of carcinoma colon
  - – For follow-up after resection
  - – Early knowledge about tumor recurrence and metastasis
  - – Levels of CEA are elevated in 70% of patients but are poorly correlated with cancer stage.
  - – After complete surgical resection, CEA level should be normalized, persistent levels imply a poor prognosis.

Diagnosis of colon carcinoma is confirmed by colonoscopy and biopsy as some benign and other malignant conditions also show high values of CEA:
- • Pancreatic, breast and stomach carcinoma
- • Alcoholic cirrhosis
- • Hepatitis
- • IBD

98. **Ans. (c) Ovarian carcinoma** *(Ref: Harrison 16th/439, Robbins 9/e p337)*

99. **Ans. (b) Hand and feet bones:** *(Ref: Robbins 7th/1303, 9/e 1207)*
    - • Metastasis may occur any bone but most commonly involve axial skeleton (e.g. vertebra, pelvis, ribs. skull. sternum) > Proximal femur > humerus.
    - • Metastasis in small bone of hand and feet are uncommon and usually originates in cancer of lung, kidney and colon

    - • *Skeletal metastasis are typically multifocal,* however **carcinoma of kidney and thyroid** produce **solitary lesions.**

100. **Ans. (d) A technique for raising monoclonal antibodies** *(Ref: Harsh Mohan 6th/15)*

101. **Ans. (a) Follicular lymphoma** *(Ref: Robbin 7th/675, 9/e 594-595)*
     - • The hallmark of follicular lymphoma is a (14; 18) translocation, which leads to the juxtaposition of the IgH locus on chromosome 14 and BCL 2 locus on chromosome 18.
     - • This translocation is seen in most but not all follicular lymphomas and leads to over-expression of BCL2 protein.

     - • *B-cell lymphoma* is associated with breakpoint involving the BCL 6 locus on chromosome 3.
     - • *Mantle cell lymphoma* is associated with a locus on chromosome 11 variously known as BCL1 or PRAD1.

102. **Ans. (c) Hepatoma** *(Ref: Robbins 7th/338, 9/e p337)*
     AFP is glycoprotein synthesized in fetal life by yolk sac, fetal liver and fetal GIT. It is a **marker of HCC, hepatoma and non-seminomatous germ cell tumors of testes**.

103. **Ans. (a) Yolk sac tumor** *(Ref: Robbins 8th/990, 1049; 7th/1041, 1043, 9/e p977)*

104. **Ans. (a) Disseminated cancer; (**this is known as **Trosseau sign^Q)** *(Ref: Robbins 8th/322, 7th/335, 9/e p332)*

105. **Ans. (b) Parathyroid hormone related peptide** *(Ref: Robbins 8th/728, 7th/333, 9/e p330)*

106. **Ans. (c) Cerebellar hemangioblastoma** *(Ref: Robbins 8th/665, 7th/334, 9/e p331)*

107. **Ans. (d) Bladder carcinoma** *(Ref: Robbins 8th/327, 7th/338, 9/e p338)*

108. **Ans. (c) Ulcerative colitis** *(Ref: Robbins 8th/327, 7th/1339, 9/e p338)*

109. **Ans. (b) Anterior abdominal wall** *(Ref: Robbins 8th/1251-1252; 7th/1319, 9/e p1222)*

110. **Ans. (d) Both b and c** *(Ref: Robbins 8th/326-327; 7th/338-339, 825-826, 9/e p337)*

111. **Ans. (b) Carcinoma colon** *(Ref: Robbins 8th/327; 7th/339, 9/e p337)*

112. **Ans. (b) AFP** *(Ref: Robbins 8th/327, 7th/338, 9/e p873)*

113. **Ans. (b) Neuroblastoma** *(Ref: Robbins 8th/475, 7th/502, 9/e p476)*

114. **Ans. (d) Cholangiocarcinoma - AFP** *(Ref: Robbins 8th/880-881, 7th/926-927, 9/e p337)*

115. **Ans. (a) Chondrosarcoma** *(Ref: Robbins 8th/1230, 7th/1299)*

116. **Ans. (b) Hepatocellular carcinoma of liver** *(Ref: Robbins 8th/876, 7th/338, 9/e p873)*

117. **Ans. (d) Kidney tumor** *(Ref: Robbins 8th/326-327; 7th/338, 9/e p337)*

118. **Ans. (a) Neuroblastoma** *(Ref: Robbins 8th/478; 7th/504, 9/e p476)*

119. **Ans. (b) Parathyroid hormone related peptide** *(Ref: Robbins 7th/333-335, 9/e p330)*

Neoplasia

- Bronchogenic carcinomas are associated with the development of many different types of paraneoplastic syndrome.
- Ectopic secretion of ACTH may produce Cushing's syndrome
- Ectopic secretion of anti-diuretic hormone may produce hyponatremia
- Hypocalcemia may result from the production of parathyroid hormone- related peptide, patients with this type of paraneoplastic syndrome have increased calcium levels and decreased PTH levels.
- Other tumors associated with the production of PTHrP include clear cell carcinomas of the kidney, endometrial adenocarcinomas, and transitional carcinomas of the urinary bladder.

120. Ans. (c) Kidney *(Ref: Robbins 8th/665, 9/e p331)*

Renal cell carcinoma can lead to overproduction of erythropoietin and thereby cause secondary polycythemia. Other causes of secondary polycythemia are diseases that impair oxygenation, including pulmonary diseases (including smoking) and congestive heart failure.

Colon cancer (option B) and stomach cancer (option D) can present with anemia secondary to blood loss.

121. Ans. (a) Adrenal gland *(Ref: Robbins 8th/1156-1157, 9/e p1130)*

This is Addison disease, in which severe adrenal disease produces adrenocortical insufficiency. Causes include autoimmune destruction, congenital adrenal hyperplasia, hemorrhagic necrosis, and replacement of the glands by either tumor (usually metastatic) or granulomatous disease *(usually tuberculosis being the commonest cause in India)*. The symptoms can be subtle and nonspecific (such as those illustrated), so a high clinical index of suspicion is warranted. Skin hyperpigmentation is a specific clue that may be present on physical examination, suggesting excess pituitary ACTH secretion. **(The ACTH precursor has an amino acid sequence similar to MSH, melanocyte stimulating hormone.)** Most patients have symptoms (fatigue, gastrointestinal distress) related principally to glucocorticoid deficiency. In some cases, however, mineralocorticoid replacement may also be needed for symptoms of salt wasting with lower circulating volume.

Except in the case of primary pancreatic cancer, complete tumor replacement of the endocrine pancreas (option B) would be uncommon. In any event, pancreatic involvement would be associated with diabetes mellitus.

Involvement of the ovaries (option C) by metastatic tumor (classically gastric adenocarcinoma) would produce failure of menstruation.

Involvement of the pituitary gland (option D) could produce Addisonian symptoms, but the pigmented skin suggests a primary adrenal problem rather than pituitary involvement.

122. Ans. (a) Pancreatic cancer *(Ref: Robbins 8th/321, 903, 9/e p332)*

Pancreatic carcinoma often presents with vague abdominal, back, and gastrointestinal complaints; and physical examination is generally normal. The significant weight loss and the migrating thrombophlebitis (Trousseau's sign) is pointing towards the diagnosis, which should be confirmed with ultrasonography or CT. **Migratory thrombophlebitis is mostly associated with tumors of the pancreas, lung, and colon.**

123. Ans. (a) Breast *(Ref: Robbins 8th/1235, 9/e p1207)*

Breast cancer is unusual in that it produces both lytic and blastic metastases to bone. Breast and prostate cancers are the most common sources of bone metastases, but *prostate metastases* are usually *blastic*.

Colon cancer (choice B) does not usually metastasize to bone.

Kidney cancer (choice C), **lung cancer** (choice D), GIT and malignant melanoma produce **lytic lesions** when they metastasize to bone.

123.1. Ans. (a) Pheochromocytoma *(Ref: Robbins 8/e p1159, 9/e p1134)*

Pheochromocytomas have been associated with a *"rule of 10s"*.

- *10% of pheochromocytomas are* extra-adrenal[Q], occurring in sites such as the organs of Zuckerkandl and the carotid body.
- *10% of sporadic adrenal pheochromocytomas are* bilateral[Q].
- *10% of adrenal pheochromocytomas are* biologically malignant[Q], defined by the presence of metastatic disease.
- *10% of adrenal pheochromocytomas are* not associated with hypertension[Q].
- One "traditional" 10% rule that has now been modified pertains to familial cases. Now almost 25% of individuals with pheochromocytomas and paragangliomas harbor a germline mutation in the *succinate dehydrogenase* genes.

Also note that
  - Notably, **malignancy** is **more common** (20% to 40%) in **extra-adrenal paragangliomas,** and in tumors arising in the setting of certain germline mutations.
  - Patients with *germline mutations* are typically *younger at presentation* than those with sporadic tumors and more often *harbor bilateral disease*. Pheochromocytoma is associated with germline mutation.

123.2. Ans. (c) Cytokeratin *(Ref: Robbins 8/e p324, 9/e p334)*

Tumors and associated filaments

Intermediate Filament	Normal Tissue Expression	Tumor
Cytokeration	All epithelial cells	Carcinoma
Vimentin	Mesenchymal cells	Sarcomas
Desmin	Muscle cells	Leiomyoma Rhabdomyosarcoma
Glial fibrillary acidic protein (GFAP)	Glial cells	Astrocytoma ependymoma
Neurofilamnet	Neurons and neural crest derivatives	Pheochromocytoma neuroblastoma

123.3. Ans. (a) CA-125 *(Ref: Robbins 8/e p327, 9/e p337)*

HORMONES	
Human chorionic gonadotropin	Trophoblastic tumors, nonseminomatous testicular tumors
Calcitonin	Medullary carcinoma of thyroid
Catecholamine and metabolites	Pheochromocytoma and related tumors
ONCOFETAL ANTIGENS	
α-Fetoprotein	Liver cell cancer, non-seminomatous germ cell tumors of testis
Carcinoembryonic antigen (CEA)	Carcinomas of the colon, pancreas, lung, stomach, and heart
ISOENZYMES	
Prostatic acid phosphatase	Prostate cancer
Neuron-specific enolase	Small-cell cancer of lung, neuroblastoma
SPECIFIC PROTEINS	
Immunoglobulins	Multiple myeloma and other gammopathies
Prostate-specific antigen and prostate-specific membrane antigen	Prostate cancer
MUCINS AND OTHER GLYCOPROTEINS	
CA-125	Ovarian cancer
CA-19-9	Colon cancer, pancreatic cancer
CA-15-3	Breast cancer
NEW MOLECULAR MARKERS	
p53, APC, RAS mutants in stool and serum	Colon cancer
p53 and RAS mutants in stool and serum	Pancreatic cancer
p53 and RAS mutants in sputum and serum	Lung cancer
p53 mutants in urine	Bladder cancer

123.4. Ans. (a) CEA..........See table above *(Ref: Robbins 9/e p337)*

123.5. Ans. (a) Prostate *(Ref: Robbins 8/e p1235, 9/e p1207)*
- Carcinomas of the **kidney, lung, and gastrointestinal tract and malignant melanoma** produce **lytic bone destruction**.
- Other metastases elicit a sclerotic response, particularly **prostate adenocarcinoma**, which may do so by secreting WNT proteins that stimulate **osteoblastic bone formation**.
- Most metastases induce a mixed lytic and blastic reaction

123.6. Ans. (b) β- HCG *(Ref: Robbins 8/e p474, 9/e p474-475 The Essentials of Clinical Oncology p490)*
- *Sacrococcygeal teratomas* are the most common teratomas of childhood, accounting for 40% or more of cases). They occur with a frequency of 1 in 20,000 to 40,000 live births, and are four times more common in girls than boys
- Serum alpha fetoprotein is a useful marker for sacrococcygeal teratoma. Some books mention that even beta HCG is elevated in some patients.

123.7. Ans. (b) CDKN2A *(Ref: Robbins 8/e p1174, 9/e p1147)*
Please do not get confused with the first option friends. *Melanomas are associated with N-Ras and not N-myc.*
Coming to the other options,

Direct quote from Robbins…. "The *CDKN2A* gene (is mutated in approximately 40% of pedigrees with **autosomal dominant familial melanoma**".

123.8. Ans. (a) Chromogranin *(Ref: Robbins 8/e p726-727, 9/e p717)*

Direct quote from Robbins.. "The occurrence of **neurosecretory granules**, the ability of some of these tumors to secrete polypeptide hormones, and the presence of neuroendocrine markers such as **chromogranin, synaptophysin** and **CD57** (in 75% of cases) and parathormone-like and other hormonally active products suggest derivation of this tumor from neuroendocrine progenitor cells of the lining bronchial epithelium.

123.9. Ans. (c) PLAP *(Ref: Robbin 8/e p988-9)*

Robbins … "*Seminoma cells* are diffusely *positive* for *c-KIT*, **OCT4** and *placental alkaline phosphatase* (PLAP), with sometimes scattered keratin-positive cells"

123.10. Ans. (c) Desmin *(Ref: Robbin 8/e p1253)*

- Rhabdomyosarcoma is the most common soft-tissue sarcoma of childhood and adolescence. It usually appears before age 20
- Ultrastructurally, rhabdomyoblasts contain sarcomeres, and immunohistochemically they stain with antibodies to the myogenic markers **desmin, MYOD1** and **myogenin.**

Other questions from same topic: for AIIMS/NEET

- Most common location is the *head and neck or genitourinary tract,* where there is little if any skeletal muscle as a normal constituent.
- Rhabdomyoblasts are also known as *tadpole or strap cells*
- Rhabdomyosarcoma is histologically subclassified into **embryonal**, **alveolar**, and **pleomorphic** variants. The *embryonal variant is the commonest.*

123.11. Ans. (c) Metastasis from another solid tissue tumor *(Ref: Robbin 9/e p 1133)*

Metastases to the adrenal cortex are significantly more common than primary adrenocortical carcinomas.

Even Harrison says… "The most common cause of adrenal tumors is metastasis from another solid tumor like breast cancer and lung cancer".

Malignant	Prevalence
Adrenocortical carcinoma	2-5
Malignant pheochromocytoma	<1
Adrenal neuroblastoma	<0.1
Lymphoma (incl primary adrenal lymphoma)	<1
Metastases (most frequent: breast, lung)	15

123.12. Ans. (b) Lung *(Ref: Robbin 9/e p 1315)*

123.13. Ans. (d) Urine contains 5H.I.A.A *(Ref: Robbin 9/e p 478)*

- *Neuroblastoma* is the *most common extracranial solid cancer in childhood* and the most common cancer in infancy.
- *About 90% of neuroblastomas, regardless of location, produce catecholamines,* which are an important diagnostic feature (i.e., elevated blood levels of catecholamines and elevated urine levels of the metabolites vanillylmandelic acid and homovanillic acid.

Increased urinary 5HIAA is a feature of carcinoid tumour and not neuroblastoma.

GOLDEN POINTS FOR QUICK REVISION / UPDATED INFORMATION FROM 9TH EDITION OF ROBBINS

(NEOPLASIA)

- **Chromosomal translocation** *is the* commonest cause *of* activation of proto-oncogenes.
- *Blood cancers* (the leukemias and lymphomas, sometimes called *liquid tumors*) are derived from blood-forming cells that normally have the capacity to enter the bloodstream and travel to distant sites. So, they are always considered as malignant…….pg 272-3

Carcinogenesis…..pg 281

Carcinogenesis results from the accumulation of complementary mutations in a stepwise fashion over time:

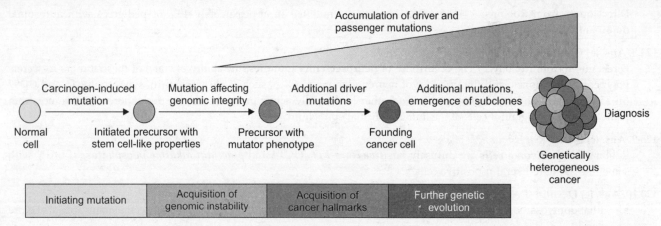

a. Mutations that contribute to the development of the malignant phenotype are referred to as ***driver mutations.*** The first driver mutation that starts a cell on the path to malignancy is the initiating mutation, which is typically maintained in all of the cells of the subsequent cancer.

b. Loss-of-function mutations in genes that maintain genomic integrity is a common early step in carcinogenesis, particularly in solid tumors. There is also increased frequency of the mutations that have no phenotypic consequence, so-called ***passenger mutations.*** The latter are more common than driver mutations.

c. During oncogenesis, there is competition among tumor cells for access to nutrients and microenvironmental niches. This leads to formation of subclones with the capacity to overgrow their predecessors. Thus, the tumors tend to become more aggressive over a period of time and are referred to as ***tumor progression.***

d. By the time the tumours are clinically evident, their constituent cells are often extremely heterogeneous genetically.

Clinical importance

This also leads to an important clinical consequence: cancer cells after a cycle of effective chemotherapy or radiotherapy becomes resistant because of the survival advantage of those cells which were intrinsically resistant to the drugs/radiotherapy.

Warburg effect.....pg 283

It is the phenomenon in which rapidly growing cells (both benign and malignant) upregulate **glucose and glutamine uptake** and decreases their production of ATP per glucose molecule. This is responsible for providing metabolic intermediates which are useful for cellular growth and maintenance.
This is due to the fact that rapidly growing cells have the ***M2 isoform of pyruvate kinase***.

Oncogene addiction

Oncogene addiction is a phenomenon in which tumor cells are highly dependent on the activity of one or more oncogenes. This is exemplified by the *BCR-ABL tyrosine kinase activity required for most CML tumor cells* to proliferate and survive. Hence, inhibition of this activity is a highly effective therapy.

Lewis Thomas and **Macfarlane Burnet** coined the term ***immune surveillance***, which implies that a normal function of the immune system is to constantly "scan" the body for emerging malignant cells and destroy them.

Robbins 9th/ 315...

After encountering antigen mature B cells express a specialized enzyme called ***antigen-induced cytosine deaminase*** (AID), which catalyzes both immunoglobulin gene class switch recombination and somatic hypermutation. Errors during antigen receptor gene assembly and diversification are responsible for many of the mutations that cause ***lymphoid neoplasms.***

Cancer-Enabling Inflammation.....315-6

Inflammatory cells increase the risk of cancers by different mechanisms like:
i. Release of factors that promote proliferation
ii. Removal of growth suppressors,

iii. Enhanced resistance to cell death,
iv. Inducing angiogenesis,
v. Activating invasion and metastasis
vi. Evading immune destruction

Previous AIIMS Question!

- The detachment of epithelial cells from basement membranes and from cell-cell interactions can lead to a particular form of cell death called *anoikis*.
- **COX2 inhibitors** decrease the incidence of colonic adenomas and are now approved for treatment of patients with **familial adenomatous polyposis**

Potential Future Exam Questions from New Data!

- **All trans retinoic acid** is a highly effective therapy is **the first example** of *differentiation therapy*, in which immortal tumor cells are induced to differentiate into their mature progeny, which have limited life spans. It is used for treating patients with **acute promyelocytic leukemia**. ....Robbins 9th/ 317

- **Chromothrypsis** is a process in which a chromosome is "shattered" and then re-assembled in a haphazard way. It is seen in is found in up to 25% of **osteosarcomas** and at a relatively high frequency in **gliomas** as well.... Robbins/9th 318

Epigenetics in cancer

"Epigenetics" refers to factors other than the sequence of DNA that regulate gene expression (and, thereby, cellular phenotype). These factors include histones modifications catalyzed by

enzymes associated with chromatin regulatory complexes; DNA methylation, and other less well characterized proteins that regulate the higher order organization of DNA (e.g., looping of enhancer elements onto gene promoters).

Epigenetic changes have important roles in many aspects of the malignant phenotype, including the expression of cancer genes, the control of differentiation and self renewal, and even drug sensitivity and drug resistance.

Cancers Showing Epigenetic Changes

Gene(s)	Function	Tumor (Approximate Frequency of Mutation)
DNMT3A	DNA methylation	Acute myeloid leukemia (20%)
MLL1	Histone methylation	Acute leukemia in infants (90%)
MLL2	Histone methylation	Follicular lymphoma (90%)
CREBBP/EP 300	Histone acetylation	Diffuse large B cell lymphoma (40%)
ARD1A	Nucleosome Positioning/chromatin remodeling	Ovarian deer cell carcinoma (60%) endometrial carcinoma (30%-40%)
SNF5	Nucleosome Positioning/chromatin remodeling	Malignant rhaboid tumor (100%)
PERM1	Nucleosome Positioning/chromatin remodeling	Renal carcinoma (30%)

At a glance: Mechanism of Action of Major Tumor Suppressor Genes

APC

It encodes a factor that negatively regulates the WNT pathway in colonic epithelium by promoting the formation of a complex that degrades β-catenin.

- It gets mutated in familial adenomatous polyposis, autosomal dominant disorder associated with development of thousands of colonic polyps and early onset colon carcinoma; tumor development associated with loss of the single normal APC allele. It is also mutated in about 70% of sporadic colon carcinomas; tumor development associated with acquired biallelic defects in APC

E-cadherin:

It is a cell adhesion molecule that plays an important role in contact-mediated growth inhibition of epithelial cells. It also binds and sequesters β-catenin which is a signaling protein that functions in the WNT pathway.

- Germline loss-of-function mutations in the E-cadherin gene (CDH1) associated with autosomal dominant *familial gastric carcinoma*.

CDKN2A:

It encodes two tumor suppressive proteins, p16/INK4a, a cyclin-dependent kinase inhibitor that augments RB function, and ARF, which stabilizes p53
- Germline loss-of-function mutations are associated with autosomal dominant *familial melanoma*
- Biallelic loss-of-function seen in leukemias, melanomas, and carcinomas

TGF-β pathway

It is an inhibitor of cellular proliferation in normal tissues
- Frequent loss-of-function mutations involving TGF-β receptors (colon, stomach, endometrium) or downstream signal transducers (SMADs, pancreas) in diverse carcinomas

PTEN

It encodes a lipid phosphatase that is an important negative regulator of PI3K/AKT signaling
- Germline loss-of-function mutations associated with Cowden syndrome, autosomal dominant disorder associated with a high risk of breast and endometrial carcinoma

NF1

It encodes neurofibromin 1 which is a GTPase that acts as a negative regulator of RAS
- Germline loss-of-function mutations cause neurofibromatosis type 1 (autosomal dominant disorder associated with neurofibromas and malignant peripheral nerve sheath tumors)

NF2

It encodes neurofibromin 2 (also called merlin), a cytoskeletal protein involved in contact inhibition
- Germline loss-of-function mutations cause neurofibromatosis type 2, autosomal dominant disorder associated with a high risk of bilateral schwannomas

WT1: encodes a transcription factor that is required for normal development of genitourinary tissues
- Germline loss-of-function mutations associated with Wilms tumor, a pediatric kidney cancer; similar WT1 mutations also found in sporadic Wilms tumor

PTCH1: encodes membrane receptor that is a negative regulator of the Hedgehog signaling pathway
- Germline loss-of-function mutations cause Gorlin syndrome (AD disease with a high risk of basal cell carcinoma and medulloblastoma)

VHL

It is responsible for degradation of hypoxia-induced factors (HIFs), transcription factors that alter gene expression in response to hypoxia
- Germline mutation is associated with von Hippel-Lindau syndrome, autosomal dominant disorder associated with a high risk of renal cell carcinoma and pheochromocytoma
- Acquired biallelic loss-of mutations are common in sporadic renal cell carcinoma

Neoplasia

Immunity is the defensive power of the body (protecting the body from various infections). It can be of **two types**: innate immunity and adaptive immunity. **Innate immunity** (also known as natural or native immunity) refers to defense mechanisms that are **present since birth** and have evolved to recognize microbes. It is the **first line of defense**. It is **non-specific** and has **no memory**. *Adaptive immunity* (also called acquired or specific immunity) consists of mechanisms that are stimulated by microbes and are capable of recognizing non-microbial substances also. Adaptive immunity develops later (*after exposure to antigens*). It is *more specific* as well as powerful as well as has *memory*.

The major components of innate immunity are
1. Epithelial barriers like intact skin that blocks entry of environmental microbes
2. Cells like phagocytic cells (mainly neutrophils and macrophages), Natural killer (NK) cells, Dendritic cells
3. Plasma proteins (proteins of the complement system, mannose binding lectin and C-reactive protein)

The innate immunity is due to presence of **pattern recognition receptors (PRR)**. These are peptide molecules on the leukocytes which recognize particular structural pattern on a micro-organism called **p**athogen **a**ssociated **m**olecular **p**atterns (**PAMP**s). A similar group of molecules released by injured cells is called **d**anger **a**ssociated **m**olecular **p**atterns (**DAMP**, uric acid is an example). The PRR can be of two types:

Soluble pattern recognition receptors	Surface pattern recognition receptors
• Mannose receptors (for mannose binding lectin) • C-reactive protein	• Scavenger receptors (on macrophages) • Toll like receptors • NOD-like receptors • RIG-like receptors

Some important Toll like receptors (TLR) and the molecules they recognize are:
- **TLR-2**: peptidoglycan of gram + bacteria; lipopolysaccharide of **leptospira**[Q]
- **TLR-3**: dsRNA viruses
- **TLR-4**[Q]: Chlamydia and lipopolysaccharide **of Gram (–) bacteria**[Q] except leptospira

Signaling by Toll-like receptors causes the activation of nuclear transcription factors (NF-κβ and AP-1). This result in recruitment of inflammatory cytokines, endothelial adhesion molecules (E-selectin) and proteins involved in microbial killing mechanisms (inducible nitric oxide synthase).

The **adaptive immune system consists** of lymphocytes and their products like antibodies. It has two components: *cellular (or cell mediated) and humoral immunity. The former is protective against intracellular microbes whereas the latter is effective against extracellular microbes.*

IMMUNE CELLS

Apart from the leucocytes, our focus here would be to discuss the other important immune cells (lymphocytes and antigen presenting cells) in detail.

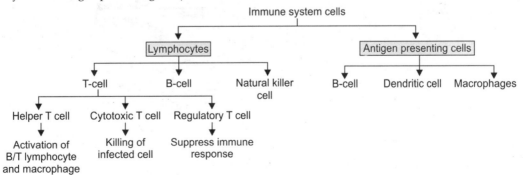

Sidebar notes:

Innate immunity
* Present **from birth**
* **First line of defense**
* **No prior exposure** to antigen
* **Non-specific**
* **No memory**[Q] is seen

Adaptive/Acquired immunity
* Acquired in nature
* **Second line of defense**
* **Prior exposure** to antigen is **present**[Q]
* **Specific**
* **Memory**[Q] is seen

Toll-like receptors causes the activation of NF-κβ ("master switch" to the nuclear factor) and AP-1.

All Gram (–) bacteria recognize **TLR-4** *except leptospira* which recognises *TLR-2*

1. T-lymphocytes (Thymus Derived)

> **CD-3** is known as pan T-cell **marker**. It is also involved in T-cell activation.

They constitute 60-70% of peripheral blood lymphocytes and are located in the *paracortical areas of lymph node and the periarteriolar sheaths of spleen*. These cells have an antigen specific T cell receptor (TCR) [composed of α and β polypeptide chains in 95% cases] to bind with the antigen. The $\alpha\beta$ T cells are present in blood and tissues. The other 5% cells have TCR composed of γ/δ chains and are present mostly at the epithelial/mucosal surface. A large number of TCRs can be generated because of rearrangement of genes coding for α and β polypeptide chains. When an antigenic peptide comes in contact with TCR, it activates a particular T cell only and not all the cells. This is called as **clonal selection**.

> Demonstration of TCR gene rearrangement by southern blot is a molecular marker of T cell lineage.

> The ratio of CD4 and CD8 T-cell is normally **2:1**

The cells have on their surface cluster differentiating (CD) molecules by which they can be readily identified. **The CD molecules present on T cells are CD1, CD2, CD3, CD4, CD5, CD7, CD8 and CD28.** The T cell having CD4 molecule is called **CD4+ T cell or the Helper T cell** and that having CD8 molecule is called as **CD8+ T cell or Cytotoxic/Killer T cell**. CD4+ T cells secrete cytokines and help macrophages and B cells to fight infections whereas CD8+ T cells destroy host cells having microbes like viruses and tumor cells.

> **Helper T cell** (or CD4+ T cell) is known as the '**master regulator**' of the immune system.

CD3 is involved in **signal transduction** and is also called as a **Pan T cell marker**. The T cells also have presence of CD40 ligand on their surface which is required for B cell activation and induction of immunoglobulin 'isotype switching'. (Described later).

The activation of T cells requires two signals

> *Signal 1:* Comes from binding of the TCR to MHC bound antigen. The CD4 or CD8 act as co-receptors and enhance this signal.
> *Signal 2:* Comes from the interaction of CD28 with co-stimulatory molecules B7-1 and B7-2 present on the antigen presenting cells.

> **CD 45** is called as Leukocyte common antigen (**LCA**)

The activated T cells gives rise to two groups of cells: effector T cells which manage the antigen at that time only and some differentiate into long lived memory cells (for future exposure to the same antigen).

Location of cell	Molecular marker
All leucocytes	CD45 and CD45RB
Medullary thymocytes ('**Naive**' T- cells)	CD45 RA and CD45RC
Cortical thymocytes (**Memory T-cells**)	CD45RO

> *m*
>
> Short Story: T-cell activation is like starting a vehicle. We put in a key and turn on the ignition of the car engine (Signal 1). But the car would move only when we put the gear (signal 2). If we don't put the car in gear, the engine will make the car lose its fuel and the car will stop without moving (anergy).

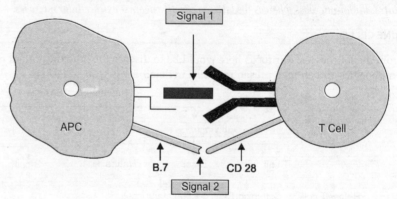

Interaction between APC and T cell

Importance of signal 2 in immunity

- Signal 2 ensures that the activation of the T cells is not taking place by chance. It is due to a particular antigen only. So, it acts like a safety signal.
- Secondly, if by any mistake, the APC present a self antigen (normal body tissue), signal 2 is not generated. In the absence of signal 2, T cell undergoes anergy. This is an important mechanism of **peripheral immunological tolerance**.

Concept of Superantigen

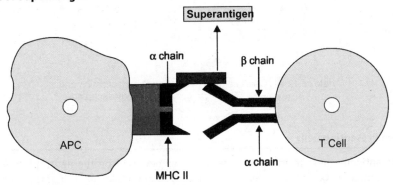

- Antigen which **does not**^{Q} require antigenic processing and not specific for a T cell receptor (TCR)
- Attaches itself **outside**^{Q} the antigen binding cleft
- Attaches to α **chain of MHC II with** β **chain of T cell receptor**^{Q} (TCR)
- Causes T cell activation and **massive release of cytokines** like TNF-α and IL-1
- Examples include **staphylococcal toxic shock syndrome toxin 1**^{Q} (TSST-1), **Streptococcal erythrogenic exotoxin**^{Q}

Types of CD4+ Helper Cells

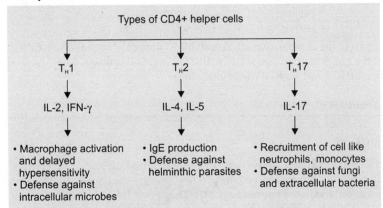

- Recently a new group of T cells have been discovered called as **NK-T cells**. These T cells express markers normally present on Natural Killer cells and recognize glycolipid antigens displayed by MHC-like molecule CD1. These are important defense mechanisms against microorganisms like *Listeria monocytogenes* and *M tuberculosis*.

Naive T cell (TH0) can get differentiated into either TH1 cell or TH2 cell. The differentiation towards TH1 cell is driven by strong innate response and intracellular organisms (TB, Listeria). TH1 cells release IL-2 and IFN-γ which causes cytotoxic T cell activation and granuloma formation. Constitutively which means most of the times physiologically, TH0 cell differentiates into TH2 cell. TH2 cells release IL-4 and IL-5 which cause B cell activation and multiplication leading to antibody formation.

Concept ____

Cytotoxic T cell (or **CD8+ T cell**) binds only to antigens presented with Class I MHC molecules. So, they are called as **MHC-I restricted**. These recognize endogenous peptides.

Concept ____

Helper T cell binds only to antigens presented with Class II MHC molecules. So, they are called as **MHC-II restricted**. These recognize *exogenous peptides*.

Diagram of different T helper cells

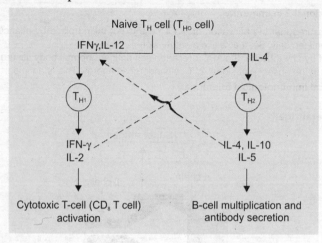

2. Antigen Presenting Cells

> Antigene presenting cells include B cell, macrophages and dendritic cells.

When an antigen enters inside the body, it is phagocytosed by the neutrophils following which the antigenic peptides are released in the circulation. However, if antigen presenting cells phagocytose the antigen, they process it inside themselves and present on their surface in association with MHC molecule. This processed antigen is now presented to the T cells.

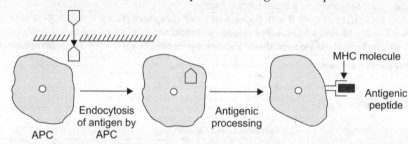

> The part of the antigen associated with MHC molecule on the APC is called as **aggretope**.
>
> The antigenic part in contact with TCR is called **epitope**.

The part of the antigen associated with MHC molecule on the APC is called as **aggretope** whereas the antigenic part in contact with TCR is called **epitope**. MHC molecules can be of two types: MHC I and MHC II (described later).

Details about APCs

> Macrophage associated markers include CD13, CD14, CD15 and CD33. **CD133** induces formation of **glioma**

MACROPHAGES

These cells have a role in induction (in cellular immunity) and the effector (in humoral immunity) phase of immune response. They process and present antigen to T cells for induction of cell mediated immunity (CMI). They get activated by the presence of *IFN-γ* and are the effector cells in humoral immunity as they phagocytose opsonised microbes.

DENDRITIC CELLS

> **Langerhan's cells** are Immature dendritic cells within the epidermis.

These are important antigen presenting cells in the body and can be of the following types:

a. **Interdigitating dendritic cells** (*dendritic cells*[Q]) are the **most important antigen-presenting cells** for initiating primary immune responses against protein antigens.

Why is the dendritic cell most important antigen presenting cell?

1. These cells are located under epithelia (a common site of entry of microbes and foreign antigens) and in the interstitia of all tissues (site of antigen production).

Immunity

2. Dendritic cells express many receptors (like TLRs and mannose receptors) for capturing and responding to antigens. These cells also express the same chemokine receptor as do naive T cells. They are *recruited to the T-cell zones of lymphoid organs* because of *specialised post capillary venules called high endothelial venules (HEV)*, where they are ideally located to present antigens to recirculating T cells.

3. Dendritic cells express high levels of MHC class II molecules as well as the co-stimulatory molecules B7-1 (CD80) and B7-2(CD86). Thus, they have all the necessary molecules required for presenting antigens to and activating CD4+ T cells.

Concept

HEV are lined by simple cuboidal cells as opposed to regular venules lined by endothelial cells.

b. **Follicular dendritic cells** are present in the germinal centers of lymphoid follicles in the spleen and lymph nodes.
   - These cells bear Fc receptors for IgG and receptors for C3b and can trap antigen bound to antibodies or complement proteins. Such cells are required for the process of '*Affinity Maturation*' (**production of antibodies having high affinity for antigens**).

Follicular dendritic cells act as reservoir for HIV in acquired immunodeficiency syndrome (AIDS).

3. B-lymphocytes (Bone Marrow Derived)

They constitute 10-20% of peripheral blood lymphocytes and are located in the *cortical areas of lymph node, white pulp of spleen and mucosa associated lymphoid tissue of pharyngeal tonsils and Peyer's patches of GIT.*

These cells have a B cell receptor (BCR) composed of IgM and IgD on their surface to bind with the antigen. BCR has unique antigen specificity. The rearrangement of immunoglobulin gene can give rise to different types of BCRs. The antigen however binds to the complementary BCR only (clonal selection).

The presence of rearranged immunoglobulin genes in a lymphoid cell is used as a molecular marker of B-lineage cells.

B cell associated markers are CD10 (CALLA), CD19, CD20, CD21 (EBV receptor), CD22, CD23.

B cells have Igα and Igβ on their cell membrane which are required for signal transduction (similar to CD3 of the T cells). They also have CD 40 molecule on its surface.

Detail of antigenic interaction with B cells and T cells

The activation of T cells requires two signals

Signal 1: Comes from binding of the TCR to MHC bound antigen.
Signal 2: Comes from the interaction of CD28 with *co-stimulatory* molecules B7-1 and B7-2 present on the antigen presenting cells.

CD19 is involved in signal transduction and is called as a Pan B cell **marker**.

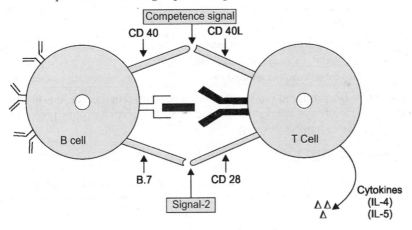

Competence signal (CD40-CD40L interaction) is required for the following functions:

1. *B cell mitogen*
2. Required for *isotype switching.*
3. *Affinity maturation*

In addition to these two, there is a **Competence signal** is due to interaction between CD40 molecules on B cells with CD 40 ligand on T helper cells. It results in the release of cytokines like IL-4 and IL-5. These cytokines cause B cell proliferation resulting in formation of plasma cells and memory cells.

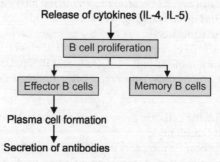

> The change in the class of the antibody being produced by the plasma cell is called as **Isotype Switching**

Concept

Hyper- IgM immunodeficiency is a paradoxical T-cell disorder in which a defect in CD40 ligand (normally present on Tcells) prevents isotype switching in B lymphocytes. So, these patients have reduced levels of IgG, IgE and IgA but **increased levels of IgM**. It is an **X linked** disorder. Patients have recurrent infections with *P. jiroveci* affecting respiratory tract.

The plasma cells secrete immunoglobulins. These can of different classes or isotypes like IgG, IgM, IgD, IgA and IgE. Initially, the first antibody produced by the plasma cell is IgM and later, other antibodies like IgG, IgA etc. are produced due to change in the nature of heavy chains. **Isotype Switching** is due to IFN-γ and IL-4. Polysaccharide and lipid antigens produce mainly IgM whereas protein antigens induce production of different isotypes of antibodies (IgG, IgA, IgE etc.).

$$\text{Isotype/Class Switching}$$
$$\text{IgM} \xrightarrow{\hspace{2cm}} \text{IgA, IgE, IgG}$$
(Due to change in heavy chain)

IMPORTANT POINTS ABOUT ANTIBODIES

Ig G	• Present in **maximum concentration**[Q] the human body • Important for **secondary immune response**[Q] • Can **cross the placenta**[Q]
Ig A	• Resent in **physiological secretions**[Q] of the body • Present in **monomer form in serum** and as **dimer**[Q] form in glandular secretions • Responsible for activation **alternate pathway**[Q]
Ig M	• Important for **primary immune response**[Q] • Having **maximum molecular weight**[Q] • Having **maximum size**[Q] • Present as a **pentamer**[Q] • Also known as '**Millionaire's antibody**'[Q] • Functions as **B cell receptor**[Q] • **IgM**[Q] and IgG (**IgM**[Q] > IgG) are responsible for activation of **classical pathway**[Q]
Ig D	• Functions as **B cell receptor**[Q]
Ig E	• Increased in **allergic conditions**[Q] • Also known as '**homocytotropic antibody**[Q]' • Also called '**reaginic antibody**'[Q]

> One antibody has **two heavy chains** and **two light chains**. Within light and heavy chains, **three hypervariable regions** exist – HV 1, 2 and 3

> The **efficiency of immunoglobulin transfer** across placenta: **Ig G1>** Ig G3> Ig G4> **Ig G2**

The antibodies produced remove the antigen by different mechanisms like complement activation (by membrane attack complex formation), opsonisation (for preferential killing) and antibody dependent cytotoxicity.

Cell Mediated Immunity

It is for more important for intracellular pathogens, virus infected/malignant cells and endogenous antigens. It is mediated by CD8 T cells, macrophages and natural killer cells.

Endogenous antigen is expressed with MHC I molecule by the nucleated cells. These cells are also destroyed in the process, so, the preferred name for them is Target cells and not APCs.

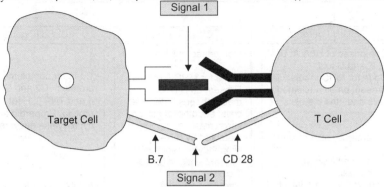

Antigen activated CD8T cells undergo proliferation. They release perforin-granzyme molecules and express Fas Ligand both of which initiate apoptosis of Target cells.

NATURAL KILLER CELLS (NK CELLS) OR NULL CELLS OR NON-T, NON-B LYMPHOCYTES

NK cells are also called 'Large granular lymphocytes' as they are *morphologically larger* than both T and B lymphocytes and *contain azurophillic granules* (which are absent in both T and B lymphocytes). They constitute 5-10% of peripheral blood lymphocytes. They arise in both bone marrow and thymic microenvironments. NK cells are activated in presence of IL-2 to Lymphocyte activated killer (LAK) cells. These cells express the following molecules:

CD16^Q: Surface receptors for Fc portion of IgG
CD56^Q: Surface receptors for NCAM – 1
CD8 and CD2: Some T-cell lineage markers (less common)

They are first line defense against cancer and virus infected cells. So, functionally NK cells share features of both monocyte-macrophages and neutrophils. The hyporesponsiveness of NK cells is seen in patients of Chediak-Higashi syndrome.

The NK cells express activating and inhibitory receptors. The functional activity of the NK cells is regulated by a balance between signals from these receptors. Normal cells are not killed because inhibitory signals from normal MHC class I molecules override activating signals. **The ability of NK cells to kill target cells is inversely related to target cell expression of MHC class I molecules**. If virus infection or neoplastic transformation disturbs or reduces the expression of class I MHC molecules, inhibitory signals delivered to NK cells are interrupted and lysis occurs. IL 2 and IL 15 stimulate proliferation of NK cells whereas IL 12 stimulates NK cells to secrete IFN-γ.

Major Histocompatibility Complex (MHC) or Human Leucocyte Antigen (HLA) Complex

MHC is a cluster of genes located on short arm of **chromosome 6** (*6p^Q*) whose main physiologic function is to bind peptide fragments of foreign proteins for presentation to antigen-specific T cells.

It is classified into **three classes namely class I, II and III genes**. The class I genes includes HLA-A, -B, -C, - E, -F and -G. HLA-A,-B and -C gene codes for MHC I molecule and the **HLA-E** molecule is the major **self-recognition target** for the natural killer (NK) cell inhibitory receptors. **HLA-G** is expressed selectively in extravillous trophoblasts, the fetal cell population directly in contact with maternal tissues. It provides inhibitory signals to both NK cells and T cells and maintains **maternofetal tolerance** and the function of *HLA-F* remains largely *unknown*. The class II genes include HLA-D and code for MHC II molecule whereas the class III gene codes for the complement and other proteins.

NK cells are unique as they are capable of direct cell lysis which is:
- Not mediated by an immune response
- *MHC – unrestricted*
- Does *not* involve an antigen antibody interaction

MHC is a cluster of genes located on **short arm of chromosome** 6 (6p).

Immunity

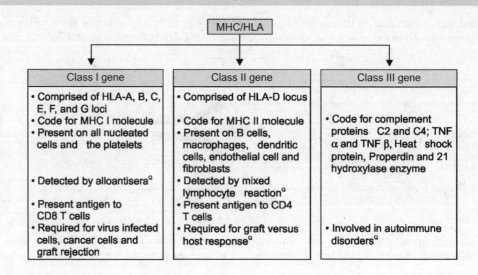

Class III genes code for:
- Complement components C2 and C4 of classical pathway (Not C3)
- Properdin factor B of alternate pathway
- Tumor necrosis factor: Alpha and Beta
- Heat shock protein 70
- Enzyme tyrosine hydroxylase

Class I gene	Class II gene	Class III gene
• Comprised of HLA-A, B, C, E, F, and G loci • Code for MHC I molecule • Present on all nucleated cells and the platelets • Detected by alloantisera^Q • Present antigen to CD8 T cells • Required for virus infected cells, cancer cells and graft rejection	• Comprised of HLA-D locus • Code for MHC II molecule • Present on B cells, macrophages, dendritic cells, endothelial cell and fibroblasts • Detected by mixed lymphocyte reaction^Q • Present antigen to CD4 T cells • Required for graft versus host response^Q	• Code for complement proteins C2 and C4; TNF α and TNF β, Heat shock protein, Properdin and 21 hydroxylase enzyme • Involved in autoimmune disorders^Q

MHC I molecule is present on all the nucleated cells and platelets It is **not** present on **mature RBCs.**

MHC-I MOLECULE

It consists of α *chain (heavy chain) linked to* $β_2$ *microglobulin (light chain; not encoded within MHC)* and binds to peptides that are derived from proteins *synthesized within the cell* like the viral antigens. The antigen binding cleft is formed by α**1and** α**2 chain** of the MHC molecule (**distal α domains of MHC**^{Q}). The antigens binding with MHC I molecule are presented to CD8+ T cells. As discussed earlier, cytotoxic T cells/**CD8+ T cells are MHC-I restricted**.

Structure of antigen binding cleft of MHC molecule on the surface of APC

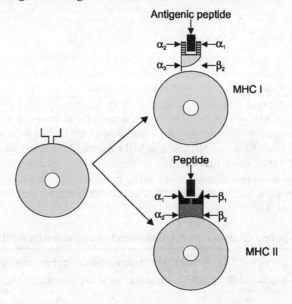

MHC-II molecule

It consists of α chain linked to β-chain. The antigen binding cleft is formed by $α_1$ and $β_1$ chain of the MHC molecule (**distal α and β domains of MHC**^{Q}). The antigens binding with MHC II molecule are presented to CD4+ T cells. As discussed earlier, helper T cells/**CD4+ T cells are MHC-II restricted**.

MHC II molecule is present on **macrophages, dendritic cells, B cells** and their expression can be induced on *endothelial cells* and *fibroblasts* by IFN-γ

Mnemonic

Normal CD4: CD8T cell ratio is 2:1. So, MHC 2 with CD4 and MHC 1 with CD8.

Concept

As described earlier, MHCII molecule is required for the development of graft versus host disease. In a condition associated with a congenital deficiency of MHC II molecule as '***Bare Lymphocyte Syndrome***', the affected individuals would never develop Graft versus host disease even on being given mismatched bone marrow transplantation. They also have absence or deficiency of CD4T cells and so, also have hypogammaglobulinemia. These individuals have normal number of CD8T cells.

HLA and Disease Association

HLA- class I	
B-27	Spondyloarthropathies Ankylosing spondylitis Reiter's syndrome Acute anterior uveitis Reactive arthritis Psoriatic arthritis
B-8	Hyperthyroidism [Graves' disease] Myasthenia gravis
B-51	Behcet's disease
B-47	Congenital adrenal hyperplasia
CW6	Psoriasis vulgaris
HLA- class II	
DR-2	- Japanese SLE - Multiple sclerosis - Narcolepsy - Goodpasture's syndrome
DR-3	- Myasthenia gravis - Graves' disease - Type I DM - Dermatitis herpetiformis - Chronic active hepatitis - Caucasian SLE - Sjogren's syndrome
DR-4	Type 1 DM Pemphigus vulgaris Rheumatoid arthritis
DR-5	Juvenile (pauciarticular) arthritis
DR-8	Type I DM
DQ-1	Pemphigus vulgaris
DQ -	Gluten sensitive enteropathy [celiac sprue]
DQ-7	Bullous pemphigoid
DQ-8	Type 1 DM

DR-2 has negative association with type 1 DM i.e. genetic association with protection from DM

DISORDERS OF THE IMMUNE SYSTEM

Hypersensitivity Reactions

These are caused by the activity of the immune system detrimental to the host in response to exposure of the antigens.

TYPE I HYPERSENSITIVITY REACTION/ANAPHYLACTIC TYPE/IMMEDIATE TYPE OF HYPERSENSITIVITY REACTION

It is defined as a rapidly developing immunologic reaction *occurring within minutes* after the combination of an antigen with antibody bound to mast cells in individuals previously sensitized to the antigen. It is commonly referred to as *allergy*.

> The clinical features are usually seen during the second time antigen exposure subsequent to sensitization or priming

> The cell critical in the pathogenesis is the mast cell whereas TH2 also plays an important role in the pathogenesis.

> **Histamine** is responsible for the **early** clinical features because it is **preformed mediator**.
> *PAF* is the major mediator of the *late* phase reaction

> **IgE** is the most important antibody to cause **type I** hypersensitivity reactions.

> **IL-4** is responsible for the **secretion of IgE** from the B cells.
>
> **IL-5** is the most potent **eosinophil-activating cytokine** known.

Concept

> If there is presence of low concentration of antibodies on the cells then they are killed by 'phagocyte and complement independent' process known as antibody dependent cellular cytotoxicity (ADCC). It is mediated by neutrophils, macrophages and NK cells.

PATHOGENESIS

The first step is the **stage of sensitization** or priming in which there is entry of the antigen inside the body for the first time where it is captured by the antigen presenting cells and presented to the T cell which then differentiates into TH2 cell. The TH2 cell releases mediators like IL-3, IL-4 and IL-5. *IL-4 causes activation of B cell leading to the release of IgE from them whereas IL-5 is responsible for activating the eosinophils.* The secreted IgE then binds to mast cells in the circulation because of presence of Fc receptors on the mast cells. So, in the initial exposure or sensitization, there is *presence of mast cells* in the circulation having the presence of IgE on their surface.

The **subsequent exposure** to the same antigen causes the features in two phases. In the *initial phase* (within minutes of antigen exposure), there is *release of preformed mediators* of the mast cell due to their degranulation causing the *release of histamine, proteases and chemotactic factors*. Histamine causes vasodilation, bronchoconstriction and increased permeability. Late phase (2-24 hours after antigen exposure) is marked by the release of *secondary mediators* from the mast cells that include *prostaglandins, leukotrienes, cytokines and platelet activating factor (PAF)*. PGD2 is abundant in lung mast cells and causes bronchoconstriction as well as increased mucus production. The secondary mediators are responsible for the effects like bronchospasm, increased mucus production and recruitment of the inflammatory cells at the site of inflammation. *PAF causes bronchospasm, increased permeability and release of histamine and is considered to be* important in the initiation of the late-phase response. The release of various mediators is responsible for the clinical features seen in type I hypersensitivity reaction.

CONCEPT

Anaphylactic hypersensitivity reaction should **not be** confused with **anaphylactoid reaction.** The important differences are:
*Anaphylactoid reaction occurs on **first antigenic exposure**
*It is also **short lived** because its pathogenesis involves only degranulation of the mast cells and not cytokine synthesis.

Examples of type I hypersensitivity includes:

Localized hypersensitivity	Systemic hypersensitivity
- Bronchial asthma - Hay fever/allergic rhinitis - Food allergies - Atopic dermatitis - Urticaria - Angioedema	Anaphylaxis due to: - Antibiotics: Most commonly penicillin (therefore, a test dose should always be given before administration of penicillin to any patient) - Bee stings - Insect bites

TYPE II HYPERSENSITIVITY REACTION/ANTIBODY MEDIATED/CYTOLYTIC HYPERSENSITIVITY REACTION

Type II hypersensitivity is mediated by antibodies directed toward endogenous or exogenous specific antigens present on cell surfaces or extracellular matrix. The effector mechanisms for this reaction include:

I. Opsonisation and Complement- and Fc Receptor-Mediated Phagocytosis
   The antibodies are formed against the antigens and these are responsible for complement system activation resulting in the formation of membrane attack complex (MAC) leading to destruction of the antigen. The antibodies may also cause opsonisation (through C3b and C4b) and Fc receptor mediated phagocytosis.

II. Complement and Fc Receptor-Mediated Inflammation
   When antibodies deposit in *extracellular tissues*, the injury is because of inflammation and not phagocytosis or lysis of cells. The deposited antibodies activate complement system leading to recruitment of neutrophils and monocytes. These cells also bind to the deposited antibodies via their Fc receptors. The activated leukocytes release enzymes resulting in tissue damage.

III. Antibody mediated cellular dysfunction

In this mechanism, the antibodies directed against *cell-surface receptors* impair or dysregulate function without causing cell injury or inflammation.

Examples of type II hypersensitivity reaction

Opsonization and Complement- and Fc Receptor-Mediated Phagocytosis	• Transfusion reactions • Erythroblastosis fetalis • Autoimmune hemolytic anemia • Autoimmune thrombocytopenic purpura
Complement and Fc Receptor-Mediated Inflammation	• Goodpasture syndrome • Vasculitis due to ANCA • Acute rheumatic fever • Vascular rejection in organ grafts
Antibody mediated cellular dysfunction	• Myasthenia gravis (against acetylcholine receptor) • Graves' disease (against TSH receptor) • Pemphigus vulgaris (against epidermal cadherin) • Pernicious anemia (against intrinsic factor) • Insulin resistant diabetes (against insulin receptor)

𝓜

My-	**My**asthenia gravis
Blood-	**Blood** transfusion reactions
Group-	**G**oodpasture syndrome and **G**raves' disease
Is-	**I**nsulin resistant diabetes, **ITP**
R -	**R**heumatic fever
h-	**H**yperacute graft rejection
Positive-	**P**ernicious anemia and **P**emphigus vulgaris

TYPE III HYPERSENSITIVITY REACTION OR IMMUNE COMPLEX DISEASE

Antigen-antibody complexes produce tissue damage mainly by eliciting inflammation at the sites of deposition. The antigen can be either endogenous or exogenous. The immune complexes once formed may be present in the circulation (*circulating immune complexes*) or may get deposited inside the vessels or extravascular sites (*in situ immune complex*). They may either be generalized or localized. Systemic or generalized immune complex disease has the following phases:

Phase I or Immune Complex Formation

It is characterized by the formation of the antibody *about 5 days* **after** introduction of the antigen. The small or intermediate immune complexes are most pathogenic. The large complexes are rapidly removed by the macrophages.

Phase II or Immune Complex Deposition

In this phase, the immune complexes get deposited in the glomeruli, joints, skin, heart, serosal surfaces and the blood vessels.

Phase III

Immune complex mediated inflammation is *seen 10 days* **after antigen administration** and results in the development of vasculitis, glomerulonephritis and arthritis. The immune complexes cause inflammation by activation of the complement system resulting in the neutrophilic infiltration, vasodilation and edema. They also cause activation of the intrinsic pathway of coagulation system and microthrombi formation contributing to tissue ischemia and necrosis.

The blood vessels show intense neutrophilic infiltration and necrotizing vasculitis having the presence of **fibrinoid necrosis**.

𝓜

S	:**S**erum sickness, **S**chick test and **S**LE
H	:**H**ypersensitivity pneumonitis and **H**enoch Schonlein Purpura
A	:**A**rthus reaction
R	:**R**eactive arthritis and **R**heumatoid arthritis, **R**aji assay
P	:**P**olyarteritis nodosa (PAN) and **P**ost Streptococcal glomerulonephritis (PSGN)

Examples of type III hypersensitivity include:

Localized hypersensitivity	Systemic hypersensitivity
*Arthus reaction *Farmer's lung *Hypersensitivity pneumonitis *Polyarteritis nodosa	*SLE *Reactive arthritis *Henoch Schonlein purpura *Post streptococcal glomerulonephritis *Serum sickness *Type II lepra reaction

CONCEPT

> The difference between type II and type III hypersensitivity reactions is that in the former, the antigen is tissue specific whereas in type III it is non-specific. In type II reaction, the tissue injury is direct (because antigen is intrinsic component of target cell) whereas in type III, it is mediated by the deposition of antigen antibody complexes in different tissues.

TYPE IV OR CELL MEDIATED HYPERSENSITIVITY REACTION

The cell-mediated type of hypersensitivity is initiated by antigen-activated (sensitized) T lymphocytes. It includes the *delayed type hypersensitivity reactions* mediated by CD4+ T cells, and *direct cell cytotoxicity* mediated by CD8+ T cells.

1. **Pathogenesis of delayed type hypersensitivity reactions** (mediated by CD4+ T cells)

   The first step is the entry of the antigen inside the body where it is captured by the APCs and presented to the T cell which then **differentiates into TH1 cell** (*remember that in type I hypersensitivity, the naïve T-cells differentiate into TH2 cells*). The sensitized TH1 cells enter the circulation and remain in the memory pool of the body. When there is re-exposure of the same individual to the antigen for the subsequent time, there is release of cytokines like TNF-α, lymphotoxin, IFN-γ, IL-2 and IL-12.

   > - TNF-α and lymphotoxins have effects on endothelial cells leading to extravasation of lymphocytes and monocytes.
   > - IL-2 causes proliferation of antigen specific T-cells.

   The collective release of these mediators recruits a lot of inflammatory cells at the site of inflammation. The activated macrophages give rise to epithelioid cells and these cells surrounded by a collar of lymphocytes all around lead to **formation of a granuloma**. This granuloma formation is seen with tuberculin test, and other intracellular pathogens like mycobacterium, fungi and some parasites. Delayed type hypersensitivity reaction is also important in transplant rejection.

2. **Pathogenesis of T cell mediated cytotoxicity** (mediated by CD8+ T cells)

   Cytotoxic T lymphocytes (CTL) cause destruction of antigen bearing target cells particularly the tumor cells, the virus infected cells and allogeneic tissue during graft rejection. There are two mechanisms involved in this:
   - *Perforin granzyme dependent killing:* The mediators present in the lysosomal granules of the CTLs like perforin cause pore formation and the granzyme activates apoptosis on entering the cells via these pores.
   - *Fas-Fas ligand dependent killing:* Activated CTL express Fas ligand which can bind to Fas expressed on the target cells leading to apoptosis.

Antibody-mediated hypersensitvity reactions types **I, II and III.**
Type IV hypersensitivity: *cellular immunity*

IFN-γ causes activation of macrophages.

IL-12 is produced by macrophages and dendritic cells and is critical in the pathogenesis of delayed hypersensitivity because it induces the TH1 response.

Examples of Type IV Hypersensitivity Include:

*Tuberculin reaction	*Lepromin test	*Multiple sclerosis
*Chronic graft rejection	*Contact dermatitis	*Sarcoidosis
*Temporal arteritis	*Primary biliary cirrhosis	*Type I lepra reaction
*Tumor immunity	*Resistance to viral infections	*Crohn's disease

TRANSPLANT REJECTION

It is a complex process in which both cellular and humoral immunity plays a role.

T cell Mediated Rejection

The T cell mediated rejection is also called as cellular rejection and it has two pathways:

- *Direct pathway* in which the interstitial dendritic cells of the donor present the antigen to the CD4 and CD8 T cells of the host. The host CD4 Tcells differentiate into TH1 cells and similar to delayed hypersensitivity cause graft injury. CD8 T cells differentiate into cytotoxic T lymphocytes and cause graft tissue damage by perforin-granzyme and Fas–Fas ligand pathways.

Immunity

- *Indirect pathway* in which the dendritic cells of the recipient present the antigen to CD4 Tcells. There is *no involvement of the CD8 T cells.*

Antibody Mediated Rejection or Humoral Rejection

It is also known as **rejection vasculitis** and takes place by two mechanisms:
- *Hyperacute rejection* takes place when there is preformed anti-donor antibodies present in the circulation of the recipient. It takes place within minutes to hours and is associated with previous blood transfusions, multiparous lady or already rejected transplant. It is an example of **type II hypersensitivity** reaction.
- *Acute rejection* is seen within days to months after transplantation. The mechanisms involved include inflammation, complement dependent cytotoxicity and ADCC.

MORPHOLOGY OF TRANSPLANT REJECTION

Hyperacute rejection

It takes place in individuals with preformed antibodies usually **within minutes to hours** of transplantation. The preformed antibodies result in immune complex disease with the presence of neutrophils within arterioles, glomeruli and peritubular capillaries and fibrin-platelet thrombi in vessel wall. There is presence of necrosis of the renal cortex.

Acute rejection

It is seen **days to months** after transplantation. It can be acute humoral rejection or acute cellular rejection.

The *acute cellular rejection* is seen within few months after transplantation. There is presence of endothelitis with the presence of CD4 and CD8 T cells in the interstitium along with the mononuclear cells in the glomerular and peritubular capillaries.

The *acute humoral rejection* or rejection vasculitis is mediated primarily by anti-donor antibodies and it manifests mainly as damage to the blood vessels in the form of necrotizing vasculitis with endothelial cell necrosis, neutrophilic infiltration, deposition of immunoglobulins, complement, and fibrin, and thrombosis. There is associated necrosis of the renal parenchyma.

Chronic rejection

It occurs **months to years** after transplantation. In this, the vascular changes consist of *dense, obliterative intimal fibrosis in the cortical arteries* resulting in glomerular loss, interstitial fibrosis and tubular atrophy, duplication of basement membranes of the glomeruli (also called as chronic transplant glomerulopathy). The renal interstitium also has mononuclear cell infiltrates containing large numbers of plasma cells and eosinophils.

GRAFT VERSUS HOST DISEASE (GVHD)/RUNT DISEASE (in animals)

Graft versus host disease occurs in any situation in which **immunologically competent cells** or their precursors are transplanted into **immunologically crippled patients** and the transferred cells recognize **alloantigens** in the host. It occurs most commonly in the setting of **allogenic bone marrow transplantation.** The recipients of bone marrow transplants are **immunodeficient** because of either their primary disease or prior treatment of the disease with drugs or irradiation. When such recipients receive normal bone marrow cells from allogenic donors, the *immunocompetent T cells* present in the donor marrow recognize the *recipient's HLA antigen* as foreign *antigen* and reacts against them. Both **CD4$^+$** and **CD8$^+$T** cells recognize and attack host tissues.

ACUTE GVHD

- It is characterized by an erythematous maculopapular rash; persistent anorexia or diarrhea, or both; and by liver disease with increased serum levels of bilirubin, alanine and aspartate aminotransferase, and alkaline phosphatase.
- *Diagnosis usually requires skin, liver, or endoscopic intestinal biopsy for confirmation.* In all these organs, endothelial damage and lymphocytic infiltrates are seen.

The **direct pathway** is important for **acute graft rejection**

The **indirect pathway** is important for **chronic graft rejection**.

The **initial target of the anti-bodies** is the **graft vasculature**.

Hyperacute rejection is **type II** hypersensitivity reaction.

Acute rejection is **type II + type IV** reactions **hypersensitivity reaction.**

Concept

Acute rejection can be reversed with immunosuppressive drugs like cyclosporine, muromonab and steroids.

Both acute as well as chronic rejection are usually irreversible

GVH reaction: skin rash/dermatitis, jaundice and diarrhea.

Immunity

*Skin: Epidermis and hair follicles are damaged.
*Liver: Small bile ducts show segmental disruption.
*Intestines: Destruction of the crypts and mucosal ulceration may be noted.

GVHD developing **within the first 3 months** post transplant is termed **acute GVHD**.

Clinical Staging and Grading of Acute Graft-versus-Host Disease

Clinical Stage	Skin	Liver—Bilirubin (mg/dL)	Gut
1	Rash <25% body surface	2–3	Diarrhea 500–1000 mL/d
2	Rash 25–50% body surface	3–6	Diarrhea 1000–1500 mL/d
3	Generalized erythroderma	6–15	Diarrhea >1500 mL/d
4	Desquamation and bullae	> 15	Ileus
Overall Clinical Grade	Skin Stage	Liver Stage	Gut Stage
I	1–2	0	0
II	1–3	1	1
III	1–3	2–3	2–3
IV	2–4	2–4	2–4

The **risk** of graft versus host can be **decreased** by **Depletion of T cells from graft**

*Grade I acute GVHD is of little clinical significance, does not affect the likelihood of survival, and does not require treatment. In contrast, grades II to IV GVHD are associated with significant symptoms and a poorer probability of survival, and they require aggressive therapy.

CHRONIC GVHD

GVHD developing or persisting **beyond 3 months** post-transplant is termed **chronic GVHD**.

Chronic GVHD resembles an autoimmune disorder with malar rash, sicca syndrome, arthritis, obliterative bronchiolitis, and bile duct degeneration and cholestasis.
- Because patients with chronic GVHD are susceptible to significant infections, they should receive *prophylactic trimethoprim-sulfamethoxazole.*
- Infection with cytomegalovirus is particularly important.

Autoimmune Disorders

Tolerance (unresponsiveness) to self-antigens is an important fundamental property of the immune system. The breakdown of tolerance is the basis of autoimmune diseases. Tolerance can be of the following subtypes:

1. ***Central tolerance:*** immature lymphocytes that recognize self-antigens in the central (generative) lymphoid organs are killed by apoptosis; in the B-cell lineage, some of the self-reactive lymphocytes switch to new antigen receptors that are not self-reactive.

PTPN-22 is the most frequently implicated gene in autoimmunity.

2. ***Peripheral tolerance:*** mature lymphocytes that recognize self-antigens in peripheral tissues become functionally inactive (anergic), or are suppressed by regulatory T lymphocytes, or die by apoptosis.

The causes of a failure of self-tolerance and the development of autoimmunity include:
1. Inheritance of susceptibility genes that may disrupt different tolerance pathways,
2. Infections and tissue alterations that may expose self-antigens and activate APCs and lymphocytes in the tissues due to molecular mimicry between microbial antigens and self molecules.

In rheumatic heart disease, streptococcal proteins cross react with myocardial proteins causing myocarditis.

Detailed Role of infections in autoimmunity.
1. Antigenic cross reactivity: this is due to similarity is the microbial antigenic structure and the self antigens. This is also known as 'molecular mimicry'.
2. Upregulation of co-stimulatory molecules by infectious organisms.
3. Polyclonal B cell activation: caused by EBV[Q] and HIV[Q] resulting in production of autoantibodies.

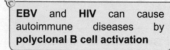

EBV and HIV can cause autoimmune diseases by **polyclonal B cell activation**

Immunity

4. Alteration of tissue antigens: infections may alter tissue self antigens so that they activate T cells and loose the property of self tolerance.

SYSTEMIC LUPUS ERYTHEMATOSUS (SLE)

SLE is an autoimmune multi-system disorder of unknown etiology characterised by loss of self tolerance and production of auto-antibodies. It is more commonly seen in the females affecting them around the age of 20-30's. The *deficiency of early complement proteins (C1, C2 and C4) has been postulated to be associated with increased incidence of SLE*. The auto-antibodies in this condition are formed against DNA, histones, non histone proteins bound to RNA and nucleolar antigens. These are collectively called as antinuclear antibodies (ANA).

Clinical significance of anti nuclear antibodies

Antiphospholipid antibody syndrome is characterized by antibodies against plasma proteins in complex with phospholipid. In **primary antiphospholipd antibody syndrome** there is hypercoagulable state without evidence of autoimmune disorders. In association with SLE or lupus, the name given is **secondary antiphospholipd antibody syndrome.** There is formation of antibody against **phospholipid beta– 2-glycoprotein 1 complex**[Q]. It also binds to cardiolipin antigen and lead to **false positive test for syphilis**[Q]. It also interferes with in vitro clotting time and so, called as lupus anticoagulant. In vivo, these patients have hypercoagulable state resulting in **arterial and venous thrombosis** resulting **spontaneous recurrent miscarriage** and focal or cerebral ischemia.

The **clinical criteria** for the diagnosis of SLE include **any 4 of the following mentioned 11 criteria**:

• Malar rash	• Serositis- Pleuritis or pericarditis
• Discoid rash	• Renal disorder
• Photosensitivity	• Hematological disorder
• Oral ulcer	• Immunological disorder
• Arthritis	• Antinuclear antibody

• Neurological disorder- Seizure or psychosis in the absence of known drug/metabolic abnormality.

ORGAN INVOLVEMENT

Kidney: WHO classification of renal involvement or **'lupus nephritis'** is as follows:
- Class I - Minimal or no change
- Class II - Mesangial lupus glomerulonephritis
- Class III - Focal proliferative glomerulonephritis
- Class IV - Diffuse proliferative glomerulonephritis.
- Class V - Membranous glomerulonephritis

Heart	There is development of **Libman-Sacks endocarditis**[Q] having vegetations on both the sides of the valvular surface. There is also presence of pericarditis.
Mouth	**Oral ulcers** are usually **painless**
Joints	**Non-erosive arthritis** involving 2 or more peripheral joints with tenderness and effusion.
Skin	Erythematous rash present over malar region is also called **'butterfly rash'**. Exposure to sunlight **accentuates the erythema.**
Blood	Presence of autoimmune cytopenia (anemia, neutropenia or thrombocytopenia). The presence of **LE cell or hematoxylin body** is also seen.

• If ANAs can bind to exposed cell nuclei, the nuclei may lose their chromatin pattern, and ecome homogeneous to produce lupus erythematosus (LE) bodies.
• *Almost all the patients having SLE have hematological manifestations clinically.*
• **SLE Nephropathy**[Q] has the findings called as "full house phenomenon"

SJOGREN SYNDROME

It is an autoimmune disorder characterised by the destruction of lacrimal and salivary glands resulting in the *inability to produce tears and saliva*. It is more commonly seen in females. It can be **primary** when it is called **sicca syndrome** and it may also be secondary to other autoimmune disorders; rheumatoid arthritis being most commonly associated disorder.

Anti-double stranded DNA antibody and the antibody against Smith **(Sm)** antigen **Highly specific** for SLE.

Antinuclear antibody **(ANA) Highly sensitive** for SLE

Anti Ro Antibody – Neonatal lupus

Anti-P antibody – Associated with **lupus psychosis**

Anti-SS-A and Anti-SS-B antibody- Associated with **congenital heart block** and **cutaneous lupus**

Anticardiolipin antibodies may produce a **false positive** VDRL test for syphilis.

Diffuse proliferative or type IV glomerulonephritis is the **most common** and **most serious** renal lesion

The presence of subendothelial deposits gives rise to **'wire loop' lesions** on light microscopy in **SLE.**

The **LE cell** is any phagocytic leukocyte (**neutrophil** or **macrophage**) that has engulfed the denatured nucleus of an injured cell.

Tart Cell is usually a **monocyte** which has ingested another cell or nucleus of another cell.

SLE is an example of both **type II** (hematological features) and **type III** (visceral lesions) hypersensitivity reactions.

Sjogren syndrome: dry eyes; dry mouth.
Diagnosis is confirmed with **lip biospy**

Sjogren syndrome: presence of anti-ribonucleoprotein antibodies like SS-A (Ro) and SS-B (La).

Sjogren syndrome: presence of anti-ribonucleoprotein antibodies like SS-A (Ro) and SS-B (La).

Diffuse Scleroderma: anti-DNA topoisomerase^Q antibodies

Limited scleroderma: anti-centromere^Q antibodies

CREST Syndrome= Calcinosis, Raynaud phenomenon, Esophageal dysmotility, Sclerodactyly and Telangiectasia.

There is *presence of anti-ribonucleoprotein antibodies like SS-A (Ro) and SS-B (La)*. The presence of former is associated with early disease onset, longer disease duration, and extraglandular manifestations, such as cutaneous vasculitis and nephritis.

Clinical features include dry mouth (*xerostomia*) and dry eyes (*keratoconjunctivitis sicca*), the latter due to lymphocytic infiltration and destruction of the lacrimal gland. *Mickulicz syndrome* include lacrimal and salivary gland enlargement of whatever cause. Patients with Sjogren syndrome have an *increased risk of developing lymphoid malignancies*.

MIXED CONNECTIVE TISSUE DISEASE (MCTD)

It is a disease seen in a group of patients who are identified clinically by the coexistence of features suggestive of SLE, polymyositis, rheumatoid arthritis, and systemic sclerosis. These patients have *high titers of antibodies to RNP particle-containing U1 RNP*. The factors lending distinctiveness to mixed connective tissue disease include the *reduced incidence of renal involvement and a good response to corticosteroids*.

SCLERODERMA

- It is an autoimmune disorder characterised by fibroblast stimulation and collagen deposition in the skin and internal rgans. The **skin is most commonly affected**, but the gastrointestinal tract, kidneys, heart, muscles, and lungs also are frequently involved.
- It is more commonly seen in the females and is due to release of growth factors acting on the fibroblasts like fibroblast growth factor (*FGF*), platelet derived growth factor (*PDGF*) and cytokines like *IL-1*.

The disease has two categories:

- *Diffuse Scleroderma* is characterized by presence of **anti-DNA topoisomerase^Q antibodies (Scl-70)**. There is widespread skin involvement at onset, with rapid progression and early visceral involvement. The symptoms include dysphagia, malabsorption, arrhythmia (due to cardiac fibrosis), exertional dyspnea and renal insufficiency.
- *Limited scleroderma* is characterized by the presence of **anti-centromere^Q antibodies**. The skin involvement is often confined to fingers, forearms, and face. Since the visceral involvement occurs late; so, the clinical course is relatively benign. Some patients develop *CREST syndrome^Q* whose features include Calcinosis, Raynaud phenomenon, Esophageal dysmotility, Sclerodactyly, and Telangiectasia.

ANA: the sensitivity of antinuclear antibodies determination is higher than 95% for systemic lupus erythematosus although specificity is fairly low. The different patterns which are seen are:

Homogeneous: systemic lupus erythematosus.
Peripheral: connective tissue diseases.
Speckled: systemic lupus erythematosus, mixed connective tissue disease, Sjögren's syndrome, polymyositis or scleroderma.
Nucleolar: approximately 50-70% of the patients with overlapping scleroderma and polymyositis/ dermatomyositis syndromes and in 1/3rd patients with systemic scleroderma, especially those with renal complications.

X-LINKED AGAMMAGLOBULINEMIA OF BRUTON

It is an X-linked immunodeficiency disorder *characterized by the failure of B-cell precursors (pro-B cells and pre-B cells) to mature into B cells* due to *mutation of B-cell tyrosine kinase (Btk)*. Btk is required for the maturation of pre-B cell to mature B cell. The disease is **seen almost entirely in males**. In most cases, recurrent bacterial infections of the respiratory tract, such as acute and chronic pharyngitis, sinusitis, otitis media, bronchitis, and pneumonia, are present. The causative organisms are *Haemophilus influenzae, Streptococcus pneumoniae*, or *Staphylococcus aureus* in most of the patients.

The classic form of this disease has the following characteristics:

- B cells are absent or markedly decreased in the circulation and the serum levels of all classes of immunoglobulins are reduced.
- Absence of plasma cells.
- T cell mediated reactions are normal.

It is associated with an increased risk of other autoimmune disorders.

Concept

Bruton's disease usually does not become apparent until about 6 months, when maternal immunoglobulins are depleted.

Germinal centers of lymph nodes, Peyer patches, the appendix, and tonsils are under developed or rudimentary

WISKOTT - ALDRICH SYNDROME

- Wiskott-Aldrich syndrome (WAS) is a rare X-linked recessive disease[Q].
- It is caused by mutations in the WASP gene located on short arm of chromosome X. The WASP protein is expressed in cells of all hematopoietic lineages. It is required for cytoskeletal integrity and signal transduction that are particularly important in platelets and T cells.
- The disorder is seen in male patients[Q] and becomes symptomatic in children. It is characterized by bruising caused by thrombocytopenia[Q], eczema[Q] (itchy rash), recurrent infections[Q], bloody diarrhea (due to thrombocytopenia)and a propensity for autoimmune disorders and malignancies[Q] (mainly lymphoma and leukemia).
- In Wiskott-Aldrich syndrome, the platelets are small[Q], have a shortened half life and do not function properly. They are removed by the spleen, which leads to low platelet counts. Splenomegaly may be seen.

Triad of WAS= thrombocytopenia+eczema+ recurrent infections

In WAS, ↓ IgM, ↑IgA and IgE, normal IgG levels may be elevated.

Diagnosis

- The diagnosis is made on the basis of clinical parameters, the blood film and low immunoglobulin levels.

Decreased levels of Wiskott-Aldrich syndrome protein (WASP) and/or confirmation of a causative mutation provide the most definitive diagnosis.

Treatment

It is done with **bone marrow transplantation**. The alternatives include intravenous immunoglobulin infusions or splenectomy.

COMMON VARIABLE IMMUNODEFICIENCY

Most patients with common variable immunodeficiency have normal or near-normal numbers of B cells in the blood and lymphoid tissues which are not able to differentiate into plasma cells. Patients have intrinsic B-cell defects (**defective cytokine receptor called BAFF** which normally promotes B cell differentiation and survival) as well as abnormalities of T cell-mediated regulation of B cells. The clinical manifestations include recurrent sinopulmonary pyogenic infections, recurrent herpesvirus infections and persistent diarrhea caused by *G. lamblia*. It affects **both sexes equally**, and the onset of symptoms is relatively **late (in childhood or adolescence)**. These patients have a high frequency of autoimmune diseases like rheumatoid arthritis and increased risk of lymphoid malignancy (particularly in women).

Common variable immuno-deficiency: characterized by *hypogammaglobulinemia* affecting all the antibody classes (but sometimes only IgG) even with *near-normal numbers of B Cells.*

DIGEORGE SYNDROME OR VELOCARDIOFACIAL SYNDROME

It is a *T-cell deficiency due to* deletion of chromosome 22q11.2. The patients have a **loss of T cell-mediated immunity** (owing to hypoplasia or lack of the thymus), tetany (owing to lack of the parathyroids), and congenital defects of the heart and great vessels. They may also have abnormal facies with defects in the mouth and ears. The absence of cell-mediated immunity results in the development of recurrent fungal and viral infections.

DiGeorge syndrome: failure of development of the **third** and **fourth** pharyngeal pouches

Absence of the parathyroid glands and the thymus.

Mnemonic: (CATCH 22)	
C	Cardiac abnormalities (especially tetralogy of Fallot)
A	Abnormal facies
T	Thymic aplasia
C	Cleft palate
H	Hypocalcemia (due to hypoplasia or lack of parathyroids)
22	22q11 deletion

ACQUIRED IMMUNODEFICIENCY SYNDROME (AIDS)

This retroviral disease is caused by the human immunodeficiency virus (HIV). It is characterized by the triad of immunosuppression associated with opportunistic infections, secondary neoplasms, and neurologic manifestations. The major routes of HIV infection are:

1. *Sexual contact*

   It is the *most common* **mode of spread of the infection** throughout the world. It is usually through heterosexual contact. The virus is present in semen, both extracellularly in the seminal fluid (called as free form of the virus) and within the lymphocytes. It enters the recipient's body through abrasions in mucosa. The transmission of the virus can occur by either direct entry of virus into the blood vessels or into the mucosal dendritic cells. The presence of any other concomitant sexually transmitted disease causing genital ulcerations increases the risk of transmission of HIV also. *Gonorrhea and Chlamydia also act as cofactors for HIV transmission primarily by increasing the seminal fluid content of inflammatory cells carrying HIV.*

2. *Parenteral inoculation*

Parenteral transmission of HIV is a broad term which includes transmission through:

a. Intravenous drug abusers (the largest group): transmission occurs through shared needles, syringes etc.

b. Patients receiving blood or blood components (like hemophiliacs receiving factor VIII or IX concentrates)

c. Infected patient to the physician through *needle stick injury:*

The transmission through the parenteral route can be prevented with the screening of the blood and taking precautions like the universal precautions like not recapping the needle after taking blood sample of a patient and use of disinfectants like hypochlorite for blood spillages.

3. Passage of the virus from **infected *mother to newborn*** (mother to child transmission or *vertical transmission*)

The transmission from an infected to the child can take place through:

a. Transplacental spread

b. **Infected birth canal during normal vaginal delivery**[Q]: it is the MC route for vertical transmission.

c. Ingestion of breast milk

The transmission through the vertical route can be reduced by the use of elective caesarean section and the use of antiviral drugs like nevirapine and zidovudine. (For details, refer to *Review of Pharmacology* by the same authors.)

Note: HIV infection cannot be transmitted by casual personal contact in the home, workplace, or school, and insect bites. HIV is most efficaciously transmitted by contaminated blood transfusion and least efficaciously by sexual contact.

ETIOLOGY AND PATHOGENESIS

HIV is a retrovirus belonging to the lentivirus family and is of two types HIV-1 and HIV-2. There are two strains of HIV which are:

a. Macrophage-tropic (R5 virus) strain: it infects both monocytes/macrophages and T cells

b. T-cell tropic (X4 virus) strain: it infects only activated T cell lines.

The HIV-1 virion is spherical and contains an electron-dense, cone-shaped core containing the major capsid protein p24, nucleocapsid protein p7/p9, the viral RNA, and viral enzymes (protease, reverse transcriptase, and integrase) surrounded by a lipid envelope derived from the host cell membrane. p24 is the most readily detected viral antigen and is the target for the antibodies used to diagnose HIV infection in blood screening. The viral envelope has two glycoproteins (gp120 and gp41) required for HIV infection of cells. The HIV-1 proviral genome contains the genes *gag, pol* and *env* which encode for large proteins which must be broken down to form small mature proteins.

The other genes which regulate the replication of HIV include:

- **tat** (transactivator) gene is critical for virus replication
- **vpr** protein facilitates HIV infection of macrophages. Although most retroviruses require cell division for their replication, still HIV-1 can multiply in differentiated nondividing macrophages because of vpr gene.
- **nef** protein affects T-cell activation, viral replication, and viral infectivity and reduces surface expression of CD4 and MHC molecules on infected cells.
- **vpu** promotes CD4 degradation and affects virion release.

Immunity

AIDS is the commonest **secondary** immunodeficiency disorder

---

Sexual contact: Least efficacious yet most common mode of spread of HIV infection.

The **male to female** transmission is **more common** as compared to transmission from females to males

---

The risk of transmission of **HIV is 0.3%** with needle stick injury whereas the risk of hepatitis B is 30%.

Vertical transmission is the commonest cause for AIDS in the pediatric population.

The commonest cause of AIDS in India is **HIV-1 group M subtype C**

Concept

R5 strains use CCR5 as their coreceptor which is expressed on both monocytes and T cells,

X4 strains bind to CXCR4 expressed on T cells and not on monocytes/macrophages.

Almost 90% of HIV infections are **initially transmitted by R5 strains.** However, during the course of infection, X4 viruses replace R5 strains due to mutations in genes that encode gp120.

The **two major targets** of HIV infection are the **immune system and the CNS.** The profound immunodeficiency is the hallmark of AIDS. The viral envelope gp120 interacts with CD 4 molecule. The commonly affected CD 4 cells in the human body include **helper T cells**[Q] **(worst affected)**, **monocyte-macropahges** and **dendritic cells**. This binding leads to a conformational change causing exposure of a new recognition site gp 41 for the co-receptors. The virus then fuses with the host cell membrane.

Defective CCR5 receptors lead to protective effect of providing resistance to the development of AIDS.

Once inside the cell, the reverse transcriptase of the HIV forms a single stranded DNA which is used for the formation of double stranded DNA (dsDNA) by DNA polymerase enzyme. The dsDNA then integrates into host cell by the enzymatic action of integrase. The viral particle is now called as HIV provirus. The provirus may remain non transcribed for sometime (*latent infection*) or the proviral DNA may be transcribed to form complete viral particles budding from the cell membrane. This is responsible for causing damage to host cell membrane followed by their apoptosis. The released viral particles spread through circulation and usually enter lymphoid organs which act as reservoir sites. Macrophages are also infected by the virus early; they are not lysed by HIV and they transport the virus to tissues specially the brain.

The viremia is controlled by the host immune response and the patient then enters a phase of clinical latency. During this phase, viral replication in both T cells and macrophages continues unchecked. There continues a gradual erosion of CD4+ cells by the cytopathic effects of the virus, apoptosis of the infected cells and killing of virus infected cells by virus specific cytotoxic T lymphocytes. This is leading to decline in CD4+ cell count and the patient developing clinical symptoms.

Acute Stage : Macrophage affected
Chronic Stage : T_{H1} cells affected

HIV: cytotoxic to CD4 T Cells leading to loss of cell-meditated immunity.

Follicular dendritic cell in germinal center of lymph node is a potential reservor of HIV

Major Abnormalities of Immune Function in AIDS

Lymphopenia	Decreased T-Cell Function In Vivo	Altered T-Cell Function In Vitro	Polyclonal B-Cell Activation	Altered Monocyte Functions
Predominantly due to selective loss of the CD4+ helper-inducer T-cell subset; **inversion of CD4:CD8 ratio**[Q]	Preferential **loss of memory T cells** and **Decreased delayed-type hypersensitivity**	Decreased proliferative response to mitogens, alloantigens, and soluble antigens	**Hypergamma-globulinemia** and circulating immune complexes	Decreased chemotaxis and phagocytosis
	Susceptibility to neoplasms and opportunistic infections	Decreased helper function for **pokeweed mitogen-induced B-cell** immunoglobulin production	Inability to mount de novo antibody response to a new antigen or vaccine	Decreased HLA class II antigen expression and reduced antigen presentation to T cells

Natural History of HIV

The acute retroviral syndrome

It is seen for 3-12 weeks and is characterized by high levels of plasma viremia, and *widespread seeding of the lymphoid tissues*. The initial infection is controlled by the development of an antiviral immune response. Clinically, this stage is associated with a self-limited acute illness with nonspecific symptoms, including sore throat, myalgias, fever, rash, weight loss, and fatigue, and clinical features, such as rash, cervical adenopathy, diarrhea, and vomiting.

The middle chronic phase

This is characterized by a period of clinical latency. It is usually lasting for an average duration of 10 years. In this phase, there is a continuous battle between the virus and the host immune cells. The immune system is intact, but *there is continuous HIV replication, predominantly in the lymphoid tissues, which may last for several years*. Patients are either asymptomatic or develop persistent generalized lymphadenopathy. The patients may have minor opportunistic infections as thrush and herpes zoster. Persistent lymphadenopathy with significant constitutional symptoms (fever, rash, fatigue) reflects the onset of the *crisis* phase.

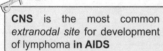

The weight loss is so severe that AIDS is also known as **"Slim's disease"**

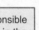

*M. tuberculosis** is the most common infection with HIV in *India*

Candidiasis is the most common fungal infection in AIDS in *India*

Pneumocystis jiroveci is the most common fungal infection in AIDS in *World*

Kaposi's sarcoma is the most common cancer seen in patients having AIDS

Stomach is the most common **extranodal site** for development of lymphoma in **non HIV** patients.

CNS is the most common *extranodal site* for development of lymphoma **in AIDS**

Toxoplasma gondii is responsible for 50% of all mass lesions in the CNS

AIDS-dementia complex is the most common **neurological manifestation** of HIV infection

Inflammatory myopathy is the commonest **skeletal muscle disorder** in HIV.

The final phase or the stage of crisis

It is associated with the loss of host immune cells in the battle and the *progression to AIDS*. It is characterized by the patient presenting with a long-lasting fever (>1 month), fatigue, weight loss, and diarrhea.

CLINICAL FEATURES

The typical adult patient with AIDS presents with fever, weight loss, diarrhea, generalized lymphadenopathy, multiple opportunistic infections, neurologic disease and secondary neoplasms.

The opportunistic infections seen are:

Bacterial infections	Viral infections	Fungal infections	Protozoal infections
• M. tuberculosis • Salmonella • Nocardiosis • Atypical myco-bacterial infections	• Cytomegalovirus • Herpes simplex virus • Varicella zoster virus • JC virus causing Progressive multifocal leukoencephalopahty	• Candidiasis • Pneumocystis jiroveci • Cryptococcosis • Histoplasmosis • Coccidiomycosis	• Cryptosporidium • Isosporidium • Toxoplasmosis

Neoplasms in AIDS

1. **Kaposi's sarcoma[Q]**: It is caused due to infection with *Kaposi sarcoma herpesvirus* (KSHV) or *human herpes virus -8* (HHV8). It is characterized by the proliferation of spindle-shaped cells that express markers of **both endothelial (vascular or lymphatic) and smooth muscle cells[Q]**. KSHV infection is related to rare B cell lymphomas in AIDS patients known as body cavity based primary effusion lymphoma and to a multicentric B-cell lymphoproliferative disorder called as **Castleman disease**.

2. **Lymphomas**: AIDS related lymphomas include
   i. Systemic lymphomas having the **CNS as the *most common extranodal site* for development of lymphoma[Q]**,
   ii. Primary CNS lymphoma found more commonly in AIDS than in general population
   iii. Body cavity lymphomas present as pleural, peritoneal or pericardial effusions.
   These tumors are more frequently seen in patients with CD4+ T cell count <50 per microlitre.

3. **Genital cancers** including cancer of the cervix and the anal cancers due to infection with human papilloma virus (HPV).

Neurological Manifestations in AIDS

The neurological manifestations are due to the involvement of the **microglia[Q]**. These include

1.	Opportunistic infections
2.	Neoplasms
3.	Aseptic meningitis
4.	Peripheral neuropathies
5.	AIDS-dementia complex[Q]
6.	Vacuolar myelopathy: It is a disorder of the spinal cord found in 20% to 30% of patients with AIDS. The findings resemble those of subacute combined degeneration, though serum levels of vitamin B12 are normal.
7.	Meningoencephalitis: HIV encephalitis is characterized microscopically as a chronic inflammatory reaction with widely distributed infiltrates of microglial nodules around the small blood vessels showing abnormally prominent endothelial cells and perivascular foamy or pigment-laden macrophages. These nodules also contain the macrophage-derived multinucleated giant cell.
8.	Inflammatory myopathy[Q]: The histological findings include muscle fiber necrosis and phagocytosis, interstitial infiltration with HIV-positive macrophages. Characteristically vasculitis is absent[Q].

Diagnosis of HIV infection or AIDS

The diagnosis of HIV is established with the following tests:

- **ELISA**[Q] is used for the detection of antibodies against viral proteins. This is the **most sensitive** and the best screening test for the diagnosis of AIDS.
- **Western blot**[Q] is the **most specific** or the confirmatory test for HIV.
- Direct detection of the viral infection is with p24 antigen capture assay, reverse transcriptase polymerase chain reaction (RT-PCR), DNA-PCR and culture of the virus from the monocytes and CD4+ T cells.

The management of the disease is done by the Highly active antiretroviral therapy (HAART) details of which can be referred from 'Review of Pharmacology' by the same authors.

Some patients with advanced disease in HIV paradoxically deteriorate on initiating the antiviral therapy. This ironical disorder whose basis in not understood is called **Immune reconstitution inflammatory syndrome**.

Amyloidosis (Beta-Fibrillosis)

It is a group of diseases having in common the deposition of amyloid (a pathologic proteinaceous substance, deposited between cells in various tissues and organs of the body). Amyloid appears as an amorphous, eosinophilic, hyaline, extracellular substance with the light microscope. Its progressive accumulation can cause pressure atrophy of adjacent cells.

Nature of Amyloid

Amyloid is seen to be made up of *nonbranching fibrils of indefinite length and a diameter of approximately 7.5 to 10 nm by the electron microscope*. X-ray crystallography and infrared spectroscopy demonstrate a characteristic cross-β-pleated sheet conformation responsible for the birefringence. Chemically, 95% of the amyloid is made up of fibril proteins.

CLASSIFICATION OF AMYLOIDOSIS

Primary Amyloidosis

It is associated with immunocyte dyscrasias like *multiple myeloma* or any other B cell neoplasm.

The tumor cells in multiple myeloma secrete *light chains of the immunoglobulins* of either lamda or kappa type which get deposited in the tissues as amyloid. The chemical nature of the amyloid is **AL**[Q] (A for amyloid and L for light chain).

Secondary Amyloidosis *(also called as **Reactive Systemic Amyloidosis**)*

It is usually seen *secondary* to chronic inflammatory conditions like *rheumatoid arthritis*[Q] *(**most commonly**)*, tuberculosis, bronchiectasis, chronic osteomyelitis, inflammatory bowel disease, ankylosing spondylitis and two cancers namely renal cell cancer and Hodgkin's disease. There is release of IL-1 and IL-6 which act on the liver cells leading to the secretion of SAA protein which gives rise to AA protein being deposited in this condition. The chemical nature of amyloid is **AA**[Q].

Hemodialysis associated Amyloidosis

It is caused by the deposition of the β_2 microglobulin which is a **component of MHC class I molecule** and can not be filtered through the cuprophane dialysis membrane. It gets deposited in the synovium, joints and the tendon sheaths. The chemical nature of the amyloid is **Aβ_2**[Q].

Heredofamilial Amyloidosis

i. *Familial Mediterranean fever* is an autosomal recessive condition characterized by development of attacks of fever associated with inflammation of serosal surfaces (pleura, peritoneum and synovial membrane). The amyloid protein deposited is AA protein and the protein associated with this condition is called **pyrin**[Q].

Concept

Window period is the term used for initial 2-4 weeks when the patient is infectious and the screening test is negative during which the investigation of HIV is made using *polymerase chain reaction for detection of viral nucleic acids.*

Amyloid

EM: *nonbranching fibrils* of indefinite length

X-ray crystallography and **infrared spectroscopy**: characteristic cross-β-**pleated** sheet conformation

Primary Amyloidosis: B cell neoplasm; AL

Secondary Amyloidosis: Chronic inflammation: AA

Chronic renal failure: $A\beta_2$

Alzheimer disease: $A\beta$

Familial Mediterranean fever: AA; involvement of pyrin.

Medullary thyroid cancer: **calcitonin** is the tumor marker and also forms amyloid; **ACal**

Spleen involvement in amyloidosis
Red pulp: Lardaceous spleen
White pulp: Sago spleen

'Remember, *red is called Lal in hindi*; so, when red pulp is involved, remember it is lardaceous spleen'

ii. *Familial amyloidotic neuropathies (several types):*
This is a group of ***autosomal dominant*** conditions in which both peripheral and autonomic nerves are involved. There is deposition of **ATTR** (A for amyloid and TTR is for transthyretin, a protein which transports thyroxine and retinol). The transthyretin deposited in this condition is a **mutant form of the normal protein**[Q].

iii. *Systemic senile Amyloidosis*
This is a condition characterized by the deposition of **structurally normal transthyretin**[Q], the chemical nature of amyloid is **ATTR** and it is usually deposited in the heart of aged individuals leading sometimes to the development of restrictive cardiomyopathy.

LOCALIZED AMYLOIDOSIS

There is presence of nodular deposits most often in lung, larynx, skin, urinary bladder, tongue and around the eyes.

i. *Senile cerebral amyloidosis*
It is seen in **Alzheimer's disease** in which there is deposition of β-amyloid protein. So, chemical nature of amyloid is **Aβ**[Q].

ii. *Endocrine*
It is associated with:
– *Medullary carcinoma of thyroid* having the deposition of **ACal**[Q] derived from calcitonin
– *Islet of Langerhans* in Type II DM having deposits of **AIAPP**[Q] derived from Islet Amyloid Peptide

iii. *Isolated Atrial Amyloidosis*
In this condition, there is deposition of **AANF** derived from Atrial natriuretic factor.

iv. *Prion disease*
In this condition, there is deposition of misfolded prion proteins **PrPsc** derived from normal prion protein PrP.

Summary of clinical conditions and the chemical nature of amyloid

S.No.	Amyloid protein	Precursor	Disease
1.	AL	Ig light chain	Multiple myeloma (primary amyloidosis)
2.	AA	SAA	Secondary or reactive amyloidosis
3.	Aβ₂m	β_2 microglobulin	Hemodialysis Associated amyloidosis
4.	Aβ	Aβ precursor protein	Senile cerebral Alzheimer's
5.	ATTR	Mutant Transthyretin Normal Transthyretin	Familial amyloidotic neuropathy Systemic senile amyloidosis
6.	ACal	Calcitonin	Medullary carcinoma of thyroid
7.	AIAPP	Islet amyloid polypeptide	Type II diabetes
8.	AANF	ANP	Isolated atrial amyloidosis Misfolded prion protein (PrPsc) disease
9.	**Aα**	**Fibrinogen**	**Familial renal amyloidosis**

Morphology in Amyloidosis

Kidney
It is the *most common* and *most serious* form of organ involvement and is usully involved in **secondary amyloidosis**. There is deposition primarily in the glomerular basement membrane, mesangium and the interstitial peritubular tissue. Arteries and arterioles are also affected.

Spleen
There is splenomegaly. If there is involvement of splenic follicles, it is called as **Sago spleen** and if there is involvement of splenic sinuses and red pulp it is called as **Lardaceous spleen**.

Liver
It is **first deposited in the space of Disse** and later result in hepatomegaly. The liver function tests are usually normal.

Heart
It is more commonly associated with **primary amyloidosis**. It is the most important organ involved in senile systemic amyloidosis. Clinically, there may be development of arrhythmia and it is also the most important cause of restrictive cardiomyopathy. There is deposition in the focal subendocardial region.

Adrenals
The intercellular deposits begin initially in zona glomerulosa.

GIT
The GI tract may be involved through the gingiva to the anus. The deposition of the amyloid in the tongue results in the nodular enlargement of tongue called *macroglossia* or the tumor forming amyloid of the tongue.

> **Macroglossia** is the *most specific* feature of **AL** type of amyloidosis. (Ref Wintrobe 12th/2442)

Clinical features are non-specific and the symptoms are seen depending on the organ predominantly affected in the disease. Deposition of the amyloid in **long term hemodialysis** takes place in joints and in the carpal ligament of the wrist, the latter leading to development of *'carpal tunnel syndrome'*.

Diagnosis

The diagnosis is made by the microscopic examination of the *biopsy from renal tissue, rectum, abdominal fat aspiration and gingiva.* The **rectum is the best site for taking the biopsy[Q]**. The staining of **abdominal fat aspirate[Q]** is quite specific but has low sensitivity. Grossly, the organs are enlarged and firm with a waxy appearance. The cut surface on painting with iodine imparts a yellow color which on application of sulfuric acid (H_2SO_4) gives a blue violet color.

STAINING FOR AMYLOID

- **Congo red**: It is the most widely used specific stain for amyloid.
- **Iodine staining: It is used for unfixed specimen or histological section. Amyloid stains mahogany brown and if sulfuric acid is added, it turns violet.**
- **Thioflavin 'T' and 'S'** give secondary immunofluorescence with ultraviolet light. *Thioflavin T is more useful for demonstrating juxtaglomerular apparatus of the* kidney.
- **Metachromatic stains** like crystal violet and methyl violet give rose pink appearance.
- Amyloid is **PAS** positive.

The condition has usually poor prognosis.

> **Congo red**
> *Pink red* color under normal *light microscopy*
>
> *'Apple green birefringence'* in the *polarized* light.

Appearance of Amyloid	
On light microscopy and standard tissue stains (H and E)	Amorphous eosinophilic extracellular substance
Congo red stain on ordinary light	Pink or red color to tissue deposits
Congo red stain on polarizing microscopy	Apple green birefringence[Q]
Fluorescent stains (thioflavin T and S)	Yellow color under UV light
Electron microscopy	Nonbranching fibrils[Q] of indefinite length and a diameter of approximately 7.5 to 10 nm.
X-ray crystallography and infrared spectroscopy	Characteristic cross b pleated[Q] sheet conformation

MULTIPLE CHOICE QUESTIONS

IMMUNE CELL: GENERAL ASPECTS

1. Which of the following features is not shared between 'T cells' and B cells'? *(AIIMS Nov 2012)*
   (a) Antigen Specific Receptors
   (b) Class I MHC Expression
   (c) Positive selection during development
   (d) All of the above

2. CD4 is not important for which of the following?
   (a) Antibody production *(AIIMS May 2011)*
   (b) Cytotoxicity of T cells
   (c) Memory B cells
   (d) Opsonisation

3. Type 1 MHC presents peptide antigen to T cell , so that peptide binding site is formed by: *(AI 2010)*
   (a) Alfa and Beta chain
   (b) Distal domain alfa 1 and 2
   (c) Alfa and beta microglobulin
   (d) Proximal domain alfa 1 and 2

4. Function of CD4 is all except: *(AI 2009)*
   (a) Memory
   (b) Immunoglobin production
   (c) Activation of macrophages
   (d) Cytotoxicity

5. A super-antigen is a bacterial product that *(AI 2008)*
   (a) Binds to B7 and CD28 co-stimulatory molecules
   (b) Binds to the beta chain of TCR and MHC class II molecules of APC stimulating T cell activation
   (c) Binds to the CD4 + molecule causing T cell activation
   (d) Is presented by macrophages to a larger-than-normal number of T helper CD4 + lymphocytes

6. Memory T cells can be identified by using the following marker: *(AI 2003)*
   (a) CD45RA
   (b) CD45RB
   (c) CD45RC
   (d) CD45RO

7. All of the following statements about NK cells are true except: *(AI 2003)*
   (a) They are derived from large granular cells
   (b) They comprise about 5% of human peripheral lymphoid cells
   (c) They are MHC restricted cytotoxic cells
   (d) They express IgG Fc receptors

8. The following feature is common to both cytotoxic T-cells and NK cells: *(AI 2002)*
   (a) Synthesize antibody
   (b) Require antibodies to be present for action
   (c) Effective against virus infected cells
   (d) Recognize antigen in association with HLA class II markers

9. MHC restriction to antigen presentation is not done for: *(AIIMS May 2009)*
   (a) Killing of viruses by cytotoxic cells
   (b) Killing of bacteria by helper cells
   (c) T cell activation in autoimmunity
   (d) Graft rejection

10. Most potent stimulator of naive T cell is?
    (a) Mature dendritic cell *(AI 2011, AIIMS Nov 08)*
    (b) Follicular dendritic cell
    (c) Macrophages
    (d) B cell

11. Natural killer cells attacks which of the following cells: *(AIIMS Nov 2006)*
    (a) Cells which express MHC1
    (b) Cells which are not able to express MHC1
    (c) MHC cells which express MHC2
    (d) Cells which are not able to express MHC

12. Toll like receptors, recognize bacterial products and stimulates immune response by: *(AIIMS Nov 2006)*
    (a) Perforin and granzyme mediated apoptosis
    (b) FADD ligand apoptosis
    (c) Transcription of nuclear factor mediated by NFκB which recruits cytokines
    (d) Cyclin

13. The following interleukin is characteristically produced in a TH_1 response: *(AIIMS Nov 2004)*
    (a) IL-2   (b) IL-4
    (c) IL-5   (d) IL-10

14. CD-95 has a major role in: *(AIIMS Nov 2003)*
    (a) Apoptosis
    (b) Cell necrosis
    (c) Interferon activation
    (d) Proteolysis

15. Which of the following chemical mediators of inflammation is an example of a C-X-C or alpha Chemokine? *(AIIMS Nov 2003)*
    (a) Lipoxin LXA4
    (b) Interleukin IL-8
    (c) Interleukin IL-6
    (d) Monocyte Chemo-attractant Protein MCP-1

Immunity

16. The complement is fixed best by which of the following immunoglobulins: *(AIIMS May 2002)*
    (a) IgG
    (b) IgM
    (c) IgA
    (d) IgD

17. Antigen presenting cells are which of the following:
    (a) Astrocytes *(AIIMS May 2002)*
    (b) Endothelial cells
    (c) Epithelial cells
    (d) Langerhan's cells

18. Antigen presenting cells are: *(PGI June 2006)*
    (a) Langerhan's cell
    (b) Macrophage
    (c) Cytotoxic T cells
    (d) Helper T cells
    (e) B lymphocyte

19. Perforins are produced by: *(PGI Dec 2001)*
    (a) Cytotoxic T cells
    (b) Suppressor T cells
    (c) Memory helper T cells
    (d) Plasma cells
    (e) NK cells

20. Cell surface molecules involved in peripheral tolerance induction are: *(PGI Dec 2003)*
    (a) B_7 and CD_{28}
    (b) CD_{40} and CD_{40L}
    (c) CD_{34} and CD_{51}
    (d) B_7 and CD_3

21. Marker for B-Lymphocyte: *(PGI Dec 2004)*
    (a) CD34
    (b) CD33
    (c) CD19
    (d) CD20
    (e) CD22

22. IL-1 causes *(Delhi PG-2008)*
    (a) Increased leukocyte adherence
    (b) Fibroblast proliferation
    (c) Increased collagen synthesis
    (d) All of the above

23. Antigen presenting cells present in skin are called
    (a) Langerhan's cells *(Delhi PG-2004)*
    (b) Kupffer's cells
    (c) Microglia
    (d) Melanocytes

24. Plasma cells *(UP 2004)*
    (a) Contain nucleus
    (b) Helps in the formation of antibody
    (c) Are deficient in cytoplasm
    (d) Are derived from T-cells

25. The normal ratio of CD4 to CD8 is *(UP 2005)*
    (a) 1: 1
    (b) 2: 1
    (c) 8: 1
    (d) 10: 1

26. CD4 cells is used to identify which of the following
    (a) MHC I *(AP 2007)*
    (b) MHC II
    (c) T cells
    (d) B cells

27. CD3 is marker for: *(Jharkhand 2006)*
    (a) Monocyte   (b) T cell
    (c) B cell   (d) None

28. Which of the following is not true about innate immunity?
    (a) It is present prior to antigenic exposure
    (b) It is relatively non-specific
    (c) Memory is seen
    (d) It is the first line of defense

29. Which one of the listed receptors is the type of receptor on leukocytes that binds to pathogen-associated molecular patterns (PAMPs) and mediates immune response to bacterial lipopolysaccharide?
    (a) Cytokine receptor
    (b) G-protein-coupled receptor
    (c) Mannose receptor
    (d) Toll-like receptor

Most Recent Questions

29.1. NK cell CD marker is:
    (a) 16   (b) 60
    (c) 32   (d) 25

29.2. Immunity against cancer cells:
    (a) Basophills   (b) Eosinophils
    (c) NK cells   (d) Neutrophils

29.3. NK cells express:
    (a) CD 15, CD 55   (b) CD 16, CD 56
    (c) CD 16, CD 57   (d) CD 21, CD 66

29.4. Which of the following immune cells have the expression of CD8 on their surface?
    (a) T-cells   (b) B-cells
    (c) Null cells   (d) Macrophages

29.5. The following interleukin is characteristically produced in a TH1 response?
    (a) IL-2   (b) IL-4
    (c) IL-5   (d) IL-10

29.6. Most potent stimulator of Naïve T-cells:
    (a) Mature dentritic cells
    (b) Follicular dendritic cells
    (c) Macrophages
    (d) B-cell

29.7. Macroglobulin is derived from:
(a) B cells   (b) T cells
(c) Both   (d) Natural killer cells

29.8. Kupffer cells are found in:
(a) Heart   (b) Lungs
(c) Liver   (d) Spleen

29.9. Birbeck granules are present in
(a) Merkel cell   (b) Langerhans cell
(c) Langhans cell   (d) Melanocyte

29.10. Which of the following immunoglobulin does not fix complement?
(a) IgA   (b) IgG
(c) IgM   (d) IgE

MHC

30. MHC class III genes encode: *(AI 2003)*
(a) Complement component C3
(b) Tumor necrosis factor
(c) Interleukin 2
(d) Beta 2 microglobulin

31. The HLA class III region genes are important elements in: *(AI 2003)*
(a) Transplant rejection phenomenon
(b) Governing susceptibility to autoimmune diseases
(c) Immune surveillance
(d) Antigen presentation and elimination

32. HLA is located on: *(AIIMS Nov 2009)*
(a) Long arm of chromosome 6   *(DNB 05,09)*
(b) Long arm of chromosome 3
(c) Short arm of chromosome 6
(d) Short arm of chromosome 3

33. HLA B27 is positive in: *(AIIMS Nov 2009)*
(a) Ankylosing spondylitis
(b) Rheumatoid arthritis
(c) SLE
(d) Behçet syndrome

34. Mixed lymphocyte culture is used to identify:
(a) MHC class I antigen   *(AIIMS Nov 2002)*
(b) MHC class II antigen
(c) B lymphocytes
(d) T helper cells

35. HLA typing is useful in: *(PGI June 2006)*
(a) Disputed paternity
(b) Thanatology
(c) Organ transplant
(d) Dactylography

36. True about MHC-class II: *(PGI June 2006)*
(a) Not involved in innate immunity
(b) Cytotoxic T-cell involved
(c) Present in nucleated cells
(d) Present in B-cells

37. MHC-II positive cells are all except: *(PGI Dec 2000)*
(a) B cells   (b) T cells
(c) Macrophages   (d) Platelets
(e) RBCs

38. True about MHC: *(PGI June 2003)*
(a) Transplantation reaction
(b) Autoimmune disease
(c) Immunosuppression
(d) Involved in T-cell function
(e) Situated at long arm of chromosome 6

39. Epitope binding floor of the MHC molecule conists of
(a) Alpha helices   *(Karnataka 2007)*
(b) Beta pleated structure
(c) Alpha and beta-1 chain
(d) Beta-2 microglobin

Most Recent Questions

39.1. MHC class I are present on all except
(a) Platelets   (b) All nucleated cells
(c) RBCs   (d) WBCs

39.2. HLA B27 is not seen in which of the following?
(a) Ankylosing spondylitis
(b) Reiter's syndrome
(c) Rheumatoid arthritis
(d) Psoriatic arthritis

39.3. The role played by Major Histocompatibility Complex 1 and 2: *(AIIMS May 2013)*
(a) Transduce the signal to T cells following antigen recognition
(b) Mediate immunogenic class switching
(c) Present antigens for recognition by T cell antigen receptors
(d) Enhance the secretion of cytokines

39.4. Antigen presented along with HLA class II stimulate
(a) CD8 cell
(b) CD4 cell
(c) CD2 cell
(d) CD19 cell

39.5. Major histocompatibility complex class I is seen on which of the following cell?
(a) Macrophages only
(b) All body cells
(c) B cell only
(d) All blood cells except erythrocytes

HYPERSENSITIVITY REACTIONS

40. What type of hypersensitivity reaction is seen in myasthenia gravis? *(AI 2012)*
(a) Type 1 hypersensitivity reaction
(b) Type 2 hypersensitivity reaction
(c) Type 3 hypersensitivity reaction
(d) Type 4 hypersensitivity reaction

Immunity

41. **Hemolytic disease of newborn is an example of:**
    (a) Type 3 hypersensitivity reaction   *(DPG 2011)*
    (b) Type 2 hypersensitivity reaction
    (c) Arthus reaction
    (d) Type 4 hypersensitivity reaction

42. **Raji cell assays are used to quantitate:**   *(DPG 2011)*
    (a) Complement levels
    (b) Immune complexes
    (c) T cells
    (d) Interferon levels

43. **Hypersensitivity pneumonitis is classically a/an:**
    (a) Allergic reaction   *(AI 2009)*
    (b) Type II hypersensitivity
    (c) Immune complex mediated hypersensitivity
    (d) Cell mediated hypersensitivity

44. **The immunoglobulin involved in type I hypersensitivity reaction is:**   *(AI 2007)*
    (a) IgE   (b) IgM
    (c) IgA   (d) IgG

45. **Arthus reaction is what type of hypersensitivity reaction:**   *(AI 2007), (UP'03)*
    (a) Localized immune complex
    (b) Ag-Ab reaction
    (c) Complement mediated
    (d) Ab mediated

46. **A 40 year old man has chronic cough with fever for several months. The chest radiograph reveals a diffuse reticulondular pattern. Microscopically on transbronchial biopsy there are focal areas of inflammation containing epitheloid cell granuloma, Langhans giant cells, and lymphocytes. These findings are typical for which of the following type of hypersensitivity immunologic responses:**
    (a) Type I   *(AIIMS May 2003)*
    (b) Type II
    (c) Type III
    (d) Type IV

47. **Ram Devi presented with generalized edema sweating and flushing tachycardia and fever after bee sting. This is:**   *(AIIMS Nov 2001)*
    (a) T cell mediated cytotoxicity
    (b) IgE mediated reaction
    (c) IgG mediated reaction
    (d) IgA mediated hypersensitivity reaction

48. **Example of Type IV Hypersensitivity is/are:**
    (a) Farmer's lung   *(PGI June 2006)*
    (b) Contact hypersensitivity
    (c) Immediate hypersensitivity
    (d) Myasthenia gravis

49. **Example of Type II Hypersensitivity is/are:**
    (a) Blood transfusion reaction   *(PGI June 2006)*
    (b) Arthus reaction
    (c) Hay Fever
    (d) Post-streptococcal glomerulonephritis

50. **Which of the following diseases is/are mediated through complement activation:**   *(PGI Dec 03)*
    (a) Atopic dermatitis
    (b) Graft versus Host disease
    (c) Photoallergy
    (d) Necrotizing vasculitis
    (e) Urticaria

51. **Which of following statements is not true about Mycobacterium tuberculosis infection?**   *(Delhi PG 2009 RP)*
    (a) M. tuberculosis leads to development of delayed hypersensitivity
    (b) Lymphocytes are the primary cells infected by M. tuberculosis
    (c) Positive tuberculin test signifies cell mediated hypersensitivity
    (d) Tuberculin test does not differentiate between infection and disease.

52. **A man after consuming sea food develops rashes. It is due to:**   *(Delhi PG-2008)*
    (a) IgE mediated response
    (b) Complement activation
    (c) Cell mediated response
    (d) None of the above

53. **Granuloma in Sarcoidosis is called**   *(Delhi PG-2004)*
    (a) Hard sore   (b) Soft sore
    (c) Hard tubercle   (d) Caseating granuloma

54. **Myasthenia gravis may be associated with**
    (a) Thymoma   *(Karnataka 2004)*
    (b) Systemic lupus erythematosus
    (c) Hyperthyroidism
    (d) All of the above

55. **Which of the following type of hypersensitivity reaction is found in blood transfusion reaction?**
    (a) Anaphylactic type   *(UP 2001)*
    (b) Cytotoxic type
    (c) Type III hypersensitivity
    (d) Cell mediated hypersensitivity

56. **Which of the following type of hypersensitivity reactions occurs in Farmer's lung**   *(UP 2008)*
    (a) Type I   (b) Type II
    (c) Type III   (d) Type IV

57. **Tuberculin test positivity indicates**   *(AP 2005)*
    (a) Good humoral immunity
    (b) Infection with mycobacterium
    (c) Good cell mediated immunity
    (d) None

Most Recent Questions

57.1. **Myasthenia gravis is most commonly associated with which of the following?**
    (a) Thymoma
    (b) Thymic carcinoma
    (c) Thymic hyperplasia
    (d) Lymphoma

57.2. Cell mediated immunity is:
(a) Type I (b) Type II
(c) Type III (d) Type IV

57.3. Antibody found in patients with myasthenia gravis is directed against
(a) Acetylcholine
(b) Acetylcholine receptors
(c) Acetylcholine vesicles in nerve terminal
(d) Actin-myosin complex of the muscle

TRANSPLANT REJECTION, GVHD

58. Hyperacute rejection is due to *(AIIMS Nov 2012)*
(a) Preformed antibodies
(b) Cytotoxic T-lymphocyte mediated injury
(c) Circulating macrophage mediated injury
(d) Endothelitis caused by donor antibodies

59. All are affected in Graft-Versus host reaction:
(a) Skin *(AIIMS May 2007)*
(b) GIT
(c) Liver
(d) Lung

60. Preformed antibodies cause: *(PGI June 2006)*
(a) Hyperacute rejection
(b) Acute rejection
(c) Chronic rejection
(d) Acute humoral rejection

61. True about graft versus host disease is: *(PGI Dec 2005)*
(a) Associated with solid organ transplantation
(b) Graft must contains immunocompetent T cell
(c) It is seen in immunosuppressed persons
(d) Also called as Runt disease in animals

62. Acute humoral renal transplant rejection is characterized by the following, except: *(Delhi PG 2009 RP)*
(a) Presence of anti-donor antibodies
(b) Interstitial and tubular mononuclear cell infiltrate
(c) Necrotizing vasculitis
(d) Acute cortical necrosis

63. Transfer of the graft of different species are called as
(a) Isograft *(UP 2002)*
(b) Allograft
(c) Homograft
(d) Xenograft

64. Acute graft versus host disease reaction occurs in all except *(UP 2007)*
(a) Liver (b) Adrenal
(c) Gut (d) Skin

Most Recent Questions

64.1. Preformed antibodies cause:
(a) Hyperacute rejection
(b) Acute rejection

(c) Chronic rejection
(d) Acute humoral rejection

64.2. Principal cause of death in renal transplant patient is
(a) Uraemia
(b) Malignancy
(c) Rejection
(d) Infection

AUTO IMMUNE AND IMMUNODEFICIENCY DISEASES

65. Autoimmunity in EBV infection is the result of
(a) Molecular mimicry *(AI 2012)*
(b) Polyclonal B cell activation
(c) Expressing sequestrated antigens
(d) Antigenic cross reactivity

66. A 14 yrs. old girl on exposure to cold has pallor of extremities followed by pain and cyanosis. In later ages of life she is prone to develop? *(AIIMS May 2011)*
(a) Systemic lupus eryhtematosis
(b) Scleroderma
(c) Rheumatoid arthritis
(d) Hisiocytosis

67. Which is not autoimmune disease? *(AI 2011)*
(a) Systemic Lupus Erythematosis
(b) Grave's Disease
(c) Myasthenia Gravis
(d) Sickle Cell Disease

68. Which among the following is seen in antiphospholipid antibody syndrome? *(AI 2011)*
(a) Beta 2 microglobulin antibody
(b) Anti nuclear antibody
(c) Anti centromere antibody
(d) Anti glycoprotein antibody

69. Necrotizing lymphadenitis is seen in *(AI 2011)*
(a) Kimura disease
(b) Kikuchi Fujimoto disease
(c) Hodgkin disease
(d) Castelman disease

70. Wire loop lesions are seen in: *(DPG 2011)*
(a) SLE
(b) Diabetic nephropathy
(c) Benign nephrosclerosis
(d) Wegener's granulomatosis

71. Tissue from rat used for detection of antinuclear antibodies? *(AIIMS Nov 2009)*
(a) Kidney (b) Brain
(c) Stomach (d) Liver

72. Which is not found in CNS in a case of AIDS?
(a) Perivascular giant cell *(AIIMS May 2009)*
(b) Vacuolization
(c) Inclusion bodies
(d) Microglial nodule

73. **A person present with recurrent swelling on face and lips due to emotional stress. Likely cause is:**
    (a) C1 esterase inhibitor deficiency   *(AIIMS May 2009)*
    (b) Allergy
    (c) Anaphylaxis
    (d) None of the above

74. **All of the following statements are true about Wiskott Aldrich syndrome except?**   *(AIIMS Nov 2008)*
    (a) It is an autosomal recessive disorder
    (b) There is failure of aggregation of platelets in response to agonists
    (c) Thrombocytopenia is seen
    (d) Patient presents with eczema

75. **Hematoxylin bodies seen in:**   *(AIIMS May 2008)*
    (a) SLE
    (b) PAN
    (c) Rheumatoid arthritis
    (d) Wegener's granulomatosis

76. **Wire loop lesions are often characteristic for the following class of lupus nephritis:**   *(AIIMS May 2004)*
    (a) Mesangial proliferative glomerulonephritis (WHO class II)
    (b) Focal proliferative glomerulonephritis (WHO class III)
    (c) Diffuse proliferative glomerulonephritis (WHO class IV)
    (d) Membranous glomerulonephritis (WHO class V)

77. **A renal biopsy from a 56 year old woman with progressive renal failure for the past 3 years shows glomerular and vascular deposition of pink amorphous material. It shows apple-green birefringence under polarized light after Congo red staining. These deposits are positive for lambda light chains. The person is most likely to suffer from:**
    (a) Rheumatoid arthritis   *(AIIMS May 2003)*
    (b) Tuberculosis
    (c) Systemic lupus erythematosus
    (d) Multiple myeloma

78. **A young lady presented with bilateral nodular lesions on shins. She was also found to have bi-lateral hilar lymphadenopathy on chest X-ray. Mantoux test reveals indurations of 5 mms. Skin biopsy would reveal:**
    (a) Non caseating Granuloma   *(AIIMS May 2002)*
    (b) Vasculitis
    (c) Caseating Granuloma
    (d) Malignant cells

79. **Anti ds-DNA antibodies are commonly seen in:**
    (a) SLE   *(PGI June 01)*
    (b) Scleroderma
    (c) PAN
    (d) Dermatomyositis
    (e) Rheumatoid arthritis

80. **Low complement levels seen in:**   *(PGI Dec 2006)*
    (a) PSGN
    (b) MPGN
    (c) Good pasture's syndrome
    (d) Wegner's granulomatosis
    (e) Infective endocarditis.

81. **Which is seen in Chediak-Higashi syndrome:**
    (a) Leucocytosis   *(PGI Dec 2001)*
    (b) Neutropenia
    (c) Defective microbial killing
    (d) Presence of large granules in neutrophil
    (e) Immunodeficiency

82. **Adenosine deaminase deficiency is seen in:**
    (a) Severe combined immunodeficiency.
    (b) Wiskott Aldrich Syndrome   *(PGI Dec 2003)*
    (c) Agammaglobulinemia as HIV

83. **True about alpha-1 antitrypsin deficiency, is/are:**
    (a) Autosomal dominant   *(PGI June 01)*
    (b) Pulmonary emphysema
    (c) Diastase resistant hepatic cells
    (d) Hepatic cells are orcein stain positive
    (e) Associated with berry aneurysm

84. **All are true regarding Hyper IgE syndrome exept:**   *(Delhi PG 2009)*
    (a) Inheritance is as a single locus autosomal dominant trait with variable expression
    (b) Coarse facial features
    (c) Recurrent staphylococcal abscesses involving skin, lungs
    (d) High serum IgE with low IgG, IgA and IgM

85. **All are true about Wiskott- Aldrich Syndrome except:**
    (a) Bloody diarrhea during infancy   *(Delhi PG 2009)*
    (b) Low IgM and elevated IgA and IgE
    (c) Large size platelets
    (d) Atopic dermatitis

86. **Diagnosis of X linked Agammaglobulinemia should be suspected if:**   *(Delhi PG 2009)*
    (a) Absent tonsils and no palpable lymph nodes on physical examination
    (b) Female sex
    (c) High isohemagglutinins titers
    (d) Low CD3

87. **Which of the following cell types is not a target for initiation and maintenance of HIV infection?**
    (a) CD4 T cell   *(Delhi PG 2009 RP)*
    (b) Macrophage
    (c) Dendritic cell
    (d) Neutrophil

88. **All of the following are found in SLE except:**
    (a) Oral ulcers   *(Delhi PG-2006)*
    (b) Psychosis
    (c) Discoid rash
    (d) Leucocytosis

89. Which of the following immunoglobulin is absent in Ataxia telangiectasia: *(Delhi PG-2005)*
    (a) IgG
    (b) IgM
    (c) IgA
    (d) IgD

90. Scl-70 antibody is characteristic of
    (a) Systemic lupus erythematosus *(Karnataka 2007)*
    (b) Scleroderma
    (c) Dermatomyositis
    (d) Sjogren's syndrome

91. LE cell phenomenon is seen in *(Karnataka 2005)*
    (a) Lymphocyte
    (b) Neutrophil
    (c) Monocyte
    (d) Eosinophil

92. Most sensitive test for screening of "Systemic Lupus Erythematosus" (SLE) is *(Karnataka 2005, RJ 2002)*
    (a) LE phenomenon
    (b) Rheumatoid factor
    (c) Anti nuclear factor (ANF)
    (d) Double stranded DNA test

93. According to WHO, the feature of class II lupus is
    (a) Transient proteinuria *(UP 2000)*
    (b) Massive proteinuria
    (c) Hematuria
    (d) RBC casts

94. ANCA antibody with peripheral rim distribution is indicative of *(UP 2000)*
    (a) Antihistone antibody
    (b) Anti smith antibody
    (c) Anti double stranded DNA antibody
    (d) Anti double stranded RNA antibody

95. Basic pathology in cystic fibrosis is *(UP 2001)*
    (a) Defect in the transport of chloride across epithelia
    (b) Defect in the transport of sodium across epithelia
    (c) Defect in the transport of potassium across epithelia
    (d) Defect in the transport of bicarbonate across epithelia

96. Besbuer Boeck Schaumann disease is also called as
    (a) Sarcoidosis *(UP 2003)*
    (b) Crohn's disease
    (c) Whipple's disease
    (d) Hodgkin's disease

97. Most common viral antigen used for diagnosis of HIV in blood before transfusion is *(UP 2005)*
    (a) p24   (b) p17
    (c) p7   (d) p14

98. Most common vascular tumor in AIDS patients is
    (a) Kaposi's sarcoma *(UP 2000) (UP 2007)*
    (b) Angiosarcoma
    (c) Lymphangioma
    (d) Lymphoma

99. Which in not an autoimmune disease *(RJ 2001)*
    (a) Syphilis
    (b) SLE
    (c) Systemic sclerosis
    (d) RA

100. Bilateral parotid gland enlargement is seen in all except. *(RJ 2001)*
    (a) Sarcoidosis
    (b) Sjogren's syndrome
    (c) SLE
    (d) Viral infections

101. Sarcoidosis does not involve *(RJ 2004)*
    (a) Brain
    (b) Heart
    (c) Lung
    (d) Kidney

102. Characteristic of SLE of kidney is *(RJ 2004, Jharkhand 05)*
    (a) Focal sclerosis
    (b) Focal necrosis
    (c) Wire loop lesions
    (d) Diffuse glomerulosclerosis

103. Libman-Sacks endocarditis is seen in *(AP 2001)*
    (a) Rheumatoid arthritis
    (b) SLE
    (c) Infective endocarditis
    (d) Nonbacterial thrombotic endocarditis

104. Chediak-Higashi syndrome is due to defect in:
    (a) Opsonisation *(Kolkata 2003)*
    (b) Chemotaxis
    (c) LAD
    (d) Extracellular microbicidal killing

105. Anti-double stranded DNA is highly specific for:
    (a) Systemic sclerosis *(Bihar 2004)*
    (b) SLE
    (c) Polymyositis
    (d) Rheumatic sclerosis

106. Anti-topoisomerase I is marker of: *(Bihar 2004)*
    (a) Systemic sclerosis
    (b) Classic polyarteritis nodosa
    (c) Nephrotic syndrome
    (d) Rheumatoid arthritis

107. An 8-year-old boy presents with sarcoidosis. Which of the following is correct? *(Bihar 2005)*
    (a) Hilar lymphadenopathy with perihilar calcification
    (b) Basal infiltrates
    (c) Rubbery lymph nodes
    (d) Egg-shell-calcification

108. Most common site for lymphoma in AIDS patients is
    (a) CNS *(Jharkhand 2004, 05)*
    (b) Spleen
    (c) Thymus
    (d) Abdomen

Immunity

109. All are true about histological features of Kaposi's sarcoma except: *(Jharkhand 2005)*
    (a) Microscopically lesion similar to granulation tissue
    (b) Dilated and irregular blood vessels with interspersed infiltrate of lymphocyte and plasma cells
    (c) Atypical blood vessels have solid spindle cell appearance
    (d) Nodule is the initial lesion of Kaposi's sarcoma

110. HIV affects which of the following most commonly?
    (a) Helper cells *(Jharkhand 2006)*
    (b) Suppressor cell
    (c) RBCs
    (d) Platelets

111. Which of the following lesions/conditions shows most specific anatomic changes in HIV infection?
    (a) Lymph nodes
    (b) Opportunistic infections
    (c) CNS lesions
    (d) Kaposi's sarcoma (blood vessels)

112. A 21-year-old female Pallavi Kumari comes to the physician because of migratory arthralgia and a skin rash that is exacerbated by sun exposure. Her urinalysis shows moderate proteinuria and red blood cell casts. Serum auto-antibodies with high specificity for this patient's condition react with
    (a) Mitochondrial extract
    (b) Fc portion of human IgG
    (c) Centromere
    (d) Double stranded DNA

113. A 50-year-old woman, Seeta presents with dry eyes, a dry mouth, and difficulty swallowing solid food. Physical examination finds enlargement of her parotid glands along with marked dryness of her buccal mucosa. Laboratory examination finds the presence of both SS-A and SS-B anti bodies. A biopsy of her lip is likely to show infiltration of minor salivary glands by what type of inflammatory cell?
    (a) Basophil
    (b) Eosinophil
    (c) Epithelioid cell
    (d) Lymphocyte
    (e) Neutrophil

114. A 16-year-old boy, Raju is being evaluated for failure to have a growth spurt and the recent development of signs of premature aging. Physical examination finds the boy to be short with thin skin and muscle autopsy. The skin of his face is wrinkled and his lips appear atrophic. In the last year, he also has developed bilateral cataracts and early signs of osteoporosis. None of these signs were present in his first decade of life. Which of the following is the most likely diagnosis?
    (a) DiGeorge's syndrome
    (b) Hutchinson-Gilford syndrome
    (c) Leukocyte adhesion deficiency
    (d) Werner syndrome

115. A 7-month-old baby boy Guddu is evaluated because of repeated episodes of pneumococcal pneumonia. Serum studies demonstrate very low levels of IgM, IgG, and IgA. This patient's condition is thought to be related to a deficiency of which of the following proteins?
    (a) Adenosine deaminase
    (b) Class III MHC gene
    (c) Gamma chain of the IL-2 receptor
    (d) Tyrosine kinase

116. A patient with systemic lupus erythematosus very much wants to become pregnant. What should her physician tell her regarding pregnancy in lupus patients?
    (a) There is no increased risk to the baby.
    (b) There may be an increase in cardiovascular malformations
    (c) There may be an increase in nervous system malformations.
    (d) There may be an increase in spontaneous abortions and prematurity

117. A woman Kamlesh with swelling of the oral mucosa and dry mouth is found to have intense destructive inflammation of the salivary glands and antibodies against the ribonucleoprotein La. Which of the following clinical findings would most likely be associated with this syndrome?
    (a) Conjunctivitis
    (b) Goiter
    (c) Hemolytic anemia
    (d) Proximal muscle weakness

118. A female being diagnosed with SLE has undergone a biopsy of 'butterfly rash'. Which is most likely to demonstrate which of the following?
    (a) Fibroblastic-like cells in a storiform pattern
    (b) Granular complement and IgG at the dermal-epidermal junction
    (c) Sawtooth dermal/epidermal junction
    (d) Pautrier microabscesses

119. A terminally ill HIV infected patient develops focal neurologic signs, dementia, and coma. Amoebic parasites are demonstrated in CSF. Which of the following organisms is most likely to be the causative agent?
    (a) Acanthamoeba sp.
    (b) Entamoeba histolytica
    (c) Giardia lamblia
    (d) Naegleria fowleri

120. A 21-year-old male Rohan presents with complaints of dull lower back pain and morning stiffness. There is tenderness over the costosternal junctions, spinous processes of the vertebrae, and the iliac crests. Which of the following tests be helpful in establishing a diagnosis of ankylosing spondylitis?
    (a) serum IgA
    (b) Erythrocyte sedimentation rate

(c) HLA typing

(d) Serum alkaline phosphatase

121. A 27-year-old man Alok Kumar with AIDS develops a reddish, slightly raised rash on his face, neck, and mouth, consistent in appearance with Kaposi's sarcoma. Microscopically, the proliferating cells in this malignancy most closely resemble which of the following?

(a) Angiosarcoma

(b) Carcinosarcoma

(c) Lymphoma

(d) Malignant fibrous histiocytoma

Most Recent Questions

121.1. Which of the following autoantibody is specific for SLE?

(a) ds DNA (b) Anti RO

(c) Anticentromere (d) Anti topoisomerase

121.2. Which of the following autoantibody isleast likely associated with SLE?

(a) Anti ds DNA

(b) Anti Sm

(c) Anti topoisomerase

(d) Anti histone

121.3. Most common CNS neoplasm in HIV patient is:

(a) Meduloblastoma

(b) Astrocytoma

(c) Primary CNS Iymphoma

(d) Ependymoma

121.4. Regarding severe combined immunodeficiency disease, which of the following statement is true?

(a) Adenosine deaminase deficiency

(b) Decreased circulating lymphocytes

(c) NADPH oxidase deficiency

(d) C1 esterase deficiency

121.5. Which of the following is a finding in lymphoid tissues in individuals with common variable hypogammaglobulinemia?

(a) Decreased B cell count

(b) Increased B cell count

(c) Normal B cell count

(d) Absent B cells

121.6. Thymic hypoplasia is seen in which of the following?

(a) Wiskott-Aldrich syndrome

(b) Digeorge syndrome

(c) IgA deficiency

(d) Agammaglobulinemia

121.7. Onion peel appearance of splenic capsule is seen in:

(a) SLE

(b) Scleroderma

(c) Rheumatoid arthritis

(d) Sjogren syndrome

121.8. Following is not a feature of AIDS related lymphadenopathy:

(a) Florid reactive hyperplasia

(b) Follicle lysis

(c) Haematoxylin bodies

(d) Collection of monocytoid B – Cells in sinuses

121.9. A false negative tuberculin reaction may be obtained in all of the following situations EXCEPT:

(a) Children previously tested with tuberculin test

(b) Post – measles test

(c) Corticosteroid therapy

(d) Miliary tuberculosis

121.10. Risk of HIV transmission is not seen with

(a) Whole blood

(b) Platelets

(c) Plasma derived Hepatitis B vaccine

(d) Leucocytes

121.11. All of the following methods are used for the diagnosis of HIV infection in a 2months old child, except

(a) DNA –PCR (b) Viral culture

(c) HIV ELISA (d) P 24 antigen assay

121.12. Mantoux test reading of less than 5 mm indicates:

(a) Tuberculous infections

(b) Disseminated TB

(c) Susceptibility to TB

(d) Immunity to TB

121.13. The poly-arthritic condition that is NOT common in males

(a) Gout

(b) Psoriatic arthritis

(c) Ankylosing spondylitis

(d) Systemic lupus erythematosus

121.14. Epitope spreading refers to

(a) A type of mechanism of spread of malignant tumors

(b) One type of mechanism of HIV dissemination

(c) A mechanism for the persistence and evolution of autoimmune disease

(d) One of the mechanisms of apoptosis

121.15. Heerfordt's syndrome consists of fever, parotid enlargement, facial palsy and

(a) Arthralgia

(b) Bilateral hilar adenopathy

(c) Erythema nodosum

(d) Anterior uveitis

121.16. HIV affects CD4 cells by which protein

(a) Gp 120 (b) Gp 41

(c) CCR5 (d) CXCR4

121.17. Treatment for Asymptomatic HIV is done when CD4 count is below

(a) 200 (b) 350

(c) 400 (d) 500

Immunity

121.18 Hodgkins lymphoma caused for by
- (a) EBV
- (b) CMV
- (c) HHV6
- (d) HHV8

AMYLOIDOSIS

122. Secondary amyloidosis is associated with   *(AI 2012)*
- (a) Aβ
- (b) AL
- (c) AA
- (d) APrP

123. A 60 year old female is suffering from renal failure and is on hemodialysis since last 8 years. She developed carpal tunnel syndrome. Which of the following finding will be associated?   *(AIIMS Nov 2011)*
- (a) AL
- (b) AA
- (c) ATTR
- (d) β_2 microglobulin

124. The best investigation for the diagnosis of amyloidosis is   *(AIIMS May 2010)*
- (a) Colonoscopy
- (b) Rectal biopsy
- (c) Upper GI endoscopy
- (d) CT scan

125. Which type of amyloidosis is caused by mutations in transthyretin gene?   *(DPG 2011, AI 2005)*
- (a) Familial Mediterranean fever
- (b) Familial amyloidosis polyneuropathy
- (c) Dialysis associated amyloidosis
- (d) Prion protein associated amyloidosis

126. In Hemodialysis associated amyloidosis, which of the following is seen: *(AI 2008)*
- (a) Transthyretin
- (b) β_2 Microglobulin
- (c) SAA
- (c) α_2 Microglobulin

127. Bone marrow in AL amyloidosis shows:
- (a) Bone marrow plasmacytosis   *(AI 2007)*
- (b) Granulomatous reaction
- (c) Fibrosis
- (d) Giant cell formation

128. A diabetic patient is undergoing dialysis. Aspiration done around the knee joint would show:
- (a) A beta 2 microglobulin   *(AI 2007)*
- (b) AA
- (c) AL
- (d) Lactoferin

129. What is the best method for confirming amyloidosis?
- (a) Colonoscopy   *(AI 2007)*
- (b) Sigmoidoscopy
- (c) Rectal biopsy
- (d) Tongue biopsy

130. Neointimal hyperplasia causes vascular graft failure as a result of hypertrophy of: *(AI 2006)*
- (a) Endothelial cells
- (b) Collagen fibers
- (c) Smooth muscle cells
- (d) Elastic fibers

131. Which one of the following stains is specific for Amyloid?   *(AI 2005)*
- (a) Periodic Acid Schiff (PAS)
- (b) Alizarin red
- (c) Congo red
- (d) Von-Kossa

132. In amyloidosis Beta pleated sheet will be seen in:
- (a) X-ray crystallography   *(AIIMS Nov 2006)*
- (b) Electron microscope
- (c) Spiral electron microscope
- (d) Congo red stain

133. A 50-year-old presented with signs and symptoms of restrictive heart disease. A right ventricular endo-myocardial biopsy revealed deposition of extracellular eosinophilic hyaline material. On transmission electron microscopy, this material is most likely to reveal the presence of: *(AIIMS May 2006)*
- (a) Non branching filaments of indefinite length
- (b) Cross banded fibers with 67 m periodicity
- (c) Weibel Palade bodies
- (d) Concentric whorls of lamellar structures

134. Amyloid deposits stain positively with all of the following EXCEPT: *(AIIMS May 2006)*
- (a) Congo-red
- (b) Crystal violet
- (c) Methanamine silver
- (d) Thioflavin T

135. On electron microscopy amyloid characteristically exhibits: *(AIIMS Nov 2005)*
- (a) Beta-pleated sheat
- (b) Hyaline globules
- (c) 7.5-10 nm fibrils
- (d) 20-25 nm fibrils

136. Familial amyloidotic polyneuropathy is due to amyloidosis of nerves caused by deposition of:
- (a) Amyloid associated protein   *(AIIMS Nov 2002)*
- (b) Mutant calcitonin
- (c) Mutant transthyretin
- (d) Normal transthyretin

137. Lardaceous spleen is due to deposition of amyloid in:
- (a) Sinusoids of red pulp   *(AIIMS Nov 2002)*
- (b) White pulp
- (c) Pencillary artery
- (d) Splenic trabeculae

138. What are the stains used for Amyloid?   *(PGI Dec 2007)*
- (a) Thioflavin
- (b) Congo red
- (c) Eosin
- (d) Auramine
- (e) Rhodamine

139. Gingival biopsy is useful in the diagnosis of:
- (a) Sarcoidosis   *(Delhi PG 2010)*
- (b) Amyloidosis
- (c) Histoplasmosis
- (d) Scurvy

140. Amyloid is   *(UP 2000)*
    (a) Mucopolysaccharide
    (b) Lipoprotein
    (c) Glycoprotein
    (d) Intermediate filament

141. Serum amyloid associated protein is found in
    (a) Alzheimer's disease   *(UP 2007)*
    (b) Chronic inflammatory states
    (c) Chronic renal failure
    (d) Malignant hypertension

142. Most common site of biopsy in amyloidosis *(RJ 2002)*
    (a) Liver
    (b) Spleen
    (c) Kidney
    (d) Lung

143. T-lymphocytes from a 6-year-old female Ramya with severe recurrent respiratory infections are found to lack the IL-12 receptor. Supplementation with which of the following substances would be most helpful in treating this patient's disease?
    (a) Immunoglobulins
    (b) Interferon-γ (IFN-γ)
    (c) Interleukin-2 (IL-2)
    (d) GM-CSF

144. A 43-year-old women Kanata Devi presents with a several year history of progressive abdominal colic and constipation. Colonic biopsy stained with Congo red reveals the acellular material exhibiting green birefringence. The birefringence is thought to be most closely related to which of the following protein properties?
    (a) Ability to bind to oxygen
    (b) Beta-pleated sheet tertiary structure
    (c) Electrophoretic mobility
    (d) Hydroxyproline content

145. Correctly matched pairs in amyloidosis are:
    (a) Multiple myeloma - light chain   *(PGI June 2006)*
    (b) Chronic inflammation - AA
    (c) Cardiac - ATTR
    (d) Neural – Beta-2 microglobulin

Most Recent Questions

145.1. Which of the following is the chemical nature of Hemodialysis associated with amyloid?
    (a) AA
    (b) AL
    (c) Beta – 2-microglobulin
    (d) ATTR

145.2. A diabetic patient is undergoing dialysis. Aspiration done around the knee joint would show:
    (a) A-β2 Microglobulin
    (b) AA
    (c) AL
    (d) Lactoferrin

145.3. Amyloidosis is most commonly seen in:
    (a) Maturity onset DM
    (b) Type 1 DM
    (c) Type 2 DM
    (d) Equally seen with all forms of DM

145.4. Which of the following is the most serious organ involvement in amyloidosis?
    (a) Cardiac tissue
    (b) Renal tissue
    (c) Splenic tissue
    (d) Hepatic tissue

145.5. Which type of Amyloidosis is caused by mutation of the transthyretin protein?
    (a) Familial Mediterranean fever
    (b) Familial amyloidotic polyneuropathy
    (c) Dialysis associated amyloidosis
    (d) Prion protein associated amyloidosis

145.6. Cause of death in amyloidosis involving kidney:
    (a) Cardiac failure
    (b) Renal failure
    (c) Sepsis
    (d) Liver failure

145.7. Secondary amyloidosis complicates which of the following:
    (a) Pneumonia
    (b) Chronic glomerulonephritis
    (c) Irritable bowel syndrome
    (d) Chronic osteomyelitis

145.8. On Congo- red staining, amyloid is seen as:
    (a) Dark brown color
    (b) Blue color
    (c) Brilliant pink color
    (d) Khaki color

145.9. Lardaceous spleen is due to deposition of amyloid in:
    (a) Sinusoids of red pulp
    (b) White pulp
    (c) Pencillary artery
    (d) Splenic trabeculae

EXPLANATIONS

1. **Ans. (c) Positive selection during development** *(Ref: Immunology by SK Gupta 1st/142-150, Robbins 8th/209)*
   This appeared to be a tough question but let us analyze all the options step wise.
   - Both B cells and T cells have antigen specific receptors. T cells have an antigen specific T cell receptor (TCR) composed of α and β polypeptide chains in 95% cases to bind with the antigen. B cells have a B cell receptor (BCR) having unique antigen specificity composed of IgM and IgD on their surface to bind with the antigen.
   - Since **MHC I** is expressed on **all the nucleated cells**, so, it is likely to be present on both 'B' as well as 'T' cells.

   As discussed in our accompanying DVD on Immunology, the T cells undergo both negative and positive selection. Both these are described below:

   - **Positive selection:** T cells in the *thymic cortex* are allowed to survive only if their T cell receptor has affinity for the MHC molecule. If the T cells do not have any affinity for the MHC molecule, they are programmed to die. This is important because only if this affinity is present, the T cells can interact with the antigen presenting cells. So, positive selection is required for **self MHC restriction**.
   - **Negative selection:** T cells come in the *thymic medulla* after being already positively selected in the thymic cortex. In the medulla, if a T cell has affinity for 'self antigens', they are eliminated. This is called as negative selection. It is therefore required for the **self tolerance**.
   - Similar to the negative selection of the T cells, the B cells may also recognize *'self antigens'* in the bone marrow. In this situation, the B cell undergoes antigen receptor gene rearrangement so as to express new antigen receptors. These new receptors are designed as to not recognize 'self antigens'. This process is described as '**receptor editing**'. If because of any reason receptor editing does not take place, the B cells undergo apoptosis. This is the **negative selection of B cells** in the **bone marrow**.

   Thus, it can be concluded that **both T and B cells undergo negative selection** but *only the T cells undergo positive selection*.

2. **Ans. (c) None** *(Ref: Robbins 8th/194-5, 9/e 198)*
   It is recommended to go through the chapter review for the best understanding of this question. However, I would try to summarize the important points as follows;
   Option 'a' and 'd'....CD4 is present on helper T cell and is required for antibody production because it is interacts with B cells for causing activation, conversion into plasma cells and antibody production. The antibody IgG is required for opsonisation (making the bacteria coated for preferential killing).
   Option 'b'....Helper T cell subtype 1 is responsible for the secretion of cytokines like IFN-γ and IL-2 which cause naïve T cells to get converted into cytotoxic T cells.
   Option 'c'....CD 4 is also important for the following:

• B cell mitogen[Q]
• Required for isotype switching[Q].
• Affinity maturation[Q]
• Presence of memory in immune cells[Q]

   So, the answer is none in this question.

3. **Ans. (b) Distal domain alfa 1 and 2** *(Ref: Robbins 8th/190-191, 9/e 195 see the adjoining diagram below)*
   The antigen binding cleft is made up α_1 and α_2 chains of **MHC I** molecule which is *structurally the distal domain of these chains*....Kuby immunology.

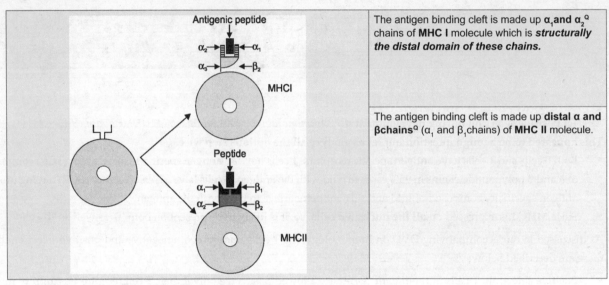

	The antigen binding cleft is made up α_1 and α_2[Q] chains of **MHC I** molecule which is *structurally the distal domain of these chains.*
	The antigen binding cleft is made up **distal α and βchains**[Q] (α_1 and β_1 chains) of **MHC II** molecule.

4. **Ans. (b) Immunoglobulin production** *(Ref: Robbins 8th/186-187, 9/e 190-191)*
   - On antigenic stimulation, the **naïve helper T cells** get differentiated into either **effector cells or memory cells**. The T helper cells can be of two types (either TH1 or TH2 cells).
   - The **TH1** cells can secrete cytokines like **IL-2 and IFN-γ** which cause **activation of macrophages** and cause **activation of CD8+T** cells **into cytotoxic** T cells.
   - The **TH2** cell can **secrete IL-4 and IL-5** which cause **B cell proliferation and differentiation** into plasma cells which **secrete antibodies** or immunoglobulins.
   - So, we need to understand that the *helper T cells is only helping in the production of immunoglobulins by plasma cells (they themselves don't produce antibodies).*

5. **Ans. (B) Binds to the beta chain of TCR and MHC class II molecules of APC stimulating T cell activation** *(Ref: Harrison 16th/1920)*

Concept of superantigen

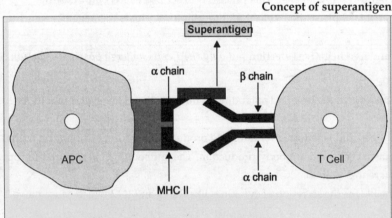

*A superantigen, such as **staphylococcal enterotoxin,** cross-links the variable domain of the **TCR beta chain to the MHC class II** molecule and specifically induces massive T cell activation. (**choice B**)
*The superantigen **does not** bind the B7 and CD28 co-stimulatory molecules (**choice A**). Instead, the costimulatory molecules bind to each other to stimulate the reaction between the antigen-presenting cell and T cell.
*The superantigen does not bind the CD 4 molecules (**choice C**) but instead binds on the other side of the TCR receptor complex.
*The term superantigen has nothing to do with the antigen being presented by macrophages to T cells (**choice D**).

6. **Ans. (d) CD 45 RO** *(Ref: Harrison 17th/2021)*
   CD 45 is called as Leukocyte common antigen (LCA)[Q]

Location of cell	Molecular marker
All leucocytes	CD45 and CD45RB
Medullary thymocytes (**'Naive' T- cells**)	CD45 RA and CD45RC
Cortical thymocytes (**Memory T-cells**)	CD45RO

7. **Ans. (c) They are MHC restricted cytotoxic cells** *(Ref: Harrison's 17th/2024-2028, 9/e 192)*
   NK cells are also called '**Large granular lymphocytes**' as they are *morphologically larger* than both T and B lymphocytes and **contain azurophillic granules** (which are absent in both T and B lymphocytes).

Immunity

They **constitute 5-10%** of peripheral blood lymphocytes. These cells express CD16 and CD 56:

•	CD16^Q: Surface receptors for **Fc portion of IgG**
•	CD56^Q: Surface receptors for NCAM – 1

*NK cells are unique** as they are capable of MHC – unrestricted^Q **direct cell lysis** which is not mediated by an immune response^Q

8. **Ans. (c) Effective against virus infected cells** *(Ref: Harrison 17th/2024 – 2028, 9/e 192)*
   • **NK cell** activity is **non-immune** (i.e. effector cells never having had previous contact with the target), **MHC– unrestricted, non-antibody mediated** killing of target cells usually malignant cells, transplanted foreign cells or virus-infected cells.
   • **Cytotoxic T-cell's** function is to produce antigen specific lysis of target cells (usually virus infected cells and cancer cells) by direct cell-to-cell contact.

   > **The common feature** to both **cytotoxic T-cells and NK cells** is **effectivity against virus-infected cells**.
   > **The difference** is however that **cytotoxic T-cell is MHC- I restricted while NK cell is MHC unrestricted**.

9. **Ans. (D) Graft rejection** *(Ref: Robbins 8th/226-230, 9/e 231-233)*
   • CD8+ cytotoxic T lymphocytes (CTLs) recognize cell-bound antigens only in association with class I MHC molecules, so, CD8+ T cells are said to be *class I MHC-restricted.*
   • CD4+ T cells can recognize antigens only in the context of self-class II MHC molecules; they are referred to as *class II MHC-restricted.*
   • So, killing of viruses by cytotoxic cells, killing of bacteria by helper cells and T cell activation in autoimmunity all require MHC molecules for their normal function.
   • Talking now about option 'D' i.e. graft rejection;
   Rejection is a complex process in which both cell-mediated immunity and circulating antibodies play a role. T cell-mediated graft rejection is called *cellular rejection,* and it is induced by two mechanisms: destruction of graft cells by CD8+ CTLs and delayed hypersensitivity reactions triggered by activated CD4+ helper cells. Both these as discussed above would require MHC molecules.
   Antibodies evoked against alloantigens in the graft can also mediate rejection. This process is called *humoral rejection.* It can be of two types
   1. Hyperacute rejection occurs when preformed antidonor antibodies are present in the circulation of the recipient
   2. In recipients not previously sensitized to transplantation antigens, exposure to the class I and class II HLA antigens of the donor may evoke antibodies which are usually formed against graft vasculature. So, in this type of graft rejection, T cells are not required and so, it becomes the answer here.

10. **Ans. (a) Mature Dendritic Cell** *(Ref: Robbins 7th/199, 8th/187, 9/e 191)*

11. **Ans. (b) Cells which are not able to express MHC I** *(Ref: Robbins 7th/201, 8th/188, 9/e 192)*
   • The **NK cells express activating and inhibitory receptors**. The functional activity of the NK cells is regulated by a balance between signals from these receptors. Normal cells are not killed because inhibitory signals from normal MHC class I molecules override activating signals. **The ability of NK cells to kill target cells is inversely related to target cell expression of MHC class I molecules^Q.** If virus infection or neoplastic transformation disturbs or reduces the expression of class I MHC molecules, inhibitory signals delivered to NK cells are interrupted and lysis occurs.

12. **Ans. (c) Transcription of nuclear factor mediated by NF-κβ which recruits cytokines** *(Ref: Robbins 7th/195, 9/e 187)*
   The Toll-like receptors are **membrane proteins** that recognize a variety of *microbe-derived molecules* and stimulate innate immune responses against the microbes. These derive there name due to homology to a *Drosophila* protein called 'Toll'. The Toll-like receptors are expressed on many immune cells of the body. *Signaling by Toll-like receptors results in the activation of transcription factors, notably NF-κB and AP-1.*

13. **Ans. (a) IL-2** *(Ref: Robbins 7th/198, 8th/195, 9/e 198)*
   T-helper cells can be divided in three distinct types on the basis of **different cytokines they produce.**
   • **T-helper – 1 (T$_H$1) secretes:** *IL-2 and interferon γ, these cells are important for type IV hypersensitivity*
   • **T-helper– 2 (T$_H$2) secretes:** *IL-4, IL-5, these cells are* important for type I hypersensitivity reaction.
   • **TH 17 Cells:** Secrete IL-17, IL-22, these cells provide defense against extracellular bacteria and fungi.

14. **Ans. (a) Apoptosis** *(Ref: Robbins 8th/29, 7th/29, 9/e 56)*

15. **Ans. (b) Interleukin IL – 8** *(Ref: Robbins 8th/62, 7th/71-72, 9/e 87)*

16. **Ans. (b) IgM** *(Ref: Harrison, 17th/2036)*

17. **Ans. (b) endothelial cells (c) epithelial cells and (d) Langerhans cells** *(Ref: Robbins Illustrated 7th/204, 9/e 195)*
As already discussed in the text also, the antigen presenting cells include macrophages, Dendritic Cells (found in lymphoid organs) and Langerhans' cells (found in epidermis). The question ideally should have been ...with 'all except'

18. **Ans. (a) Langerhan's cell; (b) Macrophages; (e) B-lymphocyte** *(Ref: Robbins 7th/197, 9/e 195)*
Antigen presenting cells are:
- B-cell
- Langerhan's cell in skin
- Macrophages

19. **Ans. (a) Cytotoxic T cells:** *(Ref: Robbins 7th-218, 8th/208, 9/e p210)*
- Perforins are hole forming proteins synthesized by cytotoxic T-cells. They can perforate the plasma membrane of the target cells that are under attack by CD8+ lymphocytes. Granzymes are delivered into the target cells through these holes formed by perforins. In addition the perforin pores allow water to enter the cells, thus causing osmotic lysis.

20. **Ans. (a) B7 and CD28;** *(Ref: Robbins 7th/225, Harrison 16th/1907, 9/e p213)*
Immunological tolerance is a state in which the individual is incapable of developing an immune response to a specific antigen. It is of two types:
- **Central:** deletion or negative selection of self reactive cell clones during their maturation in bone marrow and thymus.
- **Peripheral:** In peripheral lymphoid organs.
CD28 molecules (co-stimulatory molecule) are constitutively expressed on certain T-cells. These co-stimulatory molecules bind to their ligands-CD80 (B7-l) and/or CD86 (B7-2) and get activated and deliver upregulating function of T-cell thereby preventing tolerance and enhancing CD40$_L$ expression. If the antigen presented by cell do not bear CD28 ligand, a negative signal is delivered and cell become tolerant and anergic.
Thus the balance of co-stimulatory signal affects immune homeostasis and self-tolerance
Other mechanism of peripheral tolerance:
- **Clonal deletion** by activation induced cell death (via Fas and Fas L)
- **Peripheral suppression by regulatory T-cells.**

21. **Ans. (c) CD19; (d) CD20; (e) CD22** *(Ref: Immunology by Roitt, 6th/29, 30, 19 9/e p191)*

CD19, 20 and 22 are main markers of human B cells. Other B cell markers are CD72 to CD78.
CD33: present in monocyte.
CD34: marker of hematopoetic stem cell

22. **Ans. (d) All of the above** *(Ref: Robbins 7th/71, 9/e p87)*

23. **Ans. (a) Langerhan's cells** *(Ref: Robbins 7th/1228, 9/e p192)*

24. **Ans. (b) Helps in the formation of antibody** *(Ref: Robbins 8th/183-184; 7th/82 , 9/e p191)*

25. **Ans. (b) 2: 1** *(Ref: Robbins 8th/186; 7th/197, 9/e p190-191)*

26. **Ans. (c) T cells** *(Ref: Robbins 8th/192, 7th/204, 9/e p191)*

27. **Ans. (b) T cell** *(Ref: Robbins 7th/670 , 9/e p191)*

28. **Ans (c) Memory is seen** *(Ref: Robbins 8th/184, 9/e p186-188)*

Innate immunity	Adaptive/Acquired immunity
Present **from birth**[Q]	**Acquired**[Q] in nature
First line of defense[Q]	**Second line**[Q] of defense
No prior exposure to antigen[Q]	**Prior exposure** to antigen is **present**[Q]
Non-specific[Q]	**Specific**[Q]
No memory[Q] is seen	**Memory**[Q] is seen

29. **Ans. (d) Toll like receptor** *(Ref: Robbins 7th/, 57- 60, 194-196, 9/e p187-188)*

Toll-like receptors (TLRs), stimulate one of the immune responses directed against microbes,
TLRs bind to pathogen-associated molecular patterns (PAMPs), which are small molecular sequences found commonly on pathogens.
Examples of PAMPs include *bacterial lipopolysaccharide (LPS), lipoteichoic acid, and peptidoglycan.*
LPS is probably the prototypical PAMP[Q].
TLRs, in conjunction with CD14, bind to LPS (endotoxin), and activate leukocytes to produce cytokines and reactive leukocytes to produce cytokines and reactive oxygen intermediates (ROIs).

29.1. Ans. (a)16 *(Ref: Robbins 8/e p188, 9/e p192)*
- **Natural Killer cell** is identified with the molecules as **CD16 and CD56**[Q].
- **CD16** is an Fc receptor for IgG, and it confers on NK cells the ability to lyse IgG-coated target cells. This phenomenon is known as *antibody-dependent cell-mediated cytotoxicity (ADCC)*[Q].

29.2. Ans. (c) NK cells *(Ref: Robbins 8/e p188, 9/e p192)*
- The NK cells are also known as *large granular lymphocytes* as they have a larger size and contain abundant azurophilic granules.
- NK cells are endowed with the ability to kill a variety of **infected** and **tumor cells, without prior exposure** to or activation by these microbes or tumors.

29.3. Ans. (b) CD 16, CD 56...explained earlier *(Ref: Robbins 9/e p192)*

29.4. Ans. (a) T-cells *(Ref: Robbins 8/e p186, 9/e p191)*
- The CD molecules present on **T cells** are CD1, CD2, **CD3, CD4,** CD5, CD7, **CD8** and CD28. The T cell having CD4 molecule is called **CD4+ T cell or the Helper T cell**[Q] and that having CD8 molecule is called as **CD8+ T cell or Cytotoxic/ Killer T cell**[Q].
- **B cell** associated markers are **CD10 (CALLA), CD19 (*pan B cell marker*[Q]),** CD20, **CD21 (*EBV receptor*[Q]),** CD22, CD23.

29.5. Ans. (a) IL-2 *(Ref: Robbins 8/e p195, 9/e p198)*

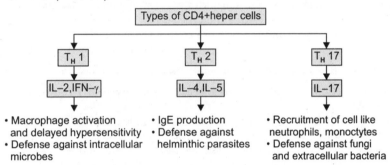

After coming in contact with antigen presenting cells, CD4+ helper T cells secrete IL-2 and expresses high-affinity receptors for IL-2. **IL-2** is a growth factor that acts on these T lymphocytes and stimulates their proliferation, leading to an **increase in the number of antigen-specific lymphocytes.**

29.6. Ans. (a) Mature dentritic cells *(Ref: Robbins 8/e p187, 9/e p191)*
Direct quote.. *"interdigitating dendritic cells,* or just *dendritic cells* are the most important *antigen-presenting cells (APCs) for initiating primary T-cell responses against protein antigens'*

29.7. Ans. (a) B cells *(Ref: Robbins 8/e p187, 7/e p198-199, 9/e p191)*
Macroglobulin is the other name for antibodies. So, the answer becomes obvious. i.e. B cells. The activated B cells are called as plasma cells and are responsible for secretion of antibodies.

29.8. Ans. (c) Liver...refer to text for details *(Ref: Robbins 8/e p834, 7/e p79, 9/e p102)*

29.9. Ans. (b) Langerhans cell *(Ref: Robbins 9/e p622)*

29.10. Ans. (d) IgE... see text table for details

30. Ans. (b) Tumor necrosis factor *(Ref: Ananthanarayan 6th/121, Harrison 17th/2047, 9/e p194-195)*
*HLA class III contains genes for

- **Complement components C_2 and C_4**[Q] of classical pathway **(Not C_3[Q])**
- **Properdin factor B**[Q] of alternate pathway
- **Tumor necrosis factor**[Q]: Alpha and Beta
- Heat shock protein 70[Q]
- Enzyme **tyrosine hydroxylase**[Q]
- Genes for **MHC** (also known as HLA) are located on **short arm of chromosome 6**[Q].

31. Ans. (b) Governing susceptibility to autoimmune disease *(Ref: Ananthanarayan 6th/108, Roilt's Essential Immunology – 262, Robbins 9/e p215)*
*HLA class III** region contains genes for **early complement components C_2 and C_4** of classical pathway.
*Deficiency** of these early components of the classical pathway viz C_1, C_2 and C_4 is associated with **autoimmune diseases** like SLE and other collagen vascular diseases.

- These genes are thus, important in regulating susceptibility to autoimmune disease
- **Class III genes do not participate in MHC restriction or graft rejection components.**

32. **Ans. (c) Short arm of chromosome 6** *(Ref: Robbins 8th/190, 7th/203, 9/e p194)*

33. **Ans. (a) Ankylosing spondylitis** *(Ref: Robbins 8th/193, Harrison 17th/2051, 9/e p215)*

34. **Ans. (b) MHC class II antigen** *(Ref: Harrison 16th/1933, 17th/2047, 9/e p194)*
    - The MHC **class II region** was originally termed the *D-region*. The allelic gene products were first detected by their ability to stimulate lymphocyte proliferation by *mixed lymphocyte reaction.* So, mixed lymphocyte culture is used to identify HLA II. It is present on all antigen presenting cells (B cells, dendritic cells and macrophages) and can be induced on endothelial cells and fibroblasts.

35. **Ans. (a) Disputed paternity, (c) Organ transplantation** *(Ref: Robbins, 9/e p195, 215)*
    Uses of MHC/HLA typing

Anthropology	Transfusion
Paternity Testing	Forensic science
Transplantation	Disease Correlation

36. **Ans. (a) Not involved in innate immunity; (c) Present in nucleated cells; (d) Present in B-cells** *(Ref: Robbins 7th/203, 9/eP194-195)*
    - Class II MHC Proteins are glycoprotein present on the surface of certain cells including **macrophages, B-lymphocytes, dendritic cells of the spleen and Langerhan's cells of the skin.**
    - Endothelial cells and fibroblasts can be induced to express Class II MHC by IFN-γ.

37. **Ans. (b) T cells, (d) Platelets; (e) RBCs** *(Ref: Ananthanarayan' 7th/130, Robbins 7th/203, 9/e p194)*

38. **Ans. (a) Transplantation reaction; (b) Autoimmune disease; (d) Involved in T-cell function** *(Ref: Harrison 16th-1930, 1934; Robbins 7th-204-205)*
    The principal physiologic function of Major histocompatibility complex (MHC) is to bind peptide fragments of foreign proteins for presentation to appropriate *antigen specific T-cells.* Thus MHC is involved in *transplantation reaction, disease susceptibility (i.e. autoimmune disease, inflammatory disease, infections, etc.), immune response* and *tolerance.*

39. **Ans. (a) Alpha helices and (c) Alpha and beta1 chain** *(Ref: Robbins 7th/203-204, 9/e p195)*
    Friends, the examiner should have specified the type of MHC molecule so that question becomes clear.

    α_1 and α_2 domains form a cleft/groove where the peptides bind to MHC I molecule.
    The antigen binding cleft in MHC II is formed by an interaction of α_1 and β_1 domains of both chains.

39.1. **Ans. (c) RBCs** *(Ref: Robbins 8/e p190, 9/e p194)*
    - *Class I MHC molecules* are expressed on **all nucleated cells**[Q] and **platelets**[Q]

39.2. **Ans. (c) Rheumatoid arthritis** *(Ref: Robbins 8/e p193, 9/e p215)*
    HLA B27 is associated with **Seronegative spondyloarthropathies.** Please revise the following important features about these.

Seronegative spondyloarthropathies (Mnemonic: PAIR)	Salient features of these diseases
P: Psoriatic arthritis **A: A**nkylosing spondylitis (AS) **I: I**nflammatory bowel disease arthritis **R: R**eactive arthritis (**R**eiter syndrome)	* **Absence of serum auto-antibodies** * Associated with **HLA B27** (MC **AS**) * **Onset before** the age of **40 years** * Presence of **uveitis, spine/large peripheral joint arthritis**

39.3. **Ans. (c) Present antigens for recognition by T cell antigen receptors** *(Ref: Robbin 8/e p191)*
    The physiologic function of MHC molecules is to display peptide fragments of proteins for recognition by antigen-specific T cells.... *(Ref: Robbin 8/e p190)*
    Also now that:
    - **Class I MHC** molecules are required to display antigens to **CD8 T cells**
    - **Class II MHC** molecules are required to display antigens to **CD4 T cells.**

39.4. **Ans. (b) CD4 cell** *(Ref: Robbins 9/e p195)*

39.5. **Ans. (d) All blood cells except erythrocytes** *(Ref: Robbins 9/e p194)*

40. **Ans. (b) Type 2 hypersensitivity reaction** *(Ref: Robbins 8th/203, 9/e p206)*
    Myasthenia gravis is a type 2 hypersensitivity reaction. Other important examples can be remembered from the mnemonic *"My blood group is R h positive".* For details see text.

Immunity

41. Ans. (b) Type 2 hypersensitivity reaction *(Ref: Robbins 7th/211, 9/e p206)*

42. Ans. (b) Immune complexes *(Ref: Internet, 9/e p207)*
A Raji cell assay identifies the presence of circulating immune complexes. A positive result suggests the presence of antigen-nonspecific immune complexes in the circulation. The raji cell assay may be helpful in differentiating diseases. Additionally, raji cell tests may assist with the assessment of disease activity. A positive raji cell assay that turns negative may suggest that the disease activity has improved.

43. Ans. (c) Immune complex mediated hypersensitivity *(Ref: Robbins 8th/703, 9/e p207)*
Hypersensitivity pneumonitis (*allergic alveolitis*) is ideally an example of **type III and type IV** hypersensitivity. Complement and immunoglobulins demonstrated within vessel walls by immunofluorescence as well as presence of specific antibodies in the serum of affected patients indicate type III (immune complex) hypersensitivity. The presence of non-caseating granulomas in 2/3rd patients suggest the development of a T cell-mediated (type IV) delayed-type hypersensitivity against the implicated antigen(s).
However, the single best answer to be marked would be type III hypersensitivity reaction because immune complex formation plays a relatively more important role in hypersensitivity pneumonitis.

44. Ans. (a) IgE *(Ref: Robbins 8th/198, 7th/207-208, 9/e p202)*

45. Ans. (a) Localized immune complex *(Ref: Robbins 8th/205, 7th/215, 9/e p207)*
The Arthus reaction is a localized area of tissue necrosis resulting from acute immune complex vasculitis, usually elicited in the skin. Revise the mnemonics "SHARP" from the text.

46. Ans. (d) Type IV *(Ref: Robbins 8th/207, 7th/216-217, 9/e p210)*
- Presence of epitheloid cell granuloma, langhans giant cells and lymphocytes is characteristic of chronic granulomatous inflammation, which is associated with type IV hypersensitivity action.

47. Ans. (b) IgE mediated reaction *(Ref: Robbins 7th/210, 8th/197, 9/e p202)*
- The symptoms of the patient are due to hypersensitivity type I reaction Type I is mediated by IgE and it flairs up within minutes.
- The symptoms range form rashes to anaphylactic shock with vasodilation hypotension and bronchiolar spasm.

Type I	Type II
• The symptoms range form rashes to anaphylactic shock with vasodilation hypotension and bronchiolar spasm • Mediated by IgE **Examples of Type I** • Eczema* • Hay Fever* • Asthma* • Anaphylactic shock* • Urticaria* • Acute dermatitis* • Theobald Smith Reaction*	• Is characterized by an antigen antibody reaction on the surface of a host cell* • Mediated by IgG or IgM **Examples of Type II** • Blood transfusion reactions* • Transplant rejection* • Autoimmune hemolytic anemia* • Good Pasture's syndrome* • Graves disease* • Myasthenia gravis* • Pemphigus vulgaris • Pernicious anemia* • Rheumatic fever*

Type III	Type IV
• Mediated by antigen/antibody complex* **Examples of type III** • **S**: **S**erum sickness, Post - streptococcal glomerulonephritis, **SLE**, **S**chick test • **H**: **H**ypersensitivity pneumonitis • **A**: **A**rthus reaction, **A**cute viral hepatitis • **R**: **R**eactive arthritis, **R**heumatoid arthritis • **P**: **P**enicillamine toxicity, • **P**olyarteritis nodosa (PAN)	• Cell mediated reaction (delayed hypersensitivity)* **Examples of type IV** • Tuberculosis • Sarcoidosis* • Temporal arteritis • Contact dermatitis* • Lepromin test and PPD (Mantoux test)* • Patch test* • Type I DM

48. Ans. (b) Contact hypersensitivity *(Ref: Robbins 7th/215, 8th/197, 9/e p209)*

49. Ans. (a) Blood transfusion reaction *(Ref: Robbins 6th/212, 8th/197, 9/e p206)*

50. **Ans. (d) Necrotizing vasculitis** *(Ref: Harrison's 16th/327, 328, Robbins 7th/212, 213, 1253, 9/e p207)*
    - Acute necrotizing vasculitis is the dominant morphological consequences of immune complex injury *[Type-III hypersensitivity reaction]*. The immune complexes incite an activation of complement and produce inflammatory reaction and necrosis.

• Atopic dermatitis and urticaria –Type I.
• Photoallergy- type IV hypersensitivity or delayed hypersensitivity
• Graft versus host disease is mediated by T-cells.

51. **Ans. (B) Lymphocytes are the primary cells affected by *M. tuberculosis*** *(Ref: Robbins 8th/368, 9/e p371)*
    - *Macrophages* are the primary cells infected by *M. tuberculosis*.

52. **Ans. (a) IgE mediated response** *(Ref: Robbins 7th/199-200, 8th/198-200, 9/e p202)*

53. **Ans. (a) Hard sore** *(Ref: Robbins 7th/738, 9/e p693)*
    - Granulomas found in sarcoidosis are non-caseating and so, refered to as *"Hard sore."* They contain.
        - **Asteroid Bodies**
        - **Schaumann bodies and**
        - **Birefringent crystals**

54. **Ans. (d) All of the above** *(Ref: Robbins 7th/1344, 9/e p1235-1236; Harrison's 16th/2521 table 366-3)*
    Myasthenia gravis: revision of key points

Autoimmune mediated neuromuscular disease example of **type II hypersensitivity reaction**
Distinct finding: ↓ ACh receptors (in muscles) and **circulating antibodies to ACh receptors**
Associations 1. Hyperthyroidism 2. Thymic hyperplasia – 65% 3. Thymoma – 15% 4. Autoimmune disorders (Hashimoto's thyroiditis, Graves' disease, RA/SLE, positive family history of autoimmune diseases)
In severe cases **muscle biopsy shows type 2 fiber atrophy**[Q]
Most sensitive test: **Single fiber electromyography**[Q]
Most specific test: antibodies to ACh receptors[Q]
Electrophysiological studies: ↓ in motor response[Q] **on repeated stimulation**
Nerve conduction studies: Normal[Q]
Treatment is done with drugs **(neostigmine with atropine**[Q]**) and thymectomy**[Q]

55. **Ans. (b) Cytotoxic type** *(Ref: Robbins 8th/198-202; 7th/206, 9/e 205)*

56. **Ans. (d) Type III** *(Ref: Robbins 8th/703, 7th/739, 9/e 207)*

57. **Ans. (c) Good cell mediated immunity** *(Ref: Robbins 8th/207, 7 th/381, 9/e 210)*

57.1. **Ans. (c) Thymic hyperplasia** *(Ref: Robbins 8/e p635, 9/e 1235-1236)*
    Direct quote... **"Thymic hyperplasia** is found in **65%** and *thymoma in 15%* of affected patients".

    Myasthenia gravis: revision of key points for NEET/AIIMS!

• Autoimmune mediated neuromuscular disease example of **type II hypersensitivity reaction** • When arising *before age 40 years* it is most commonly seen in *women*, but it occurs **equally in both sexes in older patients**. • Distinct finding: ↓ ACh receptors (in muscles) and **circulating antibodies to ACh receptors** • **Most specific test: antibodies to ACh receptors**[Q] • **Electrophysiological studies: ↓ in motor response**[Q] **on repeated stimulation** • **Nerve conduction studies: Normal**[Q] • **Treatment** is done with drugs **(neostigmine with atropine**[Q]**) and thymectomy**[Q]

    Frequently observed associations asked in exams (PGI)!
    - Hyperthyroidism
    - Thymic hyperplasia – 65%
    - Thymoma – 15%
    - Autoimmune disorders (Hashimoto's thyroiditis, Graves' disease, RA/SLE, positive family history of autoimmune diseases).

Immunity

57.2. Ans. (d) Type IV *(Ref: Robbins 8/e p197, 9/e 24)*

The hypersensitivity reactions have been given the following names:

- **Immediate** or **(type I) hypersensitivity**
- **Antibody-mediated** or **(type II) hypersensitivity**
- **Immune complex–mediated** or **(type III) hypersensitivity**
- **Cell-mediated** or **(type IV) hypersensitivity**

57.3. Ans. (b) Acetylcholine receptors *(Ref: Robbins 9/e 195)*

58. Ans. (a) Preformed antibodies *(Ref: Robbins 8th/228, 9/e 233-234)*

*Direct quote from Robbins. '**Hyperacute rejection** occurs when **preformed antidonor antibodies** are present in the circulation of the recipient'.* Such antibodies may be present:

- In a recipient who has previously rejected a kidney transplant
- Multiparous women who develop anti-HLA antibodies against paternal antigens shed from the fetus may have preformed antibodies to grafts taken from their husbands or children
- Prior blood transfusions
- In recipients not previously sensitized to transplantation antigens, exposure to the class I and class II HLA antigens of the donor graft may evoke antibodies. *The initial target of these antibodies in rejection seems to be the graft vasculature.* Thus, antibody-dependent *acute humoral rejection* is usually manifested by a vasculitis, sometimes referred to as *rejection vasculitis*

Also know that endothelitis is caused by injury to the vascular endothelial cells *mediated by CD8+ T cells*. **This is a component of acute cellular rejection.**

59. Ans. (d) Lung *(Ref: Robbin 7th/222-3, 9/e 236, Harrison's 17th/717)*

- *GVHD affects skin (earliest organ), intestine and liver*
- Lungs are **not** affected in GVHD. For details see text.

60. Ans. (a) Hyperacute rejection. *(Ref: Robbins 7th/219, 220, 8th/197, 9/e 233-234)*

Hyperacute rejection takes place when there are preformed antibodies in the circulation of the recipient. It can be due to:

Patient who has already rejected a transplant
Multiparous females
Prior blood transfusions

61. Ans. (a) Associated with solid organ transplantation; (b) Graft must contains immunocompetent T cell (c) It is seen in immunosuppressed persons; (d) Also called as Runt disease in animals *(Ref: Robbins 7th/222, 9/e 232-233; Harrison 16th/670; Ananthanarayan 7th/180)*

Graft versus host reaction (GVH) occurs in any situation in **which immunologically competent cells** or there precursors are transplanted into **immunologically crippled recipient** cells and the transferred cells recognize alloantigens in the host. GVHD occurs **most commonly in allogenic bone marrow transplantation**[Q] but may also follow transplantation of **solid organs** rich in lymphoid cells.

62. Ans. (b) Interstitial and tubular mononuclear cell infiltrate *(Ref: Robbins 8th/228-229 , 9/e 232-233)*

63. Ans. (d) Xenograft *(Ref: Harsh Mohan 6th/65)*

- **Isograft:** Is a graft from a different individual genetically identical with recipient e.g. identical twin
- **Autograft:** Is to self
- **Allograft:** Graft from same species but different genotype (from one human to another human)
- **Xenograft:** Graft from different species (from animal to human)

64. Ans. (b) Adrenal *(Ref: Robbins 9/e 236, 8th/230; 7th/125)*

64.1. Ans. (a) Hyperacute rejection *(Ref: Robbins 8/e p201-2, 9/e 233-234)*

Hyperacute rejection	Acute rejection	Chronic rejection
*Takes place in individuals with **preformed antibodies**[Q] usually **within minutes to hours** of transplantation	*Seen **days to months** after transplantation. It can be acute humoral rejection or acute cellular rejection	*Occurs **months to years** after transplantation

64.2. Ans. (d) Infection *(Ref Cambell's Urology, 8/e p346,349)*

Principal causes of death in renal transplant patients (in decreasing order)
- Heart disease
- **Infection**
- Stroke

65. **Ans. (b) Polyclonal B cell activation** *(Ref: Robbins 8th 212, 9/e 216)*
   Role of infections in autoimmunity is exemplified by the following:
   1. Antigenic cross reactivity: this is due to similarity is the microbial antigenic structure and the self antigens. This is also known as 'molecular mimicry'. The classical example is rheumatic heart disease[Q] in which streptococcal proteins cross react with myocardial proteins causing myocarditis.
   2. Upregulation of co-stimulatory molecules by infectious organisms.
   3. Polyclonal B cell activation: caused by EBV[Q] and HIV[Q] resulting in production of autoantibodies
   4. Alteration of tissue antigens: infections may alter tissue self antigens so that they activate T cells and loose the property of self tolerance

   - Even **HIV** can cause autoimmune diseases by polyclonal B cell activation
   - **Robbins** *page 212* also mentions the *paradoxical protective effect of infections against some autoimmune diseases* because infections promote *low level IL-2 production* and this is essential for maintaining regulatory T cells.

66. **Ans. (b) Scleroderma** *(Ref: Robbins 8th/225, 518, Harrison 18th/2096, 9/e 228-229)*
   The symptoms present in this girl are suggestive of Raynaud's phenomenon (pallor and cyanosis of the digits of hands and feet due to exaggerated vasoconstriction of digital arteries and arterioles). It can either be:
   - Primary Raynaud's phenomenon or
   - Secondary Raynaud's phenomenon (due to SLE, scleroderma, Buerger's disease, atherosclerosis). Since, Raynaud's phenomenon may the first manifestation of these diseases, the patient with new symptoms need to be evaluated.
   Direct quote Robbins 8th/225.... 'though systemic sclerosis shares many features with SLE, rheumatoid arthritis and polymyositis, *its distinctive features are the striking cutaneous changes*, notably skin thickening. *Raynaud phenomenon,* manifested as episodic vasoconstriction of the arteries and arterioles of the extremities, is *seen in virtually all patients* and **precedes other symptoms in 70% of cases.' Dysphagia** is seen in **50%** patients.
   Ruling out SLE, the presentation in SLE is....'*Typically, the patient is a young woman with some of the following features: a butterfly rash over the face, fever, pain but no deformity in one or more peripheral joints (feet, ankles, knees, hips, fingers, wrists, elbows, shoulders), pleuritic chest pain, and photosensitivity.*'

67. **Ans. (d) Sickle Cell Disease** *(Ref: Harrison 17th/2074)*
   Sickle cell disease is caused by a point mutation in the β_6 chain of hemoglobin. It is **not** an auto immune disease.

68. **Ans. (d) Anti glycoprotein antibody** *(Ref: Robbins 8th/215, Harrison 17th/2073, 9/e 219)*
   Antiphospholipid antibody syndrome is characterized by antibodies against **phospholipid beta– 2-glycoprotein 1 complex**[Q]. For detail, see text under SLE.

69. **Ans. (b) Kikuchi Fujimoto disease** *(Ref: Harrison 17th/1011)*
   The other name of Kikuchi Fujimoto disease is histiocytic necrotizing lymphadenitis. This will answer our question.
   Kikuchi-Fujimoto disease (KFD)/Histiocytic necrotizing lymphadenitis

   - Benign and self-limited disorder in young individuals characterized by regional cervical lymphadenopathy with tenderness, usually accompanied with mild fever and night sweats.
   - May be viral in etiology
   - Diagnosed on the basis of an excisional biopsy of affected lymph nodes which shows fragmentation, necrosis and karyorrhexis, presenting with posterior cervical lymphadenopathy.
   - Patients should be followed-up because of increased chances of development of SLE (systemic lupus erythematosus).

   Castleman disease (CD)

   - Defined by lymph node hypertrophy with angiofollicular lymphoid hyperplasia.
   - Has localised form or multicentric form (several Lymph nodes are affected).
   - Clinical features inlcude Peripheral lymphadenopathy, hepatomegaly and/or splenomegaly and POEMS syndrome (polyneuropathy, organomegaly, endocrinopathy, monoclonal gammopathy, skin changes)
   - Human herpes virus 8 (HHV-8) is the etiological agent
   - Lymph node histological analysis with immunohistochemical staining, shows polyclonal angiofollicular lymphoid hyperplasia, most often of the hyalinovascular type (especially in localised CD) and more rarely of the plasma-cell type (particularly in multicentric CD) or mixed/intermediate type.

Immunity

70. **Ans. (a) SLE** *(Ref: Harrison 17th/2077, Robbins 8th/218, 9/e 224)*
Subendothelial deposits create a homogeneous thickening of the capillary wall **called wire loop lesion**, which can be seen by means of light microscopy when they are extensive. They usually *reflect active disease.*

71. **Ans. (d) Liver** *(Ref: Immunofluorescence Methods for Microscopic Analysis in Methods in Nonradioactive Detection, Lange Publications/247)*
Quote from the book…. *"Serum anti-nuclear antibodies (ANA) bind to the corresponding antigens present in rat liver sections.* The antigen-antibody complexes are detected by means of a fluorescein labeled anti-human immunoglobulin, and visualized with the aid of a fluorescence microscope".

72. **Ans. (c) Inclusion bodies** *(Ref: Robbins 9/e 250-255, 8th/1305, 7th/1375-76)*

73. **Ans. (a) C1 esterase inhibitor deficiency** *(Ref: Robbins 8th/235, 9/e 238)*
A **deficiency of C1 esterase inhibitor** gives rise to an **autosomal dominant** disorder *hereditary angioedema.* The C1 esterase inhibitor is a protease inhibitor whose target enzymes are C1r and C1s of the complement cascade, factor XII of the coagulation pathway, and the kallikrein system. So, any individual having the deficiency of C1 esterase inhibitor would have excessive complement activation.
This causes the release of anaphylatoxins (C3a, C5a) and other inflammatory mediators. These patients therefore have episodes of edema affecting skin and mucosal surfaces such as the larynx and the gastrointestinal tract. This may result in life-threatening *asphyxia or nausea, vomiting,* and *diarrhea* after minor trauma or emotional stress.

74. **Ans. (a) It is an autosomal recessive disorder** *(Ref: Robbins 9/ p242)*

75. **Ans. (a) SLE** *(Ref: Robbins 7th/230, 8th/220, 9/e 218)*
In **SLE,** if antinuclear antibodies (ANAs) can bind to exposed cell nuclei, the nuclei may lose their chromatin pattern, and become homogeneous to produce lupus erythematosus (LE) bodies. The **LE** body is also know as hematoxylin body.

76. **Ans. (c) Diffuse proliferative Glomerulonephritis (WHO class IV)** *(Ref: Harrison 17th/2077, Robbins illustrated 8th/218, 9/e p224)*
   • **Wire loop lesions**[Q] are characteristic of **type IV or diffuse proliferative glomerulonephritis**[Q].
   • It is associated with extensive subendothelial deposits in this type of glomerulonephritis.
   • It is the **most serious of the renal lesions** in SLE.

77. **Ans. (d) Multiple myeloma** *(Ref: Robbins 9/e p258-259, 8th/252-254, 7th/261)*
Pink and amorphous material that shows apple green birefringence under polarized light confirms the diagnosis of Amyloidosis. The presence of Lambda light chains is suggestive of multiple myeloma.

78. **Ans. (a) Non caseating granulomas** *(Ref: Robbins 9/e p693, Harrison, 17th/2135)*
   • The presence of **bilateral nodules on the shin; bilateral hilar lymphadenopathy** and **negative Mantoux test** in a female patient point to a probable diagnosis of **Sarcoidosis.**
   • The skin lesions characteristically show the presence of **non – caseating granulomas**[Q] in **sarcoidosis.**

79. **Ans. (a) SLE:** *(Ref: Robbins 7th/229, 234, 9/e p218)*
Antibodies to ds DNA and the so called Smith (Sm) antigens are virtually diagnostic of SLE. Anti ds-DNA is common in SLE (40-60%).
Anti nuclear antibody is present in all the mentioned diseases but anti double stranded DNA is very specific for SLE.

80. **Ans. (a) PSGN; (b) MPGN; (e) Infective endocarditis** *(Ref: Harrison 16th-/680)*
Causes of hypocomplementemia
   • Glomerulonephritis
     – Idiopathic proliferative GN
     – Cresenteric GN
     – MPGN
     – Post-infectious GN
   • Lupus nephritis
   • Cryoglobulinemia
   • Bacterial endocarditis
   • Shunt nephritis
   • Atheroembolic renal disease
   • Sepsis
   • Acute pancreatitis
   • Advanced liver disease

81. **Ans. (b) Neutropenia; (c) Defective microbial killing; (d) Presence of large granules in neutrophils; (e) Immunodeficiency:** *(Ref: Harrison' 16th/353, 354, Robbins 7th/61, 62, 9/e p238)*

Chediak-Higashi syndrome

- **Autosomal recessive** inheritance
- Due to **defect in lysosomal transport** protein LYST.
- Clinical features include: primary immune deficiency, neutropenia, defective microbial killing, impaired chemotaxis, hypopigmentation of skin, eyes and hair, photophobia and nystagmus
- Microscopic examination shows **giant peroxidase positive inclusions** in the cytoplasm of leukocytes.

82. **Ans. (a) Severe combined immune deficiency.** *(Ref: Robbins 7th/244, 9/e p239)*

83. **Ans. (b) Pulmonary emphysema; (c) Diastase resistant hepatic cells:** *(Ref: Robbins 7th/911-912, 9/e p850-851)*

- α_1-anti-trypsin deficiency is an **autosomal recessive** disease having abnormally low levels of α_1-anti-trypsin
- Deficiency of the enzyme leads to pulmonary **panacinar emphysema**
- Gene located on Chr 14.
- Characterized by **PAS positive** and **diastase resistant** inclusions in hepatocytes.

84. **Ans. (d) High serum IgE, with low IgG, IgA and IgM** *(Ref: Robbins 9/e p242, Harrison 17th/384, 2061, 2056, 381)*

Hyper IgE syndrome is also known as **Job's syndrome**
Abnormal chemotaxis is a variable feature.
Patients have characteristic facies with **broad nose, kyphoscoliosis, osteoporosis and eczema.**
Recurrent abscesses (known as **cold abscesses**) involving skin, lungs and other organs is a prominent feature
Serum IgE level is significantly elevated whereas IgM, IgG and IgA level are normal.

Note: In Hyper- IgM syndrome, IgM is elevated and IgG, IgA are normal.

85. **Ans. (c) Large size platelet** *(Ref: Robbins 9e/p242, 8th/235, Harrison 17th/2060, OP Ghai pediatrics 6th/326)*

86. **Ans. (a) Absent tonsils and no palpable lymph nodes on physical examination** *(Ref: Robbins 9/e p240-241, 8th/231-233)*

87. **Ans. (d) Neutrophil** *(Ref: Robbins 8th/238, 9/e p248)*

88. **Ans. (d) Leucocytosis** *(Ref: Robbins 7th/228, 9/e p218)*

89. **Ans. (c) IgA** *(Ref: Harrison 16th/2423, 9/e p242-243)*

- Patients with ataxia telangiectasia (AT) present in the first decade of life with progressive telangiectatic lesions associated with deficits in cerebellar function and nystagmus. There is a high incidence of recurrent pulmonary infections (**bronchiectasis**[Q]) and neoplasms of the lymphatic and reticuloendothelial system.
- It is caused due to **defect in DNA repair genes**[Q].
- Thymic hypoplasia with **cellular and humoral (IgA**[Q] **and IgG$_2$) immunodeficiencies, premature aging**[Q] and endocrine disorders such as **insulin resistance or type-I DM**[Q].
- The most striking neuropathologic changes include **loss of Purkinje, granule and basket cells** in the cerebellar cortex as well as of neurons in the deep cerebellar nuclei.
- A **poorly developed or absent thymus gland** is the most consistent defect of the lymphoid system.

90. **Ans. (b) Scleroderma:** *(Ref: Robbins 7th/229)*

91. **Ans. (b) Neutrophil** *(Ref: Robbins 7th/230, 9/e p222)*
LE cell or hematoxylin body is a phagocytic leukocyte (**neutrophil or macrophage**) that has engulfed the denatured nucleus of an injured cell.

Tart Cell is usually a **monocyte** which has ingested another cell or nucleus of another cell.

92. **Ans. (c) Antinuclear factor** *(Ref: Robbins 7th/229, 9/e p218-219)*

Most sensitive test for SLE – antinuclear antibody (ANA)
Most specific test for SLE – anti-ds DNA antibody; anti-Smith antibody

93. **Ans. (c) Hematuria** *(Ref: Robbins 9/e p222, 8th/217; 7th/23)*

94. **Ans. (c) Anti double stranded DNA antibody** *(Ref: Robbins 9/e p219, 8th/214; 7th/228)*

95. **Ans. (a) Defect in the transport of chloride across epithelia** *(Ref: Robbins 9/e p466-467, 8th/465; 7th/489-490)*

Immunity

96. **Ans. (a) Sarcoidosis** *(Ref: Harsh Mohan 6th/164-165)*

97. **Ans. (a) P24** *(Ref: Robbins 7th/246, 9/e p245)*

98. **Ans. (a) Kaposi's sarcoma** *(Ref: Robbins 8th/523-524; 7th/256)*

99. **Ans. (a) Syphilis** *(Ref: Robbins 9/e p217, 8th/374, 7th/223)*

100. **Ans. (c) SLE** *(Ref: Robbins 9/e p225-227, 8th/22, 7th/231,236,239)*

101. **Ans. (a) Brain** *(Ref: Robbins 9/e p693, 8th/701-703, 7th/738)*

102. **Ans. (c) Wire loop lesions** *(Ref: Robbins 9/e p224 8th/218, 7th/232)*

103. **Ans. (b) SLE** *(Ref: Robbins 9/e p224, 8th/215; 7th/233-234, 597-598)*

104. **Ans. (b) Chemotaxis** *(Ref: Walter and Israel 7th/150)*
The direct quote from the book is *"Chediak Higashi syndrome is an autosomal recessive condition in which polymorphs exhibit defective random movements, **defective chemotaxis** and impaired degranulation on phagocytosing particles.*

105. **Ans. (b) SLE** *(Ref: Robbins 9/e p219, 8th/215; 7th/234)*

106. **Ans. (a) Systemic sclerosis** *(Ref: Robbins 9/e p228 8th/215,223; 7th/229)*

107. **Ans. (a) Hilar lymphadenopathy with perihilar calcification** *(Ref: Robbins 9/e p693, 8th/703, 7th/738)*

108. **Ans. (a) CNS** *(Ref: Robbins 9/e p254-255, 8th/247; 7th/257)*

109. **Ans. (d) Nodule is the initial lesion of Kaposi's sarcoma** *(Ref: Robbins 9/e p254, 8th/529; 7th/549)*

110. **Ans. (a) Helper cells** *(Ref: Robbins 9/e p246, 8th/239, 7th/248)*

111. **Ans. (c) CNS** *(Ref: Robbins 8th/249, 9/e p254-255)*
Direct quote from Robbins…. *"The anatomic changes in the tissues (**except of lesions in the brain**[Q]) are neither specific nor diagnostic".*

112. **Ans. (d) Double stranded DNA** *(Ref: Robbins 8th/215, 9/e p219)*
Explanation:

Skin rash, photosensitivity, arthralgia and renal disease in a young woman are suggestive of systemic lupus erythematosus (SLE); an autoimmune multisystem vasculitis.
Antibodies against double-stranded DNA (**anti-dsDNA**) are **specific** for SLE. However they are only present in 60% of cases. So absence of anti-dsDNA does not rule out the diagnosis. Antibodies against small nuclear ribonucleoproteins (**anti-snRNPs**), also called **Anti-Smith antibodies** are **also specific** for **SLE**.

(Choice A) **Anti-mitochondrial antibodies** are specific for **primary biliary cirrhosis**[Q], a disease that affects mainly middle- aged women and presents with jaundice, pruritus, hepatosplenomegaly, and hypercholesterolemia.

(Choice B) **Rheumatoid factor** is an IgM[Q] antibody directed against the Fc fragment of self IgG[Q] found in patients with rheumatoid arthritis. It is also found in other collagen tissue disorders.

(Choice C) **Anti-centromere antibodies** are present in the majority of patients with **CREST syndrome**[Q].

113. **Ans. (d) Lymphocyte** *(Ref: Robbins 7th/235-236, 9/e p227)*

The combination of **dry eyes (keratoconjunctivitis)** and **dry mouth (xerostomia)** in an adult woman is suggestive of **Sjogren's syndrome**, an autoimmune disorder characterized by immunologic destruction of the lacrimal and salivary glands. This disorder is characterized by the **presence of SS-A and SS-B auto-antibodies**, but the diagnosis of Sjogren's syndrome is confirmed by finding a **lymphocytic infiltrate** are characteristic of organs affected by autoimmune diseases. In addition to enlargement of the salivary glands, the lymph nodes of patients with Sjogren's syndrome may be enlarged due to a pleomorphic infiltrate of B-lymphocytes.
Patients with Sjogren's syndrome have an **increased risk** for developing **non- Hodgkin's lymphoma, especially marginal zone lymphoma**[Q].

Biopsy of the lip (to examine minor salivary glands) is essential for making a diagnosis of **Sjogren syndrome**[Q].

114. **Ans. (d) Werner's syndrome** *(Ref: Robbins 7th/, 42-43, 8th/39-40, 9/e p66-67)*

> **Progeria (or Hutchinson-Gilford syndrome)** is a disease characterized by symptoms of premature aging; symptoms **begin around the age of 6-12 months** of age.
> **Werner's syndrome** is a similar appearing disease that first causes symptoms in affected individuals in their **late teens**. Werner's syndrome is caused by a mutation in the WS gene which results in the production of a **defective DNA helicase[Q]**.
> **Mnemonic:** remember the legendry **Amitabh Bachchan** as Auro in 'Paa'

115. Ans. is (d) i.e. Tyrosine kinase *(Ref: Robbins 8th/231-232, 9/e p240-241)*

> This patient has **X-linked[Q] (Bruton's) agammaglobulinemia**, which is due to a **deficiency in a tyrosine kinase[Q]**, leading to a B cell maturation arrest at the pre-B cell level.

> **Selective IgA deficiency** has been linked to defective **class III MHC** genes (option B).

> **Severe combined immunodeficiency** is apparently a heterogeneous disease, and different subgroups have been linked to abnormalities of **adenosine deaminase** (option A), the **gamma chain of the IL-2 receptor[Q]** (option C), and **purine nucleotide phosphorylase**.

116. Ans. is (d) i.e. There may be an increase in spontaneous abortions and prematurity *(Ref: Robbins 8th/220, 9/e p222)*

> **Systemic lupus erythematosus** (SLE) predominantly affects **younger women**, and these patients have an **increased incidence of spontaneous abortion, fetal death in utero, and prematurity**. The mother may experience an exacerbation in the activity of her disease in the third trimester or peripartum period.
> Congenital malformations (options B and C) are not a complication of pregnancies in patients with SLE.

117. Ans. is (a) i.e. Conjunctivitis *(Ref: Robbins 9/e p226-227, 8th/221)*
The patient has Sjögren's syndrome, characterized by dry eyes (keratoconjunctivitis) and a dry mouth (xerostomia) due to destruction of the lacrimal and salivary glands. The most diagnostic autoantibodies are those against ribonucleoproteins Ro (SS-A) and La (SS-B), although co-existing rheumatoid factor and lupus antibodies are also seen.

118. Ans. is (b) i.e. Granular complement and IgG at the dermal-epidermal junction *(Ref: Robbins 8th/219, 9/e p224)*

> The disease SLE having the characteristic "butterfly" facial rash of lupus is due to deposition of antibodies and complement at the dermal/pidermal junction.

> Cells similar to fibroblasts growing in a **storiform ("pinwheel") pattern** (option A) are characteristic of **dermatofibrosarcoma protuberans[Q]**, a slow-growing type of fibrosarcoma.

> A **sawtooth dermoepidermal junction** (option C) is a feature of the skin condition **lichen planus[Q]**.

> **Pautrier microabscesses** (option D) are a feature of a cutaneous T-cell lymphoma called **mycosis fungoides**.

119. Ans. is (a) i.e. Acanthamoeba sp. (No reference..........read explanation below)
Two types of free-living amoeba can infect the brain and meninges: Naegleria fowleri and **Acanthamoeba sp**.
The former affects healthy adolescent or adult divers, while the latter causes **infection in patients with immunosuppression** (*diabetes, alcoholism, cancer, or HIV infection*).
The brain infection characteristically has a *prominent perivascular character*, which causes a multifocal hemorrhagic necrotizing meningoencephalitis. Skin ulcers, nasal infection, or pneumonia may also be present. It is thought that the organisms may release a toxin causing host tissue necrosis.
Naegleria fowleri (choice D) is an amoebic cause of meningoencephalitis in **previously healthy swimmers[Q]** and divers.

120. Ans. is (c) i.e. HLA typing *(Ref: Robbins 8th/193, 9/e p215)*
Ankylosing spondylitis is a seronegative spondyloarthropathy primarily affecting the vertebrae and the sacroiliac joints, usually beginning in late adolescence or early adulthood. Majority 90-100% of these patients are HLA-B27 positive. So, tests for this HLA type are the most helpful of those given as options in confirming the diagnosis.

Seronegative spondyloarthropathies (Mnemonic: PAIR)	Salient features of these diseases
P: Psoriatic arthritis **A:** Ankylosing spondylitis (AS) **I:** Inflammatory bowel disease arthritis **R:** Reactive arthritis (Reiter syndrome)	*Absence of serum auto-antibodies *Associated with **HLA B27 (most commonly AS)** *Onset before** the age of **40 years** *Presence of **uveitis, spine/large peripheral joint arthritis**

- C-reactive protein and erythrocyte sedimentation rate (choice B) are non-specific markers of inflammation that can be elevated in active ankylosing spondylitis.
- Serum alkaline phosphatase (choice D) and serum IgA (choice E) can also be (usually mildly) elevated, but do not specifically suggest ankylosing spondylitis.

Immunity

121. Ans. is. (a) i.e. Angiosarcoma *(Ref: Robbins 8th/246, 9/e p254)*

> **Kaposi's sarcoma** is a spindle cell neoplasm that is highly associated with AIDS (infact, it is the **commonest**[Q] malignancy in AIDS). It is caused due to **Herpes simplex virus type 8**[Q]. The tumor has an appearance very **similar to that of angiosarcoma**[Q]-proliferating **stromal cells and endothelium** creating vascular channels that contain blood cells.

Malignant fibrous histiocytoma (MFH); (choice D) is an extremely poorly differentiated (anaplastic) stromal malignancy. MFH does not produce any recognizable mesenchymal structures-thus, the production of vascular structures by Kaposi's sarcoma differentiates the two tumors.

121.1. Ans. (a) ds DNA *(Ref: Robbins 8/e p214-215, 9/e p218-219)*

Revise the important features of antibodies in SLE

•	**Anti-double stranded DNA antibody** and the antiSmith **(Sm)** antibody:**Highly specific** for SLE.
•	Antinuclear antibody (**ANA**):**Highly sensitive** for SLE
•	**Anti-P antibody** – Associated with **lupus psychosis**
•	**Anti-SS-A** and **Anti-SS-B** antibody- Associated with **congenital heart block** and **cutaneous lupus**
•	**Anticardiolipin antibodies** may produce a **false positive** VDRL test for syphilis

121.2. Ans. (c) Anti topoisomerase *(Ref: Robbins 8/e p215 , 9/e p219)*

Anti topoisomerase is least commonly associated with SLE amongst the given options. The following is a modified table given for a reference from Robbins.

Nature of Antigen	Antibody System	% Positive in SLE
Many nuclear antigens (DNA, RNA, proteins)	Generic ANA (indirect IF)	>95
Native DNA	Anti–double-stranded DNA	40–60
Histones	Antihistone	50–70
Core proteins of small nuclear RNP particles (Smith antigen)	Anti-Sm	20–30
RNP (U1RNP)	Nuclear RNP	30–40
RNP	SS-A(Ro)	30–50
RNP	SS-B(La)	10–15
DNA topoisomerase I	Scl-70	<5
Centromeric proteins	Anticentromere	<5
Histidyl-tRNA synthetase	Jo-1	<5

121.3. Ans. (c) Primary CNS lymphoma *(Ref: Robbins 8/e p247, 9/e p254-255)*
- **Primary CNS lymphoma**[Q] is the most common CNS neoplasm in immunosuppressed individuals, including those with **AIDS** and **immunosuppression after transplantation.**
- The term *primary* emphasizes the distinction between these lesions and secondary involvement of the CNS by lymphoma arising elsewhere in the body.
- Primary brain lymphoma is **often multifocal** within the brain parenchyma
- Most primary brain lymphomas are of **B-cell origin**[Q] and most have infection caused by **EBV**[Q] in the setting of immunosuppression.
- Histologically, reticulin stains demonstrate that the infiltrating cells are separated from one another by silver-staining material; this pattern, referred to as **"hooping,"** is **characteristic of primary brain lymphoma**.
- In addition to expressing B-cell markers, most of the cells also express **BCL-6**; when tumors arise in the setting of immunosuppression,

121.4. Ans. (a) Adenosine deaminase deficiency *(Ref: Robbins 8/e p234, 9/e p239)*
- Severe combined immunodeficiency (SCID) represents a constellation of genetically distinct syndromes, all having in common *defects in both humoral and cell-mediated immune responses*
- **The most common form**, accounting for 50% to 60% of cases, is **X-linked**, and hence SCID is more common in boys than in girls. The genetic defect in the X-linked form is a *mutation in the common γ-chain (γc) subunit of cytokine receptors*
- The **remaining cases** of SCID are inherited as **autosomal recessive**. The most common cause of autosomal recessive SCID is a *deficiency of the enzyme adenosine deaminase (ADA).*

121.5. Ans. (c) Normal B cell count *(Ref: Robbins 8/e p233, 9/e p241)*

Common Variable Immunodeficiency

- Rare disease characterised by hypogammaglobulinemia, generally affecting all the antibody classes but sometimes only IgG.
- The diagnosis of common variable immunodeficiency is based on exclusion of other well-defined causes of decreased antibody production.
- *In contrast to X-linked agammaglobulinemia*, most individuals with **common variable immunodeficiency** have **normal or near-normal numbers of B cells in the blood and lymphoid tissues**. These B cells, however, are not able to differentiate into plasma cells.
- Clinical manifestations include *recurrent sinopulmonary pyogenic infections*. The patients with the disease are prone to the development of persistent diarrhea caused by *G. lamblia*[Q].
- It affects **both sexes equally** (In contrast to X-linked agammaglobulinemia)
- Histologically the B-cell areas of the lymphoid tissues (i.e., lymphoid follicles in nodes, spleen, and gut) are hyperplastic.
- Associated with high frequency of autoimmune diseases like rheumatoid arthritis and malignancies (lymphoid cancer and gastric cancer)

121.6. Ans. (b) Digeorge syndrome *(Ref: Robbins 8/e p234, 9/e p241)*

Digeorge syndrome/ Thymic hypoplasia/Velocardiofacial syndrome

- *DiGeorge syndrome is a T-cell deficiency that results from failure of development of the third and fourth pharyngeal pouches.*
- Individuals with this syndrome have a **variable loss of T cell–mediated immunity** (resulting from **hypoplasia or lack of the thymus**), **tetany** (resulting from lack of the parathyroids), and *congenital defects of the heart and great vessels.*
- The T-cell zones of lymphoid organs (paracortical areas of the lymph nodes and the periarteriolar sheaths of the spleen) are depleted.
- DiGeorge syndrome results from the deletion of a gene mapped to chromosomes **22q11**.

Mnemonic: (CATCH 22)

C	Cardiac abnormalities (especially tetralogy of Fallot)
A	Abnormal facies
T	Thymic aplasia
C	Cleft palate
H	Hypocalcemia (due to hypoplasia or lack of parathyroids)
22	22q11 deletion

121.7. Ans. (a) SLE *(Ref: Robbins 9/e p224, 8/e p220, 7/e p234)*

In the splenic tissue involvement in SLE, splenomegaly, capsular thickening, and follicular hyperplasia are common features. Central penicilliary arteries may show concentric intimal and smooth muscle cell hyperplasia, producing so-called **onion-skin lesions**[Q].

121.8. Ans. (c) Haematoxylin bodies *(Ref: Robbins 9/e p256)*

- Biopsy specimens from enlarged lymph nodes in the early stages of HIV infection reveal a **marked follicular hyperplasia**
- **Monocytoid cells** along the blood vessels can be seen in acute lymphadenitis.
- With disease progression, the frenzy of B-cell proliferation subsides and gives way to a pattern of **severe follicular involution**. The follicles are depleted of cells, and the **organized network of follicular dendritic cells is disrupted**. The germinal centers may even become hyalinized.
- During this advanced stage viral burden in the nodes is reduced, in part because of the disruption of the follicular dendritic cells. These **"burnt-out" lymph nodes**[Q] are atrophic and small

121.9. Ans. (a) Children previously tested with tuberculin test *(Ref: Robbins 9/e p371)*

Children previously tested with tuberculin test may show a *FALSE POSITIVE TUBERULIN TEST.*

False-negative Mantoux test	False-positive Mantoux test
• Sarcoidosis[Q] • Malnutrition[Q] • Hodgkin disease[Q] • Immunosuppression[Q] • Fulminant tuberculosis[Q]	• Infection by atypical mycobacteria[Q] • Previous vaccination with BCG[Q]

121.10. Ans. (c) Plasma derived Hepatitis B vaccine

Blood products which can transmit HIV	Blood products which can NOT transmit HIV
• Whole blood • Packed red blood cells • Platelets • Leukocytes • Plasma • All are capable of transmitting HIV infection.	• Hyperimmune gamma globulin • Hepatitis B immune globulin • Plasma-derived hepatitis B vaccine • Rho immune globulin • The procedures involved in processing these products either inactivate or remove the virus.

121.11. Ans. (c) HIV ELISA

Excellent question testing your basics buddies!
- HIV ELISA is required for detection of antibodies against the virus. The antibodies may be present in the infant because of maternal infection also because IgG antibodies can cross the placental barrier. So, the presence of anti HIV antibodies is not reliable for diagnosis of HIV in a 2 month old child.
- Please don't get foxed by the option viral culture friends. There is indeed a HIV culture method being used which is called as *'peripheral blood mononuclear cells'* (PBMC) using the virus microculture in macrophages concept. PBMC are drawn in high concentration from centrifugation of freshly drawn anticoagulated venous blood.
- Viral DNA detection using DNA-PCR andp24 antigen assay are standard techniques used for viral detection.

121.12. Ans. (b) Disseminated TB *(Ref: Robbins 9/e p371)*
- Mantoux test is simply able to predict the presence or absence of cell mediated immunity against the tubercular antigens. It **CANNOT** differentiate between infection and disease.
- Negative Mantoux test just indicates that the individual has never been exposed to tubercle bacilli earlier; it can't indicate the susceptibility to the disease.

121.13. Ans. (d) Systemic lupus erythematosus *(Ref: Robbins 9/e p218)*

Similar to many autoimmune diseases, SLE predominantly affects women. A female-to-male ratio of 9:1 is seen during the reproductive age group. By comparison, the female-to-male ratio is only 2:1 for disease developing during childhood or after the age of 65.

121.14. Ans. (d) A mechanism for the persistence and evolution of autoimmune disease *(Ref: Robbins 9/e p217)*

Epitope spreading is a phenomenon in which an immune response against one self antigen causes tissue damage, releasing other antigens, and resulting in the activation of lymphocytes by these newly encountered epitopes. This is responsible for the persistence and progression of autoimmune diseases.

121.15. Ans. (d) Anterior uveitis *(Ref: Harrison 18th/2806)*

- *Löfgren's syndrome* consists of erythema nodosum, hilar adenopathy on chest X ray and uveitis.
- Heerfordt's syndrome: fever, parotid enlargement, facial palsy and uveitis.

121.16. Ans. (a) Gp 120 *(Ref: Robbins 8th/246-7)*

HIV-1 uses CD4 to gain entry into host T-cells and achieves this through its viral envelope protein known as gp120.

121.17. Ans. (b) 350

Under the revised guidelines the treatment of AIDS patients with respect to opportunistic infections has undergone a change with H.A.A.R.T being initiated at a threshold of CD4 count <350 cells/cu.mm instead of previous 200 cells/cu.mm.

121.18. Ans. (a) EBV *(Ref: Robbins 9th/607)*

122. Ans. (c) AA *(Ref: Robbins 8th/252-3, 9/e p257)*

123. Ans. (d) β_2 microglobulin *(Ref: Robbins 8th/254, 9/e p258)*

Hemodialysis associated amyloidosis is caused by the deposition of the β_2 microglobulin which is a **component of MHC class I molecule** and cannot be filtered through the cuprophane dialysis membrane. It gets deposited in the synovium, joints and the tendon sheaths.
Deposition of the amyloid in long term hemodialysis takes place in joints and in the carpal ligament of the wrist, the latter leading to development of 'carpal tunnel syndrome'

124. Ans. (b) Rectal biopsy *(Ref: Harrison 17th/2145-6; Robbins 8th/255, 9/e p262, Harsh Mohan 6th/88)*

The histological examination of the biopsy material is the commonest and confirmatory method for the diagnosis in a suspected case of amyloidosis. The sites for the biopsy can be the *renal tissue, rectum, abdominal fat aspiration and gingiva.* The **rectum**Q is the **best site for taking the biopsy** in the options provided.

Note: Congo red staining of **aspirated abdominal fat** is **initial test of choice** in most cases. If it is found to be negative, more invasive biopsy of other affected organ can be taken. The staining of abdominal fat aspirate is quite specific but has low sensitivity.

125. **Ans. (b) Familial amyloidosis polyneuropathy** *(Ref: Robbins 8th/252-253, 9/e p259)*

Transthyretin is a normal serum protein that binds and transports thyroxine and retinol (transthyretin). A mutant form of transthyretin is deposited in a group of genetically determined disorders referred to as familial amyloid polyneuropathies'.
- **Inherited amyloidosis** *due to* **ATTR is autosomal dominant**
- *Even* **normal transthyretin** *(pre-albumin) can form fibrils and lead to* **senile systemic amyloidosis.**

126. **Ans. (b) β_2 microglobulin** *(Ref: Robbins 7th/159-160, 9/e p258)*

β_2 microglobulin, a component of MHC-1 molecule complicates the course of patients on long term hemodialysis. It is similar to the normal β_2 microglobulin protein which is retained in circulation of patients with renal failure because it cannot be filtered through the cuprophane dialysis membrane.

127. **Ans. (a) Bone marrow plasmacytosis** *(Ref: Robbins 7th/pg 260, 8th/252, 9/e p257)*
AL (Amyloid Light chain) protein is produced by immunoglobulin secreting plasma cells and their deposition is associated with some form of monoclonal B cell proliferation. **These patients have a modest increase in the number of plasma cells in the bone marrow (plasmacytosis) which presumably secrete the precursors of AL protein.**

128. **Ans. (a) A beta 2 Microglobulin** *(Ref: Robbins 7th/260, 261, 8th/253, 9/e p258)*

129. **Ans. (c) Rectal biopsy** *(Ref: Harrison 16th/2028, 17th/2145 Robbins 9/e p262)*

130. **Ans. (c) Smooth muscle cells** *(Ref: Robbins 7th/515)*
The proliferation of smooth muscle cells is a critical event in the neointimal hyperplastic response. Several studies have clearly demonstrated that blockade of smooth muscle cell proliferation resulted in preservation of normal vessel phenotype and function, causing the reduction of neointimal hyperplasia and graft failure.

131. **Ans. (c) Congo red** *(Ref: Robbins 7th/259, 8th/255, 9/e p257 Harrison 17th/2145)*

132. **Ans. (a) X-ray crystallography** *(Ref: Robbin 7th/259, 8th/250, 9/e p257)*

- β Pleated structure is seen on X-ray crystallography
- Electro Microscope shows non branching fibrils of indefinite length.

133. **Ans. (a) Nonbranching filaments of indefinite length** *(Ref: Robbins 7th/259, 9/e p257)*

134. **Ans. (c) Methanamine silver** *(Ref: Harsh Mohan 5th/89, 6th/87, Robbins 9/e p262)*

135. **Ans. (c) 7.5-10 nm fibrils** *(Ref: Robbins 6th/259, 8th/249, 9/e p257)*
Remember β-pleated structure of amyloid is seen on X-ray crystallography, whereas it is seen as a non-branching fibril of 7.5-10 nm diameter and infinite length on electron microscopy.

136. **Ans. (c) Mutant transthyretin** *(Ref: Robbin's 7th/260, 9/e p259)*

137. **Ans. (a) Sinusoids of red pulp** *(Ref: Robbins 7th/263, 9/e p261)*
Amyloidosis of spleen

Sago spleen	Lardaceous spleen
Amyloid deposition is largely limited to splenic follicles	Amyloid deposition spares the follicles and involve the walls of the splenic sinuses in **red pulp**

Mnemonic: Red is 'lal' in hindi, so, similar sounding **lardaceous**.

138. **Ans. (a) Thioflavin; (b) Congo red.** *(Ref: Robbins 7th/254, 9/e p262)*

139. **Ans. is b i.e. Amyloidosis** *(Ref: Harrison 17th/2146; Robbins 7th/264, 9/e p262)*

140. **Ans. (c) Glycoprotein** *(Ref: Robbins 9/e p256, 8th/250, 7th/259)*

141. **Ans. (b) Chronic inflammatory states** *(Ref: Robbins 9/e p257, 8th/251-252; 7th/159)*

142. **Ans. (c) Kidney** *(Ref: Robbins 8th/254, 9/e p261)*

143. **Ans. (b) Interferon-γ (IFN- γ)** *(Ref: Robbins 8th/195, 206-8)*

IL-12 stimulates differentiation of "naive" T-helper cells into the T_H1 subpopulation. Patients with IL-12 receptor deficiency suffer from severe mycobacterial infections due to the inability to mount a strong cell-mediated granulomatous immune response. They are treated with IFN-γ.

The differences between the T_H1 and T_H2 subpopulations of helper T-cells are presented below:

	T_H1	T_H2
Type of immunity	Cell mediated	Humoral/antibody mediated
Function	Activate macrophages and cytotoxic T cells	Activated B cells
Cytokines secreted	IL-2, IFN-γ	IL-4, 5
Result	Cytotoxicity, Delayed hypersensitivity	Secretion of antibodies

(Choice A) B-cell differentiation into plasma cells and secretion of immunoglobulins is dependent on the T_H2 subpopulation of helper T-cells.

(Choice C) Synthesis of IL-2 is diminished in patients with IL-12 receptor deficiency. This interleukin activates both T and B-lymphocytes but does not activate macrophages. It is not directly responsible for delayed hypersensitivity reactions.

144. **Ans. (b) i.e. Beta-pleated sheet tertiary structure** *(Ref: Robbins 8th/250, 9/e p257)*
The patient has amyloidosis and this protein has a beta-pleated sheet tertiary structure that apparently is reflected in the apple-green birefringence. Other mentioned properties do not contribute to birefringence.

> The **ability to bind oxygen** (option A) is important to **hemoglobin.**
> **Electrophoretic mobility** (option C) is used to **separate serum proteins.**
> **Hydroxyproline content** (option D) is important to **collagen structure.**

145. **Ans. (a) Multiple myeloma-Light chain; (b) Chronic inflammation- AA; (c) Cardiac-ATTR** *(Ref: Harsh Mohan 5th/87, Robbins 7th/260, 8th/252, 9/e p259)*

145.1. **Ans (c) Beta – 2-microglobulin** *(Ref: Robbins 8/e p252, 9/e p258)*

Hemodialysis associated Amyloidosis
- It is caused by the deposition of the β2 microglobulin which is a **component of MHC class I molecule** and cannot be filtered through the cuprophane dialysis membrane. It gets deposited in the synovium, joints and the tendon sheaths. The chemical nature of the amyloid is $A\beta_2^Q$.
- Patients often present with **carpal tunnel syndrome** because of β_2-microglobulin deposition.

145.2. **Ans. (a) A-β_2 Microglobulin………….See earlier explanation** *(Ref: Robbins 9/e p258)*

145.3. **Ans. (c) Type 2 DM** *(Ref: Robbins 8/e p253, 9/e p259)*
Amyloid replacement of islets is a **characteristic finding** in individuals with **long-standing type 2 diabetes[Q]**. It is believed that the islet amyloid protein is directly cytotoxic to islets, analogous to the role played by amyloid plaques implicated in the pathogenesis of Alzheimer disease.

145.4. **Ans. (b) Renal tissue** *(Ref: Robbins 8/e p254, 9/e p261)*
- Amyloidosis of the **kidney** is the **most common** and potentially the **most serious form** of organ involvement

145.5. **Ans. (b) Familial amyloidotic polyneuropathy** *(Ref: Robbins 8/e p253, 9/e p259)*

Clinical conditions and the chemical nature of amyloid

S.No.	Amyloid protein	Precursor	Disease
1.	AL	Ig light chain	Multtiple myeloma (primary amyloidosis)
2.	AA	SAA	Secondary or reactive amyloidosis
3.	$A\beta_2m$	$\beta_2$microglobulin	Hemodialysis Associated amyloidosis
4.	Aβ	Aβ precursor protein	Senile cerebral Alzhemimer's
5.	ATTR	Mutant Transthyretin / Normal Transthyretin	Familial amyloidotic neuropathy / Systemic senile amyloidosis
6.	ACal	Calcitionin	Medullary carcinoma of thyroid
7.	AIAPP	Islet amyloid polypeptide	Type II diabetes
8.	AANF	ANP	Isolated atrial amyloidosis / Misfolded prion protein (PrPsc) disease
9.	Aα	Fibrinogen	Familial renal amyloidosis

145.6. Ans. (b) Renal failure *(Ref: Robbins 8/e p254, 9/e p261)*
"Amyloidosis of the kidney is the most common and potentially the most serious form of organ involvement".....direct lines from Robbins.
Renal involvement gives rise to proteinuria that may be severe enough to cause the nephrotic syndrome. Progressive obliteration of glomeruli in advanced cases ultimately leads to renal failure and uremia. Renal failure is a common cause of death.

145.7. Ans. (d) Chronic osteomyelitis *(Ref: Robbins 9/e p257, 8/e p253, 7/e p261)*
Direct quote... "tuberculosis, bronchiectasis, and chronic osteomyelitis were the most important underlying conditions, but with the advent of effective antimicrobial chemotherapy the connective tissue disorders such as **rheumatoid arthritis**[Q] (**most common**), ankylosing spondylitis, and inflammatory bowel disease, particularly Crohn disease and ulcerative colitis. Among these the most frequent associated condition is."

145.8. Ans. (c) Brilliant pink color *(Ref: Robbins 9/e p257, 8/e p253, 7/e p263)*
Congo red under *ordinary light* imparts a *pink or red color to amyloid deposits*. Under polarized light, the Congo red–stained amyloid shows a green birefringence.

145.9. Ans. (a) Sinusoids of red pulp *(Ref: Robbins 9/e p261, 8/e p254, 7/e p263)*
Spleen involvement in amyloidosis
- **Red pulp** like splenic sinuses: **Lardaceous spleen**
- *White pulp* like splenic follicles : *Sago spleen*

GOLDEN POINTS FOR QUICK REVISION / UPDATED INFORMATION FROM 9TH EDITION OF ROBBINS

(IMMUNITY)

Pattern Recognition Receptors (Page 187 of Robbins)

Cells that participate in innate immunity are capable of recognizing certain microbial components that are shared among related microbes and are often essential for infectivity. These microbial structures are called *pathogen-associated molecular patterns*.
Pattern recognition receptors are the cellular receptors that recognize these molecules and include:
a. **Toll-Like Receptors:** The TLRs are present in the plasma membrane and endosomal vesicles. All these receptors activates either *NF-κB* (stimulating the synthesis and secretion of cytokines) or *interferon regulatory factors* (IRFs; stimulate the production of the antiviral cytokines)
b. **NOD-Like Receptors and the Inflammasome.** NOD-like receptors (NLRs) are cytosolic receptors which recognize a wide variety of substances like products of necrotic cells (e.g., uric acid and released ATP), ion disturbances (e.g., loss of K+), and some microbial products. Some NLRs signal via a cytosolic multiprotein complex called the *inflammasome* to produce the biologically active form of IL-1.

> The NLR-inflammasome pathway may also play a role in many common conditions like gout, atherosclerosis and type 2 diabetes.

c. **RIG-like receptors** (RLRs): they are located in the cytosol of most cell types and detect nucleic acids of viruses that replicate in the cytoplasm of infected cells. These receptors stimulate the production of antiviral cytokines.

Innate Lymphoid Cells (ILCs); (Page 193)

ILCs belong to a population of lymphocytes that lack TCRs but produce cytokines similar to those that are made by T cells. **NK cells are considered the first defined ILC**. Different subsets of ILCs produce IFN-γ, IL-5, IL-17, and IL-22. Their functions include:

> - Early defense against infections
> - Recognition and elimination of stressed cells (so-called **stress surveillance**)
> - Shaping the later adaptive immune response, by providing cytokines that influence the differentiation of T lymphocytes.

Immunologic Tolerance and Autoimmunity (Page 213)

Tolerance (unresponsiveness) to self antigens is a fundamental property of the immune system, and breakdown of tolerance is the basis of autoimmune diseases. It can be of the following subtypes:

> - **Central tolerance:** immature lymphocytes that recognize self antigens in the central (generative) lymphoid organs are killed by **apoptosis.** Similarly in the B-cell lineage, some of the self-reactive lymphocytes switch to new antigen receptors that are not self-reactive. This is called as **receptor editing.**
> - **Peripheral tolerance:** mature lymphocytes that recognize self antigens in peripheral tissues become functionally inactive **(anergic)**, or are suppressed by **regulatory T lymphocytes**, or die by **apoptosis.**

The factors that lead to a failure of self-tolerance and the development of autoimmunity include
- Inheritance of susceptibility genes that may disrupt different tolerance pathways, and
- Infections and tissue injury that may expose self antigens and activate APCs and lymphocytes in the tissues.

Autoimmune diseases are usually chronic and progressive, and the type of tissue injury is determined by the nature of the dominant immune response.

Non HLA genes associated with autoimmune diseases....Robbins 9th/ 216

Putative Gene Involved	Diseases	Postulated Function of Encoded Protein and Role of Mutation/ Polymorphism in Disease
Genes involved in immune regulation:		
PTPN22	RA, T1 D, IBD	Protein tyrosine phosphatase, may affect signalling in lymphocytes and may after negative selection or activation of self-reactive T cells
IL23R	IBD, PS, AS	Receptor for the T$_1$17-includeing cytokine IL-23; may after differentiation of CD4+ T cells into pathogenic T$_1$ 17 effector cells
CTLA4	T1D, RA	Inhibits T cell responses by terminating activation and promoting activity of regulatory T cells; may interfere with self-tolerance
IL2RA	MS, T1D	a chain of the receptor for IL-2, which is a growth and survival factor for activated and regulatory T cells; may affect development of effector cells and/or regulation of immune responses
Genes involved in immune responses to microbes:		
NOD2	IBD	Cytoplasmic sensor of bacteria expressed in Paneth and other intestinal epithelial cells; may control resistance to gut commensal bacteria
AT616	IBD	Involved in autophagy; possible role in defense against microbes and maintenance of epithelial barrier function
IRF5, IFIH1	SLE	Role in type 1 interferon production; type I IFN is involved the pathogenesis of SLE (See text)

AUTOANTIBODIES IN AUTOIMMUNE DISORDERS....Robbins 9th/ 219

Disease	Specificity of Autoanti Body	Association with specific Disease Features
Systemic lupus erythernatosus (SLE)	Double-stranded DNA	Nephritis; specific for SLE
	U1-RNP	
	Smith (Sm) antigen (Core protein of small RNP particles)	Specific for SLE
	Ro (SS-A)/La (SS-B) nucleoproteins	Congenital heart block; neonatal lupus
	Phospholipid-protein complexes (anti-PL)	Antiphospholipid syndrome (in~10% of SLE patients)
	Multiple nuclear antigen ("generic ANAs")	Found in other autoimmune diseases, not specific.
Systemic scleroids	DNA topoisornerase 1	Diffuse skin disease, lung disease; specific for systemic sclerosis
	Centromeric proteins (CENPs) A, B, C	Limited skin disease, ischemic digital loss, putomonery hypertension
	RNA polymerase III	Acute onse, aclerodema renal crisis, cancer
Sjögren syndrome	Ro/SS-A La/SS-B	
Autoimmune myositis	Histidyl-tRNA synthetase, Jo1	Interstitial lung disease, Raynaud phenomenon
	Mi-2 nuclear antigen	Dermatomyositis, skin rash
	MDAS (cytoplasmic receptor for viral RNA)	Vascular skin lesions, interstitial lung disease
	TF1y nuclear protein	Dermatomyositis, cancer
Rheumetold arthritis	CCP (cyclic citrullinated peptides); various citrullinated proteins	Specific for rheumatoid arthritis
	Rheumatoid factor (not specific)	

For Special Attention...Potential Future AIIMS Question

- *Anti RNA polymerase III antibody* is associated with *Acute onset, scleroderma renal crisis* and *cancer.*
- *Autoimmune myositis* is associated with antibody against *Histidyl aminoacyl-tRNA synthetase, Jo1 25, Mi-2 nuclear antigen, MDA5 (cytoplasmic receptor for viral RNA)* and *TIF1γ nuclear protein*

IgG4-RELATED DISEASE....Robbins 9th/ 231

- IgG4-related disease (IgG4-RD) is an idiopathic newly recognized constellation of disorders affecting middle aged to old men characterized by tissue infiltrates dominated by IgG4 antibody-producing plasma cells and T lymphocytes, storiform fibrosis, obliterative phlebitis, and usually increased serum IgG4. Autoimmune myositis is associated with antibody against Histidyl aminoacyl-tRNA synthetase, Jo1 25, Mi-2 nuclear antigen, MDA5 (cytoplasmic receptor for viral RNA) and TIF1γ nuclear protein.
- It includes disorders like Mikulicz syndrome (enlargement and fibrosis of salivary and lacrimal glands), Riedel thyroiditis, idiopathic retroperitoneal fibrosis, autoimmune pancreatitis, and inflammatory pseudotumors of the orbit, lungs, and kidneys.

X-linked Lymphoproliferative Disease..... Robbins 9th/242

It is characterized by an *inability to eliminate Epstein-Barr virus* (EBV), eventually leading to **fulminant infectious mononucleosis** and the development of **B-cell tumors.**

In most of the cases it is caused by mutations in the gene for *SLAM-associated protein (SAP)* that are associated with the activation of NK cells and T and B lymphocytes. This leads to attenuated NK and T cell activation and result in increased susceptibility to viral infections. SAP is also required for the development of follicular helper T cells, and so, XLP patients are unable to form germinal centers or produce high affinity antibodies.

CHAPTER 7

Anemia and Red Blood Cells

Hematology is the study of the various cells and components of the blood. Hematopoeisis is the process of production of blood cells which primarily takes place in the following organs:

SALIENT FEATURES OF BONE MARROW

- The ratio of the fat cells and the hematopoeitic cells in an adult is 1:1. The number of the myeloid cells is more than the number of the erythroid cells (normal M:E ratio is 3 to 15:1).
- The investigations for the information about bone marrow are bone marrow aspiration and bone marrow biopsy.

Hematopoietic stem cells are pluripotent stem cells which are *CD34+ cells*. They give rise to the trilineage myeloid cells, lymphoblasts and monoblasts. The trilineage myeloid cell gives rise to the following three cells:

- Normoblast (Gives rise to RBCs)
- Myeloblast (Gives rise to neutrophils, eosinophils and basophils)
- Megakaryocyte (Gives rise to platelets).

Monoblast gives rise to monocytes whereas lymphoblast gives rise to lymphocytes.

> ### Sites of Hematopoeisis
>
> Till **3rd week** of intrauterine life: Yolk sac.
>
> By **3rd month** of intrauterine life: **Liver** is the main site of blood formation.
>
> At **4th month** of intrauterine life: **Bone marrow** is the main site of hematopoiesis.
>
> Finally **by birth**, the **bone marrow** in whole of the skeleton is hematopoietically active and is the chief source of blood cells and it remains so till puberty.
>
> **After puberty**, the **red marrow** is present in vertebrae, ribs, sternum, skull, pelvis and proximal epiphyseal regions of humerus and femur.

Stages of Erythropoiesis

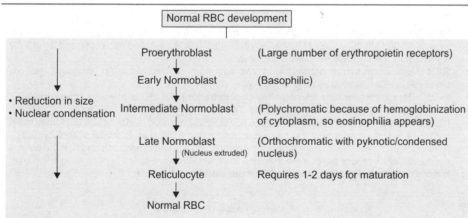

> **Hemoglobinization** takes place during the stage of **intermediate normoblast**.

General Information About RBCs

The normal red cell is biconcave in shape and has a diameter of 7-8 mm. The cytoskeleton of the RBC is made up of proteins like spectrin, ankyrin, band 2.1, band 3, band 4.1, etc. that provide deformability to the RBCs so that they can cross through tiny blood vessels like capillaries. Importance of these proteins can be appreciated in disorders like hereditary spherocytosis. When the RBCs are of unequal size, this is referred to as *anisocytosis* and when of different shapes, it is called *poikilocytosis*.

> The **normal reticulocyte count** is **0.2-2%**.

> **Spectrin** is the chief protein responsible for **biconcave shape** of normal red blood cell.

- **Reticulocytes** are nonnucleated spherical cells bigger than normal RBCs and are polychromatic (having a blue color) due to the presence of free ribosomes and RNA.
- **Reticulocyte count:** Percentage of reticulocytes among the red cells present in the peripheral blood is called reticulocyte count. Normal value is around 1.5% in adults and 1.7% in the cord blood cells.

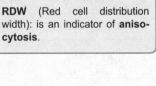

The **reticulocyte count** is an *indicator of erythropoetic activity* of the bone marrow.

- **Absolute reticulocyte count (ARC):** Number of reticulocytes present in 1 mm3 of blood.
  ARC = (Reticulocyte %) X Erythrocyte Count/100.
- **Reticulocyte Index (RI):** It adjusts reticulocyte count for hematocrit. It reflects bone marrow activity and is also known as *"Poor man's Bone Marrow Aspirate"*. Normal reticulocyte index is 1-3%.
  RI = Reticulocyte Count X (Hb/Age and sex adjusted normal Hb level).

Reticulocyte Index: Reflects bone marrow activity and is also known as *"Poor man's Bone Marrow Aspirate"*.

Reticulocytosis (Increased RBC production)	Reticulocytopenia (Decreased RBC production)
*Criteria Reticulocyte Index > 3% Reticulocyte Count > 1.5%	*Criteria Reticulocyte Index < 1% Reticulocyte Count < 0.5%
Conditions • Acute blood loss or hemorrhage • Postsplenectomy • Microangiopathic Anemia • Autoimmune Hemolytic Anemia • Hemoglobinopathy (Sickle cell anemia and Thalassemia) • Post anemia Treatment like Folate Supplementation, Iron Supplementation and vitamin B$_{12}$ Supplementation.	**Conditions** • Aplastic anemia • Bone marrow infiltration • Bone marrow suppression (Sepsis/Chemotherapy radiotherapy) • Blood transfusion • Liver disease • Disordered RBC maturation (Iron, B$_{12}$, Folate Deficiency, Hypothyroidism, Sideroblastic Anemia or Anemia of Chronic Disease)

Reticulocytes are stained in living state in vitro so staining with dyes like *brilliant cresyl blue and new methylene* blue is referred to as **supravital staining**.

ANEMIAS

Anemia is defined as any reduction below normal limits of the total circulating red cell mass which is characterized by the clinical features of pallor of skin and nails, dizziness, palpitations, lethargy and fatigue.

Some of the important terms used in context of anemias are as follows:

- **MCV (Mean cell volume):** It is the average volume (in femtolitres) of a red blood cell (normal value is 82-96 fl). If the value of MCV is less than 80 fl, RBCs are called *microcytic* and if the MCV is more than 100 fl, RBCs are called *macrocytic*.
- **MCH (Mean corpuscular hemoglobin):** Average mass of hemoglobin (in picograms) per red blood cell is MCH. *Normal value is 27-33 pg.*
- **MCHC (Mean corpuscular hemoglobin concentration):** MCHC is average concentration of hemoglobin in a given volume of packed red blood cells. *Normal value is 33-37g/dl.*
- **RDW (Red cell distribution width):** It is the coefficient of variation of size of RBCs. Normal value is 11.5-14.5. The important point to be kept in mind is that RDW is an *indicator of anisocytosis*.
- Normal RBCs have *central pallor of around a third of the diameter* (normochromic). If the color is decreased which means pallor more than one-third, the RBCs are called *hypochromic* and if color is increased (central pallor is lost), the RBCs are called *hyperchromic*.

RDW (Red cell distribution width): is an indicator of **anisocytosis**.

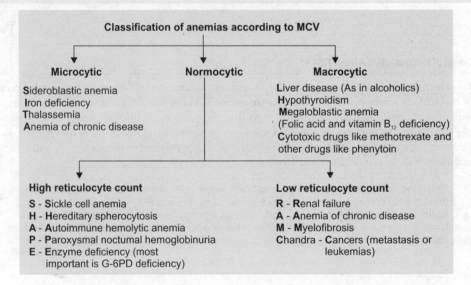

Classification of anemias according to MCV

Microcytic
Sideroblastic anemia
Iron deficiency
Thalassemia
Anemia of chronic disease

Normocytic

Macrocytic
Liver disease (As in alcoholics)
Hypothyroidism
Megaloblastic anemia
(Folic acid and vitamin B$_{12}$ deficiency)
Cytotoxic drugs like methotrexate and other drugs like phenytoin

High reticulocyte count
S - Sickle cell anemia
H - Hereditary spherocytosis
A - Autoimmune hemolytic anemia
P - Paroxysmal noctunal hemoglobinuria
E - Enzyme deficiency (most important is G-6PD deficiency)

Low reticulocyte count
R - Renal failure
A - Anemia of chronic disease
M - Myelofibrosis
Chandra - Cancers (metastasis or leukemias)

Anemia and Red Blood Cells

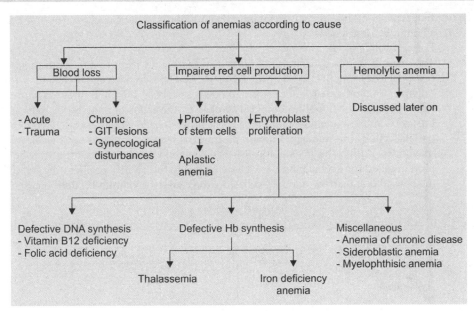

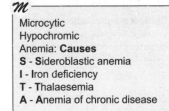

Microcytic
Hypochromic
Anemia: **Causes**
S - **S**ideroblastic anemia
I - **I**ron deficiency
T - **T**halaesemia
A - **A**nemia of chronic disease

Macrocytic
Anemia: **Causes**
L - **L**iver disease (As in alcoholics)
H - **H**ypothyroidism
M - **M**egaloblastic anemia (Folic acid and vitamin B_{12} deficiency)
C - **C**ytotoxic drugs like methotrexate and other drugs like phenytoin.

A. BLOOD LOSS

Blood loss causes decrease in hematocrit resulting in compensatory increased release of erythropoietin from the renal juxtaglomerular cells. Erythropoietin stimulates increased bone marrow activity. However, the *earliest change* in the peripheral blood is *leucocytosis* (caused by increased mobilization from the marginal pools) followed by reticulocytosis and thrombocytosis. Chronic blood loss is usually due to GIT lesions and gynecological disturbances.

B. IMPAIRED RBC PRODUCTION

1. DUE TO DECREASED ERYTHROPOIESIS

This category of anemias may result from the defective DNA synthesis due to vitamin B_{12} or folic acid deficiency (called megaloblastic anemia) or impaired heme synthesis due to iron deficiency.

a. Megaloblastic Anemia

The chief feature in this anemia is impaired DNA synthesis resulting in delayed mitosis while RNA and protein synthesis is not impaired. This leads to *nuclear/cytoplasmic asynchrony* which affects all proliferating cell lines particularly cells of bone marrow and GIT cells. The chief findings are a *hypercellular bone marrow* with megaloblasts in the bone marrow along with presence of abnormal granulocytic precursors (*giant metamyelocyte and band forms*) and *large megakaryocytes* with bizarre multilobated nuclei. The presence of *ineffective erythropoiesis* can result in *pancytopenia* associated with features of hemolytic anemia including jaundice and increased levels of serum bilirubin and LDH enzyme. In the peripheral smear, there is pancytopenia with presence of macrocytes (RBCs having MCV >100 fl) lacking a central pallor. There is characteristically presence of **large and hypersegmented neutrophils** (neutrophils having **> 5 lobes**). The *earliest manifestation* of megaloblastic anemia is *presence of hypersegmented neutrophils*. **Diagnosis is made if even a single neutrophil with ≥ 6 lobes is seen or > 5% neutrophils with 5 lobes are seen.**

*Earliest change in the peripheral blood after acute blood loss is **leucocytosis** followed by reticulocytosis and thrombocytosis.*

Note:
- **Triad** of megaloblastic anemia includes **oval macrocytes, Howell Jolly bodies and hypersegmented neutrophils.**
- MCHC is **not elevated** because hemoglobin increases proportionately to the increased volume of the RBCs.

The two main causes of this anemia are vitamin B_{12} and folic acid deficiency.

(i) Vitamin B_{12} deficiency

Normal vitamin B_{12} metabolism

The vitamin B_{12} (or cobalamin) is present in the bound form (bound with dietary proteins) in the diet. It is freed by the action of pepsin in stomach and then binds with salivary proteins called *R-binders* (also known as cobalaphilins). In the duodenum, this cobalamin-cobalaphilin complex is broken by the action of pancreatic proteases. Free cobalamin now binds with the intrinsic factor (*Castle's factor*) secreted from the parietal cells of the stomach. Vitamin B_{12}-intrinsic factor complex is *taken by the ileal enterocytes*. Within the intestinal cells, the cobalamin gets bound with a transport protein called transcobalamin II which delivers it to the rapidly proliferating cells of the body (bone marrow and GIT cells). So, the causes of vitamin B_{12} deficiency can be:

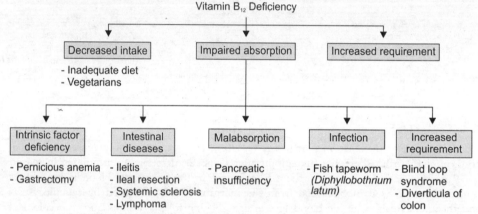

Biochemical functions of vitamin B_{12}

- It is required for the conversion of *homocysteine to methionine*
- It is also involved in the conversion of *methylmalonyl CoA to succinyl CoA* which is required for the formation of normal neuronal lipids. So, any deficiency of vitamin B_{12} results in neurological features. Also, there are increased levels of methylmalonic acid in the serum and urine of the patient with deficiency of this vitamin.

Pernicious anemia

It is an autoimmune disorder against parietal cells of the stomach by auto-reactive T cells resulting in chronic atrophic gastritis and parietal cells loss (responsible for decreased intrinsic factor production). The antibodies which are present in the patients are:

- Type I antibodies (most common): Block binding of vitamin B_{12} to IF (in 75% patients).
- Type II antibodies: Prevent cobalamin-IF binding with ileal receptors.
- Type III antibodies: formed against the α and β subunits of gastric proton pump (seen in 90% patients but not specific as it also seen in idiopathic chronic gastritis).

It is also associated with other autoimmune disorders like autoimmune thyroiditis and adrenalitis.

Morphology

The principal organs affected are the bone marrow, GIT and CNS which show the following features:

Bone marrow

Megaloblasts, hypersegmented neutrophils and precursors of granulocytes along with megakaryocytes are seen.

Earliest manifestation of megaloblastic anemia is presence of **hypersegmented neutrophils**.

MCHC is **not elevated** in megaloblastic anemia because hemoglobin increases proportionately to the increased volume of the RBCs.

Vitamin B_{12}-intrinsic factor complex is taken by the **ileal enterocytes**.

Concept

Vitamin B_{12}
- It is required for the conversion of *homocysteine to methionine*.
- It is also involved in the conversion of **methylmalonyl CoA to succinyl CoA** which is required for the formation of normal neuronal lipids. So, any deficiency of vitamin B_{12} results in neurological features.

GIT
There is presence of shiny and *"beefy" tongue* due to atrophic glossitis, almost complete loss of parietal cells and replacement of gastric mucosa by mucus secreting goblet cells *(intestinalization)*.

CNS
There is principally demyelination of the *dorsal and lateral spinal cord tracts* which can also be associated with degenerative changes in the posterior root ganglia and peripheral nerves in severe deficiency cases. Latter can result in involvement of both motor and sensory pathways. The combined involvement of the axons in the ascending tracts of posterior column and the descending pyramidal tract is a characteristic feature of vitamin B$_{12}$ deficiency giving the term as *subacute combined degeneration of the spinal cord*.

Clinical Features

They are as follows:
- Megaloblastic anemia
- Pancytopenia (Leucopenia with hypersegmented neutrophils, thrombocytopenia)
- Jaundice due to ineffective hematopoiesis and peripheral hemolysis
- Neurological features due to posterolateral spinal tract involvement.

Laboratory tests

- Serum antibodies against intrinsic factor are present.
- *Achlorhydria even after histamine stimulation*.
- Increased serum levels of methylmalonic acid and homocysteine.
- **Schilling test:** It is performed to distinguish between different causes of vitamin B$_{12}$ deficiency.

(ii) *Folic acid deficiency*

Megaloblastic anemia caused due to folic acid deficiency is clinically indistinguishable from vitamin B$_{12}$ deficiency anemia. However, folic acid deficiency is **NOT** associated with neurological abnormalities.

b. **Due to Defective Hemoglobin Synthesis**

(i) **Iron deficiency**

It is the *commonest cause of anemia worldwide*.

Normal iron metabolism

The metabolism of iron can be divided in the following headings:

Absorption

Iron is present in two forms in the food: heme and nonheme iron. The iron is absorbed more completely from the heme form (present in the nonvegetarian food) as compared to nonheme form. The factors affecting absorption of iron include:

Factors increasing absorption	Factors decreasing absorption
• Ferrous form (Fe^{2+})	• Ferric form (Fe^{3+})
• Acid (HCl) in the stomach	• Achlorhydria (absence of HCl secretion)
• Ascorbic acid	• Alkaline food (pancreatic secretions)
• Amino acid and sugars in the food	• Phytates, tannates and phosphates in diet
• Iron deficiency	• Iron overload
• Physiological conditions (pregnancy and hypoxia)	• Tetracyclines and EDTA
	• Inflammatory disorders

Iron is *absorbed primarily from the duodenum* in the ferrous form. It is transported inside the enterocytes by an apical transporter called DMT1 (Divalent Metal Transporter 1) and from here, it enters the plasma by two basal membrane transporters **(ferroportin and hephaestin)**. A fraction of ferrous iron gets converted into ferric state by intracellular oxidation. Most of the iron absorbed from the gut is lost because of mucosal lining shedding whereas in increased requirements it is absorbed in a greater percentage.

The combined involvement of the axons in the **ascending tracts of posterior column** and the **descending pyramidal tract** is a characteristic feature of vitamin B$_{12}$ deficiency giving the term as **subacute combined degeneration of the spinal cord**.

Schilling test: It is performed to distinguish between different causes of vitamin B$_{12}$ deficiency. It is **NOT USED** for the diagnosis of vitamin B$_{12}$ deficiency.

Diphyllobothrium latum is associated with megaloblastic anemia^Q

Ankylostoma duodenale is associated with *iron deficiency anemia*^{Q}.

Megaloblastic anemia caused due to folic acid deficiency is **NOT** associated with neurological abnormalities.

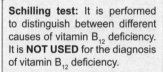

Concept

Pernicious anemia is associated with increased risk of **gastric cancer** and increased chances of **atherosclerosis** and **thrombosis** (because of elevated homocysteine levels).

CONCEPT

A regulatory protein called **hepcidin** regulates the absorption of iron from the gut. In case of iron depletion the level of this negative regulatory protein is decreased thereby increasing the absorption of iron and vice versa. **Mutation** of the gene coding for hepcidin is implicated in the causation of **hemochromatosis.**

Transport and storage of iron

From the enterocytes, the absorbed iron is transferred to a plasma protein called **transferrin** that delivers it to different cells of the body expressing high levels of transferrin receptors on their surface. These cells include *hepatocytes and the developing erythroblasts* in the bone marrow. The serum transferrin saturation is an indicator of serum iron concentration. Normally, transferrin is 33% saturated (one-third saturation) with iron. Since, the serum transferrin concentration is nearly 300-350 µg/dl (also called as total iron binding capacity or TIBC), the normal serum iron levels are in the range of 100-120 µg/dl. The iron which is not immediately required by the cells is stored in the form of **ferritin** which is a protein iron complex present in all the tissues especially liver, spleen and bone marrow. It is the *ferric form of iron which is present in ferritin.* A small amount of ferritin is also present in the plasma which is derived from the storage pools of the body iron; so, **serum ferritin is an indicator of body iron stores.** Intracellular iron is converted into hemosiderin which stains positively with potassium ferrocyanide giving a positive Prussian blue stain.

The normal requirement of iron in the diet is nearly 1 mg/d. The causes of iron deficiency anemia include the following:

Dietary lack	Impaired absorption	Increased requirement	Chronic blood loss
• Infants • Children • Low socio-economic status • Elderly	• Steatorrhea • Sprue • Chronic diarrhea • Gastrectomy	• Growing infants and children • Pregnant females • Premenopausal women	• GIT (peptic ulcer, gastric cancer, hemorrhoids, hookworm disease) • Urinary tract (renal, pelvic or bladder cancers) • Genital tract (uterine cancer, menorrhagia)

Features of Iron Deficiency Anemia

It is characterized by the following stages:

Stage I or stage of negative iron balance

This is a stage characterized by decreased amount of storage iron manifesting as decreased serum ferritin concentration and reduced amount of bone marrow iron staining with Prussian blue stain. *The serum iron and red cell protoporphyrin levels are absolutely normal.* Though TIBC is marginally increased, the *red cell indices and morphology are normal.*

Stage II or stage of iron deficient erythropoeisis

This is a stage of reduced circulating iron in addition to decrease storage form of iron. So, this stage is characterized by deficient iron stores, *reduced serum ferritin, decreased % saturation of serum transferrin and increased TIBC.* The *red cell morphology is normal.*

Stage III or stage of iron deficiency anemia

It is characterized by all features of stage II and in addition *abnormal morphology of the red cells,* i.e. the presence of microcytic and hypochromic cells.

Clinical features include fatigue, impaired growth and development, pica (eating noedible substances like mud, etc. in children), koilonychia (angular or spoon shaped nails), angular stomatitis (ulceration at the angle of mouth), dysphagia (as in Plummer Vinson syndrome) and palpitations (because of hyperdynamic circulation which can even precipitate congestive heart failure).

Iron is absorbed primarily from the **duodenum** in the **ferrous** form.

Absorbed iron is transferred to a plasma protein called transferrin.

Each molecule of **transferrin** can transport **two** molecules of iron to the desired areas.

Iron is stored in **ferritin** in the **ferric** form.

Most of the body's iron is contained in **hemoglobin** and *not ferritin.*

Serum ferritin is an *indicator* of body **iron stores**.

Peripheral blood
Microcytic and hypochromic red cells with slight reticulocytosis whereas TLC is normal. Usually, microcytosis is seen before appearance of hypochromia. Poikilocytosis is seen in form of small and elongated red cells called *pencil cells*. It is also characteristic feature of this disease. There is increased red cell distribution width also.

Bone marrow
Hypercellular bone marrow (having increased erythroid progenitors) with depleted bone marrow iron stores. • **Serum** *ferritin and serum iron are decreased whereas serum transferrin and TIBC are increased.* • **Red cell protoporphyrin levels** *are increased* because there is decrease in the availability of heme (due to reduced iron availability) resulting in elevated free erythrocytic protoporphyrin levels. RBC free protoporphyrin is normally 30-50 µg/dl whereas its value reaches > 200 µg/dl in iron deficiency anemia.

The normal requirement of iron in the diet is nearly **1 mg/d**.

The treatment of anemia is with the help of either oral or parenteral iron therapy the response of which is clinically assessed with the reticulocyte count on **about 8th - 9th day** which demonstrates reticulocytosis.

Differential diagnosis of microcytic hypochromic anemia

Tests	Iron deficiency	Inflammation	Thalassemia	Sideroblastic anemia
Peripheral smear	Micro/hypo	Normal micro/hypo	Micro/hypo with targeting	Variable
SI	< 30	< 50	Normal to high	Normal to high
TIBC	> 360	< 300	Normal	Normal
Percent TS	< 10	10-20	30-80	30-80
Ferritin(mcg/L)	< 15	30-200	50-300	50-300
Hemoglobin pattern	Normal	Normal	Abnormal	Normal

SI, serum iron; TIBC, total iron-binding capacity; TS, transferrin saturation.

In **iron deficiency anemia, microcytosis** is seen *before* appearance of *hypochromia*.

(*ii*) Thalassemia
It is discussed in detail with other hemolytic diseases.

There are many indices to differentiate between iron deficiency anemia (IDA) and beta-thalassemia (BT):

Index	Formula	Value for Iron deficiency anemia	Value for beta-thalassemia
Mentzer index	MCV/RBC count	> 13	< 13
Shine and Lal index	MCV^2 X MCH X 0.01	> 1530	< 1530
England and Fraser index	MCV – RBC – (5 X Hb) – 5.19	> 0	< 0
Srivastava index	MCH/RBC	> 3.8	< 3.8
Green and king index	MCV^2 X RDW X Hb/100	> 65	< 65
Red Cell Distribution Width index	MCV X RDW/RBC	> 220	< 220

TIBC levels at
Top = **I**ron deficiency (In iron deficiency anemia, TIBC is raised)
Bottom = **C**hronic disease (In Anemia of Chronic Disease, TIBC is low).

a. **Miscellaneous**
i. **Anemia of Chronic Disease (AOCD)**
It is characterized by the *decreased utilization of iron* from the storage from of iron, i.e. ferritin. In chronic inflammatory conditions, there is increased secretion of cytokines like IL-1, TNF, IFN-γ, etc. that cause release of the ***protein hepcidin*** because of which release of iron from the storage pool is inhibited. This result in the high serum ferritin levels, reduced TIBC, reduced % transferrin saturation and decreased serum iron levels.

Anemia of chronic disease is caused by **hepcidin**.

Anemia and Red Blood Cells

- In the **peripheral blood smear** there is presence of microcytic and hypochromic red cells.
- In the **bone marrow** there is absence of hypercellularity because of inhibition of erythropoetin secretion by renal cells due to the action of cytokines like IL-1, etc.
- Common clinical conditions having AOCD include diseases like rheumatoid arthritis, regional enteritis, osteomyelitis, lung abscess and cancers like Hodgkin's lymphoma, carcinomas of breast and lung.

Mnemonic: During a chronic inflammation (microbial or RA)… the microbes want iron, so our body reacts by locking all of its iron within the macrophages and loosing the key
The good news is that the microbe does not get any iron… However, the bad news is that our body doesn't get iron either, which reduces the amount of heme (no iron, no heme), which reduces the amount of hemoglobin. hence, microcytic anemia.

Concept

Anemia of chronic disease is differentiated from iron deficiency anemia morphologically by the fact that **microcytosis follows hypochromia** *(microcytosis precedes hypochromia in IDA).*

Sideroblastic anemia is characterized by the presence of **ringed sideroblasts**.

There is increase in serum iron, serum ferritin, % transferrin saturation and free erythrocyte porphyrin whereas TIBC is decreased.

(ii) **Anemia due to marrow infiltration**

This type of anemia is caused due to *infiltration of the bone marrow* resulting in *myelophthisic anemia.* It is characterized by presence of immature erythroid and myeloid precursors in the blood (this is called as leukoerythroblastosis). Metastasis from cancers like breast, lung and prostate are the most common cause of marrow infiltration.

(iii) **Sideroblastic anemia**

Sideroblastic anemia is characterized by the *presence of ringed sideroblasts.* These are normoblasts having pin point iron granules (easily demonstrable with the help of Prussian blue dye) in the cytoplasm or perinuclear region. Sideroblastic anemia can be *hereditary* (due to decreased ALA synthase activity) *or acquired* (secondary to leukemias, myelodysplastic syndrome, alcoholism, copper deficiency, pyridoxine deficiency or lead poisoning). The pathogenesis of the diseases involves defective heme synthesis resulting in ineffective erythropoiesis which thereby contributes to iron overload.

- Peripheral smear is characterized by presence of *microcytic hypochromic cells* which also demonstrate the presence of anisopoikilocytosis. There is *increase in serum iron, serum ferritin, % transferrin saturation and free erythrocyte porphyrin whereas TIBC is decreased.*

Note: Abnormal sideroblasts are also seen in *thalassemia, megaloblastic anemia and hemolytic anemias.*

2. DUE TO DECREASED STEM CELLS PROLIFERATION

a. **Aplastic anemia**

This is a disorder characterized by marrow failure associated with pancytopenia (anemia, thrombocytopenia and leukopenia). The causes are:

Acquired	Inherited
• Primary stem cell defect • Irradiation • Viral infections [hepatitis (non A, non B , non C, non G), CMV, EBV, varicella zoster virus] • Chemical agents (alkylating agents, antimetabolites, benzene, chloramphenicol, phenylbutazone, arsenicals, insecticides like DDT, parathion)	• Fanconi anemia

It has been postulated that the etiological agents cause alteration in the stem cells thereby activating the T cells of the body against them resulting in destruction of the stem cells contributing to the pancytopenia.

Bone marrow aspiration in aplastic anemia reveals "dry tap".

The **bone marrow** biopsy shows it is characteristically hypocellular being replaced by fat cells (in contrast to aleukemic leukemia and myelodysplastic syndrome in which we have pancytopenia associated with hypercellular marrow) whereas *bone marrow aspiration reveals "dry tap".*

Clinical features are caused because of anemia (pallor, weakness and dyspnea), thrombocytopenia (petechiae) and neutropenia (recurrent infections). *Red cells are normocytic and normochromic.*

Characteristically, **splenomegaly is absent and reticulocytopenia is the rule.**

It is treated with either bone marrow transplantation (in young patients) or antithymocyte globulin (in old patients).

b. **Anemia of chronic disease (**has been discussed above)

c. **Anemia of renal failure**

It is characterized by inadequate release of erythropoetin resulting in development of anemia. The other contributory factors are:
- Iron deficiency secondary to increased bleeding tendency (seen in uremia)
- Extracorpuscular defect induced hemolysis

The severity of anemia is proportional to uremia and is usually managed with recombinant erythropoetin.

> Features of **Shwachman–Diamond syndrome** are exocrine pancreatic insufficiency, bone marrow dysfunction, skeletal abnormalities, **neutropenia** and short stature.

C. HEMOLYTIC ANEMIA

This type of anemia can be due to intracorpuscular or extracorpuscular defects.

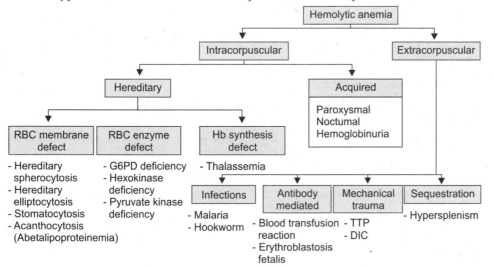

Hemolysis can result due to destruction of RBCs inside the circulation (intravascular) or outside the blood vessels (extravascular).

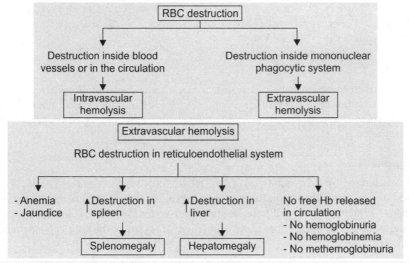

> **Haptoglobin followed by hemopexin** form the defense against free heme in the plasma.

Note: Serum haptoglobin decrease but not as much as in intravascular hemolysis.

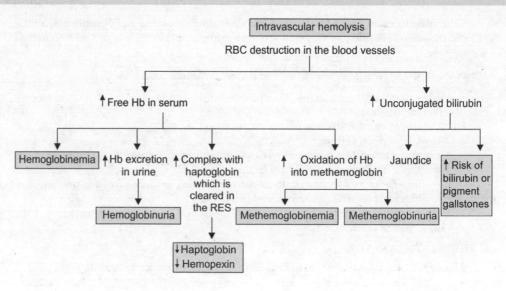

1. Hereditary Spherocytosis

Hereditary spherocytosis (HS), an **autosomal dominant**[Q] disorder, is an important cause of hemolytic anemia.

Normal RBC membrane skeleton

Normally, RBC membrane consists of a protein **spectrin**, which has *two subunits α and β*. This spectrin is attached to cell membrane at two sites. At head region, spectrin binds to ion transporter, band 3 of membrane with the help of ankyrin and band 4.2 whereas at the tail region, spectrin binds to glycophorin A of the membrane by protein 4.1 and actin.

> Mostly the mutations in HS are seen in head region most commonly in **ankyrin**[Q].

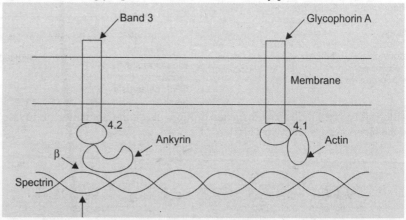

> **Maximum** amount of **H antigen: O** blood group

Mutations in these proteins can result in HS. Mostly the **mutations** are seen in head region **most commonly in ankyrin**[Q] [*Robbins 8th/e pg 642*] and the next common mutation is in band 3 (Anion channel). Rarely, the mutations can be seen in band 4.2 (Palladin), spectrin and glycophorin A.

Pathogenesis

> **Minimum** amount of **H antigen: AB** blood group

HS is characterized by *reduced life span of RBC* [10-20 days as compared to 120 days] and has increased osmotic fragility (the pathogenesis is explained above). The main clinical findings are *jaundice, splenomegaly and gallstones*. A characteristic feature of HS is **increase in MCHC**[Q] due to dehydration caused by loss of K⁺ and water. It is almost the *only condition where high MCHC is seen.*

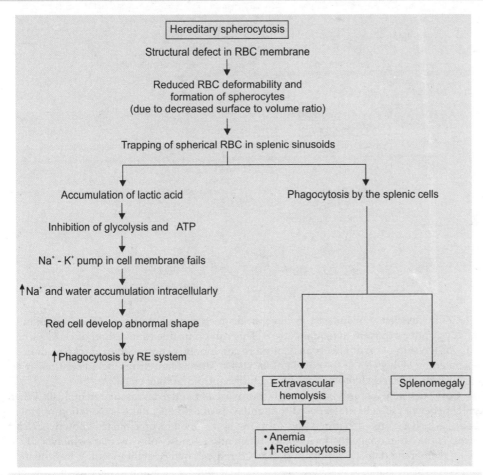

A *characteristic feature* of HS is increase in **MCHC**^Q due to dehydration caused by loss of K⁺ and water.

Note:
- *Mutations in a spectrin are most common cause of hereditary elliptocytosis* [65% cases] and β spectrin mutation is responsible for another 30% cases. Some of the cases of HE occur due to mutation in band 4.1.
- Please note that **spherocytosis** on peripheral smear is not pathognomic of HS because **autoimmune hemolytic anemias, infections/burns, ABO hemolytic disease (NOT with Rh hemolytic disease) of new born and G6PD deficiency can** also result in formation of spherocytes.
- Unlike hereditary spherocytosis, Autohemolysis in ABO HDN is not corrected by addition of **glucose**^Q

Osmotic fragility is **increased** in HS.

Pink test^Q is done to measure the osmotic fragility. **Splenectomy**^Q is almost always beneficial in HS. After splenectomy anemia is corrected but spherocytes will remain in blood. The vaccination against encapsulated organisms like pneumococccus and H. influenza is also must.

2. Glucose 6-Phosphate Dehydrogenase Deficiency (G-6PD Deficiency)

Abnormalities in the hexose monophosphate shunt or glutathione metabolism resulting from deficient or impaired enzyme function reduce the ability of red cells to protect themselves against oxidative injuries. This results in hemolytic disease. The most important of these is G6PD deficiency. Normal G6PD functioning is required to decrease oxidative damage to RBCs.

Most common mutation in **HS** is in **ankyrin** and in *HE* is in a *spectrin*.
To rememeber: S is not for S means spectrin is not in spherocytosis.

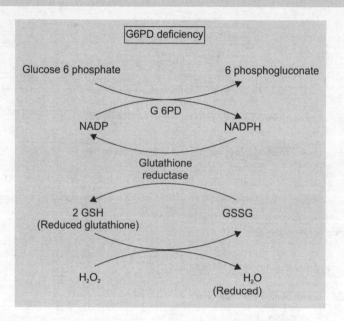

G6PD deficiency manifests in several distinct clinical patterns. Most common is hemolysis after exposure to oxidant stress. This can occur due to ingestion of certain *drugs* or foods (consumption of fava beans), or more commonly, exposure to oxidant free radicals generated by leukocytes in the course of *infections*. The oxidant drugs include antimalarials (e.g., primaquine and chloroquine), sulfonamides, nitrofurantoin, etc.

G6PD deficiency causes both episodic intravascular and extravascular hemolysis. When G6PD-deficient red cells are exposed to high levels of oxidants, there is oxidation of globin chains, which become denatured and form membrane-bound precipitates known as *Heinz bodies*. These can damage the membrane sufficiently to cause intravascular hemolysis. Less severe membrane damage results in decreased red cell deformability leading to formation of spherocytes or removal of membrane by the macrophages leading to the presence of "bite cells". Both **bite cells and spherocytes** are trapped in splenic circulation resulting in their removal by erythrophagocytosis.

> The episode is **self-limited**, as hemolysis stops when only the **younger red cells** remain (even if administration of an offending drug continues).

> Features of chronic hemolytic anemias like **splenomegaly** and **cholelithiasis** are **absent** because the hemolytic episodes occur intermittently.

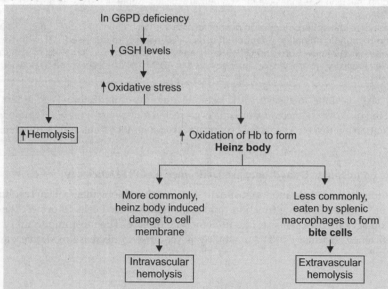

Acute intravascular hemolysis with anemia, hemoglobinemia, and hemoglobinuria usually begins 2 to 3 days following exposure of G6PD-deficient individuals to oxidants. Since only older red cells are at risk for lysis, the episode is *self-limited*, as **hemolysis stops when only**

the younger red cells remain. Reticulocytosis is seen in the recovery phase. The **features of chronic hemolytic anemias like splenomegaly and cholelithiasis are absent** because the hemolytic episodes occur intermittently.

3. Paroxysmal Nocturnal Hemoglobinuria

Paroxysmal nocturnal hemoglobinuria (PNH) is the **only hemolytic anemia caused by an acquired intrinsic defect in the cell membrane.** The stem cells of the bone marrow acquire *mutations in Phosphatidyl inositol glycan A (PIGA) gene, which is essential for the synthesis of the glycosylphosphatidyl inositol (GPI) anchor.* GPI is responsible for providing an anchor for cell membrane attachment of some proteins. These proteins are also required for inactivating the complement. The examples of these proteins include:

- Decay-accelerating factor or CD55
- Membrane inhibitor of reactive lysis, or CD59
- C8 binding protein

Out of the above mentioned proteins, *CD 59 is most important.* It is a potent inhibitor of C3 convertase, and thereby prevents spontaneous activation of the alternative complement pathway in vivo. These defects are not limited to red blood cells, as deficient platelets and granulocytes are also more sensitive to lysis by complement.

Clinical features include intravascular hemolysis with hemoglobinuria. The complement system is activated by acidotic conditions like exercise (accumulation of lactic acid) or sleep (due to decreased respiratory rate). Since the respiration decreases at night, so, patient experiences intermittent attacks (**paroxysmal**) of hemolysis at night (**nocturnal**) resulting in passage of red urine (**hemoglobinuria**) in the morning. The dysfunction of the GPI linked proteins on the platelets is responsible for the prothrombotic state. *Thrombosis is the leading cause of disease related death* in PNH patients as it can affect cerebral, hepatic or portal veins.

Diagnosis

- It is best made with **flow cytometry** in which there is presence of **bimodal distribution of the red cells** i.e. cells which are deficient in CD55/CD59 as well normal cells which are CD55+/CD59+.
- Other tests demonstrating increased susceptibility to the complement system which can be used for diagnosis include:
  1. *Ham's acidified serum test:* lysis of erythrocytes on addition of acidified serum.
  2. *Sucrose lysis test:* complement system is increased by the presence of sucrose.

4. Immune Hemolytic Anemias

Immune hemolytic anemias are caused because of the formation of anti-RBC antibodies.

Types of Immune Hemolytic Anemia

Warm antibody type	Cold antibody type
Mostly IgG^Q; rarely IgA	Mostly IgM^Q, rarely IgG
Causes	**Causes**
• Primary (Idiopathic) • **SLE^Q** , rheumatoid arthritis • **B cell** lymphoid neoplasms • Drugs (α-methyldopa, penicillin)	• Primary (Idiopathic) • **M**ycoplasma infection, • Infectious **M**ononucleosis • Lymphoid neoplasms • **Paroxysmal cold hemoglobinuria (IgG)**
Mechanism of hemolysis	**Mechanism of hemolysis**
Extravascular hemolysis (in spleen)	Extravascular hemolysis in cold agglutinin Intravascular hemolysis in cold hemolysins
The antibody does not usually fix complement, and is active at 37°C.	Antibodies reacts at 4-6°C, dissociate at 30°C or above

PNH is the **only hemolytic anemia** caused by an **acquired intrinsic defect** in the cell membrane.

The stem cells of the bone marrow acquire mutations in Phosphatidyl inositol glycan A (PIGA) gene.

The **triad** of **hemolysis, pancytopenia and thrombosis** is *unique to PNH.*

Thrombosis is the *leading cause of disease related death* in PNH.

PNH is best diagnosed with **flow cytometry** in which there is presence of **bimodal distribution** of the red cells.

Cold-antibody autoimmune hemolytic anemia (cold AIHA) is subdivided into two clinical categories based on the type of antibodies involved. These two types of cold antibodies are:

1. *Cold agglutinins*: these are monoclonal IgM antibodies that react at 4 to 6°C. They are called agglutinins because the IgM directed against the I antigen present on the RBCs can agglutinate red cells due to its large size (pentamer). In addition IgM can activate complement resulting in the cells being coated with C3b followed by **extravascular hemolysis**. Examples include *Mycoplasma* pneumonitits and *infectious monoucleosis*. Vascular obstruction by the red cell agglutination can produce Raynaud's pheonomenon, which is characterized by ischemia in the fingers when expose to the cold.

2. *Cold hemolysins*: these are seen in patients with *paroxysmal cold hemolglobinuria* (PCH). They are unique because they are *biphasic antierythrocyte autoantibodies*. These antibodies are IgG that is directed against the P blood group antigen. They are called biphasic because they attach to red cells and bind complement at 4°C but the complement activation takes place when the temperature is increased. This is followed by **intravascular hemolysis.** The antibody is called the **Donath-Landsteiner antibody** (previously associated with syphilis, but also with mycoplasma pneumonia measles, mumps, and ill defined viral and "flu" syndromes[Q].

3. **Microangiopathic hemolytic anemia (MAHA)**

MAHA is a microangiopathic subgroup of hemolytic anemia (anemia, loss of red blood cells through destruction) caused by factors in the small blood vessels. The endothelial layer of small vessels is damaged with resulting fibrin deposition and platelet aggregation. As red blood cells travel through these damaged vessels, they are fragmented resulting in intravascular hemolysis. It is identified by the finding of anemia and **schistocytes, "burr cells," "helmet cells," and "triangle cells"on microscopy (should be > 3/5000 cells) and these should have 1-3 sharp spicules.** It is associated with conditions like **DIC[Q] (most commonly)**, malignant hypertension, SLE, thrombotic thrombocytopenic purpura (TTP), hemolytic-uremic syndrome (HUS), and disseminated cancer.

4. **Hemoglobinopathies**
   - The normal hemoglobin is composed of *heme* (consisting of iron and protoporphyrin) *and globin* (having two pairs of polypeptide chains).
   - The adult hemoglobin (HbA) forms about 95-96% of total hemoglobin and is composed of two identical α and two β chains.
   - The other hemoglobin seen in the adults is HbA2 (normally less than 3.5% of total hemoglobin) consisting of two identical α and two δ chains.
   - The hemoglobin in the fetal life is HbF consisting of two identical α and two γ chains.

A. Sickle cell anemia

This is characterized by the presence of an abnormal type of hemoglobin called HbS. It results from a point mutation that causes the glutamic acid to be replaced by valine at the $\beta 6$ position of the globin chain. If the individual is homozygous, it is represented as HbSS (1 gene each from both the parents) whereas the heterozygous is HbAS (1 gene from one parent is for HbS and the other gene is for HbA). Heterozygotes are *protected against falciparum malaria*.

Mnemonic: Glutamic acid can **G**o and **V**aline is **W**elcome

Pathogenesis

When deoxygenated, HbS molecules becomes insoluble, undergoes aggregation and *polymerization* producing a sickle cell or holly leaf shape of the RBCs. Initially, this process is reversible (on getting oxygenated, the cells attain there normal shape) but repeated attacks of aggregation can cause irreversible sickling of the RBCs which also causes oxidative damage to the red cells.

Cold agglutinins: Are associated with **Mycoplasma** pneumonitits and **infectious mononucleosis**.

Paroxysmal cold hemolglobinuria (PCM) has the presence of **Donath-Landsteiner antibody**.

Microangiopathic hemolytic anemia **(MAHA)** is identified by the finding of anemia and **schistocytes, "burr cells," "helmet cells," and "triangle cells"** on microscopy.

HbA is $\alpha_2\beta_2$ (95-96%)
HbA$_2$ is $\alpha_2\beta_2$ (3-3.5%)
HbF is $\alpha_2\gamma_2$ (present in the fetal life). As gestational age increases, the γ chains are replaced by the β chains, resulting in formation of adult hemoglobin, HbA.

Anemia and Red Blood Cells

Reversible sickled cells exhibit increased adhesiveness within the microcirculation of organs with sluggish blood flow thereby causing episodes of hypoxia and infarction called as *vasoocclusive crisis or pain crisis*. Hemoglobin released from the lysed red cells causes inactivation of NO thereby increasing the severity of ischemia.

Irreversible sickled cells get sequestrated in the spleen thereby contributing to *extravascular hemolysis*.

Factors Affecting Sickling of the Hemoglobin

Amount of HbS (most important factor) and its interaction with other hemoglobins
The presence of relatively low concentration of HbS (25-40%) and the presence of HbA in heterozygotes prevents efficient HbS sickling thereby contributing to decreased severity of the disease in them. In comparison, the homozygotes have full blown disease. Other hemoglobins like *fetal hemoglobin (HbF) and HbC* (having a substitution of lysine for glutamic acid at β6 position) *have inhibitory effect* on the disease. HbF inhibits the polymerization of HbS, so, newborns do not manifest the disease till 5-6 months of age when their HbF levels fall. This finding is utilized in the management of the disease with hydroxyurea which actually increases the HbF concentration. HbC has increased tendency to aggregate than HbS so the disease is milder in patients with HbSC disease.

Hemoglobin concentration of the red cell
Hb concentration of the cell, i.e. MCHC affects polymerization to a great extent. Hence, intracellular dehydration which increases MCHC facilitates sickling and vaso-occlusion. On the other hand, in patients with thalassemia, there is reduced severity of the disease because these patients usually have low Hb concentration (due to reduced globin chain formation) in their RBCs.

Decrease in pH
Acidosis decreases the affinity of hemoglobin for oxygen, so, there is more deoxygenated hemoglobin and increased chances of sickling.

Duration of time red cells are exposed to decreased oxygen tension
Normal transit time for RBCs is not sufficient for significant aggregation of deoxygenated HbS to occur but in organs having slow or sluggish circulation, there is an increased chance of sickling. This is particularly important in organs like bone and spleen.

Clinical features

- Severe anemia results in *jaundice and pigment gallstone formation* and is associated with *reticulocytosis*. Vaso-occlusive crisis clinically manifests as painful episodes in affected organs of the body. In the bone, it presents as dactylitis or inflammation of the bones of hands and feet, so called *Hand foot syndrome*, increased chances of *Salmonella* osteomyelitis, avascular necrosis of femoral head, *fish mouth appearance of vertebra* (due to occlusion of vertebral arteries) and prominent cheek bones and *crew cut appearance of skull* (both because of extramedullary hematopoeisis).
- Other organs of the body may also be affected, e.g. lungs (*acute chest syndrome* characterized by cough, fever and chest pain), brain (seizures or stroke), skin (leg ulcers), penis (stagnation in corpora cavernosa leads to priapism) or spleen. In the initial stages, there is splenomegaly due to congestion and trapping of red cells in the vascular sinusoids (**Gamma gandy bodies;** consisting of *foci of fibrosis having iron or calcium salts* deposited in connective tissue are seen).
- In the later stages, hypoxia and infarction induced progressive shrinkage of the spleen results in reduced splenic mass that may be replaced by fibrous tissue called **autosplenectomy**. This also increases susceptibility to infection with capsulated organisms like *Hemophilus influenzae, Pneumococcus, etc.*
- Parvovirus infection can precipitate an attack of aplastic crisis also. Chronic anemia can cause hyperdynamic circulation resulting in cardiomegaly.

Peripheral smear shows anisopoikilocytosis, presence of sickle cells, **target cells**, polychromatophilia and ovalocytes. **Howell Jolly bodies** (composed of chromatin aggregates in red cells) are *seen particularly after autosplenectomy*. **ESR is low** because roleaux formation is not seen with sickle cells.

Sickling of hemoglobin affects its **solubility** and **NOT** its *function/stability/affinity*.

Sequestration crisis is the **most dangerous** crisis in sickle cell anemia because it can cause heart failure.

Vaso occlusive crisis are the **most common** type of crisis in sickle cell disease.

Sickle cell anemia shows splenomegaly and later **auto-splenectomy** because it can cause heart failure.

In most other causes of anemia, ESR is high **except** in sickle cell disease. *ESR is less is sickle cell disease*.

Management of sickle cell anemia is done by ensuring that the patient should be properly hydrated and with the help of drugs like **hydroxyurea** (it increases HbF and NO and acts as an anti-inflammatory agent), **5'azacytidine**, etc.

Diagnosis is done with the help of the following:

- **Sickling test**: Sickling is induced by a reducing agent like **2% metabisulfite or dithionite** to blood. However, this test cannot differentiate between sickle cell disease and sickle cell trait.
- **Hb electrophoresis:** It is carried out on a cellulose acetate membrane (pH 8.6). HbS is slower moving as compared to normal HbA, so, heterozygotes show 2 bands of hemoglobin.
- **HbF estimation** (by alkali denaturation method) shows HbF to be 10-30% in homozygotes.
- **Prenatal genetic testing** can be done using the enzyme **MstII endonuclease**. **Chorionic villus sampling** at **10-12 weeks of gestation** is used to estimate fetal DNA abnormality.

B. Thalassemia

It is a group of autosomal recessive inherited disorders characterized by decreased synthesis of either α or β globin chain of HbA. It is the most common *type of hemoglobinopathy in the world*. β and α thalassemia is caused by deficient synthesis of β and α chains respectively.

The a globin chain is coded by a gene on chromosome 16 and the gene for β globin chain is located on chromosome 11. The clinical features therefore result from deficiency of one chain and the relative excess of the other chain.

> **Thalassemia** is the *most common* type of *hemoglobinopathy* in the world.

Pathogenesis of β thalassemia

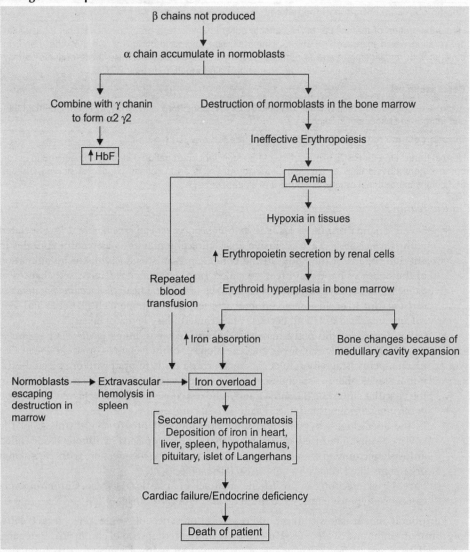

i. **β thalassemia syndromes**

This type of thalassemia is caused by point mutations. These are of two types:

1. *β⁰ thalassemia* – Characterized by total absence of β chains in the homozygous state.
2. *β⁺ thalassemia* – Characterized by reduced synthesis of β chains in the homozygous state.

Mutations can be caused due to the following mechanisms:

a. *Promoter region mutation*: Causes reduced transcription of the β chains leading to β⁺ thalassemia.
b. *Chain terminator mutations*: Either creation of a stop codon in exon or frameshift mutation inducing a downstream stop codon leads to premature chain termination resulting in β° thalassemia.
c. *Splicing mutation*: They are the most common *cause* of thalassemia resulting in unspliced mRNA being degraded in the nucleus leading to the development of either β⁺ thalassemia or β° thalassemia.

> **Splicing mutations:** Are the *most common* cause of β **thalassemia**.

Clinical features

Clinically β, thalassemia is of three types: thalassemia major, thalassemia intermedia and thalassemia minor.

a. **Thalassemia major** (also called **Cooley anemia**): It is seen in individuals *homozygous for the β thalassemia genes* (β⁺/β⁺or β°/β°); these individuals have a severe *transfusion dependent anemia* which manifests at usually 6 to 9 months after birth. There is presence of prominent frontal and cheek bones, hepatosplenomegaly (due to extramedullary hemopoiesis), jaundice, increased risk of pigment stones and endocrinological manifestations as delayed puberty (due to GH deficiency), bone fractures (hypoparathyroidism) and/or diabetes mellitus (iron in islet of Langerhans).

Peripheral smear shows moderate to *severe anemia, anisocytosis, microcytic hypochromic red cells, target cells, nucleated red cells, basophilic stippling, Howell Jolly bodies*, etc. There is reticulocytosis and **left shift in the leukocytes**. Since β chains are not produced but γ chains are synthesized normally, **HbF is markedly increased and is the major constituent of red cells (90%).** MCH, MCV and MCHC are reduced.

Bone marrow is hypercellular with erythroid hyperplasia causing **reversal of normal M:E ratio** (it becomes 1:3 in thalassemia). Pink inclusions are seen in the normoblasts (caused by α chain accumulation). Widening of the diploe gives rise to *crew cut appearance* on skull X-ray.

> **Thalassemia major** (also called **Cooley anemia**): is a severe transfusion dependent anemia in this condition **HbF** is **markedly increased**.

b. **Thalassemia minor or trait:** It is seen in individuals heterozygous with one β thalassemia gene and one normal gene (β⁺/β or β°/β). It is more common clinically than the major variant and offers resistance against falciparum malaria. These patients are usually asymptomatic with only mild anemia.

Peripheral smear shows *microcytic, hypochromic cells with basophilic stippling and presence of target cells*. MCH, MCV and MCHC are reduced. The levels of **HbA₂ are characteristically elevated** (It is normally 3-3.5% but in thalassemia trait, the level is *3.6-8%*; this is a *diagnostic feature* of this disease). HbF is mildly increased (5%).

> **Thalassemia minor** (also called **Thalassemia trait**): HbA₂ is characteristically elevated.

NESTROF Test

A Screening test used for this condition is **N**aked **E**ye **S**ingle **T**ube **R**ed cell **O**smotic **F**ragility **(NESTROF)** test. In this test 2 blood samples (1of a normal person serving as control and 1 of patient) are added to 2 tubes with 0.35% saline. After 30 min a white paper with a black line is placed behind both the tubes. The RBCs in control sample undergo hemolysis so the black line is visible whereas cells in thalassemia trait are resistant so black line is not clearly visible.

> Naked Eye Single Tube Red cell Osmotic Fragility (NESTROF) is a **Screening test** and *NOT a diagnostic* test used for this condition.

c. **Thalassemia intermedia:** The patients show anemia but do not require transfusions. The features of the disease are intermediate between the two other types of thalassemia discussed above.

Important Investigations

- Apart from the above mentioned investigations, the thalassemia patients must undergo **Hb electrophoresis** to determine the nature of the hemoglobin present. **HbA$_2$^{Q}** is characteristically elevated in a patient of **thalassemia minor^Q**.
- Globin chain synthesis can be studied by calculating α: β **ratio**. It is normally 1:1 but in thalassemia, it is **5-30:1.**
- **Alkali denaturation method^Q** is done to determine the concentration of HbF which is relatively resistant to denaturation by strong alkali like NaOH/KOH as compared to HbA. In the RBCs, HbF is shown by acid elution method (**Kleihauer's cytochemical method^Q**).

> **HbF** is shown by acid elution method (**Kleihauer's** cytochemical method^Q).

Concept

- **Qualitative** estimation of HbF is done by **Apt test^Q**
- **Quantitive** estimation of HbF is done by **Kleihauer test^Q**

Management of these patients is done with **blood transfusions** (to maintain hemoglobin concentration), **iron chelators** like desferrioxamine, deferiprone and defrasirox (to chelate excessive iron) and **bone marrow transplantation** (if HLA matched donor is available).

Preventive measures include marriage counseling and chorionic villus sampling at 9-10 weeks followed by PCR analysis. All antenatal females with Hb <11 gm% should undergo NESTROF test.

ii. α **thalassemia syndromes**

This type of thalassemia is **caused by gene deletion^Q**. These are of four types.

In the **silent carrier** state, the patients are clinically asymptomatic. The clinical picture in β-**thalassemia trait** is similar to that discussed in β-thalassemia minor which means there is presence of microcytosis, minimal or no anemia, and no abnormal physical signs. **HbH^Q** is a major cause of anemia, as precipitates of oxidized HbH form in older red cells, which are then removed by splenic macrophages. This produces a moderately severe anemia resembling β-thalassemia intermedia. **Hydrops fetalis** is the *most dangerous form of a-thalassemia* and severe tissue anoxia leads to intrauterine fetal death. The fetus shows severe pallor, generalized edema, and massive hepatosplenomegaly.

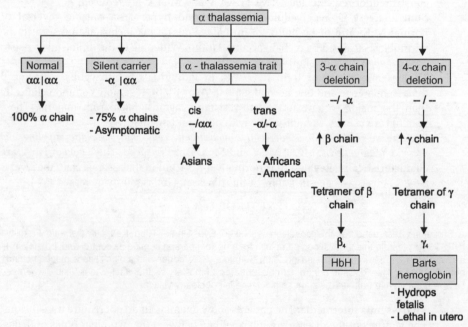

(side tab) Anemia and Red Blood Cells

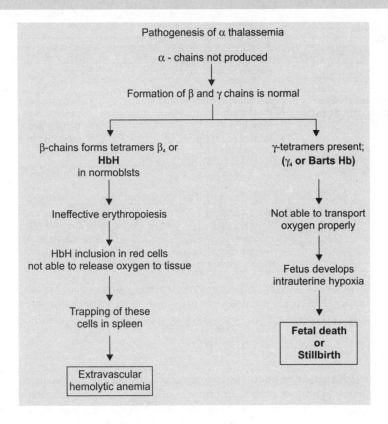

SPECIAL TOPICS FOR EXAMS

Massive Blood Transfusion

Massive Transfusion is defined as the need to transfuse from one to two times the patient's normal blood volume. In a normal adult, this is equivalent to 10-20 units.

Complications of massive blood transfusion are:

- *Coagulopathy:* Most common cause of bleeding after massive transfusion is dilutional thrombocytopenia.
- *Citrate toxicity:* Citrate in the transfused blood may bind calcium. Clinically, significant hypocalcemia usually do not develop because citrate is metabolized by liver to bicarbonate. In hepatic dysfunction, this effect can be pronounced.
- *Hypothermia*: Massive transfusion is an absolute indication for warming of all blood and fluids to body temperature to avoid hypothermia.
- *Acid Base Imbalance:* Most common abnormality is metabolic alkalosis. It results from conversion of citrate (present in stored blood) and lactate (accumulated due to hypoperfusion) to bicarbonate.
- Serum potassium can rise because K^+ concentration in stored blood increases steadily with time.

Anticoagulants

Agents	Trisodium EDTA	3.2% Trisodium Citrate	Heparin	Potassium Oxalate
Mechanism of action	Remove calcium	Remove calcium	Activation of antithrombin III	Binds calcium
Preferred Uses	• **Blood cell counts and morphology**[Q]	• **Platelet studies**[Q] • **Coagulation studies**[Q] • **ESR**[Q]	• **Osmotic fragility test**[Q] • **WBC Functional or immunophenotyping**[Q] • **Red cell testing**[Q]	• **Anticoagulant (not preferred because labile factors are unstable in oxalate)**
Advantages	Complete anticoagulation with **minimal morphologic and physical effects on the cell**	Preserves the labile coagulation factors	Does **not** affect shape and size	Cheap Easily available
Disadvantages			• Not suitable for blood counts because it cannot inhibit platelet and leucocyte clumping • *Bluish discoloration* to blood smear slide on applying Wright Giemsa stain.	• **Distorts cell morphology** • Shrinks red cell size, so, **not used for hematocrit estimation**

- **Anticoagulated blood** may be **stored at 4°C**[Q] for **24 hour period** without significantly altering cell counts or cellular morphology but hematologic analysis should be done as soon as possible.
- **Any anticoagulant**[Q] can be used for collecting blood for **Flow cytometry**[Q].

Splenectomy

- Indications of splenectomy include traumatic or iatrogenic splenic rupture (most common), symptom control in patient with massive splenomegaly, correction of cytopenias in patients with hypersplenism, staging of patients with Hodgkin's disease, treatment of hairy cell leukemia and prolymphocytic leukemia.
- The **only contraindication to splenectomy is the presence of marrow failure**, in which the enlarged spleen is the only source of hematopoietic tissue.
- Most serious consequence of splenectomy is increased susceptibility to capsulated bacterial infections like *Streptococcus. Pneumoniae, H. influenzae* and some gram-negative enteric organisms.
- Increased susceptibility to Babesisis (intra-RBC parasite) is also noted in splenectomized patients
- Pneumococcal vaccine and vaccine against *Neisseria meningitides* are recommended for patients in whom elective splenectomy is planned. *H. influenza* type B vaccine may also be given.
- **Acute manifestations** of splenectomy include *leukocytosis* (up to 25000/µl) and *thrombocytosis* (up to 1×10^6/µl) but return back to normal levels within 2-3 weeks.

Chronic Manifestations of splenectomy include:
- Anisocytosis and poikilocytosis
- Howell-Jolly bodies (nuclear remnants)
- Heinz bodies (denatured hemoglobin)
- Basophilic stippling
- Target cells
- Pappenheimer bodies (contain sideroblastic granules)
- Irregular contracted red cells. (WBC count usually normal but there may be mild lymphocytosis and monocytosis. Thrombocytosis persists in about 30% of cases.
- Occasional nucleated erythrocyte in peripheral blood.

When such erythrocyte abnormalities are seen without splenectomy, splenic infiltration by tumor should be suspected.

SPLENOSIS: It is the presence of multiple rests of spleen tissue not connected to portal circulation it occur in patients with splenic rupture causing peritoneal seeding of splenic fragments. This condition is similar to endometriosis (presence of endometrial tissue at non-endometrial sites).

MULTIPLE CHOICE QUESTIONS

RBC: GENERAL ASPECTS

1. **Which of the following is associated with an intrinsic defect in the RBC membrane?** *(AIIMS May 2012)*
   (a) Autoimmune hemolytic anemia
   (b) Hereditary spherocytosis
   (c) Microangiopathic haemolytic anemia
   (d) Thermal injury causing anemia

2. **Which of the following is not a stem cell of the bone marrow?** *(AI 2012)*
   (a) Lymphoblast (b) Myeloblast
   (c) Myoblast (d) Normoblast

3. **Which of the following surface glycoproteins is most often expressed in human hematopoietic stem cell?**
   (a) CD 22 *(AIIMS May 2008)*
   (b) CD 40
   (c) CD 15
   (d) CD 34

4. **Reticulocytosis is seen in all except:**
   (a) P.N.H. *(AIIMS May 2007)*
   (b) Hemolysis
   (c) Nutritional anemia
   (d) Dyserythropoietic syndrome

5. **Which of these are seen on Romanowsky stain:**
   (a) Reticulocytes *(PGI Dec 2004)*
   (b) Basophilic stippling
   (c) Heinz bodies
   (d) Howell-Jolly bodies
   (e) Cabot ring

6. **Which of the following surface glycoproteins is most often expressed in human hematopoietic stem cell?**
   (a) CD22 *(Delhi PG 2010)*
   (b) CD40
   (c) CD15
   (d) CD34

7. **Inappropriate erythropoietin level is found in all except** *(UP 2001)*
   (a) Renal cell carcinoma
   (b) Lung disease
   (c) High altitude
   (d) Benign liver tumor

8. **The size of the red blood cells is measured by:**
   (a) MCV *(UP 2007)*
   (b) MCHC
   (c) ESR
   (d) MCH

9. **Anemia which is associated with pancytopenia is**
   (a) Hemolytic *(RJ 2002)*
   (b) Iron deficiency
   (c) Megaloblastic
   (d) All

10. **Hematuria with dysmorphic RBCs are seen in:**
    (a) Acute glomerulonephritis *(RJ 2002)*
    (b) Renal TB
    (c) Renal calculi
    (d) Chronic renal failure

11. **MCHC is increased in:** *(RJ 2005)*
    (a) Iron deficiency anemia
    (b) Spherocytosis
    (c) Thalassemia
    (d) All

12. **In polycythemia vera, all are raised except:**
    (a) Hematocrit *(RJ 2006)*
    (b) Platelet count
    (c) RBCs
    (d) Erythropoietin

13. **The type of anemia seen in chronic renal failure is:**
    (a) Microcytic *(AP 2008)*
    (b) Normocytic
    (c) Macrocytic
    (d) All of the above

14. **Burr cell is seen in:** *(Jharkhand 2003)*
    (a) Uremia
    (b) Hepatocellular carcinoma
    (c) Gastric carcinoma
    (d) Ovarian carcinoma

15. **Acanthocytes are seen in:** *(Jharkhand 2003)*
    (a) Abetalipoproteinemia
    (b) Hartnup disease
    (c) Whipple disease
    (d) None

16. **A 74 year-old female Lajo Devi with renal failure presents for hemodialysis. She complains of weakness and palpitations for about a month. On further investigations, she is found to be anemic and is given a dose of erythropoietin. Erythropoietin stimulates which of the following intermediates in hematopoiesis?**
    (a) Basophilic erythroblasts
    (b) Colony forming units-erythroid
    (c) Proerythroblasts
    (d) Reticulocytes

Most Recent Questions

16.1. Progenitor hematopoetic stem cells originate in which of the following?
(a) Bone marrow
(b) Thymus
(c) Lymph node
(d) Spleen

16.2. The anaemia associated with leukaemia is ?
(a) Iron deficiency
(b) Megaloblastic type
(c) Myelophthisic type
(d) None of the above

16.3. Linzenmeyer is used to measure:
(a) Bleeding time
(b) Clotting time
(c) Prothrombin time
(d) ESR

16.4. Normal platelet count is found in:
(a) Wiskott Aldrich syndrome
(b) Henoch Schonlein purpura
(c) Immune thrombocytopenia
(d) Dengue fever

16.5. Thrombosthenin is:
(a) Coagulation protein
(b) Contractile protein
(c) Thrombus inhibiting protein
(d) Protein for platelet production

16.6. The longest living WBC is which one of the following
(a) Lymphocyte
(b) Eosinophil
(c) Neutrophil
(d) Monocyte

16.7. Freezing point of normal human plasma is:
(a) $4°$ C
(b) $0°$ C
(c) $-0.54°$ C
(d) $-1.54°$ C

16.8. The normal albumin: globulin (A/G) ratio blood is
(a) 5:1
(b) 2:1
(c) 1:2
(d) 1:1

16.9. In an adult man, there is about how much grams of hemoglobin in the circulating blood?
(a) 350
(b) 500
(c) 900
(d) 1000

16.10. The best method for estimation of hemoglobin concentration in blood is
(a) Acid hematin method
(b) Alkali hematin method

(c) Cyanmethemoglobin method
(d) Any of the above

16.11. The number of Fe^{2+} atoms in one Hb molecule
(a) 1
(b) 2
(c) 4
(d) 8

16.12. Hb is a good buffer because of:
(a) Histidine residues
(b) Protein nature
(c) Acidic nature
(d) Iron molecule

16.13. Serum contains all the clotting factors except
(a) Plasma thromboplastin
(b) Labile factor
(c) Hageman factor
(d) Christmas factor

16.14. Reticulocytes are stained with
(a) Methyl violet
(b) Brilliant Cresyl blue
(c) Sudan black
(d) Indigo carmine

16.15. Haematocrit is the ratio of:
(a) WBC to whole blood
(b) Platelets to whole blood
(c) RBCs to whole blood
(d) Total blood cells to plasma

16.16. Storage form of iron
(a) Ferritin
(b) Transferrin
(c) Hepcidin
(d) Ferroportin

16.17. Reticulocytes are stained with which of the following stains?
(a) Brilliant cresyl blue
(b) Sudan black
(c) Warthin starry
(d) Hemotoxylin-eosin stain

MEGALOBLASTIC ANEMIA, APLASTIC ANEMIA

17. Which of these does not indicate megaloblastic anemia?
(a) Increased reticulocyte count   *(AIIMS Nov 2012)*
(b) Raised Bilirubin
(c) Mild splenomegaly
(d) Nucleated RBC

18. A patient with Hb-6 gm%, TLC 1200, platelet-60,000, MCV 12fl, what is the diagnosis?
(a) Aplastic anemia   *(AIIMS May 2008)*
(b) Megaloblastic anemia
(c) PNH
(d) Myelofibrosis

19. Macrocytosis in complete blood count can be diagnosed by: *(PGI Dec 2006)*
    (a) ↑ MCV
    (b) ↑ MCHC
    (c) ↑ Hematocrit
    (d) ↑ Red cell distribution width

20. Which is the true statement regarding megaloblastic anemia: *(PGI Dec 01)*
    (a) Megaloblastic precursors are present in bone marrow
    (b) Mean corpuscular volume is increased
    (c) Serum LDH is increased
    (d) Thrombocytosis occurs
    (e) Target cells are found

21. Macrocytic anemia may be seen in all of these *except:*
    (a) Liver disease *(PGI June 2002)*
    (b) Copper deficiency
    (c) Thiamine deficiency
    (d) Vitamin B_{12} deficiency
    (e) Orotic aciduria

22. Causes of vitamin B12 deficiency megaloblastic anemia are: *(PGI June 2005)*
    (a) Fish tap worm infestation
    (b) Dilantin therapy
    (c) Gastrectomy
    (d) Ileal resection
    (e) Methotrexate

23. Aplastic anemia can progress to all except:
    (a) AML *(Delhi PG 2010)*
    (b) Myelodysplastic anemia
    (c) Pure red cell aplasia
    (d) Paroxysmal nocturnal hemoglobinuria

24. Serum vitamin B_{12} level is increased in all except:
    (a) Hepatitis *(UP 2000)*
    (b) Cirrhosis of liver
    (c) Hepatocellular carcinoma
    (d) Cholestatic jaundice

25. Normocytic normochromic anemia is seen in all except: *(UP 2000)*
    (a) Aplastic anemia
    (b) Chronic renal disease
    (c) Pure red cell aplasia
    (d) Thalassemia

26. A 76 years old male presented with anemia with splenomegaly. PBS shows tear drop shaped cells and bone marrow examination was normal. The diagnosis is: *(UP 2000)*
    (a) Myelofibrosis
    (b) Iron deficiency anemia
    (c) Folic acid deficiency
    (d) CML

27. TRUE about Schilling test is all except:
    (a) B_{12} deficiency *(UP 2001)*
    (b) Folic acid deficiency
    (c) Ileal disease
    (d) Bacterial overgrowth

28. Cause of macrocytic anemia is: *(UP 2002)*
    (a) Sideroblastic anemia
    (b) Iron deficiency
    (c) Thalassemia
    (d) Hypothyroidism

29. Pure red cell aplasia is associated with:
    (a) Thymoma *(UP 2004)*
    (b) Renal cell carcinoma
    (c) Hepatocellular carcinoma
    (d) Prostate carcinoma

30. Vitamin B_{12} malabsorption is caused by:
    (a) Ankylostoma duodenale *(UP 2005)*
    (b) Diphyllobothrium latum
    (c) Giardiasis
    (d) Taenia solium

31. Maturation failure in poor absorption of the vitamin B_{12} is associated with *(UP 2006)*
    (a) Microcytic hypochromic anemia
    (b) Sickle cell anemia
    (c) Anemia occurs after 3-4 months of poor absorption
    (d) Causes polycythemia

32. FIGLU test is done for: *(UP 2008)*
    (a) Cyanocobalamin deficiency
    (b) Folic acid deficiency
    (c) Thiamine deficiency
    (d) Riboflavin deficiency

33. Hypersegmented neutrophils are present in which of the following anemia? *(RJ 2000)*
    (a) Hemolytic
    (b) Iron deficiency
    (c) Megaloblastic
    (d) Aplastic

34. Hypersegmented neutrophils are seen in:
    (a) Thalassemia *(RJ 2002)*
    (b) Iron deficiency
    (c) Megaloblastic anemia
    (d) All

35. Howell-Jolly bodies are seen in: *(RJ 2002)*
    (a) Alcoholics
    (b) Cirrhosis
    (c) Nephrotic syndrome
    (d) Postsplenectomy

36. Macrocytic anemia is caused by: *(AP 2004)*
    (a) Hookworm infestation
    (b) Iron deficiency
    (c) Diphyllobothrium latum infestation
    (d) All of the above

37. An adult who develops pure red cell aplasia should be explicitly evaluated for which of the following?
    (a) Gastric adenocarcinoma
    (b) Pancreatic adenocarcinoma
    (c) Papillary thyroid cancer
    (d) Thymoma

38. A 50-year-old female Ramya with megaloblastic anemia and ataxia is given radiolabeled cobalamin by mouth followed by an intramuscular injection of unlabeled cobalamin. The urine radioactivity level measured afterwards is determined to be normal. Which of the following is the most likely cause of this patient's symptoms?
    (a) Dietary cobalamin deficiency
    (b) Atrophic gastritis
    (c) Nontropical sprue
    (d) Fish tapeworm infestation

39. A 50-year-old male Pandey undergoing evaluation for fatigue and exertional dyspnea is diagnosed with macrocytic anemia. Upper gastrointestinal endoscopy is consistent with atrophic gastritis. Some blood parameter changes after the first dose of cyanocobalamin are shown in the graph on the left side of the page. The first curve most likely corresponds to which of the following parameters?
    (a) RBC count   (b) Reticulocyte count
    (c) Haptoglobin   (d) Gastrin

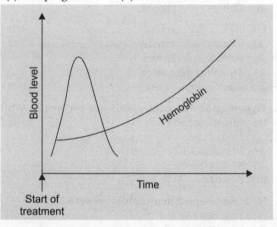

Most Recent Questions

39.1. Hb A2 is raised in which of the following conditions?
    (a) Beta thalassemia trait
    (b) Sickle cell anemia
    (c) Hereditory spherocytosis
    (d) G6 PD deficiency

39.2. Schilling test is used for identification of which of the following?
    (a) Fat absorption
    (b) Vit K absorption
    (c) Vitamin B12 absorption
    (d) Vitamin D absorption

39.3. Which of the does not indicate megaloblastic anemia?
    (a) Raised bilirubin
    (b) Mild splenomegaly
    (c) Increased reticulocyte count
    (d) Nucleated red cells

39.4. All of the following can cause reticulocytosis except
    (a) Aplastic anemia
    (b) Thalassemia
    (c) Sickle cell anemia
    (d) Chronic blood loss

39.5. Reticulocytosis is not seen in which of the following conditions?
    (a) Thalassemia
    (b) Hereditary spherocytosis
    (c) Chronic renal failure
    (d) Sickle cell anemia

39.6 Which of following viruses causes hemolysis of red blood cells?
    (a) Rubella   (b) Human parvo virus B19
    (c) Measles   (d) Dengue virus

MICROCYTIC ANEMIA: IDA, AOCD, SIDEROBLASTIC ANEMIA

40. A 60-year old male patient with history of rheumatoid arthritis presents with the following: Hb:4.5g/dL. platelet count is 2 lakh/mm³. TLC: 6000/mL, serum ferritin is 200µg/dL, serum iron 30mg/dL and TIBC 280ng/L. Which of the following is the most likely diagnosis?
    (a) Anaemia of chronic disease   (AIIMS Nov 2011)
    (b) Thalassemia minor
    (c) Iron deficiency anemia
    (d) Autoimmune haemolytic anemia

41. A 20 year old female presents with the following laboratory values: hemoglobin 9gm%, MCV is 55%, RBC is 4.5 million/mm³. There is no history of blood transfusion. What is the most likely diagnosis out of the following?   (AIIMS Nov 2011)
    (a) Thalassemia major
    (b) Thalassemia minor
    (c) Iron deficiency anemia
    (d) Anemia of chronic disease

42. A 13 yr girl with fatigue and weakness was found to be having reduced hemoglobin. Her MCV 70fl, MCH 22pg and RDW was 28. What is her most likely diagnosis?
    (a) Iron deficiency anemia   (AI 2010)
    (b) Thalassemia minor
    (c) Sideroblastic anemia
    (d) Thalassemia major

43. Ringed sideroblasts are seen in: (AI 2008)
    (a) Iron deficiency anemia
    (b) Myelodysplastic syndrome
    (c) Thalassemia
    (d) Anemia of chronic disease

44. A 30 years old female, RBC count 4.5 million, MCV 55fl, TLC 8000/mm3. There is no history of blood transfusion. What is the likely diagnosis?
    (a) Iron deficiency anemia   (AIIMS May 2008)
    (b) Thalassemia major

Anemia and Red Blood Cells

(c) Thalassemia minor
(d) Megaloblastic anemia

45. **The pathogenesis of hypochromic anemia in lead poisoning is due to:** *(AIIMS Nov 2002)*
    (a) Inhibition of enzymes involved in heme biosynthesis
    (b) Binding of lead to transferrin, inhibiting the transport of iron
    (c) Binding of lead to cell membrane of erythroid precursors.
    (d) Binding of lead to ferritin inhibiting their breakdown into hemosiderin

46. **A patient presents with increased serum ferritin, decreased TIBC, increased serum iron, % saturation increased. Most probable diagnosis is:**
    (a) Anemia of chronic disease *(AIIMS Nov 2006)*
    (b) Sideroblastic anemia
    (c) Iron deficiency anemia
    (d) Thalassemia minor

47. **Anemia in CRF is due to:** *(PGI Dec 2006)*
    (a) ↓ erythropoietin
    (b) ↓RBC survival
    (c) ↓ folate
    (d) Bone marrow hypoplasia
    (e) Iron deficiency

48. **Iron deficiency anemia is seen in:** *(PGI Dec 2006)*
    (a) Chronic renal failure
    (b) Billroth II operation
    (c) Hookworm infection
    (d) Celiac sprue
    (e) Carcinoma cecum

49. **Bone marrow iron is increased in:** *(PGI Dec 2003)*
    (a) Thalassemi(a)
    (b) Iron deficiency anemi(a)
    (c) Anemia in chronic disease.
    (d) PNH
    (e) Megaloblastic anemi(a)

50. **Microcytosis is seen in:** *(PGI June 2004)*
    (a) Thalassemia   (b) Hb Lepore
    (c) Hb Barts   (d) Gastrectomy
    (e) Systemic sclerosis

51. **True about iron deficiency anemia is:** *(PGI June 2005)*
    (a) Microcytic hypochromic anemia
    (b) Decreased TIBC
    (c) Increased ferritin
    (d) Bone marrow iron decreased earlier than serum iron

52. **In Anemia of chronic disease, what is seen?**
    (a) TIBC ↑ *(Delhi PG-2008)*
    (b) S. Iron ↑
    (c) BM iron ↓
    (d) S. ferritin ↑

53. **A 30 years old female asymptomatic not requiring blood transfusion has Hb-13 gm%, HbF-95%, HbA₂ 1.5%. Which of the following is the most likely diagnosis?**

(a) Beta-Heterozygous thalassemia *(Delhi PG-2008)*
(b) Beta-Homozygous thalassemia
(c) Intermediate thalassemia
(d) Persistently raised HbF

54. **The condition which does not cause microcytic hypochromic anemia is:** *(Karnataka 2008)*
    (a) Iron deficiency
    (b) Hookworm infestation
    (c) Absence of intrinsic factor
    (d) Prolonged bleeding episodes

55. **Hypochromic microcytic blood picture is seen in all of the following conditions except:**
    (a) Iron deficiency anemia *(Karnataka 2007)*
    (b) Lead poisoning
    (c) Rheumatoid arthritis
    (d) Sideroblastic anemia

56. **Lead poisoning is associated with:**
    (a) Microcytic hypochromic anemia
    (b) Macrocytic anemia *(Karnataka 2005)*
    (c) Decreased levels of zinc protoporphyrin
    (d) Howell-Jolly bodies

57. **Microspherocytes in peripheral blood smear are seen in:** *(Karnataka 2005)*
    (a) Congenital spherocytosis
    (b) Autoimmune acquired hemolytic anemia
    (c) Thalassemia
    (d) All of the above

58. **"Macropolycytes" in peripheral smear is a feature of:**
    (a) Hereditary spherocytosis *(Karnataka 2004)*
    (b) Iron deficiency anemia
    (c) Sickle cell anemia
    (d) Megaloblastic anemia

59. **Anemia of chronic disease is characterized by of all except:** *(UP 2000)*
    (a) ↓ Serum iron level
    (b) ↓ TIBC
    (c) ↓ Serum ferritin level
    (d) Increased macrophages iron in marrow

60. **Most common cause of anemia is:** *(UP 2003)*
    (a) Iron deficiency
    (b) Folic acid deficiency
    (c) Sideroblastic anemia
    (d) Pernicious anemia

61. **A patient of anemia due to chronic inflammation, the positive finding is**
    (a) Serum iron is increased *(UP-2000) (UP 2004)*
    (b) S. ferritin is decreased
    (c) TIBC is decreased
    (d) Presence of normal iron in blasts

62. **Which of the following glycoproteins is transported in plasma in iron metabolism:** *(UP 2006)*
    (a) Spectrin   (b) Transferrin
    (c) Ferritin   (d) Hemosiderin

63. **All are laboratory finding in iron deficiency anemia except:** *(UP 2006)*
    (a) Decreased serum iron
    (b) Increased total iron binding capacity
    (c) Decreased serum ferritin
    (d) Increased mean corpuscular volume

64. **Best parameter for assessment of body iron stores is**
    (a) Serum iron *(RJ 2002)*
    (b) Serum TIBC
    (c) Serum ferritin
    (d) Serum transferin

65. **Hemochromatosis affects all of the following organs except:** *(RJ 2002)*
    (a) Liver   (b) Pancreas
    (c) Heart   (d) Salivary gland

66. **Skin pigmentation in hemochromatosis occurs due to:**
    (a) Melanin *(RJ 2002)*
    (b) Ferritin
    (c) Hemosiderin
    (d) All

67. **Storage form of iron in body is:** *(RJ 2005)*
    (a) Ferritin   (b) Transferrin
    (c) Ceruloplasmin (d) Ferriportin

68. **Microcytic hypochromic anemia is seen in:**
    (a) Hereditary spherocytosis *(AP 2001)*
    (b) Thalassemia major
    (c) Iron deficiency anemia
    (d) Pernicious anemia

69. **A 68 year-old man Babu Rao Apte presents with skin pigmentation, cirrhosis and diabetes mellitus. Which pattern for serum iron and total iron-binding capacity (TIBC) is most consistent with the familial illness suggested by these findings?**
    (a) Increased Serum iron, Increased TIBC
    (b) Increased Serum iron, Decreased TIBC
    (c) Decreased Serum iron, Decreased TIBC
    (d) Decreased Serum iron, Increased TIBC

Most Recent Questions

69.1. **Sideroblastic anemia is caused by all except:**
    (a) Collagen vascular disease
    (b) Erythropoetic porphyria
    (c) Lead poisoning
    (d) Cutaneous porphyria

69.2. **Lead causes following except:**
    (a) Uroporphyrinuria
    (b) Sideroblastic anemia
    (c) Basophilic stippling
    (d) Macrocytic anemia

69.3. **All of the following if present provide protection against malaria except:**
    (a) Duffy blood group
    (b) Sickle cell anemia

    (c) Thalassemia
    (d) G6PD deficiency

69.4. **Response of iron therapy in a patient with iron deficiency anemia is denoted by:**
    (a) Restoration of enzymes
    (b) Reticulocytosis
    (c) Increase in iron binding capacity
    (d) Increase in hemoglobin

69.5. **Sideroblastic anemia is seen in chronic poisoning with:**
    (a) Lead   (b) Arsenic
    (c) Copper   (d) Mercury

69.6. **Echinocytes are types of:**
    (a) RBCs   (b) Lymphocytes
    (c) Monocytes   (d) Platelets

69.7. **Anemia in humans can be caused by which of the following worm?**
    (a) Roundworm   (b) Hookworm
    (c) Strongyloides (d) Tapeworm

69.8. **Earliest feature of correction of iron deficiency anemia is:**
    (a) Reticulocytosis
    (b) Increase in serum ferritin
    (c) Increase in RBC count
    (d) Increase in serum iron level immediately

69.9. **Rate of iron uptake is regulated by which one of the following:**
    (a) Mucosal cell iron stores
    (b) Route of administration
    (c) Preparation administered
    (d) Age of the patient

69.10. **Low iron and low TIBC is seen in**
    (a) Anaemia of chronic disease
    (b) Sideroblasticanaemia
    (c) Iron deficiency anaemia
    (d) Aplastic anemia

HEMOLYTIC ANEMIA: PNH, HS, G6PD, IMMUNE HEMOLYTIC ANEMIA

---

70. **A 23-year-old female presented with jaundice and pallor for 2 months. Her peripheral blood smear shows the presence of spherocytes. The most relevant investigation to arrive at a diagnosis is which of the following?** *(AIIMS May 2012)*
    (a) Tests for PNH
    (b) Osmotic fragility test
    (c) Coombs test
    (d) Reticulocyte count

71. **An abnormal Ham test is most likely associated with which of the following?** *(AIIMS Nov 2011)*
    (a) Spectrin
    (b) Defect in complement activating proteins

(c) Defective GPI anchor

(d) Mannose-binding residue effect

72. **A 5 year old male child presents with episodic anemia and jaundice since birth. He is least likely to have which of the following?** *(AIIMS Nov 2011)*
(a) Hereditary spherocytosis
(b) Sickle cell disease
(c) G6PD deficiency
(d) Paroxysmal nocturnal hemoglobinuria

73. **Thrombotic event is seen in all of following except:** *(AIIMS May 2011)*
(a) Paroxysmal nocturnal hemogloninuria
(b) Disseminated intravascular coagulation
(c) Idiopathic thrombocytopenic purpura
(d) Heparin induced thrombocytopenia

74. **PNH associated with somatic mutation affecting:**
(a) Decay accelerating factor (DAF) *(AI 2010)*
(b) Membrane inhibitor of reactive lysis (MIRL)
(c) Glycosylphosphatidylinositol (GPI)
(d) C8 binding protein

75. **Cold hemagglutinin is associated with:** *(AI 2008)*
(a) Anti IgM
(b) Anti IgG
(c) Anti IgA
(d) Donath-Landsteiner antibody

76. **The following protein defects can cause hereditary spherocytosis except:** *(AI 2007)*
(a) Ankyrin   (b) Palladin
(c) Glycophorin C   (d) Anion transport protein

77. **Autoimmune hemolytic anemia is seen in:** *(AI 2001)*
(a) ALL   (b) AML
(c) CLL   (d) CML

78. **Microangiopathic hemolytic anemia is seen in all of the following diseases except** *(AIIMS Nov 2008)*
(a) Antiphospholipid antibody syndrome
(b) Thrombotic thrombocytopenic purpura
(c) Microscopic polyangiitis
(d) Metallic cardiac valves

79. **An Rh -ve woman became pregnant with Rh +ve fetus. Within few days after birth, the infant developed jaundice, ascites, hepatomegaly and edema. The likely substance(s) deposited in skin and sclera in jaundice is/ are given below. Which is the best possible answer?**
(a) Biliverdin *(AIIMS Nov 2003)*
(b) Conjugated and unconjugated bilirubin
(c) Unconjugated bilirubin
(d) Conjugated bilirubin

80. **Features seen in hemolytic anemia are all except:**
(a) Teardrop and Burr cells
(b) ↓ Haptoglobin
(c) Reticulocytosis
(d) Hemoglobinuria

81. **Intravascular hemolysis occurs in:**
(a) Hereditary spherocytosis *(PGI Dec 2000)*
(b) Acute G6PD deficiency
(c) Sickle cell disease
(d) Thalassemia
(e) PNH

82. **Microangiopathic hemolytic anemia is seen in:**
(a) HUS *(PGI June 01)*
(b) ITP
(c) Malignant hypertension
(d) Prosthetic valves
(e) TTP

83. **Spherocytosis in blood smear is seen in:**
(a) Hemoglobin C *(PGI June 2004)*
(b) Mechanical trauma
(c) Hereditary spherocytosis
(d) Hereditary elliptosis

84. **Cause of fragmented RBC in peripheral blood:**
(a) Microangiopathic hemolytic anemia
(b) DIC *(PGI June 2005)*
(c) Hemophilia-A
(d) Malignant hypertension
(e) HELLP syndrome

85. **Intravascular hemolysis is seen in:** *(PGI June 2005)*
(a) Glucose-6 phosphate dehydrogenase deficiency
(b) Thalassemia
(c) Sickle cell anemia
(d) Hemophilia

86. **The peripheral smear of hereditary spherocytosis will show spherocytes:** *(PGI Dec 2006)*
(a) Usually of same size
(b) Reticulocytosis seen
(c) Smaller size
(d) Anemia is negligible
(e) Always associated with ↑ MCHC

87. **Microangiopathic hemolytic anemia seen in:**
(a) Thrombotic thrombocytopenic purpura
(b) Hemolytic uremic syndrome *(PGI Dec 2003)*
(c) Henoch-Schonlein purpura
(d) DIC
(e) IgA nephropathy

88. **Donath-Landsteiner antibodies are seen in:**
(a) Warm agglutination *(Delhi PG 2010)*
(b) Cold agglutination
(c) Paroxysmal nocturnal hemoglobinuria
(d) ITP

89. **In hereditary spherocytosis an inherited abnormality is seen in which of the following red blood cell component:** *(Delhi PG 2009)*
(a) α-globin chain
(b) β-globin chain
(c) Phosphatidyl inositol glycan A
(d) Spectrin

265

90. **Hereditary spherocytosis is due to:** *(UP 2001)*
    (a) Acquired membrane defect
    (b) Ankyrin deficiency
    (c) Defective hemoglobin synthesis
    (d) Mechanical trauma to red cells

91. **Not seen in paroxysmal nocturnal hemoglobinuria is:**
    (a) LDH levels are raised *(AP 2000)*
    (b) Increased hemosiderin in urine
    (c) Decreased leukocyte alkaline phosphatase
    (d) Increased platelets

92. **'Warm' autoantibodies are seen in:** *(AP 2003)*
    (a) SLE
    (b) Mycoplasma
    (c) Syphilis
    (d) Varicella

93. **Hot agglutinin is found in all except:**
    (a) Mycoplasma infection *(Bihar 2006)*
    (b) SLE
    (c) Methyl dopa
    (d) Rheumatoid arthritis

94. **A 20-year-old man John Abraham is transported to the emergency department within 20 minutes of sustaining a road traffic accident on his bike. The patient is poorly responsive. If it is presumed that he may have lost about 1.5 liters of blood at the scene, which of the following is the most likely finding in this patient?**
    (a) Increased mean corpuscular hemoglobin concentration
    (b) Decreased hematocrit
    (c) Decreased blood pressure
    (d) Decreased red blood cell count

95. **Rahul Singh migrates from UP to Bihar to work under the NREGA scheme as a daily wage labourer. The district has high endemicity of malaria. So, his physician Dr. Dubey gives him primaquine chemoprophylaxis for Plasmodium vivax malaria. Several days after beginning such a regimen, Mr. Singh develops anemia, hemoglobinemia, and hemoglobinuria. Special studies will likely reveal an abnormality in which of the following?**
    (a) Duffy antigen
    (b) Glucose-6-phospate dehydrogenase
    (c) Intrinsic factor
    (d) PIG-A

96. **A 38-year-old male Kritesh presents to his physician with the complaints of sudden onset of fever, chills and dysuria. He has no significant past medical history. A per-rectal examination reveals tenderness. The prostatic secretions are collected and on microscopic examination, it demonstrates >15 WBCs/hpf. A diagnosis of acute prostatitis is made. He was started on treatment with trimethoprim-sulfamethoxazole, but subsequently developed dark urine and anemia with a high reticulocyte count. Which of the following is the best explanation for the observed findings?**
    (a) Anti body-mediated erythrocyte destruction
    (b) Hereditary erythrocyte membrane defect
    (c) Hereditary erythrocyte enzyme deficiency
    (d) Microangiopathic hemolytic anemia

97. **A young male photographer Alok Nath from Bangalore is evaluated for recurrent episodes of jaundice. He has no history of recent travel. Past medical history is insignificant and the person is not on any medication. He does admit to unprotected sex with multiple sexual partners. His blood pressure is 120/80 mmHg, pulse is 72/mm, temperature is 36.7C (98F) and respiratory rate is 14/min. Physical examination shows pallor, icterus and mild splenomegaly. There is no lymphadenopathy or hepatomegaly. Laboratory studies are shown below**
    - Hemoglobin   9.1 g/L
    - Platelets   188,000/mm3
    - Leukocyte count   6,400/mm3
    - LDH   Increased
    - Total bilirubin   3.5 mg/dL
    - Direct bilirubin   1.1 mg/dL
    - Aspartate aminotransferase (AST)   27 U/L
    - Alanine aminotransferase (ALT)   32 U/L

    When red blood cells are incubated in hypotonic saline, hemoglobin is released. The control sample does not release hemoglobin. This patient is at highest risk of developing which of the following?
    (a) Cirrhosis and hepatocellular carcinoma
    (b) Pigmented gallstones
    (c) Avascular necrosis of the femur
    (d) Episodic venous thrombosis

98. **A 16-year-old female Gitika notices that her urine becomes red after she is given sulfonamides for treatment of a urinary tract infection. Both urine and serum test positive for free hemoglobin, and the urine red cell count is 1.2 million/mm3. A peripheral blood smear shows normocytic and normochromic red cells and a few "bite cells." Deficiency of which of the following substances is most likely responsible for these symptoms?**
    (a) Alpha-chain of hemoglobin
    (b) Beta-chain of hemoglobin
    (c) Glucose-6-phosphate dehydrogenase
    (d) Glycoprotein IIb/IIIa

99. **An infant presents with mild anemia, jaundice, and splenomegaly. A complete blood count with differential reveals spherocytosis; with elevated reticulocyte count. The parents state that several relatives have also suffered from a similar illness. The infant's condition is most likely caused by defective**
    (a) Clathrin   (b) Connexon
    (c) Ankyrin   (d) Spectrin

100. **A 30-year-old woman A. Jolie with SLE and chronic renal failure manifests rapidly progressive weakness. She appears pale and has slightly yellow sclerae and an enlarged spleen. Blood tests reveal severe anemia and mild, mostly unconjugated, hyperbilirubinemia. Coombs test is positive at 37°C but negative at 0-4°C.**

This patient developed anemia because of
(a) Bone marrow aplasia
(b) IgG directed against red blood cells
(c) IgM directed against red blood cells
(d) Spleen sequestration

Most Recent Questions

100.1. In DIC, following are seen except –
(a) Fibrinogen decreased
(b) Thrombocytopenia
(c) Normal APTT
(d) PT elevation

100.2. D.I.C is seen in:
(a) Acute promyelocytic leukemia
(b) Acute myelomonocytic leukemia
(c) CML
(d) Autoimmune haemolytic anemia

100.3. Intravascular hemolysis occurs in:
(a) Hereditary spherocytosis
(b) Autoimmune haemolytic anemia
(c) Paroxysmal nocturnal hemoglobinuria
(d) Thalassemia

100.4. Bite cells are seen in:
(a) G6PD deficiency
(b) Sickle cell anemia
(c) Hereditary spherocytosis
(d) Trauma

100.5. Cold agglutinin is:
(a) IgG
(b) IgM
(c) IgA
(d) IgD

100.6. Helmet cells are characteristic of anemia of:
(a) Hemolytic uremic syndrome
(b) Polysplenia
(c) Spherocytosis
(d) Acanthocytosis

100.7. Schistocyte is/are found in:
(a) TTP
(b) March hemoglobinuria
(c) Severe iron deficiency
(d) All of the above

100.8. PNH due to defect in:
(a) CD 59
(b) CD 15
(c) CD 100
(d) CD 20

100.9. All are the features of hemolytic anemia except:
(a) Hemoglobinuria
(b) Jaundice
(c) Increased haptoglobin
(d) Hemosiderinuria

100.10. G6PD help in maintaining the integrity of RBC by?
(a) Controlling reduction stress on RBC
(b) Controlling oxidative stress on RBC
(c) Maintaining flexibility of cell membrane
(d) Component of electron transport chain

HEMOGLOBINOPATHIES: SICKLE CELL ANEMIA, THALASSEMIA

101. Person having heterozygous sickle cell trait are protected from infection of? *(AIIMS Nov 2012)*
(a) P. falciparum (b) P. vivax
(c) Pneumococcous (d) Salmonella

102. A 6yrs old child belonging to Punjabi family with past history of blood transfusions presented with hemoglobin 3.5 g/dl, MCV – 30 fl, MCHC – 20. Peripheral smear findings of microcytic hypochromic anemia with target cell and reduced osmotic fragility. What is the he probable diagnosis of patient? *(AIIMS Nov 2012)*
(a) Alpha thalassemia
(b) Beta thalassemia
(c) Sickle cell anemia
(d) G6PD deficiency

103. NESTROF test is a screening test for which of the following conditions? *(AIIMS Nov 2011)*
(a) β- thalassemia
(b) Hereditary spherocytosis
(c) Autoimmune haemolytic anaemia
(d) Megaloblastic anaemia

104. Which of the following is the cause of alpha thalassemia?
(a) Deletion of alpha genes *(AIIMS May 2011)*
(b) Deletion of beta genes
(c) Excess of alpha genes
(d) Single amino acid substitution in alpha chain

105. HbH is formed due to which of the following?
(a) Deletion of 4 alpha chains *(AI 2011)*
(b) Deletion of 3 alpha chains
(c) Deletion of 2 alpha chains
(d) Deletion of 1 alpha chain

106. Mutation causing sickle cell anemia is protective for which of the following? *(AI 2010)*
(a) Malaria (b) Filaria
(c) Leishmania (d) None of the above

107. What is affected in HbS (Hemoglobin S)? *(AI 2009)*
(a) Stability (b) Function
(c) Affinity (d) Solubility

108. A couple, with a family history of beta thalassemia major in a distant relative, has come for counseling. The husband has HbA2 of 4.8% and the wife has HbA2 of 2.3%. The risk of having a child with beta thalassemia major is: *(AI 2003)*
(a) 50%
(b) 25%
(c) 5%
(d) 0%

109. **The primary defect which leads to sickle cell anemia is:** *(AI 2003)*
    (a) An abnormality in porphyrin part of hemoglobin
    (b) Replacement of glutamate by valine in b-chain of HbA
    (c) A nonsense mutation in the b-chain of HbA
    (d) Substitution of valine by glutamate in the a-chain of HbA

110. **Which one of the following statements about hemoglobin S (HbS) is not true:** *(AIIMS Nov 2004)*
    (a) Hemoglobin HbS differs from hemoglobin HbA by the substitution of Val for Glu in position 6 of the beta chain
    (b) One altered peptide of HbS migrates faster towards the cathode (–) than the corresponding peptide of HbA
    (c) Binding of HbS to the deoxygenated HbA can extend the polymer and cause sickling of the red blood cells
    (d) Lowering the concentration of deoxygenated HbS can prevent sickling

111. **Sickle cell trait patient do not have manifest-tations of sickle cell disease, because:** *(AIIMS Nov 2001)*
    (a) 50% HbS is required for occurrence of sickling
    (b) HbA prevents sickling
    (c) 50% sickles
    (d) HbA prevents polymerization of HbS

112. **True about Sickle cell anemia are all except:**
    (a) Commonly seen in blacks *(PGI June 2004)*
    (b) R.(b)(c) size is altered
    (c) Valine is substituted for glutamic acid in beta chain of globin.
    (d) Deletion of gene
    (e) Target cell are present

113. **True about beta-thalassemia trait is:**
    (a) Increased HbF *(PGI June 2004)*
    (b) Increased HbA2
    (c) Microcytosis
    (d) Severe anemia
    (e) Target cell

114. **Sickle cell anemia is the clinical manifestation of homozygous genes for an abnormal haemoglobin molecule. The event responsible for the mutation in the β chain is** *(Delhi PG 2010)*
    (a) Insertion   (b) Deletion
    (c) Non- disjunction (d) Point mutation

115. **Hemoglobin H disease is caused by deletion of:**
    (a) A single α globin gene *(Karnataka 2009)*
    (b) Two α globin genes
    (c) Three α globin genes
    (d) All four α globin genes

116. **All of the following aggravate sickling phenomenon in sickle cell disease EXCEPT:** *(Karnataka 2008)*
    (a) Higher concentration of HbS
    (b) Higher concentration of HbF
    (c) Lower concentration of HbC
    (d) A fall in blood pH

117. **Sickle cell anemia is due to:** *(UP 2001)*
    (a) Presence of a structurally abnormal Hb
    (b) Red cell enzyme deficiency
    (c) Unknown multiple mechanisms
    (d) Disturbance of proliferation and differentiation of stem cells

118. **In sickle cell disease, the defect is in:** *(AP 2000)*
    (a) α-chain *(Jipmer 1997, TN 1989),*
    (b) β-chain
    (c) γ-chain
    (d) Hb formation

119. **A 14-year-old male Kaalu is brought to the emergency room with high grade fever, chest pain, and dyspnea. His past medical history is significant for two prior hospitalizations for abdominal pain, which resolved with analgesics and hydration. Evaluation today reveals a hematocrit of 23% and reticulocyte count of 9%. Several hours after being admitted, the patient dies in the hospital. At autopsy, the patient's spleen is firm and brown; this finding is most likely related to:**
    (a) Work hypertrophy
    (b) Follicular hyperplasia
    (c) Vascular occlusion
    (d) Pressure atrophy

120. **A 23-year-old male Subhas Raj presents to the medicine OPD with complaint of hematuria. There is no burning sensation during urination. He also has no history suggestive of respiratory tract infection. He gives a history of two of his relatives suffering from 'some blood disease'. His coagulation studies are within normal limits. The hemoglobin electrophoresis shows the following: Hb A 60% and Hb S 40%. Which of the following is most likely true about this patient?**
    (a) Irreversible sickle cells are present on the peripheral smear.
    (b) Reticulocyte count is elevate(d)
    (c) He is protected from *Plasmodium falciparum.*
    (d) MCHC is decrease(d)

121. **Which of the following manifestations is common to sickle cell anemia and thalassemia major?**
    (a) Autosplenectomy
    (b) Bone marrow expansion in the calvarium
    (c) Ineffective erythropoiesis
    (d) Predisposition to *Hemophilus influenzae* infections

Most Recent Questions

121.1 **The primary defect which lead to sickle cell anemia is ?**
    (a) An abnormality in porphyrin part of haemoglobin
    (b) Substitution of valine by glutamate in the β-chain of HbA
    (c) Replacement of glutamate by valine in β-chain of HbA
    (d) A nonsense mutation in the β-chain of HbA

121.2. In α-thalassemia, which of the following is a finding?
(a) No β-chain
(b) Excess α-chain
(c) No α-chain
(d) Relative excess of β, γ, and δ chains

121.3. In sickle cell anemia defect is in which chain:
(a) Alpha chain   (b) Beta chain
(c) Both the chains   (d) None of these

121.4. Sickle cell red blood cells have:
(a) Altered stability
(b) Altered functions
(c) Decreased oxygen carrying capacity
(d) Protective action against adult malaria

121.5. Bone infarcts are seen in:
(a) Iron deficiency anemia
(b) Thalassemia
(c) Sickle cell anemia
(d) Hereditary spherocytosis

121.6. Ideally children with thalassemia should be transfused with
(a) Packed RBC
(b) Platelet rich plasma
(c) Saline washed packed RBC
(d) Whole blood

121.7. A 18 year old Afro American boy presenting with a non healing ulcer of the foot, with recurrent pneumonia and chronic hemolytic anemia. The peripheral blood erythrocytes showed some peculiar appearance. Most likely cause is:
(a) Trinucleotide repeat
(b) Genomic imprinting
(c) Single amino acid base substitution
(d) Antibody to red cell membrane

121.8. Molecular pathogenesis of α thalassemia involves
(a) Mutation in transcription sequence
(b) Gene deletion
(c) Codon termination mutation
(d) mRNA splicing defect

121.9. One of the common variants of sickle cell anemia frequently marked by lesser degree of haemolytic anemia and greater propensity for the development of retinopathy and aseptic necrosis of bones is
(a) Sickle cell trait
(b) Haemoglobin SC disease
(c) Sickle thalassaemia
(d) Sickle –Hb E disease

121.10. All are seen in Thalasemia major except-
(a) Transfusion dependency
(b) Splenoheptatomegaly
(c) Ineffective erythropoiesis
(d) Macrocytic anaemia

BLOOD GROUPING, BLOOD TRANSFUSION, ANTI COAGULANTS

122. Which of the following regarding Bombay blood group is false? *(AIIMS May 2012)*
(a) Lack of H, A and B antigen on RBCs
(b) Lack of H, A and B substance in saliva
(c) Lack of antigens of several blood group systems
(d) H, A and B antibody will always be present in serum

123. Which of the following is the genotype of a person with blood group A? *(AI 2012)*
(a) BO   (b) AO
(c) AB   (d) OO

124. Secondary hemochromatosis is associated with all except: *(AI 2012)*
(a) Thalassemia
(b) Sideroblastic anemia
(c) Multiple drug transfusions
(d) Paroxysmal nocturnal hemoglobinuria

125. The anticoagulant of choice for anticoagulation testing
(a) Heparin   *(AIIMS Nov 2011)*
(b) EDTA
(c) Sodium oxalate
(d) 3.2% trisodium citrate

126. You are working in a PHC and have to send a sample for blood glucose estimation. Which of the following anticoagulant will you use for sending your sample?
(a) EDTA   *(AIIMS Nov 2011)*
(b) Heparin
(c) Potassium oxalate + sodium fluoride
(d) Tri Sodium citrate

127. A newborn with ABO incompatibility, the characteristic feature on peripheral smear is the presence of
(a) Microspherocytes   *(AIIMS Nov. 2010)*
(b) Fragmented RBC
(c) Polychromasia
(d) Elliptocytosis

128. Most common blood transfusion reaction is:
(a) Febrile non-hemolytic transfusion reaction
(b) Hemolysis   *(AI 2008)*
(c) Transmission of infections
(d) Electrolyte imbalance

129. Rh antigen is a/an: *(AI 2008)*
(a) Antibody
(b) Mucopolysaccharide
(c) Protein
(d) Fatty acid

130. A 40 years old male had undergone splenectomy 20 years ago. Peripheral blood smear examination would show the presence of: *(AI 2003)*
(a) Dohle bodies
(b) Hypersegmented neutrophils
(c) Spherocytes
(d) Howell-Jolly bodies

131. **Which of the following complications is likely to result after several units of blood have been transferred?**
    (a) Metabolic alkalosis *(AI 2001)*
    (b) Metabolic acidosis
    (c) Respiratory alkalosis
    (d) Respiratory acidosis

132. **ABO incompatibility not seen with:**
    (a) Fresh frozen plasma *(AIIMS Nov 2009)*
    (b) Platelet rich plasma
    (c) Single donor platelets
    (d) Cryoprecipitate

133. **A 55 years old male accident victim in casualty urgently needs blood. The blood bank is unable to determine his ABO group, as his red cell group and plasma group do not match. Emergency transfusion of the patient should be with:** *(AIIMS Nov 2002)*
    (a) RBC corresponding to his red cell group and colloids/crystalloid
    (b) Whole blood corresponding to his plasma group
    (c) O positive RBC and colloids/crystalloid
    (d) AB negative whole blood

134. **Although more than 400 blood groups have been identified, the ABO blood system re-mains the most important in clinical medicine because:**
    (a) It was the first blood group system to be discovered
    (b) It has four different blood group A, B, AB, O (H)
    (c) ABO (H) antigens are present in most body tissues and fluids *(AIIMS Nov 2002)*
    (d) ABO (H) antibodies are invariably present in plasma when persons RBC lack the corres-ponding antigen

135. **Which of the following is seen in peripheral smear of a patient who has underwent splenectomy:**
    (a) Howell-Jolly bodies *(PGI Dec 2001)*
    (b) Eosinophilia
    (c) Macrocytosis
    (d) Thrombocytopenia
    (e) Neutrophilia

136. **Blood component products are all except?**
    (a) Whole blood *(PGI Dec 2005)*
    (b) Platelets
    (c) Fresh frozen plasma
    (d) Packed red blood cells
    (e) Leukocyte reduced RBC

137. **The anticoagulant of choice for performing coagulation studies is:** *(Delhi PG 2010)*
    (a) EDTA
    (b) Heparin
    (c) Trisodium citrate
    (d) Double oxalate

138. **Howell Jolly bodies are seen in:** *(Karnataka 2009)*
    (a) Liver disease
    (b) Postsplenectomy
    (c) Hemolysis
    (d) DIC

139. **Spur cell anemia is caused by:** *(UP 2003)*
    (a) Chronic liver disease
    (b) Acute blood loss
    (c) Chronic blood loss
    (d) None

140. **Hypersplenism is characterized by all except:** *(UP 2006)*
    (a) Leukemoid reaction
    (b) Thrombocytopenia
    (c) Splenomegaly
    (d) Responds to splenectomy

141. **The antigen lacking in Rh negative person is:** *(UP 2006)*
    (a) C   b) D
    (c) d   (d) E

Most Recent Questions

141.1. **Hemophilia is associated with :**
    (a) X chromosome   (b) Y Chromosome
    (c) Chromosome 3   (d) Chromosome 16

141.2. **Hemophilia B is due to deficiency of:**
    (a) Factor VIII   (b) Factor VII
    (c) Factor IX   (d) Factor X

141.3. **All are true about polycythemia vera except:**
    (a) Increased LAP score
    (b) Increased erythropoietin level
    (c) Splenomegaly
    (d) May cause Budd-Chiari syndrome

141.4. **Elevated ESR is seen in following conditions except:**
    (a) Polymyositis rheumatica
    (b) Multiple myeloma
    (c) Temporal arteritis
    (d) Polycythemia rubra

141.5. **True about von Willebrand factor are all except**
    (a) Component of factor VIII
    (b) Synthesized by hepatocytes
    (c) Facilitate the adhesion of platelets
    (d) None

141.6. **Patient with hemophilia A have bleeding disorder because of:**
    (a) Lack of platelet aggregation
    (b) Lack of reaction accelerator during activation of factor X in coagulation cascade
    (c) Neutralization of antithrombin III
    (d) Release of Thromboxane A2

141.7. **A 7-year-old girl presents with bleeding in joints. She has prolonged aPTT, normal PT and platelet counts. What could be the deficiency?**
    (a) Factor IX   (b) Factor VIII
    (c) Factor VII   (d) von Willebrand Factor

141.8. Hemophilia A is characterized by:
   (a) Prolonged PTT
   (b) Prolonged PT
   (c) Low platelet count
   (d) Abnormal BT

141.9. True about hemophilia is:
   (a) If the male is affected, it will transmit to male
   (b) Normal PT
   (c) Low PT
   (d) Low aPTT

141.10. The major hemoglobin present in an adult is
   (a) HbA_2 (b) HbA_1
   (c) HbA_{1c} (d) HbA_{1b}

141.11. Bence Jones protein in urine are due to the presence of
   (a) Light chain of monoclonal immunoglobulins
   (b) Heavy chain of monoclonal immunoglobulins
   (c) Light chain of polyclonal immunoglobulins
   (d) Heavy chain of polyclonal immunoglobulins

141.12. "Starry Sky" pattern is seen in all of these except:
   (a) Burkitt's lymphoma
   (b) Large B cell lymphoma
   (c) Small cleaved cell lymphoma
   (d) Lymphoblast lymphoma

141.13. Platelets growth factor are synthesized by:
   (a) Glial cells
   (b) Endothelium
   (c) Fibroblasts
   (d) All of the above

141.14. Blood group antigens are
   (a) Carried by sex chromosomes
   (b) Attached to plasma proteins
   (c) Attached to hemoglobin molecule
   (d) Sometimes found in saliva

141.15. Stored plasma is deficient in
   (a) Factors 7 and 8
   (b) Factors 5 and 7
   (c) Factors 5 and 8
   (d) Factors 5, 7 and 8

141.16. Carbohydrate present in blood group substance is
   (a) Fucose   (b) Deoxyribose
   (c) Ribulose   (d) Ribose

141.17. All cause pseudohyperkalemia, except
   (a) Thrombocytopenia
   (b) Leucocytosis
   (c) Clenching of fists
   (d) Hemolysis

EXPLANATIONS

1. **Ans. (b) Hereditary spherocytosis** *(Ref: Robbins 8th/640-2, 9/e p632)*
   Regarding Hereditary spherocytosis;
   Direct quote from Robbins....*'this inherited disorder is caused by* intrinsic defects in the red cell membrane *that render red cells spheroid, less deformable, and vulnerab le to splenic sequestration and destruction'*
   Other disorders with intrinsic defect in red cell membrane are hereditary elliptocytosis and abetalipoproteinemia.

2. **Ans. (c) Myoblast** *(Ref: Robbins 8th/85, 9/e p580)*

   ### Bone marrow cells include

   - **Hematopoietic stem cells** include **lymphoblast, myeloblast** and **normoblast**.
   - **Marrow stromal cell**/multipotent stem cells (MSC) including **myoblast, osteoblasts, chondrocytes, adipocytes** and **endothelial cell precursors**. Myoblast is an example of MSC giving rise to muscle cells or myocytes.

3. **Ans. (d) CD 34** *(Ref: Robbins 7th/670, 9th/590)*

   CD34 is expressed on pluripotent hematopoietic stem cells and progenitor cells of many lineages

4. **Ans. (c) Nutritional anemia** *(Ref: Harrison 18th/454, 17th/359-361 and Ghai 6th/306)*

   Reticulocytes are nonnucleated spherical cells bigger than normal RBCs and are polychromatic (having a blue color) due to the presence of free ribosomes and RNA.

Reticulocytosis (Increased RBC production)	Reticulocytopenia (Decreased RBC production)
*Conditions	*Conditions
• Acute blood loss or hemorrhage • Postsplenectomy • Microangiopathic Anemia • Autoimmune Hemolytic Anemia • Hemoglobinopathy (Sickle cell anemia and Thalassemia) • Post anemia treatment like folate supplementation, iron supplementation & vitamin B_{12} supplementation.	• Aplastic anemia • Bone marrow infiltration • Bone marrow suppression (Sepsis/Chemo/radiotherapy) • Blood transfusion • Liver disease • Disordered RBC maturation (Iron, B_{12}, Folate Deficiency, Hypothyroidism, Sideroblastic Anemia or Anemia of Chronic Disease)

5. **Ans. (b) Basophilic stippling; (d) Howell-Jolly bodies; (e) Cabot ring.** *(Ref: PJ Mehta 16th/372, T. Singh 1st/34)*
   - **Romanowsky dyes** are used for staining blood films. They are made up of combination of acid and basic dyes. The nucleus and neutrophilic granules are basophilic and stains blue. Hemoglobin is acidophilic and stains red.
   - Various modifications available are **Leishman's stain, Wright's stain, Giemsa and Jenner's stain.**
   - Basophilic stippling, Howell-Jolly body and Cabot rings are seen by Romanowsky stain.

   - **Basophilic stippling:** These are small blue or black granules in red cells seen in megaloblastic anemia, heavy metal poisonings, etc.
   - **Howell-Jolly Body:** These are remnants of the nucleus seen as small, round dark blue particles near the periphery of the cells; found in postsplenectomy, asplenia and severe hemolytic anemia.
   - **Cabot ring:** These are pale staining nuclear remnants in the form of rings or figure of eight seen in hemolytic anemia, megaloblastic anemia, leukemia and after splenectomy. These are arginine rich and acidophilic.
   - Heinz bodies are denatured hemoglobin which does not stained with Romanowsky stain. It is demonstrated by supravital stains such as crystal violets. Reticulocytes also require Supravital staining.

6. **Ans. (d) CD 34** *(Ref: Robbins 7th/670, 9/e p590)*

7. **Ans. (d) Benign liver tumor** *(Ref: Robbins 7th/334, 649 9/e p331)*

8. **Ans. (a) MCV** *(Ref: Robbins 9/e p630, 8th/289, 7th/623 9/e p630)*

9. **Ans. (c) Megaloblastic** *(Ref: Robbins 9/e p645, 8th/655, 7th/638)*

Anemia and Red Blood Cells

10. **Ans. (a) Acute glomerulonephritis** *(Ref: Robbins 9/e p898, 8th/941, 7th/973-974)*

11. **Ans. (b) Spherocytosis** *(Ref: Robbins 9/e p633, 8th/642-644, 7th/627)*

12. **Ans. (d) Erythropoietin** *(Ref: Robbins 9/e p656, 8th/628, 7th/699)*

13. **Ans. (b) All of the above** *(Ref: Robbins 8th/665; 7th/960, Harrison 18 Table 280 (5))*

14. **Ans. (a) Uremia** *(Ref: Tejinder Singh 1st/38)*

15. **Ans. (a) Abetalipoproteinemia** *(Ref: Tejinder Singh 1st/38)*

16. **Ans. (b) Colony forming units-erythroid** *(Ref: Robbins 9/e p580, 8th/641)*
    The colony forming unit-erythroid (CFU-E) is a unipotential stem cell that develops from a burst forming unit-erythroid (BFU-E), which develops eventually from the multipotential stem cell. The CFU-E is completely dependent on erythropoietin. Erythropoietin is normally released from the kidney in response to hypoxic or anemic conditions.
    The basophilic erythroblast (option a) differentiates from the proerythroblast. It has a dark basophilic staining due to hemoglobin synthesis. The proerythroblast (option c) is the first recognizable cell in the red cell lineage. It develops from the CFU-E cell. The basophilic erythroblast and the proerythroblast are not affected directly by erythropoietin, but instead increases in number from the increased CFU-E cells.
    The reticulocyte (option d) is the enucleated cell just before the mature red blood cell. It is not directly stimulated by erythropoietin, but increases in number as a result of the increase in precursors.

16.1. **Ans. (a) Bone marrow** *(Ref: Robbins 8/e p590, 9/e p580)*
    By birth, marrow throughout the skeleton is hematopoietically active and hepatic hematopoiesis dwindles to a trickle, persisting only in widely scattered foci that become inactive soon after birth.

16.2. **Ans. (c) Myelophthisic type** *(Ref: Robbins 8/e p665, 9/e p655)*
    - *Myelophthisic anemia* describes a form of marrow failure in which space-occupying lesions replace normal marrow elements. The commonest cause is metastatic cancer, most often carcinomas arising in the breast, lung, and prostate.
    - *There is presence of leukoerythroblastosis* (nucleated erythroid precursors) and the appearance of **teardrop-shaped red cells**. This is due to disturbance of mechanisms regulating the egress of red cells and granulocytes from the marrow.

16.3. **Ans. (d) ESR ....** *(Ref: A Textbook of Hematology p133)*

16.4. **Ans. (b) Henoch Schonlein purpura** *(Ref: Robbins, 9/e p526-527 8/e p666; 7/e p986-987)*
    All other options have decreased platelet count except Henoch Schonlein purpura. Though it has the name purpura, but the *platelet count in this condition is normal*. The skin manifestations in HSP are due to **small vessel vasculitis**.

16.5. **Ans. (b) Contractile protein** *(Ref: Harsh Mohan 5th/ 177, The Circulating Platelet/ 215-8)*
    - Thrombosthenin is a contractile protein in platelets that is active in the formation of blood clots.

16.6. **Ans. (a) Lymphocyte** *(Read below)*
    - **Lymphocyte** is the **longest living**[Q] white blood cell.
    - **Neutrophil** is the most **numerous**[Q] white blood cell.

16.7. **Ans. (c) –0.54° C** *(See below)*

• The **freezing point** of normal **human plasma** averages **-0.54 °C**[Q], which corresponds to an osmolal concentration in plasma of **290 mOsm/L**[Q].
• The term **tonicity** is used to describe the osmolality of a solution relative to plasma
• A **0.9% saline solution** and **5% glucose solution is isotonic** when initially infused intravenously.

    Also know how to calculate osmolality: medicine link!

    $$\text{Osmolality (mOsm/L)} = 2[\text{Na}^+]\text{ (mEq/L)} + 0.055[\text{Glucose}]\text{ (mg/dL)} + 0.36[\text{BUN}]\text{ (mg/dL)}$$

16.8. **Ans. (b) 2:1** *(Read below)*
    - Normal **albumin-globulin ratio** is **1.8 : 1 to 2 : 1**[Q].
    - Synthesis of **albumin exclusively occurs in liver** but many *globulins (immunoglobulins) are synthesized by B-lymphocyte.*

    Conditions with altered albumin globulin ratio

High Albumin Globulin Ratio	Low Albumin Globulin Ratio
• Hypothyroidism • Hypogammaglobulinemia • Leukemia • Glucocorticoid excess	• Overproduction of globulins in conditions like **multiple myeloma, chronic infections** and in some autoimmune diseases. • Under production of albumin in conditions like **liver cirrhosis, malnutrition and nephrotic syndrome**.

16.9. Ans. (c) 900 *(Read below)*
About **900 g**[Q] **of hemoglobin** is present in the circulating blood of an **adult man**
Also know:
- The **erythrocytes** carry hemoglobin in the circulation. They are *biconcave disks* because of the protein called as **spectrin**[Q].
- In humans, the RBCs survive in the circulation for an average of **120 days**.[Q]
- The average normal red blood cell count is 5.4 million/ L in men and 4.8 million/ L in women.
- 1 g of hemoglobin yields **35 mg of bilirubin**[Q].

16.10. Ans. (c) Cyanmethemoglobin method *(Read below)*

Hemoglobin estimation		
Visual Colorimetric method	Sahli's (acid hematin method) Alkali hematin method	Most popular method
Photocolorimetric method	Cyanmethemoglobin method	**Most accurate** and currently used

16.11. Ans. (c) 4
Hemoglobin is a globular molecule made up of four subunits. Each subunit contains a **heme** moiety conjugated to a polypeptide. Heme is an iron-containing porphyrin derivative. So, **hemoglobin = 4 globins + 4 heme groups**
Since each heme molecule contains an iron, so total iron atoms present in hemoglobin are 4 in number.
- **70%** of the iron in the body is in **hemoglobin**, 3% in myoglobin, and the rest in ferritin, which is present not only in enterocytes, but also in many other cells.

16.12. Ans. (a) Histidine residues
Harper mentions …'Hemoglobin also functions in CO_2 and proton transport from tissues to lungs. Release of O_2 from oxy Hb at the tissues is accompanied by uptake of protons due to lowering of the pKa of *histidine residues*.'
- Decarboxylation of histidine to *histamine* is catalyzed by a broad-specificity *aromatic L-amino acid decarboxylase*[Q]
- Histidine compounds present in the human body include *ergothioneine, carnosine, and dietary anserine*

16.13. Ans. (b) labile factor.
If whole blood is allowed to clot and the clot is removed, the remaining fluid is called **serum.** Serum has essentially the same composition as plasma, except that:
- **Fibrinogen (factor I)** and clotting factors **II, V, and VIII** have been **removed** and
- Has **higher serotonin content** because of the breakdown of platelets during clotting.
Also know that **factor 5** is called as **labile factor**[Q].

16.14. Ans. (b) Brilliant Cresyl blue *(Ref: Robbins, 9/e 635)*
- **Reticulocytes** are stained in **living state** *in vitro* so staining with dyes like brilliant cresyl blue and new methylene blue is referred to as *supravital staining*.

16.15. Ans. (c) RBCs to whole blood *(Ref: Robbins, 9/e 631)*
Haematocrit (also known as packed cell volume) is the volume percentage (%) of red blood cells in blood.

16.16. Ans. (a) Ferritin *(Ref: Robbins, 9/e 650)*
Ferritin is the storage and transferring the transport form of iron.
Ferroportin is a transmembrane protein that transports iron from the inside of a cell to the outside of it.
Hepcidin is released by liver in setting of anaemia of chronic disease. It is the "master regulator" of human iron metabolism.

16.17. Ans. (a) Brilliant cresyl blue *(Ref: Robbins, 9/e)*
The most common supravital stain is performed on reticulocytes using new methylene blue or brilliant cresyl blue. It makes it possible to see the reticulofilamentous pattern of ribosomes characteristically precipitated in these live immature red blood cells.

17. Ans. (a) Increased reticulocyte Count *(Ref: Robbins 9/e 645, 8th/655, Wintrobe's 12th/1151-3)*
Direct quote from Robbins … *'The reticulocyte count is low'*.
Please be clear of the concept friends that the *reticulocyte count is increased* when the megaloblastic anemia is being treated with *vitamin B12 and folate supplementation* i.e. after the initiation of the treatment in these patients.

- The marrow is usually markedly hypercellular as a result of increased hematopoietic precursors, which often completely replace the fatty marrow. Certain peripheral blood findings are shared by all megaloblastic anemias. The presence of red cells that are macrocytic and oval (macro-ovalocytes) is highly characteristic. There is presence of marked variation in the size (anisocytosis) and shape (poikilocytosis) of red cells. The reticulocyte count is low. Nucleated red cell progenitors occasionally appear in the circulating blood when anemia is severe. Granulocytic precursors also display dysmaturation in the form of giant metamyelocytes and band forms. Neutrophils are also larger than normal and are hypersegmented (having five or more nuclear lobules instead of the normal three to four). Megakaryocytes, too, can be abnormally large and have bizarre, multilobate nuclei.
- The derangement in DNA synthesis causes most precursors to undergo apoptosis in the marrow (ineffective hematopoiesis) and leads to pancytopenia. The anemia is further exacerbated by a mild degree of red cell hemolysis. This leads to raised bilirubin.
- Wintrobe mentions ... 'Mild reversible splenomegaly is present in megaloblastic anemia'.

18. **Ans. (d) Myelofibrosis** *(Ref: Harrison 17th/661, 674, 646)*
The findings in the given question are:
Anemia (Hb = 6g)
Reduced leukocyte count (TLC= 1200)
Reduced platelet count (60000)
Reduced MCV (12fL)

- Normal value of MCV is 80-100 fL. It is the measure of size of RBC. Reduced MCV means microcytic and increased MCV means macrocytic RBCs. Normal TLC is 4000-11000, normal platelet count is 1,50,000 to 4,50,000 and normal Hb is above 12 g/dL.
- Now, considering the options one by one:

  - **Aplastic anemia** has reduced RBC, WBC as well as platelet counts. Anemia is normocytic normochromic, thus it can be easily ruled out.
  - **Paroxysomal nocturnal hemoglobinuria (PNH)** typically presents with anemia which is usually normomacrocytic. If MCV is high, it is due to reticulocytosis. Neutropenia and thrombocytopenia may or may not be present. Therefore, this option also cannot be the answer.
  - **Megaloblastic anemia** presents with raised MCV. There may be leukopenia as well as thrombocytopenia. Severity of these changes parallels the degree of anemia.
  - **Myelofibrosis** usually presents with anemia, leukopenia and thrombocytopenia. Mostly anemia is normocytic but in 30% cases microcytic anemia can be present.

Based on the above discussion, the most probable answer is 'Myelofibrosis'.
However, the value of MCV given is 12 fL which is practically not possible. Normal value of MCV is 80-100 fL. MCV < 50 fL is considered to be extremely low. Therefore, one possibility is that it may be 112 fL and due to typographical error in the question, written as 12 fL. If this is the case, then the answer will become megaloblastic anemia.

As we cannot say for sure that it is a printing mistake, so we will go for 'Myelofibrosis'.

19. **Ans. (a) ↑MCV.** *(Ref: T. Singh 1st/35, Harrison 17th/357, Robbins 9/e 629-630)*
MCV > 100fL indicates *macrocytosis*.

20. **Ans. (a) Megaloblastic precursors are present in bone marrow; (b) Mean corpuscular volume is increased; (c) Serum LDH is increased:** *(Ref: Robbins 9/e 645, Harrison' 17th/645-646)*
- Megaloblastic anemia is a maturation disorder of red cells
- **Cells are macrocytic and hyperchromic. Anisocytosis and** hypersegmented neutrophils are also seen.
- Bone marrow shows hypercellularity, erythrocyte precursors at different stages of development is found. Increased megaloblast causes ineffective erythropoiesis.
- In severe anemia as many as 90% of RBC precursors may be destroyed before their release into the circulation (Normal 10-15%). Thereby **increased unconjugated bilirubin and lactic acid dehydrogenase**.
- *Target cells* result due to increased ratio of RBC surface area to volume, seen in *hemoglobin disorders, thalassemia, liver disease*. **Reticulocytes, platelet count and leukocyte count decreased**.

21. **Ans. (b) Copper deficiency:** *(Ref: Harrison 17th/449)*

Copper deficiency is manifested by hypochromic normocytic anemia, osteopenia, depigmentation, mental retardation and psychomotor abnormalities.

Thiamine, pyridoxine and B_{12} deficiency leads to megaloblastic anemia.

Classification of megaloblastic anemia

	Drugs	Diseases	Unknown etiology
Cobalamin deficiency Folic acid deficiency	Purine and Pyrimidine antagonists Others-procarbazine, zidovudine hydroxyurea, acyclovir	Hereditary orotic aciduria Lesch-Nyhan syndrome	Refractory megaloblastic anemia. Di-Gueglielmo syndrome Congenital dyserythropoietic anemia

- Causes of anemia in Liver diseases are gastrointestinal bleeding, folate deficiency and hypersplenism.

22. **Ans. (a) Fish tapeworm infestation; (c) Gastrectomy; (d) Ileal resection.** *(Ref: Robbins 7th/640, 9/e 645)*
The other two cause megaloblastic anemia by interfering with folic acid metabolism.

23. **Ans. (c) Pure Red Cell Aplasia** *(Ref: T. Singh 1st/140; Robbins 7th/648, 636, 9/e 642)*
PNH is the only hemolytic anemia caused by an acquired intrinsic defect in the cell membrane. PNH arises in the setting of aplastic anemia and these patients are at increased risk of developing acute myelogenous leukemia.
Aplastic anemia may progress to PNH and MDS.

24. **Ans. (d) Cholestatic jaundice** *(Ref: Robbins 7th/640, 9/e 645)*

25. **Ans. (d) Thalassemia** *(Ref: Robbins 9/e 639, 8th/649, 7th/635)*

26. **Ans. (a) Myelofibrosis** *(Ref: Robbins 9/e 620-621, 8th/630-631; 7th/700-701)*

27. **Ans. (b) Folic acid deficiency** *(Ref: Robbins 9/e 648, 8th/659; 7th/642)*

28. **Ans. (d) Hypothyroidism** *(Ref: Tejinder Singh 1st/66, Robbins 9/e 645)*

29. **Ans. (a) Thymoma** *(Ref: Robbins 9/e 627, 8th/636-637; 7th/707-708)*

30. **Ans. (b) Diphyllobothrium latum** *(Ref: Robbins 9/e 648, 8th/655, 7th/640)*

31. **Ans. (c) Anemia occurs after 3-4 months of poor absorption** *(Ref: Robbins 9/e 648, 8th/657; 7th/682)*

32. **Ans. (b) Folic acid deficiency** *(Ref: Harsh Mohan 6th/308, Robbins 9/e 647)*

33. **Ans. (c) Megaloblastic** *(Ref: Robbins Robbins 9/e 645, 8th/655, 7th/638)*

34. **Ans. (c) Megaloblastic anemia** *(Ref: Robbins 9/e 645, 8th/655, 7th/638)*

35. **Ans. (d) Postsplenectomy** *(Ref: Robbins 9/e 627, 633, 8th/646, 7th/627, Harrison 17th/375)*

36. **Ans. (c) Diphyllobothrium latum infestation** *(Ref: Robbins 9/e 648, 8th/655)*

37. **Ans. (d) Thymoma** *(Ref: Robbins 9/e 627, 8th/664)*
In the rare pure red cell aplasia, the erythroid marrow elements are absent or nearly absent, while granulopoiesis and thrombopoiesis remain unaltered. This condition occurs in both primary and secondary forms, both of which are thought to be related to autoimmune destruction of erythroid precursors. There is a specific association between thymic tumors (thymoma) and autoimmune hematologic diseases, specifically including pure red cell aplasia.

38. **Ans. (a) Dietary cobalamin deficiency** *(Ref: Robbins 9/e 648, 8th/656-8)*
Vitamin B_{12} deficiency may occur due to low dietary intake of this vitamin, the presence of antibodies against intrinsic factor (pernicious anemia) or malabsorption.

The **Schilling test** helps to differentiate between different causes of vitamin B_{12} deficiency. The patient is first given a dose of radiolabeled oral vitamin B_{12} and an intramuscular injection of unlabeled Vitamin B_{12}. The urinary excretion of radioactive B_{12} is then measured. Normal urinary excretion of radiolabeled vitamin B_{12} suggests normal absorption, and B_{12} deficiency in this setting is most likely due to poor intake of Vitamin B_{12} in the diet (choice A).

Diminished urinary excretion of radiolabeled vitamin B_{12} is a sign of impaired intestinal absorption. To differentiate between pernicious anemia and malabsorption, the next dose of radiolabeled B_{12} is given with intrinsic factor. Normal excretion after the addition of intrinsic factor is diagnostic of pernicious anemia. Low excretion of B_{12} after administration of intrinsic factor rules out pernicious anemia and suggests a malabsorption syndrome such as pancreatic insufficiency, bacterial overgrowth, or short gut syndrome.

(Choice B) Pernicious anemia is associated with atrophic gastritis and the presence of antibodies against gastric parietal cells and intrinsic factor. Administration of vitamin B_{12} without intrinsic factor will show low urinary radioactive vitamin B12 excretion on the Schilling test.
(Choices C and D) Nontropical sprue (celiac disease) and *Diphyllobothrium latum* infestation are examples of malabsorption syndromes. They are characterized by impaired absorption of vitamin B12 on the Schilling test that is not corrected by oral intrinsic factor supplementation.

39. **Ans. (b) Reticulocyte count** *(Ref: Robbins 8th/641)*

The graph describes the treatment response to vitamin B$_{12}$ (cyanocobalamin) in a patient with vitamin B$_{12}$-deficiency anemia secondary to atrophic gastritis. Once vitamin B$_{12}$ replacement therapy is begun the rate of effective erythropoiesis increases immediately. Immature erythrocytes are released from the bone marrow into the bloodstream. The peripheral count of these reticulocytes may rise within one week as indicated by the Gaussian curve on the graph. The anemia typically takes as long as six weeks to correct as indicated by the exponential curve on the graph.

(Choice A) The RBC count curve would be expected to follow the contour of the total hemoglobin curve.

(Choice C) Since this patient is suffering from a vitamin B12-deficiency anemia (which is non-hemolytic in nature) we would not expect serum haptoglobin levels to be affected by the anemia or its treatment.

(Choice D) In chronic atrophic gastritis, parietal cell loss results in profound hypochlorhydria, increased serum gastrin levels (antral G cell gastrin secretion is inhibited by the presence of hydrochloric acid) and inadequate intrinsic factor production. The vitamin B$_{12}$ deficiency in this patient is a consequence — not a cause — of his parietal cell atrophy.

> **Atrophic gastritis** can result in profound **hypochlorhydria** inadequate intrinsic factor production, vitamin B12 deficiency, megaloblastic anemia and **elevated serum gastrin and methylmalonic acid** (MMA) levels. Once vitamin B12 replacement therapy is initiated in an individual with atrophic gastritis the reticulocyte count increases dramatically. **Hemoglobin and RBC count** levels **gradually rise** while the **methylmalonic acid level decreases**.

39.1. Ans. (a) Beta thalassemia trait *(Ref: Robbins 9/e 641, 8/e p649)*

Hemoglobin electrophoresis usually reveals an **increase in HbA$_2$** ($\alpha_2\delta_2$) **to 4% to 8%** of the total hemoglobin (normal, 2.5% ± 0.3%), which is a reflection of an elevated ratio of δ-chain to β-chain synthesis. *HbF levels are generally normal or occasionally slightly increased.*

39.2. Ans. (c) Vitamin B$_{12}$ absorption *(Ref: Robbins 9/e 648, 8/e p657-8)*

The **Schilling test** is performed to determine the cause for **cobalamin malabsorption**. Since cobalamin absorption requires multiple steps, including gastric, pancreatic, and ileal processes, the Schilling test also can be used to assess the integrity of those other organs.

Differential Results of Schilling Test in Several Diseases with Cobalamin (Cbl) Malabsorption

	^{58}Co-Cbl	With Intrinsic Factor	With Pancreatic Enzymes	After 5 Days of Antibiotics
Pernicious anemia	Reduced	Normal	Reduced	Reduced
Chronic pancreatitis	Reduced	Reduced	Normal	Reduced
Bacterialovergrowth	Reduced	Reduced	Reduced	Normal
Ileal disease	Reduced	Reduced	Reduced	Reduced

39.3. Ans. (c) Increased reticulocyte count..... *(Ref: Robbin 8/e p655, Wintrobe's 12/e p1151-3)*

Repeat from AIIMS Nov 12 see earlier explanation

39.4. Ans. (a) Aplastic anemia..... *(Ref: Robbin 9/e p653)*

Aplastic anemia refers to a syndrome of chronic primary hematopoietic failure and attendant *pancytopenia* (anemia, neutropenia, and thrombocytopenia).

39.5. Ans. (c) Chronic renal failure..... read below

The same question was asked in different sets with different choices. Choices a,b,d are examples of hemolytic anemias and hence the answer by exclusion is chronic renal failure. CRF has low erythropoietin levels due to less production and has normocytic normochromic anaemia.

39.6. Ans. (b) Human parvo virus B19 *(Ref: Robbin 9/e p460)*

Parvovirus B19 causes erythema infectiosum or "fifth disease of childhood" in immunocompetent older children. Parvovirus B19 has a particular *tropism for erythroid* cells, and diagnostic viral inclusions can be seen in early erythroid progenitors in infected infants.

Parvovirus infection in pregnant women is associated with hydrops fetalis due to severe fetal anemia, sometimes leading to miscarriage or stillbirth.

40. Ans. (a) Anaemia of chronic disease *(Ref: Robbins 9/e 652-653, Wintrobe 12th/1221-2)*

Looking at the data one by one friends, we infer that:

• We have an old patient with chronic inflammatory condition. In addition,

Parameter with value in question	Normal range	Inference in our patient
Hemoglobin 4.5gm/dl	13-17g/dl	Decreased
Platelet count 2 lakh/ml	1.5-4.5lakh/ml	Normal
TLC 6000/mm^3	4000-11000/mm^3	Normal

Contd...

Contd...

Parameter with value in question	Normal range	Inference in our patient
Serum ferritin 200 µg/L	15-300 µg/L	Normal
Serum iron 30 mg/L	50-150 µg/L	Reduced
TIBC 280 ng/L	300-400 mg/L	Reduced

Final conclusion, *decreased serum iron, increased storage iron i.e. serum ferritin, decreased serum transferring and decreased total iron binding capacity suggest the diagnosis of anaemia of chronic disease.*

41. **Ans. (b) Thalassemia minor** *(Ref: Hematology by Renu Saxena 1st/174)*
Thalassemia major patient presents with *severe anemia* and cannot survive without blood transfusion, so this option can be easily ruled out. For other options, **Mentzer index** is useful for differentiating between thalassemia minor and iron deficiency anemia.
Mentzer index is calculated as MCV/RBC count. Its value is >13 in iron deficiency anemia and <13 in thalassemia minor. For our given question, the value on calculation comes out to be 55/4.5 = 12.22.
As the value is < 13, so it is a case of thalassemia minor.

42. **Ans. (a) Iron deficiency anemia** *(Ref: Robbins 8th/651, 9/e 652, T.Singh 1st/34)*
   - Decreased hemoglobin with the clinical features of fatigue and weakness is diagnostic of anemia
   - MCV is 70 fl, so, microcytosis is present (normal MCV is 82-96fl)
   - MCH is 22pg, so, decreased MCH is suggestive of hypochromic anemia (normal MCH is 27-33pg)
   - Red cell distribution width (RDW) is the coefficient of variation of size of RBCs. Normal value is 11.5-14.5. It is an indicator of anisocytosis which may present in IDA as well as hemolytic anemias.
   - In early iron deficiency anemia, RDW increases along with low MCV while in beta thalassemia trait, RDW is normal with low MCV, thus distinguishing from each other.

Increased reticulocytosis is a feature of iron deficiency anemia.

43. **Ans. (b) Myelodysplastic syndrome** *(Ref: Robbins 9/e 615, Wintrobe's 10th/1022-25)*
Sideroblastic anemia can be *hereditary* (due to decreased ALA synthase activity) *or acquired* (secondary to leukemias, myelodysplastic syndrome, alcoholism, copper deficiency, pyridoxine deficiency or lead poisoning).

44. **Ans. (c) Thalassemia minor** *(Ref: Robbins 9/e 641, 8th/651, 7th/633-634)*
   - Thalassemia major patient presents with *severe anemia* and **cannot survive** without blood transfusion, so this option can be easily ruled out.
   - This cannot be a case of megaloblastic anemia because in megaloblastic anemia, **M.C.V. is increased** (> 100 fL)
   - So, we are left with two options, i.e. Iron deficiency anemia and thalassemia minor. Both of these presents with **microcytic hypochromic anemia.**
The key point in the differential diagnosis of these two conditions is the RBC count.
   - In thalassemia minor, the **RBC count is near normal and** only the hemoglobin is reduced. *In this condition the R.B.C. count is not reduced as much as the hemoglobin and hematocrit in fact it is usually normal.* This due to the fact that the marrow can keep on producing the cell at normal rate but it cannot fill them with hemoglobin. Hence, the hemoglobin is low and the empty cells occupy less space thus lowering the hematocrit relative to the erythrocyte count.
   - On the other hand, in Iron deficiency anemia, the **RBC** *production is also impaired.*
There are many indices to differentiate between iron deficiency anemia (IDA) and beta-thalassemia (BT):

Index	Formula	Value for iron Deficiency anemia	Value for beta-thalassemia
Mentzer index	MCV/RBC count	> 13	< 13
Shine and Lal Index	MCV^2 X MCH X 0.01	> 1530	< 1530
England and fraser index	MCV – RBC – (5 X Hb) – 5.19	> 0	< 0
Srivastava Index	MCH/RBC	> 3.8	< 3.8
Green and King index	MCV^2 X RDW X Hb/100	> 65	< 65
Red Cell Distribution Width index	MCV X RDW/RBC	> 220	< 220

In the given question, only the value of MCV and RBC are given, so we can utilize **Mentzer index**. The Mentzer index in the given question is 55/4.5 = 12.22
As the value is < 13, so it is a case of thalassemia minor.

45. **Ans. (a) Inhibition of enzymes involved in heme biosynthesis** *(Ref: Robbins 9/e 411, Tejinder Singh 1st/147)*

Anemia and Red Blood Cells

- **Lead inhibits** the enzymes **δ aminolevulinic acid dehydrase**, red cell **pyrimidine 5' nucleotidase** and **ferrochelatase** which are involved in the synthesis of heme.
- Deficiency of heme causes microcytic hypochromic anemia because heme is an integral part of hemoglobin and hemoglobin deficiency causes microcytic hypochromic anemia.

46. **Ans. (b) Sideroblastic anemia** *(Ref: Harrison 17th/631-32 (t) 98-4)*
    The hematological findings suggest the diagnosis of **sideroblastic anemia.**
    Differential diagnosis of microcytic hypochromic anemia (Very Important for exams)

Tests	Iron deficiency	Inflammation	Thalassemia	Sideroblastic anemia
Peripheral smear	Micro/hypo	Normal micro/hypo	Micro/hypo with targeting	Variable
SI	↓	↓	Normal to high	Normal to high
TIBC	↑	↓	Normal	Normal
Percent TS	↓	↓	↑	↑
Ferritin (mcg/L)	↓	↑	↑	↑
Hemoglobin pattern	Normal	Normal	Abnormal	Normal

SI, serum iron; TIBC, total iron-binding capacity; TS, transferrin saturation.

47. **Ans. (a) ↓ Erythropoietin; (b) ↓ RBC survival; (c) ↓ folate; (d) Bone marrow hypoplasia; (e) Iron deficiency.** *(Ref: Harrison 17th/633-634, 18th/e (t) 280 (5))*

48. **Ans. All.** *(Ref: Robbins 9th/651, Harrison' 17th/631; (t) 98(2))*

49. **Ans. (a) Thalassemia; (c) Anemia in chronic disease (e) Megaloblastic anemia** *(Ref: Harsh Mohan 6th/302, 307)*
    - Increased bone marrow iron is seen in:
      - Sideroblastic anemia
      - Anemia of chronic disease
      - Megaloblastic anemia
      - Pernicious anemia
      - Thalassemia.

50. **Ans. (a) Thalassemia; (b) Hb Lepore; (c) Hb Bart's.** *(Ref: Harsh Mohan 6th/323-324)*
    Causes of microcytosis (MCV < 80fl)
    - Iron deficiency anemia
    - Thalassemia
    - Sideroblastic anemia
    - Anemia of chronic disease
    In *Hb Barts,* all the four α chain genes are deleted resulting in formation of Barts Hb.

    In Hb Lepore, there is nonhomologus *fusion* of β and δ genes and forms an abnormal hemoglobin with total *absence* of normal β *chain.* It is one of the form of β *thalassemia minor.*

51. **Ans. (a) Microcytic hypochromic anemia; (d) Bone marrow iron decrease earlier than serum iron.** *(Ref: Robbins 7th/645, de Gruchy's 5th/42)*

52. **Ans. (d) S. ferritin ↑** *(Ref: Harrison 17th/632-4, Robbins 9/e 625-653, 8th/662)*

53. **Ans. (d) Persistently raised HbF** *(Ref: Wintrobes 11th/1326; Nelson 17th/1630)*
    It is a case of persistently raised HbF.
    Characteristics
    - There is persistence of fetal Hb in adult life so that almost whole of the Hb of patient is HbF.
    - Patient remains asymptomatic even without blood transfusion.
    - No anemia or splenomegaly seen.

	Beta-globin genes	HbA	HbA2	HbF
Normal	Homozygous β	97-99%	1-3%	< 1%
Thalassemia major	Homozygous β⁰	0%	4-10%	90-96%
	Homozygous β⁺(mild)	0-30%	0-10%	60-100%
Thalassemia intermedia	Homozygous β⁺ (mild)	0-30%	0-10%	60-100%
Thalassemia minor	Homozygous β⁰	80-95%	4-8%	1-5%
	Homozygous β⁺	80-95%	4-89%	1-5%

- From the values given in question it can be thalassemia major or thalassemia intermedia.
- In thalassemia major patient presents with severe hemolytic anemia at the age of 6 months and cannot survive without blood transfusions.
- In thalassemia intermedia patient can survive without transfusion but they are not asymptomatic.

54. **Ans. (c) Absence of intrinsic factor** *(Ref: Robbins 9/e 645, 7th/639-640)*
Absence of IF causes *Pernicious anemia* which is an example of *megaloblastic anemia*.

55. **Ans. (c) Rheumatoid arthritis** *(Ref: Robbins 7th/639-640)*
Hypochromic/microcytic blood picture is seen in: (mnemonic: **SITA**)
S - Sideroblastic anemia shows presence of ringed sideroblasts (Lead poisoning has basophilic stippling), **I** - Iron deficiency anemia, **T** - Thalassemia major, **A** - Anemia of chronic disease

Note: In anemia of chronic disease (of Rheumatoid Arthritis, TB, UTI, etc), the red cells are mainly normocytic; normochromic red cells. In some cases, red cells may be hypochromic. So, we would go with **RA** as the best answer in this question.

How to differentiate feature between IDA and AOCD is:
- In IDA → microcytosis precedes development of hypochromia.
- In Anemia of chronic disease → hypochromia precedes microcytosis.

56. **Ans. (a) Microcytic hypochromic anemia** *(Ref: Hematology by Tejinder Singh/83)*
Explained in text.

57. **Ans. (a) Congenital spherocytosis** *(Ref: Robbins 7th/625)*
Hereditary spherocytosis – Small RBCs are seen without central pallor (normal RBCs have central 1/3rd pallor). It is also seen conditions where spherocytes are present in peripheral blood like:

• Hereditary spherocytosis • Autoimmune hemolytic anemia • Cirrhosis • Clostridial sepsis	• Burns • G6PD deficiency • ABO incompatibility

58. **Ans. (d) Megaloblastic anemia** *(Ref: Robbins 9/e 645, 7th/639/643/626/629)*
- Megaloblastic anemia: Two principal types
- **Pathology:** Defective DNA synthesis and diminished erythropoiesis
- **Morphology** - Anisocytosis (various size + shape), Macrocytosis (MCV > 100 fl), MCHC is normal and, Macropolymorphonuclear (hyper segmented) neutrophils

59. **Ans. (c) ↓ Serum ferritin level** *(Ref: Robbins 9/e 652-653, 8th/662, 7th/646)*

60. **Ans. (a) Iron deficiency** *(Ref: Robbins 9/e 652-653, 8th/659; 7th/643)*

61. **Ans. (c) TIBC is decreased** *(Ref: Robbins 9/e 652-653, 8th/662; Harrison 17th/632)*

62. **Ans. (b) Transferrin** *(Ref: Robbins 9/e 650, 8th/659; 7th/644)*

63. **Ans. (d) Increased mean corpuscular volume** *(Ref: Robbins 9/e 652, 8th/660-661, 7th/645)*

64. **Ans. (c) Serum Ferritin** *(Ref: Robbins 9/e 652, 8th/659-660)*

65. **Ans. (d) Salivary gland** *(Ref: Robbins 9/e 848-849, 8th/660, 7th/909)*

66. **Ans. (a) Melanin** *(Ref: Robbins 9/e 849, 8th/660-661, 7th/910)*

67. **Ans. (a) Ferritin** *(Ref: Robbins 9/e 650, 8th/659-660, 7th/644)*

68. **Ans. (c) Iron deficiency anemia** *(Ref: Robbins 9/e 652, 8th/659-662; 7 th/634, 646)*

69. **Ans. (b) Serum iron increased, TIBC decreased** *(Ref: Robbins 9/e 849, 8th/862-3)*
The stem of the question is suggestive of long-standing, late stage hereditary hemochromatosis, and the expected findings would include markedly increased serum iron and moderately reduced TIBC. This combination often results in almost 100% saturation of iron-binding capacity.

69.1. **Ans. (d) Cutaneous porphyria** *(Ref: Hematology: Diagnosis and Treatment p467)*
Sideroblastic anemia is associated with the following

Hereditary: X linked, autosomal recessive, autosomal dominant
Acquired: previous chemotherapy, irradiation, myelodysplasia, myelproliferative disorders

Drugs: alcohol isoanizid, choramphenicol, pyridoxine deficiency, lead poisoning

Rare causes: copper deficiency, zinc overload, hypothermia, **erythropoetic porphyria**

Hereditary syndromic: Pearson syndrome, thiamine responsive megaloblastic anemia,

69.2. Ans. (d) Macrocytic anemia *(Ref: Robbins 9/e 411, 8/e p406-7)*

- **Lead inhibits** the activity of enzymes involved in heme synthesis; δ-aminolevulinic acid dehydratase[Q] **and ferrochelatase**[Q] (BIOCHEMISTRY NEET QUESTION INFO)
- Ferrochelatase catalyzes the incorporation of iron into protoporphyrin, and its inhibition causes a **rise in protoporphyrin** levels as well as appearance of scattered **ringed sideroblasts**[Q]. The elevated levels of protoporphyrin may appear in the urine of an individual.
- There is a distinctive **punctate basophilic stippling**[Q] **of the red cells** and the presence of *microcytic, hypochromic anemia*[Q].
- Also know that in lead poisoning is associated with reduction in uric acid excretion which can lead to gout ("**saturnine gout**"[Q])

69.3. Ans. (a) Duffy blood group *(Ref: Robbins 9/e 391, 8/e p387)*

Conditions providing protection against malaria with the reasons

- **Sickle cell disease**: *P falciparum* can not multiply properly in the presence of HbS
- α and β thalassemia:
- **Absence** of **duffy blood group**: duffy antigen is required for parasite to enter the RBCs
- **G6 PD deficiency**: G6PD is required for respiration of plasmodium

69.4. Ans. (b) Reticulocytosis *(Ref: Robbins 9/e 652, 8/e p662, 7/e p624)*

In uncomplicated cases, oral iron supplementation produces an increase in reticulocytosis in about 5-7 days that is followed by a steady increase in blood counts and normalization of red cell indices.

69.5. Ans. (a) Lead *(Ref: Robbins 9/e 411, 8/e p406-407, 7/e p432-433)*

Lead is associated with sideroblastic anemia.....details are discussed in a separate question.

69.6. Ans. (a) RBCs *(Ref: Harrison 17/e p77)*

You must know: Different type of red blood cells are:

- Echinocytes/Burr cells : Regular spine-like projections on cell surface; in Megaloblastic anemia/burns/hemolytic anemia
- Acanthocytes/Spur cells : irregular thorn-like projections; in liver disease, abetalipoproteinemia
- Stomatocytes : Slit-like (mouth like) area of pallor
- Schistocytes : Fragmented RBCs; triangular, comma-shaped or helmet shaped
- Leptocytes : Thin flat cells
- Codocytes : Mexican hat cells
- Dacrocytes : Tear drop cells or Target cells (red cells with central dark area; in liver disease, anemia of chronic disease)
- Drepanocytes : Sickle cells
- Elliptocytes : Pencil cells or cigar cells
- Keratocytes : Helmet cells
- Knizocytes : Cells with more than one concavities

69.7. Ans. (b) Hookworm *(Ref: Robbins 9/e 651, 8/e p336, 7/e p623)*

Hookworm infestation can cause chronic blood loss and therefore may cause iron deficiency anemia.

69.8. Ans. (a) Reticulocytosis...explained earlier *(Ref: Robbins 9/e 652, 8/e p641, 7/e p624)*

69.9. Ans. (a) Mucosal cell iron stores *(Ref: Robbins 9/e 650)*

Rate of iron uptake is dependent on the levels of a protein called hepcidin. This protein functions to regulate (inhibit) iron transport across the gut mucosa, thereby preventing excess iron absorption and maintaining normal iron levels within the body. Hepcidin also inhibits transport of iron out of macrophages (where iron is stored).

- **Mutation** of the gene coding for hepcidin is implicated in the causation of **hemochromatosis.**

69.10. Ans. (a) Anaemia of chronic disease.... see text for details

Revision of iron profile table

Parameter	Iron deficiency anemia	Sideroblastic anaemia	Anemia of chronic disease
Serum iron	Low	High	**Low**
Serum ferritin	Low	High	**High**
T.I.B.C	Increased	decreased	**Low**
Homozygous b+ (mild)	0-30%	0-10%	**60-100%**

70. Ans. (c) Coombs test *(Ref: Robbins 9/e 643, 8th/653)*

The presence of spherocytes can be seen in the following conditions:

- *Hereditary spherocytosis*
- *Autoimmune hemlolytic anemia*
- *G6PD deficiency*
- *Infections*
- *Burns*
- *Hemolytic disease of new born*

- PNH is not a cause for the presence of spherocytes; so, no test for this condition is required.
- Osmotic fragility is increased with spherocytes. So, it does not add anything to our existing information about the disease causing spherocyte formation.
- Reticulocyte count is expected to be elevated in the setting of haemolytic anemia (suggested by jaundice and pallor).

Coombs test is done for detection of the antibodies formed against the normal antigens present on the surface of cells like platelets and red blood cells. So, it is going to be positive in autoimmune hemolytic anemia whereas negative in hereditary spherocytosis. Thus, a differentiation between these conditions can be done.

71. Ans. (b) Defective GPI anchor *(Ref: Robbins 9/e 642, 8th/65, Harrison 17th/660)*

Ham's acidified serum test is the lysis of erythrocytes on addition of acidified serum. It demonstrates increased susceptibility to the complement system and is seen in paroxysmal nocturnal hemoglobinuria (PNH).

PNH is caused due to acquired *mutations in Phosphatidyl inositol glycan A (PIGA) gene*. Normally, this gene is *essential for the synthesis of the glycosylphosphatidyl inositol (GPI) molecule* which provides an anchor for cell membrane attachment of some proteins. These **proteins are also required for inactivating the complement (***not for activating complement as was given in the option***)**. The examples of these proteins include:

- Decay-accelerating factor or CD55
- Membrane inhibitor of reactive lysis, or CD59
- C8 binding protein

Thus it is easy for us to understand that in PNH, the defective GPI anchor prevents the attachment of the above mentioned proteins.

72. Ans. (d) Paroxysmal nocturnal hemoglobinuria *(Ref Wintrobe's 12th/1007, 1044-5, Nathan and Oski's Hematology of infancy and childhood 7th/45, Guha's NEONATOLOGY Principles and Practice vol 2, 3rd/910)*

- G6PD and Hereditary spherocytosis can cause anemia and jaundice since birth and are causes of haemolytic anemias. So, they are easily ruled out.
- Friends I got some worthy information after spending few days and multiple book searching which should bring a smile on your face.
- These are the lines from **Oski's Hematology** "β chain mutations generally produce no clinical symptomatology in the newborn period. This does not mean that chain variants are never a problem in the neonate. *Sickle cell hemoglobinopathies are the most commmonly encountered β chain variants in the newborn period*. Several cases of *homozygous sickle cell disease have been seen in neoanates*. In infants in whom sickle cell anemia has been diagnosed in first days of life because of some specific symptoms specifcally jaundice, fever, pallor, respiratory distress and abdominal distension".
- *'Hyperbilirubinemia appears to be more common in newborns with sickle cell anemia.'*.. **Nathan and Oski 7th/45**
- *'β chain defects do not manifest in newborn. An important exception is sickle cell disease which can manifest in newborn as up to 30% of hemoglobin at birth may be adult hemoglobin*. Sickling and hemolytic jaundice may result and is best treated with exchange transfusion.'... Guha 3rd/910*, Jaypee

Therefore the answer of exclusion is option 'd' .. paroxysmal nocturnal hemogloninuria. Its mean age of presentation is in the 30's. Even after extensive search, I could not get hold of any material which supports presence of symptomatic PNH in infancy.

73. Ans. (c) Idiopathic thrombocytopenic purpura *(Ref: Robbins 9/e 658-659, 8th/668, Harrison 17th/367)*

Primary or idiopathic ITP has two clinical subtypes: acute and chronic. Both of them are autoimmune disorders in which platelet destruction results from the formation of antiplatelet autoantibodies. The opsonized platelets are rendered susceptible to phagocytosis by the cells of the mononuclear phagocyte system.

Option 'a': The triad of hemolysis, pancytopenia and **thrombosis** *is* **unique** *to this condition. Thrombosis is the leading cause of death in individuals with PNH....Robbins 8th/653*

Option 'b': DIC is an acute, subacute, or chronic thrombohemorrhagic disorder occurring as a secondary complication in a variety of diseases. It is characterized by activation of the coagulation sequence that leads to the formation of **microthrombi throughout the microcirculation** *of the body.. Robbins 8th/673*

Option 'd': Heparin Induced Thrombocytopenia can be two types; type I thrombocytopenia which occurs rapidly after onset of therapy, is moderately severe, clinically insignificant and may resolve despite continuation of heparin therapy. Type II thrombocytopenia is more severe and occurs 5 to 14 days after initiation of therapy. It can, **paradoxically**, lead to life-threatening **venous and arterial thrombosis.**

Why do we have paradoxical thrombosis in HIT type II?

It is caused by an immune reaction against a complex of heparin and platelet factor 4 (a normal component of platelet granules). The attachment of *antibody to platelet factor 4 produces immune complexes that activate platelets, promoting thrombosis even in the setting of marked thrombocytopenia.*

Additional important features of Heparin Induced Thrombocytopenia

- Platelet count < 100,000/µL or decreased by > 50%.
- Starts 5-10 days after starting heparin.
- More common with unfractionated heparin (than LMW heparin), Surgical patients (than medical patients) and females (than males)
- Venous thrombosis is more common than arterial.

74. Ans. (c) Glycosylphosphatidylinositol (GPI) *(Ref: Robbins 9/e 642, 8th/65, Harrison 17th/660)*

Paroxysmal nocturnal hemoglobinuria (PNH) *results from acquired mutations in Phosphatidyl inositol glycan A (PIGA) gene, which is essential for the synthesis of the glycosylphosphatidyl inositol (GPI) anchor.* GPI is responsible for providing an anchor for cell membrane attachment of some proteins like CD59 (most important), CD55 and C8 binding protein which are also required for inactivating the complement.

It is the **only hemolytic anemia** caused by an acquired intrinsic defect in the cell membrane. The triad of **hemolysis, pancytopenia** and thrombosis is unique to this condition.

75. Ans. (d) Donath-Landsteiner antibody *(Ref: Robbins 9/e 644, 7th/407-408; Harrison 16th/611-614)*

Cold hemagglutinin is associated with more commonly **IgM** or rarely **IgG** antibodies. These are not to be confused with anti-IgM or anti-IgG antibodies given as other options in the question. An important example of cold hemagglutinin disease is paroxysmal cold hemoglobinuria. For details, see text

76. Ans. (c) Glycophorin C *(Ref: Harrison 17th/653-655, Robbins 9/e 632, 8th/642-644, 7th/625)*

- Normally, RBC membrane consists of a protein **spectrin**, ion transporter called band 3 of membrane with the help of ankyrin and band 4.2.
- Mutations in glycophorin A has **not** been reported.

Mutations in α-spectrin are most common cause of hereditary elliptocytosis [65% cases] and β-spectrin mutation is responsible for another 30% cases. Some of the cases of HE occur due to mutation in band 4.1.

77. Ans. (c) CLL *(Ref: Harrison 17th/693, Robbins 9/e 643)*

Leukemias especially of the CLL type are associated with warm autoimmune hemolytic anemia.

78. Ans. (d) Metallic cardiac valves *(Ref: Rubin's pathology 5th/878, Nathan and Oski hematology 7th/643, Goljan pathology edn 2013/ 314)*

Microangiopathic hemolytic anemia is associated with fragmentation of the red cells in the microcirculation. It is associated with antiphospholoid antibody syndrome... NMS Medicine 5th/348

Pathologically, macroangiopathic hemolytic anemia is associated with prosthetic cardiac valves.

Macroangiopathic hemolytic anemia may be caused by:

•	Direct red cell trauma from abnormal valvular surface: prosthetic valve grafts, tight aortic stenosis and synthetic vascular grafts.
•	Large vessel disorders that may cause shearing of red cells: cavernous hemangioma (Kasabach Merrit syndrome),
•	Other causes include coarctation of aorta, ruptured sinus of valsalva, ruptured chordae tendinae and aortic aneurysm.

Causes of Microangiopathic hemolytic anemia

1. Vasculitis like microscopic polyangiitis	5. Scleroderma
2. Malignant hypertension	6. Thrombotic thrombocytopenic purpura (TTP) and Hemolytic uremic Syndrome (HUS)
3. Eclampsia	7. DIC
4. Renal graft rejection	8. March hemoglobinuria

79. **Ans. (b) Conjugated and unconjugated bilirubin** (*Ref: Robbins illustrated, 9/e 853, 8th/840-841, 7th/886-887*)
    - It is a case of *erythroblastosis fetalis*. (**type II Hypersensitivity reaction**)
    - In erythroblastosis fetalis there is excessive breakdown of RBC's leading to increased production of bilirubin in the blood. This **increased** bilirubin is predominantly **unconjugated** but the level of **conjugated bilirubin** will also increase because of compensatory increase in bilirubin conjugation process by the liver. So, both unconjugated bilirubin and bilirubin glucuronides may accumulate systemically and deposit in tissues, giving rise to the yellow discoloration of jaundice. This is particularly seen in yellowing of the **sclera** (because of presence of **elastin fibers**).

80. **Ans. (a) Teardrop and Burr cells** (*Ref: Robbins 7th/766, 687, 9/e 620*)
    - Teardrop cells also known as dacryocytes are seen in *myelofibrosis*. Rest of the features are seen in hemolytic anemia.

81. **Ans. (b) Acute G6PD deficiency; (e) PNH** (*Ref: Robbins' 7th/624, 625, 9/e 631-632*)
    Intravascular hemolysis occurs due to disruption of red cell membrane in circulation. The RBCs are damaged mechanically, by *complement fixation, malaria, toxins and drugs*. **It is seen in:** Acute G6PD deficiency and PNH
    - In Sickle cell disease and hereditary spherocytosis, RBC destruction occurs in spleen (extravascular hemolysis)
    - Thalassemia is a hemoglobinopathy.

82. **Ans. (a) HUS; (c) Malignant hypertension; (d) Prosthetic valves; (e) TTP:** (*Ref: Robbins' 7th/638, 9/e 630*)

83. **Ans. (a) Hemoglobin C; (c) Hereditary spherocytosis** (*Ref: de Gruchy's 5th/184, Robbins 9/e 632*)
    Spherocytosis is the anomaly due to abnormal ion permeability of the red cell membrane.
    This results in higher level of Na⁺ and low level of K⁺ in the cell, thus making the cell hyperosmotic. Interior of the cell takes up water and the cell becomes macrocytic and hypochromic and thus osmotic fragility is increased.
    Acquired causes of spherocytosis:

    - Autoimmune acquired hemolytic anemia.
    - Infections/burnchemicals
    - Water dilution hemolytic anemia
    - Hemolytic disease of the newborn (ABO incompatibility)
    - Heinz body hemolytic anemia.

    Hb C disease – associated with compensated hemolysis with normal hemoglobin level or mild anemia. In this disease in peripheral smear, target cells and microspherocytes are seen.

84. **Ans. (a) Microangiopathic hemolytic anemia; (b) DIC; (d) Malignant hypertension; (e) HELLP syndrome** (*Ref: de Gruchy's 5th/209 , Wintrobes 11th/1236, Robbins 9/e 630*)
    Schistocytosis or fragmented RBCs are found in

Thalassemia	Severe burn	DIC
Hereditary elliptocytosis	Microangiopathic hemolytic anemia	Malignant hypertension
Megaloblastic anemia	Iron deficiency anemia	HUS
HELLP syndrome		

85. **Ans. (a) Glucose-6 phosphate dehydrogenase deficiency:** (*Ref: Robbins 7th/624, 628, 9/e 631*)

86. **Ans. (b) Reticulocytosis seen; (c) Smaller size; (d) Always associated with ↑ MCHC.** (*Ref: Robbins 7th/626, 9/e 633*)
    Hereditary spherocytosis is an usually autosomal dominant condition in which the ratio of surface area to volume decreases and hence the RBC becomes rounded. Spherocytes are **small** densely staining RBC without central pallor. Mean cell Hb concentration **(MCHC) is always increased** in this disease because the size is decreased. Reticulocytosis would be seen because HS is an important cause of hemolytic anemia.

Anemia and Red Blood Cells

RBCs are macrocytic; hyperchromic and show anisocytosis. Hypersegmented neutrophils are also seen.

87. **Ans. (a) Thrombotic Thrombocytopenic purpura; (b) Hemolytic uremic syndrome; (d) DIC** *(Ref: Robbins 7th/638, 9/e 630)*
    - In Henoch-Schonlein purpura, there is hematuria and palpable purpura.

    DIC is the commonest cause of Microangiopathic hemolytic anemia.

88. **Ans. (b) Cold agglutination** *(Ref: Harrison 17th/660, Robbins 7th/657, Robbins 9/e 644)*
    Paroxysomal cold hemoglobinuria is characterized by the presence of Donath-Landsteiner antibody. It has anti-P specificity and bind to red cells only at low temperature (Optimally at 4°C)

89. **Ans. (D) Spectrin** *(Ref: Robbins 9/e 632, 8th/642)*
    Ideal answer is ankyrin (most commonly) but in the given options, spectrin is the best option.

90. **Ans. (b) Ankyrin deficiency** *(Ref: Robbins 9/e 632, 8th/642; 7th/625)*

91. **Ans. (d) Increased platelets** *(Ref: Robbins 9/e 642, 8th/654; 7 th/636)*

92. **Ans. (a) SLE** *(Ref: Robbins 9/e 642-644, 8th/653-654; 7 th/230)*

93. **Ans. (a) Mycoplasma infection** *(Ref: Robbins 9/e 643-644, 8th/653-654; 7th/637)*

94. **Ans. (c) Decreased blood pressure**
    Read explanation below:
    Within the first few hours of acute blood loss, findings of hypovolemia predominate, especially with signs of hypovolemic shock, such as decreased blood pressure. It is likely that red cell indices (red blood cell counts, hemoglobin, and hematocrit) eventually decrease as a result of hemodilution.

    Increased mean corpuscular hemoglobin concentration (MCHC) is a rare finding but is seen in hereditary spherocytosis.

95. **Ans. (b) Glucose-6-phospate dehydrogenase** *(Ref: Robbins 8th/643-4, 9/e 634-635)*
    Explanation
    Drugs that cause oxidative stress (e.g., primaquine, sulfa-containing drugs) result in intravascular hemolytic anemia in individuals (most often male) with glucose-6-phosphate dehydrogenase (G6PD) deficiency.
    Duffy antigen is a minor red blood cell antigen, the **absence** of which provides **resistance to malarial infection**. Intrinsic factor may be absent in pernicious anemia. PIG-A deficiency results in paroxysmal nocturnal hemoglobinuria.

96. **Ans. (c) Hereditary erythrocyte enzyme deficiency** *(Ref: Robbins 9/e 634-635, 8th/644)*
    The patient has signs of hemolysis induced by trimethoprim-sulfamethoxazole. It is a common scenario for glucose-6-phosphate dehydrogenase (G6PD) deficiency to present.
    Glucose-6-phosphate dehydrogenase deficiency is an **X-linked disorder**[Q] of the hexose monophosphate (pentose phosphate) pathway. In affected individuals, the amount of NADPH produced in RBCs is low, which impairs glutathione-mediated inactivation of free radicals. Hemolytic episodes are induced by **infections**[Q], **medications**[Q] (e.g. TMP-SMX, dapsone, antimalarials, nitrofurantoin), and other **oxidants**[Q] (e.g. fava beans).
    Hemolytic episodes manifest with symptoms of anemia such as malaise and pallor, indirect bilirubinemia (jaundice), hemoglobinemia and hemoglobinuria (dark-red urine). The level of serum haptoglobin decreases and a reticulocytosis develops to compensate for the increased destruction of RBCs. Patients are **generally asymptomatic between episodes.**

    (Choice A) **Autoimmune hemolytic anemias** result from extrinsic antibody-mediated hemolysis and are associated with a **positive Coombs test**[Q]. These anemias often accompany SLE, Hodgkin and non-Hodgkin lymphomas, mycoplasma infections (cold agglutinins) and infectious mononucleosis.

    (Choice B) **Hereditary spherocytosis** is an **autosomal dominant**[Q] defect in RBC structural proteins (spectrin, ankyrin, or protein 4.1) characterized by **increased erythrocyte osmotic fragility**[Q] and MCHC[Q] > 36 g/dL.

    (Choice D) **Microangiopathic hemolytic anemia** (MAHA) occurs when there is destruction of RBCs within small vessels due to widespread thrombosis. MAHA is associated with **disseminated intravascular coagulation**[Q] (DIC), **thrombotic thrombocytopenic purpura**[Q] (TTP) and **hemolytic-uremic syndrome**[Q] (HUS).

97. **Ans. (b) Pigmented gallstones** *(Ref: Robbins 8th/644, 9/e 632-633)*
    The patient has anemia, an elevated LDH, and indirect bilirubinemia, suggesting hemolytic anemia. The lysing of blood cells when incubated in hypotonic saline describes a **positive osmotic fragility test, the diagnostic test for spherocytosis**. Here, the sexual history is deliberately given just to confuse you friends, it is not related to the cause of this patient's anemia. You may find such questions in NEET-PG more frequently.

Pigmented gallstones are a complication of any hemolytic anemia. In chronic hemolysis, the increased bilirubin from lysed red blood cells precipitates as calcium bilirubinate, forming pigmented stones in gallbladder.

(Choice A) **Cirrhosis of the liver** may result from chronic alcohol use, hepatitis B or C infection, hemochromatosis, Wilson disease, and alpa-1 antitrypsin deficiency. The sexual history of this patient might make you suspect blood-borne hepatitis, but then the **AST/ALT would have been abnormal**.

(Choices C and D) The abnormal adhesion of sickle-cell red blood cells to the endothelium may cause episodic venous thrombosis and avascular necrosis of the femur. The unique anatomy of the femoral head makes it exceptionally susceptible to avascular necrosis from a range of causes, including sickle cell anemia.

> **Hereditary spherocytosis** is an **autosomal dominant**[Q] defect in RBC structural proteins (**ankyrin**[Q] most commonly) characterized by **increased erythrocyte osmotic fragility**[Q] and **MCHC**[Q]

98. Ans. (c) Glucose-6-phosphate dehydrogenase *(Ref: Robbins 9/e 634, 8th/644)*

The presence of free hemoglobin in the serum and urine, and "bite cells" due to splenic removal of Heinz bodies (oxidized hemoglobin) all point to hemolysis. Hemolysis following oxidant injury by drugs (sulfonamides, for example) or infection suggests glucose-6-phosphate dehydrogenase deficiency or the related deficiencies of glutathione synthetase, pyruvate kinase, and hexokinase. These conditions are typically asymptomatic between episodes of hemolysis.

Deficiencies of glycoprotein IIb/IIIa (choice D) produce thrombasthenia, a platelet aggregation defect.

99. Ans. (c) Ankyrin *(Ref: Harrison 17th/653-655, Robbins 9/e 632)*

100. Ans. (b) IgG directed against red blood cells *(Ref: Robbins 8th/653, 9/e 643-644)*

100.1. Ans. (c) Normal APTT *(Ref: Robbins 8/e p673-4, 9/e 665, Harrison 18/e p)*

DIC is an acute, subacute, or chronic thrombohemorrhagic disorder characterized by the excessive activation of coagulation, which leads to the formation of thrombi in the microvasculature of the body.

Harrison 18/e pmentions… "Common findings include the **prolongation of PT and/or aPTT**; **platelet counts ≤100,000/μL³**, or a rapid decline in platelet numbers; the presence of **schistocytes** (fragmented red cells) in the blood smear; and **elevated levels of FDP**.

- The D-dimer test is more specific for detection of fibrin—but not fibrinogen—degradation products and indicates that the cross-linked fibrin has been digested by plasmin. Because *fibrinogen has a prolonged half-life, plasma levels diminish acutely only in severe cases of DIC*.

The **most sensitive test** for DIC is the **FDP level**[Q]. *DIC is an unlikely diagnosis in the presence of normal levels of FDP.*

100.2. Ans. (a) Acute promyelocytic leukemia *(Ref: Robbins 9/e 664, 8/e p673-4, Harrison 18/e p)*

The most common causes are **bacterial sepsis**, malignant disorders such as solid tumors or **acute promyelocytic leukemia**[Q], and obstetric causes (pregnant women with **abruptio placentae**, or with **amniotic fluid embolism**).

100.3. Ans. (c) Paroxysmal nocturnal hemoglobinuria (PNH) *(Ref: Robbins 9/e 642, 8/e p652)*

- PNH is a disease that results from **acquired**[Q] **mutations** in the phosphatidylinositol glycan complementation group A gene (**PIGA**[Q]), an enzyme that is essential for the synthesis of certain cell surface proteins.
- Red cells, platelets, and granulocytes deficient in these GPI-linked factors are abnormally susceptible to lysis by complement. In red cells this manifests as *intravascular hemolysis*[Q], caused by the C5b-C9 membrane attack complex.

Also revise

- The **triad** of **hemolysis, pancytopenia and thrombosis** is *unique to PNH*.
- **Thrombosis** is the *leading cause of disease related death* in PNH.
- PNH is best made with **flow cytometry** in which there is presence of **bimodal distribution** of the red cells

100.4. Ans. (a) G6PD deficiency *(Ref: Robbins 9/e 634, 8/e p645)*

Direct lines … "*Oxidants cause both intravascular and extravascular hemolysis in G6PD-deficient individuals. Exposure of G6PD-deficient red cells to high levels of oxidants causes the globin chains to get denatured and form membrane-bound precipitates known as Heinz bodies. These can damage the membrane sufficiently to cause intravascular hemolysis.*

As inclusion-bearing red cells pass through the splenic cords, macrophages pluck out the Heinz bodies. As a result of membrane damage, some of these partially devoured cells retain an abnormal shape, appearing to have a bite taken out of them. These **bite cells** and spherocytes are trapped in splenic cords and removed rapidly by phagocytes.

100.5. Ans. (b) IgM *(Ref: Robbins 9/e 644, 8/e p653)*

Cold agglutinins are monoclonal IgM antibodies that react at **4 to 6°C**. They are called agglutinins because the IgM directed against the 'I' antigen present on the RBCs can agglutinate red cells due to its large size (pentamer).

100.6. Ans. (a) Hemolytic uremic syndrome *(Ref: Robbins 9/e 660, 8/e p952)*

Schistocytes are typically irregularly shaped, jagged, and have two pointed ends. *A true schistocyte does **not** have central pallor.* **Helmet cells** are also known as **schistocytes/triangle cells/burr cells** are a feature of microangiopathic diseasesincluding disseminated intravascular coagulation (**DIC**), thrombotic microangiopathies (**TTP**), **mechanical artificial heart valves** and hemolytic uremic syndrome (**HUS**).

100.7. Ans. (d) All of the above *(Ref: Robbins 8/e p952)*

Yes friends, only additional important thing that you need to be aware of is that schistocytes can also be seen in severe iron deficiency anemia.

Echinocytes/Burr cells Acanthocytes/Spur cells Stomatocytes Schistocytes Leptocytes Codocytes Dacrocytes Drepanocytes Elliptocytes Keratocytes Knizocytes	• Regular spine-like projections on cell surface; • irregular thorn-like projections; • Slit-like (mouth like) area of pallor • Fragmented RBCs; triangular, comma-shaped or helmet shaped • Thin flat cells • Mexican hat cells • Tear drop cells or Target cells (red cells with central dark area; • Sickle cells • Pencil cells or cigar cells • Helmet cells	• **Megaloblastic anemia/ hemolytic anemia /burns** • in **liver disease, abetalipoproteinemia** • in liver disease, anemia of chronic disease)

100.8. Ans. (a) CD 59 *(Ref: Robbins 9/e 642, 8/e p652)*

PNH blood cells are deficient in three GPI-linked proteins that regulate complement activity:

- Decay accelerating factor, or CD**55**;
- Membrane inhibitor of reactive lysis, or **CD59**; and
- **C8 binding protein.**

Of these factors, the **most important is CD59,** a potent *inhibitor of C3 convertase* that prevents the spontaneous activation of the alternative complement pathway.

100.9. Ans. (c) Increased haptoglobin *(Ref: Robbins 9/e 631, 8/e p641-642, 7/e p624)*

Hemolytic anemia is characterized by a reduction in the free haptoglobin levels because the hemoglobin released by destruction of red cells binds to the serum haptoglobin decreasing its levels.

100.10. Ans. (b) Controlling oxidative stress on RBC *(Ref: Robbins 9/e 634)*

G6PD helps in neutralizing the effect of oxidative stress on the RBC. Oxidative stress is induced by drugs like primaquine and hence in patients of G6PD there is accelerated hemolysis (intravascular during the hemolytic episode) resulting in hemoglobinuria and passage of shockingly black urine by the patient.

101. Ans. (a) P. Falciparum *(Ref: Robbins 9/e 391, 8th/387, 645)*

- People who are heterozygous for the **sickle cell trait (HbS)** become infected with *P. falciparum*, but they are less likely to die from infection. The HbS trait causes the parasites to grow poorly or die because *of the low oxygen concentrations.*
- **HbC**, another common hemoglobin mutation, also protects against severe malaria *by reducing parasite proliferation.*
- People can also be resistant to malaria due to the absence of proteins to which the parasites bind. **P. vivax enters red cells by binding to the Duffy blood group antigen.** Many individuals (usually Africans), are not susceptible to infection by *P. vivax* because they do not have the Duffy antigen.

102. Ans. (b) Beta Thalassemia *(Ref: Robbind 9/e 640-641, 8th/648-652, Textbook of Hematology 1st/89)*

Friends, let's get the answer of this question in a methodical manner. The clues in the question:

- Reduced values of MCV and MCHC: microcytic hypochromic anemia (G6PD deficiency is ruled out)
- Age of presentation and ethnicity: 6 year old and Punjabi ethnicity
- History of repeated blood transfusion: in favour of thalassemia
- Osmotic fragility is reduced: in favour of thalassemia again though it may be seen in sickle cell also

If we compare the above mentioned points, we can deduce that the stem talks about a patient suffering from thalassemia. Now comparing the incidence of alpha and beta thalassemia, it is clear that beta thalassemia is far more common than alpha thalassemia. Hence, it is a better option than alpha thalassemia.

Also, the hemoglobin is the question is more suggestive of **severe anemia** with **positive history of multiple blood transfusions** both being important pointers towards **thalassemia major.**

Please note that apart from Punjabis, other ethnic groups having high prevalence of thalassemia are Sindhis, Gujaratis, Parsis, Begalis and Lohanas. The clinical importance of knowing this fact is the application of screening test like **N**aked **E**ye **S**ingle **T**ube **R**ed cell **O**smotic **F**ragility (NESTROF) in these groups before marriage so as to avoid complications like having kids with thalassemia major/intermedia later on.

103. **Ans. (a) β- thalassemia** *(Ref Recent Advances in Hematology -3, 1st/173)*

104. **Ans. (a) Deletion of alpha genes** *(Ref: Robbins 8th/651, T. Singh 2nd/95)*

105. **Ans. (b) Deletion of 3 alpha chains** *(Ref: Robbins 8th/652, 9/e 642)*
    α **thalassemia** is caused by **gene deletion.**when there is deletion of 3 α chains, it results in the formation of tetramers of β chain called as HbH. Note that γ chain tetramers are responsible for the formation of barts hemoglobin.

106. **Ans. (a) Malaria** *(Ref: Robbins 9/e 638, 8th/645, T. singh 1st/270)*
    Sickle cell trait patients are *protected against falciparum malaria* because the sickled RBCs with parasites inside them are sequestered in the reticuloendothelial cells of the spleen providing protection against malaria.

    A similar protection against malaria is also seen in patients having G6PD deficiency as the parasites needs G6PD enzyme for survival. Protection against malaria is also seen in conditions like Thalassemia, pyruvate kinase deficiency; HbC and duffy negative RBcs.

107. **Ans. (d) Solubility** *(Ref: Robbins 9/e 635-636, 8th/645-648)*

108. **Ans. (d) 0%** *(Ref: Robbins 7e/632-33, Harrison – 17th/641)*
    Normal percentage of HbA2 ranges from 1.5 to 3%.
    - In thalassemia trait (β thalassemia minor), HbA2 level may be elevated (3.5-7.5%).
    - Thus, wife in this question has normal genotype (bb) whereas husband has thalassemia – trait (β+β).
    - β-Thalassemia is an **autosomal recessive** disease

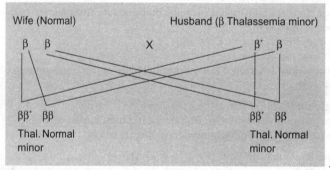

    - None of the offsprings thus will have thalassemia major (β+ β+), thus, the risk of having a child with thalassemia major is therefore 0%.
    - 50% of the offspring (β+β) will be carriers like father.

109. **Ans. (b) Replacement of glutamate by valine in β chain of HbA** *(Ref: Robbins 9/e 635, Harrison 17th/637)*
    - Sickle cell anemia results due to a missense point mutation.
    - Normally, glutamic acid is present at 6th position of β chain. It is replaced by valine due to missense mutation.

    Valine is Welcome and Glutamic acid can Go

110. **Ans. (c) Binding to HbS to the deoxygenated HbA can extend the polymer and cause sickling of the red blood cells**
    (Ref: Harper 25th/71, Robbins 7th/628, 630, 8th/645-646, 9/e 636)
    - **Sickle cell anemia** is caused by a point mutation is which there is *replacement of glutamine by valine* at *position 6* of the *beta chain* generating a **sticky patch on** the surface of HbS.
    - The sticky patch on the surface of adjacent HbS molecules cause their polymerization resulting in formation of long fibrous precipitates.
    - HbA molecule can complementarily bind with the sticky patch by HbS but cannot promote the formation of long fibers because it does not have a patch itself. So, the option *c* is false in the given question.
    Other hemoglobins which also weakly interact with HbS and prevent its polymerization include *HbF* and *HbC*.

111. **Ans. (a) 50% HbS is required for occurrence of sickling** *(Ref: Robbins 7th/628-629, 9/e 635-636)*
    - Sickle cell disease is a hemoglobinopathy in which HbS due to point mutation. If an individual is homozygous for sickle mutation almost all the Hb in erythrocyte is HbS, if he is heterozygote only 40% is HbS the remainder being normal.
    - In addition, Nelson also mentions that '**persons with sickle cell trait have totally benign clinical course because the low level of HbS present in them (35-40% of total) is insufficient to produce sickling manifestation'**. So, option 'a' is a better answer than option 'b'.

112. Ans. (d) Deletion of gene *(Ref: Robbin 9/e 635, 7th/628-629)*

113. Ans. (a) Increased HbF; (b) Increased HbA$_2$; (c) Microcytosis; (e) Target cell *(Ref: Harrison 17th/641, Robbins 7th/634-635, 9/e 641)*

Characteristics of thalassemia minor (trait):
- Microcytosis and hypochromia
- Target cells
- Mild to moderate anemia (MCV > 75 fL and Hematocrit < 30 to 33%).

Hemoglobin electrophoresis classically reveals **increased HbA2 (3.5-7.5%)** and *HbF is normal or elevated*. Patients with beta thalassemia trait are resistant against falciparum malaria, making it more prevalent disease in areas where malaria is endemic.

114. Ans. (d) Point Mutation *(Ref: Harrison 17th/637 Robbins 7th/628, 9/e 635)*

115. Ans. (c) Three α globin genes *(Ref: Robbins 7th/636, 9/e 642)*

116. Ans. (b) Higher concentration of HbF *(Ref: Robbins 7th/629, 9/e 642)*

117. Ans. (a) Presence of a structurally abnormal Hb *(Ref: Robbins 8th/645; 7th/628)*

118. Ans. (b) β-chain *(Ref: Robbins 8th/645; 7 th/628, 9/e 635)*

119. Ans. (c) Vascular occlusion *(Ref: Robbins 8th/645-8, 9/e 637-638)*

In a patient with the hematologic findings described above and recurrent episodes of abdominal pain that resolve with hydration, sickle cell anemia is the most likely diagnosis. The patient has presented with symptoms of "acute chest syndrome" (ACS), which is vaso-occlusive crisis localized to the pulmonary vasculature that can occur in patients with sickle cell anemia. ACS is commonly precipitated by pulmonary infection..

In patients with homozygous hemoglobin S disease vaso-occlusive crises can also cause splenic infarctions. Repeated infarctions produce a spleen that is shrunken, discolored, and fibrotic. By the time they reach adulthood, most patients with sickle cell anemia have undergone "**autosplenectomy**"^{Q} as a result of these infarcts and are left with only a small, scarred splenic remnant. The spleen may demonstrate brownish discoloration (hemosiderosis) due to extensive ingestion of sickled RBCs by splenic macrophages (extravascular hemolysis).

- (Choices A and B) There may be **hyperplasia** and hypertrophy of normal splenic elements (especially macrophages and lymphoid cells) **in systemic infections and various other disease states**.
- (Choice D) Pressure atrophy of the splenic parenchyma can be seen when there is **a tumor infiltrating the spleen**.
- **Autonephrectomy**^{Q} is seen with tubercular infection of the urinary tract.

120. Ans. (c) He is protected from *Plasmodium falciparum* *(Ref: Robbins 8th/645, 9/e 638)*

Patients who are heterozygous for the sickle cell trait (Hb AS) have hemoglobin composed of 35 to 40% hemoglobin S (HbS); they are generally protected from sickle cell crisis, aplastic crisis and sequestration crisis by the presence of > 50% normal hemoglobin (Hb A).

Amount of HbS^Q is the most important factor **affecting sickling** of the RBCs

The alteration of the hemoglobin (from **HbA to HbS**) reduces its **solubility**.

Patients with sickle cell trait are usually asymptomatic, although they may develop hematuria and a limited ability to concentrate urine. A high incidence of UTI and splenic infarction at high altitude may be seen. The heterozygotes enjoy relative protection from *Plasmodium falciparum* (malaria) because of increased sickling of parasitized sickle-cell trait red blood cells and accelerated removal of these cells by the splenic monocyte macrophage system.

(Choices A, B and D) Peripheral smears are usually normal in sickle cell trait patients; irreversibly sickled cells are not seen. Furthermore, red cell indices and red cell morphology are normal; the reticulate count is not elevated. However, the sickling test will be positive (RBCs will sickle when sodium metabisulfite is added). Increased MCHC, which represents intracellular dehydration, is seen only with homozygous SS (i.e. full-blown sickle cell anemia).

Sickling test: Sickling is induced by a reducing agent like 2% *metabisulfite or dithionite* to blood.
Hb electrophoresis is *the best investigation* for diagnosis of sickle cell disease and trait.

121. Ans. (b) Bone marrow expansion in the calvarium *(Ref: Robbins 8th/646-651, 9/e 636-638)*

Sickle cell anemia is caused by a point mutation leading to substitution of valine for glutamate at the 6th position of the β-globin chain. Thalassemia major refers to the clinical picture of patients with homozygous β-thalassemia, leading to severely deficient or absent synthesis of β globin chains. Sickle cell anemia results in shortening of erythrocyte life by causing hemolysis of irreversibly sickled cells. β-thalassemia causes formation of excess free α-globin chains, which precipitate within the normoblasts, resulting in premature apoptosis of red cell precursors (ineffective erythropoiesis). Compensatory increases of erythroid precursors occur in both conditions, leading to expansion of bone marrow with resultant bone deformities. The radiologic "crew haircut" appearance of the skull is due to bone marrow expansion in the calvarium and is seen in both sickle cell anemia and thalassemia major patients.

Autosplenectomy (choice A) and increased predisposition for infections by capsulated organisms (H. influenzae and Streptococcus pneumoniae) is characteristic of sickle cell anemia.

121.1. Ans. (c) Replacement of glutamate by valine in β-chain of HbA *(Ref: Robbins 8/e p645, 9/e 635)*
Direct lines from Robbins... "Sickle cell disease is caused by a **point mutation** in the sixth codon of β-globin that leads to the **replacement of a glutamate residue with a valine residue**."

121.2. Ans. (d) Relative excess of β, γ, and δ chains *(Ref: Robbins 8/e p651, 9/e 635-636)*
- *The α-thalassemias are caused by inherited deletions that result in reduced or absent synthesis of α-globin chains.*
- As in β-thalassemias, the anemia stems both from a lack of adequate hemoglobin and the effects of excess unpaired non-α chains (β, γ, and δ), which vary in type at different ages.
- **In newborns** with α-thalassemia, excess unpaired γ-globin chains form $γ_4$ tetramers known as **hemoglobin Barts**, whereas in *older children and adults* excess β-globin chains form $β_4$ tetramers known as *HbH*.
- Since free β and γ chains are more soluble than free α chains and form fairly stable homotetramers, hemolysis and ineffective erythropoiesis are **less severe** than in β-thalassemias.
- Also, remember that **gene deletion** is the most common cause of **reduced α-chain synthesis**.

The options which created confusion were options "c" and "d".

Total absence of α-chains is a feature of most severe form of α-thalassemia resulting in **hydrops fetalis**.

Every patient having *α-thalassemia* would **not** be having total absence of α- *chains but all patients would be having relative excess of β, γ, and δ chains as per their age of presentation.* Hence, we prefer option "d" as the answer for this question.

121.3. Ans. (b) Beta chain....too obvious friends *(Ref: Robbins 9/e 635, 8/e p645, 7/e p628)*

121.4. Ans. (d) Protective action against adult malaria *(Ref: Robbins 9/e 638, 8/e p645-648, 7/e p629)*

121.5. Ans. (c) Sickle cell anemia *(Ref: Robbins 9/e 635, 8/e p645-648, 7/e p402)*
Sickled cells can cause microvascular occlusion affecting bones, brain, kidney, liver, retina and pulmonary vessels.

121.6. Ans. (c) Saline washed packed RBC *Ref: Choudhary p80*
- *Saline washed RBCs* are specially indicated in conditions requiring repeated transfusion when the chances of urticarial reactions due to plasma is high. These have negligible plasma proteins and just 10% leucocytes. It is also preferred in the management of babies suffering from **thalassemia** and **paroxysmal nocturnal hemoglobinuria**.

121.7. Ans. (c) Single amino acid base substitution *(Ref: Robbin 8/e p645-6)*
Afro American male presenting with the mentioned features is suggestive of sickle cell anemia is due to vaso-occlusion caused by sickled cells. Sickle cell anemia can cause chronic hemolytic anemia, recurrent pneumonia and non haling painful ulcer.

"Sickle cell anemia is caused by a point mutation in the sixth codon of β-globin that leads to the replacement of a glutamate residue with a valine residue"... (Ref: Robbind 8/e p645)

121.8. Ans. (b) Gene deletion *(Ref: Robbin 9/e p641)*
The α-thalassemias are caused by inherited deletions that result in reduced or absent synthesis of α-globin chains.

121.9. Ans. (c) Sickle thalassemia *(Ref: Robbin 9/e and Harrison chapter 104, disorders of hemoglobin synthesis)*

Condition	Clinical Abnormalities	Hemogblobin Level g/l (g/dL)	MCV. fL	Hemoglobin Electrophoresis
Sickle cell trait	Non: rare painless hematunia	Normal	Normal	Hb S/A: 40/60
Sickle cell anemia	Vasooclusive crises; aseptic necrosis of bone	70-100 (7-10)	80-100	Hb S/A: 100/0 Hb F:2-25%
S/ B0 thalassemia	Vasoocclusive crises: aseptic necrosis of bone	70-100 (7-10)	60-80	Hb S/A: 100/0 Hb F;1-10%
S/B+ thalassemia	Rare crises and aseptic necrosis	100-140 (10-14)	70-80	Hb S/A: 60/40
Hemoglobin SC	Rare crises and aseptic necrosis; painless hematuria	100-140 (10-14)	80-100	Hb S/A:50/0

121.10. Ans. (d) Macrocytic Anaemia *(Ref: Robbin 9/e)*
Thalassemia major presents before 1 yr of age with severe anemia which necessitates packed RBC transfusions every 2-3 months. The child is said to be transfusion dependent as survival is decided by RBC being transfused.

The ineffective erythropoiesis in bone marrow results in shift of hematopoiesis to liver and the bone marrow. Hence the liver and spleen enlarge in size. But the net result is defective microcytes being produced. The type of anaemia is microcytic hypochromic anaemia.

Mnemonic to remember causes of macrocytic anemia: ABCDEF

- **A**lcohol + liver disease
- **B**12 deficiency
- **C**ompensatory reticulocytosis (blood loss and hemolysis)
- **D**rug (cytotoxic and AZT)/ **D**ysplasia (marrow problems)
- **E**ndocrine (hypothyroidism)
- **F**olate deficieny/ **F**etus (pregnancy)

122. **Ans. (c) Lack of antigens of several blood group systems** *(Ref: Wintrobe's hematology 12th/635-6 ; Harrison 18th/951)*
- Red cells of **group O** individuals lack A and B antigens but carry **H substance**
- The enzyme in **group A** individuals is **N-acetylgalactosaminosyl transferase**
- The enzyme in **group B** individuals is **D-galactosyltransferase**

- People with Bombay phenotype (rarest blood group in the world) express no A, B or H antigens on the red blood cells. These are homozygous for the silent h allele (being represented hh). So, these antigens are not present in the saliva also. As the antigens are not expressed, so, the H, A and B antibody will always be present in serum.
- ABO antigens are present not only on the red blood cells abut *also on the other blood cells, in most body fluids* (**except CSF**), cell membrane of tissues such as intestine, urothelium and vascular endothelium.

- Clinical significance of knowing about Bombay blood group is that in case of requirement of blood transfusion, these people would be compatible only with Bombay blood from another individual.

123. **Ans. (b) AO**
Too obvious to explain friends.

124. **Ans. (d) Paroxysmal nocturnal hemoglobinuria** *(Ref: Robbins 8th/861 (table 18-6, 9/e 847)*

I. Hereditary Hemochromatosis
• Mutation in the gene coding for HFE, transferring receptor 2 or hepcidin • Mutation in the gene coding for hemojuvilin:juvenile hemochromatosis
II. Secondary Hemochromatosis
A.Parenteral iron overload: Transfusions, Long-term hemodialysis, Aplastic anemia, Sickle cell disease, Leukemias, Myelodysplastic syndromes Iron-dextran injections
B.Ineffective erythropoiesis with increased erythroid activity β-Thalassemia, Sideroblastic anemia and Pyruvate kinase deficiency
C.Increased oral intake of iron: African iron overload (Bantu siderosis)
D. Congenital atransferrinemia
E. Chronic liver disease: Chronic alcoholic liver disease and Porphyria cutanea tarda.

125. **Ans. (d) Trisodium citrate 3.2%** *(Ref: Henry's Clinical Diagnosis and Management by Laboratory Methods 21st/188, Clinical Chemistry Theory, Analysis and Correlation (Mosby) 4th/23-4, 71,Wintrobe 12th/1, Dacie and Lewis practical hematology 10th/7, 391)*
See text.

126. **Ans. (c) Potassium oxalate + sodium fluoride** *(Ref: Henry's Clinical Diagnosis and Management by Laboratory Methods 21st/188, Clinical Chemistry Theory, Analysis and Correlation (Mosby) 4th/23-4, 71, Harper 27th/152)*
Direct quote from Harper.... *'enolase enzyme in the glycolysis is inhibited by fluoride, and when blood samples are taken for measurement of glucose, it is collected in tubes containing fluoride to inhibit glycolysis.'*
The standard clinical sample for glucose estimation is *venous plasma glucose*. Glucose is metabolized at room temperature. The *rate of metabolism is higher with leucocytosis.* To inhibit the glycolysis, sodium fluoride is added.... **Henry 21st/188**
Biochemistry concept: Source *Clinical Chemistry*

Lithium Iodoacetate[Q] is another anticoagulant which can be used for blood glucose estimation. However, it acts by inhibiting the enzyme **glyceraldehyde 3 phosphate dehydrogenase**[Q]. It inhibits glycolysis for 24 hours in contrast to sodium fluoride which inhibits glycolysis for 3 days.

127. **Ans. (a) Microspherocytes** *(Ref: Wintrobe's 12th/982-3, T. Singh Hematology 2nd/32-3, Handbook of pediatric transfusion medicine by Hillyer 1st/198)*
- Wintrobe's mentions 'spherocytes predominate in the peripheral blood smear of infants with ABO hemolytic disease of newborn.' Peripheral blood smear shows numerous spherocytes, occasional nucleated red cells, anisocytosis and polychromasia.

- The blood film in ABO hemolytic disease of the newborn (ABO HDN) is marked by the presence of microspherocytes (a feature not usually seen in Rh hemolytic disease of the newborn). The spherocytosis is attributed to loss of membrane surface area when the spleen removes antigen-antibody complexes from the affected cell.
- **Handbook of pediatric transfusion** medicine writes clearly 'The peripheral blod smear in ABO hemolytic disease of new born is marked by the presence of microspherocytes. Increased osmotic fragility and autohemolysis may be demonstrated just like hereditary spherocytosis'.

Concept: potential future question

Unlike hereditary spherocytosis, Autohemolysis in ABO HDN is not corrected by addition of glucose^Q.

Other options

Option B... Fragmented RBC or schistocytes are feature of microangiopathic hemolytic anemia, DIC and cardiac hemolytic anemia.

Option C...polychromasia is the term used for red cells staining bluish red with Roamnowsky stains. These cells are larger than normal and show fine reticulin network in supravital staining. They are commonly observed in response to therapy in deficiency anemias and hemolytic anemia. So, is not specific for ABO incompatibility.

Option D... Elliptocytosis is a feature of hereditary elliptocytosis and macrocytic anemias.

128. **Ans. (a) Febrile nonhemolytic transfusion reaction** *(Ref: Harrison 16th/665-666, Robbin 9/e 665)*
The **most frequent reaction** associated with the transfusion of cellular blood components is a **febrile non-hemolytic transfusion reaction**.

FNHTR is characterized by chills and rigor and > 1°C rise in temperature.

129. **Ans. (c) Protein** *(Ref: Wintrobe's hematology, 11th/797; Harrison 17th/708)*
- Unlike other red cell antigens, **Rh antigens do not contain any sugar**. The Rh proteins are multipass membrane proteins that traverse the RBC membrane 12 times. The Rh proteins form a complex with other membrane glycoproteins.

- Red cells of group O individuals lack A and B antigens but carry H substance
- The enzyme in group A individuals is N-acetylgalactosaminosyl transferase
- The enzyme in group B individuals is D-galactosyltransferase
- People with Bombay phenotype (rarest blood group in the world) express no A, B or H antigens

Please remember friends that the Rh antigen should not be confused with Rh factor which is an antibody (Ig) against the Fc portion of IgG seen in patients of rheumatoid arthritis.

130. **Ans. (d) Howell-Jolly bodies** *(Ref: Harrison's 17th/374-375, 9/e 623, 636)*
Howell-Jolly bodies are spherical or ovoid eccentrically located granules in stroma of erythrocytes in stained preparations. These represent nuclear remnants and these occur most frequently after:

1. Splenectomy 2. Megaloblastic anemia 3. Severe hemolytic anemia

Acute manifestations of splenectomy include *leukocytosis* (up to 25000/µl) and *thrombocytosis* (up to 1 × 106/µl) but these return back to baseline levels within 2-3 weeks.
Chronic Manifestations of splenectomy include:
- Anisocytosis and poikilocytosis
- Howell-Jolly bodies (nuclear remnants)
- Heinz bodies (denatured hemoglobin)
- Basophilic stippling
- Occasional nucleated erythrocyte in peripheral blood

When such erythrocyte abnormalities are seen without splenectomy, splenic infiltration by tumor should be suspected.

Other options
- **Dohle bodies** are discrete round or oval bodies. These represent rough ER and glycogen granules and are found in neutrophils. These may be seen in patients with infections, burns, trauma, pregnancy or cancer.
- **Hypersegmented neutrophills** are seen in **megaloblastic anemia.**
- **Spherocyte** result from acquired or inherited defect in erythrocyte membrane. It *may be seen in hypersplenism and not following splenectomy.*

131. **Ans. (a) Metabolic Alkalosis** *(Ref: Harrison 17th/293, 9/e 666)*
Massive Transfusion is defined as the need to transfuse from one to two times the patient's normal blood volume. In a normal adult, this is equivalent to **10-20 units**. Most common abnormality is metabolic alkalosis. It results from conversion of citrate (present in stored blood) and lactate (accumulated due to hypoperfusion) to bicarbonate

132. Ans. (d) Cryoprecipitate: *(Ref: Harrison 17th/708-710, Wintrobes 11th/846-8)*
Donated blood is processed into components: PRBCs, platelets, and fresh-frozen plasma (FFP) or cryoprecipitate. Whole blood is first separated into PRBCs and platelet-rich plasma by slow centrifugation. The platelet-rich plasma is then centrifuged at high speed to yield one unit of random donor (RD) platelets and one unit of FFP. Cryoprecipitate is produced by thawing FFP to precipitate the plasma proteins, and then separated by centrifugation.
Wintrobe's clearly mentions that 'ABO incompatible plasma carries high risk of transfusion reactions, therefore, plasma transfusions should always be ABO incompatible'. So, option 'a' and 'b' are ruled out.
The platelets bear the intrinsic ABO antigens. So, platelet rich plasma and single donor platelets also should be preferably ABO compatible. So, **answer of exclusion is cryoprecipitate.** It is not carrying ABO antigens but should preferably be ABO compatible to avoid even the minimal risk of hemolytic reaction.
Apheresis technology is used for the collection of multiple units of platelets from a single donor. These single-donor apheresis platelets (SDAP) contain the equivalent of at least six units of RD platelets and have fewer contaminating leukocytes than pooled RD platelets. Still **the risk of severe hemolytic reactions is much more with single donor incompatible platelets than pooled plasma because the dose of incompatible plasma is also increased.**

> FFP is an acellular component and does not transmit intracellular infections, e.g. CMV

133. Ans. (c) O positive RBC and colloids/crystalloids *(Ref: Wintrobes Clinical Hematology vol.I, 10th/833, CMDT 2010/477)*
Selection of blood for emergency transfusion

- **If patient's blood group is known,** unmatched blood group of the same group may be used.
- **If the patient's blood cannot be determined,** Group O red blood cells should be chosen. The use of such unmatched blood should be Rh (–ve) when used in woman of child-bearing age in whom we do not want sensitization to Rh antigen. As Rh negative blood is often in limited supply, Rh positive blood is used in the emergency transfusion of older females and males of unknown blood group. In such cases sensitization may occur but the risk of an immediate hemolytic reaction is low. O blood group is the universal donor and therefore, should be given to this patient.

134. Ans. (d) ABO (H) antibodies are invariably present in plasma when persons RBC lacks the corresponding antigen. *(Ref: Harrison 17th/708, CMDT 2010/477)*
- In clinical transfusion practice the ABO blood groups are the most important and can never be ignored in red cell transfusion, because individuals, who genetically lack any antigen, have antibodies against the red cell types that they have not inherited. These antibodies can destroy red cells rapidly in circulation.
- The same is not the case with other blood groups where antibodies are formed only after exposure to the sensitive antigen (**Preformed antibodies are absent**).

135. Ans. (a) Howell-Jolly bodies; (c) Macrocytosis: *(Ref: Harrison' 17th/374-375, 9/e 623-636)*
Chronic manifestations of splenectomy (Postsplenectomy hematological features) are:
- Red cells: Marked variation in size and shape (**anisocytosis, poikilocytosis**)
- **Macrocytosis**
- Presence of **Howell-Jolly bodies** (nuclear remnants)
- **Heinz bodies** (denatured hemoglobin)
- **Basophilic stippling**
- Occasional nucleated red cells in the peripheral blood
- **Target cells**
- **Pappenheimer bodies** (contain sideroblastic granules)
- Irregular contracted red cells.
  - WBC count usually normal but there may be mild lymphocytosis and monocytosis.
  - Thrombocytosis persists in about 30% of cases.

136. Ans. (a) Whole blood. *(Ref: Harrison 17th/709)*
Whole blood is processed into its components intended for transfusion. The blood component products are:

Packed RBC	FFP
Platelets	Cryoprecipitate
Plasma derivatives, e.g. albumin, antithrombin, coagulation factors	Leukocyte reduced RBC

137. Ans. is c i.e. Trisodium citrate *(Ref: Wintrobe's Clinical Hematology 11th/4)*

138. Ans. (b) Postsplenectomy >> (c) hemolysis *(Ref: Tejinder singh's 1st/38-39, internet)*
Friends, in hemolytic anemia Howell Jolly body is seen only if anemia is very severe. So, the preferred answer is **post splenectomy**[Q]

Howell-Jolly bodies are nuclear remnants seen in red cells, intermediate or late normoblasts. They are seen in:

- Normally in neonates (spleen is immature)
- Megaloblastic anemia is due to dyserythropoiesis
- Post splenectomy due to absence of pitting function of the spleen
- Acute severe hemolytic anemias
- Hyposplenia (radiation exposure, splenic trauma, autosplenectomy due to sickle cells disease)
- Myelodysplastic syndrome

139. **Ans. (a) Chronic liver disease** (*Ref: Harrison 17th/359, T. Singh 1st/86*)

140. **Ans. (a) Leukemoid reaction** (*Ref: Robbins 8th/633; 7th/704, 9/e 719*)

141. **Ans. (b) D** (*Ref: Robbins 8th/460, 7th/485*)

141.1. **Ans. (a) X chromosome** (*Ref: Robbins 8/e p672, 9/e 662*)
Hemophilia A is caused by mutations in factor VIII, which is an essential cofactor for factor IX in the coagulation cascade. It is inherited as an **X-linked recessive trait[Q]** and thus affects **mainly males** and *homozygous females*.
Read the following lines carefully for a future NEET question!
- *Hemophilia A is the most common hereditary disease associated **with life-threatening bleeding**.*
- **Von Willebrand disease** *is the* **most common inherited bleeding disorder** *of humans*

141.2. **Ans. (c) Factor IX** (*Ref: Robbins 8/e p672, 9/e 662-663*)

Disorder	Deficiency
• Hemophilia A	• Factor **8**
• Hemophilia B (Christmas disease)	• Factor **9 (Christmas factor)**
• Hemophilia C	• Factor **11**
• Parahemophilia	• Factor **5 (labile factor)**

141.3. **Ans. (b) Increased erythropoietin level** (*Ref: Robbins 9/e 656, 8/e p628, 7/e p699*)
Polycythemia vera progenitor cells have markedly decreased requirements for erythropoietin and other hematopoietic growth factors. Accordingly, *serum erythropoietin levels in polycythemia vera are very low*, whereas almost all other forms of absolute polycythemia are caused by elevated erythropoietin levels.

141.4. **Ans. (d) Polycythemia rubra** (*Ref: Robbins 9/e 619, 656, 8/e p665, 7/e p699*)
Lab manifestations in polycythemia rubra (CMDT)
- Elevated hemoglobin level and hematocrit: due to increased number of red blood cells
- Platelet count or white blood cell count may also be increased.
- Erythrocyte sedimentation rate (ESR) is **decreased** due to an increase in zeta potential.
- Low erythropoietin (EPO) levels.

141.5. **Ans. (b) Synthesized by hepatocytes** (*Ref: Robbins 9/e 661, 8/e p878; 7/e p654-655*)
von Willebrand factor is synthesized by endothelial cells and megakaryocytes. It has the following functions:
- **It facilitates platelet adhesion** by linking platelet membrane receptors to vascular endothelium (*most important function*).
- It serves as the **plasma carrier for the factor VIII**, the anti-hemophilic factor and increases its shelf life in circulation.

141.6. **Ans. (b) Lack of reaction accelerator during activation of factor X in coagulation cascade.** (*Ref: Robbins 9/e 662, 8/e p672*)
- Hemophilia A is caused by the deficiency of clotting factor 8.
- The chief role of the extrinsic pathway in hemostasis is to initiate a limited burst of thrombin activation upon tissue injury. This initial procoagulant stimulus is reinforced and amplified by a critical feedback loop in which thrombin activates factors XI and IX of the intrinsic pathway. *In the absence of factor VIII, this feedback loop is inactive and insufficient thrombin (and fibrin) is generated* to create a stable clot.

141.7. **Ans. (d) von Willebrand Factor** (*Ref: Robbins 9/e 661-662, 8/e p671, 672*)
The clues given in the stem of the question are:
- Female patient
- Bleeding tendency
- Prolonged aPTT
- Normal PT
- Normal platelet count

- As platelet count is normal, thrombocytopenia as a cause of bleeding can be easily ruled out.
- PT is prolonged in defects of extrinsic pathway of coagulation whereas aPTT increases in defective intrinsic pathway. Therefore, deficiency of factor VII can be ruled out, because it is involved in extrinsic pathway and its deficiency will prolong PT.
- Factor VIII and IX are involved in intrinsic coagulation pathway and vWF stabilizes factor VIII. Therefore, deficiency of any of these will prolong aPTT with PT remaining normal. However, both Hemophilia A (factor VIII deficiency) and Hemophilia B (Christmas disease; factor IX deficiency) are X-linked recessive diseases and commonly affect males. Females are affected only in homozygous state, which is rare.
- So, the answer is **vWF deficiency** which is mostly inherited as **autosomal dominant disorder**.

141.8. Ans. (a) Prolonged PTT *(Ref: Robbins 9/e 662, 8/e p672; 7/e p 655)*
- aPTT is prolonged by **deficiency** of factors **XII, XI, IX, III, X, V, prothrombin and fibrinogen**[Q] and drugs like **heparin**[Q]
- **Hemophilia A** is characterized by the deficiency of **factor 8** and decreased activity of intrinsic pathway. This is associated with prolongation of **partial thromboplastin time**[Q].

141.9. Ans. (b) Normal PT *(Ref: Robbins 9/e 662, 8/e p672; 7/e p656)*
As discussed earlier, hemophilia A is an X linked disorder, so, if a male is affected, he cannot transmit it to his son (option 'a' is false). In this sdiorder, there is an **increase in the activated partial thrombolastin time** and **normal values of prothrombin time**.

141.10. Ans. (b) HbA$_1$ *(Read below)*
- **HbA** is $\alpha_2\beta_2$ (95-96%)
- **HbA$_2$** is $\alpha_2\delta_2$ (3-3.5%)
- **HbF** is $\alpha_2\gamma_2$ (present in the fetal life). As gestational age increases, the γ chains are replaced by the β chains, resulting in formation of adult hemoglobin, HbA.

HbA1c is glycated hemoglobin and is used for both diagnosis and checking the compliance of a patient having diabetes mellitus.

141.11. Ans. (a) Light chain of monoclonal immunoglobulins *(Ref: Robbins 9/e p600)*
Bence Jones proteins are made up of light chains of the immunoglobulin and are monoclonal in nature.

141.12. Ans. (c) Small cleaved cell lymphoma *(Ref : Pattern Approach to Lymph Node Diagnosis by Anthony S-Y Leong)*
Friends, I know people would require reference for this question for believing the answer! JJ The tumor cells, which are large with minimal cytoplasm, are closely apposed to each other, forming a dark blue background (the "sky"). These cells have a *very high turnover rate*, so the macrophages that happen to be hanging around get stuffed with cellular debris (they are at this point called "tingible body macrophages"), and upon fixation, the cytoplasm falls away, leaving round white spaces filled with debris (the "stars"). This pattern can be seen on both bone marrow or lymph node sections. It is seen with:
- Burkitt's lymphoma (earlier called as *small non cleaved lymphoma*)
- Mantle cell lymphoma
- Large B cell lymphoma (including plasmablastic lymphoma)
- T lymphoblastic lymphoma

141.13. Ans. (b) endothelium *(Ref: Robbins 8/e p434, 9/e p19-20)*
Platelet-derived growth factor (PDGF) is present in the following:
- The alpha granules of the **platelets**
- **Macrophages**
- **Endothelial cells**
- **Keratinocytes and**
- **Smooth muscle cells.**

141.14. Ans. (d) Sometimes found in saliva *(Read below)*
- The A and B antigens are inherited as mendelian allelomorphs, A and B being dominants and they are located on **chromosome 9**.
- They are located on the **membranes of human red cells**
- Antigens very similar to A and B are common in intestinal bacteria and possibly in foods to which newborn individuals are exposed. Therefore, infants rapidly develop antibodies against the antigens not present in their own cells. Thus, type A individuals develop anti-B antibodies, type B individuals develop anti-A antibodies, type O individuals develop both, and type AB individuals develop neither
- **Secretors** are individuals who secrete ABH antigens in body fluids like **saliva** and **plasma**.

141.15. Ans (c) Factor 5 and 8 *(Ref: Internet)*

FFP contains an average of 1 IU/mL of each coagulation factor, including the labile factors V and VIII. In the question it was asked regarding stored plasma.

By day 5 of storage the amount of factor VIII (8) is reduced by up to 40% and factors V (5) and VII (7) may be reduced by up to 20%

141.16. Ans (a) Fucose *(Ref: Harrison 18th/ 951)*

The first blood group antigen system was ABO and is the most important in transfusion medicine. The major blood groups of this system are A, B, AB, and O. H substance is the immediate precursor on which the A and B antigens are added. This H substance is formed by the addition of fucose to the glycolipid or glycoprotein backbone. The subsequent addition of N-acetylgalactosamine creates the A antigen, while the addition of galactose produces the B antigen.

141.17. Ans (d) Hemolysis……… *(Ref: Hematology manual)*

Conditions with pseudohyperkalemia

- Excessive muscle activity during venipuncture (fist clenching),
- Thrombocytosis, leukocytosis, and/or erythrocytosis
- Acute anxiety
- Cooling of blood after venipuncture
- Gene defects leading to hereditary pseudohyperkalemia

Hemolysis causes real hyperkalemia.

GOLDEN POINTS FOR QUICK REVISION / UPDATED INFORMATION FROM 9TH EDITION OF ROBBINS
(ANEMIA AND RED BLOOD CELLS)

Complications of Blood Transfusion ……..Page 665

Blood products are often responsible for saving lives of individuals but may be associated with the development of the complications. These include:

- *Febrile nonhemolytic reaction:* this is the ***most common complication*** leading to fever and chills, sometimes with mild dyspnea, within 6 hours of a transfusion of red cells or platelets. It is caused by the release of inflammatory chemicals from the donor leukocytes. It is treated symptomatically with antipyretics.
- *Allergic Reactions:* Severe, potentially fatal allergic reactions may occur when blood products containing certain antigens are given to previously sensitized recipients. These occur more commonly in patients with IgA deficiency. *Urticarial allergic reactions* may be triggered by the presence an allergen in the donated blood product that is recognized by IgE antibodies in the recipient. This is more common. The condition is managed with antihistaminic drugs.
- *Hemolytic Reactions:* Acute hemolytic reactions are usually caused by preformed IgM antibodies against donor red cells that fix complement. They occur due to improper labeling in the blood bank **(ABO incompatibility)**. Clinical features include fever with chills, flank pain, intravascular hemolysis, and hemoglobinuria. It is diagnosed with a positive direct Coombs test. It may be fatal in rare cases.
- *Delayed hemolytic reactions:* they are caused by **antibodies that recognize red cell antigens that the recipient was sensitized to previously,** for example, through a prior blood transfusion. These are typically caused by IgG antibodies to foreign protein antigens and are associated with a positive direct Coombs test.
- *Transfusion-Related Acute Lung Injury:* **TRALI** is a severe, frequently fatal complication in which factors in a transfused blood product trigger the activation of neutrophils in the lung microvasculature. It is associated with a *two hit hypothesis* (priming event that leads to increased neutrophils in the lung microvasculature followed by activation of the primed neutrophils). TRALI is associated with antibodies that bind major histocompatibility complex (MHC) antigens, particularly MHC class I antigens. It is more common in multiparous women receiving plasma derived blood products. Clinically, there is a sudden onset of respiratory failure, fever, hypotension and hypoxemia. The treatment is largely supportive.
- *Infectious Complications:* though any infection can be transmitted through blood products, but bacterial and viral infections are relatively more commonly seen. It is also more common with platelet preparations. Donor screening and infectious disease testing have reduced the incidence of viral transmission by blood products.

CHAPTER 8

White Blood Cells and Platelets

HEMATOGENOUS NEOPLASMS

Leukemia is a term used to describe the widespread **involvement of the bone marrow accompanied with large number of cancer cells in the peripheral blood** whereas *lymphoma* is a term used for *proliferation of lymphoid cells arising as discrete tissue masses.*

> According to **WHO** classification, *blasts should be* **>20%** in bone marrow for diagnosis of acute leukemia.

WHO Classification of the Lymphoid Neoplasms

I. Precursor B-Cell Neoplasms	II. Peripheral B-Cell Neoplasms	III. Precursor T-Cell Neoplasms	IV. Peripheral T-Cell Neoplasms
* Precursor-B lymphoblastic leukemia or lymphoma	Chronic lymphocytic leukemia/small lymphocytic lymphoma	*Precursor-T lymphoblastic leukemia or lymphoma	Angioimmunoblastic T-cell lymphoma
	B-cell prolymphocytic leukemia		Large granular lymphocytic leukemia
	Lymphoplasmacytic lymphoma		T-cell prolymphocytic leukemia
	Splenic and nodal marginal zone lymphomas		Peripheral T-cell lymphoma, unspecified
	Extranodal marginal zone lymphoma		Anaplastic large cell lymphoma
	Mantle cell lymphoma		Mycosis fungoides/ Sezary syndrome
	Follicular lymphoma		Enteropathy-associated T-cell lymphoma
	Marginal zone lymphoma		Panniculitis-like T-cell lymphoma
	Hairy cell leukemia		Hepatosplenic γδ T-cell lymphoma
	Plasmacytoma/plasma cell myeloma		Adult T-cell leukemia/ lymphoma
	Diffuse large B-cell lymphoma		NK/T-cell lymphoma, nasal type
	Burkitt lymphoma		NK-cell leukemia

V. HODGKIN LYMPHOMA

Classic subtypes	Non classical
• Nodular sclerosis	• Lymphocyte predominant
• Mixed cellularity	
• Lymphocyte-rich	
• Lymphocyte depletion	

- **The FAB** (French-American-British Classification) diagnostic criteria for acute leukemia is the **presence of >30% blasts** in the bone marrow (normally, they are <5%) and increased number of cells in the blood.
- Note that according to **WHO classification**, blasts **should be >20% in** bone marrow for diagnosis of acute leukemia.

For broad understanding, WBC neoplasms can be classified as:

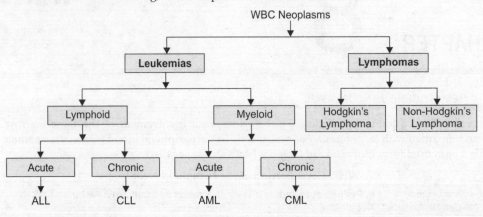

> ALL is the commonest leukemia seen in childhood[Q].

- **Acute leukemias** have a **high rate of proliferation without differentiation** and their clinical course is **rapid**.
- *Chronic leukemias* have a *low rate* of proliferation of tumor cells with *good differentiation* and their clinical course is *slow*.

LEUKEMIAS

1. Acute Lymphoblastic Leukemia (ALL)

It is the *commonest leukemia seen in childhood*[Q] having slight predilection for males. The etiological agents include exposure to ionizing radiations as X rays, chemical like benzene, genetic disorders like Down syndrome, ataxia telangiectasia and acquire disorders like paroxysmal nocturnal hemoglobinuria and aplastic anemia.

> Lymphoblast[Q] staining positively with PAS and (TdT).

The *predominant cell seen in this leukemia is lymphoblast*[Q] characterized by coarse nuclear chromatin, 1-2 nucleoli, high N:C (nuclear:cytoplasmic) ratio and *staining positively with PAS (block positivity) and terminal deoxynucleotidyltransferase (TdT)*.

FAB (French-American-British) classification of ALL (Older classification)

> **L1 ALL** is the **Commonest**[Q] type of ALL having the **best prognosis**.

> **L3 ALL** is the **rarest** type of ALL having the **worst prognosis**.

L1 ALL	L2 ALL	L3 ALL
Commonest[Q] type of ALL having the *best prognosis*.	Next common type having worse prognosis.	Rarest type of ALL with the worst[Q] prognosis.
Small homogenous blast, scanty cytoplasm, indistinct nucleoli	Large, heterogenous blast, indented nuclei, one or more nucleoli, moderately abundant cytoplasm, minimal cytoplasmic vacuolation	Large homogenous blast, abundant basophilic cytoplasm with prominent cytoplasmic vacuolation staining positive with Oil Red 'O'.

Immunological classification of ALL (**Latest WHO classification**)

B-cell lineage

- More common
- B-lymphoblasts have surface markers like immunoglobulins, CD19, CD20
- Associate with pancytopenia due to marrow involvement

T-cell lineage

- Less common
- T-lymphoblasts have markers including CD1, CD2, CD5, CD7 (more commonly) and even CD3, CD4 and CD8 may be present
- Associated with mediastinal mass, lymphadenopathy and splenomegaly and CD8 may be present

Clinical features

- ALL is characterized by *sudden onset* of symptoms that arise due to replacement of the normal bone marrow cells with blast cells, thereby causing features/symptoms due to decreased number of RBC, WBC and platelets (*anemia, infections and increased bleeding tendency* respectively). The leukemic cells also infiltrate the organs of the body like spleen, liver and lymph nodes causing *splenomegaly, hepatomegaly and lymphadenopathy.*
- Bone marrow expansion is responsible for bone *pain and tenderness* (usually sternal tenderness) in these patients. *Testicular involvement and CNS features* like headache, vomiting and nerve palsies are also seen in these patients. This leukemia can either be a precursor B-cell or T-cell type (these are the two predominant types of lymphocytes). In the pre-T-cell type, there is presence of mediastinal mass due to thymus involvement which can compress either the vessels or airways in the region.

Aleukemic leukemia is diagnosed by the presence of **>20% blasts** in the **bone marrow.**

Testicular involvement and is seen with **T type ALL** and is associated with **bad prognosis.**

Investigations

Blood findings
They include *markedly elevated WBC count.* Uncommonly, some patients may show *pancytopenia with few or no blast cells in peripheral blood* which is called as **aleukemic leukemia**. *However,* diagnosis is made in this condition by the presence of *>20% blasts in the bone marrow.* Blast cells with Periodic Acid Schiff (PAS) positivity are seen. There is presence of anemia, neutropenia and thrombocytopenia.

Bone marrow
It is hypercellular with *blast cells >20%* of the marrow cells.

Biochemical investigations
It include *elevated serum uric acid and phosphate* levels accompanied by *hypocalcemia* (because of hyperphoshatemia). *Serum LDH is also increased* as a result of increased turnover of the cancer cells.

Prognostic factors in ALL

Good Prognosis	Bad Prognosis
• Age 2-10 years	• Age <1 year or > 10 years
• Female sex	• Male sex
• L1 cell	• L2 or L3 cell
• Peripheral blast count <1,00,000	• Peripheral blast count >1,00,000
• Pre B-cell phenotype	• Pre T-cell phenotype
• Absence of mediastinal mass	• Mediastinal mass
• Hyperdiploidy (>50 chromosomes) or t(12;21)	• Pseudodiploidy or t (9;22) (Philadelphia chromosome) or t (8;14) or t (4;11)
• Trisomy 4,7 and 10	

Genetic associations of ALL

- **T cell ALL** is associated with *gain of function* mutation in **NOTCH 1 gene** (normally required for T cell development)
- **B cell ALL** is associated with *loss of function* mutation in **PAX5, E2A** and **EBF** or balanced t (12; 21) affecting TEL and AML1 genes (normally required for B cell development).

Treatment of choice for ALL is **allogenic bone marrow transplantation** and cancer drug regime used for *induction* is VAPD (*vincristine + asparaginase + prednisolone +daunoribicin*) with *intrathecal methotrexate.*

Treatment of choice for ALL is **allogenic bone marrow transplantation** and cancer drug regime used for induction is **VAPD** (vincristine + asparaginase + prednisolone + daunoribicin) with **intrathecal methotrexate.**

2. Acute Myelogenous Leukemia (AML)

It is the leukemia affecting adults seen most commonly between the ages of 15-39 years. The etiological agents include exposure to ionizing radiations such as X-rays, chemicals like benzene, secondary to myelodysplastic syndrome, drugs like anti-cancer drugs and genetic disorders like Down's syndrome and Fanconi's anemia.

The *predominant cell* seen in this leukemia is *myeloblast* characterized by fine nuclear chromatin, 3-5 nucleoli, high N: C (nuclear: cytoplasmic) ratio, presence of *Auer rods* (these

Myeloblast stains positively with **Sudan black B**, myeloperoxidase **(MPO)** and Non Specific Esterase **(NSE).**

are abnormal azurophilic granules) and *staining positively with Sudan black B, myeloperoxidase (MPO) and Non Specific Esterase (NSE).*

FAB (French-American-British) classification of AML

Class	Salient Features
M0: Minimally differentiated AML M1: AM L without maturation	Myeloid lineage blasts Myeloblasts without maturation (> 3% blasts MPO or SBB positive)
M2: AML with maturation	t (8;21)^Q is present, *maximum incidence of chloroma*^{Q}, Auer rods are seen
M3: Acute (Hypergranular) promyelocytic leukemia	t (15;17)^Q seen, Associated with disseminated intravascular coagulation (DIC)^Q, Auer rods are seen
M4: Acute myelomonocytic leukemia *(Naegli type)*	*Inversion 16*^{Q} present, Presence of both myeloblasts and monoblasts (blasts > 20%; neutrophil and its precursors > 20%; monocyte and precursors > 20%)
M5: Acute monocytic leukemia *(Schilling type)*	t (9;11) seen, Highest incidence of *tissue infiltration*^{Q}, organomegaly, and lymphadenopathy
M6: Acute erythroleukemia *(Di Gugliemo disease)*	Abnormal erythroid precursors are seen
M7: Acute megakaryocytic leukemia	Least common type of AML, Megakaryocytes are seen, Release of platelet derived growth factor (PDGF) causes **myelofibrosis**

MPO: Myeloperoxidase; SBB: Sudan black B

ADDITIONAL SALIENT POINTS

- Generally AML following myelodysplastic syndrome (MDS) is associated with monosomy involving chromosomes 5 and 7 and lack chromosomal translocation **except** AML following treatment with topoisomerase II inhibitors (which is associated with translocation on chromosome 11 involving MLL gene).
- Cells with multiple Auer rods are called "faggot cells" and are seen in M3- AML.
- Some authorities mention **AML-M8 as acute basophilic leukemia**.

Clinical features

They are similar to ALL i.e. fatigue due to anemia, bleeding and infections in oral cavity, lungs etc. Patients may develop bleeding diathesis due to DIC which results from release of thromboplastic substances in the granules (most common with M3 AML). Infiltration of these cells into the organs is relatively less common as compared to ALL resulting in only mild hepatosplenomegaly and lymphadenopathy.

However, *gum hypertrophy and infiltration in the skin (called as leukemia cutis) is common with* **particularly M5 AML**. Less frequently, patients may present with localized masses in absence of marrow or peripheral blood involvement called **myeloblastoma, granulocytic sarcoma or chloroma** (most commonly with *M2 AML* and so named as they turn green in presence of dilute acid due to the presence of MPO). **Lysozyme, CD43, CD45, CD117** and *MPO* are positive markers of granulocytic sarcoma. These manifest as **proptosis**^{Q} (due to orbital involvement) **most commonly** or may present as bone or periosteal masses.

INVESTIGATIONS

Blood findings
It includes markedly elevated WBC count. Findings are similar to that in ALL except that the blast cells show positivity with MPO, NSE or Sudan black. There is presence of anemia, neutropenia and thrombocytopenia.

Bone marrow
It is hypercellular with blast cells >20% of the marrow cells.

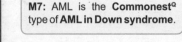

M2: AML is the **Commonest**^{Q} type of AML.

M3: AML is associated with disseminated intravascular coagulation (*DIC*).

M7: AML is the **Commonest**^{Q} type of **AML in Down syndrome**.

Cells with multiple Auer rods are called **"faggot cells"** and are seen in M3- AML.

Therapy in M3 AML specifically can be done with all trans retinoic acid^Q (ATRA) or arsenic oxide^Q.

Biochemical investigations

These show elevated serum uric acid and phosphate levels accompanied by hypocalcemia (because of hyperphosphatemia). Serum Muramidase levels is also increased in M4 and M5 AML. The fibrin degradation products (FDPs) are elevated in M3 AML due to DIC.

PROGNOSTIC FACTORS IN AML

Good prognosis	Bad prognosis
• Age <40 years	• Age <2 years or >55 years
• M2,M3,M4 forms of AML	• M0,M6,M7 forms of AML
• Blast cell with Auer rods	• Complex karyotypes
• TLC < 25 X 10⁹/L	• TLC > 100 X10⁹/L
• t(15;17), t (8;21), inv 16	• Deletions 5q, 7q
• Rapid response to therapy	• Delayed response to therapy
• Leukemia without preceding MDS	• AML with preceding MDS or anticancer drug exposure

Therapy in **M3 AML** specifically can be done with **all trans retinoic acid**^{Q} (ATRA) or **arsenic oxide**^{Q}. In M3 AML or Acute promyelocytic leukemia, the translocation between chromosomes 15 and 17 results in fusion of a gene encoding retinoic acid receptor α (RAR α) with another protein PML and this fusion gene blocks the differentiation of the myeloid cells. So, trans retinoic acid provided from external source is beneficial in these patients. For other types of AML, the drugs used are **cytarabine with daunorubicin**.

However, *treatment of choice* of AML is *allogenic bone marrow transplantation*.

LEUKEMOID REACTION

It is defined as the presence of leucocytes in the peripheral blood resembling leukemia in an individual who actually does not have leukemia.

Myeloid leukemoid reaction	Lymphoid leukemoid reaction
Seen in conditions like:	Seen in conditions like:
• Infections (sepsis, TB, endocarditis)	• Infections (usually viral like measles, chicken pox, CMV, infectious mononucleosis or bacterial like TB, pertussis)
• Severe hemorrhage and hemolysis	
• Malignancies (Hodgkin's, multiple myeloma, metastasis, myelofibrosis)	
• Miscellaneous (burns, eclampsia, mercury poisoning).	• Rare with malignancies.

CONCEPT

Leukemoid reaction is *differentiated from leukemia* by:
- **Absence** of hepatosplenomegaly, lymphadenopathy and hemorrhage
- Presence of immature cells/**blasts to <5%** (in leukemia, blasts are >20%)
- Presence of **increased leukocyte alkaline phosphatase** score (in leukemia, LAP score is decreased)
- Presence of toxic granulations and **Dohle bodies** (cytoplasmic small round bodies) in neutrophils {in leukemia, Dohle bodies are absent}

MYELODYSPLASTIC SYNDROMES (MDS)

Myelodysplastic syndromes refer to a *clonal stem cell disorder* resulting in *ineffective hematopoiesis and increased risk of* development into acute myelogenous leukemia (*AML*). The bone marrow is replaced with multipotent stem cells which can differentiate but in an unorganized and ineffective manner only.

It has been linked to the exposure to radiation, benzene, alkylating agents and some chromosomal abnormalities. MDS can be classified into:

1. **Primary MDS** – Develops slowly usually after 50 years of age.
2. **Secondary or Therapy related MDS (t-MDS)** – Usually 2 to 8 years after toxic drug or radiation exposure. The secondary MDS *gets transformed to AML* most frequently and so *has a poorer prognosis*.

Deletions in the long arm of **chromosome 5** are the most frequent cytogenetic changes in **MDS in adults**^{Q}.

Monosomy 7 is the most frequent cytogenetic change in **MDS in children**^{Q}.

The *bone marrow is usually hypercellular* in this condition but the myelodysplastic precursor cells undergo apoptosis at a fast rate resulting in *ineffective hematopoiesis*. MDS is frequently associated with chromosomal abnormalities including monosomy 5 and 7, deletion of 5q and 7q, trisomy 8 and deletion of 20 q.

Bone marrow findings

Cells affected	Features seen
Erythroid cells	**Ringed sideroblasts**[Q] (Iron laden mitochondria in erythroblasts) with increased iron stores Megaloblasts, nuclear budding, intranuclear bridging, irregular nuclei
Megakaryocytes	**Pawn ball megakaryocytes**[Q] (Megakaryocytes with multiple separate nuclei)
Neutrophils	**Dohle bodies**[Q] (toxic granulations) are seen, **Pseudo-Pelger-Huet cells**[Q] (Neutrophils with two nuclear lobes) are also seen

Peripheral blood shows the presence of Pseudo-Pelger-Huet cells, giant platelets, macrocytes, poikilocytes and monocytosis.

Clinical features are seen in only 50% patients including weakness, infection and hemorrhage due to pancytopenia. Usually patients are of an old age (mean age of onset is >60 years). The prognosis is poor.

3. Chronic Myelogenous Leukemia (CML)

It is a type of myeloproliferative disorder characterized by the increased number of immature leukocytes, basophilia and splenomegaly seen in adults between the ages of 25-60 years. An increased risk of CML is seen in people exposed to ionizing radiation (survivors of nuclear bombs). There is presence of ABL gene (a proto-oncogene) on chromosome 9 and BCR (break point cluster) gene on chromosome 22. A reciprocal translocation between these two chromosomes causes formation of BCR-ABL fusion gene on chromosome 22 (called **Philadelphia chromosome**[Q] or Ph). This fused gene causes synthesis of a 210 kDa fusion protein.

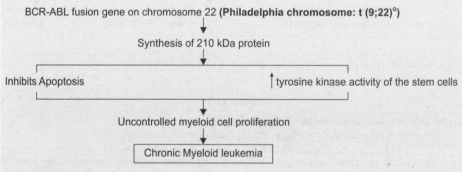

Clinical features

CML has a gradual onset with fatigue, anorexia and weight loss as the initial complaints. Characteristically, there is presence of **splenomegaly**[Q] caused by infiltration of leukemic cells as well as extramedullary hematopoiesis. *Hepatomegaly* is also seen but lymphadenopathy is uncommon in these patients. Leukocytic infiltration and hypercellularity can cause *sternal tenderness* whereas leukostasis can cause priapism, venous thrombosis and visual disturbances.

Bone marrow

It is 100% cellular in these patients (in normal individuals, the marrow is 50% cellular and 50% fat is present). *The erythroid precursors are decreased* (due to replacement by myeloid precursors) whereas *abnormal megakaryocytes are commonly seen*. The presence of scattered histiocytes with blue granules (sea-blue histiocytes or **pseudo-Gaucher cells**[Q]) is characteristically seen. There is also increased deposition of reticulin fibres.

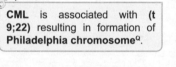

Juvenile myelomonocytic leukemia[Q] is a childhood myelodysplastic syndrome. It is the commonest leukemia seen in children suffering from **neurofibromatosis-1**[Q].

CML is associated with (t 9;22) resulting in formation of **Philadelphia chromosome**[Q].

The **Neutrophil Alkaline Phosphate** (NAP or LAP) is **decreased** (in chronic phase) in **CML**.

White Blood Cells and Platelets

PERIPHERAL SMEAR

It shows the presence of *thrombocytosis and marked leukocytosis* with presence of immature white cells, eosinophilia and basophilia. The *Neutrophil Alkaline Phosphate (NAP or LAP)* **is decreased (in chronic phase)** in these patients.

BIOCHEMICALLY

There are increased levels of uric acid, serum B_{12} levels (due to increased transcobalamin) serum LDH and serum alkaline phosphatase.

PHASES OF CML

1.	**Chronic phase**
	• Lasting for about 3-6 years having **<10% blasts** in the blood or bone marrow.
2.	**Accelerated phase**
	• Aggressive phase lasting for few months showing increased anemia and thrombocytopenia.
	• Number of *blasts are >10% but <20%.*
	• Cytogenetic abnormalities like trisomy 8, isochromosome 17q, duplication of Ph chromosome may develop.
3.	**Blast phase**
	• Resembles AML
	• Characterized by the presence of *>20% blasts* in the blood/bone marrow.
	• Two third of the blasts are of myeloid lineage whereas the remaining 1/3rd are of lymphoid lineage (expressing CD10 & CD19; TdT).

Management

• **Drug as well as treatment of choice** for CML is a *tyrosine kinase inhibitor Imatinib mesylate*.

Concept

•	**LAP score** is reduced in CML but it often **increases** when CML transforms to a **blast crisis or accelerated phase**.
•	A variant of CML is seen in children called as **juvenile CML**. It is characterized by *presence of skin rash, absence of Philadelphia chromosome, increased levels of HbF and a poor prognosis*.

4. Chronic Lymphocytic Leukemia (CLL)/Small Lymphocytic Lymphoma (SLL)

It is a proliferation of mature lymphocytes seen in the **old patients (mean age is 60 years)** having a chronic course of onset which means that in this cancer, replacement of the bone marrow hematopoietic cells occurs after a period of few years. So, anemia, thrombocytopenia and granulocytopenia occur late in this disease.

The exact cause of this cancer is unknown but the role of TNF-α and TGF-β is demonstrable which are produced by the cancer cells. These are responsible for suppression of the proliferation of normal lymphocytes and bone marrow cells.

The chromosomal defects are rare in CLL but the ones still seen include **deletion of 13q[Q]** (commonest and has good prognosis) and 11q trisomy 12q and deletion of 17p (have poor prognosis). (Ref Wintrobes 12th edn **2222**).

CLINICAL FEATURES

The cancer is more commonly seen in males and is asymptomatic in a large number of cases. **Fatigue**[Q] is the commonest presenting complaint associated with lymphadenopathy (initially, cervical followed by a generalized lymphadenopathy). There is also presence of pallor, mild

Drug of choice as well as **treatment of choice** for CML is a *tyrosine kinase inhibitor* **Imatinib mesylate**.

Mean age of patients having **CLL** is **60 years**.

> **CLL** is the only blood cancer **NOT** associated with **radiation exposure**.

hepatosplenomegaly, skin rash and petechiae. However, *sternal tenderness is absent* (it is seen in acute leukemia). These cells are not able to produce normal immunoglobulins resulting in the increased susceptibility to infections. As already discussed above, the presence of anemia, thrombocytopenia and granulocytopenia signify the late stage of the disease.

Investigations

The **diagnostic criteria** for CLL are:

- Peripheral blood lymphocyte count >5000 cells/mm3with <55% cells being atypical.
- Bone marrow aspirate showing >30 % lymphocytes.

Blood investigation

It reveals **low Hb, elevated TLC with lymphocytosis** being the hallmark of the disease. Peripheral smear shows increased number of lymphocytes with scanty cytoplasm. These cells are fragile, so they get disrupted while making a smear and are called as **'smudge' cells or 'basket' cells or 'parachute' cells**.

> **CLL** is also associated with *Autoimmune Hemolytic anemia* (so, **Coombs test is positive** in this condition.

Bone marrow

It is hypercellular with >30% *of the nucleated cells being lymphocytes* as the diagnostic feature of the leukemia. The aggregation of small lymphocytes and larger cells called 'prolymphocytes' is called **proliferation center** which is a characteristic finding of CLL.

Immunophenotyping

The cancer cells are positive for **CD19, CD20, CD23 and CD5.** There is also low level expression of **surface immunoglobulin** heavy and light chains.

Additional points

- The distinguishing feature of **CLL** and SLL is that in the former **blood involvement is predominant** presenting feature whereas in **SLL** the patients usually have **lymph node findings**.

NON-HODGKIN LYMPHOMA (NHL)

1. Follicular Lymphoma

It is the commonest NHL in the US **(otherwise the commonest NHL is Diffuse large B cell lymphoma)** derived from the **B-lymphocytes** usually presenting in the middle age. It shows the presence of translocation **t(14;18)[Q]**. Normally chromosome 14 has immunoglobulin heavy chain gene whereas the chromosome 18 has bcl-2 gene. The translocation results in the increased expression of **bcl-2[Q]**. The bcl-2 being the inhibitor of apoptosis causes promotion of the follicular lymphoma cells resulting in the cancer.

Clinical features

> **Follicular lymphoma** has the presence of translocation t(14;18)[Q].

The cancer presents usually as painless generalized lymphadenopathy with less commonly the involvement of CNS, GIT or testes. The median survival is for 7-9 years. In almost 50% of patients, this cancer gets transformed to diffuse large B-cell lymphoma.

Investigations

> The cells in **follicular lymphoma** express **bcl-2** protein, **surface Ig**, CD19, CD20 and CD10 (CALLA). **CD5 is negative** in these cells.

Immunophenotyping
The cells expressing *bcl-2 protein, surface Ig*, CD19, CD20 and CD10 (CALLA). CD5 is negative in these cells (*differentiating feature from mantle cell lymphoma and CLL*).
Lymph node biopsy
There is presence of *centrocytes* (small cell with cleaved nucleus and scant cytoplasm) and *centroblasts* (large cell with open nuclear chromatin and multiple nucleoli).

Peripheral blood
Presence of lymphocytosis.
Bone marrow
It shows the presence of characteristic *para-trabecular lymphoid aggregates.*

2. Mantle Cell Lymphoma

It is a neoplasm in which the tumor cells resemble the normal mantle zone B-cells which surround germinal centers. These have the translocation t(11; 14)^Q. Normally chromosome 11 has cyclin D1 (bcl-1) locus whereas the chromosome 14 has immunoglobulin heavy chain gene. This translocation leads to in the increased expression of cyclin D1^Q which promotes the G1 to S phase progression in the cell cycle resulting in development of neoplasia.

Clinical features

The cancer usually presents as painless generalized lymphadenopathy, splenomegaly or involvement of the GIT. Uncommonly, multifocal mucosal involvement of the small bowel and colon produces **lymphomatoid polyposis.**

> Mantle cell lymphoma has the presence of translocation t(11;14)^Q.

Investigations

Immunophenotyping reveals the cells expressing *cyclin D1, surface Ig and CD 5.* **CD23 is negative** in these cells. **Lymph node biopsy** reveals typically the presence of small cleaved cells with diffuse effacement of lymph nodes.

- *Centroblasts are absent^Q* (differentiating feature from mantle cell lymphoma and CLL).
- **CD23 is negative^Q** in these cells (differentiating feature from CLL)

3. Burkitt's Lymphoma/Small Non Cleaved Lymphoma

It is a cancer of the germinal center B cell origin characterized by the presence of hallmark translocation **t(8;14)^Q.** The other translocations which may be present include t (2;8) or t (8;22). Normally chromosome 8 has c-MYC gene whereas the chromosome 14 has immunoglobulin heavy chain gene. The translocation results in the increased expression of c-MYC resulting in development of neoplasia. It has the following 3 categories:

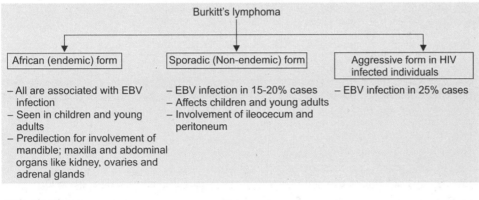

> **Burkitt's** lymphoma has the presence of translocation t(8;14)^Q.

> **Burkitt's** lymphoma has the presence of **starry sky** pattern in the *lymph node biopsy.*

Investigations

Immunophenotyping reveals the cells expressing *bcl-6^Q protein, surface Ig, CD19, CD20 and CD10* (CALLA).

Lymph node biopsy reveals typically the *presence of a high mitotic index* of lymphoid cells associated with apoptotic cell death. The presence of tissue macrophages with clear cytoplasm distributed with tumor cells creates the typical **starry sky^Q** pattern.

> Unlike the other tumors arising from the germinal centre, there is failure of expression of the anti-apoptotic gene bcl-2 in Burkitt's lymphoma.

4. MARGINAL ZONE LYMPHOMA (MALToma)

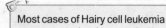

> Marginal zone lymphoma has the presence of translocation t(11;18)^Q. It is associated with *H. pylori* infection.

It is a group of **B-cell** tumors arising within the lymph nodes, spleen or extranodal tissues in which the tumor cells resemble the normal marginal zone B cells. They are associated with mucosa associated lymphoid tissue, so, are called maltoma. Their salient features include:

- Begin as polyclonal activation associated with autoimmune disorders, chronic inflammatory conditions or having infectious etiology.
- Remain localized for a long duration of time.
- May regress if causative agent is removed.
- Splenic marginal zone lymphomas are TRAP +ve (like hairy cell leukemia)

The extranodal lymphomas can occur in stomach (H. pylori), orbit (Chlamydia), skin (Borrelia), lung, salivary gland, intestine, etc. Tumors may respond to antibiotic therapy. If they have cytogenetic abnormality **t (11;18)^Q** as in extranodal marginal zone lymphoma, they are refractory to antibiotic therapy.

5. Hairy Cell Leukemia

> Most cases of Hairy cell leukemia are caused by activating mutations in BRAF (Serine/ threonine kinase)

It is a misnomer because it is not a leukemia but a *B cell NHL* of the old age predominantly affecting males (M:F ratio is 4:1) characterized by the presence of hairy cells in the peripheral blood, splenomegaly and pancytopenia. The exact cause of this cancer is unknown but the role of TNF- α is postulated which is responsible for proliferation of hairy cells and are responsible for the suppression of the proliferation of the normal bone marrow cells resulting in pancytopenia. The chromosomal abnormalities associated with this leukemia like trisomy 5 etc have been detected.

Clinical features are *massive splenomegaly* and less commonly there is presence of hepatomegaly (note that *lymphadenopathy is distinctly rare* in this disorder). Marrow failure contributes to pancytopenia resulting in increased chances of infection, fatigue and easy bruisability in these patients.

> Cytochemistry reveals the diagnostic feature of presence of **TRAP** (Tartarate resistant acid phosphate) cells in **Hairy cell leukemia**.

Investigations

Blood
There is presence of *pancytopenia* with the presence of atypical lymphoid cells despite the presence of neutropenia. Characteristic cells are hairy cells which are leukemic cells having hair-like projections due to fine cytoplasmic processes seen best *under phase contrast microscope*. Electron microscope shows the presence of ribosomal lamellar complexes in the cytoplasm. Peripheral blood shows hairy cells with nuclei of different shapes.

> All **NHLs** involve **white pulp** of the spleen *except* Hairy cell leukemia and hepatosplenic lymphoma which involve red pulp of the spleen. In hairy cell leukemia, the white pulp is atrophic.

Bone marrow aspirate
There is presence of **dry tap**^{Q} due to presence of reticulin fibrils along with the leukemic cells.

Bone marrow biopsy
It reveals infiltration by the cancer cells called as **honeycomb appearance**^{Q} and leukemic cells have nucleus surrounded by cytoplasmic halo called as **fried egg appearance**^{Q} which is diagnostic of hairy cell leukemia.

Immunophenotyping
Tumor cells have the presence of pan B cell markers like positivity for surface Ig, CD19, CD20, CD11c, CD25 and CD103. **Presence of CD11c, CD25 and CD103 positivity is characteristic of hairy cell leukemia.** Cytochemistry reveals the diagnostic feature of **presence of TRAP+**^{Q} **(Tartarate resistant acid phosphate) cells** in Hairy cell leukemia.

> Drug of choice for Hairy cell leukemia is **cladribine**.

CONCEPT

- TRAP is also **positive** in some cases of **splenic marginal zone lymphoma**.
- Hairy cell leukemia appears benign even though it is malignant because it is having less mitotic rate resulting in reduced N:C ratio (normally malignant cells have increased N:C ratio) and there is ample space between tumor cells (normally malignant cells are overcrowded).

Characteristic Immunophenotypes of Major Subtypes of Lymphoma

Lymphoma	Immunophenotype
Follicular	CD20+, CD3−, CD10+, CD5−
Small lymphocytic	CD20+, CD3−, CD10−, CD5+, CD23+
Marginal zone/MALT	CD20+, CD3−, CD10−, CD5−, CD23−
Mantle cell	CD20+, CD3−, CD10−, CD5+, CD23−, CD43+, PRADI+
Diffuse large B-cell	CD20+, CD3−, CD5−, CD45+
Burkitt	CD20+, CD3−, CD10+, CD5−; Tdt−
Lymphoblastic	CD20−, CD3+, Tdt+
Anaplastic large cell	CD20−, CD3+, CD30+, CD15−, EMA+, ALK+
Peripheral T-cell	CD20−, CD3+
Hodgkin	CD30+, CD15+

CD135 is an important cell surface marker used to identify hematopoietic progenitors in the bone marrow. Specifically, multipotent progenitors (MPP) and common lymphoid progenitors (CLP) express high surface levels of CD135. This marker is therefore used to differentiate hematopoietic stem cells (HSC), which are CD135 negative, from MPPs, which are CD135 positive. HSC are CD 34 positive.

HODGKIN'S LYMPHOMA (HL)

It is a group of lymphoid neoplasms arising in a single node and spreads from the nodes to spleen, then liver and finally bone marrow. Clinical importance of this predictable route of spread is highlighted by the importance of staging which determines prognosis as well guides the choice of therapy of HL.

It is differentiated from non- Hodgkin's lymphoma by the following features:

Hodgkin's Lymphoma	Non-Hodgkin's Lymphoma
• More often localized to a single axial group of nodes (cervical, mediastinal, para-aortic)	• More frequent involvement of multiple peripheral nodes
• Orderly spread by contiguity	• Non contiguous spread
• Mesenteric nodes and Waldeyer ring rarely involved	• Waldeyer ring and mesenteric nodes commonly involved
• Extra nodal involvement uncommon	• Extranodal involvement common

There is presence of neoplastic giant cell called **Reed-Sternberg cell** (*derived from the germinal center B cell*) which induces the accumulation of reactive lymphocytes, macrophages and granulocytes.

The cause for the development of HL is inappropriate *activation of NF-κB* usually induced by the latent membrane protein-1 of Ebstein Barr virus (EBV) in majority of the cases.

The malignant cell is Reed Sternberg (RS) cell which is having an **"owl-eye" appearance** due to the presence of symmetric (mirror image) bilobed nucleus with prominent nucleoli surrounded by clear space. The **RS cells are positive for CD15 and CD30 for most subtypes except in lymphocyte predominant HL** in which the neoplastic cells *stain for CD20 and BCL-6* and are negative for CD15 and CD30.

Important points about Reed Sternberg cell

- **Lacunar cell** is a variant of RS cell having a clear space surrounding the cell.
- **Popcorn cell** is a *lymphohistiocytic (L-H) variant of RS cell* having a multilobed nucleus resembling a popcorn kernel.
- **CD 30** is the **most sensitive** marker of Reed Sternberg cell.
- Cells similar or identical in appearance to Reed-Sternberg cells are also seen in other conditions like *infectious mononucleosis, solid tissue cancers*, and NHL (*Immunoblastic lymphoma*). Thus, although Reed-Sternberg cells are requisite for the diagnosis, they must be present in an appropriate background of non-neoplastic inflammatory cells (lymphocytes, plasma cells, eosinophils).

The malignant cell in **Hodgkin's lymphoma** is a **Reed Sternberg** (RS) cell which is having an "owl-eye" appearance

WHO Classification of Hodgkin Lymphoma				
Nodular sclerosis	**Mixed cellularity**	**Lymphocyte rich**	**Lymphocyte depleted**	**Lymphocyte predominant (non classical HL)**
– MC type of HL	– MC type of HL **in India**		– Associated with HIV	
– Incidence equal in M and F	– M > F	– M>F	– M>F	– M > F
– RS cell variant in **lacunar cell** (clear space surrounding cell)	– Has eosinophils and plasma cells – **Maximum number** of RS cell	– Mononuclear and RS cell – **Lowest number** of RS cells	– 3 unique RS cell (pleomorphic, mummified, necrobiotic type) – Maximum area of necrosis	– LH cells **(popcorn cells)** in background – Other cells scanty or absence of B cells
– Cells are CD15 + CD30+	– Cells are CD15 + CD30+	– Cells are CD15 + CD30 + and CD20–	– Cells are CD15 + CD30+	– RS cell are **CD20 + CD15–, CD30 – BCL6 +, EMA +**[Q]
– No association with EBV	– Associated with EBV	– Associated with EBV	– Associated with EBV	– Not associated with EBV
– **Excellent prognosis**	– Prognosis very good	– Good to excellent prognosis	– Poor prognosis	– Excellent prognosis
– Adolescent and young adult	– **Biphasic incidence**[Q] (young adults as well as > 55 years)	–Old age group	–Old age group	–Young males

*EMA is Epithelial Membrane Antigen

> **Lymphocyte predominant** Hodgkin's lymphoma is also called as **Non classical Hodgkin's lymphoma**.

> **PAX 5** is the most specific marker of Reed Sternberg cell.

> Treatment of Hodgkin's lymphoma is done with **ABVD** (**A**driamycine, **B**leomycin, **V**inblastine and **D**acarbazine.

CLINICAL FEATURES

Presence of painless enlargement of lymph nodes is the common presenting symptom and is associated with fever (**Pel Ebstein fever**) and night sweats in disseminated disease. A strange paraneoplastic syndrome in HL is *pain in the affected lymph nodes on consumption of alcohol*. The prognosis is directly related to the number of RS cells present.

CHRONIC MYELOPROLIFERATIVE DISORDERS

The common pathogenic feature of the myeloproliferative disorders is the presence of mutated, constitutively activated tyrosine kinases which lead to growth factor independent proliferation and survival of marrow progenitor cells. These arise from the *clonal proliferation of multipotent stem cells* which proliferate along the three cell lines (erythroid, megakaryocytic and granulocytic) except in CML in which with the pluripotent cell gives rise to myeloid cells.

Depending on the predominant cell in the myeloproliferative disorder, following disorders can be seen:

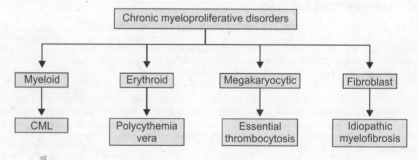

1. Chronic Myelogenous Leukemia (CML)

It has been discussed earlier with other leukemias.

2. Polycythemia Vera

This is a myeloproliferative disorder characterized by the increased number of erythroid, granulocytic and megakaryocytic cells. The presence of erythrocytosis or polycythemia is responsible for the development of the symptoms. Polycythemia vera progenitor cells have markedly decreased requirements for erythropoietin and other hematopoietic growth factors. Accordingly, serum erythropoietin levels in polycythemia vera are very low, whereas almost all other forms of absolute polycythemia are caused by elevated erythropoietin levels.

Clinical features are primarily caused by increase in hematocrit and red cell mass contributing to *sluggish blood flow* and even *increased chances of thrombosis*. These manifest in the form of dusky cyanosis, visual disturbances, headache, dizziness, venous thrombosis (causes Budd Chiari syndrome due to hepatic vein thrombosis), bowel infarction and stroke. The increased basophils in the circulation (release histamine) are responsible for the development of *intense itching and increased incidence of peptic ulcer* in these patients. *Hyperuricemia* is seen due to increased cell turnover. The patients also have *splenomegaly* due to extramedullary hematopoiesis.

Investigations

- Blood shows **elevated hemoglobin** (Hb > 18 g %) **and red cell count** (> 6 million/mm³; normal is 3.5-5.0 million/mm³), **increased hematocrit** with **decreased levels of erythropoietin**. The last differentiate it from secondary polycythemia in which serum erythropoietin is elevated.
- Peripheral blood shows **increased basophils and abnormal platelets**.
- Bone marrow is hypercellular having increased number of erythroid, granulocytic and megakaryocytic cells. In later stage, there is presence of myelofibrosis.

Recent info in exams

Proposed Revised WHO Criteria for Diagnosis of Polycythemia Vera*	
Major criteria	1. Hemoglobin > 18.5 g/dL in men or > 16.5 g/dL in women or evidence of increased red cell volume 2. Presence of JAK2 mutation
Minor criteria	1. Hypercellular bone marrow biopsy with panmyelosis with prominent erythroid, granulocytic, and megakaryocytic hyperplasia 2. Low serum erythropoietin level 3. Endogenous erythroid colony formation **in vitro**

Polycythemia vera is the most common of the chronic myeloproliferative disorders. Its diagnosis requires presence of both the major criteria and one minor criterion or the presence of the first major criterion plus 2 minor criteria.

3. Essential Thrombocytosis

It is associated with **activating mutation in JAK2** (more commonly) or MPL, a receptor tyrosine kinase normally activated by thrombopoietin. This is the stem cell disorder having increased proliferation of the megakaryocytes in bone marrow and *high platelet count* in the blood (> 6 lakh/mm³; normal level is 1.5-4.5 lakh/mm³). It is usually a *diagnosis of exclusion*.

It is strongly associated with activating point mutation in the tyrosine kinase JAK2 or MPL, the latter is receptor tyrosine kinase activated by thrombopoietin.

Clinical features arise because of *non-functioning platelets* resulting in *bleeding* (mucosal bleeding, skin bleeding or spontaneous bleeding following trauma) and occlusion by these dysfunctional platelets can result in *thrombotic manifestations* (arterial thrombosis occurs more commonly as compared to deep venous thrombosis resulting in headache, dizziness or ischemia of the digits).

Polycythemia Vera is strongly associated with activating point mutation in the **tyrosine kinase JAK2**.

Transformation to AML is **uncommon** in polycythemia vera.

Management of polycythemia vera is done with **venesection** or **alpha interferon**.

White Blood Cells and Platelets

309

Investigations

Erythromelalgia is a characteristic symptom caused by throbbing pain and burning of hands and feet due to occlusion of small arterioles by platelet aggregates.

- **Bone marrow** is *hypercellular* with increase in number of giant megakaryocytes along with dysmegakaryopoeisis. Erythroid and myeloid cell show only mild hyperplasia, if at all.
- **Blood** shows elevated platelet count in the blood *(diagnostic criteria is > 6 lakh/mm³)*, normal Hb levels and *elevated LAP scores*.

Management is done with *aspirin* or *hydroxyurea* or *anagrelide*.

4. IDIOPATHIC OR PRIMARY MYELOFIBROSIS

It is characterized by the presence of marrow fibrosis associated with extramedullary hemopoeisis in the spleen in old patients (usually more than 60 years of age). It is associated with **activating mutation in JAK2** (more commonly) or MPL. There is presence of *neoplastic megakaryocytes* which are *responsible for the release of fibrogenic factors like PDGF* (platelet derived growth factor) *and TGF-β*. These factors cause progression of marrow fibrosis. This results in:

- Replacement of normal hematopoietic stem cells by fibrous tissue.
- Movement of hematopoietic stem cells to spleen and liver (responsible for hepatosplenomegaly).

Both the above contribute to development of decreased cell count resulting in the symptoms of fatigue, weight loss or bleeding episodes along with hepatosplenomegaly. Hyperuricemia is seen due to increased cell turnover.

Bone marrow aspiration reveals **dry tap** due to fibrosis of the bone marrow.

Concept

The fibrosis of the bone marrow can occur as a primary hematological process (called **primary myelofibrosis** or **myeloid metaplasia**).

So, bone marrow biopsy is the investigation of choice for the diagnosis *which shows the presence of* **hypocellularity** *with increased deposition of reticulin inside the marrow, abnormal megakaryocytes and the characteristic finding of* dilated marrow sinusoids.

Peripheral blood findings include presence of nucleated red cells and immature white cells (called as **leukoerythroblastosis**).

There is also presence of abnormal red cells called *dacryocytes* (or *tear drop RBC*) formed due to damage to red cell membrane caused by fibrous tissue in the marrow. Blood shows mild leukocytosis, decreased Hb and hematocrit levels and *elevated LAP scores*.

PLASMA CELL DYSCRASIAS

Myelophthisis ia a term used for *secondary myelofibrosis* due to tumors (breast/lung/prostate cancers or neuroblastoma) or granulomatous processes (infections like TB/fungi/HIV) or radiation therapy.

These are characterized by proliferation of B-cell clone which synthesizes and secretes a single homogenous immunoglobulin or its fragments. The entity includes the following conditions:

- **Multiple myeloma** (Plasma cell myeloma) – presents as multiple masses in the skeletal system. Smoldering myeloma is an asymptomatic subtype with high plasma M component.
- **Waldenstrom's macroglobulinemia** – Caused by blood hyperviscosity due to high level of *IgM*. It is seen in adults with *lymphoplasmacytic lymphoma*.
- **Heavy chain disease** – Characterized by synthesis and secretion of free heavy chain fragments and is seen in association with CLL/SLL, Mediterranean lymphoma, lymphoplasmacytic lymphoma.
- **Primary or immunocyte associated amyloidosis** – Results from a monoclonal proliferation of plasma cell secreting free light chains (most commonly α isotype).
- **Monoclonal Gammopathy of Undetermined Significance (MGUS)** – It is the *most common* symptomatic monoclonal gammopathy. Usually asymptomatic disease seen in elderly patients. Rarely, it may progress to symptomatic monoclonal gammopathy (most often multiple myeloma).

*Hyperviscosity is defined on the basis of the relative viscosity of serum as compared with water.

*Normal relative viscosity of serum is 1.8

*Hyperviscosity is seen in
- Multiple myeloma
- Waldenstrom's macroglobulinemia
- Cryoglobulinemia
- Myeloproliferative disorders

Multiple Myeloma is a **monoclonal** plasma cell disorder[Q].

1. Multiple Myeloma

It is a plasma cell cancer having skeletal involvement at multiple sites. The most common karyotypic abnormalities in this condition are *deletions of 13q and translocation involving Ig heavy chain locus on 14q.*

IL-6 is the **most important cytokine** for the proliferation of the plasma cells.

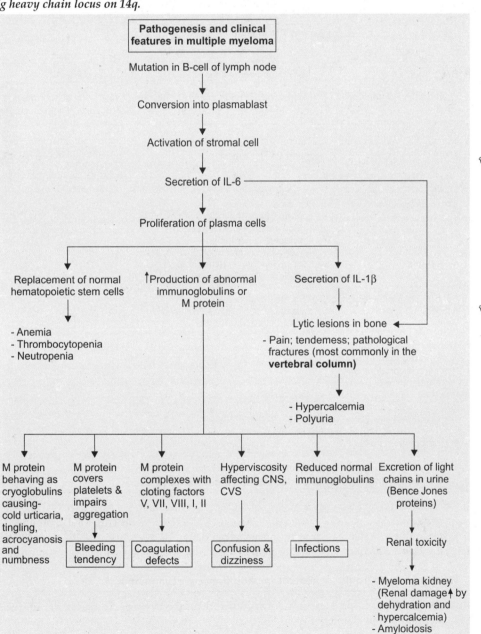

Infections are the *commonest cause* of death.

Serum β_2 **microglobulin** is the most important **prognostic marker**.

Note: Commonest cause of Death in Multiple Myeloma is infections[Q].

DIAGNOSIS

In 2008 WHO diagnostic criteria for diagnosis of plasma cell myeloma are

Symptomatic plasma cell myeloma
- M-protein in serum or urine (No level is included). M-protein in most cases is > 30 g/L if IgG, > 25g/L for IgA or 1g/dL urine light chain.
- Bone marrow clonal plasma cell or plasmacytoma (monoclonal plasma cell usually **exceed 10%** of nucleated cells in the marrow).
- Related organ or tissue impairment (**CRAB:** hypercalcemia, renal failure, anemia and bone lesions).

The diagnosis can be made on the basis of blood, bone marrow and urine findings as described the following flowchart:

Investigations in Multiple Myeloma

Blood findings	Bone marrow findings	Electrophoresis
1. Normocytic, normochronic anemia	1. Hypercellular bone marrow	1. Urine (> 6g/dL of protein) - Presence of light chains in urine
2. Normal TLC and platelet count	2. Increased number of plasma cells usually >30%	2. Serum (> 3g/dL protein) - Presence of M band or monoclonal band of immunoglobulins (most commonly of IgG)
3. ↑Globulin levels cause↑ESR and rouleaux formation	3. Presence of plasma cells or its modified forms - **Flame cells** (have fiery red cytoplasm) - Mott cell (have blue grape like cytoplasmic droplets) - Cell having immunoglobulin inclusions in the cytoplasm (**Russell body**) or nucleus (**Dutcher body**)	
4. ↑Serum uric acid, creatinine and ↑ blood urea	4. Normal myelopoiesis and megakaryopoiesis with reduced erythropoiesis	
5. ↑Serum β_2 microglobulin - **prognostic marker of MM** - high levels correlate with poor prognosis		

> **X-ray** shows the presence of **punched out lytic lesions** in flat bones like skull, ribs, pelvis and vertebra.

Note:
- Definitive diagnosis is by **Bone marrow examination**[Q].
- Treatment is done with **melphalan**, bortezomib and lenalidomide[Q] (refer to *Review of Pharmacology* for details)

2. Monoclonal Gammopathy of Undetermined Significance (MGUS)

> MGUS is the commonest cause of monoclonal gammopathy.

It is characterized by the *presence of M spike without associated disease of the B cells*. MGUS is the *commonest cause of monoclonal gammopathy*. Around 1% of the patients with MGUS progress to develop multiple myeloma per year. It is usually a diagnosis of exclusion. Patients of MGUS have *less than 3 g/dL* of monoclonal protein in the serum and no Bence Jones proteinuria.

3. Waldenstrom Macroglobulinemia/Lymphoplasmacytic Lymphoma

> In **Waldenstrom Macroglobulinemia**, there is presence of a 'M' or **monoclonal spike** caused due to **IgM**.

It is a B cell neoplasm presenting in 6th or 7th decade of life having features similar to CLL/SLL and multiple myeloma.

- Like MM, there is presence of a *'M' or monoclonal spike (caused due to IgM* whereas in MM, it is caused by IgG)
- Like SLL (unlike MM), the neoplastic cell *infiltrates into organs* like spleen, lymph node and bone marrow.
- Unlike multiple myeloma, there is *absence of lytic lesions and serum calcium levels are normal.*
- Unlike multiple myeloma, there is *balanced production of light and heavy chains* thereby decreasing the development of renal failure and amyloidosis.

Clinical features

These include non specific symptoms like fatigue, weakness, weight loss, hepatosplenomegaly and cervical lymphadenopathy. The immunoglobulin increases viscosity of the blood resulting in hyperviscosity syndrome affecting CNS and retina characterized by the headache, dizziness, visual disturbances etc. Abnormal globulins may interfere with platelet function resulting in bleeding and cryoglobulins may lead to acrocyanosis and cold urticaria.

Investigations

- **Bone marrow** reveals the presence of *plasmacytoid lymphocytes' infiltration.* PAS + inclusions containing immunoglobulins are seen in the cytoplasm (called *Russell bodies*) or in the nucleus (called *Dutcher bodies*) of the plasmacytoid cells.
- **Blood** investigations show *anemia with atypical plasmacytoid lymphocytes.* ESR is elevated and rouleaux formation is seen. Immunoelectrophoresis reveals the presence of 'M' spike composed of IgM.
- **Immunophenotyping** reveals the lymphocytic cells expressing *B-cell markers like CD20.* These cells are negative for CD5 and CD10. The plasma cell secretes a monoclonal immunoglobulin.

Deletion involving chromosome 6q is the commonest abnormality in **Waldendtrom's macroglobulinemia.**

Langerhans Cell Histiocytosis (LCH)

The term histiocytosis is a broad term for a variety of proliferative disorders of dendritic cells (DCs) or macrophages. Langerhans cell is a special type of dendritic cell in the skin functioning as antigen presenting cell. Langerhans cell histiocytosis (LCH) has the following entities:

1. Letterer-Siwe syndrome (multifocal multisystem LCH)
2. Pulmonary Langerhans' cell histiocytosis: seen in adult smokers and may regress on cessation of smoking.
3. Eosinophilic granuloma.

- These three conditions are now considered different expressions of the same basic disorder. The tumor cells in each are derived from dendritic cells and express **HLA-DR, S-100, and CD1a.** They have abundant, often vacuolated cytoplasm and vesicular nuclei containing linear grooves or folds.
- *The presence of **Birbeck's granules** in the cytoplasm is characteristic. These granules,* under the electron microscope, have a pentalaminar, rod like, tubular appearance and a dilated terminal end (**tennis-racket appearance**) which contains the protein *langerin.*
- The reason for the involvement of the organs like skin, bone, lymph node is that while *normal epidermal cells* express CCR6, their neoplastic counterparts co-express CCR6 and CCR7, and this allows the abnormal DCs to migrate into tissues that express the relevant chemokines—CCL20 in skin and bone (the ligand for CCR6) and CCL19 and 21 in lymphoid organs (ligands for CCR7).

The presence of **Birbeck's granules** in the cytoplasm is characteristic.

Hand-Schuller-Christian triad is composed of *calavrial bone defects, diabetes insipidus and exophthalmos.*

PLATELETS

Platelets are enucleated cells in the circulation released from the megakaryocyte, likely under the influence of flow in the capillary sinuses. The normal blood platelet count is 1.5- 4.5 lakhs/mm³. The production of the platelets is regulated by the hormone thrombopoietin produced in the liver.

The platelet synthesis is also specifically increased by interleukin 6. The average life span of the platelets is 7–10 days.

Normal hemostasis is a process that maintains blood in a fluid, clot-free state in normal vessels while inducing the rapid formation of a localized *hemostatic plug* at the site of vascular injury. After initial injury a brief period of *arteriolar vasoconstriction* occurs followed by the formation of a temporary hemostatic plug due to platelets. This platelet plug formation requires the following steps:

1. **Platelet adhesion**
   On vascular injury, platelets adhere to the site of injury and this is mediated primarily by two collagen receptors glycoprotein (Gp) Ia/IIa, and GpVI. This interaction with collagen is stabilized by the von Willebrand factor (vWF) which is an adhesive glycoprotein helping in the attachment of the platelets to the vessel wall. The vWF forms a link between a platelet receptor site on Gp Ib/IX and collagen fibrils.

2. **Platelet activation**
   The adherent platelets get activated, undergo a shape change and degranulate. The granules in the platelets can be
   a. *Alpha granules* having P-selectin, fibrinogen, fibronectin, factors V and VIII, platelet factor 4, platelet-derived growth factor, and transforming growth factor-β.
   b. *Delta granules* or *delta bodies* having ADP, ATP, ionized calcium, histamine, serotonin, and epinephrine.

3. **Platelet aggregation**
   The release of mediators in granule result in release of calcium (required in the coagulation cascade), ADP and the surface expression of *phospholipid complexes*, which provide the platform for the coagulation cascade. The platelets also synthesize thromboxane A_2 (TXA_2) which is a potent vasoconstrictor and is also responsible for platelet aggregation. The released ADP binds to platelet-specific purinergic receptor P_2Y_{12} which result in change in the conformation of the GpIIb/IIIa complex so that it binds fibrinogen, linking adjacent platelets into a hemostatic plug. During platelet aggregation (platelet-platelet interaction), additional platelets are recruited from the circulation to the site of vascular injury, leading to the formation of an occlusive platelet thrombus. The platelet plug is anchored and stabilized by the developing fibrin mesh.

A defect in the **glycoprotein Ib** factor results in defective platelet adhesion known as **Bernard-Soulier syndrome**

A deficiency of **Gp IIb-IIIa** lead to **Glanzmann thrombasthenia**, a disorder having defective platelet aggregation.

Glanzmann is a defect in platelet aggregation (both have 'g' in them).
Bernard Soulier syndrome is a defect in platelet adhesion (both have 'd' in them).

A deficiency of vWF results in von Willebrand's disease.

Ristocetin is an antibiotic which increase the interaction between VWF and GpIb receptor on platelets.

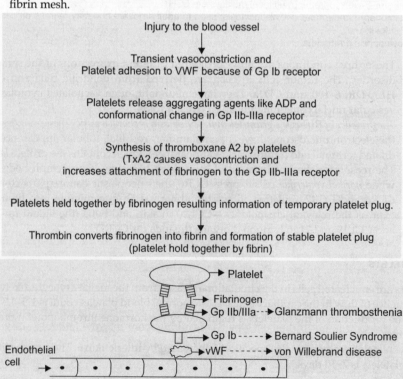

White Blood Cells and Platelets

314

Classification of functional platelet disorders	
Disorders of adhesion	
Inherited Bernard-Soulier syndrome von Willebrand disease	**Acquired** Uremia Acquired vWD
Disorders of aggregation	
Inherited Glanzmann thrombasthenia Afibrinogenemia	**Acquired** FDP inhibition Dysproteinemias Drugs-Ticlopidine, GpIIb/IIIa inhibitors
Disorders of granule release	
Inherited Oculocutaneous albinism Chediak-Higashi syndrome Isolated dense granule deficiency Gray platelet syndrome (combined α and β granule deficiency)	**Acquired** Cardiopulmonary bypass Myeloproliferative disease Drugs- NSAIDs

Bleeding time represents the time taken for a standardized skin puncture to stop bleeding and it gives an in vivo assessment of platelet response to limited vascular injury. The value varies from 2 to 9 minutes. It is abnormal when there is a defect in platelet numbers or function. Currently, quantitative measures of platelet function are being introduced by using an electronic particle counter.

> *Thrombocytopenia is characterized by spontaneous bleeding a prolonged bleeding time and a normal PT and PTT.*

Immune Thrombocytopenic Purpura (ITP)

ITP can be either primary (idiopathic) or secondary (SLE, AIDS, viral infections and drug induced). The primary ITP can be dependent on the duration of the disease, acute (less than 6 months) or chronic (> 6 months). The platelet destruction in both of them results from the formation of antiplatelet autoantibodies (type II hypersensitivity reaction).

Pathogenesis

Chronic ITP is caused by the formation of autoantibodies mostly of the **IgG** class against platelet membrane glycoproteins, most often **IIb-IIIa** or **Ib-IX**. The opsonized platelets are rendered susceptible to phagocytosis by the cells of the mononuclear phagocyte system. The spleen is the major site of removal of sensitized platelets.

Clinical features

Chronic ITP occurs most commonly in **adult women** younger than age 40 years. The female-to-male ratio is 3:1. This disorder is often insidious in onset and is characterized by bleeding into the skin (*pinpoint hemorrhages* called petechiae, especially in the dependent areas where the capillary pressure is higher or ecchymoses), mucosal surfaces (nose bleed, post brushing gum bleeds and hematuria), menorrhagia (menstrual bleeding in females) and intracranial bleeds. *Splenomegaly and lymphadenopathy are uncommon in primary ITP, and their presence should make one consider other possible diagnoses.*

Findings: The blood smear shows abnormally large platelets (**megathrombocytes**). The spleen is normal in size and sinusoidal congestion with prominent germinal centers. Bone marrow is hypercellular and shows megakaryocytic hyperplasia. The bone marrow should be examined to rule out thrombocytopenias resulting from marrow failure. A decrease in the number of megakaryocytes argues against the diagnosis of ITP. The bleeding time is prolonged, but PT and PTT are normal.

> **Thrombocytopenia** is defined as a platelet count of **1 lakh cells/µL or less** though spontaneous bleeding is seen usually when the count falls below 20000 cells/µL.

> Immune Thrombocytopenic Purpura (**ITP**) is a **type II** hypersensitivity reaction.

The management is done with immunosuppressive therapy like glucocorticoids and intravenous immunoglobulins. Splenectomy is beneficial because it is the site of destruction of the platelets and is also an important site of autoantibody synthesis which are reduced after its removal.

Acute Immune Thrombocytopenic Purpura

It is similar to chronic ITP (caused by anti platelet antibodies) but is differentiated from the same by the following:

- Seen in **children**
- **Less** duration (2-6 weeks)
- Occurs with **equal frequency** in both sexes
- **Abrupt onset** of thrombocytopenia
- Preceded by a **viral illness** and is
- **Self-limiting** (resolving spontaneously within 6 months). Steroids may be required in few cases only.

The diagnosis of Idiopathic Thrombocytopenic Purpura should be made only after exclusion of other known causes of thrombocytopenia.

Thrombotic Thrombocytopenic Purpura (TTP)/Moschcowitz Disease

It is a rare disorder of the blood-coagulation system, causing extensive microscopic blood clots to form in the small blood vessels throughout the body. It arises from deficiency of the vWF metalloprotease enzyme *ADAMTS13* which is responsible for cleaving large multimers of von Willebrand factor (vWF). In the absence of this enzyme, very high molecular weight multimers of vWF accumulate in plasma and promote platelet aggregation. This is also associated with activation of coagulation in the small blood vessels. Platelets are consumed in the coagulation process, and bind fibrin, the end product of the coagulation pathway. These platelet-fibrin complexes form microthrombi which circulate in the vasculature and cause shearing of red blood cells, resulting in hemolysis. Any additional endothelial cell injury further increases microaggregate formation. Reduced blood flow and cellular injury result in end organ damage.

Classically, the following five features ("**pentad**") are indicative of TTP:

- Fluctuating neurological symptoms, such as bizarre behavior, altered mental status, stroke or headaches
- Kidney failure
- Fever
- Thrombocytopenia (low platelet count), leading to bruising or purpura
- Microangiopathic hemolytic anemia (anemia, jaundice and a characteristic blood film)

If coagulation tests indicate a major consumption of procoagulants, the diagnosis of TTP is doubtful .The inherited inherited deficiency of ADAMTS13, known as the **Upshaw-Schulman syndrome**. The management of these patients is done with plasmapheresis (plasma exchange) and sometimes additional immunosuppressive therapy.

The combination of **hemolytic anemia with fragmented RBCs, thrombocytopenia, normal coagulation tests, fever, neurological disorders** and **renal dysfunction** is virtually pathognomic of TTP.

Hemolytic Uremic Syndrome (HUS)

HUS is also associated with microangiopathic hemolytic anemia and thrombocytopenia but is distinguished from TTP by
- Normal ADAMTS13 levels
- Absence of neurological symptoms
- Dominance of acute renal failure
- Childhood onset of disease

White Blood Cells and Platelets

It can be of the following types:

1. **Epidemic or typical HUS:** It is associated with infectious gastroenteritis caused by *E. coli* strain O157: H7. This bacterium releases a Shiga-like toxin damaging endothelial cells followed by platelet activation and aggregation. The patients presents with bloody diarrhea followed by HUS after few days.

2. **Non-epidemic or atypical HUS:** It is associated with mutations in the gene encoding complement regulatory proteins like *factor H, factor I or membrane cofactor protein CD46*. These proteins normally prevent excessive activation of alternate pathway of the complement system. So, their deficiency is associated leads to uncontrolled complement activation after minor endothelial injury, resulting in thrombosis. The patients have a relapsing remitting course.

HUS can also be seen due to other factors (e.g., certain drugs, radiation therapy) that damage endothelial cells.

> Activation of the coagulation cascade is not of primary importance in HUS and TTP and so, the laboratory tests of coagulation (such as the PT and the PTT) are usually normal.

Concept

> **In HUS, microthrombi mainly contain fibrin** *whereas in TTP these are composed of platelet aggregates, fibrin and VWF.*

Von Willebrand Disease

The von-Willebrand factor (vWF) is a heterogenous multimeric plasma glycoprotein produced by endothelial cells (*Weibel Palade bodies*) and megakaryocytes (can be shown inside platelet α-granules) with two major functions:

1. It **facilitates platelet adhesion** under conditions of high shear stress by linking platelet membrane receptors to vascular endothelium (*most important function*).

2. It serves as the **plasma carrier for the factor VIII**, the anti-hemophilic factor and increases its shelf life in circulation. Factor VIII is synthesized tissues like sinusoidal endothelial cells and Kupffer cells in the liver and glomerular and tubular epithelial cells in the kidney.

> von Willebrand disease which is the most common inherited disorder of bleeding in humans.

The disease can have the following variants:

1. Type 1 and type 3 von Willebrand disease are associated with a *reduced quantity of circulating vWF*. Type 1 (commonest variant) is an autosomal dominant disorder and is mild clinically. Type 3 (an autosomal recessive disorder) is associated with extremely low levels of functional vWF, and severe clinical manifestations. Type 1 disease is associated with missense mutations whereas Type 3 disease is associated with deletions or frameshift mutations

2. Type 2 von Willebrand disease is characterized by qualitative defects in vWF. The type 2A variant is the most common. It is inherited as an autosomal dominant disorder and is associated with missense mutations. It is associated with mild to moderate bleeding.

Clinical features in von Willebrand disease are due to

Platelet Adhesion defects
Deficiency of vWF results in defect in the adhesion of platelets to collagen preventing the formation of haemostatic plug. It leads to mucus and cutaneous bleeding in the form of epistaxis, menorrhagia and GI bleeding.

Coagulation defect
There is reduced half life of factor VIII leading to its deficiency resulting in hemorrhages and intramuscular hematoma.

LABORATORY FINDINGS

1. A *prolonged bleeding time* in the presence of a *normal platelet count*.
2. The defective platelet adhesion also results in a *positive tourniquet test* (*Hess test*).
3. In deficiency of vWF, ristocetin induced platelet aggregation does not take place. So, *ristocetin induced aggregation is defective* and is diagnostic of this disease. However, platelet aggregation with ADP, collagen and thrombin is normal.

White Blood Cells and Platelets

4. Though the synthesis of factor VIII remains normal but half life of VIII in plasma decreases due to reduced vWF (carrier) levels. This leads to secondary VIIIC deficiency in plasma. So, intrinsic pathway of coagulation is affected and thus, *aPTT is increased* in these patients.

Hemophilia A (Factor VIII Deficiency)

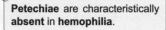

The management of these patients is done with **desmopressin** and **cryoprecipitate**.

Hemophilia A is the most common *hereditary disease associated with serious bleeding*. This X linked disorder is caused by a reduction in the amount or activity of factor VIII which is a cofactor for factor IX in the activation of factor X in the coagulation cascade. The disease can have the following variants:

1. Mild disease – levels of factor VIII activity between 6% and 50% of normal
2. Moderate disease - levels between 2% and 5% of normal
3. Severe disease- the levels less than 1% of normal activity.

The severe variant of hemophilia A is caused due to an inversion of the intron 22 sequence involving the X chromosome that completely abolishes the synthesis of factor VIII.

Clinical features: it includes easy bruising and massive hemorrhage after trauma or operative procedures. The disease is evident early in life when there is bleeding after circumcision or when the child begins to walk or crawl. The hemorrhages occur frequently in the joints (*hemarthroses*) and recurrent bleeding may lead to progressive deformities. Acute hemarthroses is painful and to avoid pain, the patient may adopt a fixed position leading to muscle contractures. It mainly affect knees, elbows, ankles, shoulders, and hips *Petechiae are characteristically absent*. Muscle hematoma can also be seen leading to a compartment syndrome. Fascial hemorrhages can result in the formation of blood filled cysts with calcification and proliferation of fibroblasts giving the appearance of a tumor (pseudotumor syndrome). Self limiting episodes of hematuria in the absence of genitourinary pathology are frequent in the patients.

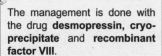

Petechiae are characteristically **absent** in **hemophilia**.

LABORATORY FINDINGS

1. Patients with hemophilia A typically have a *normal bleeding time, platelet count*, and *PT*
2. There is a *prolongation of aPTT* due to an abnormality of the intrinsic coagulation pathway.
3. Factor VIII-specific assays are required for diagnosis.

Hemophilia B (Christmas disease, Factor IX Deficiency)

The factor IX deficiency produces a disorder similar to hemophilia A. It is inherited as an X-linked recessive trait and the PTT is prolonged and the PT is normal, as is the bleeding time. The diagnosis is done only by assay of the factor IX levels.

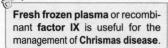

The management is done with the drug **desmopressin, cryoprecipitate** and **recombinant factor VIII**.

Fresh frozen plasma or recombinant **factor IX** is useful for the management of **Chrismas disease**.

SUMMARY OF LABORATORY FINDINGS IN HEMOSTATIC DISORDERS

Diseases	Platelet count	Bleeding time	PT	APTT	FDP
Hemophilia A	N	N	N	↑	Absent
Hemophilia B	N	N	N	↑	Absent
vWD	N	↑	N	↑	Absent
Liver failure	↓	↑	↑	↑	Absent
DIC	↓	↑	↑	↑	Present
Vascular purpura	N	N	N	N	Absent
Aspirin	N	↑	N	N	Absent
Warfarin	N	N	↑ (Even in low dose)	↑ (In high dose)	Absent

White Blood Cells and Platelets

MULTIPLE CHOICE QUESTIONS

LEUKEMIA: ALL, AML, CLL, CML

1. Flow cytometry is done in: *(AIIMS Nov 2012)*
    (a) Polycythemia
    (b) Thrombocytosis
    (c) Neutrophilia
    (d) Lymphocytosis

2. Myelofibrosis leading to a dry tap on bone marrow aspiration is seen with which of the following conditions?   *(AIIMS Nov 2012)*
    (a) Burkitt's lymphoma
    (b) Acute erythroblastic leukemia
    (c) Acute megakaryocytic leukemia
    (d) Acute undifferentiated leukemia

3. Marker of myeloid cancers: *(AIIMS Nov 2012)*
    (a) S100
    (b) HMB45
    (c) Common leukocyte antigen
    (d) Cyto-keratin

4. Adult patient presents with generalized lymphadenopathy and blood film shows 70% immature looking lymphocytes. What should be the next best investigation?
    (a) Genotyping/karyotyping   *(AIIMS Nov 2012)*
    (b) Immunophenotyping
    (c) Bone marrow
    (d) Peripheral smear study

5. Which of the following statements in context of leukemias is true?   *(AIIMS May 2012)*
    (a) Chronic myeloid leukemia occurs beyond 50 years of age
    (b) Hairy cell leukemic in less than 50 years has a good prognosis
    (c) Acute lymphoid leukemic in less than 1 year has a poor prognosis
    (d) Chronic lymphocytic leukemia occurs in less than 50 years of age

6. In an ablated animal, myeloid series cells are injected. Which of following is seen after incubation period?
    (a) Fibroblast   *(AIIMS May 2012)*
    (b) T lymphocytes
    (c) RBC
    (d) Hematopoetic stem cell

7. A young boy came with dyspnea and was found to have a mediastinal mass. Which of the following is known to produce mediastinal lymphadenopathy?   *(AI 2012)*
    (a) Diffuse large B cell Lymphoma
    (b) B cell rich T cell lymphoma
    (c) Mediastinal rich B cell lymphoma
    (d) T cell Lymphoblastic ALL

8. Which of the following is the least likely to be a pre-leukaemic condition?   *(AIIMS Nov 2011)*
    (a) Paroxysmal nocturnal haemoglobinuria
    (b) Aplastic anaemia
    (c) Paroxysmal cold haemoglobinuria
    (d) Myelodysplastic syndrome

9. A 6 year old child presents with pallor that required two blood transfusions previously. He has now developed fever and petechial haemorrhages. His hemoglobin is is 9 g/dL, platelet count is 20,000/mm³ and TLC is 60,000/mm³. Flow cytometry reveals the cells to be CD10+ve, MPO+ ve, CD 19 + ve, CD 33 – ve, CD 117 + ve, and CD3 – ve. Which of the following is the most likely diagnosis?   *(AIIMS Nov 2011)*
    (a) ALL
    (b) AML
    (c) Mixed phenotypic leukaemia
    (d) Undifferentiated leukaemia

10. Poor prognostic factor for ALL is   *(AI 2011)*
    (a) Hyperdiploidy
    (b) t(9;22) t(4;11)
    (c) Age at presentation is 2-8 yrs
    (d) Total Leucocyte count <50000

11. All the following are poor prognostic indicators in AML except   *(AIIMS Nov. 2010)*
    (a) Inv 16
    (b) Complex karyotype
    (c) AML M7
    (d) Deletion 7q

12. Most specific marker for myeloid series is
    (a) CD 34   *(AIIMS May 2010)*
    (b) CD 45
    (c) CD 99
    (d) CD 117

13. t (2,8) is associated with: *(AI 2010)*
    (a) T cell ALL
    (b) B cell ALL
    (c) CML
    (d) CLL

14. ALL L3 morphology is a malignancy arising from which cell lineage?   *(AI 2007)*
    (a) Mature B-cell
    (b) Precursor B-cell
    (c) Immature T-cell
    (d) Mixed B cell and T-cell

15. Non-specific esterase is positive in all the categories of AML except *(AI 2007)*
    (a) M3
    (b) M4
    (c) M5
    (d) M6

16. Which of the following statements pertaining to leukemia is correct? *(AI 2005)*
    (a) Blasts of acute myeloid leukemia are typically Sudan black negative
    (b) Blasts of acute lymphoblastic leukemia are typically myeloperoxidase positive
    (c) Low leucocyte alkaline phosphatase score is characteristically seen in blastic phase of chronic myeloid leukemia
    (d) Tartarate resistant acid phosphatase positivity is typically seen in hairy cell leukemia

17. Which is the most common cytogenetic abnormality in adult myelodysplastic syndrome (MDS)? *(AI 2004)*
    (a) Trisomy 8
    (b) 20q–
    (c) 5 q–
    (d) Monosomy 7

18. Which of the following is a pan-T lymphocyte marker?
    (a) CD2 *(AI 2003)*
    (b) CD3
    (c) CD19
    (d) CD25

19. B cell marker are all except: *(AIIMS Nov 09)*
    (a) CD 19
    (b) CD 20
    (c) CD 10
    (d) CD135

20. Which of the following is having poor prognosis in ALL:
    (a) TLC 4000-10000 *(AIIMS Nov 09)*
    (b) Age < 2 yrs
    (c) Presence of testicular involvement at presentation
    (d) Presence of blasts in peripheral smear

21. All of the following are good prognostic factors for acute lymphoblastic leukemia except
    (a) Age of onset between 2-8 years *(AIIMS Nov 2008)*
    (b) Initial WBC count less than 50000
    (c) Hyperdiploidy
    (d) t(9:22), t(8:14), t(4:11)

22. AML with gum infiltration, hepato- splenomegaly is most likely to be: *(AIIMS May 2008)*
    (a) ALL
    (b) M3
    (c) M2
    (d) M4

23. Marker for granulocytic sarcoma: *(AIIMS May 2008)*
    (a) CD33
    (b) CD38
    (c) CD117
    (d) CD137

24. Pancytopenia with a cellular marrow is seen in all except *(AIIMS Nov 2007)*
    (a) PNH
    (b) Megaloblastic anemia
    (c) Myelodysplastic syndrome
    (d) Congenital dyserythropoietic anemia

25. All are B-cell marker except: *(AIIMS May 2007)*
    (a) CD-15 (b) CD-19
    (c) CD-21 (d) CD-24

26. Acid phosphatase is specific to which of the following cells *(AIIMS Nov 2006)*
    (a) Monocyte
    (b) T-lymphocyte
    (c) B-lymphocyte
    (d) Myelocytes

27. A peripheral smear with increased neutrophils, basophils, eosinophils, and platelets is highly suggestive of: *(AIIMS May 2006)*
    (a) Acute myeloid leukemia
    (b) Acute lymphoblastic leukemia
    (c) Chronic myelogenous leukemia
    (d) Myelodysplastic syndrome

28. A 17-year-old boy presented with TLC of 138 × 10⁹/L with 80% blasts on the peripheral smear. Chest X-ray demonstrated a large mediastinal mass. Immunophenotyping of this patient's blasts would most likely demonstrate: *(AIIMS May 2006)*
    (a) No surface antigens (null phenotype)
    (b) An immature T-cell phenotype (Tdt/CD34/CD7 positive)
    (c) Myeloid markers, such as CD13, CD33 and CD15
    (d) B cell markers, such as CD19, CD20 and CD22

29. A 15-year-old boy presented with one day history of bleeding gums, subconjunctival bleed and purpuric rash. Investigations revealed the following results: Hb-6.4 gm/dL; TLC-26,500/mm³ Platelet 35,000 mm³; prothrombin time-20 sec with a control of 13 sec; partial thromboplastin time-50 sec; and Fibrinogen 10mg/dL. Peripheral smear was suggestive of acute myeloblastic leukemia. Which of the following is the most likely? *(AIIMS May 2006)*
    (a) Myeloblastic leukemia without maturation
    (b) Myeloblastic leukemia with maturation
    (c) Promyelocytic leukemia
    (d) Myelomonocytic leukemia

30. In a patient with acute leukemia, immunophenotype pattern is CD 19+ve, CD 10+ve, CD33+ve, CD 13+ve. He may probably have *(AIIMS May 2004)*

White Blood Cells and Platelets

(a) Biphenotypic leukemia
(b) ALL
(c) AML-M
(d) AML-M$_0^2$

31. Which of the following is not compatible with a diagnosis of chronic myelomonocytic leukemia? *(AIIMS Nov 2003)*
(a) Peripheral blood monocytosis more than $1×10^9/L$
(b) Absence of Philadelphia chromosome
(c) More than 20% blasts in blood or bone marrow
(d) Absent or minimal dysplasia in myeloid lineages

32. A 60 year old man presented with fatigue, weight loss and heaviness in left hypochondrium for 6 months. The hemogram showed Hb, 10gm/dL, TLC 5 lakhs/mm^3, platelet count 4 lakhs/mm^3, DLC, neutrophil 55%, lymphocytes 4%, monocytes 2%, basophils 6%, metamyelocytes 10%, myelocytes 18%, promyelocytes 2% and blasts 3%. The most likely cytogenetic abnormality in this case is *(AIIMS May 2003)*
(a) t (1:21)
(b) t (9:22)
(c) t (15, 17)
(d) Trisomy 21

33. A 42-year old man was referred with a 2 week history of fever weakness and bleeding gum. Peripheral smear showed pancytopenia. The bone marrow examination revealed 26% blasts frequency exhibiting Auer rods and mature myeloid cells. An occasional neutrophil with pseudo Pelger-Huet anomaly was also detected. Which of the following cytochemical stains is most likely to be positive?
(a) Acid phosphatase *(AIIMS Nov 2002)*
(b) Non-specific esterase
(c) Myeloperoxidase
(d) Toluidine blue

34. AML with worst prognosis *(AIIMS May 2007)*
(a) 8/21 translocation
(b) Inversion 16
(c) Normal cytogenetics
(d) Monosomy 7

35. Pancytopenia with cellular marrow is seen in all except
(a) Megaloblastic anemia *(AIIMS Nov 2006)*
(b) Myelodysplasia
(c) Paroxysmal nocturnal hemoglobinuria
(d) G6PD deficiency

36. Highest LAP score is seen in *(PGI Dec 2001)*
(a) CML
(b) Polycythemia vera
(c) PNH
(d) Pregnancy
(e) Lymphoma

37. Causes of eosinophilia are: *(PGI June 2004)*
(a) Hodgkin's disease
(b) Filariasis

(c) MI
(d) HIV infection

38. Sideroblasts are seen in: *(PGI Dec 2005)*
(a) Thalassemia
(b) Myelofibrosis
(c) Alcoholism
(d) Iron overload

39. Absolute monocytosis is seen in: *(PGI Dec 2006)*
(a) Infectious mononucleosis
(b) Kala-azar
(c) TB
(d) Brucellosis

40. Aplastic anemia can progress to: *(PGI Dec 01)*
(a) AML
(b) Myelodysplastic syndrome
(c) CLL
(d) PNH
(e) Iron deficiency anemia

41. True about aplastic anemia: *(PGI June 2005)*
(a) Splenomegaly
(b) Nucleated RBC in peripheral blood.
(c) Reticulocytopenia
(d) Thrombocytopenia
(e) Neutropenia

42. Leucocytosis is seen in all except: *(Delhi 2010)*
(a) Brucellosis
(b) Acute MI
(c) Typhoid
(d) Diphtheria

43. The blast cells of acute lymphocytic leukemia in childhood contain: *(Delhi PG 2005)*
(a) Surface antigen
(b) CALLA Ag
(c) Antibodies to WBC
(d) Thrombocytosis

44. "Smudge cells" in the peripheral smear are characteristic of: *(Karnataka 09)*
(a) Chronic myelogenous leukemia
(b) Chronic lymphocytic leukemia
(c) Acute myelogenous leukemia
(d) Acute lymphoblastic leukemia

45. Chromosomal translocation characteristic in acute promyelocytic leukemia is *(UP 2003)*
(a) t (15: 17)
(b) t (22: 9)
(c) t (21: 17)
(d) t (8: 21)

46. TRUE abut acute myelogenous leukemia
(a) Philadelphia chromosome is seen *(UP 2003)*
(b) Auer bodies are seen
(c) Common in childhood
(d) Peroxidase negative granules

47. In CML, serum vitamin B12 level is *(UP 2003)*
    (a) Slightly decreased
    (b) Normal
    (c) Markedly decreased
    (d) Increased

48. BCR-ABL hybrid gene is present in *(UP 2005)*
    (a) Burkitt's lymphoma
    (b) Retinoblastoma
    (c) Breast carcinoma
    (d) CML

49. The difference between leukemia and leukemoid reaction is done by: *(UP 2006)*
    (a) Total leukocyte count
    (b) Leucocyte alkaline phosphatase
    (c) Erythrocyte sedimentation rate
    (d) Immature cells

50. Neutropenia is caused by all except: *(UP 2006)*
    (a) Typhoid fever
    (b) Viral infection
    (c) Brucellosis
    (d) Glucocorticoids

51. Basophilic leucocytosis occurs in *(UP 2007)*
    (a) AML
    (b) ALL
    (c) CML
    (d) CLL

52. All are causes of splenomegaly except *(RJ 2001)*
    (a) Malaria
    (b) Kala azar
    (c) Hemolytic anemia
    (d) Aplastic anemia

53. In myelodysplastic syndrome, the following statement is incorrect *(AP 2000)*
    (a) Platelet counts are normal or elevated
    (b) Leucocyte counts are normal or elevated
    (c) Hypocellular bone marrow
    (d) Refractory anemia

54. Leukoerythroblastic picture is seen in all except
    (a) Myelofibrosis *(AP 2005)*
    (b) Secondary malignancy of bone marrow
    (c) Thalassemia
    (d) Gaucher disease

55. A round cell having, fine nuclear chromatin, prominent nucleoli and fine azurophillic granule, cell is:
    (a) Myeloblast *(Bihar 2006)*
    (b) Lymphoblast
    (c) Monoblast
    (d) None

56. Autoimmune hemolytic anemia is seen in:
    (a) ALL *(Jharkhand 2004)*
    (b) AML
    (c) CLL
    (d) CML

57. A 38 year old female Raman presented with the complaints of fever with chills and rigors for last 10 days. Her blood reports show

Hemoglobin	14.1 g/dl
Hematocrit	42.3%
MCV	90 fL
Platelet count	2.4 lac/mm3
WBC count	14,000/mm3
Differential count	
Segmented neutrophils	78%
Bands	10%
Lymphocytes	8%
Monocytes	4%

The bone marrow biopsy specimen show hyper-cellularity with a marked increase in myeloid precursors at all stages of maturation and in band neutrophils. The likely cause for the above mentioned findings would be which of the following?
    (a) Steroid (glucocorticoid) therapy
    (b) Pulmonary abscess
    (c) Vigorous exercise
    (d) Acute myelogenous leukemia

58. A 42 year woman Sunaya presents with complaints of bleeding gums for the past 20 days. The oral examination shows thickened and friable gums. Also, she has hepatosplenomegaly with generalized non tender lymphadenopathy. The blood count reveals:

Hemoglobin	11.4g/dl
Platelet count	90,000/mm3
WBC count	4600/mm3

The bone marrow biopsy shows 100% cellularity, with many large blasts that are peroxidase negative and nonspecific esterase positive. What of the following is the most likely diagnosis for this patient?
    (a) Acute lymphoblastic leukemia
    (b) Acute megakaryocytic leukemia
    (c) Acute promyelocytic leukemia
    (d) Acute monocytic leukemia

59. Akshay, an 8 years old boy presents with severe headache for 10 days. His examination revealed petechial hemorrhages, bone tenderness, hepatosplenomegaly and generalized lymphadenopathy. His CBC shows:

Hemoglobin	8.6 g/dl
Platelet count	38,000/mm3
WBC count	15,200/mm3.

A bone marrow biopsy shows 100 % cellularity, with predominance of large cells having scant cytoplasm, lacking granules, delicate nuclear chromatin, and rare nucleoli. The physician feels that the child can have a complete remission following appropriate chemotherapy. Which of the following markers is most likely to be seen in this patient?
    (a) Early pre-B (CD19+, TdT +) ; Hyperdiploidy
    (b) Early pre –B (CD 19+, TdT+) ; t(9;22)
    (c) Early pre –B (CD 5+, TdT+) ; Normal karyotype
    (d) Early pre –B (CD 5+, TdT+) ; t(9;22)

60. An experimental study performed by Ayush Medical International reveals that children with an unknown disease have blood cells with absence of surface molecules like CD1a, CD2, CD3, CD4, CD5 and CD8. Which of the following may be the karyotype anomaly seen in these children?
    (a) +21   (b) XXY
    (c) 22q11.2   (d) t (15:17)

61. The presence of the Philadelphia chromosome is associated with a worse prognosis in patients with which of the following diseases?
    (a) Acute lymphoblastic leukemia
    (b) Acute myelogenous leukemia
    (c) Chronic lymphocytic leukemia
    (d) Chronic myelogenous leukemia

62. Examination of a peripheral blood smear demonstrates leukemia composed of small mature lymphocytes without blast forms. Which of the following is the most likely age of this patient?
    (a) 1 year   (b) 20 years
    (c) 45 years   (d) 65 years

Most Recent Questions

62.1. Reed Sternberg cells are found in:
    (a) Hodkin's disease (b) Sickle cell anaemia
    (c) Thalassemia   (d) CML

62.2. Specific stain for myeloblasts is:
    (a) Sudan black
    (b) PAS
    (c) Myeloperoxidase (MPO)
    (d) LAP

62.3. Dohle bodies are seen in which of the following?
    (a) Multiple myeloma
    (b) May-Heggline anomaly
    (c) Waldenstorm Macroglobulinemia
    (d) Lymphoma

62.4. Dohle bodies in neutrophils are comprising of:
    (a) Mitochondria
    (b) Golgi apparatus
    (c) Lysosomes
    (d) Dilated endoplasmic reticulum

62.5. What is the chromosomal translocation in AML M3:
    (a) t (18, 21)   (b) t (15, 17)
    (c) t (8, 21)   (d) t (9, 11)

62.6. Which of the following is associated with good prognosis in ALL?
    (a) T cell line
    (b) Philadelphia chromosome
    (c) Hyperdiploidy
    (d) Hypodiploidy

62.7. B cell ALL is due to which of the following?
    (a) T cells   (b) Immature B cells
    (c) Immature T cells (d) Both T and B cells

62.8. CD-10 is seen in:
    (a) ALL   (b) CLL
    (c) GCL   (d) CML

62.9. Auer rods are seen in
    (a) Lymphoblast   (b) Myeloblast
    (c) Erythroblast (d) Megakaryoblast

62.10. The peripheral blood eosinophil count in Eosinophilia myalgia syndrome is usually
    (a) Between 500 to 2000 cells microilter
    (b) 2000 to 5000 cells/microliter
    (c) Less than 500 cells/microliter
    (d) More than 5000 cells/microliter

62.11. Most common ALL subtype?
    (a) Pre B cell   (b) Pre T cell
    (c) T cell   (d) B cell

NON HODGKIN LYMPHOMA

63. Progressive transformation of germinal centres (PTGC) is a precursor lesion of: (DPG 2011)
    (a) Hodgkin's Lymphoma, nodular sclerosis
    (b) Hodgkin's Lymphoma, mixed cellularity
    (c) Anaplastic large cell Lymphoma
    (d) Peripheral T cell Lymphoma

64. Eosinophilic Abscess in lymph node is characteristically seen in: (DPG 2011)
    (a) Kimura's disease
    (b) Hodgkin's Lymphoma
    (c) Tuberculosis
    (d) Sarcoidosis

65. A 50 years old male presents with massive splenomegaly. His differential diagnosis will include all, except:
    (a) Chronic myeloid leukemia   (DPG 2011)
    (b) Polycythemia rubra vera
    (c) Hairy cell leukemia
    (d) Aplastic anemia

66. Burkitt's lymphoma is associated with: (AI 2010)
    (a) t (8:14)
    (b) t (9:22)
    (c) t (11; 14)
    (d) t (8:21)

67. All of the following immunohistochemical markers are positive in the neoplastic cells of granulocytic sarcoma, except: (AI 2006)
    (a) CD 45 RO
    (b) CD 43
    (c) Myeloperoxidase
    (d) Lysozyme

68. Mantle cell lymphomas are positive for all of the following, except: (AI 2006)
    (a) CD 23   (b) CD 20
    (c) CD 5   (d) CD 43

69. The classification proposed by the International Lymphoma Study Group for non-Hodgkin lymphoma is *(AI 2005)*
    (a) Kiel classification
    (b) REAL classification
    (c) WHO classification
    (d) Rappaport classification

70. A 48 year old woman was admitted with a history of weakness for two months. On examination, cervical lymph nodes were found enlarged and spleen was palpable 2 cm below the costal margin. Her hemoglobin was 10.5 g/dl, platelet count 2.7×10⁹/L and total leukocyte count 40×10⁹/L, which included 80% mature lymphoid cells with coarse clumped chromatin. Bone marrow revealed a nodular lymphoid infiltrate. The peripheral blood lymphoid cells were positive for CD 19, CD 20 and CD 23 and were negative for CD 79B and FMC-7.

    The histopathological examination of the lymph node in this patient will most likely exhibit effacement of lymph node architecture by: *(AI 2005)*
    (a) A pseudofollicular pattern with proliferation centers
    (b) A monomorphic lymphoid proliferation with a nodular pattern
    (c) A predominantly follicular pattern
    (d) A diffuse proliferation of medium to large lymphoid cells with high mitotic rate

71. A four year old boy was admitted with a history of abdominal pain and fever for two months, maculopapular rash for ten days, and dry cough, dyspnea and wheezing for three days. On examination, liver and spleen were enlarged 4 cm and 3 cm respectively below the costal margins. His hemoglobin was 10.0 g/dl, platelet count 37×10⁹/L and total leukocyte count 70×10⁹/L, which included 80% eosinophils. Bone marrow examination revealed a cellular marrow comprising 45% blasts and 34% eosinophils and eosinophilic precursors. The blasts stained negative for myeloperoxidase and nonspecific esterase and were positive for CD 19, CD 10, CD 22 and CD 20. Which one of the following statements is not true about this disease? *(AI 2005)*
    (a) Eosinophils are not part of the neoplastic clone
    (b) t (5:14) rearrangement may be detected in blasts
    (c) Peripheral blood eosinophilia may normalize with chemotherapy
    (d) Inv (16) is often detected in the blasts and the eosinophil

72. All of the following statements about hairy cell leukemia are true except: *(AI 2004)*
    (a) Splenomegaly is conspicuous
    (b) Results from an expansion of neoplastic T lymphocytes
    (c) Cells are positive for Tartarate Resistant Acid phosphatase
    (d) The cells express CD25 consistently

73. True about Burkitt's lymphoma: *(AIIMS Nov 09)*
    (a) CD 34 and surface Ig both +ve
    (b) CD 34 negative but surface Ig+
    (c) CD 34 positive but surface Ig -
    (d) CD 34 and surface Ig both (–) ve

74. Which of the following is false? *(AIIMS Nov 09)*
    (a) Bcl-6 is associated with Burkitts lymphoma
    (b) Bcl-2 is associated with follicular lymphoma
    (c) CD-10 is associated with mantle cell lymphoma
    (d) CD 34 is associated with Diffuse large B Cell Lymphoma

75. Post transplant lymphoma occurs due to proliferation of which of the following cells
    (a) T-cell *(AIIMS Nov 2006)*
    (b) B-cell
    (c) NK cell
    (d) Monocyte

76. Which of the following statements on lymphoma is not true? *(AIIMS May 2006)*
    (a) A single classification system for Hodgkin's disease (HD) is almost universally accepted
    (b) HD more often tends to remain localized to a single group of lymph nodes and spreads by contiguity
    (c) Several types of non Hodgkin's lymphoma (NHL) may have a leukemic phase
    (d) In general follicular (nodular) NHL has worse prognosis compared to diffuse NHL

77. Mantle cell lymphomas are positive for all of the following except: *(Delhi 2010)*
    (a) CD23
    (b) CD20
    (c) CD5
    (d) Cyclin D1

78. Over-expression of BCL-2 proteins occurs in
    (a) Burkitt's lymphoma *(UP 2005)*
    (b) Follicular lymphoma
    (c) Diffuse large B-cell lymphoma
    (d) Small lymphocytic lymphoma

79. 'Starry sky' appearance is seen in *(UP 2007)*
    (a) Burkitt's lymphoma
    (b) Mantle cell lymphoma
    (c) Extra nodal marginal zone B-cell lymphoma of MALT type
    (d) Chronic myeloid leukemia

80. All are B cell lymphomas except *(AP 2005)*
    (a) Burkitt's lymphoma
    (b) Mycosis fungoides
    (c) Mantle cell lymphoma
    (d) Follicular cell lymphoma

81. True statement regarding non Hodgkin's lymphoma of follicular type is: *(Kolkata 2002)*
    (a) Increased incidence in adolescents
    (b) Predominantly in males
    (c) Prognosis is better than in diffuse type
    (d) Affects T cells only

82. MALToma is: *(Jharkhand 2006)*
    (a) B-cell lymphoma
    (b) APUDoma
    (c) NK cell tumor
    (d) T cell lymphoma

83. An old man, Amarnath presents with increasing abdominal discomfort, fatigue and easy bruising of his skin. He also has tender splenomegaly. Laboratory investigations show:

Hemoglobin	7.9 g/dl
Platelet count	35,000/mm3
WBC count	2500/mm3
Serum AST	77 U/L
Serum ALT	86 U/L.

    Which of the following is the most likely diagnosis?
    (a) Acute myelogenous leukemia
    (b) Cirrhosis
    (c) Systemic lupus erythematosus
    (d) Infectious mononucleosis

84. Molecular studies on an abdominal lymph node containing lymphoma demonstrate (2;8)(p12;q24) translocation. This is most compatible with which of the following diseases?
    (a) Burkitt's lymphoma
    (b) Mantle cell lymphoma
    (c) Multiple myeloma
    (d) Small cell lymphoma

85. A 21-year-old male Imraan Hashmi with fatigue, recurrent fever, and enlarged cervical lymph nodes has numerous atypical lymphocytes in his peripheral blood smear. Lymph node biopsy shows expansion of lymphoid follicles with preservation of the underlying architecture. Numerous atypical lymphocytes are present in the paracortical areas. This patient most likely has
    (a) AIDS
    (b) Burkitt's lymphoma
    (c) Hodgkin's Disease
    (d) Infectious mononucleosis

Most Recent Questions

85.1. Marginal lymphoma is type of:
    (a) B cell lymphoma
    (b) T cell lymphoma
    (c) NK cell lymphoma
    (d) Hodgkin lymphoma

85.2. Which of the following is the marker of mantle cell cancer?
    (a) CD5 +, CD25 –   (b) CD 5 +, CD 10 +
    (c) CD 5 +, CD 23 + (d) CD 5 +, CD 23 –

85.3. Mycosis fungoides is:
    (a) Fungal infections of skin
    (b) Leukemia
    (c) Exfoliative erythroderma
    (d) Cutaneous lymphoma

85.4. The low grade non- Hodgkin's lymphoma is:
    (a) Follicular small cleaved lymphoma
    (b) Follicular large cell lymphoma
    (c) Diffuse large cell lymphoma
    (d) Lymphoblastic lymphoma

85.5. Which of the following is the most common non Hodgkin lymphoma? *(AIIMS Nov 2013)*
    (a) Follicular lymphoma
    (b) Anaplastic large cell lymphoma
    (c) Diffuse large B cell lymphoma
    (d) Marginal zone lymphoma

85.6. Most common Non-Hodgkin's lymphoma of orbit:
    (a) B cell   *(AIIMS May 2013)*
    (b) T cell
    (c) NK cell
    (d) Plasma cell

85.7. Which of the following is the most common site for extranodal lymphoma?
    (a) Esophagus   (b) Stomach
    (c) Intestine   (d) Skin

85.8 Cell of origin of hairy cell leukemia is
    (a) T cell   (b) B cell
    (c) NK cell (d) Dendritic cell

85.9. Which one of the following Non-Hodgkin Lymphomas is aggressive?
    (a) Follicular Lymphoma
    (b) Burkitt Lymphoma
    (c) Small lymphocytic lymphoma
    (d) Lymphoplasmacytic lymphoma

85.10. Histological presence of "Hallmark Cells" with horse shoe-like or embryoid like nuclei and voluminous cytoplasm are seen in
    (a) Anaplastic large cell lymphoma (ALK positive)
    (b) Familial Medullary Carcinoma
    (c) Familial Neuroblastoma
    (d) Lymphocyte predominance type Hodgkin's lymphoma

85.11. Prevalence of burkitt lymphoma is highest in?
    (a) Australia   (b) Africa
    (c) Asia   (d) America

HODGKIN LYMPHOMA

86. A 35-year-old man is diagnosed with non-Hodgkin lymphoma. Even without knowing the specific diagnosis, it can safely be said that this patient's lymphoma is characterized by
    (a) B-lymphocytic origin
    (b) Histiocytic origin
    (c) Lymph node localization
    (d) Monoclonal origin

87. A 26-year-old man Ronit has progressive, painless enlargement of neck lymph nodes. Routine chest film

and CT scan show marked enlargement of mediastinal nodes. No nodules are seen in the liver or lungs. When evaluating the biopsy of one of the involved nodes, Dr Mohit, a pathologist would find which of the following?
(a) Abnormal plasma cells
(b) Giant platelets
(c) Immature neutrophil precursors
(d) Reed-Sternberg cells

88. Classical markers for Hodgkin's disease are:
(a) CD 15 and CD 30   *(AI 2008)*
(b) CD 15 and CD 22
(c) CD 15 and CD 20
(d) CD 20 and CD 30

89. The subtype of Hodgkin's disease, which is histogenetically distinct from all the other subtypes, is:
(a) Lymphocyte predominant   *(AI 2005)*
(b) Nodular sclerosis
(c) Mixed cellularity
(d) Lymphocyte depleted

90. All of the following are the good prognostic features for Hodgkin's disease except:
(a) Hemoglobin > 10 gm/dl   *(AI 2004)*
(b) WBC count < 15000/mm^3
(c) Absolute lymphocyte count < 600/µl
(d) Age < 45 years

91. The lymphocytic and histiocytic variant of Reed-Sternberg cell is seen in   *(AIIMS Nov 2005)*
(a) Follicular center lymphoma
(b) Lymphocyte depleted Hodgkin's disease
(c) Nodular sclerosis Hodgkin's disease
(d) Lymphocyte predominant Hodgkin's disease

92. Which cell is not seen in Hodgkins lymphoma
(a) Reed Sternberg cell   *(PGI Dec 2000)*
(b) Lacunar cell   (c) L and H cell
(d) Langerhan's cell   (e) Hodgkin cell

93. Lacunar type of Reed Sternberg cells are seen in:
          (Delhi 2009 RP)
(a) Mixed cellularity Hodgkin's lymphoma
(b) Nodular sclerosis Hodgkin's lymphoma
(c) Lymphocyte depleted Hodgkin's lymphoma
(d) Lymphocyte predominant Hodgkin's lymphoma

94. The sub-type of Hodgkin's lymphoma characteri zed by L and H cells is: *(Karnataka 09)*
(a) Nodular sclerosis
(b) Mixed cellularity
(c) Lymphocyte depletion
(d) Lymphocyte predominant

95. Lacunar cells are seen in which type of Hodgkin's lymphoma   *(PGI-99) (UP 2004) (Kolkatta & Bihar 03)*
(a) Nodular sclerosis
(b) Mixed cellularity
(c) Lymphocyte depletion
(d) Lymphocyte predominant

96. Lacunar cells are present in which Hodgkin's lymphoma?   *(RJ 2000)*
(a) Nodular sclerosis
(b) Lymphocyte predominant
(c) Mixed cellularity
(d) All

97. 'Popcorn cells' are seen in which type of Hodgkin's disease?   *(AP2003)*
(a) Lymphocyte dominant
(b) Lymphocyte depleted
(c) Nodular sclerosis
(d) Mixed type

98. An elderly patient presented with hypercellular bone marrow, peripheral blood smear shows pancytopenia, and 15% myeloblast cells. Most likely diagnosis is
(a) Myelodysplastic syndrome   *(UP 2003)*
(b) Blast crisis in CML
(c) AML
(d) Polycythemia vera

Most Recent Questions

98.1. Which Hodgkin's disease is associated with best prognosis:
(a) Lymphocyte depletion
(b) Mixed cellularity
(c) Lymphocytic predominance
(d) Nodular sclerosis

98.2. Lacunar cells are seen in which type of Hodgkin's lymphoma:
(a) Lymphocyte predominance
(b) Lyphocyte depletion
(c) Nodular sclerosis
(d) Mixed cellularity

98.3. In a 45 year old female presenting with painless supraclavicular lymphadenopathy, biopsy was taken. It revealed the presence of binucleated acidophlic owl eye appearance with clear vacuolated space. The cell was CD15 and CD30 positive. Which is the most likely diagnosis?
(a) Lymphocyte predominant Hodgkin lymphoma
(b) Nodular sclerosis Hodgkin lymphoma
(c) Mixed cellularity Hodgkin lymphoma
(d) Lymphocyte depleted Hodgkin lymphoma

MYELOPROLIFERATIVE DISORDERS

99. Splenomegaly is associated with all except: *(AI 2012)*
(a) CML
(b) Polycythemia vera
(c) Essential thrombocythemia
(d) Primary myelofibrosis

White Blood Cells and Platelets

100. **Essential criteria for polycythemia vera according to WHO is:** *(AI 2010)*
    (a) Low EPO
    (b) JAK 2 mutation
    (c) Bone marrow showing panmyelosis
    (d) MPL point mutation

101. **Which of the following is not a chronic myeloproliferative disorder?** *(Delhi PG 2006)*
    (a) Polycythemia vera
    (b) Myeloid metaplasia
    (c) CML
    (d) Essential thrombocytopenia

102. **An old man Durga Prasad presents to you with complaints of fatigue, weight loss, night sweats, and abdominal 'heaviness' for the past 10 months. Physical examination reveals marked splenomegaly but no lymphadenopathy. His investigations are given below:**

Hemoglobin	10g/dl
Platelet count	90,000/mm3
WBC count	15,250/mm3
Peripheral blood smear	teardrop cells
Serum uric acid level	9 g/dl
Bone marrow biopsy	Extensive marrow fibrosis and groups of atypical megakaryo-cytes

    Which of the following is the likely cause for the old man's splenomegaly?
    (a) Hodgkin lymphoma
    (b) Extramedullary hematopoiesis
    (c) Portal hypertension
    (d) Metastatic adenocarcinoma

103. **A child presents with seborrheic dermatitis, sinusitis and chronically draining ears. On examination child has failure to thrive with hepato-splenomegaly and exophthalmos. Probable diagnosis is**
    (a) Histiocytosis-X
    (b) Wegener's granulomatosis
    (c) Chronic grnaulomatous disease
    (d) Chediak higashi syndrome

Most Recent Questions

103.1. **Polycythemia is absolute venous haematocrit of more than:**
    (a) 45%   (b) 55%
    (c) 65%   (d) 70%

103.2. **CD marker of histiocytosis is:**
    (a) CD 1a   (b) CD 1b
    (c) CD 1c   (d) CD 1d

103.3. **Shape of Birbeck granules is which of the following?**
    (a) Hockey stick   (b) Bat
    (c) Ball   (d) Tennis racket

103.4. **Leucocyte alkaline phosphatase (LAP) is raised in all conditions except:**
    (a) Myelofibrosis
    (b) Essential thrombocythemia

    (c) Chronic myeloid leukemia
    (d) Polycythemia

103.5. **Leukoerythroblastic reaction is seen in the following except:**
    (a) Secondaries in bone
    (b) Multiple myeloma
    (c) Hemolytic anemia
    (d) Lymphoma

103.6. **Increase in alkaline phosphatase is seen in:**
    (a) Chronic myeloid leukemia; CML
    (b) Leukemoid reaction
    (c) Eosinophilia
    (d) Malaria

103.7. **One of the following is not a myelo-proliferative disorder?**
    (a) Essential thrombocytosis
    (b) Myelofibrosis with myeloid metaplasia
    (c) Acute myeloblastic leukemia
    (d) Chronic myeloid leukemia

103.8 **Isolated deletion of which chromosome is associated with myelodysplastic syndrome?**
    (a) 2q   (b) 5q
    (c) 8q   (d) 11q

PLASMA CELL DYSCRASIAS

104. **Which of the following is the least common presentation of multiple myeloma?** *(AI 2012)*
    (a) Anemia   (b) Hyperviscosity
    (c) Bone pains   (d) Infection

105. **Which of the following metabolic abnormality is seen in multiple myeloma?** *(DPG 2011)*
    (a) Hypernatremia   (b) Hypokalemia
    (c) Hypercalcemia   (d) Hyperphosphatemia

106. **Lymphoplasmacytoid lymphoma is associated with:**
    (a) IgG   *(AI 2010)*
    (b) IgA
    (c) IgD   (d) IgM

107. **Which of the following statement is not true?** *(AI 2005)*
    (a) Patients with IgD myeloma may present with no evident M-spike on serum electrophoresis.
    (b) A diagnosis of plasma cell leukemia can be made if circulating peripheral blood plasma blasts comprise 14% of peripheral blood white cells in a patient with white blood cell count of 1×10^9/L and platelet count of 88×10^9/L
    (c) In smoldering myeloma plasma cells constitute 10-30% of total bone marrow cellularity
    (d) In a patient with multiple myeloma, a monoclonal light chain may be detected in both serum and urine

108. **Which of the following is not a minor diagnostic criterion for multiple myeloma?** *(AIIMS Nov 08, 10)*
    (a) Lytic bone lesions
    (b) Plasmacytosis greater than 20%
    (c) Plasmacytoma on biopsy
    (d) Monoclonal globulin spike on serum electrophoresis of < 2.5 g/dl for IgG, < 1.5 g/dl for IgA)

109. **A 3 year old female child presented with skin papules. Which of the following is a marker of Langerhan's cell histiocytosis?** *(AIIMS Nov 2007)*
    (a) CD 1a   (b) CD 3
    (c) CD 68   (d) CD 57

110. **A 70-year-old male has a pathologic fracture of femur. The lesion appears a lytic on X-rays film with a circumscribed punched out appearance. The curetting from fracture site is most likely to show which of the following?** *(AIIMS May 2006)*
    (a) Diminished and thinned trabecular bone
    (b) Sheets of atypical plasma cells
    (c) Metastatic prostatic adenocarcinoma
    (d) Malignant cells forming osteoid bone

111. **Hyperviscosity is seen in** *(PGI Dec 2003)*
    (a) Cryoglobulinemia
    (b) Multiple myeloma
    (c) MGUS
    (d) Lymphoma
    (e) Macroglobulinemia

112. **Hyperviscosity syndrome is seen in:**
    (a) NHL   *(PGI Dec 2004)*
    (b) Waldenstrom's macroglobulinemia
    (c) Multiple myeloma
    (d) Hodgkin's lymphoma
    (e) Acute promyelocytic leukemia

113. **True about Langerhan's cell histiocytosis is:**
    (a) CD 68+   *(PGI Dec 2005)*
    (b) CD 1+
    (c) Birbeck's granules are pathognomic
    (d) Proliferation of antigen presenting cells
    (e) Resembles dendritic cells

114. **Finding of multiple myeloma in kidney are all except:**
    (a) Tubular casts   *(Delhi 2010)*
    (b) Amyloidosis
    (c) Wire loop lesions
    (d) Renal tubular necrosis

115. **Proliferation and survival of myeloma cells are dependent on which of the following cytokines?**
    (a) IL-1   *(Karnataka 2005)*
    (b) IL-6
    (c) IL-2
    (d) IL-5

116. **Plasma cell dyscrasias include all of the following except** *(Karnataka 2005)*
    (a) Waldenstorm's macroglobulinemia
    (b) Heavy chain disease

    (c) Monoclonal gammopathy of uncertain significance
    (d) Systemic lupus erythematosus

117. **Histiocytosis is NOT associated with** *(AP 2003)*
    (a) Spontaneous fractures
    (b) Cutaneous eruptions
    (c) Bone marrow suppression
    (d) No lymphadenopathy

118. **M-spike in multiple myeloma is due to?** *(Bihar 2003)*
    (a) IgM   (b) IgA
    (c) IgG   (d) None of these

119. **Birbeck's granule is found in:** *(Bihar 2006)*
    (a) Langerhans cell   (b) Langhans giant cell
    (c) Lepra cell   (d) Clue cell

120. **A 62 year old man Kuljeet developed weakness, fatigue and weight loss over the past 4 months. He also complains of decreasing vision, headache and dizziness. His hands have become sensitive to cold. On the general physical examination of this individual, the physician observes generalized lymphadenopathy and hepatosplenomegaly. The laboratory reports show hyperproteinemia with a serum protein level of 16g/dl and the serum albumin concentration of 3.4 g/dl. The treating physician performs a bone marrow biopsy that demonstrated infiltration of small plasmacytoid lymphoid cells with Russell bodies in the cytoplasm on microscopic examination. Which of the following is the most likely finding in this patient?**
    (a) Monoclonal IgM spike in serum
    (b) WBC count of 2,40,000/mm3
    (c) Hypercalcemia
    (d) Bence Jones proteinuria

121. **An old woman is seen in the emergency after fracturing her hip. She is found to have a malignant tumor. She also has a history of recurrent pneumonia over the last 6 months. Lab investigations reveal a normal white blood cell count, but decreased platelets and serum albumin with an elevated erythrocyte sedimentation rate (ESR). Serum electrophoresis indicates an M-protein spike band of IgG kappa. The urine will most likely show the presence of Bence-Jones proteins composed of**
    (a) IgG heavy chains
    (b) kappa and lambda light chains of a 60:40 ratio
    (c) kappa light chains
    (d) lambda light chains

Most Recent Questions

121.1. **Russell bodies are found in which of the following conditions?**
    (a) Multiple Myeloma
    (b) Gonadal tumor
    (c) Parkinsonism
    (d) Intracranial neoplasms

White Blood Cells and Platelets

121.2. Which histiocytosis involves the bones:
(a) Malignant
(b) Langherhans
(c) Sinus histiocytosis
(d) Option not recalled

121.3. Beta-2 microglobulin is a tumor marker for
(a) Multiple myeloma
(b) Lung cancer
(c) Colonic neoplasm
(d) Choriocarcinoma

PLATLETS AND BLEEDING DISORDERS

122. A newborn baby presented with profuse bleeding from the umbilical stump after birth. Rest of the examination and PT, APTT are within normal limits. Most likely diagnosis is which of the following?
(a) Factor X deficiency
(b) Glanzmann's thrombasthenia
(c) von Willebrand disease
(d) Bernard Soulier disease

123. A 25 years old asymptomatic female underwent a pre-op coagulation test. Her bleeding time is 3minutes, PT is 15/14sec, a PTT is 45/35 sec, platelet count is 2.5 lac/mm³ and factor VIII levels were 60IU/dL. What is her most likely diagnosis?   (AIIMS Nov 2011)
(a) Factor IX deficiency
(b) Lupus anticoagulant
(c) Factor VIII inhibitors
(d) VWD – Type III

124. True about prothrombin time to   (AIIMS Nov 2011)
(a) Immediate refrigeration to preserve factor viability
(b) Platelet-rich plasma is essential
(c) Done within 2 hours
(d) Activated with kaolin

125. A 22 year old female having a family history of autoimmune disease presents with the complaints of recurrent joint pains. She has now developed petechial hemorrhages. She is most likely to have which of the following disorders?   (AIIMS Nov 2011)
(a) Megakaryocytic thrombocytopenia
(b) Amegakaryocytic thrombocytopenia
(c) Platelet function defects/Functional platelet defect
(d) Acquired Factor VIII inhibitors

126. Patient with bleeding due to platelet function defects has which of the following features?   (AI 2011)
(a) Normal platelet count and normal bleeding time
(b) Normal platelet count and increased bleeding time
(c) Decreased platelet count and increased bleeding time
(d) Normal platelet count and decreased bleeding time

127. A 9-year-old boy presents with elevation in both PT and aPTT. What is the diagnosis?   (AIIMS Nov. 2010)
(a) Defect in extrinsic pathway

(b) Defect in intrinsic pathway
(c) Platelet function defect
(d) Defect in common pathway

128. All are true about thrombotic thrombocytopenic purpura except?   (AIIMS Nov 2008)
(a) Microangiopathic hemolytic anemia
(b) Thrombocytopenia
(c) Normal complement level
(d) Grossly abnormal coagulation tests

129. D.I.C. is seen in: (AIIMS May 2007)
(a) Acute promyelocytic leukemia
(b) Acute myelomonocytic leukemia
(c) CMC
(d) Autoimmune hemolytic anemia

130. All of the following can cause megakaryocytic thrombocytopenia, except   (AIIMS Nov 2004)
(a) Idiopathic thrombocytopenia purpura
(b) Systemic lupus erythematosus
(c) Aplastic anemia
(d) Disseminated intravascular coagulation (DIC)

131. A patient with cirrhosis of liver has the following coagulation parameters, Platelet count 2,00,000, Prothrombin time 25s/12s, Activated partial thromboplastin time 60s/35s, thrombin time 15s/15s. In this patient   (AIIMS May 2004)
(a) D-dimer will be normal
(b) Fibrinogen will be < 100 mg
(c) ATIII will be high
(d) Protein C will be elevated

132. The presence of small sized platelets on the peripheral smear is characteristic of: (AIIMS Nov 2003)
(a) Idiopathic thrombocytopenia purpura (ITP)
(b) Bernard Soulier syndrome
(c) Disseminated intravascular coagulation
(d) Wiskott Aldrich syndrome

133. Platelet aggregation in vivo is mediated by
(a) Serotonin   (PGI Dec 2003)
(b) Ig mediators.
(c) Interaction among the leukocytes
(d) Interaction among the platelets
(e) Macromolecules.

134. Conditions associated with incoagulable state:
(a) Abruption placentae   (PGI Dec 2004)
(b) Acute promyelocytic leukemia
(c) Severe falciparum malaria
(d) Snake envenomation
(e) Heparin overdose

135. In DIC, which is/are seen: (PGI June 2005)
(a) Normal aPTT
(b) Increased PT
(c) Increased factor VIII
(d) Decreased fibrinogen
(e) Decreased platelets

136. **Causes for DIC are:** *(PGI Dec 2005)*
    (a) Anaerobic sepsis (b) Malignancy
    (c) Lymphoma (d) Leukemia
    (e) Massive blood transfusion

137. **Platelet function defect is seen in:** *(PGI June 03)*
    (a) Glanzmann syndrome.
    (b) Bernard Soulier syndrome
    (c) Wiskott Aldrich syndrome
    (d) Von-Willebrand disease
    (e) Weber Christian disease

138. **VWF factor deficiency causes:** *(Delhi PG 2008)*
    (a) ↓ Platelet aggregation
    (b) ↓ Factor VIII in plasma
    (c) Defective platelet adhesion
    (d) All of the above

139. **Thrombospondin is** *(Delhi PG 2008)*
    (a) Coagulation protein
    (b) Coagulation promoting protein
    (c) Contractile protein
    (d) Angiogenesis inhibitory protein

140. **Which is must for prothrombins time (PT)?**
    (a) Thromboplastin *(Delhi PG 2007)*
    (b) Prothrombin
    (c) Fibrin
    (d) Fibrinogen

141. **Thrombocytosis is seen in:** *(Delhi PG 2005)*
    (a) Myelofibrosis
    (b) SLE
    (c) Azidothymidine therapy
    (d) Myelodysplastic syndrome

142. **All of the following are true about Willebrand factor except:** *(Delhi PG-2005)*
    (a) Synthesized by hepatocytes
    (b) Its deficiency can cause factor 8 defect also
    (c) Its deficiency may cause problem with platelet adhesion
    (d) It serves as carrier for the factor eight

143. **All of the following clotting factors are completely synthesized from liver except** *(UP 2002)*
    (a) II (b) V
    (c) VII (d) VIII

144. **Cryoprecipitate contain all except** *(UP 2002)*
    (a) Fibrinogen
    (b) Factor VIII
    (c) von Willebrand factor
    (d) Antithrombin

145. **Bleeding time is abnormal in:** *(UP 2006)*
    (a) Hemophilia
    (b) Christmas disease
    (c) von Willebrand disease
    (d) Vitamin K-deficiency

146. **The chromosomal translocation involving bcl-2 in B-cell lymphoma is** *(UP 2008)*
    (a) t (8: 14) (b) t (8: 12)
    (c) t (14: 18) (d) t (14: 22)

147. **Agranulocytosis means:** *(Kolkata 2000)*
    (a) Decrease in neutrophil count
    (b) Decrease in platelet count
    (c) Increase in RBC count
    (d) Decrease in RBC count

148. **Thrombocytopenia syndrome is caused by decrease in platelet counts below:** *(Bihar 2004)*
    (a) 50,000/cmm (b) 1,00,000/cmm
    (c) 1.2 lac/cmm (d) 20, 000/cmm

149. A 28-year-old woman Salma presents complaining of nosebleeds. She also has easy bruising and excessively heavy bleeding during her periods. There is no history of drug intake. Physical examination shows scattered petechiae with normal sized spleen. Laboratory examination shows platelet count of 37000/microliter and a bleeding time of 16 minutes. The bone marrow shows an increased number of megakaryocytes. Antinuclear antibody is negative. Autoantibodies directed against which of the following antigens would likely be found in this patient's serum?
    (a) Acetylcholine receptor
    (b) Erythrocyte membrane protein
    (c) Glycoprotein IIb/IIIa
    (d) Intrinsic factor

150. A young female Vibhuti presents with a several month history of easy bruising and increased menstrual flow is evaluated for a bleeding disorder. She has idiopathic thrombocytopenic purpura (ITP). In this disorder, the low platelet count is due to which of the following?
    (a) Antiplatelet antibodies
    (b) Defective platelet aggregation
    (c) Hypersplenism
    (d) Ineffective megakaryopoiesis

Most Recent Questions

150.1. **Glanzmann disease is characterised by which of the following?**
    (a) Congenital defect of RBCs
    (b) Defect of neutrophils
    (c) Congenital defect of platelets
    (d) Clotting factor deficiency

150.2. **All of the following are true about DIC except:**
    (a) Platelet aggregation
    (b) Fibrin deposition in microcirculation
    (c) Decreased fibrin degradation products
    (d) Release of tissue factor

150.3. All are true regarding thrombotic thrombocytopenic purpura except:
(a) Normal complement levels
(b) Microangiopathic hemolytic anemia
(c) Thrombocytopenia
(d) Thrombosis

150.4. Glycoprotein IIb-IIa complex is deficient in
(a) Bernard Soulier syndrome
(b) Glanzmann disease
(c) Von willebrand disease
(d) Gray platelet syndrome

150.5. All the following statements are correct about treatment in chronic immune thrombocytopenic purpura except
(a) Most of the patients respond to immunosuppressive doses of glucocorticoids
(b) Relapse is rare
(c) Splenectomy is the treatment of choice for relapse
(d) Minority have refractory forms of ITP and difficult to treat

150.6 Splenectomy is useful in which of the following?
(a) Chronic ITP
(b) Sickle cell anemia
(c) Tuberculosis
(d) Good pasture syndrome

150.7. Pancreatic insufficiency and cyclic neutropenia is a part of which syndrome
(a) Young syndrome
(b) Colts syndrome
(c) Shwachman syndrome
(d) Roots syndrome

EXPLANATIONS

1. **Ans. (d) Lymphocytosis** *(Ref: Robbins 8th/324)*

   Flow cytometry can rapidly and quantitatively measure several individual cell characteristics, such as membrane antigens and the DNA content of tumor cells.
   Flow cytometry has also proved useful in the identification and classification of tumors arising from **T and B lymphocytes** and from mononuclear-phagocytic cells.

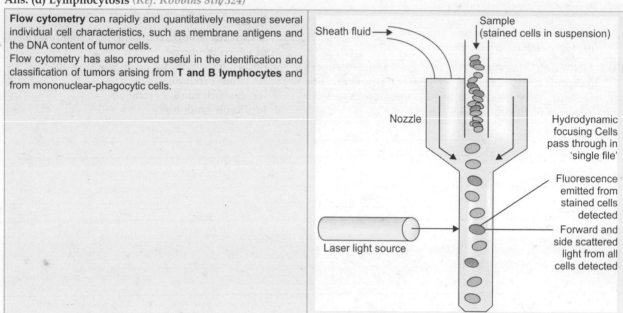

2. **Ans. (c) Acute megakaryocytic leukemia.** *(Ref: Robbins 8th/622, 9/e p612, Wintrobe's 12th/1857-8)*
   Direct quote from Robbins… *'In some AMLs, blasts show **megakaryocytic differentiation**, which is **often accompanied by marrow fibrosis** caused by the release of fibrogenic cytokines'*
   Acute megakaryocytic leukemia is the most common variant of AML associated with **Down syndrome.** The release of PDGF (platelet derived growth factor) is responsible for marrow fibrosis.

3. **Ans. (C) Common leukocyte antigen** *(Ref: Robbins 8th/600, 9/e p590)*
   • CD45 is present on all the leukocytes; it is also known as leukocyte common antigen (LCA).

4. **Ans. (b) Immunophenotyping** *(Ref: Robbins 8th /604, 9/e p593)*
   Adult patient presenting with generalized lymphadenopathy and blood film shows 70% immature looking lymphocytes is highly suggestive of chronic lymphocytic leukemia.
   Immnophenotyping can be one of the best ways to differentiate between CLL and other B cell neoplasms.
   Important points about CLL
   • Most of the patients are often asymptomatic at diagnosis. When symptoms appear, they are nonspecific and include easy fatigability, weight loss, and anorexia. Hepatosplenomegaly and generalized lymphadenopathy are present in 50% to 60% of symptomatic patients.
   • The immunophenotype of CLL is distinct. The tumor cells express the pan-B cell markers CD19 and CD20, as well as CD23 and CD5, the latter a marker that is found on a small subset of normal B cells. Low-level expression of surface Ig (usually IgM or IgM and IgD) is also typical.

5. **Ans. (c) Acute lymphoid leukemic in less than 1 year has a poor prognosis** *(Ref: Robbins 8th/603, 9/e p592, Wintrobe 12th)*
   Prognostic factors in ALL have been discuss in text

   Explaining other options,
   • Chronic myeloid leukemia occurs beyond 50 years of age…Robbins 8th/
   • Hairy cell leukemic is present in median age of 55 years and has M:F ratio of 5:1. HCL tends to follow an indolent course. For unclear reasons, the tumor cells are exceptionally sensitive to particular chemotherapeutic regimens,

which produce long-lasting remissions. The overall prognosis is excellent. So, the condition is not having additional increase in improvement with age less than 50 years.

- The median age of diagnosis of Chronic lymphocytic leukemia is 60 years and there is a 2:1 male predominance.... Robbins 8th/603

6. **Ans. (c) RBC** (*Ref: Robbins 8th/592-593, 9/e p580*)
The following flowchart is self explanatory for this question:

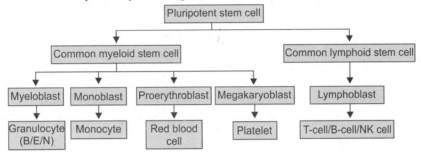

B: Basophil, E: Eosinophil, N: Neutrophil

So, on the injection of a myeloid stem cell, it can give rise to a cell of its lineage which can be either of the RBCs, monocytes, neutrophils, eosinophils, basophils and platelets. The answer is therefore, red blood cells.

7. **Ans. (d) T cell Lymphoblastic ALL** (*Ref: Robbins 8th/601-3, 9/e p592*)

8. **Ans. (c) Paroxysmal cold haemoglobinuria** (*Ref: Robbins 8th/625, 653,664, 9/e p544, Wintrobes 12th/965*)
Analyzing all the options one by one;
Option 'a'...direct quote.. 'about 5% to 10% of patients eventually develop acute myeloid leukemia or a myelodysplastic syndrome, possibly because hematopoietic stem cell have suffered some type of genetic damage'. (Robbins 8th/653)
Even PNH is associated with aplastic anemia as both the disorders have an autoimmune basis.
Option 'b'...direct quote.., aplastic anemia results from a fundamental stem cell defect supported by the presence of karyotypic aberrations in many cases; the occasional transformation of aplasias into myeloid neoplasms, typically myelodysplasia or acute myeloid leukemia; and the association with abnormally short telomeres. (Robbins 8th/664)
Option 'd'...direct quote.. The term "myelodysplastic syndrome" (MDS) refers to a group of clonal stem cell disorders characterized by maturation defects that are associated with ineffective hematopoiesis and a high risk of transformation to AML. (Robbins 8th/625).

> So the answer of exclusion is PCH (paroxysmal cold hemoglobinuria). It is an autoimmune haemolytic anemia due to IgG autoantibodies which bind to P blood group antigen and cause intravascular hemolysis and hemoglobinuria. Most cases are seen in children and have recovery within a month.....Wintrobes.

9. **Ans. (c) Mixed phenotypic leukaemia** (*Ref: Wintrobes 12th/1814-8, Dacie and Lewis hematology 10th/344-6*)
Mixed lineage acute leukemia is alternatively also known as bilineal acute leukemia. As is suggested by the name, there are 2 populations of cells which are morphologically and immunophenotypically distinct from each other. Analyzing the markers on the cells,

- B lymphoid markers: CD10, CD19 and CD79
- T lineage markers: CD2, CD3 and CD7
- Myeloid markers; CD13, CD33, CD117 and myeloperoxidase (MPO).
- Non lineage specific markers which are expressed in hematopoietic progenitor cells: CD34, HLA-DR and TdT

Comparing this with the information provided in the stem of our question, it is easy to decipher that the cells mentioned are CD10+ve, MPO +ve, CD19+ve, CD33-ve, CD117 +ve and CD3-ve which is showing both lymphoid (CD10, CD19;B lymphoid lineage) and myeloid (CD117 and MPO+-; myeloid lineage) markers. So, the answer is **Mixed phenotypic leukemia**

A word about the last option 'd', please note that in un-differentiated acute leukemia, b**lasts usually lack any evidence of lineage differentiation.** (Ref Wintrobes 12th/1814-8)

10. Ans. (b) t(9;22) t(4;11) *(Ref: Robbins 8th/603, 9/e p592-593)*
Prognostic factors in ALL

GOOD PROGNOSIS	BAD PROGNOSIS
• Age 2-10 years • Female sex • L1 cell • Peripheral blast count <1,00,000 • Pre B cell phenotype • Absence of mediastinal mass • Hyperdiploidy (>50 chromosomes) or t(12;21) • Trisomy of chromosomes 4,7,10	• Age <1 year or > 10 years • Male sex • L2 or L3 cell • Peripheral blast count >1,00,000 • Pre T cell phenotype • Mediastinal mass • Pseudodiploidy or t (9;22) or presence of Philadelphia chromosome, t (8;14), t (4;11)

11. Ans. (a) Inv 16 *(Ref: Wintrobe 12th/1859, Robbins 8th/624, 9/th 614, T. Singh 2nd/168)*
Prognostic markers for AML

Good Prognosis	Bad Prognosis
• Age <40 years • M2, M3, M4 forms of AML • Blast cell with Auer rods • TLC < 25 X 10⁹/L • t(15;17), t (8;21), inv 16 • Rapid response to therapy • Leukemia without preceding MDS	• Age <2 years or >55 years • M0, M6, M7 forms of AML • Complex karyotypes • TLC > 100 X10⁹/L • Deletions 5q, 7q • Delayed response to therapy • AML with preceding MDS or anticancer drug exposure

12. Ans. (d) CD 117 *(Ref: Wintrobes 11th/4145)*
As per Wintrobe's the markers for myeloid series are CD13, CD33, CD 11b, CD15, CD117 and cMPO.

> **c MPO** is the most lineage specific marker amongst these.

Regarding other options, • CD 34 - Myeloid and lymphoid blasts, stem cells, • CD 45 - Leukocyte common antigen (non-erythroid hematopoietic cells), • CD 99 - Ewing's sarcoma/ primitive neuroectodermal cells.

13. Ans. (b) B cell ALL *(Ref: Robbins 8th/608, 9/th/597, Harrison 17th/696)*
t (2;8) is causing translocation between immunoglobulin κ chain on chromosome 2 and the myc gene present on chromosome 8 and is seen in **Burkitt's lymphoma/leukemia**. The translocation results in the increased expression of **c-MYC** resulting in development of neoplasia.

14. Ans. (a) Mature B-cells *(Ref: Robbins 7th/677, 9th/590)*
• *Acute Lymphoblastic Leukemias (ALL) of the L3 (FAB) subtype are tumors of Mature B-cells (e.g. Burkitt's lymphoma)*

15. Ans. (d) M6 *(Ref: Robbins 7th/759, Hematology Basic Principles and Practice, Hoffman, Benz et al.4th/1080)*

> Nonspecific esterase (NSE) is characteristic of M4 (Acute myelomonocytic) and M5 (Acute monocytic) leukemia only. *NSE positivity is not a characteristic feature of other subclasses of AML.*

• However, NSE positivity may also be seen in 15-20% of cases of M3 and in some cases of M7.
• *NSE positivity is not a feature of M0, M1, M2 and M6 classes of AML.*

16. Ans. (d) Tartarate resistant acid phosphatase positivity is typically seen in hairy cell leukemia *(Ref: Wintrobe's 11th/2468, 2470, 2471, Robbin 9/e p603-604)*
• **Tartarate resistant acid phosphatase (TRAP)** is an important tool in differential diagnosis of **hairy cell leukemia** (HCL). The test is positive in 95% of cases of HCL and usually negative or weakly positive in other disorders.
• TRAP is also **positive** in some cases of **splenic marginal zone lymphoma**.
• LAP (leukocyte alkaline phosphatase) score is decreased in CML and PNH (paroxysmal nocturnal hemoglobinuria). However, LAP score often increases when CML transforms to a blast crisis or accelerated phase.

17. Ans. (c) 5q⁻ *(Ref: Wintrobe's 12th/1959-64, Ann Hematol. 2008 July; 87(7): 515–526)*
The article in the Annals of hematology *'Cytogenetic features in myelodysplastic syndromes'* by Detlef Haase gives the different causes as percentage of myelopdysplastic syndromes. This is a typical example of question where the changed data may lead to the question being repeated in the future exam friends.
'Myelodysplastic syndromes' are a group of clonal hematopoietic stem cell diseases characterized by dysplasia and ineffective hematopoiesis in one or more of the major myeloid stem lines.
Direct quote from the Haase's paper.....'Deletions within the **long arm of chromosome 5** are the **most frequent cytogenetic changes in MDS**Q accounting for **roughly 30%** of abnormal cases.'
The cytogenetic abnormalities in adult myelodysplastic syndrome are:

| 5q | 30% |
| Monosomy 7 | 20% |

Complex chromosome abnormalities are defined by the simultaneous occurrence of at least three independent abnormalities within one cell clone. They are also seen in almost 30% cases.

Direct quote from **Williams Hematology** 8th/edn *"The most common abnormalities are 5q–, -7/7q–, +8, –18/18q–, and 20q–. Monosomy 7 is the second most frequent cytogenetic abnormality in the marrow cells of patients with myelodysplasia."*

So, we would prefer to go with (c) deletion of 5q as the preferred answer.

18. **Ans. (b) CD3** *(Ref: Harrison 17th/2020, 2032, Robbins 9/e 190)*
    When a cluster of monoclonal antibodies were found to react with particular antigen it was defined as a separate marker and given a CD (cluster of differentiation) number.
    • **CD3 is used as a pan T-cell marker** (present on all stages of T-cells [Pro–T, Pre-T, Immature and mature T-cells]
    • **CD19 is a Pan B-cell marker.**

CD-1	Thymocytes and Langerhans' associated
CD - 1, 2, 3, 4, 5, 7, 8	T-cell markers
CD - 10, 19, 20, 21, 22, 23	B-cell markers
CD - 10	CALLA antigen
CD - 13, 14, 15, 33	Monocyte macrophage associated
CD - 16, 56	NK- associated
CD - 41	Platelet marker
CD - 21	EBV receptors

19. **Ans. (d) CD135** *(Ref: Robbins 9/e 590, 8th/600, 7th/670, www.wikipedia.com)*
    • B cell associated markers are CD10 (CALLA), CD19, CD20, CD21 (EBV receptor), CD22 and CD23.
    Concept of CD135

    • CD135 is a proto-oncogene. It is also the receptor for the cytokine Flt3 ligand (Flt3L) and has the presence of tyrosine kinase activity. Its mutation can lead to acute myelogenous leukemia (AML) and is associated with a poor prognosis.
    • CD135 is an important cell surface marker used to identify hematopoietic progenitors in the bone marrow. Specifically, multipotent progenitors (MPP) and common lymphoid progenitors (CLP) express high surface levels of CD135. This marker is therefore used to differentiate hematopoietic stem cells (HSC), which are CD135 negative, from MPPs, which are CD135 positive.

20. **Ans. (c) Presence of testicular involvement at presentation** *(Ref: Robbins 9/e 592, 8th/603)*
    Prognostic factors in ALL

GOOD PROGNOSIS	BAD PROGNOSIS
• Age 1-10 years	• Age <1 year or > 10 years
• Female sex	• Male sex
• L1 cell	• L2 or L3 cell
• Peripheral blast count <1,00,000	• Peripheral blast count >1,00,000
• Pre B cell phenotype	• Pre T cell phenotype
• Absence of mediastinal mass	• Mediastinal mass
• Hyperdiploidy (>50 chromosomes) or t(12;21)	• Pseudodiploidy or t (9;22) or presence of Philadelphia chromosome, t (8;14), t (4;11)
• Trisomy of chromosomes 4,7,10	

Friends, please remember age is less than 2 years is given as bad prognosis in Robbins whereas in NELSON it is mentioned that the age for bad prognosis is less than 1 year. Nelson also mentions the testicular involvement to be a bad prognostic factor. Since in the given question, both (less than 2 years as well as testicular involvement) are mentioned we would go for testicular involvement as the better answer here.

21. **Ans. (d) t(9:22), t(8:14), t(4:11) explained earlier.** *(Ref: Robbins 9/e 592, 8th/603)*

22. **Ans. (d) M4** *(Ref: Robbin 7th/693, Harrison 17th/680, Wintrobe's 12th/1857)*
    Signs and symptoms related to infiltration of tissues are usually less striking in AML than in ALL. Mild lymphadenopathy and organomegaly can occur. In tumors with monocytic differentiation M4 and M5 **(more commonly)**, infiltration of the skin (leukemia cutis) and the gingiva leading to gum hypertrophy can be observed, likely reflecting the normal tendency of non-neoplastic monocytes to extravasate into tissues.

- **M5 AML is the commonest AML** associated **with extramedullary disease**[Q] (skin lesions/gum infiltration/CNS disease/testicular involvement).
- After M3 AML, **M5 AML**[Q] **is the commonest AML** associated with the development of **DIC**.

23. **Ans. (c) CD117** *(Ref: Devita 6th/503, Robbins 7th/826, 9/e 614)*
Explained in an earlier question

24. **Ans. (d) Congenital dyserythropoietic anemia** *(Ref: Harrison 17th/663)*
Differential diagnosis of pancytopenia

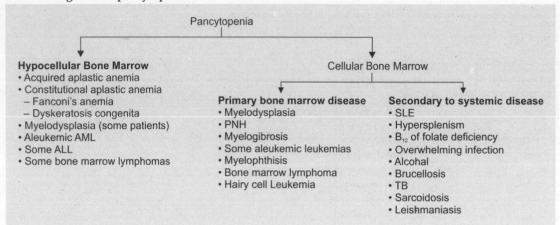

Pancytopenia

Hypocellular Bone Marrow
- Acquired aplastic anemia
- Constitutional aplastic anemia
  – Fanconi's anemia
  – Dyskeratosis congenita
- Myelodysplasia (some patients)
- Aleukemic AML
- Some ALL
- Some bone marrow lymphomas

Cellular Bone Marrow

Primary bone marrow disease
- Myelodysplasia
- PNH
- Myelogibrosis
- Some aleukemic leukemias
- Myelophthisis
- Bone marrow lymphoma
- Hairy cell Leukemia

Secondary to systemic disease
- SLE
- Hypersplenism
- B$_{12}$ of folate deficiency
- Overwhelming infection
- Alcohal
- Brucellosis
- TB
- Sarcoidosis
- Leishmaniasis

Congenital Dyserythropoietic Anemia (CDA)
CDA presents with anemia only (not pancytopenia). Anemia is normocytic or macrocytic. Bone marrow shows marked erythroid hyperplasia. Three types of CDA have been identified as:

CDA Type I: It presents with *anemia with or without jaundice*. Bone marrow shows marked erythroid hyperplasia with polychromatophilic and orthochromatophilic erythroblasts. There is distinct dissociation of nuclear and cytoplasmic maturation with immature megaloblastoid nuclei and mature cytoplasm.

CDA Type II – It is an *autosomal recessive* disorder. Recurrent or persistent *mild jaundice, hepatosplenomegaly and anemia* are the presenting features. Gall stones are common. Blood smear shows anisocytosis, poikilocytosis, tear drop cells and basophilic stippling Bone marrow shows erythroid hyperplasia with binucleated or multinucleated mature blasts. RBCs get lysed in acidic serum from normal persons but not from patient's own serum.

CDA type III: Anemia is mild and macrocytic. Bone marrow findings are similar to CDA type II. However, acid serum lysis test is negative.

Note: In PNH, RBCs get lysed in patient's own acidified serum.

25. **Ans. (a) CD-15** *(Ref: Robbins 7th/670, 9/e 590, Harrison 17th/1908, 689, Wintrobe's 12th/2507)*
Direct lines from Wintrobes hematology.....'CD-15 is expressed on neutrophils, eosinophils and monocytes but not on platelets, lymphocytes and erythrocytes'.
About option (d), CD 24 is expressed on B cells but it decreased with B cell activation and differentiation and is lost at the plasma cell stage. It is also present ion granulocytes and thymocytes but not on mature T cells. Data shows its increased levels are associated with colon/breast and pancreatic cancer.

26. **Ans. (a) Monocytes** *(Ref: Wintrobe's 12th/15)*
- *Acid phosphatase is found in all hematopoietic cells, but the highest levels are found in macrophages and osteoclasts. A dot like pattern is seen in many T lymphoblasts.*
- Tartarate resistant acid phosphatase (TRAP) is seen in osteoclasts and Hairy cell leukemia. Positive TRAP staining may be seen in activated T lymphocytes, macrophages, Gaucher cells, mast cells and some marginal zone lymphomas. Conditions associated with increased TRAP staining are:
  – **Hairy cell leukemia**
  – **Gaucher's diease**
  – **HIV-induced encephalopathy**
  – **Osteoclastoma**
  – **Osteoporosis**
  – **Metabolic bone diseases**

White Blood Cells and Platelets

27. Ans. (c) Chronic myelogenous leukemia *(Ref: Harrison 17th/683-684; Robbins 7th/697, 698, 9/e 617-618)*

The peripheral blood picture of this patient is quite characteristic of **chronic myeloid leukemia.**

> Chronic myeloid leukemia is a stem cell disease that is characterized by leukocytosis with granulocytic immaturities, basophilia, splenomegaly and distinct chromosomal abnormality Philadelphia chromosome.

28. Ans. (b) An immature T cell phenotype [Tdt/CD34/CD7 positive] *(Ref: Robbins 7th/670-673, 9/e 590-593)*

- *Increased leukocyte count in the range of 138 × 10^9/L and on peripheral blood examination 80% of them constituting blast cells indicate acute leukemia.*
- *The age group (adolescent) and the mediastinal mass suggests that this leukemia is likely to be a T-cell leukemia.*
- *"T-cell ALL tends to present in adolescent males as lymphomas often with thymic involvement"*

So, the diagnosis is **T-cell ALL.**

Immunophenotypic classification of acute lymphoblastic leukemia	
Pre-T-cell ALL	TdT, CD2, CD3, CD4, CD5, CD7, CD8, CD34
Early pre-B	TdT, DR, CD10, CD19, CD24
Pre-B-cell	TdT, DR, CD10, CD19, CD20, CD24, Surface Ig
B-cell	DR, CD19, CD20, CD24, Surface Ig

29. Ans. (c) Promyelocytic leukemia *(Ref: Robbins 7th/693, 656-658)*

The child presented with acute onset of bleeding, along with the following laboratory findings:

- *Thrombocytopenia (35000/mm^3 as compared to normal value of 1, 50,000/mm^3)*
- *Increased prothrombin time (20s as compared to control of 13s)*
- *Increased partial thromboplastin time (50s vs. normal 26-32s)*
- *Decreased fibrinogen (10 mg/dL vs. normal of 233-496 mg/dl)*

*These hematological abnormalities indicate **disseminated intravascular coagulation.***

Most common form of AML associated with DIC is M$_3$-AML (Acute promyelocytic leukemia).

30. Ans. (a) Biphenotypic leukemia *(Ref: Robbins illustrated 8th/600)*

- **CD** stands for **cluster differentiation.** These are actually group of **protein markers** present on the surface of **white blood cell.** These markers are used to **classify** the **lineage** of the **leukocytes** and are detected by **immunophenotyping.**
- *CD 10 +ve and CD 19+ve is the marker for B-cell lineage, whereas CD 33 and CD 13 is associated with monocyte and macrophages.*
- So, the patient is having **acute leukemia** with **immunophenotype** pattern of **more than one cell linkage** called as acute leukemia of ambiguous lineage. Biphenotypic leukemia is a subtype of leukemia of ambiguous lineage.

31. Ans. (c) More than 20% of blasts in blood or bone marrow. *(Ref: Wintrobe's 12th/1999-2000)*

WHO criteria for **chronic myelomonocytic leukemia** (CMML)

> 1. **Absolute monocytosis > 1 × 10^9/L** in the peripheral blood
> 2. **Blasts + monocytes < 20%** in blood and bone marrow
> 3. **Absence of philadelphia chromosome** or **BCR/ABL fusion gene**
> 4. **Dysplasia in one or more of myeloid lineages**
>   - If bone marrow blasts + monocytes > 20%, it is diagnosed as acute myeloid leukemia
>   - **Unlike** classic CML, chronic myelomonocytic leukemia has **absence** of basophilia and eosinophilia and more monocytes. Also CML does not have granulocyte dysplasia (**present in CMML**).

32. Ans. (b) t (9;22) *(Ref: Robbins 9/e 614, 8th/627-628, T. Singh 1st/186-190, Harrison 17th/683 – 84)*

- An old man having fatigue and weight loss (*due to anemia and cancer*) and heaviness in left hypochondrium (*most likely due to splenomegaly*). He also has elevated TLC (*most likely due to leukemia*). But the no. of blast cells is 3%, so it cannot be acute leukemia. Old man with leukemia and splenomegaly is suggestive of CML which is associated with t (9; 22).

Other options

- **t (15, 17)** is associated with **acute myeloid leukemia.** For the diagnosis of acute leukemia, the number of blasts in the blood should be >20%.

33. Ans. (c) Myeloperoxidase *(Ref: Robbin's illustrated 7th/692-693, 9/e p613)*

Patient here gives a short history (acute onset) of development of pancytopenia (fever; weakness and gum bleeding suggest leucopenia; anemia and thrombocytopenia respectively).

The presence of 26% blasts in the bone narrow suggests the development of acute leukemia and the presence of Auer rods means that the diagnosis is most likely AML.

Pseudo Pelger Huet cells are neutrophils having greater than 2 nuclear lobes and are usually seen in myelodysplastic syndrome. In 10% patients, MDS can give rise to AML. So, the AML in question may have developed from MDS. The chief cell in AML is myeloblast for which the staining is positive for myeloperoxidase.

Note: Acid phosphatase is useful for lymphoblasts which are seen in ALL

34. **Ans. (d) Monosomy 7** *(Ref: T. singh 1st/175, Robbins 9/e p612)*
   - There are certain factors which determine the prognosis in AML
   - In a number of studies in last 2 decades it has been observed that *cytogenetic markers are major determinants in assessment of prognosis.*

Good prognosis	t (8; 21), inv (16) or t (15; 17)
Moderately favorable outcome	No cytogenetic abnormality
Poor prognosis	inv (3), monosomy 7

For all Prognostic factors in acute myeloid leukemia, see text.

35. **Ans. (d) G6PD deficiency** *(Ref: Harrison 17th/663)*

36. **Ans. (b) Polycythemia vera** *(Ref: Wintrobe's Clinical Haematology 12th/15)*
   High levels of LAP score are found in:
   - Infection
   - Inflammatory disorder
   - Growth factor therapy
   - Pregnancy
   - OCP
   - Stress
   - Myeloproliferative disorders (*except CML*)
   - Drugs (e.g. Lithium, Corticosteroid, Estrogen)

   *Abnormally high values of LAP is seen in myeloproliferative disorder e.g. polycythemia vera and myelofibrosis
   *Decreased LAP score is seen in CML (chronic phase) and PNH (paroxysmal nocturnal hemoglobinuria).

37. **Ans. (a) Hodgkin's disease; (b) Filariasis; (d) HIV** *(Ref: Harrison 17th/383)*
   Conditions producing allergic reactions and resulting eosinophilia are:
   Drugs: Iodides, Aspirin, Sulfonamides, Nitrofurantoin, Penicillins, Cephalosporins.
   Disease conditions: Hay fever, Asthma, Eczema, Serum sickness, Allergic vasculitis, Pemphigus, All types of parasitic infections.
   Collagen vascular diseases: RA, Eosinophilic fasciitis, Allergic angiitis, Polyarteritis nodosa.
   Malignancy: Hodgkin's disease, Mycosis fungoides, CML, Carcinoma of stomach, ovary, lung, Pancreas and uterus.
   Other diseases: Job's syndrome, Sarcoidosis, Skin disease.
   Viral infection like HIV and human T-cell lymphotropic virus (HTLV-I).

   In MI polymorphonuclear leukocytosis seen.

38. **Ans. (b) Myelofibrosis; (c) Alcoholism; (d) Iron Overload;** *(Ref: de Gruchy's 5th/56)*
   Sideroblasts are erythroblasts with Prussian blue positive iron granules in their cytoplasm. They can be found in circulation in the following diseases:

*Drugs and chemicals:	*Hematological disorders:	*Inflammatory disorders:
Antitubercular drugs (INH, cycloserine)	Myelofibrosis	Rheumatoid arthritis
Lead	Polycythemia vera	SLE
Ethanol	Myeloma	Carcinoma
	Acute leukemia	Myxedema
	Hodgkin's disease	Malabsorption
	Hemolytic anemia	Iron overload.

39. **Ans. (b) Kala-azar; (c) TB; (d) Brucellosis** *(Ref: Harrison 17th/342, Harsh Mohan 6th/350)*
   CAUSES OF MONOCYTOSIS:
   - Bacterial infections: TB, sub acute bacterial endocarditis, syphilis, brucellosis.
   - Viral infections
   - Protozoa and Rickettsial infections: Malaria, typhus, trypanosomiasis, kala-azar, RMSF.

White Blood Cells and Platelets

- Hematopoietic disorder: Monocytic leukemia, lymphoma, myeloproliferative disorder, multiple myeloma, lipid storage disorder.
- Malignancies: Ca ovary, stomach and breast.
- Granulomatous diseases e.g. sarcoidosis, IBD.
- Collagen vascular diseases.

40. **Ans. (a) AML; (b) Myelodysplastic anemia; (d) Paroxysmal nocturnal hemoglobinuria** *(Ref: DeGruchy's 5th/127, Harrison 17th/663)*
    - Aplastic anemia is a pancytopenia with bone marrow hypocellularity. It can progress to –
        – Paroxysmal Nocturnal hemoglobinuria
        – Myelodysplastic anemia
        – Rarely acute leukemia

    Pure red cell aplasia is a selective disease of absence of erythrocyte progenitor cells. In contrast to aplastic anemia and MDS, the unaffected lineage (WBC and platelets) appear quantitatively and qualitatively normal.

    - Myelofibrosis is a clonal disorder of a multipotent hematopoietic progenitor cell of unknown origin and is characterized by
        – Marrow fibrosis
        – Myeloid metaplasia with extramedullary erythropoiesis
        – Splenomegaly

41. **Ans. (c) Reticulocytopenia; (d) Thrombocytopenia; (e) Neutropenia** *(Ref: Robbins 7th/647, 9/e p653)*
    Aplastic anemia is a disorder of marrow failure which stems from suppression or disappearance of multipotent myeloid stem cells. It is characterized by: Anemia, Neutropenia , Thrombocytopenia, and Reticulocytopenia. **Splenomegaly is characteristically absent**; if present, the diagnosis of aplastic anemia is almost ruled out. Bone marrow shows hypocellular marrow largely devoid of hematopoietic cells, often only fat cells, fibrous stroma, and scattered or clustered foci of lymphocytes and plasma cells.
    Nucleated RBCs in peripheral smear (**leukoerythroblastic picture**) are found in cases of marrow fibrosis.

42. **Ans. is c i.e. Typhoid** *(Ref: Harsh Mohan 6th/348)*

43. **Ans. (b) CALLA Ag** *(Ref: Robbins 7th/330)*
    - CALLA (common acute lymphoblastic leukemia antigen) is CD 10
    - CALLA positive acute leukemias have best prognosis.

44. **Ans. (B) Chronic lymphocytic leukemia** *(Ref: Robbins 7th/673, 9/e 593)*
    In CLL, the peripheral blood contains increased numbers of small, round lymphocytes with scant cytoplasm. These cells are fragile and are frequently disrupted in the process of making smears, producing so-called **smudge cells.**

45. **Ans. (a) t (15: 17)** *(Ref: Robbins 9/e 612, 8th/624; 7th/692)*

46. **Ans. (b) Auer bodies are seen** *(Ref: Robbins 9/e 613, 8th/62; 7th/692-693)*

47. **Ans. (d) Increased** *(Ref: Robbins 7th/697-698, Wintrobes 12th/205, Williams CMDT 2010/458)*
    Wintrobe's hematology mentiones….. 'granulocytes contain and release B12 binding proteins. **Markedly elevated transcobalmin I level are seen in chronic myelocytic leukemia and myeloid metaplasia** whereas **low levels are seen in chronic leucopenia and aplastic anemia'**.
    Williams hematology 8th/ adds that 'the increase is proportional to the total leukocyte count in untreated patients and falls with treatment'.

    Conditions having elevated levels of cobalamin

Hematological conditions	Non-hematological conditions
• Chronic myelogenous leukemia	• Acute hepatitis
• Promyelocytic leukemia	• Cirrhosis
• Polycythemia vera	• Hepatocellular carcinoma
• Hypereosinophilic syndrome	• Metastatic liver disease

48. **Ans. (d) CML** *(Ref: Robbins 8th/627; 7th/697-698)*

49. **Ans. (b) Leucocyte alkaline phosphatase** *(Ref: Robbins 8th/595, 9/e 584)*

50. **Ans. (d) Glucocorticoids** *(Ref: Harsh Mohan 6th/348)*

51. **Ans. (c) CML** *(Ref: Robbins 8th/627; 7th/438, 9/e 584)*

52. **Ans. (d) Aplastic anemia** *(Ref: Robbins 9/e p654, 8th/634-635, 7th/704)*

53. **Ans. (c) Hypocellular bone marrow** *(Ref: Robbins 9/e 615, 8th/625; 7th/695)*

54. **Ans. (c) Thalassemia** *(Ref: Robbins 9/e p582, 620, 653, 8th/650; 7th/701)*

55. **Ans. (c) Myeloblast** *(Ref: Robbins 8th/602, 9/e p613)*

56. **Ans. (c) CLL** *(Ref: Robbins 8th/605, 9/e p594)*

57. **Ans. (b) Pulmonary abscess Read explanation below (important concept friends)**
Chronic infections/chronic inflammatory conditions, such as pulmonary abscess may lead to an expansion of the myeloid precursor pool in the bone marrow which manifests as neutrophilic leukocytosis.

> - Steroid therapy may increase the release of marrow storage pool cells and diminish neutrophilic extravasation into tissues.
> - Even vigorous physical exercise can produce neutrophilia transiently from demargination of neutrophils.
> - In acute myelogenous leukemia, the marrow is filled with blasts, not maturing myeloid elements.

58. **Ans. (d) Acute monocytic leukemia** *(Ref: Robbins 7th/693, 9th/612)*
Sunaya has an **"aleukemic" leukemia** in which leukemic blasts fill the marrow but the peripheral blood count of leukocytes is not high. The staining of the blasts suggests presence of **monoblasts (peroxidase negative and nonspecific esterase positive)**. So, the likely diagnosis for her is M5 leukemia, which is characterized by increased chances of tissue infiltration and organomegaly.
Other options;

- **Acute lymphoblastic leukemia** is typically seen in **children and young adults**.
- **Acute megakaryocytic leukemia** is typically accompanied by **myelofibrosis** and is rare. The blasts react with platelet-specific antibodies
- **Acute promyelocytic leukemia** (M3-AML) has many promyelocytes filled with azurophilic granules, making them strongly peroxidase positive.

59. **Ans. (a) Early pre-B (CD19+TdT +); Hyperdiploidy** *(Ref: Robbins 8th/603, 9/e p592-593)*
The physician thinks the child will have remission. So, it means that this child should have ALL with good prognosis. The markers for a good prognosis for acute lymphoblastic leukemia (ALL) are:

- *Early precursor– B cell type*
- *Hyperdiploidy*
- *Age of patient between 2 and 10 years*
- *Chromosomal trisomy*
- *t(12;21)*

Marrow infiltration by the leukemic cells leads to pancytopenia.

> **Poor prognostic markers** for acute lymphoblastic leukemia/lymphoma are
> - Count >100,000
> - Presence of t(9;22)
> - Presentation in adolescents, and adulthood

60. **Ans. (c) 22q11.2** *(Ref: Robbins 8th/635, 9/e p626)*
The stem of the question describes the markers of cortical lymphocytes in the thymus of a child. The absence of these cells can be seen in the DiGeorge syndrome with 22q11.2. These patients also have parathyroid hypoplasia and congenital heart disease.

> - **Down syndrome (trisomy 21)** can have thymic abnormalities and the T-cell dysregulation that predisposes to acute leukemia, but **the thymus is typically present**.
> - Males with **Klinefelter syndrome** (XXY) **do not** have immunological abnormalities.
> - The **t(15;17)** is associated with **acute promyelocytic leukemia**.

61. **Ans. (a) Acute lymphoblastic leukmia** *(Ref: Robbins 8th/603, 9/e p593)*
The presence of the Philadelphia chromosome, a translocation from the long arm of chromosome 22 to chromosome 9 [t(9;22)], is associated with a more favorable prognosis in patients with chronic myelogenous leukemia but it associated with an unfavorable outcome in Acute lymphoblastic leukemia (ALL).

62. **Ans. (d) 65 years** *(Ref: Robbins 8th/604, 9/e p593)*
Different leukemias tend to affect populations of different ages. The disease described is chronic lymphocytic leukemia (CLL), which is a disease of older adults.

White Blood Cells and Platelets

The 1 year-old (choice A) would be most likely to have acute lymphocytic leukemia (ALL).
The 20 year-old (choice B) would be most likely to have acute myelocytic leukemia (AML).
The 45 year-old (choice C) would be likely to have either AML or chronic myelogenous leukemia (CML).

62.1. Ans. (a) Hodkin's disease *(Ref: Robbins 8/e p618-9)*
- Reed–Sternberg cells have an **"owl's eye" appearance**[Q] with prominent eosinophilic inclusion-like nucleoli.
- Reed–Sternberg cells are **CD30 and CD15 positive**, usually negative for CD20 and CD45.
- The Reed–Sternberg cells can also be found in reactive lymphadenopathy associated with infectious mononucleosis, carbamazepine associated lymphadenopathy and non-Hodgkin lymphomas.

62.2. Ans. (c) Myeloperoxidase *(Ref: Robbins 8/e p602 Pathology and Genetics of Tumours of Haematopoietic and Lymphoid Tissues p79)*
This is what we have knowledge of:
- Lymphoblast: PAS positive
- Myeloblast: Sudan black, myeloperoxidase and non-specific esterase

Please know that:
WHO manual pg 69 writes that.. "MPO is specific for myeloid differentiation. Sudan Black B reactivity is similar to MPO in myeloblasts and monoblasts. The *specificity of Sudan Black is less than MPO.*"

62.3. Ans. (b) May-Heggline anomaly *A Color Atlas and Instruction Manual of Peripheral Blood Cell Morphology pg 221,*
(Ref: Robbins 8/e p594)

Döhle bodies are basophilic leukocyte inclusions located in the peripheral cytoplasm of neutrophils. They are said to be remnants of the *rough endoplasmic reticulum.*

Conditions associated with Dohle bodies
- Burns
- Infections
- Physical trauma
- Neoplastic diseases
- Wissler's disease
- May-Hegglin anomaly (seen in neutrophil, monocyte, lymphocyte)
- Chédiak-Steinbrinck-Higashi's syndrome

62.4. Ans. (d) Dilated endoplasmic reticulum ... explained earlier

62.5. Ans. (b) t (15,17) *(Ref: Robbins 9/e p612, 8/e p624)*
Commonly asked information in NEET EXAM!

•	**t(9;22) (Philadelphia chromosome):** CML (bcr-abl hybrid)
•	t(8;14) Burkitt's lymphoma (c-myc activation)
•	**t(II ; I4):** Mantle cell lymphoma (cyclin D1 activation)
•	t(I4; 18): Follicular lymphomas (bcl-2 activation)
•	**t(I5;17):** M3 type of AML (responsive to all-trans retinoic acid)

62.6. Ans. (c) Hyperdiploidy *(Ref: Robbins 8/e p602-3, 9/e p592-593)*

Good Prognosis	Bad Prognosis
• Age 1-10 years	• Age <1 year or > 10 years
• Female sex	• Male sex
• L1 cell	• L2 or L3 cell
• Peripheral blast count <1,00,000	• Peripheral blast count >1,00,000
• Pre B-cell phenotype	• **Pre T**-cell phenotype
• Absence of mediastinal mass	• Mediastinal mass
• Hyperdiploidy (>50 chromosomes) or t(12;21)	• Pseudodiploidy or t (9;22) **(Philadelphia chromosome)** or t (8;14) or t (4;11)
• Trisomy 4,7 and 10	

62.7. Ans. (b) Immature B cells *(Ref: Robbins 8/e p600)*
As per the table given in Robbins, B cell ALL is due to **immature B cells**.

62.8. Ans. (a) ALL *(Ref: Robbins 8/e p602, 7/e p670)*
CD 10 is called as **c**ommon **a**cute **l**ymphoblastic **l**eukemia **a**ntigen or **CALLA**. It is seen in acute lymphoid leukemia (ALL).

62.9. Ans (b) Myeloblast *(Ref: Robbins 9th/612-3)*

62.10. Ans (d) More than 5000 cells/microliter *(Ref: Washington Manual 2013, table 11-4)*

62.11. Ans: (a) Pre B cell *(Ref: Robbins 9th/590)*

Most common subtype of A.L.L is L1 according to older classification and Pre B cell variety by the latest WHO classification. The recent WHO International panel on ALL recommends that the FAB classification be abandoned, since the morphological classification has no clinical or prognostic relevance. It instead advocates the use of the immunophenotypic classification.

63. Ans. (a). Hodgkin's Lymphoma, nodular sclerosis *(Ref: Loachim's lymph node pathology/186)*
Direct quote. 'Progressive transformation of germinal centers (PTGC) is a benign reaction pattern in lymph nodes. It is most often associated with reactive *follicular hyperplasia*. It is also associated with nodular sclerosis and lymphocyte predominant Hodgkin's lymphoma'.

64. Ans. (a) Kimura's disease *(Ref: Loachim's lymph node pathology/190)*
Kimura Disease is a chronic inflammatory disorder prevalent in Asians. It involves subcutaneous tissues and lymph nodes predominantly in the head and neck region and is characterized by angiolymphoid proliferation and eosinophilia.
Histopathology

- Lymphoid infiltrates with formation of follicles and germinal centers accompanied by plasma cells, mast cells and particularly large amount of eosinophils are present in subcutis.
- Lymph nodes are enlarged and show markedly hyperplastic follicles with reactive germinal centers and a well-defined peripheral mantle.
- Diffuse eosinophilia, eosinophilic abcesses and infiltration of germinal centres, sometimes resulting in folliculolysis, are part of the process.
- Polykaryocytes of the **Warthin Finkeldey type**, characterized by the overlapping, grape-like arrangement of nuclei, are common, often within the germinal centers.

65. Ans. (d) Aplastic anemia *(Ref: Harrison 17th/374, Robbins 9/e p653)*
Massive splenomegaly is labeled when spleen extends greater than 8 cm below left costal margin and/or weighs more than 1000 g.

Diseases Associated with Massive Splenomegaly	
Chronic myelogenous leukemia	Gaucher's disease
Lymphomas	Chronic lymphocytic leukemia
Hairy cell leukemia	Sarcoidosis
Myelofibrosis with myeloid metaplasia	Autoimmune hemolytic anemia
Polycythemia vera	Diffuse splenic hemangiomatosis

66. Ans. (a) t (8:14) *(Ref: Robbins 8th/608, 9/e p597)*

67. Ans. (a) CD 45 RO *(Ref: Flow Cytometry and Immunohistochemistry for Hematologic Neoplasms, Lippincott Williams and Wilkins, Tsieh Sun 1st/133; Neoplastic Hematology Daniel Knowles 2nd/1342*
Direct quote from Tsieh Sun ....."*myeloid sarcoma usually expresses CD45 but rare cases may demonstrate T cell markers, such as CD45RO, CD3 and CD7*". So, the answer of choice is CD45RO.
Salient features of Lab diagnosis of Granulocytic sarcoma

1. Screening panel for **CD45, CD19** and **CD20**.
2. **Standard flowcytometry** panel includes **CD13, 14, 15 , 33and myeloperoxidase**
3. Immunohistochemistry panel may include chloroacetate esterase (Leder stain), lysozyme, CD15, CD43 and CD 68
4. **Lysozyme[Q]** and **CD43[Q]** are the **most sensitive markers**
5. Two new markers **CD99[Q]** and **CD117[Q]** can be added in equivocal cases.
6. Common cytogenetic abnormalities include **t(8;21), inv (16)** and **t(9;11)[Q]**

Additionally, the percentage of these molecules can be derived from the data given in *Neoplastic Hematology*....

Immunohistochemistry Molecule	%
CD 45	90%
CD 43	50%
Lysozyme	75%
Leder stain (chloroacetate esterase)	>75%

No mention of staining with CD45RO is there, so, we prefer CD45 RO as the answer of choice.

68. Ans. (a) CD 23 *(Ref: Robbins 7th/683; http://www.emedicine.com/med/topic1358.htm, Robbins 9/e p603)*
Mantle cells lymphomas are usually CD23 negative. They are positive for CD5, CD20 and CD43.

Characteristic immunophenotypes of major subtypes of lymphoma

Lymphoma	Immunophenotype
Follicular	CD20$^+$, CD3$^-$, CD10$^+$, CD5$^-$
Small lymphocytic	CD20$^+$, CD3$^-$, CD10$^-$, CD5$^+$, CD23$^+$
Marginal zone/MALT	CD20$^+$, CD3$^-$, CD10$^-$, CD5$^-$, CD23$^-$
Mantle cell	CD20+, CD3−, CD10−, CD5+, CD23$^-$, CD43$^+$, PRADI$^+$
Diffuse large B-cell	CD20$^+$, CD3$^-$, CD5$^-$, CD45$^+$
Burkitt	CD20$^+$, CD3$^-$, CD10$^+$, CD5$^-$; Tdt$^-$

69. **Ans. (b) REAL Classification** *(Ref: Robbins 7th/688; AJC cancer staging handbook)*

In 1994, a group of hematopathologists, oncologists and molecular biologists came together (International Lymphoma Study Group) and introduced a new classification, called the 'Revised European- American Classification of Lymphoid Neoplasms (REAL).

WHO has reviewed and updated the REAL classification in 1999 resulting in inclusion of additional rare entities.

Non-Hodgkin's lymphoma (NHL) has been classification by many groups. Major classification systems are:

- Rappaport classification (Developed in 1966)
- Working formation classification
- REAL classification (Developed in 1994)
- WHO classification (modified REAL classification, 1999)

1. **Rappaport classification:** It is based on microscopic appearance of tumor cells.
   - Size: Lymphocytic or histiocytic
   - Growth pattern: Diffuse or nodular

2. **Working classification:** According to this system, NHL is divided according to prognostic criteria into:

Low grade	Intermediate grade	High grade
• Small lymphocytic NHL • Follicular small cleaved NHL • Follicular mixed small cleaved and large-cell NHL	• Follicular large cell NHL • Diffuse small cleaved NHL • Diffuse small cleaved NHL • Diffuse mixed small cleaved and large-cell NHL • Diffuse large-cell NHL	• Small non-cleaved NHL (Burkitt's) • Immunoblastic lymphoma • Lymphoblastic lymphoma

3. **Revised European-American classification of lymphoma (REAL) It includes:**
   - Precursor B-cell neoplasm
   - Peripheral B-cell neoplasm
   - Precursor T-cell neoplasm
   - Peripheral T-cell neoplasm
   - Hodgkin's lymphoma

4. **WHO classification:** It takes into account morphologic, clinical, immunological and genetic information. *For its details, see text.*

70. **Ans. (d) A diffuse proliferation of medium to large lymphoid cells with high mitotic rate** *(Ref: Robbins: 7th/673-674, 9th/p 593-594, several journals through internet)*

- This is a case of chronic lymphocytic leukemia (CLL) as indicated by the characteristic clinical picture and immunophenotypic characteristics. (Typically, **CLL cells express CD5, CD19, CD23 and show absence of CD79B, CD22 and FMC7**)
- Histopathological examination in a case of typical CLL shows diffuse effacement of lymphocyte architecture by small to medium sized lymphocytes with clumped chromatin, indistinct or absent nucleoli and scanty cytoplasm.
- The round lymphocytes may give way focally to paler areas consisting of larger round cells (prolymphocytes). These paler areas are often referred to as **proliferation centers** and when present are **pathognomic for CLL/SLL**. They contain relatively large number of mitotically active cells.
- Follicular lymphoma is positive for CD10, CD79b and FMC7 but negative for CD25 and CD43.
- CLL and prolymphocytic leukemia are CD23 positive.

> Mantle cell lymphoma is also CD5 positive but here the cells are CD23 negative and CD 79b and FMC7 positive.

71. **Ans. (d) Inv (16) is often detected in the blasts and the eosinophils** *(Ref: Annals of Hematology: 2000 May: 79(5): 272-4)*
This is a case of ALL with hypereosinophllic syndrome. Inv (16) is associated with AML and not ALL, and therefore represents the incorrect statement amongst the option. **About other options, the relevant points:**

> Eosinophils are not a part of this neoplasm differentiating it from eosinophilic leukemia.
> t(5;14) may be observed in about half of such patients. The symptoms may resolve after dug therapy.

For details, see the journal with the relevant article.

72. **Ans. (b) Results from an expansion of Neoplastic T-lymphocytes** *(Ref: Harrison's 17th/697; Robbins 7th/683, 9/e p588)*
Hairy cell leukemia is a type of *B-cell leukemia*. For details, see text.

73. **Ans. (b) CD 34 negative but surface Ig+** *(Ref: Robbins 9/e p597-598, 8th/608, 7th/677-678, Harrison 17th/, 696)*
    - **Burkitt's lymphoma** is a cancer characterized by the presence of hallmark translocation **t (8;14)**[Q].
    - The translocation results in the **increased expression of c-MYC**[Q] resulting in development of neoplasia.
    - **Immunophenotyping** reveals the tumor cells expressing *bcl-6 protein, surface Ig, CD19, CD20* and *CD10* (**CALLA**[Q].

74. **Ans. (d) CD 34 is associated with Diffuse large B Cell Lymphoma** *(Ref: Robbins 9/e p603 8th/605-608, 612-613, 7th/675-678, Wintrobe's 12th/2223)*

	Burkitt's lymphoma	Follicular lymphoma	Mantle cell lymphoma
Hallmark translocation	t (8;14)	t (14;18)	t (11; 14)
Over expression of gene	bcl-6	bcl-2	bcl-1
Immunophenotyping	sIgM+, CD5–, CD10+, CD19+, CD20+, CD23–, CD45+	sIg, CD5–, CD10+, CD19+, bright CD20+, CD23–/+, CD38+, CD45+	sIgM+, sIgD+, CD5+, CD10–, CD19+, CD20+, CD23–, Cyclin D1+, FMC-7+

Though *Williams hematology* mentiones (Table 92.1) and even we normally read that the **Mantle cell lymphoma** is CD10- but **WHO manual** writes that '**mantle cell lymphoma may show expression of CD10 molecule rarely'**. This is also supported by Wintrobe's 12th/pg 2223 where the table clearly mentions that Mantle cell lymphoma may be **CD10+/-**. So, option C may be assumed to be true (after all AIIMS questions can be nerve wrecking friends. This question has been altered to suit the easy goals in other MCQ books).
The answer of exclusion is therefore 'D' as CD 34 is the marker for hematopoetic stem cell. Diffuse large B cell lymphoma has the phenotype of *sIgM+, sIgD+/-, CD5-/+, CD10-/+, CD19+, CD20+, CD45+, PAX5+*. **The tumor cells** can be **BCL-6 positive** in **40%** cases when associated with **t (3;14)** or **bcl-2 positive** in 20% with **t(14;18)**.

75. **Ans. (b) B-cell** *(Ref: Harrison 17th/845, 847, Robbins 9/e p1313)*
    - 'Post-transplant Lymphoproliferative Disorders' (**PTLDs**) are lymphomas developing after solid organ transplantation e.g. kidney, liver, heart or lung transplants.
    - PTLDs are almost always related to infection by the Epstein-Barr virus (EBV) which causes a cancerous transformation of B-cells. In normal individuals immune cells can tackle the EBV infection, but in organ transplants, the high doses of drugs used suppress the immune system and the the chances of developing lymphomas increase.

    > Difference between Post transplant lymphomas and non Hodgkin's lymphomas. PTLDS have the following:

    - **Extranodal involvement** (brain, lungs and the intestines)
    - Poorer prognosis

76. **Ans. (d) In general follicular (nodular) NHL has worse prognosis compared to diffuse NHL** *(Ref: Robbins 7th/674- 6, 667-8)*
    - Hodgkin's lymphoma is clinically and histologically distinct from the non-Hodgkin's lymphoma. **While non-Hodgkin lymphomas frequently occur at extranodal sites and spreads in an unpredictable fashion, Hodgkin's lymphoma arises in a single node or chain of nodes and spreads first to anatomically contiguous nodes.** Several ways of classifying Hodgkin's lymphoma exist **Rappaport, REAL classification and now WHO (modified REAL classification).**

    > The prognosis of non Hodgkin's lymphoma varies markedly with various histological types of non Hodgkin's lymphoma, "In general lymphomas with a follicular histological pattern are of lower grade (longer survival) than those of diffuse pattern".

77. **Ans. is b i.e. CD 23** *(Ref: Harrison 17th/695, Robbins 7th/683, 9/e p602-603)*
Mantle cell lymphomas are positive for CD43, CD20, Bcl-1 Protein (Cyclin D1) and CD5.

78. **Ans. (b) Follicular lymphoma** *(Ref: Robbins 8th/605; 7th/675, 9/e p594)*

79. **Ans. (a) Burkitt's lymphoma** *(Ref: Robbins 8th/608, 7th/677 9/e p597)*

80. **Ans. (b) Mycosis fungoides** *(Ref: Robbins 9/e p605, 8th/1184-1185; 7th/685)*

81. **Ans. (c) Prognosis is better than in diffuse type** *(Ref: Robbins 9/e p594-595, 8th/619)*

82. **Ans. (a) B-cell lymphoma** *(Ref: Robbins 9/e p603, 8th/613, 7th/826)*

83. **Ans. (b) Cirrhosis** *(Ref: Robbins 8th/634)*
Pancytopenia with the splenomegaly is suggestive of hypersplenism as a cause for the patient's anemia, leucopenia and thrombocytopenia. A common cause of congestive splenomegaly is portal hypertension resulting from cirrhosis. The elevated AST and ALT is also suggestive of liver disease. Regarding other options friends, please note:

- The WBC count should be high with acute leukemias.
- SLE can lead to cytopenias from reduced bone marrow function, but there is no associated splenomegaly.
- Infectious mononucleosis may lead to splenomegaly but it is more common in younger individuals.

84. Ans. (a) Burkitt's lymphoma: *(Ref: Robbins 9/e p597, 8th/608)*

Burkitt's lymphoma is actually associated with three translocations. The common variant t(8;14)(q24;q32), involving the oncogene myc on chromosome 8, and the heavy immunoglobulin chain on chromosome 14. The other two variants are: t(8;22)(q24;q11), involving myc and the lambda light chain immunoglobulin site, and t(2;8)(p12;q24), involving the kappa light chain and myc.

85. Ans. (d) Infectious mononucleosis: *(Ref: Robbins 9/e p361, 8th/355-357)*

Infectious mononucleosis is a benign infection caused by the Epstein-Barr Virus (EBV). Although B lymphocytes are infected by the virus, the characteristic atypical cells are activated suppresser T cells explaining the paracortical location (normally a T cell zone) in the lymph node. Lymph nodes in viral infections show expansion of germinal centers without loss of normal architecture. All lymphomas, including Burkitt's, Hodgkin's and non-Hodgkin's lymphomas, destroy the normal architecture of the lymph node.

85.1. Ans. (a) B cell lymphoma *(Ref: Robbins 9/e p603, 8/e p613)*

Marginal zone lymphoma is a **B cell**[Q] **tumour** has the presence of translocation **t(11;18)** [Q]. It is associated with *H. pylori*[Q] infection. They have the following exceptional characteristics:

- Often arise within tissues involved by *chronic inflammatory disorders of autoimmune or infectious etiology*
- Remain *localized for prolonged periods, spreading systemically only late in their course*
- *May regress if the inciting agent (e.g., Helicobacter pylori) is eradicated*

85.2. Ans. (d) CD 5 +, CD 23 – *(Ref: Robbins 9/e p602-603, 8/e p612-3)*

Lymphoma	Immunophenotype
Follicular lymphoma	CD20+, CD3–, CD10+, CD5–
Small lymphocytic lymphoma	CD20+, CD3–, CD10–, CD5+, CD23+
Marginal zone/MALT	CD20+, CD3–, CD10–, CD5–, CD23–
Mantle cell lymphoma	CD20+, CD3–, CD10–, **CD5+, CD23–**, CD43+, PRADI+
Diffuse large B-cell	CD20+, CD3–, CD5–, CD45+
Hodgkin lymphoma	CD30+, CD15+

85.3. Ans. (d) Cutaneous lymphoma *(Ref: Robbins 9/e p605, 8/e p1184-1185, 7/e p1685)*

- *Mycosis fungoides* is a **T cell lymphoma** affecting **skin** which can evolve into generalized lymphoma.
- *Histological hallmark:* **Sezary Lutzner cells**[Q] which are helper T cells forming band like aggregates in superficial dermis and have **cerebriform contour**[Q].
- May invade epidermis as single cells and small clusters called as **Pautrier microabscesses**[Q].

85.4. Ans. (a) Follicular *(Ref: Robbins 8/e p605, 7/e p675)*

This was based on the working classification of NHL:

Low grade	Intermediate grade	High grade
• Small lymphocytic NHL • Follicular small cleaved NHL • Follicular mixed small cleaved and large-cell NHL	• Follicular large cell NHL • Diffuse small cleaved NHL • Diffuse small cleaved NHL • Diffuse mixed small cleaved and large-cell NHL • Diffuse large-cell NHL	• Small non-cleaved NHL (Burkitt's) • Immunoblastic lymphoma • Lymphoblastic lymphoma

85.5. Ans. (c) Diffuse large B cell lymphoma *(Ref: Robbin 8/e p606)*

"Diffuse large B-cell lymphoma (DLBCL) is the most common form of NHL"… (Ref: Robbind 8/e p606)

85.6. Ans. (a) B cell *(Ref: Robbin 8/e p1348, Eyelid, Conjunctival, and Orbital Tumors 2/e p746)*

Direct quote… ***"Non Hodgkin Lymphoma of the B cell lineage is the most common type in the orbit"***……. Eyelid, Conjunctival, and Orbital Tumors

Also know: for a future question

- *The most frequently encountered primary neoplasms of the orbit are vascular in origin like the* capillary hemangioma, the lymphangioma and the encapsulated cavernous hemangioma.
- *MC intraocular tumour in children: Retinoblastoma*
- *MC intraocular tumour in adults: choroidal malignant melanoma*

85.7. Ans. (b) Stomach *(Ref: Robbin 9th/ 773)*

Although extranodal lymphomas can arise in virtually any tissue, they do so most commonly in the GI tract, particularly the stomach.

85.8. Ans. (b) B cell *(Ref: Robbin 9/e p603)*

85.9. Ans. (b) Burkitt Lymphoma *(Ref: Robbin 9/e p597)*

"Burkitt lymphoma is believed to be the fastest growing human tumor"…direct line

The tumor exhibits a high mitotic index and contains numerous apoptotic cells, the nuclear remnants of which are phagocytosed by interspersed benign macrophages. These phagocytes have abundant clear cytoplasm, creating a characteristic **"starry sky" pattern.**

85.10. (a) Anaplastic large cell lymphoma (ALK positive) *(Ref: Robbin 8/e p605)*

Anaplastic Large-Cell Lymphoma (ALK Positive) is an uncommon entity which is defined by the presence of rearrangements in the ALK gene on chromosome 2p23.

This tumor is typically composed of large anaplastic cells, some containing horseshoe-shaped nuclei and voluminous cytoplasm (so-called *hallmark cells*).

85.11. Ans. (b) Africa…….. Indian exam asking global question*

86. Ans. (d) Monoclonal origin *(Ref: Robbins 9/e p583, 8th/599)*

All lymphomas are monoclonal, derived from neoplastic expansion of a single transformed cell clone. Gene rearrangement studies, therefore, can be used for diagnostic purposes to determine whether a lymphoid population is monoclonal (ie, neoplastic) or polyclonal (i.e., reactive).

- Most, but not all, non-Hodgkin lymphomas are of B lymphocytic origin (choice A).
- Approximately 80% of non-Hodgkin lymphomas are derived from B lymphocytes; the remaining 20% are of histiocytic (choice B) or T lymphocytic origin.
- Lymph node localization (choice C) is variably present in non-Hodgkin lymphomas. Two thirds of these lymphomas come to clinical attention with nontender nodal enlargement involving one or more lymph nodes. The remaining one third of cases present with extranodal involvement of skin, brain, and gastrointestinal tract, for example. In contrast, virtually all cases of Hodgkin lymphoma present with lymph node enlargement.

87. Ans. (d) Reed-Sternberg cells *(Ref: Robbins 9/e p610, 8th/617)*

This is a classic presentation of Hodgkin's disease, which is a form of lymphoma characterized by neoplastic proliferation of Reed-Sternberg cells admixed with variable numbers of reactive lymphocytes, neutrophils, and eosinophils.

Abnormal plasma cells (choice A) would be a feature of multiple myeloma or some B-cell leukemias and lymphomas. Giant platelets (choice B) are a feature seen in several myeloproliferative disorders (notably essential thrombocytopenia), which do not cause lymphadenopathy. Immature neutrophil precursors (choice C) would most likely be a feature of a myeloid leukemia, which would not cause a lymphadenopathy.

88. Ans. (a) CD 15 and 30 *(Ref: Robbins 9/e p608, 7th/422-423)*

In classical HL, CD15 and CD30 are the surface markers. In non classical HL, CD20 and BCL/6 are the markers.

89. Ans. (a) Lymphocyte predominance *(Ref: Robbins 9/e p609, 7th/668, 686, 689)*

'Nodular Lymphocyte Predominance Hodgkin's disease is now recognized as an entity entirely distinct from classical Hodgkin's disease.'

In lymphocyte predominant Hodgkin's disease, the **Reed Sternberg cells** have a characteristic B cell immunophenotype distinct from that of classical Hodgkin's i.e. **CD15 and CD30 negative but express J chain, CD45 and EMA (Epithelial Membrane Antigen).**

Lymphoblast	PAS positive
Myeloblast	Sudan black, myeloperoxidase and non-specific esterase

90. Ans. (c) Absolute lymphocyte count < 600/µl *(Ref: Hodgkin's lymphoma: A Comprehensive Update on Diagnostics and Clinics By Andreas Engert/2010/104)*

Seven adverse prognostic factors described for advanced Hodgkin's disease are

White Blood Cells and Platelets

1. Male gender
2. Age > 45 years
3. Stage IV disease
4. Hemoglobin < 10.5 g/dl
5. Leukocytosis with WBC > 15,000/μl
6. A serum albumin level <4 g/dl
7. Lymphocytopenia with either Absolute lymphocyte count < 600/μl or lymphocyte being < 8% of WBCs

91. **Ans. (d) Lymphocyte predominant Hodgkin's disease** *(Ref: Robbins 7th/686, 9/e p609)*
Explained in text.

92. **Ans. (d) Langerhans' cell.** *(Ref: Robbins 9/e p 608-609, 7th/686, 688)*
Langerhans' cells *are epidermal dendritic cells that take up and* process antigenic signals and communicate the information to lymphoid cells.

93. **Ans. (B) Nodular sclerosis Hodgkin's lymphoma** *(Ref: Robbins 9/e p608, 8th/618)*

94. **Ans. (D) Lymphocyte predominant** *(Ref: Robbins 7th/688, 9/e p609)*

95. **Ans. (a) Nodular sclerosis** *(Ref: Robbins 9/e p608, 8th/618; 7th/688)*

96. **Ans. (a) Nodular sclerosis** *(Ref: Robbins 9/e p608, 8th/618-619, 7th/686)*

97. **Ans. (a) Lymphocyte dominant** *(Ref: Robbins 9/e p609, 8th/619; 7th/689)*

98. **Ans. (a) Myelodysplastic syndrome** *(Ref: Robbins 9/e p614-615, 8th/625-626; 7th/695-696)*

98.1. **Ans. (c) Lymphocytic predominance** *(Ref: Robbins 9/e p608-609, 8/e p618-9)*

WHO Classification of Hodgkin Lymphoma				
Nodular sclerosis	**Mixed cellularity**	**Lymphocyte rich**	**Lymphocyte depleted**	**Lymphocyte predominant (no classical HL)**
– MC type of HL	– MC type of HL in india		– Associated with HIV	–H > F
– Incidence equal in M and F	– M > F	– M > F	– M > F	– M > F
– RS cell variant in **lacunar cell** (clear space surrounding cell)	– Has eosinophils and plasma cells – **Maximum number** of RS cell	– Mononuclear and RS cell – **Lowest number** of RS cells	– 3 unique RS cell (pleomorphic, mummified, necrobiotic type) – Maximum area of necrosis	– LH cells (**popcorn cells**) in background – Other cells scanty or absence of B cells
– Cells are CD 15 +CD30+	– Cells are CD15 + CD30+	– Cells are CD15 + CD30 + and CD20–	– Cells are CD15 + CD30+	– RS cell are **CD20 + CD15–, CD30 – BCL6 +, EMA +**[Q]
– No association with EBV	– Associated with EBV	– Associated with EBV	– Associated with EBV	– Not associated with EBV
– **Excellent prognosis**	– Prognosis very good	– Good to excellent prognosis	– Poor prognosis	– Excellent prognosis
– Adolescent and young adult	– **Biphasic incidence**[Q] (young adults as well as > 55 years)	– Old age group	– Old age group	– Young males

* EMA is Epithelial Membrane Antigen

98.2. **Ans (c) Nodular sclerosis...See earlier explanation** *(Ref: Robbins 9/e p608)*

98.3. **Ans. (b) Nodular sclerosis Hodgkin lymphoma** *(Ref: Robbin 8/e p618-9)*
Presence of binucleated acidophlic owl eye appearance with CD15 and CD 30 is suggestive of Reed Sternberg cell.

- **Lymphocyte depletion HL** occurs predominantly in the **elderly** and in **HIV+** individuals
- In **lymphocyte predominant HL**, the Reed Sternberg cells are *positive for CD20 and BCL6*, and are usually *negative for CD15 and CD30*.

- **Mixed-cellularity** HL is more common in *males*, in *elderly* with **presence of constitutional symptoms.** Involved lymph nodes are diffusely effaced by a heterogeneous cellular infiltrate, which includes T cells, eosinophils, plasma cells, and benign macrophages admixed with Reed-Sternberg cells

99. Ans. (c) Essential thrombocythemia *(Ref: Robbins 8th/629, 9/e p620 Harrison 17th/374)*

This. is a modified version of DPG2011 question. Please see the table for causes of Massive Splenomegaly given earlier.

In CML … 'first symptom of CML is a dragging sensation in the abdomen caused by splenomegaly' Robbins 8th/627-8

Polycythemia vera Robbins 8th/629, 9/e p619.. spent phase of polycythemia has extensive extramedullary hematopoeisis principally in the spleen which enlarges greatly ''

Primary myelofibrosis page 631, 9/e p621… 'it comes to attention because of progressive anemia and splenomegaly'

100. Ans. (b) JAK 2 mutation *(Ref: Robbins 9/e p618, 8th/626-8, Wintrobe's hematology 12th/1991-2; Journal Blood 110:1092, 2007)*

Polycythemia vera is the most common of the chronic myeloproliferative disorders. As discussed is text: JAK 2 mutation is a major criteria. However this mutation is not diagnostic of PV as it is also seen in essential thrombocytosis, chronic idiopathic myelofibrosis (CIMF) and atypical myeloproliferative disorders.

Other options, options "a" and "c" are minor criteria whereas Option 'd', remember friends that
- **MPL point mutation** is seen in 5-10% patients with **essential thrombocytosis** and **primary myelofibrosis.**

Burkitt's lymphoma is having the germinal B cell as the cell of origin. This condition is diagnosed with the demonstration of a very high proliferative fraction and the presence of any of the following cytogenetic abnormalities on the surface of the cells
- t (8;14) (most commonly)
- t (2;8) or
- t (8;22)

101. Ans. (d) Essential thrombocytopenia *(Ref: Robbins 7th/696, 9/e p616)*
Essential thrombocytosis (and not Essential thrombocytopenia) is a myeloproliferative disorder.

102. Ans. (b) Extramedullary hematopoiesis *(Ref: Robbins 9/e p620, 8th/630, Harrison 18th/900-1)*

The patient has the **classic features of myelofibrosis with myeloid metaplasia.** It is a stem cell disorder, in which neoplastic megakaryocytes secrete fibrogenic factors leading to marrow fibrosis. The neoplastic clone goes to spleen where it shows trilineage hematopoietic proliferation (extramedullary hematopoiesis) with prominent megakaryocytes. The peripheral blood has immature RBC and WBC precursors (**leukoerythroblastic picture**).

Teardrop RBCs are altered shaped red cells found when marrow undergoes fibrosis.

Marrow injury also can be the result of other causes (e.g. metastatic tumors or irradiation). These causes also can give rise to a leukoerythroblastic picture but splenic enlargement with trilineage proliferation usually is not seen. The other options Hodgkin lymphoma and portal hypertension can cause splenic enlargement but not marrow fibrosis. Adenocarcinoma metastases to the spleen are uncommon.

103. Ans. (a) Histiocytosis-X *(Ref: Robbins 8th/631-2, 9/e p621)*

Histiocytosis is an "umbrella" designation for a variety of proliferative disorders of dendritic cells or macrophages. It is divided into three categories: Letterer-Siwe syndrome, Hand-Schuller-Christian disease, and eosinophilic granuloma.

Letterer-Siwe disease
• Also known as Multifocal multisystem Langerhans cell histiocytosis
• Occurs *most frequently before 2 years* of age but occasionally affects adults.
• Chief clinical feature is the development of cutaneous lesions resembling a seborrheic eruption, which is caused by infiltrates of Langerhans cells over the front and back of the trunk and on the scalp.
• Affected patients also have concurrent hepatosplenomegaly, lymphadenopathy, pulmonary lesions, and, eventually, destructive osteolytic bone lesions.
• Extensive infiltration of the marrow often leads to anemia, thrombocytopenia, and *predisposition to recurrent infections such as otitis media and mastoiditis.*
• The course of untreated disease is **rapidly fatal.**

103.1. Ans. (c) 65% *(Ref: Textbook of Clinical Pediatrics 2/e p356)*

Direct lines…. "Polycythemia is defined as venous hematocrit **exceeding 65%".**

Polycythemia is not to be confused with the polycythemia vera for which the following information is asked repeatedly….

Revised WHO criteria for polycythymia vera

Major criteria	• Hemoglobin > 18.5 g/dL in men or > 16.5 g/dL in women or evidence of increased red cell volume • Presence of **JAK2 mutation**[Q]

Also know:

- Lines from Harrison…. "Unless the hemoglobin level is **≥20 g/dl (hematocrit ≥60%)**, it is not possible to distinguish true erythrocytosis from disorders causing plasma volume contraction.
- *Stress* or *spurious erythrocytosis* is called as *Gaisböck's syndrome*.

103.2. Ans. (a) CD 1a *(Ref: Robbins 9/e p622, 8/e p631)*

- In Langerhans cell histiocytosis, *the presence of Birbeck granules in the cytoplasm is characteristic.*
- In this condition, **Birbeck granules**[Q] are pentalaminar tubules, often with a dilated terminal end producing a **tennis racket–like appearance**[Q], which contain the protein langerin.
- In addition, the tumor cells also typically express **HLA-DR, S-100,** and **CD1a**[Q].

103.3. Ans. (d) Tennis racket *(Ref: Robbins 8/e p631, 9/e p622)*

Questions like this have been asked in the national board exam. So, be familiar with this fact.

103.4. Ans. (c) Chronic myeloid leukemia *(Ref: Robbins 8/e p628 , 9/e p618)*

Leukocyte alkaline phosphatase (LAP) is found within the white blood cells. Revise the following condition s asked in the exam:

High LAP score	Low LAP score
• Leukemoid reaction	• Chronic myelogenous leukemia (CML)
• Polycythemia vera (PV)	• Paroxysmal nocturnal hemoglobinuria (PNH)
• Essential thrombocytosis (ET)	• Acute myelogenous leukaemia (AML).
• Primary myelofibrosis (PM)	• Sideroblastic anemia

103.5. Ans. (c) Hemolytic anemia *(Ref: Robbins 8/e p595, Blood 2/e p255, T. Singh 1/e p198)*

Leukoerythroblastosis is a term used for "an anemia characterized by the presence in the peripheral blood of immature red cells and a few immature white cells of the myeloid series" that is erythroblasts and leukoblasts. The following are the causes of leukoerythroblastosis:

Causes of leukoerythroblastosis

Marrow invasion	**Tumors** (lymphoma, Hodgkin disease, leukemia, multiple myeloma, bony metastasis) **Infections** (sepsis, TB, osteomyelitis) **Miscellaneous** (osteopetrosis, histiocytosis, storage disease, vasculitis including rheumatoid arthritis)
Myeloproliferative disorders	Polycythemia vera Myelofibrosis CML Erythroleukemia Thrombocythemia Down syndrome
Hematological disease	Erythroblastosis fetalis Pernicious anemia Thalassemia major Severe hemolytic anemia
Hypoxia	Congestive heart failure Cyanotic congenital heart disease Respiratory disease

Please remember friends that severe hemolytic anemias may be associated with a similar picture but routinely, leukoerythroblastosis is not observed with hemolytic anemia.

103.6. Ans. (b) Leukemoid reaction.. *(Ref: Robbins 8/e p595, 9/e p584, Hematology 3/e p402)*

LAP is found in the membranes of secondary granules of neutrophils. Its activity is measured in **mature neutrophils and band cells only**[Q].

Eosinophils do not[Q] show alkaline phosphatase activity and must not be mistaken with mature neutrophils with a score of zero. **Malaria** is characterized by **monocytosis.**

Increased LAP Score	Decreased LAP Score
• Leukemoid reaction • Pregnancy IIIrd trimester • Polycythemia vera • Infection, inflammation	• PNH • Sideroblastic anemia • CML • Myelodysplastic disorders

- LAP score is **normal** in **juvenile CML.**

103.7. Ans. (c) Acute myeloblastic leukemia *(Ref: Robbins 9th/ 616)*
Myeloproliferative disorders are charcterised by an increased production of one or more types of blood cells. The common pathogenic feature is the presence of mutated, constitutively activated tyrosine kinases or other acquired mutations resulting in growth factor independence. The examples include:
- Chronic myelogenous leukemia
- Chronic neutrophilic leukemia
- Polycythemia vera
- Primary myelofibrosis
- Essential thrombocythemia
- Chronic eosinophilic leukemia
- Mastocytosis

103.8. Ans. (b) 5q *(Ref: Robbins 9/e p615)*

104. Ans. (b) Hyperviscosity *(Ref: Robbins 8th/610-1, 9/e p600, Harrison 18th/938-940, Wintrobes hematology 12th/2374-8)*
According to Harrison,
- **Bone pain** is seen in 70% patients
- **Infections** is the next common (>75% have serious infection at some time in their course)
- **Normocytic normochromic anemia** is seen in 80% patients

105. Ans. (c) Hypercalcemia *(Ref: Harrison 17th/702, 9/e p600)*

106. Ans. (d) IgM *(Ref: Robbins 8th/65, 9/e p601)*
Lymphoplasmacytoid lymphoma (or **Waldenstrom's macroglobulinemia**) is a B cell neoplasm presenting in 6th or 7th decade of life having features similar to CLL/SLL and multiple myeloma (MM). Like MM, there is presence of a 'M' or monoclonal spike (caused due to IgM whereas in MM, it is caused by IgG).

✎ Also Remember
- Deletion involving chromosome 6q is the commonest abnormality in Waldenstrom's macroglobulinemia.

107. Ans. (b) A diagnosis of plasma cell leukemia...... *(Ref: Wintrobe's haematology 11th/2620, 2593)*
Plasma cell leukemia by definition is characterized by more than 20% plasma cells in the peripheral blood.
The patient in question has 14% plasma blasts in the peripheral blood and thus does not fit into category of plasma cell leukemia.
Distinguishing Features In Various Types of Plasma Cell Disorders:

1.	**Plasma cell leukemia**
	• More than 20% plasma cells in the peripheral blood • Absolute plasma cell count of more than 2 X 10⁹/L
2.	**IgD Myeloma**
	• Presence of Monoclonal IgD in the serum usually indicates IgD myeloma • No evident M– spike on serum protein electrophoresis • Higher incidence of renal insufficiency, amyloidosis and proteinuria than IgG/IgA myeloma. • Higher incidence of extramedullary involvement and inferior survival rates.
3.	**Monoclonal gammopathy of undetermined significance (MGUS)**
	• Serum monoclonal protein <3g/dl • Clonal bone marrow plasma cells < 10% • Absence of end organ damage such as hypercalcemia, renal failure, anemia and bone lesions (**CRAB**) • No lytic bone lesions • No evidence of other B-cell proliferative lesion

4.	Smoldering multiple myeloma (Asymptomatic multiple myeloma)
	Both criteria must be met
	• Serum monoclonal protein ($\geq$ 3 g/dl) and/or $\geq$ 10% clonal bone marrow plasma cells or both • Absence of end organ damage (CRAB)
5.	**Multiple myeloma**
	All three criteria must be present * Monoclonal protein present in serum or urine * > 10% clonal bone marrow plasma cells on biopsy or histological evidence of plasmacytoma * Evidence of end organ damage **(CRAB)**: • **C**alcemia (> 11.5 g/dl) • **R**enal insufficiency (Serum creatinine > 1.73 mmol/L) • **A**nemia (Hb< 10g/dl or > 2g/dl lower than normal) • **B**one marrow plasma cell labeling index > 1% • Lytic lesions or osteoporosis and $\geq$ 30% plasma cells in marrow

108. Ans. (c) Plasmacytoma on biopsy *(Ref: T. Singh 1st/210-211, Robbins 9/e p600-601)*

The commonly used diagnostic criteria of multiple myeloma are:

MULTIPLE MYELOMA

Major criteria
1.   Plasmacytoma on tissue biopsy
2.   Bone marrow plasmacytosis with > 30% plasma cells
3.   Monoclonal globulin spike on serum electrophoresis (> 3.5g/dL for IgG, > 2 g/dL for IgA) or on urine (> 1g/24 h of Bence-Jones protein)

Minor criteria
1.   Bone marrow plasmacytosis 10 to 30% plasma cells
2.   Monoclonal globulin spike less than the level defined above
3.   Lytic bone lesions
4.   Reduced normal immunoglobulin (<50% of normal); IgM <0.05 g/dL, IgA < 0.1g/dL, IgG < 0.6 g/dL

The diagnosis of multiple myeloma requires a minimum of two major criteria or one major criteria + one minor criteria, or three minor criteria.

109. Ans. (a) CD 1a *(Ref: Robbins 9/e p622, 7th/701, 702)*

Histiocytosis is a broad term for a number of dendritic cells or macrophages proliferative disorders. Langerhans cell is a special type of dendritic cell in the skin functioning as antigen presenting cell. In the past, these disorders were called **histiocytosis X** and were subdivided into three categories:

• *Letterer-Siwe syndrome*
• *Hand-Schüller-Christian disease,*
• *Eosinophilic granuloma.*

> •   The tumor cells in each are derived from dendritic cells and express **HLA-DR, S-100, and CD1a.**
> •   They have abundant, often vacuolated cytoplasm and vesicular nuclei containing linear grooves or folds.
> •   The presence of Birbeck's granules in the cytoplasm is characteristic. Under the electron microscope, Birbeck's granules have a **tennis-racket appearance.**

110. Ans. (b) Sheets of atypical plasma cells *(Ref: Robbins 9/e p599, 7th/679)*

• Old patient along with *lytic circumscribed punched out* X-ray appearance suggests **multiple myeloma**
• **Multiple myeloma** most often presents as multifocal destructive bone tumors composed of **plasma cells** throughout the skeletal system.

111. Ans. (a) Cryoglobulinemia; (b) Multiple myeloma; (d) Lymphoma; (e) Macroglobulinemia

(Ref: William's Haemotology 6/1268)

Hyperviscosity is seen in
• Multiple myeloma
• Waldenstrom's macroglobulinemia
• Cryoglobulinemia
• Myeloproliferative disorders

MGUS (Monoclonal Gammopathy of uncertain significance): Here M Protein can be identified in the Serum of 1% of healthy individual >50 years. age and 3% in older than 70 years of it is the most common form of monoclonal gammopathy. In MGUS less than 3g/dL of monoclonal protein is present in serum and there is no Bence Jones proteinuria.

Hyperviscosity is defined on the basis of the relative viscosity of serum as compared with water. *Normal relative viscosity of serum is 1.8*

112. **Ans. (b) Waldenstrom's macroglobulinemia; (c) Multiple myeloma.** *(Ref: William's Hematology 6th-1268)*

113. **Ans. (b) CD l+ ; (c) Birbeck's granules are pathognomonic; (d) Proliferation of antigen presenting cells; (e) Resembles Dendritic cells;** *(Ref: Robbins 9/e p622, 7th/701)*

114. **Ans. is c i.e. Wire loop lesions** *(Ref: Harrison 17th/573, Robbins 7th/232 9/e p223)*
    Wire loop lesions are characteristic of **SLE** and are *not seen in multiple myeloma*.

115. **Ans. (b) IL-6** *(Ref: Robbins 7th/679, 9/e p599)*

116. **Ans. (d) Systemic lupus erythematosus** *(Ref: Robbins 7th/678-679)*
    Plasma cell dyscrasias are characterized by proliferation of B-cell clone which synthesizes and secretes a single homogenous immunoglobulin or its fragments. This entity includes **Multiple myeloma, Waldenstrom's macroglobulinemia, Heavy chain diseases, Primary or immunocyte associated amyloidosis and Monoclonal Gammopathy of Undetermined Significance (MGUS).**

117. **Ans. (d) No lymphadenopathy** *(Ref: Robbins 9/e p622, 8th/631-632, 7th/701-702)*

118. **Ans. (c) IgG** *(Ref: Robbins 9/e p600, 8th/609-611; 7th/680)*

119. **Ans. (a) Langerhan's cell** *(Ref: Robbins 9/e p622, 8th/631; 7th/701)*

120. **Ans. (a) Monoclonal IgM spike in serum** *(Ref: Robbins 8th/610-2, Harrison 18th/942-3)*
    Kuljeet has symptoms of hyperviscosity syndrome like visual disturbances, dizziness, and headache. He is also having Raynaud's phenomenon. His bone marrow is infiltrated with plasmacytoid lymphocytes having immunoglobulins in the cytoplasm (Russell bodies). These findings are suggestive of the patient suffering from lymphoplasmacytic lymphoma/Waldenstrom's macroglobulinemia. This disorder is characterized by neoplastic B cells producing IgM leading to a monoclonal IgM spike in the serum. The IgM molecules aggregate resulting in hyperviscosity.
    Concept

    - There is **no leukemia phase** in **Waldenstrom's macroglobulinemia.**
    - **Multiple myeloma** (also associated with monoclonal gammopathy) does **not** cause **enlargement of liver and spleen.** Hypercalcemia occurs with myeloma because of bone destruction, and punched out lytic lesions are typical of multiple myeloma. Light chain in urine (Bence Jones proteins) is also a feature of multiple myeloma.

121. **Ans. (c) Kappa light chains:** *(Ref: Robbins 9/e p600, 8th/610)*
    The patient suffers from multiple myeloma in which malignant cells are responsible for the production of excessive amounts of immunoglobulin (usually IgG or IgA). Plasma cells synthesize a greater amount of light chains than heavy chains. In multiple myeloma, the light chains will be monoclonal. This patient is making a monoclonal population of kappa light chains and excreting them in the urine as Bence-Jones proteins. These patients make decreased levels of normal immunoglobulins of all isotypes, thus making them susceptible to infections (also the commonest cause of death). Infiltration of bone by the myeloma cells may lead to pathological fractures.

121.1. **Ans. (a) Multiple Myeloma** *(Ref: Robbins 9/e p599, 8/e p610)*
    In multiple myeloma, cytologic variants stem from the dysregulated synthesis and secretion of immunoglobulins, which often leads to intracellular accumulation of intact or partially degraded protein. Such variants include:
    - **Flame cells:** with fiery red cytoplasm,
    - **Mott cells:** with multiple grapelike cytoplasmic droplets
    The globular inclusions are referred to as **Russell bodies** (if cytoplasmic) or **Dutcher bodies** (if nuclear).

121.2. **Ans. (b) Langherhans** *(Ref: Robbins 9/e p622, 8/e p631-2)*
    LCH has the following presentations:
    - *Multifocal multisystem Langerhans cell histiocytosis (Letterer-Siwe disease)*
        - Occurs most frequently **before 2 years** of age
        - Dominant clinical feature is the development of **cutaneous lesions** resembling a seborrheic eruption over the front and back of the trunk and on the scalp.
        - Presence of concurrent hepatosplenomegaly, lymphadenopathy, pulmonary lesions, and (eventually) destructive osteolytic bone lesions.
    - *Unifocal and multifocal unisystem Langerhans cell histiocytosis (eosinophilic granuloma)*
        - Characterized by proliferations of Langerhans cells admixed with variable numbers of eosinophils, lymphocytes, plasma cells, and neutrophils.

White Blood Cells and Platelets

- Typically arises within the *medullary cavities of bones*, most commonly the calvarium, ribs, and femur. Less commonly, unisystem lesions of identical histology arise in the skin, lungs, or stomach.
- Unifocal lesions most commonly affect the skeletal system in older children or adults. Unifocal disease is indolent and may heal spontaneously or be cured by local excision or irradiation.
- Multifocal unisystem disease usually affects young children, who present with multiple erosive bony masses that sometimes expand into adjacent soft tissue.

Hand-Schuller-Christian triad: calvarial bone defects + diabetes insipidus + exophthalmos
- Pulmonary Langerhans cell histiocytosis
  - Seen in *adult smokers*
  - *Regress spontaneously upon cessation of smoking.*

121.3. Ans. (a) Multiple myeloma *(Ref: Harsh Mohan 6th/383, Robbins 9th/)*
Increased levels of microglobulin are seen in the urine and serum of patients with multiple myeloma.
Harrison 18th/941…. *Serum β 2 -microglobulin is the single most powerful predictor of survival and can substitute for staging.*

122. Ans. (b) Glanzmann's thrombasthenia > (d) Bernard Soulier disease *(Ref: Robbins 8th/, Wintrobe's 12th/1365-1370)*
Presence of normal PT and aPTT rules out the presence of any clotting factor deficiency. So, options like factor X deficiency and von Willebrand disease are ruled out. Clinically, both Glanzmann thrombasthenia and Bernard Soulier syndrome are indistinguishable. However, most of the haematologists agreed on placing Glanzmann thrombasthenia in preference to Bernard Soulier syndrome as the answer. We got an article supporting the increased prevalence of Glanzmann in comparison to Bernard Soulier in Western India as well.

Name of disease	Bernad Soulier disease	Glanzmann's thrombasthenia
Cause of disease	Defect in the platelet GpIb-IX complex	Defect in platelet Gp IIb/IIIa
Lab findings	↑BT, mild thrombocytopenia, deficient or low levels of platelet GpIb-IX complex by flowcytometry	↑BT, deficient clot retraction time, deficient platelet aggregation with ADP, collagen, thrombin, adrenaline
	Ristocetin aggregation test is defective	Ristocetin aggregation test and coagulation tests are normal
Platelet morphology	Giant platelets under normal smear	Platelets are normal under microscope

123. Ans. (c) Factor VIII inhibitors *(Ref: Robbins 8th/672-3, Wintrobe 12th/1447-1453, Harrison 18th/982)*
This is a case of 25 year old asymptomatic female whose parametric inference is as follows:

- BT is 3min (normal)
- PT is 15 sec/14 sec (normal)
- aPTT is 45sec/35sec(raised)
- Platelet count is 2.5lac/mm^3 (normal)
- Factor VIII levels were 60IU/dL (normal i.e. between 50-150IU/dL).

Analyzing all the options one by one
Option 'a'… Factor IX deficiency would have resulted in increased aPTT. However females are less likely to suffer from hemophilia B because it is an X-linked disease.
Option 'b'….. **Lupus anticoagulant** (Wintrobe 12th/1452, Harrison 18th/982) clearly says that these patients have **thrombocytopenia** (here platelet count is normal), **prolonged PTT** and **hypoprothrombinemia** due to antibodies against prothrombin (normal in this case)
Option 'c'….Factor VIII inhibitors (Wintrobe 12th/1441-1444, Harrison 18th/982); Tejender Singh hematology page no 308)
- Acquired coagulant inhibitor is immune-mediated condition characterized by autoantibody against a specific clotting factor and factor VIII is most common target.
- In 50% of patients no underlying disease is indentified at the time of diagnosis. In remaining the causes are autoimmune disease, malignancies, dermatologic diseases, pregnancy and post partum.
- Diagnosed by **isolated prolongation of PTT with normal PT** (coagulation profile is similar to haemophilia A). Platelet count and bleeding time is normal (matches with the data given in our question).
Option 'd'…. VWD – type III (Robbins 8th/672-3):**Bleeding time** will be **prolonged** (in this patient BT is normal) with abnormal platelet count. So, option'd' is excluded.
So the likely diagnosis for the patient in the stem of the question is presence of acquired coagulation inhibitors against Factor VIII.

124. Ans. (c) Done within 2 hours *(Ref: Dacie and Lewis practical hematology 10th/392, 398)*

For Prothrombin Time estimation

- **Platelet poor plasma** is used
- Sample should be kept at **room temperature**^{Q} (if stored at room temperature, PT is shortened due to VII activation in cold)
- Activation is done with thromboplastin (derived from rabbit brain or lung)
- Activation with kaolin is done for PTT not for PT
- PT, APTT are carried out on fresh samples
- The test done **within 2 hours**^{Q}
- **Normal value** is **11-16 sec**^{Q}

Interpretation of increased prothrombin time

- Administration of oral anticoagulants (vitamin K antagonists)
- Liver disease particularly obstructive type
- Vitamin K deficiency
- Disseminated intravascular coagulation
- Rarely, previously undiagnosed factor VII, X, V or prothrombin deficiency or defect

For Activated Partial Thromboplastin Time estimation

- **Platelet poor plasma** is used
- Sample should be kept at **room temperature**^{Q}
- Activation is done with kaolin/silica/ellagic acid
- **Normal value** is **26-40 sec**^{Q}

- **Conditions with elevated aPTT**

- Seen in DIC, liver disease, massive transfusion with plasma depleted RBCs, circulating anticoagulant (inhibitor), deficiency of clotting factor other than VII, administration of or contamination of heparin or other anticoagulants.

Sample should be kept at **room temperature** for estimation for **prothrombin time, lupus anticoagulant** and **factor VII assays**.

125. Ans. (d) Acquired Factor VIII inhibitors *(Ref: Wintrobes 12th/1442-4, 1274)*

The clinical presentation in a young female of recurrent joint pains with petechial hemorrhage is suggestive of an autoimmune disease. Options 'a', 'b' and 'c' are rare because these would present with some additional symptoms apart from the ones mentioned in the question. They would also be present since birth.

Talking about option 'd',

A female patient is unlike to have hemophilia as it is an X linked disorder. However, she can have autoantibodies against factor VIII. This could be due to other conditions mentioned below in the accompanying box.

Concept of Inhibitors (updated from Wintrobes 12th, Harrison 18th/982)

*A relatively rare cause of prolonged aPTT is presence of antibodies against coagulation plasma proteins called inhibitors. It can be seen due to the following reasons:

- Hemophilia A and B patients receiving clotting factors *to control their bleeding episodes*
- Pregnancy
- Autoimmune diseases
- Malignancies (lymphoma, prostate cancer)
- Dermatologic conditions

***Clinical manifestations** include bleeding episodes in soft tissues, skin, GIT and genitourinary tract.

*The diagnosis is made with a **prolonged aPTT** with normal PT and TT which is **not corrected** with **mixing the test plasma with normal pooled plasma** for 2hrs at 37°C.

*Treatment is done with **high dose i.v. immunoglobulins** and **anti CD20 monoclonal antibody**.

126. Ans. (b) Normal platelet count and increased BT *(Ref: Harrison 17th/723, Robbins 8th/670, Robbins 9/e 656)*

The stem of the question clearly mention the fact that there is platelet function defect. **It means that the platelet count is normal with a problem in the functioning of platelets. see text for details.**

- **Bleeding time** represents the time taken for a standardized skin puncture to stop bleeding and it gives an in vivo assessment of platelet response to limited vascular injury. The value varies from 2 to 9 minutes. It is abnormal when there is a **defect in platelet numbers or function**.
- Nowadays, quantitative measures of platelet function are being introduced by using an electronic particle counter.

127. Ans. (d) Defect in common pathway *(Ref: Robbins 9th/119)*

- Defect in the **extrinsic pathway** causes elevation of **PT**
- Defect in the **intrinsic pathway** causes elevation of **aPTT**.
- Defect in **common pathway** cause elevation of **both PT and aPTT**.
- **Platelet function defect** causes elevation of **BT**.

128. Ans. (d) Grossly abnormal coagulation tests *(Ref: Harrison 17th/722, Robbins 9/e p659-660)*

Thrombotic thrombocytopenic purpura arises from deficiency or inhibition of the enzyme ADAMTS13, which is responsible for cleaving large multimers of von Willebrand factor (vWF).

The combination of hemolytic anemia with fragmented RBCs, thrombocytopenia, normal coagulation tests, fever, neurological disorders and renal dysfunction is virtually pathognomic of TTP.

If coagulation tests indicate a major consumption of procoagulants, the diagnosis of TTP is doubtful.

129. Ans. (a) Acute promyelocytic leukemia *(Ref: Harrison 17th/679, Robbins 9/e p612)*

AML is classified by French-American-British (FAB) classification into various categories from M0 to M7. This classification has already been discussed in text. In which DIC is associated with *AML-M3* or *Acute promyelocytic leukemia*.

Recently WHO has also classified AML. WHO classification includes different biologically distinct groups *based on immunophenotype, clinical features, and cytogenetic and molecular abnormalities in addition to morphology.* In contrast to the previously used French-American-British (FAB) scheme, the **WHO classification places limited reliance on cytochemistry.**

WHO CLASSIFICATION OF AML

AML with recurrent genetic abnormalities	AML with multilineage dysplasia	AML and myelodysplastic syndromes, therapy-related	AML not otherwise categorized
*t(8;21) *inv(16) *Acute promyelocytic leukemia, t(15;17)	*Following a myelodysplastic syndrome *Without antecedent myelodysplastic syndrome	*Alkylating agent related *Topoisomerase type II inhibitor-related *Other types	*AML minimally differentiated *AML without maturation *AML with maturation *Acute myelomonocytic leukemia *Acute monoblastic and monocytic leukemia *Acute erythroid leukemia *Acute megakaryoblastic leukemia *Acute basophilic leukemia *Acute panmyelosis with myelofibrosis *Myeloid sarcoma

Another important difference between the WHO and FAB systems is the blast cutoff for a diagnosis of AML as opposed to myelodysplastic syndrome (MDS);

According to FAB classification AML is diagnosed when bone marrow shows 30% blasts whereas WHO keeps this value at 20%.

130. Ans. (c) Aplastic anemia *(Ref: Harrison 17th/719,720, 667-668 & 16th/674, 622)*

- Megakaryocyte is a precursor of platelet. Any peripheral destruction of platelets causes increased activity of bone marrow resulting in **megakaryocytic thrombocytopenia** because of compensatory increase in megakaryocytes.
- However, if thrombocytopenia occurs due to any defect in the bone marrow itself, the compensatory increase in megakaryocytes will not occur. This is known as **amegakaryocytic or hypoplastic thrombocytopenia.**

Aplastic anemia is also an example of amegakaryocytic thrombocytopenia.

131. Ans. (a) D-dimer will be normal *(Ref: Wintrobe's Hematology 11th/1672)*

- Coagulation defects in severe liver disease include elevated thrombin time, prothrombin time and activated partial thromboplastin time.
- All factors procoagulant as well as anti clotting factors (antithrombin III, protein C and protein S) being synthesized in the liver are reduced in liver dysfunction.
- Fibrin degradation products are increased in patients with severe liver disease and DIC because endogenous plasminogen activators are removed by the normal liver. In severe liver disease, they circulate for long time and cause activation of the fibrinolytic system.

D-dimer is usually normal in liver disease patients. It is increased with DIC.

Wintrobe's mentions page 1396-7 that ..*Normal fibrinogen level is 150-350 mg/dl and the levels between 50-100mg/dl are required for normal hemostasis.* However, I could not find any level specifically in cirrhosis patients friends.

132. Ans. (d) Wiskott Aldrich syndrome *(Ref: Robbins 7th/244, 8th/235, 9/e p242)*

Wiskott Aldrich syndrome is characterized by the **triad** of:

- Severe eczema
- Thrombocytopenia
- Recurrent infections

The platelets are small and are reduced in number in Wiskott Aldrich syndrome.

About other options, in ITP, Bernard Soulier syndrome and Myelofibrosis, there is increase in size of platelets.

133. Ans. (a) Serotonin; (b) Ig mediators; (d) Interaction among the platelets; (e) Macromolecules; *(Ref: William's Haematology 61th/1366, Harrison 17th/363-364, Robbins 9/e p117-118)*

Agonists of platelet aggregation:

Adhesins	vWF	Plasmin	Serotonin
Thrombospondin	Fibrinogen	Immunocomplex	Vasopressin
TxA$_2$	ADP	Epinephrine	

P-selectin mediates the interaction between WBC and platelets.

134. **Ans. (a) Abruptio placentae; (b) Acute pro-myelocytic leukemia; (c) Severe falciparum malaria; (d) 'Snake envenomation; (e) Heparin overdose.** *(Ref: Robbins 7th/657, 9/e 663-664, KDT 5th- 562)*

135. **Ans. (b) Increased PT; (d) Decreased Fibrinogen; (e) Decreased platelets** *(Ref: Robbins 7th/657, 9/e 664-665)*
Laboratory findings in DIC:

*Low platelet count.
*Microangiopathic hemolytic anemia
*Elevated prothrombin time, thrombin time, and activated partial thromboplastin time
*Plasma fibrinogen level decreased
*Fibrin degradation products (FDP) are raised.
*Factor V and factor VIII decreased.

136. **Ans. (a) Anaerobic Sepsis; (b) Malignancy; (c) Leukemia.** *(Ref: Robbins 7th/657, 9/e 663-664)*

137. **Ans. (a) Glanzmann's syndrome; (b) Bernard-Soulier syndrome; (c) Wiskott Aldrich syndrome; (d) von Willebrand disease** *(Ref: Harrison 17th/723, Robbins 9th/660)*
For details, See text
Leucocytosis is seen in all of the given options i.e. brucellosis, acute MI, and diphtheria but in typhoid, there is leucopenia.

138. **Ans. (d) All of the above** *(Ref: Harrison 17th/723-724; Robbins 8th/118, 9/e p662)*

139. **Ans. (d) Angiogenesis inhibitory protein** *(Ref: Robbins 9/e p306, 8th/96, 7th/105)*
- **Thrombospondin**, is a family of large multi-functional proteins, some of which, similar to **SPARC** (secreted protein acidic and rich in cysteine), inhibit angiogenesis.
- The production of thrombospondin-I has been shown to be inversely related to the ability of a cell line to produce a tumor and vessels *in vivo*; loss of thrombospondin-I production allowed non-tumorigenic cells to become tumorigenic.
- Thrombospondin-I is regulated by wild-type p53.

140. **Ans. (a) Thromboplastin** *(Ref: Robbins, 7th/649, 9/e 656)*

141. **Ans. (a) Myelofibrosis** *(Ref: Harrison 17th/723)*

Causes of Thrombocytosis

• Iron deficiency anemia	• Myelodysplasia
• Hyposplenism	• Post surgery
• Postsplenectomy	• Infection
• Malignancy	• Polycythemia vera
• Collagen vascular disorder	• Hemolysis
• Idiopathic myelofibrosis	• Hemorrhage
• Essential thrombocytosis	• Idiopathic sideroblastic anemia
• CML	• Rebound (cessation of ethanol intake, correction of B$_{12}$ and folate deficiency).

142. **Ans. (a) Synthesized by hepatocytes** *(Ref: Robbins 8th/670-671, 9/e 661)*
- von-Willebrand factor (vWF) facilitates platelet adhesion to vascular endothelium and serves as the plasma carrier for the factor VIII.
- It is synthesized in endothelial cells and megakaryocytes.
- The *Weibel Palade bodies* are storage organelle for vWF.
- Principal site of synthesis of factor VIII is liver.

143. **Ans. (d) VIII** *(Ref: Robbins 8th/835, 9/e 661)*

144. **Ans. (d) Antithrombin** *(Ref: Harsh Mohan 6th/340)*

145. **Ans. (c) von Willebrand disease** *(Ref: Robbins 8th/672-673; 7th/649, 9/e 662)*

146. **Ans. (c) t (14: 18)** *(Ref: Robbins 9/e 591, 8th/605-606, 7th/677)*

147. **Ans. (a) Decrease in neutrophil count** *(Ref: Robbins 8th/592-593, 9/e p582)*

148. **Ans. (b) 1,00,000/cmm** *(Ref: Robbins 9/e p657, 8th/667; 7th/650)*

White Blood Cells and Platelets

149. Ans. (c) Glycoprotein IIb/IIIa *(Ref: Robbins 9/e 657-658, 8th/667-668)*

The history of nosebleeds and menorrhagia, the petechiae, thrombocytopenia and increased bleeding time all suggest a platelet disorder. The decreased platelet count suggests a thrombocytopenic disorder rather than a platelet function disorder. The absence of antinuclear antibody rules out SLE (a significant cause of thrombocytopenia). The negative drug history rules out drug-associated thrombocytopenia. So, a probable diagnosis of idiopathic thrombocytopenic purpura can be made. ITP is an acquired thrombocytopenia caused by formation of autoantibodies directed against the platelet membrane proteins glycoprotein IIb/IIIa, followed by splenic destruction of opsonized platelets. The disease typically occurs in women from 20-40 years of age.

Antibodies to erythrocyte membrane proteins (choice B) are seen in autoimmune hemolytic anemia whereas antibodies to intrinsic factor (choice D) are seen in pernicious anemia.

150. Ans. (a) Antiplatelet antibodies *(Ref: Robbins 8th/667, 9/e p657)*
- ITP is a chronic autoimmune disorder in which antibodies against platelet glycoproteins cause platelet destruction and removal by the reticuloendothelial system. Secondary thrombocytopenia can also be produced by lupus, viral infections, and drugs. The diagnosis of ITP is made only when secondary thrombocytopenia has been ruled out.
- Defective platelet aggregation (choice B) is responsible for thrombasthenia that causes prolonged bleeding time but normal platelet count.
- Hypersplenism (choice C) causes thrombocytopenia when an enlarged spleen traps normal platelets in the absence of other specific platelet disorders. This type of thrombocytopenia can be cured with splenectomy. The thrombocytopenia in ITP often improves with splenectomy, ITP does not cause splenomegaly.
- Megakaryopoiesis (choice D) is disturbed in any disorder that causes bone marrow failure, including drug toxicity, leukemia, and infections. So, thrombocytopenia is often part of a pancytopenia.

150.1. Ans. (c) Congenital defect of platelets *(Ref: Robbins 8/e p670, 9/e p660)*
- **Glanzmann *thrombasthenia*** is a defect in **platelet aggregation** (both have 'g' in them).
- *Bernard Soulier syndrome* is a defect in platelet *adhesion* (both have 'd' in them).

Glanzmann thrombasthenia, which is also transmitted as an *autosomal recessive* trait. Thrombasthenic platelets fail to aggregate in response to adenosine diphosphate (ADP), collagen, epinephrine, or thrombin because of **dysfunction of glycoprotein IIb-IIIa,** an integrin that participates in "bridge formation" between platelets by binding fibrinogen

150.2. Ans. (c) Decreased fibrin degradation products...discussed earlier *(Ref: Robbins 9/e 662-663, 8/e p673-674, 7/e p658)*
- DIC is associated with **increased** *fibrin degradation products.*

150.3. Ans. (a) Normal complement levels *(Ref: Robbins 9/e 659-660, 8/e p669-670, 7/e p652-653)*
Classically, the following five features ("**pentad**") are indicative of TTP:
- Fluctuating neurological symptoms, such as bizarre behavior, altered mental status, stroke or headaches
- Kidney failure
- Fever
- Thrombocytopenia (low platelet count), leading to bruising or purpura
- Microangiopathic hemolytic anemia (anemia, jaundice and a characteristic blood film)

HUS and TTP are both caused by insults that lead to the excessive activation of platelets, which deposit as **thrombi in microcirculatory beds**. These intravascular thrombi cause a *microangiopathic hemolytic anemia* and widespread *organ dysfunction*, and the attendant consumption of platelets leads to **thrombocytopenia**.

Wintrobe's mentions that.. "immune complex formation and activation of the complement activation has been seen in TTP."

150.4. Ans (b) Glanzmann disease *(Ref: Robbins 9th/118)*
Inherited deficiency of GpIIb-IIIa results in a bleeding disorder called Glanzmann thrombasthenia.

150.5. Ans (b) Relapse is rare *(Robbins 9th/658)*
Direct quote.... "Almost all patients respond to glucocorticoids (which inhibit phagocyte function), but many eventually relapse."
- In individuals with severe thrombocytopenia, splenectomy normalizes the platelet counts.
- Immunomodulatory agents such as intravenous immunoglobulin or anti-CD20 antibody (rituximab) are often effective in patients who relapse after splenectomy or for whom splenectomy is contraindicated.
- Peptides that mimic the effects of thrombopoietin (so-called TPO-mimetics) are also useful for improving the platelet counts of the patients.

150.6 Ans: (a) Chronic ITP...see earlier explanation

150.7. Ans (c) Shwachman syndrome................*(Ref: Harrison 18th/Ch 107)*
Shwachman-Diamond syndrome is associated with pancreatic insufficiency, marrow failure and malabsorption.

GOLDEN POINTS FOR QUICK REVISION / UPDATED INFORMATION FROM 9TH EDITION OF ROBBINS
(WHITE BLOOD CELLS & PLATELETS)

Macrophage activation syndrome/ Hemophagocytic Lymphohistiocytosis..........585-6

Hemophagocytic lymphohistiocytosis (HLH) is a reactive condition having the signs and symptoms of systemic inflammation related to macrophage activation as well as having marked by cytopenias.

The most common trigger for HLH is **infection,** particularly with **Epstein-Barr virus (EBV)**.

Pathogenesis

The condition is characterized by the **systemic activation of macrophages and CD8+ cytotoxic T cells** which phagocytose blood cell progenitors in the bone marrow. The mediators released by these cells suppress hematopoeisis and produce symptoms of systemic inflammation ('cytokine storm'). Even familial forms of the disease have activating mutations in **cytotoxic T cells and natural killer cells.**

Clinical Features

Most patients present with an acute **febrile** illness associated with **splenomegaly and hepatomegaly.** Bone marrow examination demonstrates **hemophagocytosis.** Blood picture is characterized by anemia, thrombocytopenia, and very high levels of **plasma ferritin and soluble IL-2 receptor** (the latter two indicative of severe inflammation), as well as elevated liver function tests. The disease may progress to disseminated intravascular coagulation and may be fatal.

Treatment involves the use of immunosuppressive drugs and "mild" chemotherapy. Some individuals may require hematopoietic stem cell transplantation.

Chronic lymphocytic leukemia....593

- Deep sequencing of CLL genomes has also revealed gain-of-function mutations involving the NOTCH1 receptor in 10% to 18% of tumors, as well as frequent mutations in genes that regulate RNA splicing.

Common Forms of Lymphoid Leukemia and Lymphoma.......598

Acute Lymphoblastic Leukemia/Lymphoblastic Lymphoma

- *Most common type of cancer* in **children,** may be derived from either precursor B of T cells
- Highly aggressive tumors manifest with signs and symptoms of bone marrow failure, or as rapidly growing masses.
- Tumor cells contain genetic lesions that block differentiation, leading to the accumulation of immature, nonfunctional blasts.

Small Lymphocytic Lymphoma/Chronic Lymphocytic Leukemia

- **Most common leukemia** of **adults**
- Tumor of mature B cells that usually manifests with bone marrow and lymph node involvement
- Indolent course, commonly associated with immune abnormalities, including an increased susceptibility to infection and autoimmune disorders

Follicular Lymphoma

- *Most common indolent lymphoma* of adults
- Tumor cells recapitulate the growth pattern of normal germinal center B cells; most cases are associated with a (14;18) translocation that results in the over expression of **BCL2.**

Diffuse Large B-Cell Lymphoma

- **Most common lymphoma** of adults
- Heterogeneous group of mature B-cell tumors that shares a large cell morphology and aggressive clinical behavior
- Rearrangements or mutations of **BCL6 gene** are recognized associations; one third carry a (14;18) translocation involving BCL2 and may arise from follicular lymphomas.

Burkitt Lymphoma

- Very aggressive tumor of mature B cells that usually arises at extranodal sites.
- Strongly associated with translocations involving the MYC proto-oncogene
- Tumor cells often are latently infected by EBV.

Myeloid Neoplasms

Myeloid tumors occur mainly in adults and fall into three major groups:

Acute myeloid leukemias (AMLs)

- Aggressive tumors comprised of immature myeloid lineage blasts, which replace the marrow and suppress normal hematopoiesis
  Associated with diverse acquired mutations that lead to expression of abnormal transcription factors, which interfere with myeloid differentiation
- Often also associated with mutations in genes encoding growth factor receptor signaling pathway components or regulators of the epigenome

Myeloproliferative disorders

- Myeloid tumors in which production of formed myeloid elements is initially increased, leading to high blood counts and extramedullary hematopoiesis
- Commonly associated with acquired mutations that lead to constitutive activation of tyrosine kinases, which mimic signals from normal growth factors. The most common pathogenic kinases are BCR-ABL (associated with CML) and mutated JAK2 (associated with polycythemia vera and primary myelofibrosis).
- All can transform to acute leukemia and to a spent phase of marrow fibrosis associated with anemia, thrombocytopenia, and splenomegaly.

Myelodysplastic Syndromes

- Poorly understood myeloid tumors characterized by disordered and ineffective hematopoiesis and dysmaturation
- Recently shown to frequently harbor mutations in splicing factors and epigenetic regulators
- Manifest with one or more cytopenias and progress in 10% to 40% of cases to AML

Langerhans cell histiocytosis.......621

The **most common mutation** is an activating valine to- glutamate substitution at residue 600 in a serine/threonine protein kinase called **BRAF**. The latter is also commonly involved in patients with **hairy cell leukemia.**

NOTES

CHAPTER 9

Cardiovascular System

HEART

The human heart is a muscular pump responsible for maintaining the circulation of the blood and perfusion of different organs of the body. The *thickness of the left ventricle is almost three times that of the right ventricle*. The cardiac output is about 5 liters per minute. The heart is supplied by the coronary arteries:

1. Left coronary artery: It divides into *left anterior descending artery* (LAD) and the *left circumflex artery* (LCX). The LAD is responsible for supplying the following regions of the heart:
   - Apex of the heart
   - Anterior 2/3rd of the interventricular septum
   - Anterior wall of the left ventricle

   The LCX mainly supplies the lateral wall of the left ventricle.
2. Right coronary artery: It supplies
   - The entire right ventricular free wall
   - Posterobasal wall of the left ventricle
   - Posterior 1/3rd of the interventricular septum.

Out of the three layers of the heart (pericardium, myocardium and endocardium), the least collateral perfusion is present in the endocardium. So in any conditions associated with reduced perfusion (hypotension/shock), there are increased chances of sub endocardial ischemia. The coronary artery supplying the posterior 1/3rd of the ventricular septum (by giving rise to the posterior descending branch) is called *dominant*. In majority of the individuals (~80%), this vessel arises from the RCA, so they have right dominant circulation. The myocardium or the cardiac muscle is composed of the cardiac myocytes which cannot undergo division or hyperplasia in response to stress. The only adaptation that can be seen in a cardiac muscle can be hypertrophy which can be of the following types:

- **Concentric hypertrophy/pressure overload hypertrophy:** It is due to deposition of the sarcomeres (functional intracellular contractile unit of the cardiac muscle) in parallel to the long axis of the cells. It is associated with *hypertension and aortic stenosis*.
- **Volume overload hypertrophy:** In this, dilatation with increased ventricular diameter is present. It is seen with valvular regurgitation *(mitral or aortic regurgitation), thyrotoxicosis and severe anemia*.

HEART FAILURE

It is a clinical condition characterized by the inability of the heart to pump blood in proportion with the requirements of the metabolic tissues of the body or being able to do so at increased filling pressures. It may be divided into **systolic or diastolic failure** depending on whether there is abnormality in the cardiac contractility (systolic failure; as seen in ischemic heart disease, pressure or volume overload, dilated cardiomyopathy) or in the ventricular relaxation (diastolic failure; as in constrictive pericarditis, myocardial fibrosis or amyloid deposition). We can also classify heart failure as:

LEFT VENTRICULAR FAILURE/LEFT SIDED HEART FAILURE (LVF)

It is most commonly caused by *ischemic heart disease, hypertension, aortic or mitral valvular disease and myocardial disease* (non-ischemic). The features include hypertrophy and fibrosis in the myocardium associated with secondary involvement of the atria which shows enlargement. Atrial involvement results in the development of the atrial fibrillation which is responsible for thrombus formation or embolic stroke. The other organs affected include:

The volume of the blood pumped by the heart in a single beat is called as **stroke volume** (about **70 ml**).

Normal ejection fraction is 65%

The most important **source of energy** for the cardiac myocytes is the **fatty acids**.

SA node is the "pacemaker" of the heart
AV node is the "gatekeeper" of the heart

Lungs are the **most commonly** affected organ in **LVF**.

Lungs
• It is the most commonly affected organ. The increased pressure in the pulmonary vein causes *pulmonary edema* (heavy wet lungs). The edema fluid accumulates in the alveolar space. • There is leakage of hemosiderin and other iron containing particles which are phagocytosed by macrophages. The iron gets converted to hemosiderin leading to the formation of **siderophages or heart failure cells** (*hemosiderin containing macrophages*). • The alveolar fluid impairs gaseous exchange giving rise to breathlessness or ***dyspnea (earliest feature of LVF)***, orthopnea (dyspnea on lying down) and paroxysmal nocturnal dyspnea (dyspnea at night). • There is presence of **Kerley B lines** on chest X-ray due to transudate in the interlobular septa.
Kidneys
In the early stages, decreased renal perfusion causes activation of the renin-angiotensin-aldosterone system whereas in the later stages, continued reduced renal perfusion may precipitate prerenal azotemia.
Brain
It may suffer from hypoxic ischemic encephalopathy.

> **Siderophages** or **heart failure cells** are *hemosiderin containing macrophages*.

RIGHT SIDED HEART FAILURE

> **Left ventricular failure** is the most common cause of the right sided heart failure.

Left ventricular failure is the most common cause of the right sided heart failure whereas pure right sided failure is seen in chronic severe pulmonary hypertension and is called as **cor pulmonale**.

> **Cardiac cirrhosis** is characterised by **nutmeg liver**.

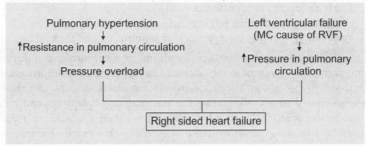

The features seen as a result of the inability of the right heart to pump blood in different organs include:

Liver
There is presence of congestive hepatomegaly. In addition, if associated LVF is present, the centrilobular necrosis is also seen which is replaced by fibrotic tissue in longstanding cases and is known as cardiac sclerosis or cardiac cirrhosis.
Spleen
Congestive splenomegaly is seen.
Kidney
These show the congestion resulting in severe azotemia. The congestion is more prominent in RVF than in LVF.

• Pleural effusion, pericardial effusion and ascites are also seen.
• The hallmark of the right sided heart failure is peripheral edema of the dependent parts of the body particularly pedal and pretibial edema.
• **Anasarca** is the *generalized massive edema* seen in heart failure.

RHEUMATIC FEVER AND RHEUMATIC HEART DISEASE (RHD)

> Most commonly affected age group in **rheumatic fever** is **5-15 years.**

Rheumatic fever is an acute *immunologically mediated* multisystem inflammatory disease that occurs few weeks after an attack of *group A β- hemolytic streptococcal pharyngitis*. It is not an infective disease. The most commonly affected age group is children between the ages of **5-15 years**[Q]. **Only 3%**[Q] of patients with group A streptococcal pharyngitis develop acute rheumatic fever.

The disease is a **type II hypersensitivity** reaction in which *antibodies against 'M' protein of some streptococcal strains (1, 3, 5, 6, and 18) cross-react with the glycoprotein antigens in the heart, joints and other tissues (molecular mimicry).*

WHO criteria for diagnosis of RF and RHD [Based on revised (1992) Jones criteria]

1.	**Major manifestations:**
	Joint involvement (Polyarthritis) **N** - **N**odules (Subcutaneous) **E** - **E**rythema marginatum **S** - **S**ydenham's chorea Criteria - **C**arditis
2.	**Minor manifestations:**
	Clinical: Fever polyarthralgia
	Laboratory: Increased ESR or C-RP
	ECG: Prolonged PR interval
3.	**Supporting evidence of a preceding streptococcal infection within last 45 days:**
	Elevated or rising ASO or other Ab titers
	Positive throat culture
	Rapid antigen test for group A streptococcus.

> **Migratory polyarthritis** is the commonest **major manifestation** of *Jones criteria* seen clinically.

Note:
1. Two major or one major and two minor manifestations plus any of the evidence of preceding group A streptococcal infection is required for diagnosis of primary episode of rheumatic fever.
2. 1992 revised Jones criteria do not include elevated TLC (total leukocyte count) as a laboratory minor manifestation [instead, it includes elevated C-reactive protein] and do not include recent scarlet fever as supporting evidence of recent streptococcal infection.

SALIENT FEATURES OF THE MAJOR CRITERIA

Carditis

All the layers of the heart namely pericardium, myocardium and endocardium are involved, so this is called **pancarditis**. The pericarditis is associated with fibrinous/serofibrinous exudate and is called as **'bread and butter' pericarditis**. Valvular involvement is common in rheumatic heart disease. The *most common valve to be affected is the mitral valve and least commonly affected is pulmonary valve.* **In acute rheumatic heart disease, the most common valvular lesion is mitral regurgitation and in chronic rheumatic heart disease, it is mitral stenosis.**

> **Pancarditis** is a characteristic manifestation of the cardiac involvement in **rheumatic fever**.

Migratory polyarthritis

There is involvement of the large joints of the body. It is more commonly seen in the adults as compared to children. The arthritis involves one joint after the other (migratory) and subsides spontaneously without any residual deformability in the joints **(non-erosive arthritis)**. Clinically, this is the *most commonly seen manifestation* and the joint pain shows dramatic response to salicylates like aspirin.

Subcutaneous nodules

These are painless subcutaneous lesions found on the **extensor surface** of the elbows, shin and the occiput.

Erythema marginatum

There is presence of red macular rash more easily appreciated in fair skinned individuals sparing the face and without residual scarring.

> The plump macrophages called **Anitschkow cells** are *pathognomonic* for rheumatic fever.

Sydenham's chorea

It is a *late manifestation* of the disease characterized by presence of involuntary, purposeless movements associated with emotional lability of the patient.

Microscopically, the characteristic feature of rheumatic heart disease is **Aschoff's body**. The latter consist of foci of swollen eosinophilic collagen surrounded by T-lymphocytes, few plasma cells and plump macrophages called **Anitschkow cells (pathognomonic for RF)**. These distinctive cells have abundant cytoplasm and central round-to-ovoid nuclei in which the chromatin is disposed in a central, slender, wavy ribbon (hence, they are also called as "caterpillar cells").

The myocardium has Aschoff's bodies in the perivascular location. The involvement of the endocardium results in **fibrinoid necrosis** within the cusps or along the tendinous cords which also have small vegetations called *verrucae* present along the lines of closure. The presence of mitral regurgitation also induces irregular thickening in the *left atrial wall* called as **MacCallum plaques**.

Chronic RHD is characterized by organization of the acute inflammation and subsequent fibrosis. The valves show leaflet thickening, commissural fusion and shortening, and thickening and fusion of the tendinous cords. There is mitral stenosis called as **'fish-mouth' or 'button-hole' stenosis**. Mitral stenosis may also lead to atrial fibrillation and thromboembolic phenomenon in these patients.

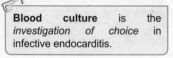

Most commonly affected valve is **mitral valve** and the *least commonly* affected is *pulmonary valve*.

INFECTIVE ENDOCARDITIS (IE)

It is colonization or invasion of heart valves and mural endocardium by microbiologic agent leading to formation of bulky, friable vegetations composed of thrombotic debris and organisms with destruction of underlying cardiac tissues. It can be

- Acute
- Subacute

Acute endocarditis	Subacute endocarditis
• Necrotizing, ulcerative, invasive valvular infection on a previously normal valve.	• Insidious infection following a protracted course on a previously damaged valve
• Highly virulent organisms	• Low virulence organisms
• Death of the patient within days to weeks	• Recover after antibiotic therapy
• MC caused by **Staph. aureus**	• MC caused by α-**hemolytic (viridans) Streptococcus**

Important Microbiology Link!

Organism in the infective endocarditis	Predisposing condition
Staphylococcus aureus	a. Intravenous drug abusers b. Native cardiac valve
Staphylococcus epididermis	Patients having prosthetic or artificial valve
Staphylococcus viridians	Previously damaged valve
Staphylococcus mutans	Patients who have had recent tooth extraction
Apart from all these enterococci and the HACEK group of bacteria (Hemophillus, Actinobacillus, Cardiobacterium, Eikenella and Kingella) can cause infective endocarditis.	

MORPHOLOGY

The aortic valve is the most commonly affected valve in **prosthetic valve endocarditis**.

The friable, bulky destructive vegetations containing fibrin, bacteria and inflammatory cells are found on the valve cusps. These can also extend on to chordae. *The aortic valve and the mitral valve are most commonly infected* whereas *the right side of heart is affected in intravenous drug abusers*. When the vegetations erode into myocardium, they can form an abscess called *Ring abscess*. The systemic embolisation can result in *septic infarcts*.

CLINICAL FEATURES

Blood culture is the *investigation of choice* in infective endocarditis.

Fever is the *most consistent sign of IE*. The other features include weight loss, flu-like syndrome, cardiac murmur, systemic emboli, **Roth spots** (due to retinal emboli), **Osler nodes** (painful, subcutaneous nodules on the fingers and toes) and **Janeway lesions** (red painless lesions on the palms and soles).

- The disease is diagnosed by **Dukes criteria**.

Cardiovascular System

COMPLICATIONS

Cardiac complications
• Valvular insufficiency or stenosis • Myocardial ring abscess • Suppurative pericarditis • Valvular dehiscence

Embolic complications
• With left sided lesion – Brain, spleen, kidney • With right sided lesion – Lung infarct, lung abscess

Renal complications
• Embolic infarct • **Focal (more common)** or *diffuse glomerulonephritis (less common)*

MARANTIC ENDOCARDITIS/NON BACTERIAL THROMBOTIC ENDOCARDITIS (NBTE)

- It is seen in patients suffering from debilitating diseases like malignancy (carcinoma pancreas and acute promyelocytic leukemia) and hypercoagulable states (DIC)
- **Vegetations on heart valves are sterile** and do not contain microorganisms. These are usually **present along the line of closure**, single or multiple.

LIBMAN-SACKS ENDOCARDITIS (SLE)

- Seen in patients of SLE
- Vegetations are small or medium sized, **sterile, granular and pink** on either or both sides of valve leaflets.
- Mitral and tricuspid valves are involved and show *fibrinoid necrosis*.

Summary of salient features of vegetations in different endocarditis

Rheumatic Fever	Non Bacterial Thrombotic (Marantic Endocarditis)	Libman Sack's Endocarditis	Infective Endocarditis
• Small, warty • Firm • Friable	• Small, warty • Friable	• Medium sized (small) • Flat, Verrucous • Irregular	• Large • Bulky • Irregular
• Along lines of closure	• Along lines of closure	• On surface of cusps • (both surfaces may be involved but the undersurface is more likely affected, less commonly mural endocardium is involved • In pockets of valves	• Vegetations on the valve cusps • Less often on mural endocardium
• Sterile (no organism)	• Sterile	• Sterile	• **Non-sterile** (bacteria)
• Embolisation is uncommon	• Embolisation is common	• Embolisation is uncommon	• Embolisation is **very common** (max chances)
• In rheumatic heart disease	• In cancers (like M3-AML, pancreatic cancer), deep vein thrombosis, Trosseau syndrome	• In SLE	• In infective endocarditis

The most frequent causes of the functional valvular lesions

- *Aortic stenosis*: *Calcification* of anatomically normal and *congenitally bicuspid aortic valves*
- *Aortic regurgitation*: Dilation of the ascending aorta due to *hypertension* and *aging*
- *Mitral stenosis*: **Rheumatic heart disease**
- *Mitral regurgitation*: **Myxomatous degeneration** (mitral valve prolapse).

BARLOW SYNDROME

- It is more common in **females**[Q]
- In this valvular abnormality, one or both mitral leaflets are "floppy" and *prolapse*, or balloon back into the left atrium during systole. This gives rise to the mid systolic click.
- Most of the patients are usually **asymptomatic**[Q]
- The condition is discovered only *on routine examination*[Q] by the presence of a *midsystolic click*[Q] as an incidental finding on physical examination.
- In those cases where mitral regurgitation occurs, there is a late systolic or sometimes holosystolic murmur
- Some patients may present with *chest pain mimicking angina, dyspnea, and fatigue* or, *psychiatric manifestations, such as depression, anxiety reactions, and personality disorders*
- *Microscopically*, The characteristic anatomic change in myxomatous degeneration is intercordal ballooning (hooding) of complete or portions of the mitral leaflets. The affected leaflets are often enlarged, redundant, thick, and rubbery. The tendinous cords are elongated, thinned, and occasionally ruptured.
- **Annular dilation** is a characteristic association(this finding is *rare in other causes of mitral insufficiency)*
- Mitral valve prolapse is defined and revealed by **echocardiography**[Q]
- The risk of complications like *Infective endocarditis, Mitral insufficiency, Stroke or other systemic infarct and Arrhythmias* is higher in men, older patients, and those with either arrhythmias or some mitral regurgitation, as evidenced by holosystolic murmurs and left-sided chamber enlargement.

ISCHEMIC HEART DISEASE

Ischemia of the heart is a result of imbalance between the perfusion and demand of the heart for oxygenated blood. Atherosclerotic narrowing resulting in coronary arterial obstruction is the cause of ischemic heart disease in almost 90% of the patients.

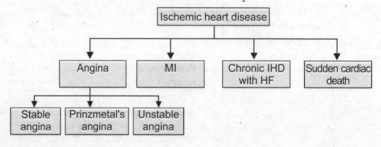

Sudden Cardiac Death

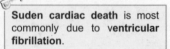

Suden cardiac death is most commonly due to **ventricular fibrillation**.

It is defined as the death of an individual *within 1 hour* of onset of symptoms. It is *most commonly due to ventricular fibrillation.*

In case of coronary vessel occlusion leading to ischemia, there is physiological compensatory vasodilation resulting in augmentation of coronary blood flow. When atherosclerotic obstruction is 75% or greater, exercise induces symptoms of ischemia and if stenosis is more than 90%, symptoms occur even at rest. The initiating event in most of these patients is disruption of partially stenosing plaque with ulceration, rupture of plaque or hemorrhage into the atheroma.

Stable Angina

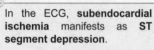
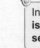

In the ECG, **subendocardial ischemia** manifests as **ST segment depression**.

Stable angina occurs when the myocardial oxygen demand is more than the supply. It takes place when the **coronary artery is occluded >75%**. Stable angina is characterized by pain on exertion which is relieved on taking rest or taking vasodilators like nitrates. There is neither any plaque disruption nor any plaque associated thrombus. ECG changes include ST segment depression and T wave inversion (subendocardial ischemia of the left ventricle).

Prinzmetal or Variant Angina

It is an episodic angina due to coronary artery spasm resulting in pain at rest. It is characterized by ST segment elevation on the ECG (due to transmural ischemia).

Unstable or Crescendo Angina

It is induced by atherosclerotic plaque disruption with superimposed partial thrombosis or vasospasm or both of them. The pain occurs with increasing frequency and for a longer duration and is characteristically precipitated by progressively less exertion.

> In the ECG, **transmural ischemia** manifests as **ST segment elevation**.

Myocardial Infarction (MI)

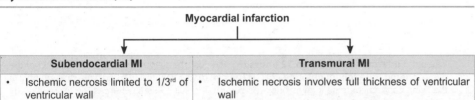

Subendocardial MI	Transmural MI
• Ischemic necrosis limited to 1/3rd of ventricular wall • Caused by incomplete coronary artery occlusion.	• Ischemic necrosis involves full thickness of ventricular wall • Caused by severe coronary atherosclerosis, with acute plaque rupture and superimoposed occlusive thrombus.

Pathogenesis of MI

Changes in atheromatous plaque (hemorrhage/ulceration/ruputre)
↓
Exposure of underlying collagen and platelet aggregation
↓
Platelets release mediators which cause vasospasm
↓
Activation of extrinsic clotting pathway and increased thrombus formation
↓
Complete occlusion of coronary vessel by thrombus

> *Concept*
>
> The main difference between angina and the MI is elevation of cardiac enzymes in the latter which is not seen usually with angina. In one third of the patients, angina may be associated with elevation of cardiac enzymes.

Myocardial Response

Feature	Time
Cessation of aerobic respiration or onset of ATP depletion	Seconds
Loss of contractility	<2 min
ATP reduced to 50% of normal	10 min
ATP reduced to 10% of normal	40 min
Irreversible cell injury	20-40 min
Microvascular injury	>1 hr

Evolution of Morphological Changes in MI

Time	Gross	Light Microscopy
Reversible injury		
0-30 min.	None	None
Irreversible injury		
30 min to 4 hr.	None	Waviness of fibers at border (earliest change)
4-12 hr.	Occasional dark mottling	Beginning of coagulative necrosis, edema and hemorrhage
12-24 hr.	Dark mottling	Ongoing coagulative necrosis, marginal contraction band necrosis, beginning of neutrophilic infiltration

> The **neutrophils** are present between **48-72 hours** but **after 72 hours, the macrophages predominate** and cause early phagocytosis.

Time	Gross	Light Microscopy
1-3 days	Mottling with yellow tan infarct center.	Coagulation necrosis, interstitial neutrophilic infiltrate
3-7 days	Hyperemic borders, central yellow tan softening	Beginning of disintegration with dying neutrophils, early phagocytosis by macrophages
7-10 days	Maximum yellow tan and soft depressed red-tan margin	Early formation of fibrovascular granulation tissue at margins
10-14 days	Red gray depressed infarct borders	Well established granulation tissue and collagen deposition
2-8 weeks	Gray-white scar progressive from border towards infarct core	Collagen deposition, ↓ Cellularity
> 2 months	Scarring complete	Dense collagenous scar

Note:
- When the **infarcts** are **less than 12 hours** old, they can be diagnosed only with the help of the dye **triphenyl tetrazolium chloride** (TTC). The dye reacts with the LDH enzyme present only in the living cardiac fibers so it gives brick-red color to the living tissue whereas the tissue already undergone **infarction shows the unstained pale zone**.
- In the case of the infarction being modified by **reperfusion**, the characteristic, microscopic feature is the presence of **necrosis with contraction band** (in irreversible injured myocytes, the increased calcium ions cause hypercontraction of the sarcomeres).

Diagnosis of MI

MI should be suspected in any patient developing severe chest pain, rapid weak pulse, sweating, dyspnea and edema. Infact, *rapid pulse is the first sign* and *dyspnea is the first symptom of acute MI*. The ECG shows the *ST segment elevation* in *acute MI* whereas '**Q' wave** indicates **old MI**.

Laboratory investigations show nonspecific markers like increased ESR, leukocytosis and elevated C-reactive protein. The specific markers include:

Enzyme	Initiation of rise	Peak	Return to baseline
CK-MB	2-4 hours	24 hours	48-72 hours
Troponin T and I (TnT, TnI)	2-4 hours	48 hours	7-10 days
AST/SGOT	In 12 hours	48 hours	4-5 days
LDH	24 hours	3-6 days	2 weeks

IMPORTANT POINTS ABOUT THE CARDIAC ENZYMES

Troponin T and Troponin I

These are the proteins that mediate calcium mediated contraction of the cardiac and the skeletal muscles. They are very specific for MI. Troponin I is more important than troponin T (remember, I for Important). If the patient has another MI (due to reinfarction within 1 week), these enzymes cannot be used for diagnosis of reinfarction because their levels remain elevated for a long time from the first attack. In that condition, we prefer an enzyme elevated for a short duration.

Creatine kinase (CK)

It is an alternative to troponin measurement. It has got 3 isoforms:
- CK-MM- Present in the skeletal muscle and heart
- CK-MB- Present in the myocardium and a small amount in skeletal muscle
- CK-BB –Present in the brain, lung and other tissues.

Elevation of the CK-MB isoforms is seen in MI. Any absence of elevation of CK-MB in the first-two days excludes the diagnosis of MI. This is the *enzyme of choice for diagnosing reinfarction*.

Myoglobin

It is a small monomer with a rapid rise and fall in serum (has a narrow window). It is the earliest enzyme to increase after MI.

MI is the leading cause of death in *diabetes mellitus*. Diabetics have '**silent MI**'.

Sequence of elevated enzymes after MI (Time to CALL emergency)
Time to   Troponin
C   CK-MB
A   AST
L   LDH1

Myoglobin: earliest enzyme to increase after MI.

Troponin: Most **sensitive** as well as **specific** for MI.

CK-MB: enzyme of choice for diagnosing **reinfarction**.

LDH

Normally, serum LDH2 is greater than LDH1 but in MI, LDH1 is more than LDH2. This is called "flipping of LDH ratio".

COMPLICATIONS OF MI

- **Contractile dysfunction** resulting in cardiogenic shock.
- **Arrhythmia-** *Ventricular fibrillation* is the most common arrhythmia *within one hour* whereas *supraventricular tachycardia* is the most common arrhythmia *after one hour* of MI.
- **Cardiac rupture syndrome:** *Rupture of ventricular free wall* is the most common cardiac rupture syndrome. It results in cardiac tamponade. The *anterolateral wall at the midventricular level* is the most common site for postinfarction free wall rupture. It is most frequent *3 to 7 days after* MI. The rupture of ventricular septum leads to formation of left to right shunt. The rupture of papillary muscles can cause mitral regurgitation.
- **Pericarditis-** It is the epicardial manifestation of the underlying myocardial injury and is also known as Dressler syndrome or post MI syndrome. It is an autoimmune reaction, which takes place around 2-3 weeks after a transmural MI. though it has been reported to occur even after 48 hrs. It is associated with pleural effusion, pleuritic chest pain and pericardial effusion.
- Right ventricular infarction.
- **Ventricular aneurysm:** This may contribute to thromboembolism also
- **Papillary muscle dysfunction:** This leads to post infarct mitral regurgitation.

> Dressler syndrome is treated with the help of **NSAIDs** with/without the use of **steroids**.

> *Concept*
>
> Rupture of the left ventricle, a complication of acute myocardial infarction, usually occurs when *the necrotic area has the least tensile strength, about 4 to 7 days after an infarction*, when repair is just beginning.

CARDIAC TUMORS

Myxoma

Myxomas are the most common primary tumor of the heart in adults. Though they may arise in any cavity of the heart but nearly *90% are located in the atria*, with a left-to-right ratio of approximately 4:1 *(atrial myxomas)*. The major clinical manifestations are due to valvular *"ball-valve" obstruction*, embolization, or a syndrome of constitutional symptoms, such as fever and malaise the latter most commonly due to the effect of interleukin-6.

Approximately 10% of patients with myxoma have a *familial cardiac myxoma syndrome* (known as *Carney syndrome*) characterized by autosomal dominant transmission, multiple cardiac and often extracardiac (e.g. skin) myxomas, spotty pigmentation, and endocrine overactivity. The familial form is associated with *mutation of the gene PRKAR1 on chromosome 17* (a tumor suppressor gene).

The tumors are almost always single. The region of the **fossa ovalis in the atrial septum is the favored site of origin.** Histologically, myxomas are composed of stellate or globular myxoma ("lepidic") cells, endothelial cells, smooth muscle cells, and undifferentiated cells embedded within an abundant acid mucopolysaccharide ground substance and covered on the surface by endothelium.

> The *most common cardiac tumor* is the *secondaries or metastasis*.

> The most common **primary** cardiac tumor in the **adults** is the **myxoma**.

Rhabdomyoma

Rhabdomyomas are the most frequent primary benign tumor of the heart in infants and children. They are actually hamartomas or malformations rather than true neoplasms. Cardiac rhabdomyoma is associated with **tuberous sclerosis** due to defect in the TSCI or TSC2 tumor suppressor gene. The TSC proteins stimulate the cell growth and are involved in myocyte overgrowth.

Rhabdomyomas are generally small, gray-white myocardial masses protruding into the ventricular chambers. Histologically they are composed of large, rounded, or polygonal cells containing numerous glycogen-laden vacuoles separated by strands of cytoplasm running from the plasma membrane to the more or less centrally located nucleus, the so-called **spider cells**.

> The most common **cardiac tumor** in the **children** is the **rhabdomyoma**.

BLOOD VESSELS

The blood vessels are responsible for the transport of blood in the circulation from the heart to the various organs and back to the heart.

The histological layers which are seen in a blood vessel (particularly arteries) are:
1. Tunica intima (Innermost layer)
2. Internal elastic lamina
3. Tunica media (Middle layer)
4. External elastic lamina
5. Tunica adventitia (Outermost layer)

The outer half of the tunica media and the whole of tunica adventitia are supplied by *vasa vasorum* whereas the other inner layers of the blood vessel get their nourishment by diffusion.

Types of blood vessels in the circulatory system and their important properties

Artery	Elastic arteries - Tunica media is rich in elastin fibers e.g. Aorta and its large branches Muscular arteries - Tunica media is rich in smooth muscle cells e.g. coronary and renal arteries^Q
Arteriole	Principle site of resistance to blood flow, so called *Resistance vessels*
Capillaries	Have maximum cross-sectional surface area^Q
Venules	Most important vessel involved in inflammation^Q
Vein	Maximum blood volume present in the veins^Q

Any injury/denudation of endothelial cells stimulate thrombosis and smooth muscle cell proliferation. The normal blood vessels particularly the arteries have an elastic recoil property referred to as the **'Windkessel effect'**. This effect is responsible for maintaining the blood flow inside the vessels during the diastolic phase of cardiac contraction. **'Sclerosis"** means loss of elasticity of vessels commonly associated with thickening. It may be of the following types:

1. **Arteriolosclerosis -** It affects small arteries and arterioles, it can be of the following types:

Hyaline arteriolosclerosis
• Pink, hyaline thickening of arteriolar walls.
• Seen in elderly, more commonly in benign hypertension, *diabetes mellitus (DM) and benign nephrosclerosis.*
Hyperplastic arteriolosclerosis
• 'Onion skinning' or concentric thickening of the arteriolar wall seen in malignant hypertension.
• Fibrinoid necrosis/necrotizing arteriolitis (inflammatory cells in vessel wall particularly in kidney)

2. **Monckeberg's medial calcific stenosis**
   – Seen is muscular arteries of people > 50 years of age.
   – Associated with *dystrophic calcification*^{Q} and is asymptomatic.

3. **Atherosclerosis**
   It is characterized by deposition of atheroma/fibrofatty plaque consisting of raised focal lesion. Plaque is present within the **intima**, has a core of lipid (cholesterol and cholesterol esters) and a covering of fibrous cap.

The histopathology shows:
1. Fibrous cap - Consists of smooth muscle cells, macrophages and foam cells.
2. 'Shoulder' - Cellular area around cap having macrophages, smooth muscle cells and T lymphocytes.
3. Necrotic core - Debris of dead cells, foam cells and cholesterol clefts.

Risk factors for atherosclerosis (Mnemonic: Atherosclerosis)

A -	**A**ge (↑ with age)
T -	**T**ype 'A' personality
H -	**H**yperhomocysteinemia (corrected by adequate folic acid and vitamin B$_{12}$ in diet)
E -	**E**xtra lipids (Hyperlipidemia); **E**xtra BP (hypertension); **E**xtra sugar (DM)

Concept

Endothelial cells contain Weibel Palade Bodies having von Willebrand factor and are identified by antibodies to CD31, CD34 and vWF.

Windkessel effect is the **elastic recoil property** of the blood vessels.

Coronary circulation is an example of **autoregulatory circulation**.

R -	Reduced physical activity
O -	Obesity
S -	Sex (More common in males, females in pre-menopausal age group are protected)
C -	CMV; Chlamydia infection; Cigarette smoking
L -	Lipoprotein 'A'

Pathogenesis

It is best explained by the **'Response to Injury Hypothesis'**[Q]

According to this hypothesis, chronic endothelial injury results in increased permeability, leukocyte adhesion and thrombotic potential. This is associated with accumulation of lipoproteins (*mainly LDL*)[Q] followed by oxidation of lipoproteins in the vessel wall. The blood monocytes initially adhere to the endothelium followed by their transformation into macrophages and foam cells inside the intima along with adhesion of platelets. The activated platelets release factors causing migration of smooth muscle cells from the media to intima and their proliferation along with release of proteoglycans and collagen. This results in enhanced accumulation of lipids. In advanced atheroma, the smooth muscle cells may undergo apoptosis and so, smooth muscle cell paucity may be observed.

Foam cells are formed because oxidized LDL is ingested by the scavenger receptors present on the macrophages and smooth muscle cells both intracellularly as well as extracellularly.

Natural History of Atherosclerosis

American Heart Association classification of human atherosclerosis:

Type	Gross	Microscopy
Clinically silent		
Type I	Fatty dot (initial lesion)	Isolated macrophage; foam cell
Type II	Fatty streak	Intracellular lipid accumulation
Type III	Intermediate lesion	Type II change + small extracellular lipid pool

Clinically silent or overt		
Type IV	Atheroma lesion	Type II + core of extracellular lipids
Type V	Fibroatheroma	Lipid core and fibrotic layer
Type VI	Complicated lesion	Surface defect, Hemorrhage and thrombus

FATTY STREAK

- *It is the earliest lesion of atherosclerosis and is composed of lipid filled foam cells. It begins as yellow flat spots less than 1 mm which gradually progress to atheroma formation.*

Significance of involved blood vessels in atherosclerosis

Abdominal Aorta	- Most common site of atherosclerotic aneurysm in body
Coronary Arteries	- Left Anterior Descending is MC coronary artery involved[Q]
Poplitial Artery	- MC peripheral vessel showing aneurysm formation[Q]
Descending Thoracic Aorta	
Internal carotid artery	
Circle of Willis	

Significance of complications of Atherosclerosis

- Aneurysm: Due to weakness of the tunica media…
- Calcification: Dystrophic calcification is seen
- Ulceration: Increases thrombus formation
- Thrombosis: Most feared complication
- Embolism: Erosion of athermanous plaque

Concept

Lipoprotein a, or Lp(a), is an altered form of LDL that contains the apolipoprotein B-100 portion of LDL linked to apolipoprotein A. It has structural similarity to plasminogen. So, it **competes with plasminogen** in clots decreasing the latter's ability to form plasmin and clear clots. Increased Lp(a) levels are associated with a higher risk of coronary and cerebrovascular disease, independent of total cholesterol or LDL levels.

Foam cells are lipid laden Smooth muscles cells/Tissue macrophages or Blood monocytes.

Leriche syndrome is **aortoiliac occlusive disease** due to atherosclerotic occlusion affecting the bifurcation of the abdominal aorta as it transitions into the common iliac arteries. It is characterised by: **buttock claudication** plus **sexual impotence** along with **reduced femoral pulses**.

Fatty streak is the **earliest lesion of atherosclerosis**.

Involvement of blood vessels affected in atherosclerosis in descending order: **ACP** of **D**elhi Traffic is **C**ute:

Abdominal Aorta
Coronary Arteries
Poplitial Artery
Descending Thoracic Aorta
Internal carotid artery
Circle of Willis

Cardiovascular System

ANEURYSM

A localized abnormal dilation of a blood vessel or the wall of the heart is called aneurysm. It is of two types:

1. **True aneurysm:** Involves intact attenuated arterial wall or thinned ventricular wall of the heart. The common causes include A*therosclerosis, syphilis and post MI ventricular aneurysms.*
2. **False/Pseudo- aneurysm:** It is characterised by a breach in the vascular wall leading to extravascular hematoma communicating with intravascular space. The two most common causes of pseudoaneurysm are *post MI rupture* and *leakage at the site of vascular anastomosis.*

Causes of True Aneurysm in Aorta

1. Atherosclerosis	*It is the most common cause of true aneurysm in aorta *The most commonly affected vessel is the abdominal aorta (below the origin of renal artery and above bifurcation into common iliac artery).
2. Syphilis	*The thoracic aorta is involved in tertiary stage of syphilis *Endarteritis of vasa vasorum results in patchy ischemia of tunica media. This is responsible for the often seen **"tree barking" appearance of the thoracic aorta**. *Aortic valve insufficiency can also occur which may result in cardiac hypertrophy. The increase in the size of heart is called as **cor bovinum**/cow heart.
3. Other causes	Trauma; infection (mycotic aneurysm; mostly due to Salmonella gastroenteritis) and systemic disease (vasculitis)

Other important points about different causes of aneurysms

- Cystic medial necrosis is characterized by weakness due to media due to degeneration of the tunica media and it affects the proximal aorta.
- Syphilitic aneurysms affect ascending aorta or aortic arch
- Tuberculous aneurysms affect the thoracic aorta.
- Traumatic aneurysms affect descending thoracic aorta just below the site of insertion of ligamentum arteriosum.

The inherited causes of aneurysm and their causes are as follows (Robbins 8th/506-7):

- **Marfan's syndrome**: defective synthesis of the protein fibrillin
- **Ehlers-Danlos syndrome**: defect in collagen type III
- **Loeys Dietz syndrome**: defect in elastin and collagen types I and III due to mutation in TGF-β receptor.

AORTIC DISSECTION

It occurs when blood splays apart the laminar planes of the media with the formation of blood-filled channel within the aortic wall. It is mostly seen in men in the age group of 40-60 years (with antecedent hypertension) and uncommonly in younger individuals with connective tissue disease (Marfan's syndrome). Medial degeneration is a characteristic pre-existing lesion in most of the patients.

Dissection is classified into two types:

1. Type A - Involves ascending aorta with/without descending aorta. It is more common and is more dangerous.
2. Type B - Does not involve ascending aorta but lesion begins distal to *subclavian artery*.

VASCULITIS

The inflammation of the vessel wall is called vasculitis. It may be classified on the basis of pathogenesis or on the basis of size of the involved vessel.

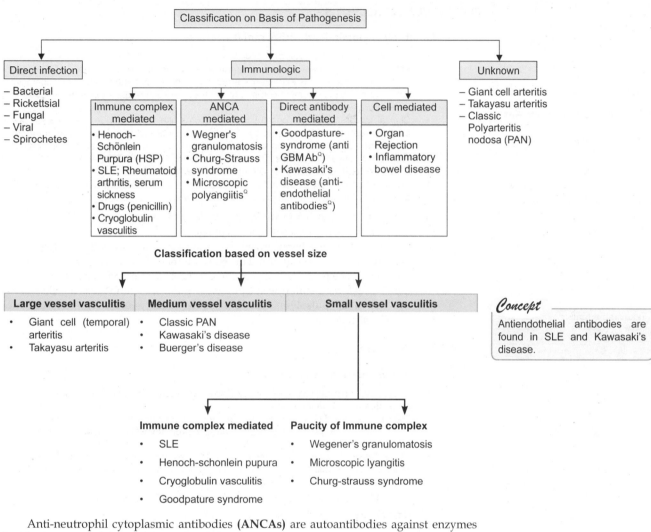

Classification on Basis of Pathogenesis

Direct infection
– Bacterial
– Rickettsial
– Fungal
– Viral
– Spirochetes

Immunologic

Immune complex mediated	ANCA mediated	Direct antibody mediated	Cell mediated
• Henoch-Schönlein Purpura (HSP) • SLE; Rheumatoid arthritis, serum sickness • Drugs (penicillin) • Cryoglobulin vasculitis	• Wegner's granulomatosis • Churg-Strauss syndrome • Microscopic polyangiitis^Q	• Goodpasture-syndrome (anti GBM Ab^Q) • Kawasaki's disease (anti-endothelial antibodies^Q)	• Organ Rejection • Inflammatory bowel disease

Unknown
– Giant cell arteritis
– Takayasu arteritis
– Classic Polyarteritis nodosa (PAN)

Classification based on vessel size

Large vessel vasculitis	Medium vessel vasculitis	Small vessel vasculitis
• Giant cell (temporal) arteritis • Takayasu arteritis	• Classic PAN • Kawasaki's disease • Buerger's disease	

Immune complex mediated
• SLE
• Henoch-schonlein pupura
• Cryoglobulin vasculitis
• Goodpature syndrome

Paucity of Immune complex
• Wegener's granulomatosis
• Microscopic lyangitis
• Churg-strauss syndrome

> **Concept**
> Antiendothelial antibodies are found in SLE and Kawasaki's disease.

Anti-neutrophil cytoplasmic antibodies **(ANCAs)** are autoantibodies against enzymes inside the neutrophils c-ANCA is formed against proteinase 3 whereas p-ANCA is formed against myeloperoxidase. These can be of the following types:

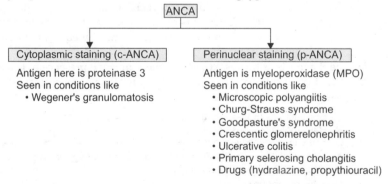

ANCA

Cytoplasmic staining (c-ANCA)
Antigen here is proteinase 3
Seen in conditions like
 • Wegener's granulomatosis

Perinuclear staining (p-ANCA)
Antigen is myeloperoxidase (MPO)
Seen in conditions like
 • Microscopic polyangiitis
 • Churg-Strauss syndrome
 • Goodpasture's syndrome
 • Crescentic glomerelonephritis
 • Ulcerative colitis
 • Primary selerosing cholangitis
 • Drugs (hydralazine, propythiouracil)

Temporal arteritis is the most common type of vasculitis in **adults**.

Lastest Information (9th Edn.)
- c-ANCA→**PR3** ANCA
- p-ANCA→**MPO** ANCA

Corticosteroids are the **drug of choice** for treatment of temporal arteritis.

The **subclavian** artery is most commonly involved vessel in Takayasu arteritis.

Glomerulonephritis and vessels of pulmonary circulation are typically not involved in PAN.

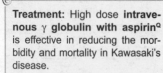

Treatment: High dose **intravenous γ globulin with aspirin**Q is effective in reducing the morbidity and mortality in Kawasaki's disease.

LARGE VESSEL VASCULITIS

1. **Giant cell (Temporal) arteritis/Cranial arteritis**
   - It is the most common type of vasculitis in adultsQ (usually >50Q years)
   - This vasculitis is characterized by granulomatous arteritis of the aorta and its major branches particularly the extracranial branches of the carotid artery. Since the superficial temporal arteryQ is the most commonly involved vessel, the giant cell arteritis is called as temporal arteritis.
   - Clinical features include constitutional symptoms like fever, fatigue, weight loss, **jaw pain**Q **(most specific symptom)**, facial pain, **localized headache**Q **(commonest symptom**; most intense along the anatomical course of the superficial temporal artery) and sudden onset of blindness (due to involvement of ophthalmic artery).
   - ***Biopsy of temporal artery***Q ***is the investigation of choice.***
   - Microscopically, there is presence of granulomatous inflammation with multinucleated giant cells and fragmentation of internal elastic lamina.

2. **Takayasu arteritis/Aortoarteritis/Aortic Arch syndrome**
   - It is seen in adult females < 50 years of age.
   - This condition is characterized by granulomatous vasculitis followed by thickening of the aortic arch and decreased lumen of the vessels arising from the aortic arch. The pulmonary, renal and coronary arteries may also be involved.
   - Clinical features include weak pulses in the upper limbs (so, the disease is also called as **pulseless disease**Q), ocular disturbances, hypertension and neurological defects.

MEDIUM VESSEL VASCULITIS

1. **Classic Polyarteritis Nodosa (PAN)**
   - It is a systemic vasculitis of medium sized muscular arteries (**no involvement of arterioles/capillaries/venules**Q).
   - The most frequently involved vessels are those of the kidney and other viscera vessels. The vessels of the **pulmonary circulation**Q **are typically NOT involved.**

   - Characteristic feature of this disease is sharp segmental lesions showing transmural inflammation of vessel wall accompanied by fibrinoid necrosis and existence of **all stages of inflammation in the same vessel.**
   - 30% patients have association with *Hepatitis B antigen*Q in their serum.
   - **No glomerulonephritis**Q is seen.
   - It is the commonest cause of **mononeuritis multiplex**Q.

2. **Kawasaki's disease (Mucocutaneous Lymph Node Syndrome)**
   - It is the vasculitis affecting children **< 5 years**Q of age. So, it was designated as *infantile polyarteritis*Q earlier. It is characterized by fever, conjunctivitis and oral erythema, skin rash often with desquamation, erythema of palms and soles and cervical lymphadenopathy.
   - For the diagnosis of Kawasaki disease, there must be presence of **fever**Q (most important constitutional symtpom) for greater than 5 days plus any 4 of the following:

     - **C - C**onjunctivitis (**non-exudative**Q; non purulent conjunctivitis)
     - **R - R**ash (polymorphous non-vesicular)
     - **E - E**dema (or erythema of hands or feet)
     - **A - A**denopathy (**cervical**Q, **often unilateral**Q and **non suppurative**Q)
     - **M - M**ucosal involvement (erythema or fissures or crusting at times referred as **strawberry tongue**Q)

   - It is the most important cause of acquired heart disease in children in USA. It may present with myocardial infarctionQ in children. It is having the presence of *anti-endothelial cell antibodies*Q. There is typically intimal proliferation and mononuclear infiltration of vessel wall. The patients also have elevated platelet count in this condition.

SMALL VESSEL VASCULITIS

1. **Microscopic Polyarteritis/Microscopic Polyangiitis/Leukocytoclastic Vasculitis**
   – Necrotizing vasculitis affecting arterioles/capillaries/venules in which **all lesions are of the same age**.
   – **Granulomatous inflammation** is **absent**[Q]
   – *Necrotizing glomerulonephritis* and capillaritis are common.
   – Fibrinoid necrosis associated with infiltration of neutrophils which become fragmented (*leukocytoclasia*).

2. **Henoch-Schönlein purpura (HSP)/Anaphylactoid purpura**[Q]
   – It is the **commonest vasculitis in childen**[Q].
   – This is a vasculitis with **IgA**[Q] deposits affecting small vessels like arterioles, capillaries and venules of the skin, gut and glomeruli and commonly associated with arthralgia.
   – Clinical features include **palpable purpura (due to vasculitis** and not reduced platelet count)[Q], **colicky abdominal pain**[Q], arthralgia in multiple joints and glomerulonephritis.
   – It is caused due to immune complex deposition but **complement levels are usually normal**[Q].

3. **Hypersensitivity vasculitis/Cutaneous vasculitis**
   - Defined as inflammation of the blood vessels of the dermis.
   - Also called as **hypersensitivity vasculitis/cutaneous leukocytoclastic angiitis**.
   - Microscopic features include presence of vasculitis of small vessels characterized by a *leukocytoclasis*[Q] (refers to the nuclear debris remaining from the neutrophils that have infiltrated in and around the vessels during the acute stages).
   - Hallmark clinical feature is **skin involvement** typically appearing as **palpable purpura**[Q] appearing on most commonly lower limbs
   - Diagnosis is best made with **biopsy** showing vasculitis.
   - Removal of offending agent (if any) and steroids help most of the patients.

4. **Churg-Strauss syndrome (Allergic granulomatosis and angiitis)**
   – Characteristically have necrotizing vasculitis accompanied by granulomas with eosinophilic necrosis.
   – p-ANCA present in 50% of patients.
   – Strong association with allergic rhinitis, bronchial asthma and eosinophilia.
   – Principal cause of death includes coronary arteritis and myocarditis.

5. **Wegener's granulomatosis (Granulomatosis with polyangitis)**
   Necrotizing vasculitis which is characterized by **triad of**
   1. Acute necrotizing *granulomas of either upper* (more commonly) *or lower respiratory tract or both.*
   2. *Focal necrotizing or granulomatous vasculitis* most commonly affecting lungs and upper airways.
   3. *Renal involvement* in the form of focal necrotizing, often crescentic glomerulonephritis.
   - Clinical features include fever, weight loss, otitis media, nasal septal perforation[Q], strawberry gums[Q], cough, hemoptyis, **palpable purpura**[Q], joint pain and ocular features (uveitis, conjunctivitis)
   - Investigations show serum **c-ANCA**[Q] positivity, **cavitatory lesions**[Q] in the chest X ray and red cell casts (indicative of glomerulonephritis) in the urine.

RAYNAUD'S PHENOMENON

Raynaud's disease or Primary Raynaud's phenomenon is seen in young females. It is characterized by intense vasospasm of *small vessels* in the digits of hands and feet induced by cold and emotional stimuli (so, *pulses are NOT affected*).
   • Characteristic sequence of color change is

---

p-ANCA is present in Microscopic Polyangiitis but is **NOT** seen with **PAN**.

Palpable purpura in **HSP** is due to **vasculitis** and not thrombocytopenia.

Lastest Information (9th Edn.) Wegener's granulomatosis is now called as **granulomatosis with polyangitis**

Concept

Limited Wegener's granulomatosis is characterized by **only respiratory tract** involvement without any renal involvement.

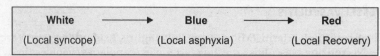

White	→	Blue	→	Red
(Local syncope)		(Local asphyxia)		(Local Recovery)

> Systemic sclerosis is the commonest cause of secondary Raynaud's phenomenon.

- Structural changes are absent *except* in later course when thickening of intima is seen.

Secondary Raynaud's phenomenon is associated with conditions like **systemic sclerosis**[Q] (commonest cause), SLE, atherosclerosis and Buerger's disease. It usually affects people of age >30 years.

Also Know

- **Secondary Raynaud's phenomenon** patients are **older in age** and have more severe symptoms and complications
- More commonly have dilatation of the capillary bed at the base of the fingernails.
- **Index and middle fingers** are more sensitive to attacks. **Thumb** is **least sensitive**.

Buerger's disease (Thromboangiitis obliterans)

> Segmental thrombosing vasculitis often extends into contiguous veins and nerves is a characteristic features of Buerger's disease.

- It is usually seen among **heavy cigarette smokers**.
- Onset is **before age 35**
- It is associated with **hypersensitivity to intradermal injections of tobacco** extracts.
- Microscopic examination demonstrates **segmental thrombosing vasculitis often extends into contiguous veins and nerves** (a *feature rarely seen in other types of vasculitis*), encasing them in fibrous tissue.
- Thrombus contains *microabscess with granulomatous inflammation*.[Q]
- This patient has distal lower extremity vascular insufficiency which may present as Calf, foot or hand intermittent claudication, superficial nodular phlebitis and cold sensitivity (Raynaud's phenomenon). Severe distal pain even at rest can result and may be due to neural involvement. Later complications include ulcerations and gangrene of the toes feet or fingers.
- **Treatment** includes **smoking cessation**, drugs (peripheral vasodilators) and may even require surgery.

VASCULAR TUMORS

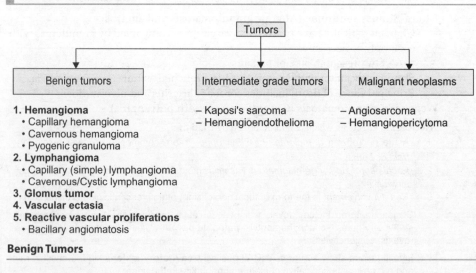

> **Strawberry gums** are seen in **Wegener's granulomatosis**.

> **Strawberry tongue** is seen in **Kawasaki disease**.

> **Strawberry hemangioma** is a type of **capillary hemagioma**.

Benign Tumors

Hemangioma

1. **Capillary hemangioma**

   - It is the most common type of vascular tumor which occurs in skin, mucus membrane and viscera.
   - "Strawberry" type of capillary hemangioma (also called as juvenile hemangioma) is very common, growing rapidly in the first few months[Q] and regresses by age 7[Q] in newborns. The child is **normal**[Q] **at birth** in almost 90% of cases.
   - Histologically, they are lobulated unencapsulated aggregates of closely packed, thin walled capillaries which are blood filled and lined by a flattened endothelium.

2. **Cavernous hemangioma**
   - It is less common than capillary hemangioma with same age and anatomic distribution. It more frequently involves deep structures as it shows no tendency to regress. So, it usually requires surgery.
   - Morphologically, Cavernous hemangiomas are made up of large, cavernous vascular spaces in which intravascular thrombosis and dystrophic calcification is common.
   - They may be life-threatening as in von Hippel Lindau disease where they occur in cerebellum, brainstem and the eye.

3. **Pyogenic granuloma**
   It is a polypoid form of capillary hemangioma seen attached by a stalk to skin or oral mucosa. It is associated with edema and inflammatory cells.
   Granuloma gravidarum is present in the gingiva of pregnant women and it regresses after delivery.

> **Cavernous lymphangioma** occurs in **Turner's syndrome** at the neck region.

LYMPHANGIOMA

1. **Cavernous lymphangioma** (also called as **cystic hygroma**)
   - This is present in the neck region of the children.
   - Made up of dilated, cystic lymphatic spaces lined by endothelial cells.
   - Lesions are non-encapsulated, so, removal is difficult.

2. **Capillary Lymphangioma**
   It is a lesion composed of small lymphatic channels occurring subcutaneously in the head and neck region and in the axilla.

Concept

Capillary lymphangioma is distinguished from the capillary channels only by the absence of blood cells.

GLOMUS TUMOR (GLOMANGIOMA)

- Benign tumor arising from the smooth muscle cells of the glomus body which is an arteriovenous anastomosis involved in thermoregulation.
- Most commonly present in the distal portion of the digits (under fingernails).
- Histologically, there is presence of branching vascular channels and stroma containing nests/aggregates of glomus cells arranged around vessels.

INTERMEDIATE/BORDERLINE TUMORS

Kaposi's Sarcoma (KS)

It is caused by **KS Herpes virus** or **Human herpes virus 8** (HHV8) and has the following 4 forms:

Type of Kaposi sarcoma	Association with HIV	Chief affected organs
Classic/Chronic/European KS	Absent	Skin plaques and nodules
African/Endemic KS	Absent	No skin lesions; lymphadenopathy present
Transplant associated/ Immunosuppression-associated KS	Absent	Lymph nodes, mucosa and visceral organs
Epidemic/AIDS associated KS	**Present**[Q]	Lymph nodes and viscera involved

The morphology is characterized by three stages:
1. Patch stage
2. Plaque stage
3. Nodular stage – Often accompanied by involvement of lymph nodes and of viscera particularly in African and AIDS-associated disease.

Hepatic **angiosarcoma** is associated with carcinogens including **arsenic**, **thorotrast** (a radioactive contrast) and **polyvinyl chloride** (PVC; a plastic).

MALIGNANT TUMORS

Angiosarcoma

- Malignant endothelial cell neoplasm most commonly seen in skin, soft tissue, breast and liver.
- May also arise from dilated lymphatic vessels (lymphangiosarcoma).
- Endothelial cell origin is demonstrated by staining for CD31, CD34 or vWF.

Hemangiopericytoma

- Tumor derived from pericytes which are the cells present along the capillaries and venules.
- These tumors most commonly arise from pelvic retroperitoneum or the lower limbs (particularly thighs).
- Capillaries are arranged in *'fish-hook pattern'* and *silver stain* is used for diagnosing this condition.

Quick review of superior vena cava and inferior vena cava syndromes

Syndromes	Associated Cancers	Clinical features
Superior Vena Cava (SVC) syndrome	• Bronchogenic cancer[Q] • Mediastinal lymphoma[Q]	• Dilation of the veins of the head, neck and arms • Cyanosis • Respiratory distress
Inferior Vena Cava (IVC) syndrome	• Renal cell carcinoma[Q] • Hepatocellular carcinoma[Q]	• Lower limb edema • Dilation of the superficial collateral veins of the lower abdomen • Massive proteinuria (if renal vein is involved)

MULTIPLE CHOICE QUESTIONS

HEART FAILURE, RHEUMATIC HEART DISEASE, ENDOCARDITIS

1. **A young female patient came for routine examination. On examination a mid systolic click was found. There is no history of rheumatic heart disease. The histopathological examination is most likely to show which of the following?** *(AIIMS May 2012)*
   - (a) Myxomatous degeneration and prolapsed of the mitral valve
   - (b) Fibrinous deposition on the tip of papillary muscle
   - (c) Rupture of chordae tendinae
   - (d) Aschoff nodule on the mitral valve

2. **Least chances of infective endocarditis is associated with** *(AI India 2012)*
   - (a) Mild MS
   - (b) Mild MR
   - (c) Small ASD
   - (d) Small VSD

3. **A 45 yrs old male had severe chest pain and was admitted to the hospital with a diagnosis of acute myocardial infarction. Four days later he died and autopsy showed transmural coagulative necrosis. Which of the following microscopic features will be seen on further examination?** *(AIIMS May 2011)*
   - (a) Fibroblasts and collagen
   - (b) Granulation tissue
   - (c) Neutrophilic infiltration surrounding coagulative necrosis
   - (d) Granulomatous inflammation

4. **Which one of the following is not included as major criteria in Jones criteria?** *(AIIMS Nov. 2010)*
   - (a) Pancarditis
   - (b) Arthritis
   - (c) Subcutaneous nodules
   - (d) Elevated ESR

5. **The mechanism of the development of Acute Rheumatic Fever is which of the following?** *(AIIMS May 2010)*
   - (a) Cross reactivity with exogenous antigen
   - (b) Innocent bystander effect
   - (c) Due to toxin secretion by streptococci
   - (d) Release of pyrogenic cytokines

6. **Cardiac involvement in carcinoid syndrome is characterized by:** *(AI 2010)*
   - (a) Calcification tricuspid valve
   - (b) Intimal fibrosis of right ventricle, tricuspid and pulmonary valve.

   - (c) Involvement of the major blood vessels is commonly seen
   - (d) Equal involvement of both the sides of the heart

7. **Most friable vegetation is seen in:** *(AI 2010)*
   - (a) Infective endocarditis
   - (b) Libman Sacks endocarditis
   - (c) Rheumatic heart disease
   - (d) Rheumatoid heart disease

8. **Aschoff's nodules are seen in:** *(AI 2005)*
   - (a) Subacute bacterial endocarditis
   - (b) Libman-Sacks endocarditis
   - (c) Rheumatic carditis
   - (d) Non-bacterial thrombotic endocarditis

9. **A 10-year-old boy, Pappu, died of acute rheumatic fever. All the following can be expected at autopsy except:**
   - (a) Aschoff's nodules *(AI 2002)*
   - (b) Rupture of Chordae tendinae
   - (c) McCallum patch
   - (d) Fibrinous pericarditis

10. **NOT true about ASO titer:** *(AIIMS Nov 2009)*
    - (a) May be positive in normal people
    - (b) Major Jones' criteria
    - (c) May be negative in post streptococcal glomerulonephritis
    - (d) May not be elevated even in presence of Carditis

11. **In mitral valve prolapse syndrome, histopathology of mitral valve shows:** *(AIIMS Nov 2007)*
    - (a) Hyaline degeneration
    - (b) Elastic degeneration
    - (c) Myxomatous degeneration
    - (d) Fibrinoid necrosis

12. **Which of the following is not a complication of infective endocarditis?** *(AIIMS Nov 2003)*
    - (a) Myocardial ring abscess
    - (b) Suppurative pericarditis
    - (c) Myocardial infarction
    - (d) Focal and diffuse glomerulonephritis

13. **Aschoff bodies in Rheumatic heart disease show all of the following features, except:** *(AIIMS Nov 2002)*
    - (a) Anitschkow cells
    - (b) Epithelioid cells
    - (c) Giant cells
    - (d) Fibrinoid necrosis

14. **Rheumatic heart disease can be diagnosed on the basis of:** *(PGI Dec 2001)*
    - (a) Aschoff bodies
    - (b) Vegetations along the lines of closure of valves

(c) Endocardial involvement only
(d) Follows skin and throat infection

15. Pathognomic feature of acute rheumatic fever is:
(a) Pericarditis *(Delhi 2009 RP)*
(b) Myocarditis
(c) Mitral stenosis
(d) Aschoff's nodules

16. Vegetations on under surface of cusps are found in:
(a) Infective endocarditis *(Delhi PG-2008, P 2006)*
(b) Libman-Sacks endocarditis
(c) SABE
(d) Rheumatic fever

17. Aschoff's nodules are seen in: *(Delhi PG-2007)*
(a) Acute rheumatic fever
(b) Bacterial endocarditis
(c) Pneumoconiosis
(d) Asbestosis

18. Anitschkow cells are pathognomonic for:
(a) Acute rheumatic fever *(Delhi PG-2006)*
(b) Yellow fever
(c) Malarial spleen
(d) ITP

19. All are the causes of myocarditis except:
(a) Trichinosis *(Karnataka 2005)*
(b) Mycobacterium tuberculosis
(c) Corynebacterium diphtheriae
(d) Systemic lupus erythematosus

20. Disarrangement of myofibrils is found in:
(a) Dilated cardiomyopathy *(UP 2001)*
(b) Constrictive cardiomyopathy
(c) Fibroelastic cardiomyopathy
(d) Hypertrophic cardiomyopathy

21. Most common cause of mitral stenosis is:
(a) Rheumatic heart disease *(UP 2002)*
(b) Infective-endocarditis
(c) Diabetes mellitus
(d) Congenital

22. Calcification of aortic valve is seen in: *(UP 2003)*
(a) Hurler's syndrome
(b) Marfan's syndrome
(c) Syphilis
(d) None

23. Most common cause of left sided cardiac failure is:
(a) Myocardial infarction *(UP 2006)*
(b) Systemic hypertension
(c) Rheumatic heart disease
(d) Infective endocarditis

24. Libman-Sacks endocarditis is found in:
(a) Rheumatoid arthritis *(UP 2001, 2007)*
(b) SLE
(c) Syphilis
(d) Lymphoma

25. Chronic constrictive pericarditis is most commonly caused by: *(RJ 2000)*
(a) Staphylococcus (b) TB
(c) Viral (d) Autoimmune

26. Aschoff's bodies are seen in: *(RJ 2006) (Jharkhand 2003)*
(a) Acute rheumatic fever
(b) SLE
(c) SABE
(d) TB

27. Diagnostic feature of rheumatic fever is:
(a) Antischkow cells *(Kolkata 2001)*
(b) Aschoff's nodule
(c) MacCallum's patch
(d) Epithelioid cells

28. Rheumatoid factor is: *(Bihar 2003)*
(a) lgM directed against lgG
(b) lgE directed against lgM
(c) lgG directed against lgM
(d) None

29. Major criteria for rheumatic fever, consists of all except: *(Bihar 2004)*
(a) Pancarditis
(b) Arthritis
(c) Subcutaneous nodule
(d) Erythema nodosum

30. An 8 year old girl, Guniya had sore throat following which she developed severe joint pains. She has been diagnosed with acute rheumatic fever. Instead of recovering as expected, her condition worsened, and she died. Which of the following is the most likely cause of death?
(a) Central nervous system involvement
(b) Endocarditis
(c) Myocarditis
(d) Streptococcal sepsis

31. Infective endocarditis is known to be caused by different bacterial species. Which of the following scenarios is most consistent with infective endocarditis caused by Staphylococcus aureus?
(a) A 34-year-old female with known mitral stenosis develops low-grade fever and negative blood culture
(b) A 28-year-old male with persistently high fever with tricuspid vegetations and tricuspid regurgitation on trans-thoracic echocardiogram
(c) A 62-year-old female has persistent fever after being diagnosed with colon cancer
(d) A 64-year-old male with fever and malaise has repeatedly negative blood culture and small mitral vegetation on trans-esophageal echocardiogram

31.1. Which of the following is the feature of vegetations in Libmann Sacks endocarditis?
(a) Large and fragile
(b) Small warty along the line of closure of valve
(c) Small or medium sized on either or both sides of valve
(d) Small bland vegetations

31.2. Which type of endocarditis has vegetation on both sides of the valves ?
(a) Infective endocarditis
(b) Libman Sack's endocarditis
(c) Rheumatic fever
(d) Non bacterial thrombotic enodcarditis

31.3. Mc Callum's patch is diagnostic of:
(a) Infective endocarditis
(b) Rheumatic endocarditis
(c) Myocardial infarction
(d) Tetralogy of Fallot (ToF)

31.4. Heart failure cells are seen in which of the following organs?
(a) Kidney   (b) Heart
(c) Lungs   (d) Brain

31.5. Tigered effect in myocardium is due to:
(a) Malignant change
(b) Fat deposition
(c) Seen in rheumatic fever
(d) Associated with myocarditis

31.6. ASLO titers are used in the diagnosis of:
(a) Acute rheumatoid arthritis
(b) Acute rheumatic fever
(c) Ankylosing spondylitis
(d) Osteoarthritis

31.7. Mitral valve vegetations do not embolise usually to:
(a) Brain   (b) Liver
(c) Spleen   (d) Lung

31.8. Which of the following cardiac valves is not commonly involved in rheumatic fever?
(a) Mitral   (b) Aortic
(c) Pulmonary (d) Tricuspid

31.9. Most common heart valve involved in IV drug user is
(a) Mitral valve
(b) Aortic valve
(c) Pulmonary valve
(d) Tricuspid valve

ISCHEMIC HEART DISEASE

32. A 70-year-old male Rohan with advanced visceral cancer dies of extensive myocardial infarction. Autopsy also reveals sterile non-destructive vegetations along the mitral leaflet edges. The pathogenesis of this patient's vegetations is most similar to that of:
(a) Hypercalcemia of malignancy
(b) Distant metastases
(c) Trousseau syndrome
(d) Raynaud's phenomenon

33. A 56-years-old male presented with sudden substernal pain, impending doom and died 4 days after. On autopsy, there was a large transmural anterior wall infarction. It would be associated with:
(a) Presence of collagen and fibroblasts   *(AI 2009)*
(b) Presence of neutrophils
(c) Granulomatous inflammation
(d) Granulation tissue

34. All of the following statements regarding subendocardial infarction are true, except:
(a) These are multifocal in nature   *(AI 2006)*
(b) These often result from hypotension or shock
(c) Epicarditis is not seen
(d) These may result in aneurysm

35. A 60-year-old male presented with acute chest pain of 4 hours duration. Electrocardiographic examination revealed new Q wave with ST segment depression. He succumbed to his illness within 24 hours of admission. The heart revealed presence of a transmural hemorrhagic area over the septum and anterior wall of the left ventricle. Light microscopic examination is most likely to reveal: *(AI 2004)*
(a) Edema in between normal myofibers
(b) Necrotic myofibers with presence of neutrophils
(c) Coagulative necrosis of the myocytes with presence of granulation tissue
(d) Infiltration by histiocytes with hemosiderin laden macrophages

36. Which of the following increases the susceptibility to coronary artery disease?   *(AI 2003)*
(a) Type V hyperlipoproteinemia
(b) von Willebrand's disease
(c) Nephrotic syndrome
(d) Systemic lupus erythematosus

37. A myocardial infarct showing early granulation tissue has most likely occurred: *(AI 2002)*
(a) Less than 1 hour
(b) Within 24 hours
(c) Within 1 week
(d) Within 1 month

38. Troponin-T is a marker of: *(AIIMS May 2004)*
(a) Renal disease
(b) Muscular dystrophy
(c) Cirrhosis of liver
(d) Myocardial infarction

39. Autopsy finding after 12 hrs in a case of death due to M.I. is   *(Delhi 2010)*
(a) Caseous pecrosis
(b) Coagulative necrosis
(c) Fat necrosis
(d) Liquefactive necrosis

40. In MI with hypothyroidism, what is the marker of choice? *(Delhi PG-2008)*
    (a) LDH
    (b) CPK-MB
    (c) Aldolase
    (d) Troponin-I

41. What is the investigation for second MI after 1 week of previous MI? *(Delhi PG-2008)*
    (a) Troponin I
    (b) Troponin T
    (c) CPK-MB
    (d) LDH

42. Earliest light microscopic change in myocardial infarction is: *(UP 04, Bihar 03)*
    (a) Waviness of the fibers
    (b) Neutrophilic infiltration
    (c) Phagocytic infiltration
    (d) Coagulative necrosis

43. Most common artery involved in myocardial infarction is: *(UP 2006)*
    (a) Right coronary artery
    (b) Left coronary artery
    (c) Left anterior descending coronary artery
    (d) Left circumflex coronary artery

44. In myocardial infarction scarring completes by:
    (a) 1 day *(RJ 2000)*
    (b) 1 week
    (c) 1 month
    (d) 3 months

45. Dressler's syndrome is: *(RJ 2000)*
    (a) Viral
    (b) Bacterial
    (c) Fungal
    (d) Autoimmune

46. Heart muscle contains the isoenzymes:
    (a) MM *(Kolkata 2001)*
    (b) MB
    (c) MM and MB
    (d) BB

47. Enzyme elevated in first 2 hours of MI is:
    (a) CPK MB *(Bihar 2004)*
    (b) LDH
    (c) SGPT
    (d) Acid phosphatase

48. A 70 year old male Kulsheen presents to your OPD with epigastric pain that typically starts about 30 minutes after meals and does not respond to antacids. He lost almost 3-4 kilograms over the last few weeks because he eats less for fear of pain. His past medical history is significant for hypertension, hyperlipidemia, coronary artery bypass grafting, and right-sided carotid endarterectomy. Upper gastrointestinal endoscopy does not reveal any abnormalities. The pathophysiology of this patient's symptoms is most close to
    (a) Peptic ulcer disease
    (b) Esophageal spasm

(c) Pulmonary embolism
(d) Stable angina

49. A 60 year old man Bhadru Kalraj is discharged after being observed in the hospital for 4 days following a myocardial infarction. He returns to his normal activities, which include sedentary work only. This point in time following a myocardial infarct is noteworthy for the special danger of which of the following?
    (a) Arrhythmia
    (b) Ventricular aneurysm
    (c) Myocardial (pump) failure
    (d) Myocardial rupture

50. A 62 year-old male Sathish is admitted following an acute ST-segment elevation myocardial infarction experiences chest pain on day four of his hospitalization. He describes the pain as sharp in quality, and adds that it increases with coughing and swallowing and radiates to his neck. The blood pressure is 130/80 mmHg, pulse is 90 beats per minute temperature is 38.3°C (101°F) and respirations are 20 per minute. Which of the following is the most likely cause of this patient's chest pain?
    (a) Recurrent thrombosis of the affected coronary vessel
    (b) Thrombosis of a new coronary vessel
    (c) Pericardial inflammation overlying the necrotic segment of myocardium
    (d) Pericardial inflammation due to autoimmune reaction to necrotic tissue

51. An old man is found dead in his home. Autopsy reveals hemopericardium secondary to ventricular wall rupture. Roughly how long before his death did the man probably have a myocardial infarction?
    (a) 2 days
    (b) 7 days
    (c) 12 days
    (d) 20 days

52. 60 year-old male smoker develops severe chest pain. He is diagnosed with MI based on his electrocardiogram and serial CK-MB levels. One week later he again complains of precordial pain and develops a fever of 101.5°F. Physical examination is remarkable for a loud friction rub. Which of the following is the most likely diagnosis?
    (a) Caseous pericarditis
    (b) Fibrinous pericarditis
    (c) Hemorrhagic pericarditis
    (d) Purulent pericarditis

Most Recent Questions

52.1. 7 day old MI the most sensitive biochemical marker:
    (a) Troponin T
    (b) CPK MB
    (c) LDH
    (d) Myoglobin

52.2. Post MI day 10 which enzyme is raised:
    (a) CPK
    (b) Troponin
    (c) LDH
    (d) Myoglobin

52.3. The cells seen after 72 hours in the infarcted area in MI are:
(a) Neutrophils
(b) Lymphocytes
(c) Macrophages
(d) Monocytes

52.4. In myocardial reperfusion injury, the maximum effect is caused due to which of the following?
(a) Neutrophil
(b) Monocytes
(c) Eosinophils
(d) Free radicals

52.5. In myocardial infarctions, microscopes picture of coagulation necrosis with neutrophilic infiltration is seen after:
(a) 4-12 hr
(b) 12-24 hr
(c) 1-3 days
(d) 3-7 days

52.6. Myocarditis is most commonly caused by
(a) Influenza
(b) Measles virus
(c) Coxsackie virus
(d) Epstein barr virus

CARDIAC TUMOUR

53. Which malignancy metastasizes to heart? *(AP 2007)*
(a) Bronchial carcinoma
(b) Prostate carcinoma
(c) Breast carcinoma
(d) Wilms' tumor

Most Recent Questions

53.1. Most common benign heart tumor is:
(a) Rhabdomyoma
(b) Hemangioma
(c) Lipoma
(d) Myxoma

53.2. Most common tumour of heart is:
(a) Myxoma
(b) Rhabdomyosarcoma
(c) Fibroma
(d) Leiomyosarcoma

53.3. Atrial myxoma commonly arises from:
(a) Left ventricle
(b) Left atrium
(c) Right ventricle
(d) Right atrium

HTN, ATHEROSCLEROSIS, ANEURYSM

54. In 2 patients with atherosclerosis, one is diabetic and the other is non diabetic. In relation to the non diabetic, the diabetic patient has 100 times risk of which of the following? *(AIIMS May 2012)*
(a) MI
(b) Stroke
(c) Lower limb ischemia
(d) Vertebrobasilar insufficiency

55. ALL of the following statements regarding athero-sclerosis are true except: *(AIIMS Nov 2012)*
(a) Omega-3 fatty acid (abundant in fish oil) decrease LDL
(b) Atherosclerosis in less important in age more than 45 years age
(c) Cigarette smoking is independent risk factor for M.I
(d) C reactive protein is independent risk factor for M.I

56. Which of the following is the commonest histological finding in benign hypertension? *(AIIMS May 2011)*
(a) Proliferative end arteritits
(b) Necrotizing arteriolitis
(c) Hyaline arteriosclerosis
(d) Cystic medial necrosis

57. The presence of stroke, peripheral vascular disease and atherosclerosis is associated with which hormone?
(a) Insulin deficiency *(AI 2010)*
(b) Hyperestrogenemia
(c) Hypothyroidism
(d) Progesterone

58. Most common cause of abdominal aortic aneurysm is:
(a) Atherosclerosis *(AI 2010)*
(b) Syphilis
(c) Trauma
(d) Congenital

59. Hallmark feature of benign HTN is: *(AI 2009)*
(a) Hyaline arteriosclerosis
(b) Cystic medial necrosis
(c) Fibrinoid necrosis
(d) Hyperplastic arteriosclerosis

60. All are seen in malignant hypertension, except:
(a) Fibrinoid necrosis *(AI 2008)*
(b) Hyaline arteriosclerosis
(c) Necrotizing glomerulonephritis
(d) Hyperplastic arteriosclerosis

61. Recurrent ischemic events following thrombolysis has been pathophysiologically linked to which of the following factors: *(AI 2003)*
(a) Antibodies to thrombolytic agents
(b) Fibrinopeptide A
(c) Lipoprotein (A)
(d) Triglycerides

62. 70-year-old man has abdominal pain with mass in abdomen. Angiography reveals aneurysm of aorta. Most likely cause is: *(AIIMS Nov 2001)*
(a) Trauma
(b) Atherosclerosis
(c) Syphilis
(d) Congenital

63. In malignant hypertension hyperplastic arteriosclerosis is seen in all except: *(AIIMS May 2001)*
    (a) Heart
    (b) Kidney
    (c) Pericardial fat
    (d) Peripancreatic fat

64. CAD predisposing factors: *(PGI Dec 2002)*
    (a) Homocysteinemia
    (b) Increased lipoprotein B
    (c) Increased fibrinogen
    (d) Increased HDL
    (e) Increased plasminogen activator inhibitors

65. Features of essential hypertension: *(PGI Dec 2002)*
    (a) Concentric hypertrophy of LV
    (b) Increased heart size
    (c) Increased size of the heart muscles
    (d) Myohypertrophy
    (e) Myohyperplasia

66. In atherosclerosis, increased LDL in monocyte macrophage is due to: *(Delhi 2010)*
    (a) LDL receptors on macrophage
    (b) LDL receptors on endothelium
    (c) Lipids in LDL get auto-oxidized
    (d) All of the above

67. Which of the following is the least common site of atherosclerotic lesions? *(Delhi 2009 RP)*
    (a) Aortic bifurcation
    (b) Pulmonary arterial trunk
    (c) Common carotid artery
    (d) Middle cerebral artery

68. Vascular pathology of benign hypertension includes:
    (a) Segmental fibrinoid necrosis *(Delhi 2009 RP)*
    (b) Hyaline arteriosclerosis
    (c) Periarteritis
    (d) Loss of internal elastic lamina

69. Accelerated phase of hypertension is characterized microscopically by: *(Delhi PG-2005)*
    (a) Fibrinoid necrosis of arteriolar wall
    (b) Hyaline arteriosclerosis
    (c) Elastosis of the intima
    (d) Marked calcification of the media

70. Most common site of atherosclerotic aneurysm is:
    (a) Coronary artery *(RJ 2006)*
    (b) Renal artery
    (c) Arch of aorta
    (d) Abdominal aorta

71. Monckeberg's calcific sclerosis affects the medium sized muscular arteries by involving the structure of:
    (a) Intima *(AFMC 2000, AP 1999, 2001)*
    (b) Media
    (c) Adventitia
    (d) All of the above

72. A 52 year old male, Puneet, presents to the emergency of a tertiary care hospital with chest pain and syncope. The physician suspects a coronary pathology. Coronary arteriography demonstrates significant atherosclerotic involvement of the left anterior descending and circumflex arteries. Which of the following cells provides major proliferative stimuli for the cellular components of atherosclerotic plaques?
    (a) Neutrophils
    (b) Eosinophils
    (c) Platelets
    (d) Erythrocytes

73. Autopsy of a 14 year-old male who died in a motor vehicle accident shows many yellow spots on the inner surface of the aorta. Which of the following best describes the lesions?
    (a) They are a very uncommon finding for a patient of this age.
    (b) Their distribution closely mimics that of future atherosclerosis.
    (c) Once formed, they inevitably progress to atheromas
    (d) They show predominantly intracellular lipid accumulation.

74. Renal biopsy in an old man Hitesh demonstrates concentric, laminated thickening of arteriolar walls due to proliferation of smooth muscle cells. This process is best described by which of the following terms?
    (a) Atherosclerosis
    (b) Hyaline arteriolosclerosis
    (c) Hyperplastic arteriolosclerosis
    (d) Mönckeberg's arteriosclerosis

Most Recent Questions

74.1. Most common site of artery of atherosclerosis:
    (a) Right coronary artery
    (b) Left anterior descending coronary artery
    (c) Left circumflex artery
    (d) Diagonal branch of LAD

74.2. Malignant hypertension causes which of the following changes in the kidney?
    (a) No change in kidney
    (b) Flea bitten kidney
    (c) Irregular granular contracted kidney
    (d) Large white kidney

74.3. Cystic medical necrosis is seen in:
    (a) Marfan syndrome
    (b) Friedrichs ataxia
    (c) Down syndrome
    (d) Kawasaki disease

74.4. Most common cause of dissecting hematoma is because of:
    (a) Hypertension
    (b) Marfan syndrome
    (c) Iatrogenic
    (d) Kawasaki

74.5. Atheromatous changes of blood vessels affects early in ?
    (a) Kidney   (b) Heart
    (c) Liver   (d) Spleen

74.6. Most common cause of aortic aneurysm is:
(a) Syphilis
(b) Marfan's syndrome
(c) Atherosclerosis
(d) Congenital

74.7. Visceral aneurysm is most commonly seen in:
(a) Splenic
(b) Renal
(c) Hepatic
(d) Coronary

74.8. Medial calcification is seen in:
(a) Atherosclerosis
(b) Arteriolosclerosis
(c) Monckeberg's sclerosis
(d) Dissecting aneurysm

74.9. Ascending aorta involvement is the commonest site of which aneurysm:
(a) Syphilitic
(b) Atherosclerotic
(c) Berry aneurysm
(d) Traumatic

74.10. Onion skin thickening of arteriolar wall is seen in:
(a) Atherosclerosis
(b) Median calcific sclerosis
(c) Hyaline arteriosclerosis
(d) Hyperplastic arteriosclerosis

74.11. Atherosclerosis is seen with which bacteria –
(a) Staph aureus
(b) Streptococcus pneumonia
(c) Chlamydia pneumoniae
(d) Chlamydia trachomatis

74.12. Commonest histological finding in benign hypertension is:
(a) Proliferating endarteritis
(b) Necrotising arteriolitis
(c) Hyaline arteriosclerosis
(d) Cystic medial necrosis

VASCULITIS, RAYNAUD DISEASE

75. Which of the following is a feature of temporal arteritis?
(a) Giant cell arteritis *(AIIMS Nov 2012)*
(b) Granulomatous vasculitis
(c) Necrotizing vasculitis
(d) Leucocytoclastic vasculitis

76. Small vessels vasculitis seen in *(AI India 2012)*
(a) Giant cell arteritis
(b) Takayasu arteritis
(c) PAN
(d) Microscopic Polyangitis

77. A 5 year old child presents with perivascular IgA deposition and neutrophilic collection. There is erythematous rash on the lower limbs and non-blanching purpura. The likely diagnosis in the child is:
(a) Henoch-Schonlein Purpura *(AIIMS Nov 2011)*
(b) Wegner's granulomatosis
(c) Giant cell Vasculitis
(d) Kawasaki's disease

78. Pathogenesis of all of the following is granulomatous, except: *(AI 2010)*
(a) Wegener's granulomatosis
(b) Buerger's disease
(c) Takayasu's arteritis
(d) Microscopic polyangiitis

79. ANCA is associated with: *(AIIMS Nov 2009)*
(a) Henoch-Schonlein Purpura
(b) Goodpasture syndrome
(c) Rheumatoid arthritis
(d) Wegener's granulomatosis

80. Which of the following is not a common cause of Vasculitis in adults? *(AIIMS Nov 2009)*
(a) Giant Cell Arteritis
(b) Polyarteritis nodosa
(c) Kawasaki disease
(d) Henoch-Schonlein Purpura

81. Hypersensitivity vasculitis most commonly involves:
(a) Arterioles *(AIIMS May 09, Nov 08, DNB 2008)*
(b) Post-capillary venules
(c) Capillaries
(d) Medium sized arteries

82. A patient presents with respiratory symptoms, i.e. cough, hemoptysis and glomerulonephritis. His c-ANCA levels in serum were found to be raised. The most likely diagnosis is: *(AIIMS Nov 2002)*
(a) Goodpasture's syndrome
(b) Classic polyarteritis nodosa
(c) Wegener's granulomatosis
(d) Kawasaki's syndrome

83. Vasculitis is seen in: *(PGI Dec 2002)*
(a) Buerger's disease
(b) HSP
(c) Gout
(d) Reiter's disease
(e) Behcet's syndrome

84. Wegener's granulomatosis involve:
(a) Lung *(PGI Dec 2003)*
(b) Liver
(c) Kidney
(d) Upper respiratory tract
(e) Heart

85. Wegener's granulomatosis: *(PGI Dec 2006)*
(a) Involve lung
(b) Involves nose
(c) Involve kidney
(d) Treated with cytotoxic agent and/or steroids

86. **All are true about ANCA associated crescentic glomeru-lonephritis, except:** *(Delhi 2009 RP)*
    (a) Seen in Wegener's granulomatosis
    (b) Seen in microscopic polyangitis
    (c) Seen in Henoch-Schönlein purpura
    (d) Is pauci immune in nature

87. **All of the following are small vessel vasculitis except:**
    (a) Kawasaki's disease *(Delhi PG-2006)*
    (b) Churg-Strauss syndrome
    (c) Wegener granulomatosis
    (d) None of the above

88. **Polyarteritis nodosa can occur in association with which of the following:** *(Delhi PG-2005)*
    (a) Hypertension   (b) Trauma
    (c) Drugs   (d) Bronchial asthma

89. **The term infantile polyarteritis nodosa was formerly used for:** *(Karnataka 2009)*
    (a) Goodpasture's disease
    (b) Henoch-Schönlein Purpura
    (c) Kawasaki disease
    (d) Takayasu's arteritis

90. **Most common organs involved in Wegener's granulomatosis are:** *(UP 2004)*
    (a) Skin and nose
    (b) Lung and kidney
    (c) Heart and kidney
    (d) Kidney and nervous system

91. **Polyarteritis nodosa does not involve:** *(AP 2003)*
    (a) Pulmonary artery
    (b) Bronchial artery
    (c) Renal artery
    (d) Cerebral artery

92. **C-ANCA antibodies are characteristic of:** *(AP 2003)*
    (a) Sjögren's syndrome
    (b) Giant cell arteritis
    (c) Wegener's granulomatosis
    (d) Kawasaki's disease

93. **ANCA is seen in all except:** *(AP 2008)*
    (a) Wegener's granulomatosis
    (b) Henoch-Schönlein purpura
    (c) Microscopic polyangiitis
    (d) Churg-Strauss disease

94. **A 30 year old male Munish with exertional calf pain and painful foot ulcers demonstrates hypersensitivity to intradermally injected tobacco extract. Which of the following pathologic processes is most likely responsible for this patient's condition?**
    (a) Lipid-filled intimal plaque
    (b) Onion-like concentric thickening of arteriolar walls
    (c) Transmural inflammation of the arterial wall with fibrinoid necrosis
    (d) Segmental vasculitis extending into contiguous veins and nerves

95. **A 57 year-old woman Beenu Dash presents with frequent headaches, which occur on one side and are throbbing. She has fever and tenderness over both temples. Investigations reveal a slightly decreased hematocrit and an elevated erythrocyte sedimentation rate. This patient should be treated immediately to prevent the development of**
    (a) Blindness
    (b) Deafness
    (c) Loss of tactile sensation
    (d) Loss of the ability to speak

96. **A 50 year-old man presents to his physician with hematuria. Renal biopsy demonstrates a focal necrotizing glomerulitis with crescent formation. The patient has a history of intermittent hemoptysis and intermittent chest pain of moderate intensity. A previous chest x-ray had demonstrated multiple opacities, some of which were cavitated. The patient also has chronic cold-like nasal symptoms. Which of the following is the most likely diagnosis?**
    (a) Aspergillosis
    (b) Wegener's granulomatosis
    (c) Renal carcinoma metastatic to the lung
    (d) Tuberculosis

Most Recent Questions

96.1. **Which of the following is not a characteristic of Wegener's granulomatosis?**
    (a) Granuloma is vessel wall
    (b) Focal necrotising glomerulonephritis
    (c) Positive for cANCA
    (d) Involves large vessels

96.2. **Which is associated with vasculitis of medium size vessels:**
    (a) Temporal arteritis
    (b) Wegners granulomatosis
    (c) Polyarteritis nodosa
    (d) Henoch Schonlein purpura

96.3. **All is true about Giant cell arteritis except:**
    (a) Involves large to small sized arteries
    (b) Granulomatous inflammation
    (c) Most commonly involved artery is abdominal aorta
    (d) Segmental nature of the involvement

96.4. **In PAN, the lesions are seen in all except:**
    (a) Lung
    (b) Pancreas
    (c) Liver
    (d) Heart

96.5. **Which of the following is abdominal angiitis?**
    (a) Giant cell arteritis
    (b) Takayasu arteritis
    (c) Kawasaki disease
    (d) Polyarteritis nodosa

96.6. **Raynaud's phenomenon what change is seen in vessels initial stage:**

(a) No change
(b) Thrombosis
(c) Fibrinoid necrosis
(d) Hyaline sclerosis

96.7. Frequency of renal involvement in Henoch Schonlein Purpura (HSP) is ?
(a) 20-40%
(b) >80%
(c) 40-60%
(d) 10%

96.8. Glomus cells are found in which of the following conditions?
(a) Carotid body tumour
(b) Thyroid carcinoma
(c) Liver carcinoma
(d) Glomus tumor

96.9. Glomus tumor is seen in:
(a) Retroperitoneum
(b) Soft tissue
(c) Distal portion of digits
(d) Proximal portion of digits

96.10. Sturge weber syndrome is associated with:
(a) Port wine stain
(b) Cavernous hemangioma
(c) Lymphangioma
(d) Hemangiosarcoma

96.11. All of the following are true about pyogenic granuloma except
(a) Bacterial infection
(b) Bleeding
(c) Benign tumour
(d) Capillary hemangioma

EXPLANATIONS

1. **Ans. (a) Myxomatous degeneration and prolapsed of the mitral valve** *(Ref: Robbins 9/e p556, 8th/563-565)*
   The important clues given in the question;
   - Female patient
   - Presenting for Routine examination (means she was asymptomatic)
   - Presence of mid systolic click on physical examination
   - Absence of history of rheumatic heart disease

   All these are significant pointers towards a diagnosis of mitral valve prolapse or Barlow syndrome. The other name of the same condition is *Myxomatous degeneration of the mitral valve. So, the answer is option 'a'*

   Direct lines from Robbins '***Most patients** with mitral valve prolapse are **asymptomatic,** and the condition is **discovered only on routine examination by the presence of a midsystolic click as an incidental finding on physical examination**'*
   Concept
   - **Commissural fusion** that *typifies rheumatic heart disease* is **absent** in mitral valve prolapse.

2. **Ans. (c) Small ASD** *(Ref: Ghai 7th/390,403, Adult congenital heart disease: a practical guide page/36-37)*
   Direct quote Ghai… *'Infective endocarditis is **very rare** in patients of ostium secundum atrial septal defect, **unless floppy mitral valve is present'.***
   Risk of infective endocarditis in various lesions

High Risk	Moderate Risk	Low Risk
• Prosthetic heart value • Tetralogy of Fallot • PDA • Aortic regurgitation • Aortic stenosis • Coarctation of Aorta • VSD • Mitral regurgitation	• MVP + M.R. • Tricuspid stenosis • Tricuspid regurgitation • Pulmonary stenosis • Mitral stenosis	• ASD • MVP without MR

3. **Ans. (c) Neutrophilic infiltration surrounding coagulative necrosis** *(Ref: Robbins 8th/550; 7th/579)*

4. **Ans. (d) Elevated ESR** *(Ref: Robbins 9/e 559, 8th/566)*

5. **Ans. (a) Cross reactivity with exogenous antigen** *(Ref: Robbins 8th/566, 9/e 558)*
   Acute rheumatic fever results from immune response to group A streptococci (Strep. pyogenes) which cross-reacts with host tissues. The antibodies directed against the M proteins of streptococci cross react with the self antigens in the heart. In addition, CD4+ T cells specific for streptococcal peptides also react with self proteins in the heart and produce macrophage activating cytokines. So, the damage to the heart tissue is a combination of antibody and T-cell mediated reactions.

6. **Ans. (b) Intimal fibrosis of right ventricle, tricuspid and pulmonary valve.** *(Ref: Robbins 8th/569, 9/e 562)*
   - Cardiac lesions are present in 50% of the patients with the *carcinoid syndrome.*
   - These are **largely right-sided** due to inactivation of both serotonin and bradykinin in the blood during passage through the lungs by the monoamine oxidase present in the pulmonary vascular endothelium.

7. **Ans. (a) Infective endocarditis** *(Ref: Robbins 9/e 560, 8th/567)*
   The *hallmark of infective endocarditis* is the presence of *friable, bulky* and *potentially destructive vegetations* containing fibrin, inflammatory cells and bacteria or other organisms on the heart valves. Do refer to the table comparing different vegetations in differrent condtions in the text.

8. **Ans. (c) Rheumatic carditis** *(Ref: Robbins 7th/593, 9/e 558, Harrison 17th/2095)*
   - **Aschoff's bodies are characteristic focal inflammatory lesion of acute rheumatic fever** *found in any of the three layers of the heart.*

9. **Ans. (b) Rupture of Chordae tendinae** *(Ref: Robbins 9/e 558-559, 7th/593-94, Harrison's 17th/2092)*

- **Acute rheumatic fever** is characterized by **Pancarditis** (i.e. endocarditis, myocarditis as well as pericarditis). **Aschoff bodies can be seen in all the three layers of heart**.
- **McCallum's patches** are irregular thickening on subendocardial region, mostly in posterior wall of left atrium. It is exacerbated by regurgitant jet and can be seen in acute rheumatic fever.
- Pericardial inflammation in rheumatoid fever is accompanied by fibrous or serofibrous exudates, described as '**Bread and Butter pericarditis**'.
- *Valvular damage is the hallmark of rheumatic carditis with the* Mitral valve being the me affected value.
- **Myocardial involvement is almost never responsible in itself for cardiac failure.**

10. **Ans. (b) Major Jones' criteria** *(Ref: Robbins 9/e 559, 8th/566, Harrison 17th/2095)*
    ASO titre may be positive due to streptococcal infection even in normal people. In some individuals with rheumatic carditis, ASO titre may **not** be elevated. In PSGN, the titre of anti DNA se B antibody is elevated more commonly than ASLO.

11. **Ans. (c) Myxomatous degeneration** *(Ref: Robbins 7th/591-2,8th/563, 9/e 556, Harrison 17th/1472)*

    ### MVP/Myxomatous degeneration/Barlow's syndrome/Floppy-valve syndrome

    - Characteristic anatomic change in **myxomatous degeneration**[Q] is interchordial ballooning of the mitral leaflets. The affected leaflets are often enlarged, redundant, thick, and rubbery.
    - **Annular dilation**[Q] is a characteristic finding. (it is rare in other causes of mitral insufficiency).
    - There is reduction in the production of type III collagen and electron microscopy has revealed fragmentation of collagen fibrils.
    - Autosomal dominant disorder seen in **females**[Q] also associated with Marfan's syndrome, Osteogenesis imperfecta, and Ehler-Danlos syndrome.
    - Clinically most patients are asymptomatic[Q], *uncommonly* they may develop chest pain, dyspnea and fatigue.
    - **Echocardiography**[Q] is the investigation of choice.

12. **Ans. (c) Myocardial infarction** *(Ref: Harrison 17th/791, Harsh Mohan 6th/448, Robbins7th 596-7, 8th/567, 9/e 561)*

Cardiac complications	Extra cardiac complications
- Valvular stenosis or insufficiency - Abscess on the myocardium **(ring abscess)** - Myocardial abscess - Suppurative pericarditis - Perforation, rupture and aneurysm of valve leaflets - Cardiac failure	- **Systemic emboli** from left side of heart affect spleen, brain and kidneys whereas those from right heart affect pulmonary abscess formation. - Antigen -antibody complexes cause focal (more commonly) and diffuse (less commonly) glomerulonephritis.

    Harrison writes that "Emboli to a coronary artery may result in myocardial infarction; nevertheless embolic transmural infarcts are rare."

13. **Ans. (b) Epithelioid cell** *(Ref: Robbins 7th/593-4, 8th/565-6, 9/e 558)*
    Aschoff bodies consist of foci of swollen eosinophilic collagen surrounded by lymphocytes (primarily T cells), occasional plasma cells, and plump macrophages called **Anitschkow cells** (*pathognomonic for rheumatic fever*). These cells are also called "caterpillar cells". Some of the larger macrophages become multinucleated to form Aschoff giant cells.

14. **Ans. (a) Aschoff bodies; (b) Vegetation along the line of closure** *(Ref: Robbins 7th/593-94, 9/e 558)*

15. **Ans. (d) Aschoff's nodule** *(Ref: Robbins 8th/565-566, 9/e 558)*

16. **Ans. (b) Libman Sack's endocarditis** *(Ref: Robbins 7th/597, 89, 9/e 562)*
    Vegetations in Libman Sack's endocarditis occur on surfaces of cusps. Both surfaces may be involved but, more commonly, the undersurface is affected.

17. **Ans. (a) Acute rheumatic fever** *(Ref: Robbin 7th/593, 9/e 558)*

18. **Ans. (a) Acute rheumatic fever** *(Ref: Robbin 8th/565, 7th/593, 9/e 558)*

19. **Ans. (b) Mycobacterium tuberculosis** *(Ref: Robbins 7th/607-609, 9/e 571)*
    - Mycobacterium tuberculosis causes involvement of pericardium (Caseous pericarditis). It is the commonest cause of **chronic constrictive pericarditis**[Q].
    - **Primary pericarditis** is unusual and is **almost always viral**[Q] **in origin**.

20. **Ans. (d) Hypertrophic cardiomyopathy** *(Ref: Robbins 9/e 569, 8th/576; 7th/604, 607)*

21. **Ans. (a) Rheumatic heart disease** *(Ref: Robbins 9/e 554, 8th/565,561; 7th/589)*

22. **Ans. (c) Syphilis** *(Ref: Robbins 9/e p554-555, 8th/375-376, 7th/532)*

23. **Ans. (a) Myocardial infarction** *(Ref: Robbins 9/e p529, 8th/535; 7th/562)*

24. **Ans. (b) SLE** *(Ref: Robbins 9/e p562, 8th/220; 7th/598)*

25. **Ans. (b) TB** *(Ref: Harrison 17th/1493, Robbins 9/e p575)*

26. **Ans. (a) Acute rheumatic fever** *(Ref: Robbins 9/e p558, 8th/565, 7th/593)*

27. **Ans. (b) Aschoff's nodule** *(Ref: Robbins 9/e p558, 8th/565-566)*

28. **Ans. (a) IgM directed against IgG** *(Ref: Robbins 9/e p1210, 8th/1238)*

29. **Ans. (d) Erythema nodosum** *(Ref: Robbins 9/e p559, 8th/566, 7th/594)*

30. **Ans. (c) Myocarditis** *(Ref: Robbins 8th/566, 9/e p559, Harrison 18th/2754)*

- The **most common** cause of death that occur during rheumatic fever is cardiac failure secondary to valvular dysfunction.
- **Microscopically**, the characteristic feature of rheumatic heart disease is **Aschoff's body**[Q]. The plump macrophages called **Anitschkow cells**[Q] are **pathognomonic for RF.**
- **Most commonly** affected valve is **mitral valve**[Q] and the **least commonly** affected is **pulmonary valve**[Q].

31. **Ans. (b) A 28-year-old male with persistently high fevers with tricuspid vegetations and tricuspid regurgitation on trans-thoracic echocardiogram** *(Ref: Robbins 9/e p560-561, 8th/567)*

- Endocarditis is an inflammation of the endocardium that can be caused by
  - Infectious agents such as S. aureus or S. viridans,
  - Inflammatory processes such as rheumatic fever or systemic lupus erythematosus (Libman-Sacks endocarditis)
  - Other processes such as metastatic cancer, carcinoid etc.
- S. aureus causes acute bacterial endocarditis with rapid onset of symptoms including shaking chills (rigors), high grade fever, dyspnea on exertion and malaise. In IV drug abusers it causes right-sided endocarditis with septic embolization into the lungs leading to pulmonary abscesses. In non- intravenous drug abuser, it causes rapid decompensation, heart failure, sepsis, septic embolization to the brain and other end organs.

(Choice A) This clinical picture is most consistent with a patient who has suffered from acute rheumatic fever in the past that has left her with mitral stenosis. It is likely that she has recently experienced yet another episode of rheumatic fever.
(Choice C) Streptococcus bovis is a part of the normal flora of the colon, and bacteremia or endocarditis caused by S. bovis is associated with colonic cancer in approximately 25% of cases.
(Choice D) This case is most consistent with culture-negative endocarditis. He has vague symptoms that can be associated with endocarditis, namely fever, fatigue, and malaise, and he has echocardiographic evidence of a valvular vegetation. Special serologies and cultures need to be sent for organisms that do not grow in standard blood culture. These organisms include Bartonella, Coxiella, Mycoplasma, Histoplasma, Chlamydia and the HACEK organisms (Haemophilus, Actinobacillus, Cardiobacterium, Eikenella and Kingella).

31.1. **Ans. (c) Small or medium sized on either or both sides of valve** *(Ref: Robbins 8/e p567, 9/e p560)*

Summary of salient features of vegetations in different endocarditis

Rheumatic Fever	Non Bacterial Thrombotic (Marantic Endocarditis)	Libman Sack's Endocarditis	Infective Endocarditis
• Small, warty • Firm • Friable	• Small, warty • Friable	• Medium sized (small) • Flat, Verrucous • Irregular	• Large • Bulky • Irregular
• Along lines of closure	• Along lines of closure	• On surface of cusps • (both surfaces may be involved but the under-surface is more likely affected, less commonly mural endocardium is involved) • In pockets of valves	• Vegetations on the valve cusps • Less often on mural endocardium
• Sterile (no organism)	• Sterile	• Sterile	• Non-sterile (bacteria)
• Embolisation is uncommon	• Embolisation is common	• Embolisation is uncommon	• Embolisation is **very common** (max chances)
• In rheumatic heart disease	• In cancers (like M3-AML, pancreatic cancer), deep vein thrombosis, Trosseau syndrome	• In SLE	• In infective endocarditis

Cardiovascular System

31.2. Ans. (b) Libman Sack's endocarditis *(Ref: Robbins 8/e p567, 9/e p562)*
Refer to the earlier question

31.3. Ans. (b) Rheumatic endocarditis *(Ref: Robbins 8/e p566, 9/e p558)*
In patients of *rheumatic heart disease*, subendocardial lesions, perhaps exacerbated by regurgitant jets, may induce irregular thickenings called **MacCallum plaques**, usually in the **left atrium**^Q.

31.4. Ans. (c) Lungs *(Ref: Robbins 8/e p 535, 9/e p529)*
Robbins... "**In patients with heart failure**, some red cells extravasate into the edema fluid **within the alveolar spaces**, where they are phagocytosed and digested by macrophages, which store the iron recovered from hemoglobin in the form of hemosiderin. These hemosiderin-laden macrophages are often referred to as **heart failure cells**".

31.5. Ans. (b) Fat deposition *(Ref: Robbins 8/e p34)*
In a pattern of lipid deposition seen with prolonged moderate hypoxia, such as that produced by profound anemia, there is intracellular deposits of fat, which create grossly apparent bands of yellowed myocardium alternating with bands of darker, red-brown, uninvolved myocardium (**tigered effect**).

31.6. Ans. (b) Acute rheumatic fever... discussed in detail earlier *(Ref: Robbins 8/e p565-566, 9/e 559)*

31.7. Ans. (d) Lung *(Ref: Robbins 9/e p561, 8/e p566, 7/e p597)*
• Mitral valve vegetations are associated with systemic embolisation which can affect brain, liver, spleen and kidney.
• *Embolisation of the lung* is associated with involvement of right heart (*tricuspid valve vegetation*) involvement.

31.8. Ans. (c) Pulmonary *(Ref: Robbins 9/e p559, 8 /e p565-567, 7/e p597)*
In **chronic rheumatic heart disease**, the *mitral valve is affected alone in 65% to 70% of cases*, and along with the aortic valve in another 25% of cases. Tricuspid valve involvement is infrequent, and the *pulmonary valve is only rarely affected*.

31.9. Ans. (d) Tricuspid valve *(Ref: Robbins 9/e p560, 8 /e p565-567, 7/e p597)*

32. Ans. (c) Trousseau syndrome *(Ref: Robbins 9/e p562, 8th/567)*

> The pathogenesis of nonbacterial thrombotic endocarditis (NBTE) often involves a hypercoagulable state. When the hypercoagulability is the result of the procoagulant effects of circulating products of cancers the resulting cardiac valve vegetations may also be called marantic endocarditis. The pathophysiology of NBTE is similar to that of Trousseau's syndrome (migratory thrombophlebitis) which may also be induced by disseminated cancers like mucinous adenocarcinoma of the pancreas and adenocarcinoma of the lung which may relate to procoagulant effects of circulating mucin.

(Choice A) Humoral hypercalcemia of malignancy, the most common cause of hypercalcemia is due to the production of a parathyroid hormone (PTH)-like substance by tumors. It would not cause a hypercoagulable state or vegetations.
(Choice B) Cancer metastases to the heart usually involve the pericardium or myocardium. Valve metastases are less frequent and would probably have shown invasive characteristics on histological examination.
(Choice D) Raynaud's phenomenon involves episodic, ischemic attacks of the digits that produce pallor and numbness. These episodes maybe induced by cold or emotional stimuli. The pathophysiology is thought to involve abnormal sensitivity of digital arteries/arterioles to vasoconstrictive influences. Raynaud's phenomenon occurs in the absence of any hypercoagulable state.

33. Ans. (b) Presence of neutrophils *(Ref: Robbins 9/e p544, 8th/550)*
As discussed in the text, granulation tissue appears between 7-10 days and collagen appears after 2 months. Between 3-7 dyas, neutrophils start disintegrating with early phagocytosis caused by macrophages. Presence of macrophages would have been a better answer but in the given question, presence of neutrophils is the best option.

34. Ans. (d) These may result in aneurysm *(Ref: Robbins 9/e p543, 7th/575)*
Ventricular aneurysms result from transmural infarcts, which involve the whole thickness of myocardium from *epicardium to endocardium. Subendocardial infarcts being limited to only the inner one-third or at most one* half of the ventricular wall do not cause ventricular aneurysms.
Aneurysm of the ventricular wall **most commonly** results from a **large transmural anteroseptal infarct**.

35. Ans. (b) Necrotic myofibers with presence of neutrophils *(Ref: Robbins 7th/578-581, 9/e p544)*
The patient in the question succumbed to myocardial infarction after about 28 hours of the attack. *After twenty-four hours of the attack light microscopy shows coagulative necrosis of myofibrils with loss of nuclei and striations along with an interstitial infiltrate of neutrophils. For details, see the table of morphological changes of MI in text.*

36. Ans. (c) Nephrotic syndrome *(Ref: Harrison 17th/272, Robbins 9/e p914)*
• Nephrotic syndrome is a clinical complex characterized by proteinuria (> 3.5 g/day), hypoalbuminemia, edema and hyperlipidemia.
• A hypercoagulable state frequently accompanies severe nephrotic syndrome due to *urinary loss of AT-III, reduced serum levels of protein C and S, hyperfibrinogenimia and enhanced platelet aggregation.*

391

• Due to increased coagulation state, predisposition to CAD is present in patients with nephrotic syndrome.
Potential future questions

Among hyperlipoproteinemias type II, III and IV are associated with increased risk of CAD whereas Type I and V are not associated with CAD.

37. **Ans. (c) Within one week** *(Ref: Robbins 7th/579, 9/e 544, Chandrasoma Taylor 3rd/364)*

38. **Ans. (d) Myocardial infarction** *(Ref: Robbins 9/e 547, 8th/555, 7th/583, Harrison 17th/1534)*
The preferred biomarkers for myocardial damage are cardiac-specific proteins, particularly Troponin-I (TnI) and Troponin-T.

39. **Ans. (b) Coagulative necrosis** *(Ref: Robbins 7th/579, 9/e 545)*

40. **Ans. (d) Troponin-I** *(Ref: Cardiovascular Imaging ; Vol. 22, No. 2, April 2006, Robbins 9/th p547)*
Hypothyroid patients have increased concentration of **CPK** that is mostly due to increased CPK MM. However CPK-MB has also been reported to increase above reference value in hypothyroid patients without myocardial damage. This may create confusion during the evaluation of myocardial injury in a hypothyroid patient presenting with chest pain. Troponin I is considered superior, marker for the diagnosis of myocardial infarction in hypothyroid patient.

41. **Ans. (c) CPK-MB** *(Ref: Harrison 17th/1535, Robbins 9/e 547)*
• Troponin levels remain elevated for 10-14 days after MI, therefore if there is reinfarction prior to that period, Troponin cannot be used for the diagnosis. As discussed is text, CPK-MB is better marker for diagnosis of reinfarction.

42. **Ans. (a) Waviness of the fibers** *(Ref: Robbins 9/e p544, 8th/550-551; 7th/581)*

43. **Ans. (c) Left anterior descending coronary artery** *(Ref: Robbins 9/e p542, 8th/551; 7th/577)*

44. **Ans. (d) 3 months** *(Ref: Robbins 9/e p544, 8th/550, 7th/579)*

45. **Ans. (d) Autoimmune** *(Ref: Robbins 9/e p549, 8th/557, 7th/584)*

46. **Ans. (c) MM and MB** *(Ref: Robbins 8th/555, 9/e p547)*

47. **Ans. (a) CPK MB** *(Ref: Robbins 9/e p547, 8th/556 ; 7th/583)*

48. **Ans. (d) Stable angina** *(Ref: Robbins 9/e p539-540, 8th/545, also read the explanation below)*
This patient's history of hypertension, hyperlipidemia, coronary artery bypass surgery, and carotid endarterectomy all indicate that he suffers from generalized atherosclerosis. When atherosclerosis involves intestinal arteries, the bowel suffers from diminished blood supply. Intestinal hypoperfusion, which can be very painful, is especially pronounced after meals when more blood is needed for the digestion and absorption of nutrients.
Chronic mesenteric ischemia is most often caused by atherosclerotic narrowing of the celiac trunk, superior mesenteric artery and inferior mesenteric artery. This **triad of symptoms** characterizes the disease:
• *Epigastric or peri-umbilical abdominal pain occurs 30-60 minutes after food intake.* Atherosclerotic arteries are not able to dilate in response to increased blood flow requirements during the digestion and absorption of food.
• *Weight loss* is common; many patients avoid the pain associated with eating. Patients report severe pain; but the physician examination will usually appear benign.
• On light microscopy, hypo-perfused areas of intestine show *mucosal atrophy and loss of villi.* Atherosclerotic plaques are found in the intestinal vessels.

Angiography is the gold standard but this method is invasive and expensive. Mesenteric duplex ultrasonography is a non- invasive alternative in assessing intestinal blood flow.

(Choice C) **Pulmonary emboli** describe the lodging of emboli (usually a blood clot) in the branches of the pulmonary artery. The most common source is blood clots in the veins of lower extremities. A similar pathogenesis accounts for **acute mesenteric ischemia associated with mural thrombus**.
(Choices A and B) The pathogenesis of peptic ulcer disease and esophageal spasm are unrelated to blood supply.

49. **Ans. (d) Myocardial rupture** *(Ref: Robbins 9/e p549, 8th/557)*
Rupture of the left ventricle, a complication of acute myocardial infarction, usually occurs when the necrotic area has the least tensile strength, about 4-7 days after an infarction, when repair is just beginning.
The anterior wall of the heart is the most frequent site of rupture, leading to fatal cardiac tamponade. Internal rupture of the interventricular septum or of a papillary muscle may also be seen.
Arrhythmias are the most important early complication of acute myocardial infarction.
Pump failure, ventricular aneurysms and mural thrombosis are other complications that may develop as a result of permanent damage to the heart after infarction.

50. Ans. (c) Pericardial inflammation overlying the necrotic segment of myocardium *(Ref: Robbins 9/e p549, 8th/557)*

The sharp and pleuritic nature of this patient's new pain suggests pericardial involvement. The exacerbation with swallowing indicates that the posterior pericardium may be involved, and the radiation into the neck suggests involvement of the inferior pericardium, which is adjacent to phrenic nerve afferents supplying the diaphragm. The patient's low-grade fever tells us that this is an inflammatory process.

> A fibrinous or serofibrinous early onset pericarditis develops in about 10-20% of patients between days 2 and 4 following a transmural myocardial infarction. This pericarditis is a reaction to the transmural necrosis.

The inflammation affects the adjacent visceral and parietal pericardium; in other words, the inflammation is usually localized to the region of the pericardium overlying the necrotic myocardial segment. This type of early post-MI pericarditis is generally short-lived and disappears with 1 to 3 days of aspirin therapy.

(Choices A and B) Thrombosis of a coronary vessel would be expected to reproduce the patient's original, anginal type pain. The pain of myocardial ischemia is not usually sharp or pleuritic in nature, but rather is constant, substernal, and "crushing."

(Choice D) This describes the late-onset post-myocardial infarction pericarditis (Dressler's syndrome). Dressler's syndrome typically begins one week to a few months after a myocardial infarction.

Typical features include fever, pleuritis, leukocytosis, pericardial friction rub, and chest radiograph evidence of new pericardial or pleural effusions. Dressler's syndrome is thought to be an autoimmune polyserositis provoked by antigens exposed or created by infarction of the cardiac muscle. Thus, the pericardium is usually diffusely inflamed. Other serosal surfaces including the lung pleura may be involved. Dressler's syndrome generally responds to aspirin, NSAIDs, and/or glucocorticoids.

51. Ans. (b) 7 days *(Ref: Robbins 8th/550, 9/e p549)*

> - A number of serious complications can occur between 5 and 10 days following infarction, due to marked weakening of the necrotic myocardium. These include rupture of the ventricular wall leading to hemopericardium and cardiac tamponade (as this patient had), rupture of the interventricular septum, and rupture of the papillary muscle.
> - Arrhythmias are the most common complication 2 days post-infarction (choice A).
> - Fibrinous pericarditis secondary to an autoimmune phenomenon (**Dressler's syndrome**) can be seen **several weeks after infarction** (choices C and D).

52. Ans. (b) Fibrinous pericarditis *(Ref: Robbins 8th/557, 9/e p549)*

> Different types of pericarditis can be seen in different settings. Fibrinous and serofibrinous pericarditis may follow acute myocardial infarction (Dressler's syndrome) and can be seen in uremia, chest radiation, rheumatic fever, systemic lupus erythematosus and following chest trauma (including chest surgery) or chest radiation.

52.1. Ans. (a) Troponin T *(Ref: Robbins 8/e p555, 9/e p547)*

Enzyme	Initiation of rise	Peak	Return to baseline
CK-MB	2-4 hours	24 hours	48-72 hours
Troponin T and I (TnT, TnI)	2-4 hours	48 hours	7-10 days
AST/SGOT	In 12 hours	48 hours	4-5 days
LDH	24 hours	3-6 days	2 weeks

52.2. Ans. (c) LDH *(Ref: Robbins 8/e p555, 9/e p547)*

52.3. Ans. (c) Macrophages *(Ref: Robbins 8/e p550, 9/e p544)*

Evolution of changes in MI

Time	Gross	Light Microscopy
Reversible injury		
0-30 min	None	None
Irreversible injury		
30 min to 4 hr.	None	Waviness of fibers at border (earliest change)
4-12 hr.	Occasional dark mottling	Beginning of coagulative necrosis, edema and hemorrhage
12-24 hr.	Dark mottling	Ongoing coagulative necrosis, marginal contraction band necrosis, beginning of neutrophilic infiltration

Time	Gross	Light Microscopy
Reversible injury		
1-3 days	Mottling with yellow tan infarct center.	Coagulation necrosis, interstitial neutrophilic infiltrate
3-7 days	Hyperemic borders, central yellow tan softening	Beginning of disintegration with dying neutrophils, early phagocytosis by macrophages
7-10 days	Maximum yellow tan and soft depressed red-tan margin	Early formation of fibrovascular granulation tissue at margins
10-14 days	Red gray depressed infarct borders	Well established granulation tissue and collagen deposition
2-8 weeks	Gray-white scar progressive from border towards infarct core	Collagen deposition, ↓ Cellularity
> 2 months	Scarring complete	Dense collagenous scar

Have a close at the table given above, the answer is undoubtedly is **macrophage**.

52.4. Ans. (d) Free radicals *(Ref: Robbins 8/e p553, 9/e p546)*

Restoration of blood flow to ischemic tissues can promote recovery of cells if they are reversibly injured. However, under certain circumstances, when blood flow is restored to cells that have been ischemic but have not died, injury is paradoxically exacerbated and proceeds at an accelerated pace. This process is called *ischemia-reperfusion injury*. The following mechanisms have been proposed for the reperfusion injury:

- New damage may be initiated during reoxygenation by increased generation of *reactive oxygen and nitrogen species* from parenchymal and endothelial cells and from infiltrating leukocytes.
- Ischemic injury is associated with *inflammation* as a result of the production of cytokines and increased expression of adhesion molecules by hypoxic parenchymal and endothelial cells, which recruit circulating neutrophils to reperfused tissue.
- Activation of the *complement system* may contribute to ischemia-reperfusion injury. Some IgM antibodies have a propensity to deposit in ischemic tissues, for unknown reasons, and when blood flow is resumed, complement proteins bind to the deposited antibodies, are activated, and cause more cell injury and inflammation.

52.5. Ans. (c) 1-3 days…. See the table in text or details *(Ref: Robbins 9/e p544, 8/e p550, 7/e p579)*

52.6. Ans. (c) Coxsackie Virus *(Ref: Robbins 7/e 610, 9/e p570)*

53. Ans. (a) Bronchial carcinoma *(Ref: Robbins 9/e p574, 8th/589, 7th/614)*

53.1. Ans. (d) Myxoma *(Ref: Robbins 9/e p575, 8/e p583-4)*

Important information about NEET

• Most common cardiac tumor: **Metastasis**[Q]
• Most common benign cardiac tumor: **atrial myxoma**[Q]
• Most common primary cardiac tumor in adults: atrial myxoma[Q]
• Most common primary cardiac tumor in children: rhabdomyoma[Q]

53.2. Ans. (a) Myxoma *(Ref: Robbind 8/e p583, 9/e 575)*

- *Myxomas* are the most common primary tumor of the heart in adults.
- Though they may arise in any cavity of the heart but nearly *90% are located in the atria,*
- The left-to-right ratio of the myxoma is approximately 4:1
- The region of the **fossa ovalis in the atrial septum is the favored site of origin.**
- Histologically, myxomas are composed of stellate or globular myxoma ("lepidic") cells,
- Major clinical manifestations: fever, malaise, features due to valvular *"ball-valve" obstruction or* embolization
- *Familial cardiac myxoma syndrome* (known as **Carney syndrome**) is characterized by autosomal dominant transmission, multiple cardiac and often extracardiac (e.g. skin) myxomas, spotty pigmentation, and endocrine overactivity.

53.3. Ans. (b) Left atrium *(Ref: Robbins 9/e 575, 8/e p583, 7/e p613)*

Atrial myxoma is most commonly located on the **left atrium**. Other important points have discussed earlier.

54. Ans. (c) Lower limb ischemia *(Ref: Robbins 8th/499, 1140)*

Direct quote from Robbins… *'Gangrene of the lower extremities as a result of advanced vascular disease is about 100 times more common in diabetics than in general population'.*

The risk of myocardial infarction (MI) is **twice** *in a diabetic as compared to a non diabetic* individual.

55. **Ans. (b) Atherosclerosis in less important in age more than 45 years age** *(Ref: Robbins 9/e p493, 8th/497)*

Risk factors for atherosclerosis

Modifiable	Non modifiable
• Hyperlipidemia • Hypertension • Cigarette smoking • Diabetes • C reactive protein	• Increasing age • Gender • Family history • Genetics

According to Robbins,

- Age is a dominant influence on atherosclerosis. Between ages 40 and 60, the incidence of myocardial infarction increases fivefold.

- Hyperlipidemia more specifically hypercholesterolemia; even in the absence of other risk factors is a major risk factor for atherosclerosis. The major component of serum cholesterol associated with increased risk is low-density lipoprotein (LDL) cholesterol. In contrast, higher levels of HDL correlate with reduced risk.

- Dietary and pharmacologic approaches that lower LDL or total serum cholesterol, and/or raise serum HDL are all of considerable interest. High dietary intake of cholesterol and saturated fats (present in egg yolks, animal fats, and butter, for example) raises plasma cholesterol levels. Conversely, diets low in cholesterol and/or with higher ratios of polyunsaturated fats lower plasma cholesterol levels.

- Omega-3 fatty acids (abundant in fish oils) are beneficial, whereas (trans) unsaturated fats produced by artificial hydrogenation of polyunsaturated oils (used in baked goods and margarine) adversely affect cholesterol profiles.

- Cigarette smoking is a well-established risk factor in both men and women. Prolonged (years) smoking of one pack of cigarettes or more daily increases the death rate from ischemic heart disease by 200%. Smoking cessation reduces that risk substantially.

- C-reactive protein (CRP) is an acute-phase reactant synthesized primarily by the liver. When locally synthesized within atherosclerotic intima, it can also regulate local endothelial adhesion and thrombotic states. Most importantly, it strongly and independently predicts the risk of myocardial infarction, stroke, peripheral arterial disease, and sudden cardiac death, even among apparently healthy individuals

56. **Ans. (c) Hyaline arteriosclerosis** *(Ref: Robbin's 8th/495-6, 9/e p490)*
Hyaline arteriosclerosis is characterized by the following:

- **Pink, hyaline thickening** of arteriolar walls (due to leaking of plasma proteins) associated with luminal narrowing.
- Seen in **elderly**[Q], more commonly in **benign hypertension**[Q], **diabetes mellitus**[Q] **(DM) and benign nephrosclerosis**[Q].

57. **Ans. (a) Insulin deficiency** *(Ref: Robbins 8th/1144-1146, 9/e p499)*
All the mentioned features in the question are the macrovascular complications of diabetes mellitus which is caused due to insulin deficiency.

58. **Ans. (a) Atherosclerosis** *(Ref: Robbins 8th/507, Harrison 18th/2060-1)*
Direct quote from Harrsion....*'atleast 90% of all abdominal aortic aneurysms >4.0 cm are related to atherosclerotic disease and most are present just below the renal arteries'.*

59. **Ans. (a) Hyaline arteriosclerosis** *(Ref: Robbins 8th/495; 507, 950, 9/e p490)*
Hyaline arteriosclerosis is characterized by the following:

- Pink, hyaline thickening of arteriolar walls (due to leaking of plasma proteins) associated with luminal narrowing.
- Seen in elderly, more commonly in benign hypertension, diabetes mellitus (DM) and benign nephrosclerosis.

Other important points

The characteristic features seen in the kidney are called benign nephrosclerosis include:
- Hyaline arterioslcerosis
- Normal or small kidney size with **leather grain appearance**[Q].
- Presence of **fibroelastic hyperplasia** (media hypertrophy, elastic lamina duplication and intimal thickening)
- Presence of patchy ischemic atrophy and glomerular sclerosis

Malignant hypertension is discussed below.

60. **Ans. (b) Hyaline arteriolosclerosis:** *(Ref: Robbins 7th/534, 8th/496, 949, 9/e p490)*
Malignant hypertension is characterized by sudden elevation of BP (diastolic BP > 120 mmHg) accompanied by papilledema, CNS manifestations, cardiac decompensation and acute progressive deterioration of renal function.

Other important points

The characteristic features include:
1. Fibrinoid necrosis^Q of the small vessels particularly the arterioles
2. Necrotizing arteriolitis^Q: Presence of inflammatory cells in the vessel wall
3. Hyperplastic arteriosclerosis^Q: Proliferation of the internal smooth muscle cells seen in the interlobular arteries giving **onion skin like appearance**^Q

Renal involvement is called malignant nephrosclerosis having the features like
a. Kidneys have a typical **"flea bitten "appearance**^Q (due to petechial hemorrhage on cortical surface)
b. Necrotizing glomerulonephritis: Necrotizing arteriolitis may involve the glomeruli also.

61. **Ans. (c) Lipoprotein 'A'** *(Ref: Robbins 7th/520-521)*
In addition to a high cholesterol level there is a positive correlation between atherosclerosis of coronary artery and other arteries and circulating levels of lipoprotein (a).

Lp (a) has structural similarity with plasminogen. It interferes with formation of plasmin and hence, fibrinolysis. This contributes to atherosclerosis.

62. **Ans. (b) Atherosclerosis** *(Ref: Harrison 17th/1563, 18th/2060-1, Robbins 7th/531, 9/e p503)*

63. **Ans. (a) Heart** *(Ref: Ultrastructural pathology/374, Robbins 8th/495-6)*
Friends, trust me this seemed to be an easy one but as i found out to my surprise, the reference pages mentioned by all MCQ books including our competitors (whom we expect to copy this info as well as has happened so many times earlier !☺) give page number from Robbins which don't have this info! But I managed to find something worthy as follows: **Ultrastructural pathology** by Cheville NF page 374 mentions that …. *'hyperplastic arteriosclerosis of the kidney has the most serious effects but this lesion is also found in the artereioles of the intestine , gall bladder and pancreas."* I was not able to found anything relevant about pericardial fat. But after discussion with many senior faculty members, the answer of consensus is option 'a' i.e. Heart.

64. **Ans. (a) Homocysteinemia; (c) Increased fibrinogen; (e) Increased plasminogen activator inhibitors.** *(Ref: Robbins 7th/520, 8th/498, 9/e p492)*

65. **Ans. (a) Concentric hypertrophy of LV; (b) Increased heart size; (c) Increased size of heart muscle; (d) Myohypertrophy:** *(Ref: Robbins 7th/587, Harrison 17th/1552)*
Features of essential hypertensions are:
• Concentric hypertrophy of the left ventricles due to pressure overload of the heart.
• Increase in weight of heart (>500 gm) is disproportionate to the increase in overall size of heart.
• Thickening of the left ventricular wall increased the ratio of its wall thickness to radius.
• Microscopically the earliest changes of systemic hypertensive heart disease is an increased transverse myocytes diameter. In advanced stage the cellular and nuclear enlargement is prominent. Electron microscopy reveals increase in number of myofilaments comprising myofibrils, mitochondrial changes and multiple intercalated disks.
• Increase total RNA and ratio of RNA to DNA contents.

66. **Ans. (c) Lipids in LDL gets auto-oxidized** *(Ref: Harrison 17th/1502 Robbins 7th/523, 9/e p496)*
Scavenger receptors and not LDL receptors on macrophages result in uptake of oxidized LDL to form foam cells contributing to atherosclerosis.

67. **Ans. (b) Pulmonary artery trunk** *(Ref: Robbins 8th/502, 9/e p498)*
See mnemonic in text.

68. **Ans. (b) Hyaline arteriosclerosis** *(Ref: Robbins 8th/495-496, 9/e p490)*

69. **Ans. (a) Fibrinoid necrosis of arteriolar wall** *(Ref: Robbins 7th/1007, 9/e p490)*
Accelerated phase of hypertension is the other name for malignant hypertension.

70. **Ans. (d) Abdominal aorta** *(Ref: Robbins 9/e p502, 8th/507, 7th/531)*

71. **Ans. (b) Media** *(Ref: Robbins 9/e p491, 8th/496; 7th/498)*

72. **Ans. (c) Platelets** *(Ref: Robbins 8th/501, 9/e p496)*
The pathogenesis of atherosclerotic plaques (atheromas) begins with endothelial cell injury, which results in endothelial cell dysfunction and/or exposure of subendothelial collagen (endothelial cell denudation). Exposure of subendothelial collagen promotes platelet adhesion, aggregation, and release of factors that promote migration of smooth muscle cells (SMC) from the media into the intima, as well as SMC proliferation. These factors include platelet-derived growth factor (PDGF) and transforming growth factor beta (TGF-β).

> PDGF is chemotactic and mitogenic for smooth muscle cells (SMC). TGF- β is chemotactic for SMC.

(Choice A) Neutrophils do not appear to play a significant role in the chronic intimal inflammatory process that generates atheromas, nor do they release growth factors.

(Choice B) Eosinophils are important in parasitic infections and IgE-mediated immune reactions.

73. Ans. (d) They show predominantly intracellular lipid accumulation. *(Ref: Robbins 9/e p496, 8th/501-4)*

> The lesions in the stem of the question are fatty streaks. These are the earliest lesions in the progression to atherosclerosis. Fatty streaks are composed of intimal lipid filled foam cells, derived from macrophages and smooth muscle cells (SMC) that have engulfed lipoprotein (predominantly LDL) which has entered the intima through an injured leaky endothelium. The foamy appearance is due to intracellular lipid containing phagolysosomes.

Fatty streaks begin as multiple yellow spots approximately 1 mm in diameter which join to form streaks approximately 1 cm long. They may contain a few lymphocytes, but foam cells are the predominant constituents. The fatty streaks are not significantly raised, so, they do not disturb normal blood flow. They can be seen in the aortas of children less than 1 year old and are present in the aortas of all children over 10. Whereas some fatty streaks maybe precursors of atheromatous plaques not all fatty streaks progress to these more advanced atherosclerotic plaques.

(Choice B) Fatty streaks often occur on regions of the vasculature not particularly prone to atheroma development later in life. Moreover, they frequently affect individuals in locations and populations with a low lifetime incidence of fully developed atheromatous plaques.

74. Ans. (c) Hyperplastic arteriolosclerosis *(Ref: Robbins 8th/496, 9/e p490)*

74.1. Ans. (b) Left anterior descending coronary artery *(Ref: Robbins 8/e p551, 9/e p542)*

The frequencies of involvement of each of the three main arterial trunks and the corresponding sites of myocardial lesions resulting in infarction (in the typical right dominant heart) are as follows:

- **Left anterior descending coronary artery (40% to 50%):** infarcts involving the anterior wall of left ventricle near the apex; the anterior portion of ventricular septum; and the apex circumferentially
- *Right coronary artery (30% to 40%):* infarcts involving the inferior/posterior wall of left ventricle; posterior portion of ventricular septum; and the inferior/posterior right ventricular free wall in some cases
- *Left circumflex coronary artery (15% to 20%):* infarcts involving the lateral wall of left ventricle except at the apex

74.2. Ans. (b) Flea bitten kidney *(Ref: Robbins 8/e p950-1, 9/e p490)*

In malignant hypertension, on gross inspection the kidney size depends on the duration and severity of the hypertensive disease. Small, pinpoint petechial hemorrhages may appear on the cortical surface from rupture of arterioles or glomerular capillaries, giving the **kidney a peculiar "flea-bitten" appearance.**

Causes of contracted kidney

Symmetric	Asymmetric
• Chronic glomerulonephritis • Benign nephrosclerosis	• Chronic pyelonephritis
Causes of enlarged kidneys	
• Amyloidosis • Rapidly progressive glomerulonephritis (RPGN) • Myeloma kidney	• Diabetic renal disease [Kimmelstiel Wilson nodules are pathognomic] • Polycystic kidney disease • Bilateral obstruction (hydronephrosis)

74.3. Ans. (a) Marfan syndrome *(Ref: Robbins 8/e p509, 9/e p502)*

The vascular wall is weakened through loss of smooth muscle cells or the inappropriate synthesis of noncollagenous or nonelastic ECM. Atherosclerosis and hypertension induced ischemia is reflected in "degenerative changes" of the aorta, whereby smooth muscle cell loss leads to scarring (and loss of elastic fibers), inadequate ECM synthesis, and production of increasing amounts of amorphous ground substance (glycosaminoglycan). Histologically these changes are collectively called *cystic medial degeneration.* Though these are nonspecific, they can be seen with **Marfan disease**[Q] and **scurvy**[Q]

74.4. Ans. (a) Hypertension *(Ref: Robbins 8/e p508, 9/e p504)*

Aortic dissection occurs when blood splays apart the laminar planes of the media to form a blood-filled channel within the aortic wall; this can be catastrophic if the dissection then ruptures through the adventitia and hemorrhages into adjacent spaces.

Aortic dissection occurs principally in two groups:

- Men aged 40 to 60, with antecedent hypertension (more than 90% of cases of dissection);
- Younger patients with systemic or localized abnormalities of connective tissue affecting the aorta (e.g., Marfan syndrome).

74.5. Ans. (b) Heart *(Ref: Robbins 8/e p502, 9/e p498)*

Coronary arteries supply the heart. They are the second most common vessel (after abdominal aorta) to be affected in atherosclerosis.

Significance of involved blood vessels in atherosclerosis

Abdominal Aorta	• – Most common site of atherosclerotic aneurysm in body
Coronary Arteries	• – Left Anterior Descending is MC coronary artery involved[o]
Poplitial Artery	• – MC peripheral vessel showing aneurysm formation[o]
Descending Thoracic Aorta	
Internal carotid artery	
Circle of Willis	

74.6. Ans. (c) Atherosclerosis *(Ref: Robbins 8/e p507, 9/e 502)*

The two most important disorders that predispose to aortic aneurysms are atherosclerosis and hypertension; **atherosclerosis** is a greater factor in **abdominal aortic aneurysms**, while *hypertension* is the most common condition associated with aneurysms of the *ascending aorta*.

An *aneurysm* is a *localized abnormal dilation of a blood vessel or the heart*); it can be congenital or acquired. When an aneurysm involves an intact attenuated arterial wall or thinned ventricular wall of the heart, it is called a *true aneurysm*.

74.7. Ans. (a) Splenic *(Ref: Peripheral Vascular Interventions chapter 15, pg 263)*
- The visceral arteries include the three main unpaired branches of the abdominal aorta namely celiac artery, superior mesenteric and inferior meseneteric arteries.
- The most common visceral vessel showing aneurysm formation is the **splenic artery**[Q] followed by the hepatic artery.

74.8. Ans. (c) Monckeberg's sclerosis *(Ref: Robbins 8/e p496, 9/e p491)*
- *Mönckeberg medial sclerosis* is characterized by **calcific deposits** in muscular arteries in persons **typically older than age 50**.
- The deposits may **undergo metaplastic change** into bone.
- Nevertheless, the lesions do not encroach on the vessel lumen and are usually **not clinically significant.**

74.9. Ans. (a) Syphilitic *(Ref: Robbins 8/e p507-508, 7/e p532)*

Direct lines… "The obliterative endarteritis characteristic of late-stage syphilis shows a predilection for small vessels, including those of the vasa vasorum of the thoracic aorta."

Atherosclerosis affects abdominal aorta most commonly. Traumatic aneurysm can affect any site of the aorta. Berry aneurysm affects the circle of Willis.

74.10. Ans. (d) Hyperplastic arteriosclerosis *(Ref: Robbins 9/e p490, 8/e p496, 7/e p530)*

Hyperplastic arteriosclerosis is associated with **malignant hypertension** in which concentric thickening of the walls and luminal narrowing leads to "**onion skin like lesions**".

74.11. Ans (c) Chlamydia *(Ref: Robbins 9/e 496, 8/e p500)*

Robbins.. "**Herpes virus, cytomegalovirus** and *Chlamydia pneumoniae* have all been detected in atherosclerotic plaques but not in normal arteries, and seroepidemiologic studies find increased antibody titers to *C. pneumoniae* in patients with more severe atherosclerosis".
- Though the book also mentions that some of these observations are confounded by the fact that *C. pneumoniae* bronchitis is also associated with smoking which is a well-established IHD risk factor. Moreover, infections with these organisms are exceedingly common (as is atherosclerosis), so that distinguishing coincidence from causality is difficult.
- Nevertheless, it is certainly possible that such organisms could infect sites of early atheroma formation; their foreign antigens could potentiate atherogenesis by driving local immune responses, or infectious agents could contribute to the local prothrombotic state.

74.12. Ans (c) Hyaline arteriosclerosis *(Ref: Robbins 9/e p490, 8/e p495)*

The following are the two patterns of vascular changes in hypertension

Hyaline Arteriolosclerosis	Hyperplastic Arteriolosclerosis
• Vascular lesion consists of a homogeneous, pink, hyaline thickening of the walls of arterioles with loss of underlying structural detail, and with narrowing of the lumen • Seen in the **elderly, hypertensive and diabetic** • Hyaline arteriolosclerosis is more generalized and more severe in patients with hypertension.	• Vascular lesion has **onionskin**, concentric, laminated thickening of the walls of arterioles with progressive narrowing of the lumina • Seen in but not exclusively in **malignant hypertension**, • Frequently accompanied by deposits of fibrinoid and acute necrosis of the vessel walls referred to as **necrotizing arteriolitis** (particularly in the kidney)

75. Ans. (a) Giant cell arteritis *(Ref: Robbins 9/e p508, 8th/512-3)*

- Giant-cell (temporal) arteritis is a chronic, typically granulomatous inflammation of large to small-sized arteries that affects principally the arteries in the head—especially the temporal arteries—but also the vertebral and ophthalmic arteries
- Histopathologically, the disease is a panarteritis with inflammatory mononuclear cell infiltrates within the vessel wall with frequent giant cell formation.
- Leukocytoclastic Vasculitis (also known as Microscopic Polyarteritis): it is a necrotizing vasculitis affecting arterioles/capillaries/venules in which all lesions are of the same age. Granulomatous inflammation is absent[Q]

76. Ans. (d) Microscopic polyangiitis *(Ref: Robbins 9/e p506, 8th/512, 515)*

It's a direct question; we just need to keep in mind the classification of vasculitis. See text for details.

77. Ans. (a) Henoch-Schonlein Purpura *(Ref: Robbins 8th/934, 9/e p926, Harrison 17th/2128, Wintrobes 12th/1343)*

- Henoch-Schonlein Purpura (HSP) is a syndrome seen in children (3-8 years of age) consisting of *purpuric skin lesions characteristically involving the extensor surfaces of arms and legs as well as buttocks; abdominal manifestations including pain, vomiting, and intestinal bleeding; nonmigratory arthralgia; and renal abnormalities.* It follows an upper respiratory infection.
- A history of atopy is present.
- The renal manifestations may include gross or microscopic hematuria, proteinuria, and nephrotic syndrome and is seen in 1/3rd of the patients. IgA is deposited in the glomerular mesangium.
- **Microscopically**
- **Kidney** has **deposition of IgA, sometimes with IgG and C3, in the mesangial region**.
- **The skin lesions** consist of subepidermal hemorrhages and a necrotizing vasculitis with IgA deposition involving the small vessels of the dermis.
- Vasculitis also occurs in other organs, such as the gastrointestinal tract, but **is rare in the kidney**[Q]

Wegner's granulomatosis and Giant cell Vasculitis are not seen in children. Options 'b' and 'c' are ruled out.

Kawasaki's disease affects children but the presentation is fever, cervical lymphadenopathy, skin rash, oral ulcers, conjunctivitis and edema of hands and feet. So, option 'd' is also ruled out.

78. Ans. (d) Microscopic polyangiitis *(Ref: Robbins 8th/513-517, 9/e p510)*

Robbins clearly mentions that "microscopic polyangiitis is characterized by segmental fibrinoid necrosis of the media with focal transmural necrotizing lesions; granulomatous inflammation is absent".

79. Ans. (d) Wegener's granulomatosis *(Ref: Robbins 8th/516-517, 9/e p507)*

- ANCA or antineutrophilic cytoplasmic antibodies are formed against certain proteins in the cytoplasm of neutrophils. Out of the given options, Wegener's granulomatosis is most strongly associated with ANCA.

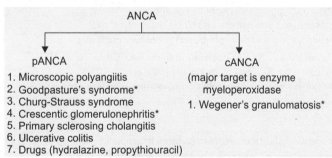

80. Ans. (c) Kawasaki's disease *(Ref: Robbins 9/e p510, 8th/515, 7th/539, Harrison 17th/2130. 18th/2800)*

Kawasaki's disease (**mucocutaneous lymph node syndrome**) is an arteritis that often involves the coronary arteries, usually in **young children** and infants (majority of the cases are seen in <5 years old). It is treated with intravenous immunoglobulin and aspirin. (For details, see text.)

81. Ans. (b) Post-capillary venules *(Ref: Harrison 17th/2128, 18th/2798, Robbins 8th/515, 9/e p510)*

Hypersensitivity vasculitis is clearly mentioned in **Harrison 18th/2798** as the other name for **cutaneous vasculitis**. However, **Robbins** confuses the issue by mentioning that *Hypersensitivity vasculitis is the other name of microscopic angiitis. However, we would prefer to go with Harrison in this context.*

Direct quote from Harrison 18th/2798… '***Post capillary venules are the most commonly involved vessels;*** *capillaries and arterioles may be involved less frequently'.*

82. **Ans. (c) Wegener's granulomatosis** *(Ref: Robbins illustrated 7th/541, 8th/516, 9/e p511-512)*
   - Both Wegener's granulomatosis and Goodpasture's syndrome can present similarly but presence of c-ANCA makes a diagnosis of **Wegener's granulomatosis.**

83. **Ans. (a) Buerger's disease; (b) HSP; (d) Reiter's disease; (e) Behcet's syndrome.** *(Ref: Harrison' 17th/2119, 1485, Robbins' 7th/535, 537)*

Vasculitis syndromes	
Primary vasculitis	**Secondary vasculitis syndrome**
• Wegener's granulomatosis • Churg-Strauss syndrome • PAN, HSP • Microscopic polyangitis • Giant cell arteritis, Takayasu's arteritis • Idiopathic cutaneous vasculitis • Essential mixed cryoglobulinemia • Behcet's syndrome, Cogan's syndrome • Kawasaki disease	• Drug induced vasculitis • Serum sickness • Infection • Malignancy • Rheumatic disease

84. **Ans. (a) Lung; (c) Kidney; (d) Upper respiratory tract; (e) Heart** *(Ref: Robbins 7th/541, 9/e p511)*

85. **Ans. (a) Involve lungs; (b) Involve nose; (c) Involve kidney; (d) Treated with cytotoxic agent and/or steroid.**
   (Ref: Robbins 7th/541, 9/e p511, Harrison 17th/2121)

   Wegener's granulomatosis is treated with steroids and cyclophosphamide. They dramatically ameliorate glomerular injury in pauci-immune glomerulonephritis.

86. **Ans. (c) Seen in Henoch Schonlein purpura** *(Ref: Robbins 8th/920-921, 9/e p926)*

87. **Ans. (a) Kawasaki disease** *(Ref: Robbin 7th/537, 9/e p506)*
   Classification of vasculitis with important points

Large vessel vasculitis
(a) *Giant cell (temporal) arteritis:* in patients older than 50. (b) *Takayasu's arteritis:* in patients younger than 50.
Medium-sized vessel vasculitis:
(a) *Polyarteritis nodosa:* Glomerulonephritis is absent (b) *Kawasaki disease:* coronary arteries are often involved, usually occurs in children.
Small vessel vasculitis:
(a) *Wegner granulomatosis:* Necrotizing glomerulonephritis is common (b) *Churg-strauss syndrome:* Associated with asthma and blood eosinophilia (c) *Microscopic polyangitis:* Necrotizing glomerulonephritis and pulmonary capillaritis
(d) *Henoch-Schonlein purpura:* Vasculitis with IgA- dominant immune deposits (e) *Essential cryoglobulinemic vasculitis:* Skin and glomeruli are often involved. (f) *Cutaneous leukocytoclastic angiitis:* Systemic vasculitis or glomerulonephritis is absent.

88. **Ans. (a) Hypertension** *(Ref: Robbins 7th/539, 9/e p509-510)*
   Polyarteritis Nodosa

   - It is a systemic vasculitis manifested by transmural necrotizing inflammation of small or medium sized muscular arteries.
   - *Renal artery* is most commonly involved whereas *Pulmonary circulation is spared*.
   - Most common manifestations are malaise, fever of unknown cause, weight loss, hypertension (rapidly developing), abdominal pain, melena, diffuse muscular pains, and peripheral neuritis (predominantly motor).

89. **Ans. (c) Kawasaki disease** *(Ref: http://emedicine.medscape.com/article/1006838, Robbins 9/e p510)*
   Clinically, infantile polyarteritis nodosa (IPAN) often is part of the spectrum of Kawasaki disease (KD).

90. **Ans. (b) Lung and kidney** *(Ref: Robbins 9/e p511-512, 8th/516; 7th/541-542)*

91. **Ans. (a) Pulmonary artery** *(Ref: Robbins 9/e p 509-510, 8th/514; 7 th/539)*

92. **Ans. (c) Wegener's granulomatosis** *(Ref: Robbins 9/e p511-512, 8th/516-517; 7 th/541)*

93. **Ans. (b) Henoch Schonlein purpura** *(Ref: Robbins 8th/920-921, 9/e p926)*

94. **Ans. (d) Segmental vasculitis extending into contiguous veins and nerves** *(Ref: Robbins 8th/517, 9/e p512)*

Cardiovascular System

Munish is most likely suffering from Buerger's disease (Young male with hypersensitivity to tobacco). Microscopically the condition shows. *Segmental thrombosing vasculitis often extending into contiguous veins and nerves* (a feature rarely seen in other types of vasculitis), encasing them in fibrous tissue.

- (Choice A) Lipid-filled intimal plaques that bulge into the arterial lumen are seen in atherosclerosis.
- (Choice B) Onion-like concentric thickening of arteriolar walls as a result of laminated smooth muscle cells and reduplicated basement membranes is seen in hyperplastic arteriolosclerosis (seen in malignant hypertension)
- (Choice C) Transmural inflammation of the arterial wall with fibrinoid necrosis is characteristic of polyarteritis nodosa.

95. Ans. (a) Blindness *(Ref: Robbins 8th/512-31, 9/e p508)*

> - Most likely diagnosis in this case is temporal (giant cell) arteritis. This is a pan-arteritis that can involve any of the branches of the aortic arch. Temporal arteritis commonly produces visual disturbances including blindness due to involvement of the ophthalmic artery. Biopsy of affected segments shows granulomatous lesions with giant cells.

- Stroke may occur in temporal arteritis, but this would not likely produce loss of all tactile sensations (choice c).
- Loss of the ability to speak (choice d) may result from stroke. *Visual disturbances are more common than stroke in temporal arteritis.*

96. Ans. (b) Wegener's granulomatosis *(Ref: Robbins 8th/516, 9/e p512)*

96.1. Ans. (d) Involves large vessels *(Ref: Robbins 8/e p516-7, 9/e p511*

Wegener's granulomatosis is a **small vessel** necrotizing vasculitis which is characterized by **triad of**

- Acute necrotizing *granulomas of either upper* (more commonly) *or lower respiratory tract or both*
- *Focal necrotizing or granulomatous vasculitis* most commonly affecting lungs and upper airways.
- *Renal involvement* in the form of focal necrotizing, often crescentic glomerulonephritis.
  - Clinical features include fever, weight loss, otitis media, nasal septal perforation[Q], strawberry gums[Q], cough, hemoptyis, **palpable purpura**[Q], joint pain and ocular features (uveitis, conjunctivitis)
  - Investigations show serum **c-ANCA**[Q] positivity, **cavitatory lesions**[Q] in the chest X ray and red cell casts (indicative of glomerulonephritis) in the urine.

96.2. Ans. (c) Polyarteritis nodosa *(Ref: Robbins 8/e p512, 9/e p506)*

Classfication based on vessel size

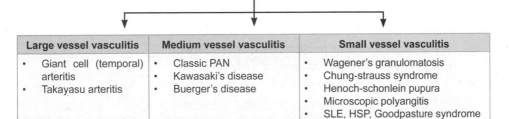

Large vessel vasculitis	Medium vessel vasculitis	Small vessel vasculitis
• Giant cell (temporal) arteritis • Takayasu arteritis	• Classic PAN • Kawasaki's disease • Buerger's disease	• Wagener's granulomatosis • Chung-strauss syndrome • Henoch-schonlein pupura • Microscopic polyangitis • SLE, HSP, Goodpasture syndrome

96.3. Ans. (c) Most commonly involved artery is abdominal aorta *(Robins 8/e p512-3, 9/e p507-508)*

Salient features of temporal arteritis/ Giant cell arteritis

- Large vessel vasculitis characterised by granulomatous arteritis of the aorta and its major branches particularly the extracranial branches of the carotid artery.
- Since the **superficial temporal artery**[Q] is the most commonly involved vessel, the giant cell arteritis is called as temporal arteritis.
- Clinical features include constitutional symptoms like fever, fatigue, weight loss, **jaw pain**[Q] **(most specific symptom)**, facial pain, **localized headache**[Q] **(commonest symptom**; most intense along the anatomical course of the superficial temporal artery) and sudden onset of blindness (due to involvement of ophthalmic artery).
- *Biopsy of temporal artery*[Q] is the *investigation of choice.*
- Since giant-cell arteritis is **extremely segmental**, adequate biopsy requires at least a 2- to 3-cm length of artery; even then, a negative biopsy result does not exclude the diagnosis
- Microscopically, there is presence of **granulomatous inflammation** with multinucleated giant cells and fragmentation of internal elastic lamina.

96.4. Ans. (a) Lung *(Ref: Robins 8/e p514-5, 9/e p509-510)*

Polyarteritis nodosa (PAN) is characterised by necrotizing inflammation typically involving renal arteries but **sparing pulmonary vessels.**

96.5. Ans. (b)Takayasu arteritis*(Ref: Internet, Robins 9/e p508)*

Takayasu arteritis is the choosen answer as it is associated with involvement of *superior mesenteric artery*. So, it may be associated with abdominal angiitis.

96.6. Ans. (a) No change*(Ref: Robbins 8/e p518, 9/e p513)*

Structural changes in the arterial walls **are absent** *except late in the course*, when intimal thickening can appear.

96.7. Ans. None or (c) 40-60%*(Ref: Robbins 8/e p Heptinstall's Pathology of the Kidney, Volume 1 p463.)*

I don't know why they frame these type of questions.

Heptinstall writes…"In different series, the degree if renal involvement in *children* with HSP (defined by the presence of hematuria) is *20-56% (overall 32%)* whereas in *adults*, it is *49-78% (overall 59%)*".

You may choose your answer friends.

96.8. Ans. (a) Carotid body tumour*(Ref: Robbins 8/e p522)*

Before we discuss the answer friends, a simple clarification that is to be kept in mind;

Glomus tumor (also known as a glomangioma) is a rare benign neoplasm arising from the *glomus body* and mainly found *under the nail*, on the fingertip or in the foot. It **DOES NOTcontain glomus cells.**

- A glomus cell (type I) is a peripheral chemoreceptor mainly located in the carotid bodies and aortic bodies helping in regulation of the breathing.
- *Neoplasms of glomus cells* are known as *paraganglioma.*
- The most common location of these tumors is **within the adrenal medulla**, where they give rise to pheochromocytomas,
- Approximately 70% of extra-adrenal paragangliomas occur in the head and neck region. Paragangliomas typically develop in two locations:
- **Paravertebral paraganglia** (e.g., organs of Zuckerkandl and, rarely, bladder). Such tumors have sympathetic connections and are **chromaffin-positive**, a stain that detects **catecholamines**.
- Paraganglia related to the great vessels of the head and neck, the so-called aorticopulmonary chain, including the *carotid bodies* (**most common**); aortic bodies; jugulotympanic ganglia; ganglion nodosum of the vagus nerve; and clusters located about the oral cavity, nose, nasopharynx, larynx, and orbit. These are innervated by the parasympathetic nervous system and **infrequently release catecholamines**

Important points about carotid body tumour

The **carotid body tumor** is a prototype of a **parasympathetic paraganglioma**.
Arisesclose to or envelops the bifurcation of the common carotid artery.
The microscopic features include presence of nests **(Zellballen)** of round to oval chief cells (neuroectodermal in origin) that are surrounded by delicate vascular septae.
The **chief cells** stain strongly for **neuroendocrine markers** such as chromogranin, synaptophysin, neuron-specific enolase, CD56, and CD57.
In addition, the supporting spindle-shaped stromal cells called *sustentacular cells* are positive for *S-100 protein*.

96.9. Ans. (c) Distal portion of digits*(Ref: Robbins 8/e p522, 9/e p517)*

- *Glomus tumor* is a biologically **benign tumor**[Q] that arises from the modified smooth muscle cells of the glomus body
- **Glomus body** is a specialized arteriovenous anastomosis that is involved in **thermoregulation**[Q].
- It is an often exquisitely painful tumor
- Glomus tumors *are most commonly found in the distal portion of the digits*[Q], especially under the fingernails.
- **Excision**[Q]is curative.

96.10. Ans (a)Port wine stain*(Ref: Robbins 8/e p522, 9/e p516)*

Sturge–Weber syndrome is usually manifested at birth by a **port-wine stain** on the forehead and upper eyelid of one side of the face.

96.11. Ans (a) Bacterial infection*(Ref: Robbins 8/e p521, 9/e p516)*

Cardiovascular System

Pyogenic granuloma: Key points

- It is a **benign**^Q tumor
- Type of **capillary hemangioma**^Q which it **bleeds**^Q easily and is often ulcerated.
- Is a rapidly growing pedunculated red nodule on the skin, or gingival or oral mucosa;
- 1/3rd of the lesions develop after trauma

Also know that;

- *Pregnancy tumor (granuloma gravidarum)* is a pyogenic granuloma that occurs infrequently (1% of patients) in the gingiva of pregnant women.
- These lesions may spontaneously regress post pregnancy) or undergo fibrosis;
- Some cases require surgical excision
- Recurrence is rare.

GOLDEN POINTS FOR QUICK REVIEW / UPDATED INFORMATION FROM 9TH EDITION OF ROBBINS (CARDIOVASCULAR SYSTEM)

9th Robbins/ 507...New Names of Antibodies

- The **c-ANCA** antibody is now called as Anti-proteinase-3 or **PR3-ANCA**. It is produced against proteinase 3 (PR3) which is a neutrophil azurophilic granule constituent. It is seen in patients having granulomatosis with polyangiitis (Wegener's granulomatosis).
- The **p-ANCA** antibody is called as Anti-myeloperoxidase or **MPO-ANCA**. It is produced against MPO which is a lysosomal granule constituent involved in oxygen free radical generation. This antibody is seen in microscopic polyangiitis and Churg-Strauss syndrome. It also develops after administration of many drugs including propylthiouracil.

Wegener's granulomatosis is now called by the new name of *granulomatosis with polyangiitis.*

Myocardial vessel spasm (concept of "Cardiac Raynaud" and "Takotsubo cardiomyopathy")

Excessive constriction of coronary arteries or myocardial arterioles may cause ischemia, and persistent vasospasm can even cause myocardial infarction. High levels of vasoactive mediators like endogenous epinephrine (in pheochromocytoma) or exogenous chemicals (cocaine or phenylephrine) can precipitate prolonged myocardial vessel contraction.

Such agents can be endogenous (e.g, epinephrine released by pheochromocytomas) or exogenous (cocaine or phenylephrine).

Extreme psychological stress can also lead to pathologic vasospasm. When vasospasm of cardiac arterial or arteriolar beds (so-called cardiac Raynaud) is of sufficient duration (20 to 30 minutes), myocardial infarction occurs. The increased catecholamines also increase heart rate and myocardial contractility exacerbating the cardiac ischemia.

Takotsubo cardiomyopathy (also called "broken heart syndrome") is an ischemic di;lated cardiomyopathy caused by emotional stress.

Robbins / 543.....Apart from transmural and subendocardial myocardial infarction, there is a new entity called as **Multifocal microinfarction.** This pattern is seen when there is pathology involving only smaller intramural vessels.

It is seen with microembolization, vasculitis, or vascular spasm, for example, due to endogenous catechols (epinephrine) or drugs (cocaine or ephedrine).

This may even lead to by a fatal arrhythmia) or an ischemic dilated cardiomyopathy, so-called takotsubo cardiomyopathy (also called "broken heart syndrome" described earlier).

NOTES

CHAPTER 10

Respiratory System

ANATOMY OF RESPIRATORY TRACT

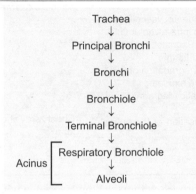

Trachea
↓
Principal Bronchi
↓
Bronchi
↓
Bronchiole
↓
Terminal Bronchiole
↓
Acinus [Respiratory Bronchiole
↓
Alveoli

> Bronchioles **DO NOT** have **cartilage** and **submucosal glands** in wall like bronchi[Q]

> Terminal bronchiole contain *maximum smooth muscle relative to the wall thickness*[Q]

- *Acinus is the functional unit of lung* whereas alveoli are the chief sites of gaseous exchange.
- *Lobule is composed of 3-5 terminal bronchioles with their acini.*
- Alveoli are lined by type I pneumocytes (forming 95% of alveolar surface) and type II pneumocytes (responsible for secretion of surfactant and repair of alveoli after type I pneumocyte destruction). The alveolar wall has the presence of **pores of Kohn**[Q] for allowing the passage of bacteria and exudate between adjacent alveoli.
- The entire respiratory tract is lined by *pseudostratified, tall, ciliated columnar epithelial cells except vocal cords* (these have stratified squamous epithelium).

Broadly, the diseases of lung may be divided into infectious, obstructive, restrictive, vascular and neoplastic etiologies.

INFECTIVE LUNG DISEASES

1. Pneumonia

Infection of the lung parenchyma is called pneumonia. It can be of two types

Pneumonia

Typical pneumonia	Atypical pneumonia
• Infection caused by extracellular organisms mainly bacteria	• Infection caused by intracellular organisms like Mycoplasma, Chlamydia pneumoniae and viruses like RSV, influenza virus, rhinovirus.
• **Characterized by neutrophilic** infilration and presence of **Intra-alveolar exudates** (leading to consolidation[Q]).	• **Characterized by lymphocytic** infiltration and presence of alveolar septal and interstitial inflammation with **absence of alveolar exudates**[Q].
• Clinical features include acute onset of high grade fever and mucopurulent cough which may also be associated with pleuritic pain.	• Clinical features include **fever, headache, dry cough and myalgia**. Productive Cough and pleural involvement is **uncommon**[Q].

Viral pneumonia result in interstitial infiltrates (therefore called interstitial pneumonia) and may result in variety of cytopathic effects. e.g. RSV shows bronchiolitis and multinucleate giant cells and CMV and herpes show inclusion bodies.

> Commonest cause of **community accquired pneumonia** is *Streptococcus pneumoniae*

> Commonest cause of **nosocomial pneumonia** is *Staphylococcus aureus*

> Most common cause of **atypical pneumonia** is *Mycoplasma pneumoniae*).

Furthermore, typical pneumonia can be of two types:

```
Typical pneumonia
```

Lobar pneumonia	Bronchopneumonia

• Condolidation of entire lobe usually caused by **Streptococcus pneumoniae**.
 • Following 4 stages of inflammation are present.
   1. **Congestion:** It is due to vasodilation. There is bacteria rich intra-alveolar fluid.
   2. **Red hepatization:** Exudate is rich in RBC, neutrophils and fibrin^Q.
   3. **Gray hepatization:** Degradation of RBC and fibrinosuppurative exudates
   4. **Resolution:** Enzymatic degradation of exudate and healing
	• Patchy consolidation in the lobe of lung.
	 • Usually **bilateral basal**^{Q} in location due to gravitation of secretions.
	 • Affects **extremes of age**^{Q} (infants or old).

• Chest X-ray show opacification of the entire lobe.	• Chest X-ray shows patchy opacification of the lobe^Q.

2. Lung Abscess

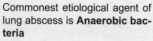
Commonest etiological agent of lung abscess is **Anaerobic bacteria**

- Local suppurative process within the lung associated with necrosis of the lung tissue is called lung abscess.
- It is most commonly caused by aspiration of infective material.
- Commonest etiological agent is Anaerobic bacteria of the oral cavity.^{Q}

```
Causes of lung abscess
```

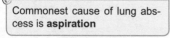
Commonest cause of lung abscess is **aspiration**

Aspiration	Post pneumonic infection	Post obstructive	Septic emboli	Miscellaneous
• Most common cause^Q. • Right lower lobe is the most frequently affected^Q.	• Infection caused by Staph aureus, klebsiella or type 3 Pneumococcus • Usually basal, multiple and diffusely scattered.	• Due to primary or secondary cancer.		• Direct hematogenous spread to lung from infection in esophagus or pleural cavity.

Clinical features: Fever, productive cough with large amount of sputum, chest pain, weight loss and presence of clubbing of the fingers and toes.

Characteristic histologic feature: Suppurative destruction of lung parenchyma within the central area of cavitation.

Complications include empyema, brain abscess or meningitis, pulmonary hemorrhage and **secondary amyloidosis**^{Q}.

3. Tuberculosis (Koch's Disease)

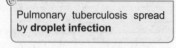
Pulmonary tuberculosis spread by **droplet infection**

Pulmonary tuberculosis is caused by **droplet infection** (coughing, sneezing etc) due to *Mycobacterium tuberculosis*. It is a strict aerobic bacteria having *mycolic acid* in its cell wall making it *acid fast* which means it resists decolourisation by a treatment with a mixture of acid and alcohol.

The reservoir of infection is a human being with active tuberculosis. However, certain clinical conditions can increase the risk of tuberculosis like diabetes mellitus, Hodgkin's lymphoma, chronic lung disease (particularly silicosis), chronic renal failure, malnutrition, alcoholism, and immunosuppression.

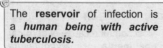
The **reservoir** of infection is a *human being with active tuberculosis.*

CONCEPT

Infection with *M. tuberculosis* is different from *disease*. Infection is the *presence of organisms*, which may or may not cause clinically significant disease. In most of the people, primary tuberculosis is asymptomatic though it may be associated with fever and pleural effusion. Infection with *M. tuberculosis* typically leads to the development of delayed hypersensitivity to *M. tuberculosis* antigens, which can be detected by the **tuberculin (Mantoux) test**. A positive tuberculin test result signifies cell mediated hypersensitivity to tubercular antigens but **does not differentiate** between infection and disease.

False-negative Mantoux test	False-positive Mantoux test
• Sarcoidosis	• Infection by atypical mycobacteria
• Malnutrition	• Previous vaccination with BCG
• Hodgkin disease	
• Immunosuppression	
• Fulminant tuberculosis	

Pathogenesis

Macrophages are the primary cells infected by *M. tuberculosis*. The bacteria enter macrophages by endocytosis. The bacterial cell wall *glycolipid lipoarabinomannan blocks the fusion of the phagosome and lysosome*. This is followed by bacterial multiplication inside the macrophages. Thus, the initial stages of primary tuberculosis (<3 weeks) in a non-sensitized individual is characterized by bacterial multiplication in the pulmonary alveolar macrophages and airspaces, with resulting bacteremia and spread to multiple sites in the body. After about 3 weeks of infection, the TH1 cells are stimulated by mycobacterial antigens and these cells differentiate into mature TH1cells by the action of IL-12.

The mature TH1 cells in the lymph nodes and lung produce IFN-γ which activates macrophages, stimulates formation of phagolysosome in them and causes nitric oxide induced oxidative damage to the mycobacteria. Activated macrophages produce TNF and recruit monocytes which then differentiate into the "epithelioid histiocytes", a characteristic feature of granulomatous inflammation. So, immunity to *M. tuberculosis* is primarily mediated by TH1 cells, which stimulate macrophages to kill the bacteria. The immune response is usually accompanied by hypersensitivity and tissue destruction. Reactivation of the infection or re-exposure to the bacilli in a previously sensitized host therefore causes activation of defense mechanism and increased tissue necrosis.

Clinical Features

Primary tuberculosis
• It *develops in a previously unexposed and unsensitized individual.* The source of the organism is usually exogenous. Most patients with primary tuberculosis develop latent disease while a minority develops progressive infection.
• Primary tuberculosis almost always begins in the lungs. Typically, the inhaled bacilli implant in the distal airspaces of the *lower part of the upper lobe or the upper part of the lower lobe* due to most of the inspired air being distributed here and form a subpleural lesion. This subpleural lesion along with the draining lymphatics and the lymph nodes is called as **Ghon's complex^Q**. During the first few weeks, there is also lymphatic and hematogenous dissemination to other parts of the body.
• At times, occult hematogenous spread occurs in primary TB where the focus is then called Simon focus.
• In majority of the people, development of cell-mediated immunity controls the infection. The Ghon's complex undergoes progressive fibrosis and calcification (detected radiologically and called as **Ranke complex^Q**).

Histologically
The sites of active disease show a characteristic granulomatous inflammatory reaction having the presence of *both caseating and non-caseating tubercles*. There is also presence of Langhans giant cells and lymphocytes.

Acid-fastness of the Mycobacterium is due to **mycolic acid**

Cord factor is a virulence factor for Mycobacterium *tuberculosis*

Both **ventilation** as well as **perfusion** per unit lung volume is **maximum at the base** of the lung.
However **ventilation perfusion ratio** is **maximum** at the **apical regions** of the lungs

Concept

Immunocompromised people **do not** form the characteristic granulomas

Respiratory System

Bronchial artery is the source of hemoptysis in TB.

Infectious aneurysms in a **pulmonary artery** secondary to pulmonary tuberculosis **(TB)** are referred to as **Rasmussen aneurysms.**

The most frequent form of **extra pulmonary** tuberculosis is **lymphadenitis** usually in the cervical region and is known as "**scrofula**".

Pott's disease is define as tubercular involvement the **vertebrae**

Clinical features in TB are drenching night sweats, fever, weight loss

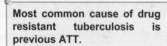

Most common cause of drug resistant tuberculosis is previous ATT.

Secondary tuberculosis

- *It is the pattern of disease that arises in a previously sensitized host.* It usually results from a reactivation of latent primary lesions after many years of an initial infection, particularly when host immunity is decreased or uncommonly may follow primary tuberculosis. Secondary pulmonary tuberculosis is classically localized to the apex of the upper lobes of the lungs called as **Puhl lesion**. The right lung is affected more commonly as compared to left because of high oxygen tension in the apices. Infraclavicular lesion of chronic pulmonary TB is called as **Assman focus**. The preexistence of hypersensitivity contributes to an immediate and marked tissue response leading to localization of the infection (the regional lymph nodes are less prominently involved in secondary tuberculosis) and cavitation followed by erosion into an airway (leading to spread of bacilli during coughing).

- **Histologically,** the active lesions show characteristic coalescent tubercles composed of epithelioid cells and Langhans cells with central caseation. The lesion of secondary pulmonary tuberculosis may heal with fibrosis either by itself or after therapy, or it may progress along the following several different pathways:

Progressive pulmonary tuberculosis

It is seen in the *elderly* and the *immunosuppressed* individuals. The apical lesion enlarges with increase in the area of caseation. The erosion of blood vessels (particularly **bronchial artery**[Q]) results in **hemoptysis**. The pleural cavity is associated with pleural effusion or empyema. If the treatment is adequate, the disease may be controlled but if it is inadequate, the infection may disseminate through airways, lymphatics or the vascular system.

Miliary disease

It occurs when organisms drain through lymphatics and blood vessels to the different organs of the body resulting in small yellow-white consolidated lesions. Miliary tuberculosis is most prominent in the liver, bone marrow, spleen, adrenals, meninges, kidneys, fallopian tubes, and epididymis.

Recent exam info: names of other healed foci

Names	Organs
• Rich focus	• Cortex of brain[Q]
• Simon focus	• Healed site of primary infection at **apex of lung**[Q]
• Simmond focus	• Liver[Q]
• Weigart focus	• Intima of **blood vessels**[Q]

Important radiological info

- Early **infraclavicular lesion - Assman Redeker** Simon[Q]
- In post primary stage (late dissemination), coarse granular dissemination is called Aschoff Puhl focus

The patients present with insidious onset of symptoms like low grade remittent fever usually associated with night sweats, productive cough, weight loss, hemoptysis, dyspnea and pleural effusion. The investigations usually reveal lymphocytosis and increased ESR (on hemogram), hilar lymphadenopathy and pleural effusion (on chest X ray), presence of acid fast bacilli with Ziehl Nielson staining. The treatment is provided with multiple drugs (for details, refer to *Review of Pharmacology* by the same authors).

Pulmonary diseases

Obstructive lung disease	Restrictive lung disease
• Characterized by increased resistance to airflow due to airway obstruction.	• Characterized by decreased expansion of the lung.
• Spirometry reveals $\frac{FEV_1}{FVC}$ ratio is **decreased**[Q].	• Spirometry reveals reduced total lung capacity and vital capacity[Q].
• Examples: Asthma, Emphysema, Chronic bronchitis, Bronchiectasis.	• Examples: 1. Chest wall disorder-polio, obesity kyphoscoliosis. 2. Interstitial/infiltrative disease: Pneumoconiosis, ARDS, Pulmonary fibrosis.

OBSTRUCTIVE LUNG DISEASES

1. Chronic Bronchitis

It is defined clinically as the presence of *productive cough for at least 3 months in at least 2 consecutive years* in absence of any other identifiable cause.

The most important initiating agent is *smoking*[Q] resulting in airway irritation leading to mucus hyper secretion; the latter may cause airway obstruction. Infection plays a secondary role particularly in maintaining chronic bronchitis and is also responsible for the acute exacerbations.

Histologic features include *chronic lymphocytic infiltration* of the airways and *submucosal gland hypertrophy*. There is also *increase in* **Reid index**[Q]. The bronchial epithelium may also have squamous metaplasia and dysplasia.

> • *Normal Reid index is 0.4* whereas its value *increases in chronic bronchitis.*

Clinical features: Late onset of dyspnea with productive cough (copious sputum), recurrent infections, hypoxemia and mild cyanosis (***BLUE BLOATERS***). Long standing chronic bronchitis can cause cor pulmonale (right sided heart failure due to pulmonary hypertension).

> Most important **initiating agent** in chronic bronchitis is **smoking**

> **Reid index** is the ratio of the mucus gland layer thickness to the thickness of the wall between epithelium and cartilage.

2. Emphysema

It is abnormal *permanent enlargement of the airspace distal to terminal bronchioles* and is associated with *destruction of their walls*.

- Most important etiological agent for emphysema is **smoking**[Q] which causes inflammation in airways resulting in increased neutrophils and macrophages. These inflammatory cells release elastase responsible for destruction of lung tissue resulting in emphysema.

- Normally, the pulmonary tissue destruction by elastase is prevented by the presence of anti-elastase activity which is primarily due to α_1-antitrypsin; α_1-AT (with minor contribution from secretory leukoprotease inhibitor in bronchial mucus and serum α_1- macroglobulin). So, any increase in neutrophils (usually in smokers) or deficiency of α_1-AT would contribute to development of emphysema. Characteristically, there is loss or reduction of elastic recoil of the lung.

- α_1-AT is synthesized in the liver. The normal α_1-AT phenotype is PiMM. The abnormal phenotype is PiZZ which is associated with α_1-AT deficiency and development of emphysema at earlier age and greater severity.

> Most important etiological agent for emphysema is **smoking**

> α**1-AT deficiency** is associated with **panacinar emphysema**

Emphysema

Centriacinar	Panacinar	Distal acinar/Paraseptal	Irregular
• Involvement of central part of acinus with **sparing of alveoli**[Q]. • Seen in smokers[Q]. • Usually more severe in **upper lobes**[Q] (due to relative deficiency of serum α1-At to this less perfused region). • MC type of emphysema seen clinically.	• Involvement of the **entire acinus**[Q]. • Seen with α1-AT deficiency. • Occurs more severely in lower lobes at **base of lung**[Q] (due to lower lung distribution of neutrophils because of more perfusion of this region).	• Distal part of acinus is affected with sparing of proximal part of acinus[Q]. • Seen in **smokers**[Q]. • Involvement of lung adjacent to pleura. • Associated with the development of spontaneous pneumothorax.	• Irregular acinar involvement associated with fibrosis/scarring[Q]. • Most common type of **emphysema histologically**[Q].

> emPhysema has letter P (and not B) so **P**ink Puffer.
> chronic **B**ronchitis has letter B (and not P) so **B**lue Bloater.

Clinical features: Progressively increasing dyspnea, weight loss, late onset of cough with scanty sputum. The patient is non-cyanotic, uses accessory muscle of respiration and shows pursed lip breathing. (*PINK PUFFERS*).

Management: Cessation of smoking and use of bronchodilators is the mainstay of the management.

3. Asthma

Hyperactivity of the airways resulting in reversible bronchoconstriction and air flow obstruction on exposure to some external stimuli is called asthma.

Pathogenesis: Primary exposure of an allergen causes T_{H2} *cell dominated* inflammatory response resulting in IgE production and eosinophil recruitment (called *sensitization*). Exposure to the same allergen causes cross linking of IgE bound to IgE receptors on mast cells in the airways which cause opening up of epithelial cells due to released mediators. Antigens then cause activation of mucosal mast cells and eosinophils and this along with neuronal reflexes (subepithelial vagal receptors) cause bronchospasm, increased vascular permeability and mucus production (**Acute or Immediate response**). Later on, leukocytic infiltration causes release of more mediators and damage to the epithelium (**Late Phase Reaction**). Eosinophils in airways release major basic protein which causes epithelial damage and more airway constriction.

Leukotrienes C_4, D_4, E_4 and acetylcholine have definite role in bronchoconstriction whereas agents like histamine, PGD_2 and platelet activating factor (PAF) may also have role in the features of the disease. The following are the two variants of asthma.

Features	Extrinsic asthma	Intrinsic asthma
Pathogenesis	Type I hyper-sensitivity reaction due to exposure to an extrinsic antigen	Initiated by non-immune mechanisms with intrinsic body stimuli
Age on presentation	Child	Adult
Family history	Present[Q]	**Absent**[Q]
Prior allergic reaction/ allergen exposure	Positive history of rhinitis, urticaria, eczema	Absent
Serum IgE levels	Increased[Q]	**Normal**[Q]
Skin test	Positive	Negative
Associated COPD	Rare	Usually present
Examples	Atopic/allergic asthma, Occupational asthma, Allergic bronchopulmonary aspergillosis	Drugs (most commonly aspirin), viral infections, cold exposure, exercise induced asthma

IMPORTANT FACT

- **IL-13 gene polymorphism** is strongly associated with **bronchial asthma**.
- **ADAM-33** is another gene causing proliferation of smooth muscle cells and fibroblasts in bronchi resulting in **bronchial hyper-reactivity** and **subepithelial fibrosis**.

Clinical features: Acute asthmatic attack is characterized by wheezing, cough and severe dyspnea.

Morphology: The most stroking macroscopic finding is occlusion of the bronchi and bronchioles by mucus plugs. Histologically, there are numerous eosinophils, **Charcot leyden crystals**[Q] (composed of eosinophil membrane protein called as galectin-10) and **Curschmann spirals**[Q] (whorls of shed airway epithelium). Structural changes in the bronchial wall called *"airway remodelling"* is characterized by presence of eosinophilic inflammation and edema of bronchial walls, increased size of submucosal glands, hypertrophy of bronchial wall smooth muscle and deposition of subepithelial collagen in the bronchial wall. Individual epithelial cells present in the sputum of the patients are called **Creola bodies**.

Management is done with bronchodilators and corticosteroids (for details, refer to the Review of Pharmacology by the same authors).

Concept

Virus induced inflammation **lowers the threshold** of the subepithelial **vagal receptors** to irritants.

Concept

Exercise causes loss of water and heat from the respiratory tract. The water loss causes **mucosal hyperosmolarity** which **stimulates release of mediators** from the mast cells. This explains the pathogenesis of exercise induced asthma

Concept

In **intrinsic asthma,** aspirin causes **shift** of the arachidonic acid metabolism **towards the lipoxygenase pathway** resulting in formation of the bronchoconstrictor leukotrienes.

Differential of **asthma** from COPD is by **Reversibility of FEV1** using bronchodilators/ oral steroids

M

3 **C's** of sputum findings in asthma;
- Charcot leyden crystals
- Curschmann spirals
- Creola bodies

Respiratory System

4. Bronchiectasis

Abnormal permanent airway dilation resulting from chronic necrotizing infections is called bronchiectasis.

Causes

Bronchial obstruction	Congenital	Necrotizing pneumonias	Miscellaneous
• Tumor • Foreign body	• Cystic fibrosis • Kartagner syndrome[Q] (Triad of Bronchiectasis + situs inversus + sinusitis).	• Mycobacterium • *Staph aureus* • Aspergillus • Influenza virus.	• SLE • Rheumatoid arthritis • Post transplatation.

Obstruction and infection are the chief contributors to the damage of airway wall associated with destruction of smooth muscle and elastic tissue fibrosis and further dilatation of bronchi.

Clinical features: Chronic cough, fever, foul smelling sputum production, recurrent pulmonary infections, sinusitis and immune deficiencies.

It usually affects vertical air passages of the *lower lobes* bilaterally with involvement of *left side*[Q] *more frequent* than right. The dilated bronchi can be followed directly out to the pleural surfaces. There is usually presence of inflammatory cells in the walls of bronchi and bronchioles which may also exhibit squamous metaplasia.

Complications include ***massive hemoptysis, amyloidosis, visceral abscess*** and ***cor pulmonale***[Q].

> **Bronchiectasis** affects vertical air passages of the **lower lobes** bilaterally with involvement of **left side** more frequent than right.

> **High Resolution CT Scan (HRCT)** is the **best investigation** for the detection of bronchiectasis

RESTRICTIVE LUNG DISEASE

1. Interstitial Lung Disease

Interstitial lung disease (ILD) is a group of heterogeneous diseases characterized by *chronic inflammation and fibrosis of the interstitium and lung parenchyma*[Q]. The interstitium of the lung (supporting structure) is the area in and around the small blood vessels and alveoli where the exchange of oxygen and carbon dioxide takes place. Inflammation and scarring of the interstitium (and eventually extension into the alveoli) will disrupt normal gas exchange. Usually, patients present with *exertional dyspnea and non-productive cough*.

The chest X-ray shows reticular or reticulonodular pattern (**"ground glass" appearance**). Pulmonary function tests show evidence of intrapulmonary *restrictive pattern*.

Earliest manifestation of the disease is inflammation in the alveolar wall called **Alveolitis**. The inflammatory cells release chemical mediators resulting in injury to parenchymal cells and stimulation of fibrosis. In advanced stages of the disease, the gross destruction and scarring of the lung results in end stage disease or **honeycomb lung.**[Q]

ILD

Fibrosis	Granulomatous	Associated with smoking	Miscellaneous
• Idiopathic pulmonary fibrosis • Collagen vascular disease associated pulmonary fibrosis (SLE, RA, Scleroderma) • Pneumoconiosis • Drug reaction • Rediation pneumonitis • Fumes and gases (SO_2 etc.)	• Sarcoidosis • Hypersensitivity pneumonitis.	• Desquamative interstitial pneumonia	• Pulmonary alveolar proteinosis.

We shall focus on each of the chief subtypes of interstitial lung disease:

A. PNEUMOCONIOSIS

Non-neoplastic lung reaction (usually fibrosis) to inhalation of mineral dust, organic and inorganic particles and chemicals and vapors is called pneumoconiosis.

The *most dangerous particle size is 1-5 μm* which reaches the terminal small airways and alveoli. These particles overwhelm the normal phagocytosis by alveolar macrophages to evoke fibroblast proliferation and collagen deposition. Some of the important pneumoconiosis includes:

(1) Coal worker's pneumoconiosis

It is due to inhalation of coal dust in coal miners and is usually present adjacent to respiratory bronchiole. It is categorized into:

Simple CWP:
(*i*) Coal macules (carbon-laden macrophages)
(*ii*) Coal nodules (*upper lobes more heavily involved*)
(*iii*) Centrilobular emphysema
Complicated CWP: Develops after many years
(*i*) Intense blackened scars larger than 2 cm in diameter
(*ii*) Center of lesion is often necrotic

(2) Silicosis

- Nodular fibrosing disease^Q due to inhalation of silica in workers engaged is sandblasting, hard rock mining, foundry work, glass and pottery making.
- *Most common chronic occupational disease* in the world^Q.
- Crystalline form of silica called *quartz is most commonly implicated in silicosis.*
- Co-inhalation of other mineral particles reduces^Q the fibrogenic effect of silicosis.
- Involvement of upper lobes of the lung.^Q
- Association with increased *susceptibility to tuberculosis^Q.*
- Chest X-ray shows presence of *Eggshell calcification^Q* (thin sheet of calcification in the lymph node surrounding a zone lacking calcification).
- *Polarized microscopy* reveals presence of *birefringent silica particles^Q.*

(3) Asbestosis

- Diffuse interstitial fibrotic disease due to inhalation of asbestos particles in workers engaged in mining, pipes, brakes, insulation and boilers.
- Initially, involvement of **lower lobes** of the lung pleurally^Q.
- In contrast to other dusts, can also *act as a tumor initiator and tumor promoter^Q.*

Two types of fibers are:
- *Serpentine (curly and flexible fibres, chrysotile):* These account for most of the asbestos used in industry.
- *Amphibole (straight, stiff and brittle fibres, crocidolite, amosite, actinolyte):* These are more pathogenic than chrysotiles, particularly with respect to induction of malignant pleural tumors (mesotheliomas).

Lesions with asbestosis

Pleural plaque^Q:
It is the most common manifestation of asbestos exposure and is composed of well circumscribed plaques of *dense collagen containing calcium*. They are usually asymptomatic and develop on anterior and posterolateral parts of parietal pleura and over the diaphragm.

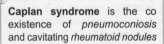

The **most dangerous** particle size for causation of pneumoconiosis is **1-5 microns.**

Dust cells are **alveolar macrophages** with *anthracotic* pigment.

Caplan syndrome is the co existence of *pneumoconiosis* and cavitating *rheumatoid nodules*

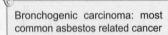

Benign pleural plaques: most common lesions in asbestosis

Bronchogenic carcinoma: most common asbestos related cancer

Respiratory System

Interstitial fibrosis
Pulmonary fibrosis with the presence of **asbestos body**[Q] (iron containing proteinaceous material coating asbestos fiber) and **ferruginous body**[Q] (iron protein complex coating other inorganic particles like talc, mica, fibre, glass and other less common materials in the lung). True asbestos bodies are clear whereas the core of these particles is dark).
Bronchogenic cancer
Most common cancer associated with asbestos[Q] whose risk is increased with concomitant smoking.
Mesothelioma
Localization of asbestos fibres in the lung close to the mesothelial layers increases the risk of development of pleural and peritoneal mesothelioma. Concomitant smoking **does not** increase the risk of mesothelioma. It is the ***most specific*** cancer associated with asbestos inhalation.
Pleural effusion, laryngeal and colon cancers.

> The presence of asbestos bodies in or adjacent to the walls of fibrotic respiratory bronchioles is the hallmark of the disease.

Other important pneumoconiosis

- **Baritosis** is caused by inhalation of *Barium sulfate* (in miners).
- **Stannosis** is caused by inhalation of *Tin oxide* (in miners).
- **Siderosis** is caused by inhalation of *Iron oxide* (in welders).
- **Byssinosis** is caused by inhalation of *cotton fibres* (in textile workers).
- **Caplan syndrome:** Coexistence of **rheumatoid arthritis with pneumoconiosis**

Clinical symptoms of pneumoconiosis include progressively increasing dyspnea, productive cough, reduced exercise tolerance which may progress to respiratory failure, cor pulmonale and ultimately death.

B. SARCOIDOSIS

It is a systematic disease of unknown etiology characterized by the presence of *non-caseating granulomas* in many organs. It is seen more commonly in *females of 20-40 years* of age. It is associated with *HLA-A1 and HLA-B8*.

> Sarcoidosis shows presence of **noncaseating** *granulomas*

Immunological abnormalities associated with sarcoidosis

- Intra-alveolar and interstitial *accumulation of CD$_4$ + T cells* resulting in CD$_4$:CD$_8$ T cell ratio ranging from 5:1 to 15:1[Q].
- Increased levels of IL-2 and IFN-γ causing *T-cell expansion and macrophage activation* respectively[Q].
- *Polyclonal hypergammaglobulinemia*[Q].
- *Anergy to skin antigens* like purified protein derivative (PPD)[Q].

Histologically, there is characteristically presence of *non-caseating granuloma*[Q] composed of aggregates of epithelioid cells and giant cells. There is also presence of *Schaumann bodies*[Q] (laminated concretions of calcium and protein) and *asteroid bodies*[Q] (stellate or star shaped inclusions in giant cells).

Concept

Sarcoidosis has **elevated ACE** levels. ACE enzyme is important even for distinguishing sarcoidosis from *bronchogenic carcinoma* as the *level* of the ACE enzyme in the latter would be *normal*.

Organs Affected

Lungs
- ***Most common site*** of organ involvement
- There is presence of **non-caseating granuloma** in the bronchial submucosa.
- ***Bronchoalveolar lavage***[Q] shows ***CD$_4$:CD$_8$ T- lymphocytes ratio of > 2.5*** is seen.
Lymph nodes
- Involvement of hilar and mediastinal nodes is seen in almost all the cases.
Liver and spleen
- Splenomegaly may be seen with sparing of capsule. Scattered granulomas are seen more in portal triads as compared to globular parenchyma.

> **Sarcoidosis** is a *diagnosis of exclusion;* rule out other granulomatous diseases.

Bone marrow
• Favored site of localization having tendency to involve *phalangeal bones of hands and feet* showing small areas of bone resorption, bony shaft widening and new bone formation.
Skin
• Lesions include erythema nodosum, subcutaneous nodules, erythematous plaques and lupus pernio[Q].
Eye, lacrimal glands and salivary glands
• Unilateral or bilateral ocular involvement resulting in iritis, glaucoma or corneal opacity may occur.
• Causes lacrimal gland inflammation (causing *dry eyes*[Q]) and salivary gland involvement (*dry mouth*[Q]).

Lofgren syndrome (has erythema nodosum, arthritis and hilar adenopathy).

Heerfordt Waldenstrom syndrome (fever, parotid enlargement, uveitis and facial palsy)

Clinical features include shortness of breath, cough, chest pain, hemoptysis, constitutional signs and symptoms (fever, fatigue, weight loss) or it may be discovered on routine X-ray as bilateral hilar lymphadenopathy. It can also manifest as Lofgren Syndrome and Heerfordt Waldenstrom Syndrome.

• Chest X-ray shows bilateral hilar and left paratracheal lymphadenopathy. There is **hypercalcemia**[Q] due to increased circulation of vitamin D by macrophages. **Elevated levels of ACE**[Q] (Angiotensin Converting Enzyme) are seen in the disease. These patients also demonstrate **skin anergy** and a **restrictive pattern** on pulmonary function tests.

• **Management:** It is done usually with corticosteroids.

C. PULMONARY ALVEOLAR PROTEINOSIS

It is a rare disease in which phospholipids accumulate within alveolar spaces. This is a condition of unknown cause characterized by auto-antibodies against granulocyte macrophage-colony stimulating factor (GM-CSF).

Some (10%) PAP cases are congenital in nature secondary to mutations in the GM-CSF gene leading to reduced or absent SP-B and intra alveolar accumulation of SP-A and SP-C.

Secondary PAP is associated with immunodeficiency, hematopoietic disorders, malignancies, acute silicosis and other inhalational syndromes.

Clinical features: Progressive dyspnea is the usual presenting symptom. Chest X-ray shows bilateral alveolar infiltrates suggestive of pulmonary edema. **Bronchoalveolar lavage shows characteristic milky appearance and PAS-positive lipoproteinaceous material**. Lung biopsy reveals amorphous intra-alveolar phospholipids.

2. Adult Respiratory Distress Syndrome (ARDS)

Sepsis is most common cause of ARDS

• Also called as *Shock lung*[Q], *Diffuse alveolar damage*[Q] *or Acute lung injury*[Q]
• Characterized by damage to alveolar cells and blood vessels resulting in oxygen refractory progressive respiratory insufficiency.

Conditions associated with ARDS

Features of ARDS severe hypoxemia, PA wedge pressure < 18 mm Hg, increased A-a (Alveolar-arterial) gradient.

Infections	Physical factors	Chemical factors	Miscellaneous
• Septicemia • Aspiration • Pulmonary infections (TB, viral, mycoplasma, etc.)	• Drowning • Head injury • Radiation exposure • Fat embolism • Smoking • Irritant gases.	• Drugs like aspirin • Heroin/Methadone • Overdose of barbiturates • Hypersensitivity by organic solvents.	• Pancreatitis • Uremia • Multiple transfusion • DIC.

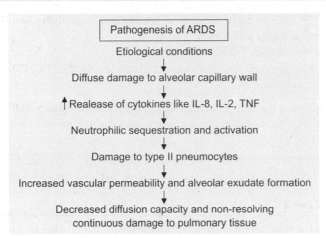

Morphological features include Interstitial and intra-alveolar edema with lining of alveoli with hyaline membrane composed of fibrin rich edema fluid and lipid remnants of epithelial cells. Later on, there is intra-alveolar fibrosis.

Clinical features include Progressively increasing dyspnea (difficulty in breathing), tachypnea resulting in respiratory failure, cyanosis and hypoxemia, chest x-ray shows bilateral diffuse infiltration **("white out" lung[Q]).** Management is done primarily with treatment of underlying cause and mechanical ventilation.

Neonatal RDS/Hyaline membrane disease

Prematurity	Infants of diabetic mothers	Cesarean section

- Results from **surfactant deficiency** which is chemically composed of lecithin (dipalmitoylphosphatidylcholine; DPPC[Q]). Due to reduced surfactant, surface tension of alveoli increases. Increased alveolar surface tension causes atelectasis resulting in hypoxemia responsible for damage to endothelial and epithelial cells. The latter contributes to formation of hyaline membrane[Q] (fibrin + necrotic cells).
- Clinical features include normal infant at birth but within 30 minutes, there is development of progressively increasing respiratory effort and cyanosis. **Chest X-ray** demonstrates multiple reticulogranular densities ("**ground glass**" appearance[Q]).

> **Prevention** of hyaline membrane disease is by delaying the onset of labor and administration of glucocorticoids to the mother. Steroids increase the formation of surfactant lipids and proteins thereby decreasing the respiratory distress. **Treatment** is by administration of artificial surfactant and oxygen using high frequency ventilation.

VASCULAR LUNG DISEASES

1. Pulmonary Emboli and Pulmonary Infarction

Most (90-95%) of the pulmonary emboli arise from deep vein thrombosis (DVT) in the leg and *only 10% of pulmonary emboli cause infarction.* The infarcts occur in patients with underlying cardiopulmonary disease. It is a wedge shaped hemorrhagic infarction. The diagnosis of pulmonary embolism is made on ventilation/perfusion scan (V/Q lung scan) which shows a mismatch. The complications associated with this condition include pulmonary hypertension, cor pulmonale, pulmonary abscess and even sudden death.

2. Pulmonary Hypertension

It is defined as increased pulmonary artery pressure, usually due to increased vascular resistance or blood flow. It is seen in association with:

> **Hyaline membrane** is made up of *fibrin* and *necrotic* cells.

> **Deep vein thrombosis** is the commonest cause of pulmonary thromboembolism.

> **Spiral CT scan** is the investigation of choice. (Ref Harrison 18th/2173)

- COPD and interstitial disease (hypoxia induced vasoconstriction is seen).
- Multiple ongoing pulmonary emboli.
- Mitral stenosis and left sided heart failure.
- Congenital heart disease with left to right shunts (ASD, VSD, PDA).
- Primary (idiopathic).

Recently **mutations in the bone morphogenetic protein receptor type 2** (BMPR2) signaling pathway have been associated with pulmonary hypertension due to increased medial hypertrophy and intimal fibrosis in small arteries.

The presence of plexogenic pulmonary arteriopathy may also be seen in primary pulmonary hypertension or congenital heart disease with left to right shunts.

3. Pulmonary Edema

It is defined as the fluid accumulation within the lungs usually due to disruption of starling forces or endothelial injury.

So, it can be due to:
1. Increased hydrostatic pressure as in left-sided heart failure, mitral valve stenosis, fluid overload, etc.
2. Decreased oncotic pressure as in nephrotic syndrome, or liver disease.
3. Increased capillary permeability as in infections, drugs (bleomycin, heroin), shock, radiation.

The lungs are wet and heavy and the fluid accumulation is more in the lower lobes. Microscopically, there is presence of intra-alveolar fluid, engorged capillaries and *hemosiderin-laden macrophages (heart-failure cells)*.

NEOPLASTIC LUNG DISEASES

1. Bronchogenic Cancer

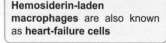

The lung is a common site of metastatic neoplasms. However, *bronchogenic cancer is the most common primary malignant tumor of the lung*. It is most frequently diagnosed major cancer in the world.

Risk factors

Non-genetic	Genetic
• Tobacco smoking (contain chemicals like benezophrene and polycyclic • Air pollution • Occupational exposure (asbestosis, uranium mining, radiation, etc.)	Mutations affecting • Tumor suppressor genes p53 and Rb gene • Oncogenes • K-ras – Adenocarcinoma • L-myc – Small cell carcinoma.

Histological variants of lung cancer

Squamous cell carcinoma	Adenocarcinoma	Small cell cancer or oat cancer	Large cell cancer
• MC type of lung cancer in smokers[Q].	• Overall MC type of cancer[Q].	• Associated with smoking	
• MC type in males[Q].	• MC type in non-smokers and females[Q].	• Commoner in smokers[Q].	

Cont...

Sidebar notes:
Mutations in the **bone morphogenetic protein receptor type 2** (BMPR2) signaling pathway have been associated with **pulmonary hypertension**.

Hemosiderin-laden macrophages are also known as **heart-failure cells**

Metastasis/Secondaries are the commonest malignant tumor of the lung.

Cont...

Cont...

• Usually central in location (arise from the segmental bronchi)	• Usually peripheral in location (arise from terminal bronchiole)	• Central in location	• Peripheral in location.
• Shows highest frequency of p53 mutation^Q.	• Associated with K-ras mutation^Q.	• Immunohistochemistry shows high expression of **Bcl-2** gene^Q in majority of tumors.	
• Intercellular bridges or junction is very specific. • Histologically, the tumor has presence of keratinization^Q.	• Glandular pattern of growth of the tumor is seen. • Cells are positive for mucin and thyroid transcription factor-1 (TTF-1)^Q.	• Cells have scanty cytoplasm, small nucleoli, granular chromatin **(salt and peper pattern^Q)**. • **Azzopardl effect** (Basophilic staining of vascular walls) is frequently present. • Electron microscopy shows presence of neurosecretory granules chromogranin, synaptophysis and leu-7^Q.	• Cells have large nuclei, prominent nucleoli and a moderate amount of cytoplasm.
		• Has best response to chemotherapy and radiotherapy. • Has the worst prognosis^Q. • Most aggressive lung cancer^Q.	
• **Hypercalcemia**^{Q} due to PTHrP is the MC paraneoplastic syndrome.	•	• Associated with maximum paraneoplastic syndrome^Q (particularly **SIADH** and **Cushing syndrome**).	• Has **gynecomastia** as paraneoplastic syndrome^Q.

SVC syndrome is most commonly caused by **small cell lung cancer**

Diagnosis of bronchogenic cancer is usually made with **sputum cytology and fibreoptic bronchoscopy**

- **Bronchoalveolar carcinoma** is a subtype of adenocarcinoma having absence of stromal, vascular or pleural invasion with growth of the tumor along the pre-existing alveolar septa. Tumors cells are present in the alveoli and tend to have *aerogenous spread^Q*. Due to involvement of the airways, the *patient usually dies by suffocation (not by metastatic spread^Q)*.

Clinical features: *Cough* is the most common symptom in these patients which is followed by *weight loss* and *dyspnea*. They also have anorexia, fatigue, hemoptysis, and chest pain.

Metastasis of the cancer causes **involvement of adrenal (most commonly^Q)** followed by liver, brain and bone. Intrathoracic spread of the cancer causes enlargement of lymph nodes (hilar, mediastinal, bronchial and tracheal), pleural involvement, hoarseness (recurrent laryngeal nerve invasion), dysphagia (esophageal obstruction), diaphragmatic paralysis (phrenic nerve paralysis), Horner syndrome and superior vena cava (SVC) syndrome.

Horner syndrome

Horner syndrome^Q is caused due to compression of sympathetic nerve plexus by an apical tumor called as *Pancoast tumor^Q*. It is usually an adenocarcinoma. Its components include: (**mnemonic: Punjabi MEAL**)

Punjabi	–	**P**tosis
M	–	**M**iosis (small pupil)
E	–	**E**nophthalmos (sunken eyes)
A	–	**A**nhidrosis (absence of sweating)
L	–	**L**oss of ciliospinal reflex (in this reflex, pinching of the skin on the nape of neck causes dilatation of the pupil of the same side)

Respiratory System

Important paraneoplastic syndromes associated with bronchogenic cancer include:

1. **Endocrinological syndrome**
   a. Cushing syndrome (Due to ACTH)
   b. Syndrome of inappropriate ADH secretion (SIADH) [Due to anti-diuretic hormone]
   c. Hypercalcemia: Due to parathyroid hormone related peptide (PTH related peptide).
   d. Hypocalcemia: Due to calcitonin
   e. Gynecomastia: Due to gonadotropins
2. **Lambert eaton syndrome:** Due to autoantibodies against neuronal calcium channel
3. **Acanthosis nigricans:** Hyperpigmentation of axillary region.
4. **Hypertrophic pulmonary osteoarthropathy** having clubbing and periosteal new born formation.

Malignant Mesothelioma is **not** associated with *smoking.*

2. Solitary (Localized) Fibrous Tumor

It was earlier referred to as '*benign mesothelioma*'. It has got *no relationship with asbestosis*^Q. Microscopically, there is presence of whorls of reticulin and collagen fibers with interspersed spindle cells resembling fibroblasts. The tumor cells characteristically show immunostaining pattern of *CD^{34(+)} and keratin-negative*^Q.

3. Malignant Mesothelioma

It is a tumor arising from visceral or parietal pleura which is seen after prolonged duration (after a latent period of 25-45 years) of *asbestos inhalation*. It is *not associated with smoking*. Unlike bronchogenic cancer, it is less commonly associated with p53 mutation. It is associated with extensive pleural effusion and local invasion of thoracic structures. Microscopically, the tumor can have the following patterns:

1. *Sarcomatoid type*: Mesenchymal stromal cell type
2. *Epithelioid type*: Consists of cuboidal, columnar or flattened cell forming tubular or papillary structure resembling adenocarcinoma.
3. *Mixed type*: It contains both epithelioid and sarcomatoid patterns.

Concept

The best marker to differentiate benign and malignant mesothelioma is p53. Its mutation is present in malignant mesothelioma and this mutation is absent in benign mesothelioma.

Concept: Epithelioid mesothelioma *is differentiated from* **pulmonary adenocarcinoma** by

- Positive staining for acid muco-polysaccharide
- **Lack of CEA** and other epithelial glycoproteins (these are expressed by adenocarcinomas)
- **Keratin positive** with accentuation of peri-nuclear halo rather than peripheral staining
- **Electron microscopy** demonstrates *long, slender,* **numerous microvilli and tonofilaments but** *absent microvillus rootlets and lamellar bodies.* This is the **gold standard** of diagnosis

Clinical features include chest pain, dyspnea and recurrent pleural effusions. Right lung is more commonly affected than left lung. It is **usually unilateral at presentation.** The lung is invaded directly, and there is often metastatic spread to the hilar lymph nodes and, eventually to the liver and other distant organs. It is associated with very poor prognosis.

ATELECTASIS

Incomplete expansion of the lungs or the collapse of previously inflated lung is known as atelectasis.

1. **Resorption Atelectasis:**
   - Due to airway obstruction leading to resorption of oxygen trapped in the alveoli.
   - Causes mediastinal shift towards affected lung.
   - Associated with chronic bronchitis/asthma/aspiration of foreign body/secretions.
2. **Compression Atelectasis:**
   - Due to presence of fluid, blood, air or tumor in pleural space.
   - Causes mediastinal shift away from the affected lung.
   - Most commonly associated with cardiac failure^Q.
3. **Contraction Atelectasis:**
   - Fibrosis in the lung or pleura preventing full expansion of pulmonary tissue.
   - Only **irreversible** cause of atelectasis^Q.

Respiratory System

MULTIPLE CHOICE QUESTIONS

INFECTIVE LUNG DISEASE: PNEUMONIA, TB, LUNG ABSCESS

1. **Infraclavicular lesion of tuberculosis is known as:**
   (a) Gohn's focus   *(AIIMS May 2011)*
   (b) Puhl's focus
   (c) Assman's focus
   (d) Simmon's focus

2. **Pulmonary tuberculosis is more common in following associated diseases, except:**   *(DPG 2011)*
   (a) Acquired immune deficiency syndrome
   (b) Diabetes
   (c) Chronic renal failure
   (d) Mitral stenosis

3. **All of the following features are seen in the viral pneumonia except**   *(AI 2005)*
   (a) Presence of interstitial inflammation
   (b) Predominance of alveolar exudate
   (c) Bronchiolitis
   (d) Multinucleate giant cells in the bronchiolar wall

4. **Atypical pneumonia can be caused by the following microbial agents except?**   *(AI 2005)*
   (a) Mycoplasma pneumoniae
   (b) Legionella pneumophila
   (c) Human corona virus
   (d) Klebsiella pneumoniae

5. **In primary tuberculosis, all of the following may be seen except:**   *(AI 2002)*
   (a) Cavitation
   (b) Caseation
   (c) Calcification
   (d) Langhans giant cell

6. **Lung granuloma with necrosis is seen in-**
   (a) PAN   *(PGI June 01)*
   (b) TB
   (c) Histoplasmosis
   (d) Cryptococcosis
   (e) Wegener's granulomatosis

7. **Predisposing factors of lung abscess are:**
   (a) Altered sensorium   *(PGI Dec 2003)*
   (b) Dental sepsis
   (c) Aggressive treatment of pneumonia
   (d) Subpulmonic effusion
   (e) Endobronchial obstruction

8. **Pulmonary, renal syndrome is seen in:**
   (a) Good pasture syndrome   *(PGI Dec 2003)*
   (b) Leptospirosis
   (c) Legionella
   (d) Wegener's granulomatosis
   (e) Hantan virus infection

9. **Lung granuloma found in A/E:**   *(PGI June 2004)*
   (a) Berylliosis
   (b) Asbestosis
   (c) SLE
   (d) Sarcoidosis

10. **True about Ghon's focus:**   *(PGI Dec 2004)*
    (a) Left apical parenchymal lesion
    (b) Right apical parenchymal lesion
    (c) Subpleural caseous lesion in right upper lobe
    (d) Subpleural caseous lesion just above or below inter-lobar fissure
    (e) Caseous hilar lymphadenopathy

11. **Which of these is seen in primary tuberculosis:**
    (a) Ghon's focus   *(PGI Dec 2006)*
    (b) Pleural effusion
    (c) Miliary mottling
    (d) Fibrosis
    (e) Cavity

12. **Characteristic histopathological feature of pneumocystis carinii pneumonia -**   *(PGI Dec 2000)*
    (a) Interstitial pneumonitis
    (b) Increased eosinophils
    (c) Foamy vacuolated exudates
    (d) Mononuclear cell in bronchoalveolar lavage
    (e) Neutrophil infiltration

13. **A 9 year old girl Bandhini developed a 10 mm area of induration on the left forearm 72 hours after intradermal injection of 0.1 ml of purified protein derivative (PPD). Though she appears healthy, a chest X ray was performed. Which of the following is most likely to be seen on the radiograph?**
    (a) Marked hilar adenopathy
    (b) Upper lobe calcifications
    (c) No abnormal findings
    (d) Reticulo-nodular densities

14. **A 60 year old smoker BD Thapa with inguinal hernia undergoes surgery under general anaesthesia. On the third post operative day, he complains of increasing difficulty in respiration. The finger probe reveals presence of pO2 of 60 mm Hg but the patient is afebrile to touch. His vitals are as follows: pulse is regular and good volume at 76/min, respiratory rate is 17/min and BP is 130/84 mm Hg. Blood investigations reveal hemoglobin is 14g/dL, TLC is 7300/mm3 and a normal DLC. One evening the resident doctor notices that Mr Thapa coughs up copious mucoid sputum following which his condition improves dramatically. What is the most likely diagnosis?**

(a) Compression atelectasis
(b) Microatelectasis
(c) Resorption atelectasis
(d) Contraction atelectasis

15. Autopsy of a person reveals a small cluster of caseating granulomas in the right lung just above the interlobar fissure and similar granulomas in the hilar lymph nodes. Acid-fast staining demonstrates acid-fast bacilli within these lesions. No other lesions were found in the remaining organs and systems. Which of the following is the most accurate interpretation of these findings?
    (a) Cavitary tuberculosis
    (b) Ghon complex
    (c) Remote healed tuberculosis
    (d) Miliary tuberculosis

Most Recent Questions

15.1. Collapse of lung is called:
    (a) Emphysema   (b) Bronchiactasis
    (c) Atelectasis   (d) Bronchitis

15.2. In the stage of Grey hepatisation, which of the following is a finding?
    (a) WBC's fill the alveoli
    (b) RBC's fill the alveoli
    (c) Organisms fill the alveoli
    (d) Accumulation of fibrin

15.3. Gray hepatization of lungs is seen on day:
    (a) 1   (b) 2-3
    (c) 3-4   (d) 5-7

15.4. The earliest feature of tuberculosis is:
    (a) Caseation
    (b) Recruitment of lymphocytes
    (c) Formation of giant cells (Langhans)
    (d) Granuloma formation

15.5. Reactivated TB is most commonly located near:
    (a) Apex   (b) Near bronchus
    (c) Subpleurally   (d) Base

15.6. Maximum smooth muscle relative to wall thickness is seen in
    (a) Terminal bronchiole
    (b) Trachea
    (c) Bronchi
    (d) Respiratory bronchioles

15.7. The alveoli are filled with exudates the air is displaced converting the lung into a solid organ this description suggests
    (a) Chronic bronchitis (b) Bronchial asthma
    (c) Bronchiectasis   (d) Lobar pneumonia

15.8. ESR is a very critical investigation is the diagnosis of TB. Which of the following is true about ESR in TB?
    (a) No change is ESR   *(AIIMS May 2013)*
    (b) Confirms recovery from TB
    (c) ESR is raised because of increased RBC aggregate
    (d) ESR is raised due to decreased RBC size

OBSTRUCTIVE LUNG DISEASE: BRONCHITIS, ASTHMA, BRONCHIECTASIS, EMPHYSEMA

16. Increased Reid's index is increased in which of the following?   *(AI 2012)*
    (a) Bronchiectasis
    (b) Bronchial asthma
    (c) Chronic bronchitis
    (d) Emphysema

17. True about alpha-1 antitrypsin deficiency, is/are -
    (a) Autosomal dominant   *(PGI June 01)*
    (b) Pulmonary emphysema
    (c) Diastase resistant hepatic cells
    (d) Hepatic cells are orcein stain positive
    (e) Associated with berry aneurysm

18. Late response in bronchial asthma is due to:
    (a) Mast cells   *(UP 2003)*
    (b) Eosinophils
    (c) Neutrophils
    (d) Macrophages

19. Charcot-Leyden crystals and Curschmann's spirals are seen in: *(UP 2006)*
    (a) Bronchial asthma
    (b) Chronic bronchitis
    (c) Bronchiectasis
    (d) Emphysema

20. Most common type of emphysema clinically is:
    (a) Panacinar   *(RJ 2006)*
    (b) Centriacinar
    (c) Paraseptal
    (d) Segmental

21. In a heavy smoker with chronic bronchiolitis, which of the following is likely to be seen:
    (a) Centrilobular emphysema   *(Kolkata 2003)*
    (b) Panacinar emphysema
    (c) Paraseptal emphysema
    (d) None of the above

22. A 37 year old male Ranjir Kapoor presents to the hospital with progressive exertional dyspnea. His symptoms began insidiously but have progressed gradually to the extent that now he has a problem even in his daily activities. Dr. Gulaeria, a respiratory medicine specialist decided to perform spirometry which shows decreased forced vital capacity (FVC). His plasma protein electrophoresis shows a markedly reduced alpha fraction. Mr Kapoor's lower lung lobes are most likely to show which of the following?
    (a) Panacinar emphysema
    (b) Centriacinar emphysema
    (c) Compensatory hyperinflation
    (d) Apical subpleural blebs

23. A 30 year old woman Chinamma has had increasing dyspnea with cough for the past week. Over the past 2 days she is having productive cough with copious sputum. On examination, she is afebrile but has extensive dullness to percussion over all the lung fields.

Respiratory System

Her chest X ray has B/L diffuse opacification. Electron microscopic examination of the biopsy tissue shows many lamellar bodies. The antibody is directed against which of the following substances in the pathogenesis of the above described condition?
(a) CFTR
(b) Granulocyte – macrophage colony stimulating factor
(c) DNA topoisomerase 1
(d) Glomerular basement membrane

24. **A 50 year old man Shahid K. John has had increasing dyspnea for the past 3 years with associated occasional cough but little sputum production. Auscultation reveals that his lungs are hyper-resonant and is associated with expiratory wheeze. Pulmonary function tests reveal increased total lung capacity (TLC) and slightly increased FVC. There is decreased FEV1 and FEV1/FVC ratio also. ABG analysis reveals pH of 7.35, pO2 of 60 mm Hg and pCO2 of 48 mm Hg. What is the most likely diagnosis?**
(a) Sarcoidosis
(b) Centriacinar emphysema
(c) Diffuse alveolar damage
(d) Chronic pulmonary embolism

25. **A 65-year-old smoker Sutta Ram with hemoptysis and weight loss undergoes a left upper lobectomy for squamous cell carcinoma. The uninvolved lung tissue shows destruction of the alveolar septae around the respiratory bronchioles, with marked enlargement of the airspaces. Anthracotic pigments deposited heavily in the walls of these tissues. These findings are most compatible with**
(a) Asthma
(b) Chronic bronchitis
(c) Emphysema
(d) Pulmonary hypertension

26. **A 52-year-old male smoker Naresh presents with fever and a cough productive of greenish-yellow sputum. The patient states that he has had a morning cough with excessive mucus production for the past 5 years. Which of the following abnormalities would most likely be found in this patient?**
(a) Apical cavitary lesions on x-ray
(b) Curschmann spirals in his sputum
(c) Increased Reid index
(d) Enlarged hilar lymph nodes on x-ray

27. **In emphysema, the destruction of many alveolar walls changes the compliance of the respiratory system. Which of the following clinical observations is directly related to this change in compliance?**
(a) Barrel chest
(b) Chronic cough
(c) Pink face
(d) Long, slow, deep breathing pattern

Most Recent Questions

27.1. **Creola bodies are seen in:**
(a) Bronchial asthma
(b) Chronic bronchitis
(c) Emphysema
(d) Bronchiectatsis

27.2. **Alpha-1-antitrypsin deficiency occurs in:**
(a) Emphysem
(b) Bronchiectasis
(c) Empyema
(d) Bronchogenic carcinoma

27.3. **Thickening of pulmonary membrane is seen in:**
(a) Asthma
(b) Emphysema
(c) Bronchitis
(d) Bronchiectasis

RESTRICTIVE LUNG DISEASE: ILD, ARDS, PNEUMOCONIOSIS

28. **Which of the following is the characteristic feature of adult respiratory distress syndrome?** *(AI 2012)*
(a) Diffuse Alveolar Damage
(b) Interstitial tissue inflammation
(c) Alveolar exudates
(d) Interstitial fibrosis

29. **All are true about phagocytosis except** *(AI 2011)*
(a) Size of the particle ingested is less than 0.5 micrometer
(b) Size of the particle ingested is more than 0.5 micrometer
(c) Combines with lysosome forming phagolysosome
(d) Amoeba and other unicellular organisms make their living out of it

30. **The following does not occur with asbestosis:**
(a) Methaemoglobinemia *(DPG 2011)*
(b) Pneumoconiosis
(c) Pleural mesothelioma
(d) Pleural calcification

31. **Ferruginous bodies are seen in:** *(AI 2008)*
(a) Silicosis (b) Byssinosis
(c) Asbestosis (d) Bagassosis

32. **All of the following are seen in asbestosis except:**
(a) Diffuse alveolar damage *(AI 2002)*
(b) Calcify pleural plaques
(c) Diffuse pulmonary interstitial fibrosis
(d) Mesothelioma

33. **Which of the following is characteristically *not* associated with the development of interstitial lung disease?** *(AIIMS May 2006)*
(a) Organic dusts
(b) Inorganic dusts
(c) Toxic gases, e.g. chlorine, sulphur dioxide
(d) Inhalation of tobacco smoke

34. All of the following features are seen in asbestosis except: *(AIIMS Nov 2002)*
    (a) Diffuse pulmonary interstitial fibrosis
    (b) Fibrous pleural thickening
    (c) Emphysema
    (d) Calcific pleural plaques

35. Asbestosis of the lung is associated with all of the following except: *(AIIMS May 2002)*
    (a) Mesothelioma
    (b) Progression of lesion even after stopping exposure to asbestos
    (c) Nodular lesions involving upper lobe
    (d) Asbestos bodies in sputum

36. Which of the following is associated with hypersensitive pneumonitis? *(AIIMS May 2002)*
    (a) Silicosis
    (b) Asbestosis
    (c) Byssinosis
    (d) Berylliosis

37. End stage lung disease is seen in: *(PGI June 2004)*
    (a) Sarcoidosis
    (b) Interstitial lung disease
    (c) Langerhan's cell histiocytosis
    (d) Aspergillosis
    (e) Asbestosis

38. Features seen in bronchiolitis obliterans with organizing pneumonia include: *(PGI Dec 2001)*
    (a) Polypoid plugs in bronchioles
    (b) Ulceration and exudation of epithelium into the lumen
    (c) Exudation of proteinaceous material in terminal airways
    (d) Bronchoconstriction
    (e) Response to steroids

39. Which of the following inhaled occupational pollutant produces extensive nodular pulmonary fibrosis?
    (a) Silica *(Delhi 2009 RP)*
    (b) Asbestos
    (c) Wood dust
    (d) Carbon

40. Earliest lesion seen in asbestosis is:
    (a) Pleural plaques *(Delhi PG-2007)*
    (b) Hilar lymphadenopathy
    (c) Adenoma lung
    (d) Mesothelioma

41. Most dangerous particles causing pneumoconiosis are of size: *(Delhi PG-2006)*
    (a) 1-5 micron   (b) < 1 micron
    (c) 5-10 micron (d) 10-20 micron

42. Asbestos exposure can cause all except:
    (a) Arthralgia *(Delhi PG-2006)*
    (b) Mesothelioma
    (c) Carcinoma larynx
    (d) Bronchogenic carcinoma

43. Predominant constituent of Hyaline membrane is:
    (a) Albumi *(Delhi PG-2005)*
    (b) Anthracotic pigment
    (c) Fibrin rich exudates
    (d) None of the above

44. "Egg-shell calcifications" are seen in: *(UP 2005)*
    (a) Silicosis
    (b) Berylliosis
    (c) Asbestosis
    (d) Bronchial asthma

45. Hyaline membrane disease is associated with:
    (a) Respiratory distress syndrome *(UP 2006)*
    (b) Bronchopulmonary dysplasia
    (c) Sudden infant death syndrome
    (d) Bronchiolitis obliterans

46. Baggasosis is caused by: *(RJ 2004)*
    (a) Cotton dust
    (b) Sugarcane
    (c) Asbestosis
    (d) None

47. Which interstitial lung disease is caused by organic dust: *(RJ 2005)*
    (a) Silicosis
    (b) Asbestosis
    (c) Byssinosis
    (d) Anthracosis

48. Lower lung involvement is common in:
    (a) TB *(RJ 2005)*
    (b) Asbestosis
    (c) Silicosis
    (d) All

49. Pleural calcification is found in all of the following except: *(Bihar 2003)*
    (a) Asbestosis
    (b) Hemothorax
    (c) Tuberculous pleural effusion
    (d) Coal worker pneumoconiosis

50. Caplan's syndrome is seen in: *(Bihar 2004)*
    (a) COPD
    (b) Pneumoconiosis
    (c) Pulmonary edema
    (d) Bronchial asthma

51. Acute pulmonary sarcoidosis is least likely to be associated with: *(Bihar 2004)*
    (a) Uveitis
    (b) Pleural effusion
    (c) Erythema nodosum
    (d) Lymphadenopathy

52. A 40 year old air-hostess man has experienced increasing respiratory difficulty for the past 18 months. She is unable to clear her annual physical fitness examination. She therefore approaches a physician. She has normal physical findings on examination but pulmonary function tests reveal a normal FEV1 and reduced FVC. Her chest X-ray is highly suggestive of

diffuse interstitial disease without any abnormal mass or hilar lymphadenopathy. Blood investigations reveal normal hemogram. Special investigations also have negative results for antibodies like ANA and anti – DNA topoisomerase I. Which of the following is the most likely diagnosis?

(a) Scleroderma
(b) Goodpasture's syndrome
(c) Silicosis
(d) Idiopathic pulmonary fibrosis

53. Just 24 hours after moving in to a new apartment in Benagaluru, a 27 years old photographer Akki develops acute onset of fever, cough, dyspnea, headache, and malaise. Surprisingly his symptoms subside over next 6 days when he visits a friend in South Gautham Nagar (a new city). When he returns, he visits his physician, Dr. Oja Jesu who finds that he is not having any abnormality on physical examination. Mr. Akki's chest X ray is also normal. Which of the following may produce these findings?

(a) Antigen – antibody complex formation
(b) Release of histamine
(c) Release of leukotrienes
(d) Toxic injury to type I pneumocytes

54. A 44-year-old woman presents with insidious onset of shortness of breath, chest pain, and fatigue. Chest x-ray films reveal bilateral pulmonary infiltrates and enlarged hilar lymph nodes. There is no history of occupational exposure to mineral dusts or organic dusts. A biopsy of one of these lesions shows non-necrotizing granulomas. Special stains for fungi and mycobacteria are negative. Which of the following is the most likely diagnosis?

(a) Asbestosis   (b) Berylliosis
(c) TB   (d) Sarcoidosis

55. Which of the following would most likely be observed in the lung during an autopsy of a 2-week-old infant who died of neonatal respiratory distress syndrome?

(a) Alveoli filled with neutrophils
(b) Dense fibrosis of the alveolar walls
(c) Enlarged air space
(d) Hyaline membranes and collapsed alveoli

Most Recent Questions

55.1. The commonest cause of death in ARDS is
(a) Hypoxemia
(b) Hypotension
(c) Non pulmonary organ failure
(d) Respiratory failure

55.2. Pneumoconiosis is seen with which particle size?
(a) 0.5-3 microns   (b) 3.5-6 microns
(c) 6.5-8 microns   (d) 10-20 microns

55.3. Which of the following increases tuberculosis?
(a) Asbestosis   (b) Sarcoidosis

(c) Silicosis
(d) Berylliosis

55.4. All are recognized causes off Adult Respiratory Distress Syndrome (ARDS), except:
(a) Smoke inhalation
(b) Malignant hypertension
(c) Gastric aspiration
(d) Viral pneumonias

VASCULAR LUNG DISEASE: INFARCT, PULMONARY EDEMA, PULMONARY HTN

56. The percentage of pulmonary emboli, that proceed to infarction, is approximately: *(AI 2006)*
(a) 0-5%
(b) 5-15%
(c) 20-30%
(d) 30-40%

57. On sectioning of an organ at the time of autopsy, a focal, wedge-shaped firm area is seen accompanied by extensive hemorrhage, with a red appearance. The lesion has a base on the surface of the organ. This findings is typically of   *(AIIMS May 2003)*
(a) Lung with pulmonary thromboembolism
(b) Heart with coronary thrombosis
(c) Liver with hypovolemic shock
(d) Kidney with septic embolus

58. All are the histological features of pulmonary hypertension: *(PGI June 2004)*
(a) Capillaritis of alveolar septa
(b) Saddle thrombi in pulmonary trunk
(c) Thrombi in pulmonary vasculature
(d) Veno-occlusive disease
(e) Thickened arterial wall

59. Bilateral exudative pleural effusion is seen in:
(a) SLE   *(PGI Dec 2006)*
(b) Lymphoma
(c) CCF
(d) Nephrotic syndrome
(e) Ascites

60. "Sudden cardio pulmonary collapse" occurring in pulmonary embolism is due to: *(UP 2005)*
(a) Peripheral embolism of the vessels
(b) 60% pulmonary circulation is obstructed by emboli
(c) Multiple small thrombi causes impaction
(d) Organization of the clot

61. Dr. Sushant Verma conducted a study in MAMC which included admitted patients hospitalized for more than 10 days and are bedridden for more than 7 days. He carries a battery of investigations on these patients including Doppler venous ultrasound of the lower limbs, arterial blood gas analysis, and radiographic ventilation and perfusion scanning of the lungs. Dr. Verma finds that a small number of patients have abnormal ultrasound (suggestive of thrombosis in lower limbs), low pO2 and pulmonary perfusion defects. Which of the following

symptoms is most likely associated with these patients?
(a) Cor pulmonale   (b) Hemoptysis
(c) Dyspnea   (d) No symptoms

Most Recent Questions

61.1. Sequestrated lobe of lung is commonly supplied by which of the following vessels?
(a) Pulmonary artery
(b) Intercostal artery
(c) Descending aorta
(d) Bronchial artery

61.2. Bronchogenic sequestration is seen in which lobe:
(a) Left lower lobe
(b) Right upper lobe
(c) Left middle lobe
(d) Left upper lobe

61.3. Which of the folloowing is not true about pulmonary embolus?
(a) Saddle embolus may cause sudden death
(b) Most lesions affect are in the lower lobes
(c) Small arterioles are blocked
(d) Most of the emboli cause infarction

■ LUNG MALIGNANCIES

62. All are true regarding mesothelioma except:
(a) Bilaterally symmetrical   *(AIIMS May 2011)*
(b) Associated with asbestos exposure
(c) Histopathalogy shows biphasic pattern
(d) Occurs in late middle age

63. A 67 yr male with history of chronic smoking hemoptysis with cough. Bronchoscopic biopsy from centrally located mass shows undifferentiated tumor histopathologically. Most useful I.H.C. (immunohistochemical) marker to make a proper diagnosis would be: *(AIIMS Nov 2009)*
(a) Cytokeratin
(b) Parvalbumin
(c) HMB-45
(d) Hep-par1

64. Which of the following is a finding in biopsy of meso-thelioma of pleura -   *(PGI Dec 01)*
(a) Myelin figures
(b) Desmosomes
(c) Weibel-Palade bodies
(d) Microvilli invasion
(e) Intense fibrosis

65. Neuroendocrine lesions of lung are:
(a) Carcinoid hamartoma   *(PGI June 2004)*
(b) Alveolar carcinoma
(c) Hamartoma
(d) Asthma

66. Hypersecretory granules are seen in which carcinoma of lung?:   *(PGI Dec 2006)*
(a) Adenocarcinoma

(b) Small cell carcinoma
(c) Large cell carcinoma
(d) Bronchoalveolar carcinoma
(e) Squamo us cell carcinoma

67. Most common site of metastasis in lung carcinoma is:
(a) Brain   *(RJ 2000)*
(b) Kidney
(c) Adrenal
(d) Testes

68. True about oat cell carcinoma of lung is:
(a) Secrete ectopic hormone   *(RJ 2001)*
(b) Variant of small cell carcinoma
(c) Cause SIADH
(d) All

69. A 42 years old woman Sugahi Ramamurty has a 3 month history of mild persistent left sided chest pain. She is a non-smoker. There is no physical finding but chest X ray shows a left side pleural mass without pleural effusion. CT scan of the chest shows a localized, circumscribed 2.5 × 6 cm mass confined to the surface of the lung. A biopsy taken after thoracotomy demonstrated the mass being composed of spindle cells resembling fibroblasts with abundant collagenous stroma. These cells were CD34 (+) but are cytokeratin negative. Which of the following is the most likely diagnosis?
(a) Hamartoma
(b) Malignant mesothelioma
(c) Metastatic breast carcinoma
(d) Solitary fibrous tumor

70. A 75-year-old man Sukhdev Singh with a significant smoking history presents to the emergency room with complaints of dyspnea and truncal, arm, and facial swelling for one week. Physical examination is remarkable for facial erythema and facial, truncal, and arm edema with prominence of thoracic and neck veins. On chest x-ray, there is a mass in the right mediastinum with adenopathy. Which of the following is the most likely diagnosis?
(a) Adenocarcinoma
(b) Hodgkin's lymphoma
(c) Large cell carcinoma
(d) Small cell carcinoma

71. A patient Rasool is brought to the emergency room following a seizure. Serum electrolyte studies demonstrate serum sodium of 128 mEq/L. The urine osmolarity is higher than the serum osmolarity. Chest x-ray demonstrates a lung mass. Which of the following forms of lung cancer is most likely to cause the described electrolyte imbalance?
(a) Adenocarcinoma
(b) Bronchioloalveolar carcinoma
(c) Large cell carcinoma
(d) Small cell carcinoma

72. A medical examination of a student reveals absence of cardiac sounds on left side of the chest but surprisingly the normal heart beat on the right side of the chest. The liver edge can be palpated on the left but not the right side of the abdomen. He also gives history of bronchiectasis and sinusitis. Which of the following should be suspected?
    (a) Down syndrome
    (b) Kartagener syndrome
    (c) Kawasaki disease
    (d) Marfan syndrome

73. A patient with small-cell carcinoma of the lung complains of muscle weakness, fatigue, confusion, and weight gain. Physical examination is unremarkable. Serum sodium is found to be 120 mEq/L. Which of the following abnormal laboratory results would also be expected in this patient?
    (a) Decreased plasma atrial natriuretic peptide (ANP) concentration
    (b) Decreased plasma vasopressin concentration
    (c) Decreased serum osmolarity
    (d) Decreased urinary sodium concentration

74. Pleural mesothelioma is associated with:
    (a) Asbestosis   (PGI Dec 2005)
    (b) Berylliosis
    (c) Silicosis
    (d) Berylliosis
    (e) Baggasosis

Most Recent Questions

74.1. APUD cells are seen in:
    (a) Bronchial adenoma
    (b) Bronchial carcinoid
    (c) Hepatic adenoma
    (d) Villous adenoma

74.2. Which of the following can develop into lung cancer?
    (a) Asbestosis
    (b) Silicosis
    (c) Byssinosis
    (d) Anthracosis

74.3. Scar in lung tissue may get transformed into:
    (a) Adenocarcinoma
    (b) Oat cell carcinoma
    (c) Squamous cell carcinoma
    (d) Columnar cell carcinoma

74.4. Cavity formation is observed in one of the following bronchogenic carcinoma:
    (a) Squamous cell
    (b) Oat cell
    (c) Adenocarcinoma
    (d) Bronchoalveolar

74.5. All give rise to malignancy except
    (a) Cholelithiasis   (b) Bronchiectasis
    (c) Ulcerative colitis (d) Paget's disease

74.6. Indoor air pollution does not lead to:
    (a) Chronic lung disease   (AIIMS Nov 2013)
    (b) Impaired neurological development
    (c) Pneumonia in child
    (d) Adverse pregnancy outcome

74.7. In a 70 year old man who was working in asbestos factory for 10-15 years. On routine X ray, a mass was seen in the right apical region of the lung. Biopsy was taken from the mass. Which of the following is seen on electron microscopic examination?   (AIIMS Nov 2013)
    (a) Numerous long slender microvilli
    (b) Melanosomes
    (c) Desmososmes with secretory endoplasmic reticulum
    (d) Neurosecretory granules in the cytoplasm

74.8. Which of the following is having the minimal chances of causing a mesothelioma?
    (a) Amphibole
    (b) Crysolite
    (c) Amesolite
    (d) Tremolite

74.9. The most common lesions in the anterior mediastinum are all except:
    (a) Thymomas
    (b) Lymphomas
    (c) Lymph node enlargement from metastasis
    (d) Teratomatous neoplasms

74.10. Least common cause of clubbing is:
    (a) Adenocarcinoma
    (b) Squamous cell cancer
    (c) Small cell cancer
    (d) Mesothelioma

74.11. Lung cancer most commonly associated with?
    (a) Asbestosis
    (b) Silicosis
    (c) Berylliosis
    (d) Coal worker pneumoconiosis

EXPLANATIONS

1. **Ans. (c) Assman's focus** *(Ref: Robbins 8th/370; OP Ghai 5th/2001-1, Radiology of chest diseases 2nd/77 Thieme)*
   Recent Advances in Pediatrics pulmonology by Suraj Gupte volume 10 page/165)

   - Most common lesion of chronic pulmonary TB is called as Puhl lesion^Q.
   - The infraclavicular lesion is called Assman Redeker Simon^Q focus.
   - In post primary stage (late dissemination), coarse granular dissemination is called Aschoff Puhl focus.

2. **Ans. (d) Mitral Stenosis** *(Ref: Robbins 8th/367-72)*
   Disease states that increase the risk of tuberculosis are:

Diabetes mellitus	Chronic lung disease (particularly silicosis)	Malnutrition
Hodgkin's lymphoma	Chronic renal failure	Alcoholism
Immunosuppression (e.g. seen in AIDS)		

3. **Ans. (b) Predominance of alveolar exudate** *(Ref: Robbins 7th/751, 8th/713-4, 9th/704; Harrison's 17th/1620)*
   Important points about viral pneumonias

   - Called as **atypical** because of **moderate amount of sputum^Q, moderate elevation of total white cell count^Q**, no finding of **consolidation^Q** and **lack of alveolar exudate^Q**.
   - Characterized by inflammatory reaction predominantly **restricted within the walls of alveoli^Q** within the interstitium.are clear whereas the core of these particles is dark.

4. **Ans. (d) *Klebsiella pneumonia*** *(Ref: Harrison 17th/838, Robbins 7th/751, 9/e p703-705)*
   *Klebsiella pneumonia presents as typical **air space pneumonia** with cough productive of purulent sputum.*
   Causes of atypical pneumonias
   - *Mycoplasma*
   - *Chlamydia pneumonia*
   - *Viral infections (Influenza, RSV, Adenovirus),*
   - *Legionella*
   - *Coxiella burnetti*
   - *Pneumocystis carinii*

   Mycoplasma^Q is the **commonest cause** of **atypical pneumonia.**

5. **Ans. (a) Cavitation** *(Ref: Robbins 7th/384–5, 9/e p373; Harrison 17th/1010)*
   - Cavitation is seen when there has been a previous sensitization of the host resulting in caseous necrotic material being present which is discharged through the cavities. So, it is associated with **secondary tuberculosis** more frequently.

   Caseous granulomas with multinuclear giant cells are present in both primary and secondary tuberculosis.

6. **Ans. (b) TB; (c) Histoplasmosis; (d) Cryptococcosis; (e) Wegener's granulomatosis**
   (Ref: Robbins' 7th/399, 754, 9/e p98,709)

   Granuloma with necrosis is seen in following conditions
   - Tuberculosis
   - Histoplasmosis
   - Wegener's granulomatosis
   - Cryptococcosis
     - Classical PAN does not involve the pulmonary artery^Q.

7. **Ans. (a) Altered Sensorium; (b) Dental sepsis; (d) Subpulmonic effusion; (e) Endobronchial obstruction.** *(Ref: Robbins 7th/753, 8th/716-7, 9/e p708)*
   Predisposing factors of lung abscess
   - **Aspiration** *of infective material:* Seen in alcoholics, during general anesthesia, sinusitis, gingivodental sepsis, coma, gastroesophageal reflux diseases.

Respiratory System

- **Antecedent primary bacterial infection**: Post pneumonic abscess.
- **Septic embolism**: Thrombophlebitis, bacterial endocarditis, IV drug abusers.
- **Carcinoma bronchus**: causing obstruction to bronchopulmonary segment.
- **Miscellaneous**: Direct spread of infection from suppuration of subphrenic space, pleural cavity, esophagus, spine, etc.

8. **Ans. (a) Goodpasture syndrome; (b) Leptospirosis; (d) Wegener's granulomatosis; (e) Hantana virus infection;** *(Ref: Harrison 17th 1793)*

Pulmonary renal syndrome is seen in:

- **Goodpasture's syndrome:** Pulmonary hemorrhage and renal failure
- **Leptospirosis:** Renal and hepatic dysfunction, hemorrhagic pneumonia, bleeding diathesis
- Hantan virus also cause pulmonary renal syndrome.
- **Wegener's granulomatosis:** Lung and kidney involvement is common.

Note: Legionella does not affect kidneys. It causes atypical pneumonia, diarrhea and hyponatremia.

9. **Ans. (b) Asbestosis; (c) SLE** *(Ref: Crofton and Douglas 5th/979,1043, 579,1437,611, Robbins 9/e p693)*
Causes of Granulomatous lung response

Known cause	Unknown cause
• Hypersensitivity pneumonitis • Inorganic dust: beryllium, silica • TB • Coccidiodomycosis • Schistosomiasis	• Sarcoidosis • Langerhan's cell granulomatosis • Granulomatous vasculitis • Wegener's granulomatosis • Churg-Strauss syndrome • Bronchocentric granulomatosis • Lymphomatoid granulomatosis

10. **Ans. (d) Subpleural caseous lesion just above or below the interlobar fissure.** *(Ref: Robbins 8th/370, 9/e p374)*
- Inhaled tubercle bacilli implanted in the distal air spaces of the *lower part of upper lobe or upper part of the lower lobe, close to the pleura* lead to formation of Ghon's focus.
- Primary complex or Ghon's complex of tuberculosis consists of 3 components
  - Pulmonary compound or Ghon's focus
  - Draining lymphatics
  - Caseating hilar lymph node
- Caseous hilar lymphadenopathy is associated with Ghon complex and not Ghon focus.

11. **Ans. (a) Ghon's focus, (b) pleural efffusion (d) Fibrosis** *(Ref: Robbins 7th/384, 9/e p374-375)*

12. **Ans. (a) Interstitial pneumonitis; (c) Foamy vacuolated exudates; (d) Mononuclear cell in bronchoalveolar lavage; (e) Neutrophil infiltration:** *(Ref: Harrison' 17th/1267-8, 18th/1671)*
Pneumocystis carinii pneumonia

- On lung sections stained with H and E, the alveoli are filled with typical foamy, vacuolated exudates.
- Severe disease may include interstitial edema, fibrosis and hyaline membrane formation.
- The host inflammatory to lung injury results in increasing neutrophil count in bronchoalveolar lavage fluid, hypertrophy of alveolar type II cells and a mild mononuclear cell infiltrate.
- Malnourished infants display an intense plasma cell infiltrate.

13. **Ans. (c) No abnormal findings** *(Ref: Robbins 8th/368-9, 9/e p373)*
Most Mycobacterium tuberculosis infections are **asymptomatic and subclinical infections**.

- Calcifications and cavitation are more frequent after re-infection or reactivation of tuberculosis infections in adults.
- Lymphadenopathy or subpleural granuloma formation is more frequent in primary tuberculosis infections.
- A diffuse reticulo-nodular pattern is suggestive of miliary tuberculosis.

14. **Ans. (c) Resorption atelectasis** *(Ref: Robbins 8th/679, 9/e p670-671)*

Resorption atelectasis
• It is the result of complete obstruction of the airway most often due to the excessive secretions or exudates in the airway wall. It may occur postoperatively, or may complicate bronchial asthma, chronic bronchitis, aspiration of foreign body etc. • Mediastinum shifts **towards** the atelectatic lung.

Compression atelectasis

- It results when the pleural cavity is partially or completely filled with fluid exudates, tumor, air or fluid as in conditions like pneumothorax, hemothorax, or pleural effusion.
- Also known as **Relaxation atelectasis**.
- Mediastinum shifts **away from** the atelectatic lung.

Microatelectasis

It can occur postoperatively, in diffuse alveolar damage, and in respiratory distress of the newborn from loss of surfactant.

Contraction atelectasis

It occurs when fibrous scar tissue surrounds the lung preventing its full expansion.

Atelectasis is a **reversible disorder** *except* for *contraction atelectasis*.

15. Ans. (b) Ghon complex *(Ref: Robbins 8th/370, 9/e p374)*

- The Ghon complex is the most frequent pathologic form of primary pulmonary tuberculosis. Mycobacterium tuberculosis first localizes in the lung parenchyma, then in the hilar lymph nodes. In both these locations, a granulomatous reaction takes place. These lesions usually heal by fibrosis, leaving only small scars at the sites of remote tuberculous infection. Reactivation of dormant bacilli in old lesions or additional re-exposure leads to secondary tuberculosis, with progression of lesions.
- Cavitary tuberculosis (choice A) and miliary tuberculosis (choice D) are expressions of secondary infection, following reactivation of old, usually clinically silent, lesions.
- The cavitary form is characterized by development of large areas of liquefactive necrosis that empty into the airspaces, leading to cavities within the lung parenchyma.
- The miliary form is due to lymphohematogenous dissemination and subsequent seeding of tubercle bacilli throughout the body.

15.1. Ans. (c) Atelectasis *(Ref: Robins 8/e p679-680, 9/e 670-671)*

Atelectasis refers either to **incomplete expansion of the lungs** (neonatal atelectasis) or to the **collapse of previously inflated lung**, producing areas of relatively airless pulmonary parenchyma.

Resorption Atelectasis	Compression Atelectasis	Contraction Atelectasis
• Due to airway obstruction leading to resorption of oxygen trapped in the alveoli.	• Due to presence of fluid, blood, air or tumor in pleural space.	• Fibrosis in the lung or pleura preventing full expansion of pulmonary tissue.
• Causes mediastinal shift towards affected lung.	• Causes mediastinal shift away from the affected lung.	• Only **irreversible** cause of atelectasis[Q].
• Associated with chronic bronchitis/asthma/ aspiration of foreign body/ secretions	• Most commonly associated with cardiac failure[Q].	

15.2. Ans. (d) Accumulation of fibrin *(Ref: Robbins 8/e p713, 9/e p704)*

The following 4 stages of inflammation are present.
- **Congestion:** It is due to vasodilation. There is bacteria rich intra-alveolar fluid.
- **Red hepatization:** Exudate is rich in RBC, neutrophils and fibrinQ.
- **Grey hepatization:** Degradation of RBC and fibrinosuppurative exudates
- **Resolution:** Enzymatic degradation of exudate and healing

15.3. Ans. (d) 5-7 *(Ref: Harsh Mohan 6/e p469)*

Stages of pneumonia

- Congestion: 1-2 days
- Red hepatization: 2-4 days
- Gray hepatization: 4-8 days
- Resolution: by 8-9 days

15.4. Ans. (b) Recruitment of lymphocytes *(Ref: Robbins 9/e p371-374, 8/e p74, 7/e p382)*

- *Macrophages are the primary cells infected by M. tuberculosis.* Early in infection, tuberculosis bacilli replicate essentially unchecked, while later in infection, the cell response stimulates macrophages to contain the proliferation of the bacteria.
- *About 3 weeks after infection*, a T-helper 1 (T_H1) response is mounted that activates macrophages to become bactericidal.

- The T_H1 response orchestrates the formation of granulomas and caseous necrosis. Macrophages activated by IFN-γ differentiate into the "epithelioid histiocytes" that characterize the granulomatous response, and may fuse to form giant cells.

15.5. Ans. (a) Apex *(Ref: Robbins 9/e p373, 8/e p370, 7/e p383)*
- *Secondary pulmonary tuberculosis* classically involves the *apex of the upper lobes* of one or both lungs

15.6. Ans. (a) Terminal bronchiole *(Read below)* *(Ref: Robbins 9/e p373)*
- The largest amount of smooth muscle relative to the thickness of the wall is present in the **terminal bronchioles**[Q].

15.7. Ans. (d) lobar pneumonia *(Ref: Robbins 9/e p704)*
- *'Bacterial invasion of the lung parenchyma causes the alveoli to be filled with an inflammatory exudate, thus causing consolidation ("solidification") of the pulmonary tissue'* .....*Robbins definition of pneumonia*

15.8. Ans. (c) ESR is raised because of increased RBC aggregate *(Ref: Wintrobe's hematology 13/e p16-7)*
ESR is a non specific test which is used as an indicator of active disease. It increases in some disease states due to increase in plasma fibrinogen, immunoglobulins and other acute phase reactants. In addition, change in red cell shape and number affect ESR.
Decreased ESR: Sickle cell disease, polycythemia, and hereditary spherocytosis.
Increased ESR: Infections, anemia, liver disease, cancer, pregnancy, collagen vascular disease
So, in a patient with TB, ESR will increase due to aggregation of red cells called rouleaux whose formation is facilitated by fibrinogen. Since, it is non specific; it cannot conform recovery from TB.

Additonal info for AIIMS

• The ESR may be measured by Wintrobe or Westergren's tube but the readings need to be corrected for the patient anemia.
• However, a variant of ESR called zeta sedimentation rate is developed which produced reproducible results and doesnot require correction for anemia.

16. Ans. (c) Chronic bronchitis *(Ref: Robbins 8th/688, 9/e p679)*

17. Ans. (b) Pulmonary emphysema; (c) Diastase resistant hepatic cells: *(Ref: Robbins 7th/911-2, 8th/865-6, 9/e p675-676)*
- Alpha 1-anti-trypsin deficiency is an *autosomal recessive* disease marked by abnormally low serum levels of α1 AT enzyme resulting in *panacinar emphysema*.
- It is characterized by presence of round to oval, *PAS positive and diastase resistant* cytoplasmic *inclusions in hepatocytes* which on H and E stain acidophilic and indistinctly demarcated from surrounding cytoplasm.

18. Ans. (b) Eosinophils *(Ref: Robbins 9/e p680, 8th/690-691; 7th/724-726)*

19. Ans. (a) Bronchial asthma *(Ref: Robbins 9/e p682, 8th/691, 7th/726)*

20. Ans. (b) Centriacinar *(Ref: Robbins 9/e p675, 8th/684, 7th/718)*

21. Ans. (a) Centrilobular emphysema *(Ref: Robbins 9/e p675, 8th/684, 7th/719)*

22. Ans. (a) Panacinar emphysema *(Ref: Robbins 8th/368-9, 9/e p675)*
Progressive exertional dyspnea with a reduction of FVC could be due to chronic obstructive or restrictive lung disease. A key clue in the stem of the question is the plasma protein electrophoresis finding suggesting α-l-antitrypsin deficiency. Deficiency of α-l-antitrypsin can cause panacinar emphysema (a form of COPD), which usually affects the lower lung lobes most severely.
- Compensatory hyperinflation refers to the expansion of normal lung parenchyma that occurs when adjacent lung segments or lobes collapse or are surgically removed.
- Rupture of apical blebs is thought to be the major cause of primary spontaneous pneumothorax.

- **α 1-antitrypsin deficiency** is associated with chronic **panacinar** emphysema preferentially localized to the **lower pulmonary lobes**.
- **Centriacinar emphysema has** a predominantly **upper lung lobe** distribution and is strongly associated with **chronic smoking.**

23. Ans. (b) Granulocyte – macrophage colony stimulating factor *(Ref: Robbins 8th/705, 9/e p696)*

The patient in the stem of the question has the acquired from of pulmonary alveolar proteinosis (PAP).

CFTR gene mutations lead to cystic fibrosis and widespread bronchiectasis.
- Anti –DNA topoisomerase I antibodies are seen in diffuse scleroderma, which produces interstitial fibrosis.

- Anti – glomerular basement membrane antibody is present in Goodpasture's syndrome with extensive alveolar hemorrhage.

- **PAP** is associated with **impaired surfactant clearance** by alveolar macrophages.
- Microscopically there is accumulation of acellular surfactant in intra-alveolar and bronchiolar spaces.

24. **Ans. (b) Centriacinar emphysema** *(Ref: Robbins 8th/684-5, 9/e p675)*
The findings of Mr. John point to an obstructive lung disease like emphysema which occurs due to airway narrowing or even from loss of elastic recoil. So, emphysema is the most likely diagnosis.

- **Sarcoidosis** is a chronic **restrictive lung disease with all lung volumes decreased, low FVC, and normal FEV1/FVC ratio.**
- Diffuse alveolar damage is an acute restrictive lung disease.
- **Chronic pulmonary embolism does not affect FVC** because the airways are not affected. It is however associated with a ventilation/perfusion mismatch.

25. **Ans. (c) Emphysema** *(Ref: Robbins 8th/684, 9/e p675-676)*
Emphysema is a pulmonary disease characterized by enlargement of the alveolar airspaces due to destruction of the septae without consequent fibrosis.
Pulmonary hypertension (choice D) affects neither the airways nor the alveoli. It is characterized by thickening of the arterial smooth muscle with intimal hyperplasia and fibrosis. Atherosclerotic changes in the normally plaque-free larger pulmonary arteries may be seen.

26. **Ans. (c) Increased Reid index** *(Ref: Robbins 8th/688, 9/e p679)*
This patient has the presentation of acute infection (elevated temperature, greenish-yellow sputum) on a background of chronic bronchitis, which is common in smokers. Hyperplasia and hypertrophy of mucous glands in chronic bronchitis causes increased Reid index in these patient.
Apical cavitary lesions (choice A) might be indicative of cavitary tuberculosis. It is not associated with excessive mucus production. Hemoptysis and weight loss might also be expected as clinical findings.
Curschmann spirals (choice B) are found in asthmatic patients and represent mucus casts of small airways. Enlarged hilar lymph nodes (choice D) might suggest bronchogenic carcinoma or a granulomatous process, which would be less likely than chronic bronchitis. In addition, patients with carcinoma often present with hemoptysis and weight loss, rather than excessive mucus production.

27. **Ans. (a) Barrel chest** *(Ref: Robbins 8th/686, 9/e p677)*
A **barrel chest** with **increased anterior/posterior diameter** is commonly observed in patients with long-standing, **severe emphysema**. This change in chest shape occurs because these patients, who have **high compliance**[Q] of the lung proper, tend to function with their lungs to some degree "over-inflated" compared to people with normal lung compliance. This over-inflation limits their ability to take further deep breaths. Patients with moderately severe emphysema are able to **maintain an adequate lung ventilation** by taking **many short breaths**[Q] (compare with choice D); this physiology is sometimes expressed by describing these patients as **"pink puffers"**[Q] (choice C). Chronic cough (choice B) in emphysema patients is not directly related to the change in compliance.

27.1. **Ans. (a)Bronchial asthma** *(Ref: Robbins 8/e p691, 9/e p682)*
Creola bodies are are clusters of ciliated epithelial cells sometimes seen in sputum samples of patients with asthma.

3 C's of sputum findings in asthma

- Charcot leyden crystals
- Curschmann spirals
- Creola bodies

27.2. **Ans. (a) Emphysema** *(Ref: Robbins 9/e p675, 8/e p685, 7/e p719)*
- **Alpha 1 anti trypsin deficiency** is associated with **panacinar emphysema**.

27.3. **Ans (a) Asthma** *(Ref: Robbins 9th/ 682)*
Thickening of the airway wall is a feature of airway remodeling and is seen in asthma.

28. **Ans. (a) Diffuse Alveolar Damage** *(Ref: Robbins 8th/680-1, 9/e p672)*

29. **Ans. (a) Size of the particle ingested is less than 0.5 micro meter** *(Ref: Robbins 8th/53, Pharmaceutical Research, Vol. 25, No. 8, August 2008)*
The article writes….Particles possessing diameters of 2-3 microns exhibits maximum phagocytosis and attachment.

30. **Ans. (a) Methaemoglobinemia** *(Ref: Harrison 17th/1612-3, Robbins 9/e p691)*

31. **Ans. (c) Asbestosis** *(Ref: Robbins 8th/700, 9/e p691)*
Robbins direct quote… *'inorganic particles may become coated with iron protein complexes and are called ferruginous bodies'*.
Asbestosis in its classical form is a diffuse fibrotic disease of the lung tissue. Typically, the fibrotic changes of asbestosis are focal and are *most prominent in the lower lung lobes*. The presence of asbestos bodies in or adjacent to the walls of fibrotic respiratory bronchioles is the hallmark of the disease. A characteristic of asbestos bodies is a core of asbestos coated by ferroprotein. (So, 'c' is the answer)

> Asbestos bodies are mimicked by "ferruginous bodies" which are formed on particles of talc, mica, fibre, glass and other less common materials in the lung. True asbestos bodies are clear whereas the core of these particles is dark.

32. **Ans. (a) Diffuse alveolar damage** *(Ref: Robbins 7th/736, 8th/700, 9/e p672)*
Diffuse alveolar damage is a characterstic feature of ARDS. As explained in the text, asbestos inhalation is associated with pleural plaque, interstitial fibrosis, bronchogenic cancer and mesothelioma.

33. **Ans. NONE** *(Ref: Harrison 17th/1643, Robbins 8th/694, 704, 9/e p685)*
All the mentioned options are associated with interstitial lung disease. Following is a table adapted from Robbins and Harrison for a quick reference.

Causes of Interstitial Lung Disease (ILD)

Fibrosing	Granulomatous	Smoking related	Miscellaneous
Usual interstitial pneumonia (idiopathic pulmonary fibrosis)	Sarcoidosis	Desquamative interstitial pneumonia	**Eosinophilic**
Associated with collagen vascular diseases, drugs and radiation	Hypersensitivity pneumonitis	Respiratory bronchiolitis-associated interstitial lung disease	**Pulmonary alveolar proteinosis**
Cryptogenic organizing pneumonia			
Nonspecific interstitial pneumonia			
Pneumoconiosis			

Directly quoting *Pneumoconiosis* as is given on page 696 of Robbins …. *'the pneumoconiosis was originally coined to describe the non-neoplastic lung reaction to inhalation of mineral dusts encountered in the workplace. Now it also includes diseases induced by organic as well as inorganic particulates and chemical fumes and vapors'*. Presented underneath is an adapted classification from Robbins table 15-6;

Causes of pneumoconiosis

Mineral dusts	Coal dust, silica, asbestos, iron oxide, barium sulfate
Organic dusts inducing hypersensitivity pneumonitis	Moldy hay, bagasse, bird droppings
Chemical fumes and vapours	Sulfur dioxide, ammonia, benzene, insecticides
Organic dusts inducing asthma	Cotton, flax, hemp

As can be concluded from both the above tables, the answer should be none in the options provided. If the question would have been containing pneumoconiosis and NOT ILD, then smoking would have been the answer of choice.

34. **Ans. (c) Emphysema** *(Ref: Robbins 7th/735-6, 8th/699-700, 9/e p691)*

35. **Ans. (c) Nodular lesions involving upper lobes** *(Ref: Robbins 7th/734-6, 8th/700, 9/e p688)*
   - In asbestosis, there is presence of lesions affecting lower lobes or base of the lungs
   - Nodular lesions involving upper lobes' is a feature of silicosis. The lesions continue to progress even after exposure to asbestos has stopped.

36. **Ans. (c) Byssinosis** *(Ref: Robbins 7/e p733, 9/3 p688)*
   - **Hypersensitivity pneumonitis** (also called **allergic alveolitis**) describes a spectrum of immunologically mediated, predominantly interstitial lung disorders caused by intense, often prolonged exposure to **inhaled organic antigens**[Q]. It is a type *III + IV hypersensitivity reaction*.
   - **Table 15-6** on page 697/8ᵗʰ Robbins mentions- **Byssinosis is an organic dust** *causing asthma*; rest of the options silicosis, asbestosis and berylliosis are given as examples of mineral dusts. So, they can be easily excluded. The best answer would therefore be option 'c' i.e. Byssinosis.

Other examples associated with hypersensitivity pneumonitis

Farmer's lung: Thermopohilic actionomycete or mouldy hay or grain dust*.
Pigeon breeder's lung: Proteins from serum, excreta or feathers of the birds.
Air conditioner lung (or Humidifier lung): Thermopohilic bacteria in heated water reservoirs.

37. **Ans. (a) Sarcoidosis; (b) Interstitial lung disease; (c) Langerhan's cell histiocytosis (e) Asbestosis.**

• Parenchymal causes of end stage lung disease: • Emphysema • Pneumoconiosis • Bronchitis • ARDS • Asbestosis • Interstitial lung disease.	• Pulmonary Langerhan's cell histiocytosis is a progressive disease, and can lead to end stage lung disease. • Sarcoidosis of the lung is an interstitial lung disease; which may lead to progressive fibrosis and end stage lung disease. • Aspergillosis causes extrinsic allergic alveolitis or hypersensitivity pneumonitis.

38. **Ans. (a) Polypoid plugs in bronchioles; (c) Exudation of proteinaceous material in terminal airways; (d) Bronchoconstriction; (e) Response to steroids** *(Ref: Robbins' 7th/731, 8th/696, 9/e p687; CMDT' 2010 243)*
Cryptogenic organizing pneumonia (earlier called as Bronchiolitis obliterans with organizing pneumonia)

- Affects men and woman equally, around 50-70 years
- Etiology is **unknown**[Q]
- Clinical features- Dry cough and dyspnea
- Chest X-ray shows **subpleural and peribronchial**[Q] patchy area of airspace consolidation.
- Histopathology: there is presence of **polypoid plugs** of loose organizing connective tissue (called as Masson bodies[Q]) within alveolar ducts, alveoli and often bronchioles[Q] (all are of same age)
- There is **no interstitial fibrosis or honey comb lung**[Q].
- Treatment is done with **steroids**[Q].

39. **Ans. (a) Silica** *(Ref: Robbins 8th/698-9, 9/e p690)*

40. **Ans. (a) Pleural plaques** *(Ref: Robbins 7th/735, 8th/700, 9/e p691)*

Pleural plaque[Q]:
It is the most common manifestation of asbestos exposure composed of plaques of dense collagen containing calcium. They are usually asymptomatic and develop on anterior and posterolateral parts of parietal pleura and over the diaphragm.

41. **Ans. (a) 1-5 micron** *(Ref: Robbins 7th/732, 8th/696, 9/e p688)*
In pneumoconiosis, the most dangerous particles range from 1-5 micron in diameter, because they may reach the terminal small airways and air sacs and settle in their linings.

Note:
- The solubility and cytotoxicity of particles, modify the nature of pulmonary response.
- In general, the smaller the particle, the higher the surface area-to-mass ratio, and the more likely and more rapidly toxic levels will appear in the pulmonary fluids.
- Larger particles resist dissolution and so may persist within lung parenchyma for years.
- Larger particles tend to evoke fibrosing collagenous pneumoconiosis, such as characteristic of silicosis.

42. **Ans. (a) Arthralgia** *(Ref: Robbins 7th/735, 8th/700, 9/e p691)*

43. **Ans. (c) Fibrin rich exudates** *(Ref: Robbins 7th/481, 8th/456-8, 9/e p457)*
- The membranes (in hyaline membrane disease) are largely made up of fibrinogen and fibrin admixed with cell debris derived chiefly from necrotic type-II pneumocytes.
- There is a remarkable paucity of neutrophilic inflammatory reaction associated with these membranes.
- The lesions of hyaline membrane disease are never seen in still born infants or in live-born infants who die within a few hours of birth.

44. **Ans. (a) Silicosis** *(Ref: Robbins 9/e p690, 8th/699, 7th/734)*

45. **Ans. (a) Respiratory distress syndrome** *(Ref: Robbins 9/e p457, 8th/680, 7th/715)*

46. **Ans. (b) Sugarcane** *(Ref: Robbins 9/e 688, 8th/697, 7th/733)*

47. Ans. (c) **Byssinosis** *(Ref: Robbins 9/e 688, 8th/697, 7th/733)*

48. Ans. (b) **Asbestosis** *(Ref: Robbins 9/e 691, 8th/700, 7th/736)*

49. Ans. (b) **Hemothorax** *(Ref: Robbins 8th/732, 9/e 722)*

50. Ans. (b) **Pneumoconiosis** *(Ref: Harrison 17th/1625, 9/e 688)*

51. Ans. (b) **Pleural effusion** *(Ref. Robbins 9/e 693, 8th/702-703, 7th/738)*

52. Ans. (d) **Idiopathic pulmonary fibrosis** *(Ref: Robbins 8th/694-5, 9/e 685)*
    - Needless to tell you the name of the airline employing a 40 year old airhostess friends, we understand that the lady has chronic restrictive lung disease. The etiology in this lady is unknown. This has to be differentiated from patients having an identifiable cause like infection, collagen vascular disease, drug use, and pneumoconiosis.
    - Scleroderma is ruled out because there is no history of skin involvement and in these, the ANA test result typically is positive.
    - Goodpasture's syndrome is a rare cause of sudden onset of severe hemoptysis but no mention of anti glomerular basement antibody is present.
    - Silicosis is due to inhalation of dust but the profession of the lady excludes that.

53. Ans. (a) **Antigen – antibody complex formation** *(Ref: Robbins 8th/703 -4, 9/e p694)*
    Mr. Akki is likely suffering from hypersensitivity pneumonitis. In this condition, the symptoms appear acutely soon after exposure to an antigen like a fungus (mould) present in ventilation or AC ducts. However, the symptoms improve if the affected individual leaves the environment having the antigen. There are minimal pathologic pulmonary changes. It is mainly a type III hypersensitivity reaction, but with more chronic exposure to the antigen, there may be a component of type IV hypersensitivity with granulomatous inflammation. Histamine release is characteristic of a type I hypersensitivity reaction that more typically occurs in allergic disease.
    Leukotrienes are important mediators in asthma produced by the lipoxygenase pathway.
    A toxic injury is more typical of inhalation of a toxic gas like sulfur dioxide (known as **silo –filler's disease**).

54. Ans. (d) **Sarcoidosis** *(Ref: Robbins 8th/702-703, 9/e 693)*
    The correct answer is D. The diagnosis of sarcoidosis is usually made by exclusion. This disease is characterized by non-necrotizing granulomas developing most frequently in the lungs, lymph nodes, retina, heart, spleen, skin, and liver. Non-necrotizing granulomas may be seen in a number of other conditions, however, such as infections and certain forms of pneumoconiosis, which must be ruled out before making a diagnosis of sarcoidosis.

55. Ans. (d) **Hyaline membranes and collapsed alveoli** *(Ref: Robbins 8th/680, 9/e 457)*
    Neonatal respiratory distress syndrome is a disease of **immaturity**. The immature lung is not able to produce sufficient surfactant to prevent collapse of many alveoli. Severe diffuse damage to alveoli causes precipitation of protein ("**hyaline membranes**") adjacent to many alveolar walls.
    Abundant neutrophils (choice A) are seen in pneumonia.
    Fibrosis (choice B) is a late, not early, feature of respiratory distress syndrome whereas the **air spaces are collapsed**, *not enlarged* (choice C), in this condition.

55.1 Ans (c) **Non pulmonary organ failure** *(Ref: Robbins 9th/ 674)*
    In ARDS, most of the deaths are attributable to sepsis or multiorgan failure and, in some cases, direct lung injury.

55.2 Ans (a) **0.5-3 microns** *(Ref: Robbins 9th/ 688)*

55.3 Ans (c) **Silicosis** *(Ref: Robbins 9/e p 690)*

55.4. Ans (b) **Malignant hypertension** *(Ref: Robbins 9th/ 672)*
    See the table of causes of acute respiratory distress syndrome. ARDS is associated with non cardiogenic pulmonary edema. Malignant hypertension will cause development of cardiogenic pulmonary edema.

    The four most important causes of ARDS:

    Sepsis, diffuse pulmonary infections, gastric aspiration and head injuries.

56. Ans. (b) **5-15%** *(Ref: Robbins 7th/742, 8th/706, 9/e 698)*
    Robbins direct quote. *'Only about 10% of pulmonary artery emboli actually cause infarction'.*

57. Ans. (a) **Lung with pulmonary thromboembolism** *(Ref: Robbins 9/e p129-130, 8th/128, 7th/138)*
    - The morphology is characteristically present as red (hemorrhagic) infarct. The red infarcts are seen in lung, liver and intestine.
    - White infarcts are seen in brain, spleen, kidney and heart.

58. Ans. (c) Thrombi in pulmonary vasculature; (d) Vaso-occlusive disease; (e) Thickened arterial wall *(Ref: Robbins 8th/708, 9/e p699-700, Harsh Mohan 6th/466)*

In pulmonary hypertension pathological changes are seen from main pulmonary arteries to arterioles. They are:

Arterioles and small pulmonary arteries (most prominently affected)	Medium sized pulmonary arteries	Large pulmonary arteries
(i) Medial hypertrophy	(i) Medial hypertrophy; which is not marked in secondary pulmonary hypertension	(i) Atheromatous deposits
(ii) Thickening and reduplication of elastic lamina.	(ii) Concentric intimal thickening	
(iii) **Plexiform pulmonary arteriopathy** in which intraluminal tuft of capillary formation occurs in dilated thin walled arteriolar branches.	(iii) Adventitial fibrosis	
	(iv) Thickening and reduplication of elastic lamina.	

The presence of many organizing or recanalizing thrombi favors recurrent pulmonary emboli as the cause and the coexistence of diffuse pulmonary fibrosis or severe emphysema and chronic bronchitis points to chronic hypoxia as the initiating event.

59. Ans. (a) SLE; *(Ref: Harrison 17th/1660)*
Transudative and exudative pleural effusion (PE) are differentiated by measuring the LDH and protein level in the pleural fluid. Exudative PE meets at least one of the following criteria:

1. Pleural fluid protein/serum protein > 0.5.
2. Pleural fluid LDH by serum LDH > 0.6.
3. Pleural fluid LDH more than 2/3rd of the normal upper limit of serum.

Transudative PE is caused by:
- CCF, cirrhosis, pulmonary embolism
- Nephrotic syndrome, peritoneal dialysis, superior vena cava obstruction
- Myxoedema

Causes of exudative pleural effusion			
Neoplastic disease	Pericardial disease	Asbestos exposure	Yellow nail syndrome
Hemothorax	Chylothorax	Uremia	Radiation therapy
Pulmonary emboli	Sarcoidosis	Meig's syndrome	Ovarian hyperstimulation syndrome
GI disease Esophageal perforation Pancreatic disease Intra-abdominal abscess Diaphragmatic hernia	**Collagen vascular disease** Rheumatoid pleuritis SLE Drug induced lupus Sjogren's syndrome Wegener's granulomatosis Churg Strauss syndrome	**Drugs** Nitrofurantoin Dantrolene Methysergide Bromocriptine Amiodarone Procarbazine	**Infections** Bacterial infections TB Fungal infections Viral infections Parasitic infections

60. Ans. (b) 60% pulmonary circulation is obstructed by emboli *(Ref: Robbins 9/e p127, 8th/126; 7th/136)*

61. Ans. (d) No symptoms *(Ref: Robbins 8th/698, 706-7)*
The stem of the question suggests that Dr. Verma's clinical study is being done on patients with pulmonary thromboembolism, and *most pulmonary emboli are small and clinically silent*. Cor pulmonale may result from repeated embolization which is associated with reduction in the pulmonary vascular bed. Hemoptysis is a rare manifestation of pulmonary embolism. It occurs usually with hemorrhagic infarction of the lung. Dyspnea occurs with medium to large emboli.

61.1. Ans. (c) Descending aorta *(Ref: Robbins 8/e p679, 9/e 670)*
- *Pulmonary sequestration* refers to the presence of a discrete mass of lung tissue *without normal connection to the airway system.*
- The blood supply to the **sequestered area** arises not from the pulmonary arteries but **from the aorta** or its branches

61.2. Ans. (a) Left lower lobe *(Ref: Fetal and Neonatal Physiology 4/e p872; Robbins 9/e p670 8/e p679; www.uptodate.com)*
Pulmonary sequestration can be either:
- *Extralobar sequestrations* are external to the lung and may be located anywhere in the thorax or mediastinum. They are seen in infants. They occur in the **lower left side of the thorax** between the left lower lobe ad the diaphragm.
- *Intralobar sequestrations* occur within the lung substance usually in older children and are often associated with recur-

rent localized infection or bronchiectasis. These are seen most commonly in the **posterior basal segment** of **left lower lobe**[Q] (**Ref.** Fetal and Neonatal Physiology).

61.3. Ans. (d) Most of the emboli cause infarction *(Ref: Robbins 8/e p706, 9/e p127)*
* Large emboli lodge in the main pulmonary artery or its major branches or at the bifurcation as a *saddle embolus*. It *may lead to sudden death.*
* *Smaller emboli travel out into the more peripheral vessels,* where they may cause hemorrhage or infarction. In patients with adequate cardiovascular function, the bronchial arterial supply can sustain the lung parenchyma. Hemorrhages may occur, but there is no infarction. The underlying pulmonary architecture is preserved, and resorption of the blood permits reconstitution of the preexisting architecture.

Also know: NEET points

•	Only about **10%**[Q] **of emboli actually cause infarction**, which occurs when the circulation is already inadequate, as in patients with heart or lung disease.
•	Pulmonaryinfarcts tend to be **uncommon** in the young.
•	About 3/4[th]of all infarcts affect the **lower lobes** [Q]
•	Inmore than half, multiple lesions occur.
•	Typically, they extend to the periphery of the lung substance as a wedge with the **apex pointing toward the hilus**[Q]of the lung.

62. Ans. (a) Bilaterally symmetrical *(Ref: Robbins 8th/733-4, Malignant Pleural Mesothelioma 1st/65, DeVita's Cancer 8th/1840, 9/e p723-724)*
Mesothelioma is an asbestos exposure releated tumor having Mean age of presentation as 50-70 years. Microscopically it may have both epithelioid and sarcomatoid patterns (**biphasic pattern).**
Option 'a'.... 'Pleural mesotheliomas are *more commonly right sided* (R:L ratio is 3:2) may be because of greater size of right sided pleural cavity. Although **usually unilateral at presentation**, it is not infrequent to find histological evidence of mesothelioma in the contralateral pleura. Macroscopic evidence of **synchronous bilateral pleural tumors is rare**'.... *Malignant Pleural Mesothelioma* 1st/65.

63. Ans. (a) Cytokeratin *(Ref: Harsh Mohan 6th/16, Robbins 8th/35, 725-726, 9/e p716)*
* The presence of chronic smoking, cough and hemoptysis in old man is a pointer towards a diagnosis of *bronchogenic cancer.* The central location suggests the possibility of a *squamous cell cancer.*
* Robbins writes "*Histologically, this tumor is characterized by the presence of keratinization and/or intercellular bridges*".
Other options

•	**HMB-45** is a specific tumor marker for **melanoma**.
•	Parvalbumin is low molecular calcium binding albumin protein localised in *fast-contracting muscles*. It is also present in the *brain* (in GABAergic interneurons) and some endocrine tissues. *Decreased PV and GAD67 expression* was found in PV+ GABAergic interneurons in **schizophrenia**.
•	**Hep-par 1** is hepatocyte paraffin 1 and is a well known marker for **hepatocellular carcinoma**.

64. Ans. (d) Microvilli invasion, (e) Intense fibrosis: *(Ref: Robbins' 7th/768-9, 8th/734, 9/e p723-724)*

	Benign mesothelioma	Malignant mesothelioma
Nature	**Solitary** fibrous tumor	**Diffuse** thick and fleshy tumor
Prior asbestos exposure	**No**[Q] relationship	**Definitive association**[Q] is present
Microscopic feature	Whorls of reticulin and collagen fibers among which interspersed spindle cells resembling fibroblasts are present	**Epithelioid type:** cuboidal/columnar cells form tubular/ papillary structures **Sarcomatoid type:** appear as spindle cell carcinoma **Mixed type**
Immunotyping	Cells are CD34(+) and keratin (-)[Q]	Cells are CD34(-) and keratin (+)[Q]

65. Ans. (a) Carcinoid hamartoma *(Ref: Robbin 7th/764, 9/e p719)*
Neoplasms of neuroendocrine cells in the lung include:
* Benign tumorlets (small tumors in areas of scarring and inflammation)
* Carcinoid
* Small cell carcinoma
* Large cell neuroendocrine carcinoma of lung.

66. **Ans. (b) Small cell carcinoma**(*Ref: Robbins 7th/762, 8th/727, 9/e p717*)
    - **Small cell carcinoma** of lung shows **dense core neurosecretory granules**. The granules are similar to those found in neuroendocrine argentaffin cells present along the bronchial epithelium.
    - Some of these tumors secrete polypeptide hormones. Presence of neuroendocrine markers such as chromogranin, synaptophysin and Leu-7 is seen.
    - *It also secretes PTH like substance.* They are most common pattern associated with ectopic hormone production.

67. **Ans. (c) Adrenal**(*Ref: Robbins 9/e p717, 8th/723, 7th/763*)

68. **Ans. (d) All**(*Ref: Robbins 9/e p717, 8th/728, 7th/762*)

69. **Ans. (d) Solitary fibrous tumor**(*Ref: Robbins 8th/732-3 9/e p723*)
    The **solitary fibrous tumor** (or *localized benign mesothelioma*) of pleura is rare neoplasm appearing as a pedunculated mass. It is **not associated with asbestos exposure**/environmental pathogens.
    A **hamartoma** is a *peripheral intra-parenchymal mass* with **cartilage tissue** and a significant component of **fibrous connective tissue**.
    Metastases are typically **multiple** and often **produce bloody effusions**.

    - The tumor cells in solitary fibrous tumor characteristically show immunostaining pattern of CD 34(+) and keratin-negative.
    - A malignant mesothelioma forms a non circumscribed pleural mass. It has atypical cells which are cytokeratin positive.

70. **Ans. (d) Small cell carcinoma**(*Ref: Robbins 8th/728-729, 9/e p718*)
    Superior vena cava (SVC) syndrome is characterized by obstruction of venous return from the head, neck, and upper extremities. Over 85% of cases of SVC syndrome are related to malignancy. Bronchogenic carcinomas (most commonly small cell cancer and squamous cell cancer) account for over 80% of these cases. Lymphomas such as Hodgkin's disease (option B) and non-Hodgkin's lymphoma are uncommon causes of SVC syndrome.

71. **Ans. (d) Small cell carcinoma**(*Ref: Robbins 8th/728-729, 9/e p717*)
    The patient has SIADH (syndrome of inappropriate antidiuretic hormone secretion), which can be caused by *ectopic ADH secretion* by **small cell carcinomas of the lung, CNS disorders, chronic pulmonary disease**, and certain drugs. Features of SIADH include excessive water retention, hyponatremia (which can lead to seizures when severe), and serum hypo-osmolarity with urine osmolarity greater than serum osmolarity.
    Bronchioloalveolar carcinoma (option B) is associated with alveolar-like spaces and **no link to smoking**.

72. **Ans. (b) Kartagener syndrome**(*Ref: Robbins 8th/692, 9/e p683*)
    - **Isolated inversion of the heart (dextrocardia) is almost always associated with cardiac defects** that may include transposition of the atria and transposition of the great arteries.
    - *However, dextrocardia as part of situs inversus totalis*, with reversal of the thoracic and abdominal organs, is *usually associated with a physiologically normal heart*. The cluster of situs inversus, sinusitis, and bronchiectasis is called **Kartagener syndrome**, which is caused by *defective ciliary function*.

    Association of cardiac defects with syndromes
    - Down syndrome - ostium primum type of atrial septal defect.
    - Kawasaki disease- coronary artery aneurysms.
    - **Marfan syndrome - aortic dissection.**
    - Turner syndrome - coarctation of the aorta.

73. **Ans. (c) Decreased serum osmolarity**(*Ref: Robbins 8th/728-729, 9/e p719*)

74. **Ans. (a) Asbestosis**(*Ref: Robbins 7th/768, 8th/700, 9/e p723*)

74.1. **Ans. (b) Bronchial carcinoid**(*Ref: Robbins 8/e p729-730, 9/e p719*)
    Amine Precursor Uptake and Decarboxylation (APUD) cells are also known as neuroendocrine cells. These cells are the cell of origin of the carcinoid tumour.

74.2. **Ans. (a) Asbestosis**(*Ref: Robbins 8/e p699-700, 7/e p735, 9/e p691*)
    Direct lines.. "In contrast to other inorganic dusts, *asbestos an also act as a tumour initiator and promoter*".

74.3. **Ans. (a) Adenocarcinoma**(*Ref: Robbins 9/e p714-715, 8/e p724, 7/e p760-761*)
    "**Peripheral adenocarcinomas** with a small central invasive component **associated with scarring** and a predominantly peripheral bronchioloalveolar growth pattern may have a better outcome than invasive carcinomas of the same size."..
    Robbins

74.4. Ans. (a) Squamous cell *(Ref: Robbins 9/e p716-717)*

Important points about Squamous cell carcinoma of lung

- MC type of lung cancer in **smokers**[Q]
- MC type in **males**[Q]
- Usually **central in location** (arise from the segmental bronchi)
- Intercellular bridges or junction is very specific.
- **Hypercalcemia**[Q] due to PTHrP is the MC paraneoplastic syndrome

74.5. Ans. (b). Bronchiectasis *(Ref: Robbins 9/e p684)*
- Bronchiectasis cannot cause malignancy. The complications which may be associated with bronchiectasis are: Cor pulmonale, metastatic brain abscesses, and amyloidosis.
- To be considered bronchiectasis, **the dilation should be permanent**; reversible bronchial dilation often accompanies viral and bacterial pneumonia.

74.6. Ans. (b) Impaired neurological development *(Ref: Robbin 8/e p 403)*

Concept: Please note friends that **impaired neurological development** can result from **lead** exposure but lead is an **outdoor air pollutant**.

Impaired lung function, lung inflammation, reduced exercise capacity; increased respiratory symptoms are associated with air pollution….

Indoor air pollution contributes to *acute respiratory infections in young children, chronic lung disease* and *cancer in adults*, and *adverse pregnancy outcomes* (such as stillbirths) for women exposed during pregnancy. Acute respiratory infections, principally pneumonia, are the chief killers of young children….Park

74.7. Ans. (c) Desmososmes with secretory endoplasmic reticulum *(Ref: Robbins 8/e p 669, Thurlbeck's Pathology of the Lung 3/e p428-435)*

Tough one friends….AIIMS guys laid the trap beautifully! Lets analyze the question…
The exposure to asbestos brings the first malignancy to our mind which is mesothelioma. However, this is not the answer for the current question because:
- Period of exposure is 10-15 years in question. However, as per Robbins.. " *there is a long latent period of 25 to 45 years for the development of asbestos-related mesothelioma*".
- More importantly, mesothelioma is a pleural tumor whereas the question clearly mentioned that the mass was seen in the right apical region. Considering that there is no history of smoking, this is more likely to an **adenocarcinoma** (and *not squamous cancer*) which is also the most common type of lung cancer associated with asbestos exposure.
- *Desmososmes with secretory endoplasmic reticulum is a feature of electrom microscopic finding of adenocarcinoma*….. Thurlbeck's Pathology table 17-7

Type	Desmosomes/Tonofilament Bundles	Microvilll	Tight Junctions	Lumina	Secretory RER	Neuro-secretory Granules
Squamous carcinomas	Many, wellformed	+	–	–	–	–
Small cell carcinoma	Small, poorly formed	Rare	–	–	–	+
Adenocarcinoma	Many, small well formed	+	+	+	+	–

For future AIIMS question!
- **Napsin A** is a **more sensitive and specific marker** than TTF-1 for **adenocarcinoma of the lung.**

Features of mesothelioma

- On electron microscopy, the presence of long microvilli and abundant tonofilaments but absent microvillous rootlets and lamellar bodies.
- **Lack of staining for carcinoembryonic antigen** (it is *positive in adenocarcinoma*)
- Positive staining for **calretinin, Wilms tumor 1 (WT-1), cytokeratin 5/6**, and D2–40

74.8. Ans (b) Crysolite *(Ref: Robbins 9/e p 691)*
The serpentine chrysotile form accounts for 90% of the asbestos used in industry. Amphiboles even though less prevalent, are more pathogenic than chrysotiles with respect to induction of mesothelioma.

74.9. Ans (c) Lymph node enlargement from metastasis *(Ref: Robbins 9/e p 721)*

Anterior Mediastinum	Middle Mediastinum	Posterior Mediastinum
• Thymoma	• Bronchogenic cyst	• Neurogenic tumors (schwannoma, neurofibroma)
• Teratoma	• Pericardial cyst	• Lymphoma
• Lymphoma	• Lymphoma	• Metastatic tumor (most are from the lung)
• Thyroid lesions		• Bronchogenic cyst
• Parathyroid tumors		• Gastroenteric hernia
• Metastatic carcinoma		

74.10. Ans (c) Small cell cancer

Principles and practice of lung cancer page 348

Clubbing is **most common with adenocarcinoma** and is least *common with small cell lung cancer*....direct quote

74.11. Ans: (a) Asbestosis *(Ref: Robbins 9/e p 713)*

GOLDEN POINTS FOR QUICK REVISION

(LUNGS)

- **"Airway remodeling"** is associated with **bronchial asthma**.
- **Pulmonary hypertension** is defined as **a mean pulmonary artery pressure greater than or equal to 25 mm Hg at rest.**
- **Cough** is the most common symptom of the bronchogenic carcinoma.
- The **lung** is the **most common site** of **metastatic neoplasms.** (Robbins 9th/721)
- The *NAB2- STAT6* **fusion gene** is virtually unique to **solitary fibrous tumor**.
- *In about 80% of mesotheliomas*, the most common is homozygous deletion of the tumor suppressor gene *CDKN2A/ INK4a*. The demonstration of this deletion (usually by **FISH**) involving chromosome 9p can be very helpful in distinguishing mesothelioma from reactive mesothelial proliferations.

UPDATED INFORMATION FROM 9TH EDITION OF ROBBINS

Acute lung injury (ALI)

- Acute lung injury (*ALI*) (also called *noncardiogenic pulmonary edema*) is characterized by the abrupt onset of significant hypoxemia and bilateral pulmonary infiltrates in the absence of cardiac failure. Acute respiratory distress syndrome (ARDS) is a manifestation of severe ALI.
- It is associated with sepsis, severe trauma, or diffuse pulmonary infection.
- The histologic manifestation of these diseases is *diffuse alveolar damage* (DAD). There is also the presence of hyaline membranes lining alveolar walls.

Pulmonary Langerhans Cell Histiocytosis

- Pulmonary Langerhans cell histiocytosis is a rare reactive inflammatory disease characterized by focal collections of Langerhans cells (often accompanied by eosinophils). It results in scarring and the appearance of irregular cystic spaces.
- Langerhans cells are immature dendritic cells with grooved, indented nuclei and abundant cytoplasm. They are positive for S100, CD1a, and CD207 (langerin) and are negative for CD68.
- Most of the affected patients are relatively young adult smokers. It is associated with acquired activating mutations in the serine/ threonine kinase BRAF.

Lymphangioleiomyomatosis

Lymphangioleiomyomatosis is a pulmonary disorder that primarily affects young woman of childbearing age. It is characterized by a proliferation of perivascular epithelioid cells that express markers of both melanocytes and smooth muscle cells. The proliferation distorts the involved lung, leading to cystic, emphysema-like dilation of terminal airspaces, thickening of the interstitium, and obstruction of lymphatic vessels. The condition is characterized by **TSC2 mutation**s. The condition affects *young women* mainly and the presenting features include dyspnea or spontaneous pneumothorax. The condition is treated with lung transplantation.

CHAPTER 11 Kidney and Urinary Bladder

Kidney is the organ of the body responsible for the removal of nitrogenous products from the blood.

SOME IMPORTANT DEFINITIONS:

1. **Azotemia** – It refers to an elevation of Blood Urea Nitrogen (BUN) and creatinine levels due to reduced glomerular filtration rate. It can be due to:
   a. *Pre-renal cause* – Associated with decreased perfusion as in shock, hemorrhage and heart failure.
   b. *Renal cause* – Due to intrinsic defect in the kidney.
   c. *Post renal cause* – Associated with obstruction to urine outflow.
   Patients **do not** require dialysis at this stage.
2. **Uremia** – Azotemia + Clinical signs and symptoms + Biochemical abnormalities
   – There is secondary presence of uremic gastroenteritis, peripheral neuropathy and uremic pericarditis.
   Patients require dialysis at this stage.

CYSTIC DISEASES OF THE KIDNEY

Polycystic Kidney Disease (PKD)

Adult PKD	Childhood PKD

• Autosomal dominant^Q inheritance
• Mutations in PKD1, PKD2 and PKD3 genes (PKD1 produces **Polycystin** protein^Q).
• Asymptomatic till middle age
• Clinical features include hematuria, hypertension, UTI and renal stones.
• Extra renal manifestations
  1. Cysts in other organs like liver^Q (most commonly), pancreas, spleen and ovary.
  2. Berry aneurysm^Q.
  3. Colonic diverticula^Q.
  4. Mitral valve prolapse and aortic regurgitation^Q.
• Grossly, bilaterally enlarged kidneys with multiple cysts containing serous or hemorrhagic fluid^Q.
	• Autosomal recessive^Q inheritance.
	• Mutation in PKHD1 gene which produces **fibrocystin** protein^Q.
	• Presents in infancy with renal insufficiency.
	• Associated with multiple hepatic cysts and congenital hepatic fibrosis^Q.
	• Grossly, bilaterally enlarged kidney with small cysts in cortex and medulla having their long axis at right angle to capsule.

MNEMONIC FOR APKD:

1. **Clinical Features:** (11 B's)
   Signs: Bloody urine
   – Bilateral pain [vs. stones, which are usually unilateral pain]
   – Blood pressure up
   – Bigger kidneys
   Complications
   – Berry aneurysm
   – Biliary cysts
   – Bicuspid valve [prolapse and other problems]

Azotemia refers to an elevation of Blood Urea Nitrogen (BUN) and creatinine levels.

Uremia = Azotemia + Clinical signs and symptoms + Biochemical abnormalities

Countercurrent mechanism of the kidney is responsible for **maintenance of osmotic gradient** in the **medulla.**

Major source of erythropoietin is **Interstitial cells in peritubular capillaries and tubular epithelial cells^Q.** It is also produced in *perisinusoidal cells in the liver*

Major source of **renin** is *JG cell of the kidney^Q*

Genetics
ADult Polycystic Kidney Disease is **A**utosomal **D**ominant
Also; **Polycystic kidney** has *16 letters* and is due to a defect on chromosome **16**.

Accelerators:
- Boys
- Blacks
- Blood pressure high.

GLOMERULAR DISEASES

PATHOGENESIS OF GLOMERULAR INJURY

1. In Situ **immune complex disease**
   1. *Anti-GBM antibody induced nephritis*

      The antibodies are directed against intrinsic fixed antigens that are normal components of the glomerular basement membrane (GBM) proper resulting in a *diffuse linear pattern* of staining for the antibodies by immunofluorescence techniques. This is the model of anti-GBM disease (Goodpasture syndrome) which is caused by antibodies against non-collagenous domain of the *alpha 3 chain of collagen type IV.*

   2. *Heymann nephritis*

      The antibodies are directed against intrinsic fixed antigen called *Heymann antigen* or *'megalin'* located on visceral epithelial cells resulting in complement activation and the formation of subepithelial deposits and a *granular pattern* of staining for the antibodies by immunofluorescence techniques.

   3. *Antibodies against planted antigens*

      Antibodies can react with antigens that are not normally present in the glomerulus but are "planted" there. These antigens include cationic molecules like DNA, nuclear proteins, bacterial, viral and parasitic products and drugs. A *granular pattern* of staining is observed by immunofluorescence techniques.

2. *Circulating immune complex disease*

   The glomerular injury is caused by entrapment of circulating antigen-antibody complex within the glomeruli. This results in complement activation, leukocytic infiltration and proliferation of glomerular and mesangial cells. The endogenous antigens include DNA and tumor antigens whereas the exogenous antigens include infectious products. Electron microscopy reveals the presence of immune complexes as electron dense deposits lying in the mesangium, between endothelial cells and the GBM (subendothelial deposits) or between the GBM and the podocytes (subepithelial deposits). By immunofluorescence microscopy, the immune complexes can be seen as granular deposits along the basement membrane, in the mesangium or both.

> Heymann antigen or **'megalin'** is located on **visceral epithelial** cells

> *Concept*
> - Anionic antigens form subendothelial deposits.
> - Cationic antigens form sub-epithelial deposits.
> - Neutral antigens form mesangial deposits.

Nephritic syndrome	Nephrotic syndrome
1. Proteinuria (1-2g/d)	1. Severe proteinuria (>3.5g/d)
2. Hematuria	2. Hypoalbuminemia (<3g/dl)
3. Hypertension	3. Edema
4. Azotemia, Oliguria	4. Hyperlipidemia, lipiduria

> **Dehydration** is the commonest cause of *primary renal vein thrombosis* in **children.**

Thrombotic and thromboembolic complications are common in nephrotic syndrome due to loss of anticoagulant factor (e.g. antithrombin III, protein C and S) combined with increased platelet activation. Renal vein thrombosis is most often a consequence of this hypercoagulative state specially in case of nephrotic syndrome associated with membranous nephropathy in adults. There is also increased synthesis of fibrinogen in the liver.

TERMINOLOGY IN GLOMERULAR DISEASES

Each region of a renal biopsy is assessed separately. By light microscopy, glomeruli **(at least 10 and ideally 20)** are reviewed individually for discrete lesions.

According to percentage of glomeruli affected
• *Focal* (Less than 50%)
• *Diffuse* (>50%)

Injury in each glomerular tuft can be
• *Segmental* (involving a portion of the tuft)
• *Global* (involving most of the glomerulus)

According to characteristic of lesion
• *Proliferative* when showing increased cellularity.
• *Endocapillary* (Proliferation of cells in the capillary tuft)
• *Extracapillary* (*Extension of proliferation* into Bowman's space)
• *Synechiae* (Epithelial podocytes attach to Bowman's capsule)
• *Crescents* (when fibrocellular/fibrin collections fill all or part of Bowman's space)
• *Sclerosis* (Acellular, amorphous accumulations of proteinaceous material throughout the tuft with loss of functional capillaries and normal mesangium)

NEPHRITIC SYNDROME

Acute Proliferative (Post Streptococcal) Glomerulonephritis

It is seen *1-4 weeks* after a **skin or pharyngeal infection** caused by *group A β hemolytic streptococci* (particularly *strains 12, 4 and 1*) usually in children. Activation of complement system results in consumption of complement proteins leading to *transiently low complement levels* (for 6-8 weeks). The antigen responsible for the development of this condition is a cytoplasmic antigen called **endostreptosin** and a cationic proteinase antigen called *nephritis strain associated protein* or **NSAP**[Q].

Clinical features
Malaise, fever, nausea, oliguria and hematuria leading to smoky or cocoa colored urine, periorbital edema and mild to moderate hypertension.

Microscopic findings
Presence of hypercellular glomeruli due to leukocytic infiltration, proliferation of endothelial and mesangial cells. **Immunofluorescence** microscopy shows the presence of IgG, IgM and C3 deposits in the mesangium and along the basement membrane giving **'starry sky' appearance.**

Investigations
There is elevated levels of antistreptolysin O or ASO and anti DNAase antibodies[Q] (indicative of streptococcal infection) and *reduced levels of serum C3*.

Management
It is done with fluid restriction. The majority of the patients recover and only a small fraction may progress to chronic glomerulonephritis.

RAPIDLY PROGRESSIVE (CRESCENTIC) GLOMERULONEPHRITIS

It is characterized by rapid and progressive loss of renal function associated with rapid development of renal failure in weeks or months.

It is of the following three types with the common feature of severe glomerular injury.

Crescentic Glomerulonephritis

Type I RPGN (Anti-GBM antibody)	Type II RPGN (Immune complex)	Type III RPGN (Pauci immune)
• Idiopathic • Goodpasture's syndrome.	• Idiopathic • Post infectious • SLE, Henoch Schonlein Purpura.	• Idiopathic. • ANCA associated. • Wegener's granulomatosis. • Microscopic polyangitis.
Immunofluorescence finding	*Immunofluorescence finding*	*Immunofluorescence finding*
• *Linear GBM deposits of IgG and C3*	• *"Lumpy bumpy" granular pattern of staining.*	• *No immunoglobulin or complement deposits in GBM.*

New Data 9/e 910
Streptococcal **pyrogenic exotoxin B** (Spe B) is the principal antigenic determinant in most cases.

Concept
There is a **transient reduction** in complement proteins in post streptococcal glomerulonephritis. The *complement levels return to normal in 6-8 weeks.* If the levels persist to be reduced, it is suggestive of another disease.

Crescents are composed of parietal cells, leukocytes and macrophage

Kidney and Urinary Bladder

The characteristic histologic feature is the presence of glomerular **crescents (in > 50% of glomeruli seen on biopsy)** which are *composed of proliferation of parietal cells, leukocytic infiltration, and monocyte and macrophage movement in the urinary space.* The fibrin is prominent within the cellular layers of the crescents. Electron microscopy shows the presence of ruptures in the glomerular basement membrane and **subepithelial deposits**.

Clinical features include hematuria with RBC casts in the urine, subnephrotic proteinuria, hypertension and edema. The prognostic features are mentioned as follows:

Poor prognostic factors	Good prognostic factors
• *Oliguria* and *azotemia* at presentation	• *Pauci immune RPGN* has best prognosis
• *More than 80% circumferential crescents* have poor response to therapy	• *Non- circumferential crescents in less than 50%* glomeruli have indolent course.
• Glomerular tuft necrosis, global glomerular sclerosis, gaps in Bowman capsule and interstitial fibrosis	• *Associated endocapillary proliferation* is a good prognostic factor

Prognosis in RPGN is related to the number of **crescents** as it corelates with oliguria.

NEPHROTIC SYNDROME

Membranoproliferative (Mesangiocapillary) Glomerulonephritis

It is characterized by the presence of basement membrane alterations, proliferation of glomerular cells (particularly in the mesangium) and leukocytic infiltration. These patients may have a nephritic or nephrotic picture.

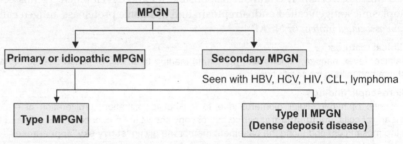

- Immune complexes in glomeruli cause activation of both classical and alternate complement pathway
- **Subendothelial** and mesangial immune complex deposits
- Granular pattern of C_3 with IgG, C_{1q} and C_4

- Immune complexes in glomeruli cause activation of alternate complement pathway
- Dense deposits in the glomerular basement membrane **(intramembranous deposits)**
- Granular and linear pattern of C_3 with absence of IgG

- In type I MPGN, the immune complexes are present in the glomeruli and they cause activation of both complement and alternate pathway.
- In type II MPGN, the immune complexes present in the glomeruli cause activation of alternate complement pathway. The serum of these patients contain C3 nephritic factor (C3NeF) which causes stabilization of alternate C3 convertase thereby causing persistent degradation of C3 and resulting hypocomplementenemia.

Light microscopy shows the lobular appearance of glomeruli which are hypercellular (due to leukocytic infiltration and proliferation of capillary endothelial cells and mesangial cells). The GBM is thickened and the synthesis of new basement membrane causes '**tram-track**' or '**double contour**' appearance appreciated with silver or PAS stains.

Electron microscopically, type I MPGN is having the presence of subendothelial electron dense deposits. Immunofluorescence studies demonstrate the deposition of C_3, IgG and early complement proteins (C_{1q} and C_4) in the glomeruli. In type II disease, there is presence of dense deposits within the GBM, so it is also called as dense deposit disease. Immunofluorescence studies demonstrate the linear or granular deposition of C_3 whereas IgG and early complement proteins are absent. C_3 may also be present in mesangial rings.

Glomerular basement membrane '**tram-track**' or '**double contour**' appearance in MPGN.

Kidney and Urinary Bladder

Clinical presentation of the patient is nephrotic syndrome with the nephritic component of hematuria. There is high incidence of recurrence in transplant patients.

Secondary MPGN is invariably type I but the exact mechanism is unknown.

Genetic Basis of Proteinuria

- **NPHS1 gene** encodes for the protein **nephrin** (component of podocyte foot process controlling glomerular permeability) and its mutation causes a hereditary form of **congenital** nephrotic syndrome **(Finnish type)**.
- **NPHS2 gene** encodes for the protein **podocin** (also a component of podocyte foot process) and its mutation results in the development of *steroid resistant* nephrotic syndrome of childhood onset or autosomal recessive focal segmental glomerulosclerosis (FSG).
- A mutation in the gene encoding podocyte actin-binding protein (α-**actinin 4**) results in **autosomal dominant** focal segmental glomerulosclerosis **(FSG)**.
- Mutations in gene encoding for **TRPC6** is implicated in *adult-onset* FSGS

M
- NPHS1 contains 1, which suggest first letter (means **N**) that stands for **N**ephrin whereas NPHS2 contains 2, which suggest second letter (means **P**) that stands for **P**odocin.
- 1 comes first, so **NPHS1** mutations cause **congenital** nephrotic syndrome whereas 2 comes later, so *NPHS2* mutations cause *acquired* disease (steroid resistant nephrotic syndrome).

LIPOID NEPHROSIS (MINIMAL CHANGE DISEASE)

It is the *commonest cause of nephrotic syndrome in the children* (peak incidence in 2-6 years) characterized by the diffuse effacement of the foot processes of epithelial cells of the glomeruli which *appear normal by light microscopy*. So, the other name of the disease is minimal change disease.

There is absence of immune deposits but presence of visceral epithelial injury due to abnormal secretion of lymphokines by T cells resulting in the loss of glomerular polyanions responsible for low molecular weight proteinuria (selective proteinuria). Mutation of the protein nephrin causes a hereditary form of congenital nephrotic syndrome (*Finnish type[Q]*).

Microscopy

Light microscopy shows the **normal glomeruli** with lipid accumulation in proximal tubular cells (lipoid nephrosis) whereas the **electron microscope** reveals the presence of *effacement of foot processes of podocytes*.

Clinical features

There is massive proteinuria particularly loss of albumin (highly selective proteinuria[Q]) in the absence of hypertension or hematuria.

The patients of lipoid nephrosis with **lipoid nephrosis** have an **excellent response to steroids**

MEMBRANOUS GLOMERULOPATHY

It is a **common cause of nephrotic syndrome in the adults** characterized by the diffuse thickening of the glomerular capillary wall and accumulation of electron dense, immunoglobulin-containing deposits along the *subepithelial side* of the basement membrane. Its causes include:

Idiopathic	Secondary
• Seen in most of the patients (in 85% patients)	• Drugs (penicillamine, captopril, NSAIDs) • Malignancies like carcinoma of colon and lung, melanoma • Infections like hepatitis B and C, syphilis, malaria, schistosomiasis • Systemic diseases like SLE, diabetes mellitus, thyroiditis

The disease has resemblance to the *Heymann nephritis model[Q]* of glomerular injury mediated by immune complex formation against a visceral epithelial antigen called Heymann antigen or *megalin*. The immune complex mediated formation of membrane attack complex C_{5b}-C_9 causes activation of glomerular epithelial and mesangial cells which release oxidants and proteases that cause vessel wall injury and protein leakage.

Microscopy

Light microscopy shows the diffuse membrane-like thickening of the glomerular capillary wall. Basement membrane projections as 'spikes'[Q] are seen on silver stains. **Electron microscopy** reveals effacement of the foot process of podocytes and presence of *subepithelial deposits*.

Immunofluorescence
It demonstrates the linear and granular deposition of C3 and IgG.

Clinical presentation
It is nephrotic syndrome with the excretion of higher weight globulins along with albumin (non selective proteinuria) which is poorly responsive to steroids.

FOCAL SEGMENTAL GLOMERULOSCLEROSIS (FSG)

This is now the **commonest** cause of nephrotic syndrome and is characterized by the presence of focal (only some glomeruli are affected) and segmental (only a part of the glomerulus is affected) sclerosis of the glomeruli.

Causes

1. Idiopathic
2. Secondary:
   - Associated with loss of renal tissue as unilateral renal agenesis or advanced stages of reflux nephropathy or hypertensive nephropathy.
   - Associated with conditions like Sickle cell anemia, HIV infection, Heroin abuse, Obesity.
   - Inherited due to mutations in genes like nephrin, podocin and α-actinin 4.

Degeneration and focal disruption of the visceral epithelial cells is the hallmark feature of focal segmental glomerulosclerosis. *The hyalinosis and sclerosis are due to protein entrapment. Mutation of the protein podocin and a-actinin 4 results in the development of autosomal recessive and autosomal **dominant** forms of focal segmental glomerulosclerosis respectively.*

Microscopy
Light microscopy reveals the focal segmental sclerosis and hyalinization of the glomeruli. **Electron microscopy** demonstrates the diffuse effacement of the podocytes, focal detachment of the epithelial cells and increased mesangial matrix in the sclerotic areas. Five mutually exclusive variants of FSGS may be distinguished by the pathological findings seen on renal biopsy
• Collapsing variant
• Glomerular tip lesion variant
• Cellular variant
• Perihilar variant
• Not otherwise specified variant (NOS)

Immunofluorescence
It demonstrates C3 and IgM deposits in the sclerotic areas and the mesangium.

It affects all age groups and is characterized by the clinical features of non-selective **proteinuria**, reduction in GFR and presence of hypertension and poor response to corticosteroids. There is high incidence of recurrence in transplant patients. Children have better prognosis than adults.

CONCEPT

- A variant of FSG is seen in HIV associated nephropathy called ***collapsing glomerulopathy***.[Q] It is characterized by the collapse and sclerosis of the entire glomerular tuft with the formation of microcysts in the renal tubules. This should be visible in atleast one glomerulus. The glomerular lesion is most specifically the result of podocyte expression of vpr and nef genes. Electron microscopy demonstrates the presence of tubuloreticular inclusions in the endothelial cells which are induced by interferon α (similar lesions are also seen in SLE). It carries a poor prognosis.

- **Most common** cause of collapsing glomerulopathy in children is **cystinosis**.

Degeneration and focal *disruption of the visceral epithelial cells* is the hallmark feature of focal segmental glomerulosclerosis.

The **NOS** variant is the **most common** subtype and *collapsing* FSGS has *worst* prognosis.

Concept

HIVAN may present clinically with nephrotic range proteinuria but is **NOT** associated with Hypertension *(HTN), edema or hyperlipidemia.* (Harrison 17th/1796)

Kidney and Urinary Bladder

IgA NEPHROPATHY (BERGER DISEASE)

This is the *commonest glomerulonephritis* in the world.[Q] It is characterized by the presence of prominent IgA deposits in the mesangial regions and clinically by gross or microscopic hematuria. It can occur either alone or secondary to liver or intestinal disease.

Pathogenesis: The patient usually develops an initial respiratory or gastrointestinal infection resulting in increased synthesis of IgA1 which gets trapped in the mesangium. Here, these immunoglobulins cause activation of alternate pathway of complement system resulting in glomerular injury. Any liver disease causes reduced clearance of IgA whereas intestinal disease causes increased mucosal production of IgA.

> **Microscopic examination** reveals the mesangial widening and proliferation which on **immunofluorescence** reveals the presence of the mesangial deposition of IgA usually with C3 and properdin. Mesangioproliferative glomerulonephritis is seen more commonly than focal proliferative and crescentic (least) glomerulonephritis.

Clinical features: Any age group of the patients (more in children and young adults) may be affected who present with **gross hematuria 3-4 days after** an infection of the respiratory, GI or urinary tract. Almost $1/3^{rd}$ of the patients have microscopic hematuria. This hematuria lasts for some days to subside and recur every few months. Recurrence of the disease in the transplanted kidneys is frequent.

Alport Syndrome

This is a nephritic disorder characterized by the involvement of the triad of **kidney, ear and eye**. There is a fundamental *defect in the α5-chain of collagen type IV* resulting in defective GBM synthesis responsible for the involvement of the organs where this collagen is found.

Microscopically
•   **Light microscopy** glomerular involvement in the form of the presence of *foam cells* in the interstitial cells.

Electron microscopy (Diagnostic for this disorder[Q])
•   It shows the presence of irregular foci of thickening and ***thinning in the GBM*** with splitting and lamination of lamina densa called as ***"basket weave appearance"***. *Absence of α5 staining is seen even on skin biopsy apart from glomerular and tubular basement membrane.*

Clinical features
•   **Males** in the age group of 5-20 years are more frequently affected presenting with gross or microscopic hematuria, nerve deafness and ocular features (posterior cataract, lens dislocation and corneal dystrophy).

Electron microscopy is diagnostic for Alport syndrome. It shows ***"basket weave appearance"*** of the GBM.

Thin Membrane Disease (Benign Familial Hematuria)

This is a disease characterized by the presence of familial asymptomatic hematuria and thinning of the basement membrane to 150-250 nm (normal GBM thickness is 300-400 nm). There is a defect in the α3 and α4 chains of collagen type IV.

Thin basement membrane disease is the most common cause of benign familial hematuria.

Goodpasture Syndrome

It is an autoimmune disorder (**type II hypersensitivity reaction**) having the presence of antibodies against non-collagenous domain of α3 chain of collagen IV causing destruction of basement membrane in *renal glomeruli and pulmonary alveoli*.

The disease affects young men more commonly and is associated with smoking, viral infections or exposure to hydrocarbon solvents (workers in dry cleaning industry).

Histologically, the alveoli show focal necrosis, intra-alveolar hemorrhage, presence of hemosiderin laden macrophages and hypertrophy of type II Pneumocytes. The renal involvement is in the form of either focal proliferative or crescentic glomerulonephritis.

Immunofluorescence studies show linear deposits of immunoglobulins along alveolar septa and GBM.

Uremia is the cause of death in Goodpasture Syndrome.

Clinical features: *Interstitial hemorrhagic inflammation* leads to the predominant symptoms of hemoptysis and hematuria. Management is done by plasmapheresis.

Goodpasture syndrome	Goodpasture disease
• Affects young males • Lungs are affected • Poor prognosis	• Affects elderly **females** • Lungs are **not affected** • **Good prognosis**

SUMMARY OF GLOMERULAR DEPOSITS

Subepithelial	Subendothelial	Basement membrane	Mesangial
*Acute GN (like PSGN) *Membranous GN *Heyman GN *RPGN (some cases) *MPGN (Type I) rarely	*MPGN (Type I) *SLE *Acute GN	*MPGN (Type II) *Membranous Glomerulopathy	*IgA nephropathy *HSP *Anti-GBM diseases like RPGN and Goodpasture syndrome

Concept: Proliferative Glomerulonephritis

Glomerular lesions with increased cells in the tufts are often known as proliferative glomerulonephritis.

It is seen in the following conditions:
• SLE (particularly class II, mesangial hypercellularity defined as >3 cells in mesangial regions)
• HIV
• Membranoproliferative glomerulonephritis
• Neoplasia (particularly CLL and MALT lymphoma)
• Post streptococcal glomerulonephritis.

CHRONIC GLOMERULONEPHRITIS

It is the final stage of many forms of glomerular disease and is characterized by progressive renal failure, uremia and ultimately death.

Clinical features include anemia, anorexia, malaise, proteinuria, hypertension and azotemia.

Grossly there is presence of *small, shrunken kidneys*. There is fine and symmetrical scars. Microscopically, there is hyalinization of glomeruli, interstitial fibrosis, atrophy of tubules, and a lymphocytic infiltrate. Management is done by dialysis and renal transplantation.

Diabetic Nephropathy

It is a disorder characterized by hyperglycemia resulting in formation of advanced glycosylation end products responsible for GBM thickening and increased mesangial matrix. There is also concomitant presence of hemodynamic changes resulting in glomerular hypertrophy with increased glomerular filtration area. Both of these contribute to the development of proteinuria.

Morphological features include:

Capillary Basement Membrane Thickening
It is the earliest morphological abnormality which is seen in *virtually all diabetics irrespective of proteinuria*. It is best detected with electron microscopy and is associated with thickening of the tubular basement membrane.

Diffuse Mesangiosclerosis
There is *diffuse increase in the mesangial matrix* usually consisting of PAS positive material associated with GBM thickening.

Nodular Glomerulosclerosis
It is a highly specific lesion of diabetes and is also known as intercapillary glomerulosclerosis or ***Kimmelsteil Wilson*** lesion. It consists of PAS positive nodules of matrix situated in the periphery of the glomeruli. It is associated with prominent accumulation of hyaline material in capillary loops and Bowman's capsule known as **"fibrin caps" and "capsular drops"** respectively.

The urinalysis in Chronic Glomerulonephritis shows broad waxy casts.

Microalbuminuria means urinary excretion of **30-300 mg** of albumin per 24 hours.

There is also presence of *hyalinizing arteriolar sclerosis* (affects characteristically *both*^Q *afferent and efferent arterioles*), pyelonephritis and *papillary necrosis*.

Clinical features: The increased GFR is associated with **microalbuminuria.**It is very important clinical predictor of development of diabetic nephropathy later on. The protein excretion then reaches subnephrotic proteinuria followed by nephrotic proteinuria. Patients of type I diabetes may also have hypertension which further aggravates the renal disease.

Concept

> Proteinuria in most adults with glomerular disease is non-selective, containing albumin and a mixture of other serum proteins while in children with minimal change disease; protein-uria is selective and largely composed of albumin.

Differences between Benign nephrosclerosis and Malignant nephrosclerosis

Features	Benign nephrosclerosis	Malignant nephrosclerosis
Condition	Benign hypertension, DM, elderly age	Malignant hypertension
Gross appearance of kidneys	**Leather grain** appearance	**Flea bitten appearance** due to tiny petechial hemorrhage
	Small or reduced kidneys	Variable size of the kidney
Microscopy	1. Narrowing of the lumens of arterioles caused by thickening and hyalinization of the walls (hyaline arteriolosclerosis) 2. Fibroelastic hyperplasia of arteries and arterioles	(i) Hyperplastic arteriolitis (onion skinning) due to proliferation and elongation of smooth muscle cells. (ii) Necrotizing glomerulitis (neutrophils infiltration and thrombosed capillaries) (iii) Fibrinoid necrosis of arterioles (iv) Necrotizing arteriolitis
Activity of renin angiotensin system	Normal	↑ed
Proteinuria	Mild	Marked
Sign of malignant hypertension	Absent	Present such as retinopathy encephalopathy
Renal failure	Rare	More common

TUBULAR DISEASES

Acute Tubular Necrosis (ATN)/Acute Kidney Injury (AKI)

- It is a disorder characterized by destruction of tubular epithelial cells resulting in loss of renal function.
- It is the *most common cause of acute renal failure* (ARF). ARF is defined as rapid and reversible deterioration of renal function leading to reduction of urine outflow to *less than 400 ml per day within 24 hours.*

> Acute Kidney Injury is the most common cause of acute renal failure (ARF).

ATN

Ischemic ATN	Nephrotoxic ATN
• Most common cause of ATN^Q. • Due to decreased blood flow (in shock, hemorrhage, hypotension or dehydration). • Presence of **focal** tubular necrosis affecting **proximal straight** tubule and ascending limb of loop of Henle^Q.	• Due to drugs (gentamicin, methicillin, radio contrast agents, organic solvents, ethylene glycol, phenol, pesticides, myoglobin). • **Diffuse** necrosis of *proximal convoluted* tubular segments and ascending Henle's loop^Q occur.

Specific features in certain poisonings

Poisoning	Features in tubular cells
Mercuric chloride	Large acidopathic inclusions^Q
Carbon tetrachloride	Accumulation of neutral lipids^Q
Ethylene glycol	Ballooning and vacuolar degeneration of PCT, Calcium oxalate crystals in tubular lumen^Q

- In both ischemic and nephrotoxic ATN, there is rupture of tubular basement membranes (*tubulorrhexis*) and occlusions of lumen by a cast mostly seen in distal convoluted tubule and collecting ducts.

Pathogenesis of ATN

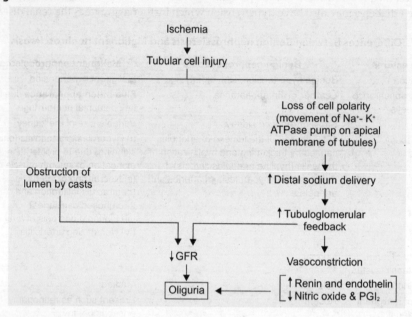

CLINICAL FEATURES OF ATN

1. **Initiation phase**–Lasts for about 36 hours and is characterized by slight decline in urine output with a rise in blood urea nitrogen (BUN).
2. **Maintenance phase**–Oliguria, salt and water overload, hyperkalemia, metabolic acidosis and rising BUN concentration.
3. **Recovery phase** – Steady increase in urine volume (upto 3L/d), hypokalemia and increased vulnerability to infections.

PYELONEPHRITIS

It is the infection involving the renal pelvis, tubules and interstitium. It can be of two types:

- *Acute Pyelonephritis* is the renal lesion associated with bacterial urinary tract infection (UTI)
- *Chronic pyelonephritis*, bacterial infection is associated with other factors including vesicoureteral reflex and obstruction.

E. coli is the commonest bacteria causing UTI[Q] followed by Proteus, Klebsiella, Enterobacter and Strep. fecalis etc.

There is initial colonization of the distal urethra followed by movement in to the bladder due to frequent instrumentation or catheterization. Bladder dysfunction or outflow obstruction causes stasis of urine promoting the bacterial multiplication. From the bladder, it is the incompetence of the vesicoureteral valve allowing retrograde urine flow in to the ureters (vesicoureteral reflux). The infected urine enters the renal pelvis more commonly in the upper and lower poles of the kidney (intrarenal reflux).

Predisposing factors include Vesicourethral reflux, urethral instrumentation, diabetes mellitus, pregnancy, urinary obstruction, benign prostatic hypertrophy and other renal pathology.

Clinical features: Females more commonly affected than males (because of shorter urethra, hormonal changes favoring bacterial adhesion to mucosa, absence of antibacterial

Ascending infection is the most common route of pyelonephritis caused by most bacteria *except TB which involves the kidney by hemtogenous spread.*

WBC casts are suggestive of renal involvement because *casts are formed only in tubules.*

Kidney and Urinary Bladder

property as in prostatic fluid and urethral trauma during sexual intercourse). There is presence of fever with chills, dysuria (painful micturition), increased frequency and urgency along with costovertebral angle tenderness.

Urinalysis reveals presence of leukocytes particularly neutrophils (pyuria) and **WBC casts**[Q] suggestive of renal involvement (because casts are formed only in tubules).

Complications include papillary necrosis (usually bilateral), pyonephrosis and perinephric abscess.

Concept of Sterile Pyuria: Causes

- Recently treated UTI
- TB, fungal infection
- Perinephric abscess
- Chronic prostatitis
- Acute interstitial nephritis
- Chronic interstitial nephritis (including analgesic nephropathy)
- Chronic pyelonephritis

Sterile pyuria is defined as 'white cells in the urine in the **absence** of significant bacterial growth'.

Differences between Chronic glomerulonephritis and Chronic pyelonephritis

Traits	Chronic glomerulonephritis	Chronic pyelonephritis
Causes	Various glomerulonephritis	Reflux nephropathy or chronic obstructive pyelonephritis
Pathogenesis	End stage glomerular disease due to specific glomerulonephritis	Chronic tubulo-interstitial inflammation and scarring associated with renal disorder
Gross appearance of surface	Diffusely, granular, cortical surfaces	Depressed area on dilated and blunted calyx
Scar	Fine and Symmetrical	Coarse and Asymmetrical
Glomeruli	Reduced in number with obliteration	Normal; may show periglomerular fibrosis
Tubules	Atrophied	Atrophy in some and hypertrophy in others filled with **colloid casts** (thyroidisation)
Renal pelvis and calyx	Normal	Dilated
Interstitial and periglomerular fibrosis	Mild	More marked
Clinical features	Insidious in onset Proteinuria, azotemia, hypertension, edema	May be asymptomatic or present with back pain, fever, polyuria, nocturia, pyuria, bacteriuria with gradual onset of hypertension and renal insufficiency

In **chronic glomerulonephritis** kidneys are **diffusely** and **symmetrically scarred** whereas in **chronic pyelonephritis**; the kidneys are irregularly and **asymmetrically scarred**.

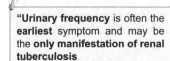

"**Urinary frequency** is often the **earliest** symptom and may be the **only manifestation of renal tuberculosis**

Xanthogranulomatous pyelonephritis (XPN)

Unusual *variant of chronic pyelonephritis*. Most cases occur in the setting of obstruction due to infected renal stones.
Grossly
• *Yellow, lobulated masses* diffusely replace the renal architecture.
Microscopically
• There is massive destruction of the kidney due to granulomatous tissue containing lipid-laden macrophages; the appearance may be *confused with renal malignancy*.
Clinical features
• It most often occurs in middle-aged women with a history of recurrent urinary tract infections. • Typical presenting symptoms include flank pain, fever, malaise, anorexia and weight loss. • A unilateral renal mass can usually be palpated on physical examination.

Diagnosis

- Examination of the urine confirms the presence of urinary tract infection. Urine culture typically demonstrates Enterobacteriaceae. The *most common organisms associated with XPN are E. coli, Proteus mirabilis, Pseudomonas, Streptococcus faecalis and Klebsiella.*

Renal Stones/Urinary Calculi

In the urinary tract, the *most common site of origin of stone is the kidney.* Males between the age group of 20-30 years are most commonly affected. Renal stones are formed either due to supersaturation of urine (constituent concentration exceeding the solubility) or deficiency of crystal formation inhibitors like pyrophosphate, diphosphonate, citrate, osteopontin and nephrocalcin.

Renal stones

Calcium oxalate	Uric acid	Magnesium ammonium phosphate	Cystine
• **Most common** stone[Q]. • **Idiopathic hyper-calciuria** is the commonest cause[Q]. • Seen in acidic urine. • Also associated with hypocitraturia[Q]. • • Radiopaque stone[Q].	• Seen with **hyper-uricemia (gout, leu-kemias)**[Q]. • Seen in acidic urine (pH < 5.5)[Q]. • **Radiolucent stone**[Q].	• Also called **"stru-vite stones"** or **"triple stones"**[Q]. • Formed in **alkaline urine** particularty in infection with **pro-teus**[Q]. • Occupy large part of renal pelvis, so, called as **"staghorn calculi"**[Q].	• Due to genetic defect in the ab-sorption of cys-tine resulting in **cystinuria**[Q]. • Formed in acid-ic urine • Change color from initial yel-low to green on air exposure[Q].

Note: Uncommon renal stones can be composed of xanthine (due to xanthine oxidase deficiency), indinavir (in AIDS patients taking this drug) or triamterene (Patients on this antihypertensive medica-tion). All these are radiolucent stones[Q].

Stones are usually unilateral (80% of patients) and are deposited in renal pelvis and bladder. If the developing stone takes the shape of the pelvicalyceal system, it is called **staghorn calculi**.

Clinical symptoms include hematuria, urinary obstruction, renal colic (if they pass into the ureters) and increased chances of infection. Most of the renal stones are managed surgically.

URINARY CASTS

Hyaline casts
• This is a **normal constituent** of urine and has no attached significance.   • Tamm Horsfall protein is a protein secreted by epithelial cells of loop of Henle[Q].   • This protein may be exerted as Hyaline cast.   • May be seen in concentrated urine, febrile disease, after heavy exercise
RBC cast
Is suggestive of glomerular injury.[Q]
White cell casts
Are suggestive of interstitial injury and may be seen in interstitial nephritis. WBC cast with bacteria indicate Pyelonephritis.[Q]
Broad granular casts
Arise in the dilated tubules of enlarged nephrons that have undergone compensatory hypertrophy in response to reduced renal mass i.e. chronic renal failure.[Q]

Kidney and Urinary Bladder (sidebar)

Patients with calcium oxalate stone are advised to maintain a **low sodium, low protein but normal calcium** diet to reduce the recurrence renal stone.

Struvite (triple) stone: **Coffin lid shaped**[Q].
Calcium oxalate: **Needle shaped/ square envelope shape**[Q]

Cystine stone: **Hexagonal**[Q]
Uric acid: **diamond / barrel shape**[Q]

Concept

Reasons why low calcium is avoided in patients with calcium oxalate are:

- *Low calcium diet increases risk of stone formation* by reducing calcium in the intestine to bind with oxalate thereby increasing oxalate levels in the urine.
- *Low calcium increases the risk of reduced bone density*.

Pigmented muddy brown granular casts
Are suggestive of ischemic or nephrotoxic injury i.e. Tubular Necrosis[Q].

Lipid cast
• Seen when there is fatty degeneration of the tubular epithelium.
• Also seen in nephrotic syndrome, lupus and toxic renal poisoning[Q].

RENAL TUMORS

Benign Tumors

- **Angiomyolipoma** – It is a hamartoma composed of fat, smooth muscle and blood vessels and is associated with tuberous sclerosis.
- **Oncocytoma**- Tumor arising from intercalated cells of collecting ducts having large, eosinophilic cells which have numerous mitochondria. The cells have expression of carbonic anhydrase C and band 3 protein.

Wilms Tumor (Nephroblastoma)

Wilms' tumor is the **most common primary renal tumor of childhood** in USA. This tumor's peak age is **2-5years**. The risk of Wilms' tumor is increased in association with at least three recognizable groups of congenital malformations:

WAGR syndrome
It is characterized by aniridia, genital anomalies, and mental *retardation* and a 33% chance of developing Wilms' tumor. Patients with WAGR syndrome carry constitutional (germline) deletions of two genes *WT1* and *PAX6* both located at chromosome **11p13**[Q].

Denys-Drash syndrome
It is characterized by *gonadal dysgenesis* (male pseudohermaphroditism) and *early-onset nephropathy* leading to renal failure. The characteristic glomerular lesion in these patients is a *diffuse mesangial sclerosis*. These patients also have germline abnormalities in *WT1*. In addition to Wilms' tumors these individuals are also at increased risk for developing germ-cell tumors called *gonadoblastomas*.

Beckwith-Wiedemann syndrome
It characterized by enlargement of body organs (organomegaly), macroglossia, hemihypertrophy, omphalocele and abnormal large cells in adrenal cortex (adrenal cytomegaly). The genetic locus involved in these patients is in band p15.5 of chromosome 11 called *"WT2"*. In addition to Wilms' tumors patients with Beckwith-Wiedemann syndrome are also *at increased risk for developing hepatoblastoma, adrenocortical tumors, rhabdomyosarcomas and pancreatic tumors*.

Concept

Anaplasia is an indicator of adverse prognosis because it is associated with p53 gene mutation and resistance to anti-cancer drugs.

MORPHOLOGY

Grossly, Wilms tumor tends to present as a large, solitary, well-circumscribed mass and on cut section, the tumor is soft, homogeneous, and tan to grey with occasional foci of hemorrhage, cyst formation, and necrosis.

Microscopically, Wilms tumors are characterized by the *classic triphasic combination of blastemal, stromal, and epithelial cell types* (immature glomeruli and tubules) seen in majority of lesions.

The tumor usually presents as a large abdominal mass, which may extend across the midline and down into the pelvis. The patient may also present with fever and abdominal pain, with hematuria, or rarely, with intestinal obstruction as a result of pressure from the tumor.

The prognosis for Wilms tumor is generally very good, and excellent results are obtained with a combination of nephrectomy and chemotherapy.

Renal Cell Carcinoma (Hypernephroma/Grawitz Tumor)

It is the **most common malignant cancer of the kidney** affecting the poles of the kidney (**more commonly upper pole**). Males are more frequently affected (M:F ratio is 2 to 3:1) in the age group of 6-7th decade.

Risk factors

Non genetic factors
• **Tobacco** (most important risk factor)[Q]
• Hypertension[Q]
• Obesity[Q]
• Tuberous sclerosis[Q]
• Estrogen therapy[Q]
• Asbestos exposure[Q]
• Chronic renal failure and acquired cystic disease[Q]
• Von Hippel Lindau syndrome

Genetic factors
• **Trisomy 7** shows increased expression of MET which is a proto-oncogene having tyrosine kinase receptor activity thereby resulting in development of **papillary type of renal cancer**.
• **t(X; 1)** causes translocation of PRCC gene to fuse with TFE-3 gene on X chromosome and fusion gene increases the risk of **papillary renal cell carcinoma** (PRCC) particularly in children.

> Triad of VHL syndrome = Cerebellar hemangioblastoma + Bilateral renal cell cancer + Retinal angiomatosis.

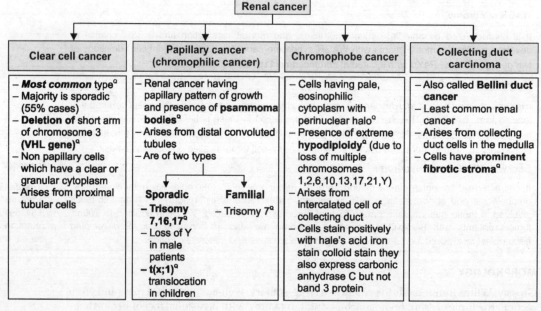

Clear cell cancer	Papillary cancer (chromophilic cancer)	Chromophobe cancer	Collecting duct carcinoma
– **Most common** type[Q] – Majority is sporadic (55% cases) – **Deletion of** short arm of chromosome 3 **(VHL gene)**[Q] – Non papillary cells which have a clear or granular cytoplasm – Arises from proximal tubular cells	– Renal cancer having papillary pattern of growth and presence of **psammoma bodies**[Q] – Arises from distal convoluted tubules – Are of two types **Sporadic** – **Trisomy 7,16,17**[Q] – Loss of Y in male patients – **t(x;1)**[Q] translocation in children **Familial** – Trisomy 7[Q]	– Cells having pale, eosinophilic cytoplasm with perinuclear halo[Q] – Presence of extreme **hypodiploidy**[Q] (due to loss of multiple chromosomes 1,2,6,10,13,17,21,Y) – Arises from intercalated cell of collecting duct – Cells stain positively with hale's acid iron stain colloid stain they also express carbonic anhydrase C but not band 3 protein	– Also called **Bellini duct cancer** – Least common renal cancer – Arises from collecting duct cells in the medulla – Cells have **prominent fibrotic stroma**[Q]

Clinical features include the classical **triad**[Q] of *hematuria* (earliest and most common symptom[Q]; usually intermittent), *palpable mass and flank pain*.

> Sarcomatoid change in any renal cancer causes **worsening of prognosis**.

Paraneoplastic syndromes associated with RCC

• Elevation of erythrocyte sedimentation rate
• Polycythemia (Due to erythropoietin)
• Stauffer syndrome (*non metastatic hepatic dysfunction*)
• Hypertension (Due to renin)
• Anemia and fever
• Hypercalcemia (Due to PTH related peptide)
• Cushing syndrome (Due to corticosteroid synthesis)
• Feminization or masculinization (Due to gonadotropin release)
• May also cause amyloidosis, eosinophilia or leukemoid reaction[Q]

> **Papillary cancer** is associated with a **strong tendency to invade the renal vein** and grow as solid column of cells. The tumor may *even extend to inferior vena cava and right side of the heart.*

Metastasis is usually by the hemotogenous route and the organs affected include **lungs**[Q] (**most common**), bones, regional lymph nodes, liver, adrenals and brain.

Management: Partial/total nephrectomy is the **treatment of choice**.

URINARY BLADDER

It is the organ (lined by transitional epithelium) responsible for the collection of urine formed by the kidney and its removal by intermittent voiding.

Inflammation of urinary bladder is called **cystitis** and it is more common in females as compared to males. It is usually due to:

1. Bacterial cause: *E.coli, Proteus, Klebsiella, Mycobacterium tuberculosis*
2. Fungal cause: *Candida albicans*, seen with immunosuppression
3. Hemorrhagic cystitis: Due to cytotoxic antitumor drugs like cyclophosphamide and Adenovirus.
4. Radiation cystitis: Due to radiation exposure.

Clinical features:

1. *Frequency* – Requirement of urination every 15-20 minutes
2. *Suprapubic pain* – Pain in anatomical location of the bladder
3. *Dysuria* - Painful or burning sensation or urination

This triad may be associated with fever and malaise.

Special cystitis

Hunner ulcer	Malacoplakia
• Painful chronic cystitis associated with hemorrhagic inflammation and fibrosis of the layers of bladder wall[Q]. • Seen frequently in **females**. • Usually idiopathic but may be associated with **SLE**. • **Mast cells**[Q] are characteristically present.	• **Chronic bacterial cystitis** having presence of soft, yellow mucosal plaques. • Most commonly associated with **E. coli** or uncommonly **proteus**. • Microscopically, there is presence of infiltration with lymphocytes and abundant epithelioid histiocytes (**Von Hansemann Histiocytes**) having PAS positive granules and characteristics 3-10μ rounded intracytoplasmic inclusions (called **Michaelis-Gutmann** bodies)[Q] that contain iron (demonstrated by prussian blue stain) **and calcium** (demonstrated by Von Kossa stain). • Similar lesions are also seen in colon, lungs, bones, kidneys and prostate etc.

URINARY BLADDER NEOPLASMS

The urinary bladder cancers usually are of epithelial origin. The commonest histological variant is the transitional cell tumors (urothelial tumors).

Risk factors of urinary bladder cancers

Transitional cell cancers	Squamous cell cancer	Adenocarcinoma
• Cigarette smoking[Q]. • Industrial exposure to arylamines as 2-napthylamine, benzidine, aniline in textile workers, dye workers and leather workers[Q]. • Pelvic irradiation for other pelvic cancer[Q]. • Long term use of analgesics. • Exposure to drugs like cyclophosphamide[Q].	• Infection with **Schistosoma hematobium**[Q]. • Chronic bladder infection and irradiation[Q]. • Diverticula in the bladder[Q].	• Usually arises from *urachal remnants*[Q] or in association with *intestinal metaplasia*[Q].

Genetic risk factors include:

- **9 p gene deletions-** Present in superficial papillary tumors.
- **17p gene deletion-** Invasive urothelial cancers.

9p and 9q have tumor suppressor gene, 17 p has the location of p53 (again tumor suppressor gene). So, any deletion of these genes increases the risk of bladder cancers.

CLINICAL FEATURES

Painless hematuria^Q (*most common symptom*), features of bladder irritability (frequency, urgency and dysuria) or uncommonly, hydronephrosis and pyelonephritis may also be seen.

The prognostic markers include grade of tumor, presence of lamina propria invasion and associated carcinoma *in situ*.

The worst prognosis is associated with tumor invading the muscularis mucosa (detrusor muscle)^Q.

> Involvement of the **detrusor muscle** is associated with the **worst prognosis**.

INVESTIGATIONS:

- *Cystoscopy and biopsy*^{Q} (**Best investigation**)
- Urine cytology of urine markers like telomerase, human complement factor H related protein, mucins, CEA, hyaluronic acid, hyaluronidase, fibrin- fibrinogen degradation products, nuclear matrix proteins and DNA content.

ISUP (International Society of Urological Pathology) Classification of Transitional Cell Tumors

- **Urothelial Papilloma** – Seen in young patients, finger like papillae covered with normal looking urothelium.
- **Urothelial neoplasm of low malignant potential** – Similar to papilloma but with thicker urothelium with diffuse nuclear enlargement.
- **Papillary urothelial carcinoma, low grade** – Almost always papillary having limited cell/nuclear pleomorphism and limited chromosomal/gene abnormalities.
- **Papillary urothelial carcinoma; high grade** – May be papillary/nodular or both having considerable anaplasia and high frequency of chromosomal/gene abnormalities.

MANAGEMENT:

1. **Intravesical BCG**^{Q}
   - Presence of lamina propria invasion
   - Carcinoma *in situ* (CIS)
2. **Radical cystectomy**
   - CIS refractory to BCG
   - Invasion of muscularis propria
   - CIS extending to prostatic urethra or down
3. **Chemotherapy (Mitomycin, thiotepa etc.)**
   - Advanced bladder cancer

Information about commonest mesenchymal tumors of urinary bladder:

- The most common **benign tumor is Leiomyoma**^{Q}
- The most common **sarcoma in infants**/children is **embryonal rhabdomyosarcoma**^{Q}
- The most common sarcoma in adults is **Leiomyosarcoma**^{Q}.

Kidney and Urinary Bladder

MULTIPLE CHOICE QUESTIONS

KIDNEY: GENERAL ASPECTS, POLYCYSTIC KIDNEY DISEASE

1. A 28 year old man has lenticonus and end stage renal disease now. His maternal uncle also died of the same illness. What is the most likely diagnosis?
   (a) Autosomal dominant polycystic kidney disease
   (b) Autosomal recessive polycystic kidney disease
   (c) Oxalosis   *(AIIMS Nov 2012)*
   (d) Alport syndrome

2. Which one of the following is not associated with adult polycystic kidney disease?   *(DPG 2011)*
   (a) Autosomal dominant inheritance
   (b) Mutations involving gene affecting cell-cell matrix interactions
   (c) Intracranial berry aneurysm may be present
   (d) Tricuspid valve prolapse

3. Which of the following is associated with adult polycystic kidney disease?
   (a) Berry aneurysms of Circle of Willis
   (b) Saccular aneurysms of aorta
   (c) Fusiform aneurysms of aorta
   (d) Leutic aneurysms

4. True about adult polycystic kidney disease is all, except: *(AIIMS Nov 2001)*
   (a) Autosomal dominant inheritance
   (b) Hypertension is rare
   (c) Can be associated with cysts in liver, lungs and pancreas
   (d) Pyelonephritis is common

5. True about autosomal dominant type of APKD:
   (a) Small kidney   *(PGI June 2004)*
   (b) Bilateral medullary cysts
   (c) Mutation of polycystin 1and 2 gene
   (d) Renal transplantation is contraindicated
   (e) Pathogenesis starts early and renal failure seen in middle life.

6. Chromosomes involved in adult polycystic kidney disease (APKD) are: *(PGI June 01)*
   (a) 6 and 11   (b) 4 and 16
   (c) 7 and 17   (d) 4 and 12
   (e) 4 and 17

7. Acquired cystic disease of kidney is associated with:
   (a) Xanthogranulomatous pyelonephritis   *(UP 2004)*
   (b) Dialysis
   (c) Renal stones
   (d) Renal dysplasia

8. A 42-year-old man Kumaran is having flank pain and hypertension. He has increased blood urea nitrogen and creatinine with hematuria. Ultrasound studies demonstrate markedly enlarged kidneys with irregular margins and many fluid-filled spaces of different sizes. Excessive secretion of which of the following hormones would be most likely responsible for the patient's hypertension?
   (a) ACTH   (b) Cortisol
   (c) Parathormone   (d) Renin

Most Recent Questions

8.1. Podocytes are seen in:
   (a) Proximal convoluted tubule
   (b) Distal convoluted tubule
   (c) Collecting tubule of the kidney
   (d) Bowman's capsule

8.2. Adult polycystic kidney disease is inherited by:
   (a) Autosomal dominant
   (b) Autosomal recessive
   (c) X-linked
   (d) Mitochondrial

8.3. Major cause of death in End Stage Renal Disease patients on display is which one of the following?
   (a) Cardiovascular disease
   (b) Infections
   (c) Uremia
   (d) Respiratory Failure

8.4. What is oliguria
   (a) Excretion of less than 300 ml in 24 hrs
   (b) Excretion of less than 500 ml in 24 hrs
   (c) Excretion of less than 300 ml in 12 hrs
   (d) Excretion of less than 100 ml in 24 hrs

8.5. What is the minimum number of red blood cells per microliter of urine required for diagnosis of hematuria?
   (a) 3
   (b) 5
   (c) 8
   (d) 10

8.6. Polycystic kidney may be associated with cysts in all the sites, except:
   (a) Lung
   (b) Liver
   (c) Pancreas
   (d) Brain

GLOMERULAR DISEASE: NEPHRITIC SYNDROME, NEPHROTIC SYNDROME, GLOMERULONEPHRITIS

9. In a specimen of kidney, fibrinoid necrosis is seen and onion peel appearance is also present. Most probable pathology is: *(AIIMS Nov 2012)*
   - (a) Hyaline degeneration
   - (b) Hyperplastic arteriosclerosis
   - (c) Glomerulosclerosis
   - (d) Fibrillary glomerulonephritis

10. Which of the following is the diagnosis for a condition having mutation in COL4A5 chain? *(AIIMS Nov 2012)*
   - (a) Alports syndrome
   - (b) Good pasture's syndrome
   - (c) Thin membrane disease
   - (d) Nodular glomerulosclerosis

11. The most common gene defect in idiopathic steroid resistance nephrotic syndrome *(AIIMS Nov 2011)*
   - (a) ACE
   - (b) NPHS 2
   - (c) HOX11
   - (d) PAX

12. A person with radiologically confirmed reflux nephropathy develops nephritic range proteinuria. Which of the following would be the most likely histological finding in this patient? *(AIIMS Nov 2011)*
   - (a) Focal segmental glomerulosclerosis
   - (b) Nodular glomerulosclerosis
   - (c) Membranous glomerulopathy
   - (d) Proliferative glomerulonephritis with crescents

13. A 7 yrs old girl is brought with complaints of generalised swelling of the body. Urinary examination reveals grade 3 proteinuria and the presence of hyaline and fatty casts. She has no history of hematuria. Which of the following statements about her condition is true? *(AIIMS May 2011)*
   - (a) IgA nephropathy is likely diagnosis
   - (b) Her C3 levels will be low
   - (c) No IgG deposits or C3 deposition on renal biopsy
   - (d) Alport syndrome is likely diagnosis

14. The pathological feature in Wegener's granulomatosis on renal biopsy is *(AIIMS Nov 2010)*
   - (a) Nodular glomerulosclerosis
   - (b) Focal necrotizing glomerulonephritis
   - (c) Granulomas in the vascular wall
   - (d) Granuloma of parenchyma of kidney

15. Fibronectin nephropathy has all of the following features except *(AIIMS Nov 2010)*
   - (a) Autosomal recessive inheritance
   - (b) Associated with mesangial expansion
   - (c) Glomeruli do not stain for immunoglobulin or complement
   - (d) PAS- positive amyloid negative deposits.

16. Pathological changes of diabetic nephropathy are all except: *(DPG 2011)*
   - (a) Fibrin caps and capsular drops
   - (b) Kimmelstein-Wilson lesion
   - (c) Basement membrane thickening
   - (d) Focal glomerular sclerosis

17. What is the cause of hypercoagulation in nephrotic syndrome: *(AI 2010)*
   - (a) Loss of antithrombin III (AT III)
   - (b) Decreased fibrinogen
   - (c) Decreased metabolism of vitamin K
   - (d) Increase in Protein C

18. Finnish type of nephrotic syndrome is associated with:
   - (a) Nephrin *(AI '09, '06)*
   - (b) Podocin
   - (c) Alpha actinin
   - (d) CD2 activated protein

19. Pauci-immune crescentic glomerulonephritis is associated with: *(AI 2009)*
   - (a) Microscopic polyangiitis
   - (b) SLE
   - (c) H S Purpura
   - (d) PAN

20. Most common mutation seen in congenital nephrotic syndrome is: *(AI 2008)*
   - (a) Nephrin
   - (b) Podocin
   - (c) α 4 actinin
   - (d) Megalin

21. Which of these does not cause crescentic glomerulonephritis? *(AI 2008)*
   - (a) Rapidly progressive glomerulonephritis
   - (b) Alport syndrome
   - (c) Goodpasture's syndrome
   - (d) Henoch-Schönlein purpura

22. All are non-proliferative glomerulonephritis, except:
   - (a) Membranous glomerulonephritis *(AI 2008)*
   - (b) Mesangiocapillary glomerulonephritis
   - (c) Diabetic glomerulosclerosis
   - (d) Amyloidosis

23. Kidney biopsy from a child with hemolytic uremic syndrome characteristically most likely presents features of: *(AI 2005)*
   - (a) Thrombotic microangiopathy
   - (b) Proliferative glomerulonephritis
   - (c) Focal segmental glomerulosclerosis
   - (d) Minimal change disease

24. Serum C3 is persistently low in the following except:
   - (a) Post streptococcal glomerulonephritis
   - (b) Membranoproliferative glomerulonephritis
   - (c) Lupus nephritis *(AI '04, DNB '07)*
   - (d) Glomerulonephritis related to bacterial endocarditis

25. **All of the following are associated with low complement levels except:** *(AI 2004)*
    (a) Lupus nephritis
    (b) Mesangiocapillary glomerulonephritis
    (c) Diarrhea-associated hemolytic uremic syndrome
    (d) Post-infections glomerulonephritis

26. **All of the following are associated with low C3 level except:** *(AI 2003)*
    (a) Post streptococcal glomerulonephritis
    (b) Membranoproliferative Glomerulonephritis
    (c) Goodpasture's disease
    (d) Systemic lupus erythematosus

27. **Which of the following is not true about Berger's disease?** *(AI 2003)*
    (a) The pathological changes are proliferative and usually confined to mesangial cells; usually focal and segmental
    (b) Hematuria may be gross or microscopic
    (c) On immunofluorescence deposits contain with IgA and IgG
    (d) Absence of associated proteinuria is pathognomic

28. **Crescent formation is characteristic of which of the following glomerular disease:** *(AI 2002)*
    (a) Minimal change disease
    (b) Rapidly progressive glomerulonephritis
    (c) Focal and segmental glomerulosclerosis
    (d) Rapidly non progressive glomerulonephritis

29. **In Wegener's granulomatosis, kidney has which of the following lesions?** *(AIIMS Nov 2009)*
    (a) Glomerular granuloma
    (b) Interstitial granuloma
    (c) Crescentic glomerulonephritis
    (d) Glomerulosclerosis

30. **The Electron Microscopy is virtually diagnostic in renal biopsy study of:** *(AIIMS May 2008)*
    (a) Goodpasture's syndrome
    (b) Churg-Strauss syndrome
    (c) Alport syndrome
    (d) Wegner's granulomatosis

31. **Which type of FSGS has worst prognosis?**
    (a) Tip variant *(AIIMS May 2008)*
    (b) Collapsing
    (c) NOS
    (d) Perihilar

32. **Steroid resistant nephrotic syndrome is caused due to mutation in the gene encoding for?**
    (a) Nephrin *(AIIMS May 2008, Nov 2006)*
    (b) Alpha-actinin-4
    (c) Podocin
    (d) Transient Receptor Potential 6

33. **Which of the following is a feature of Collapsing glomerulopathy?** *(AIIMS Nov '07)*
    (a) Tuft necrosis
    (b) Mesangiolysis

(c) Parietal epithelial proliferation
(d) Hypertrophy and necrosis of visceral epithelium

34. **The most common gene defect in idiopathic steroid resistant nephrotic syndrome** *(AIIMS May 2007)*
    (a) ACE
    (b) NPHS 2
    (c) HOX 11
    (d) PAX

35. **HIV associated nephropathy is a type of:**
    (a) Membranous glomerulonephritis *(AIIMS Nov 2004)*
    (b) Immunotaetoid glomerulopathy
    (c) Collapsing glomerulopathy
    (d) Fibrillary glomerulopathy

36. **Mesangial deposits of monoclonal kappa/Lambda light chains in indicative of** *(AIIMS May 2004)*
    (a) Mesangioproliferative glomerulonephritis
    (b) Focal and segmental glomerulosclerosis
    (c) Kimmelstiel-Wilson lesions
    (d) Amyloidosis

37. **In renal disease, Albumin is first to appear in urine because** *(AIIMS May 2004)*
    (a) Of its high concentration in plasma
    (b) Has molecular weight slightly greater than the molecules normally getting filtered
    (c) High Albumin Globulin ratio
    (d) Tubular epithelial cells are sensitive to albumin

38. **A 7 year old boy presented with generalized edema. Urine examination revealed marked albuminuria. Serum biochemical examinations showed hypoalbuminemia with hyperlipidemia. Kidney biopsy was undertaken. On light microscopic examination, the kidney appeared normal. Electron microscopic examination is most likely to reveal:** *(AIIMS Nov 2003)*
    (a) Fusion of foot processes of the glomerular epithelial cells
    (b) Rarefaction of glomerular basement membrane
    (c) Deposition of electron dense material in the basement membrane
    (d) Thin basement membrane

39. **The prognosis of rapidly proliferating glomerulonephritis (Crescentic GN) depends upon**
    (a) Number of crescents *(AIIMS Nov 2001)*
    (b) Size of crescents
    (c) Shape of crescents
    (d) Cellularity of crescents

40. **True about light microscopy in minimal change disease is:** *(AIIMS Nov 2001)*
    (a) Loss of foot process seen
    (b) Anti-GBM antibodies are seen
    (c) IgA deposits seen
    (d) No change seen

41. **A child had hematuria and nephrotic syndrome (minimal change disease) was diagnosed. True about it is:** *(AIIMS Nov 2001)*
    (a) A type of focal segmental GN
    (b) IgA deposition on basement membrane

(c) Foot process of glomerular membrane normal

(d) Glomerular function is lost due to loss of polyanionic charge on both sites of glomerular foot process

42. Mutation in alpha 5 chain of collagen type IV is seen in:

(a) Alport syndrome *(AIIMS Nov 2006)*

(b) Thin membrane disease

(c) Nodular glomerulosclerosis

(d) Good pasture syndrome

43. Persistent low C3 complement level is not found in:

(AIIMS Nov 2006)

(a) Post streptococcal glomerulonephritis

(b) Mesangiocapillary glomerulonephritis

(c) Cryoglobulinemia

(d) SLE

44. Low complement levels are seen in:

(a) PSGN *(PGI Dec 2006)*

(b) MPGN

(c) Goodpasture's syndrome

(d) Wegener's granulomatosis

(e) Infective endocarditis.

45. Subepithelial deposits in kidney are seen in:

(a) MPGN-1 *(PGI June 2001)*

(b) Goodpasture's syndrome

(c) PSGN

(d) Membranous GN

(e) RPGN

46. Nephrotic syndrome is characterized by:

(a) Proteinuria *(PGI Dec 2002)*

(b) Hyperlipidemia

(c) Edema

(d) Haematuria

(e) Lipiduria

47. In glomerular disease which of the following is mainly excreted in urine:

(PGI Dec 2003)

(a) Albumin

(b) Globulin

(c) Light chain

(d) Heavy chain

(e) Tamm-Horsfall protein

48. Which of the following is included in definition of Nephrotic syndrome?

(PGI June 2004)

(a) Microalbuminuria

(b) Massive Proteinuria

(c) Microscopic hematuria

(d) Edema

(e) Hyperlipidemia.

49. True about Heymann rat glomerulonephritis is:

(a) Heymann antigen is called megalin *(PGI Dec 2004)*

(b) Electron dense deposits in subendothelial space

(c) Electron dense deposits in mesangium

(d) Subepithelial aspect of basement membrane have deposits

(e) Antigen against bacterial and viral proteins

50. Malignant hypertension is associated with:

(a) RPGN *(PGI Dec 2004)*

(b) Malignant nephrosclerosis

(c) Membranous GN

(d) IgA nephropathy

(e) Acute pyelonephritis

51. Histology of Alport syndrome: *(PGI June 2005)*

(a) Foamy cells in interstitium

(b) Foamy cells in tubular epithelial cells

(c) Thickening of GBM > 100 nm

(d) Thinning of GBM < 100 nm

(e) Intimal proliferation.

52. RPGN is caused by: *(PGI June 2005)*

(a) FSGS

(b) Wegener's granulomatosis

(c) Goodpasture's syndrome

(d) PAN

(e) Microscopic polyangitis

53. Post streptococcal glomerulonephritis is associated with: *(PGI Dec 2006)*

(a) Subepithelial deposit

(b) Nephritis along with acute renal failure

(c) Low complement levels

(d) HTN and proteinuria

(e) Normal complement levels

54. Pauci-immune glomerulonephritis is seen in:

(a) RPGN *(Delhi PG-2007)*

(b) IgA nephropathy

(c) Microscopic polyangitis

(d) FSGS

55. Kimmelstiel Wilson lesions are characteristic of:

(a) Diabetic Nephropathy *(Delhi PG-2007)*

(b) Analgesic nephropathy

(c) RPGN

(d) Post streptococcal glomerulonephritis

56. Anti-glomerular basement membrane nephritis is seen in: *(Delhi PG-2005)*

(a) Goodpasture's syndrome

(b) SLE associated glomerulopathy

(c) MGN

(d) MPGN

57. Kimmelstiel Wilson disease is diagnostic of:

(a) Diabetic Glomerulosclerosis *(Delhi PG-2005)*

(b) Benign Hypertension

(c) Malignant Hypertension

(d) Amyloidosis

58. The following is not a feature of acute post streptococcal glomerulonephritis: *(Karnataka 2007)*
    (a) Normal C_3
    (b) Hypertension
    (c) Elevated blood urea and creatinine
    (d) Increased ASO titre

59. Visceral leishmaniasis causes *(Karnataka 2005)*
    (a) Membranous glomerulonephritis
    (b) Mesangioproliferative glomerulonephritis
    (c) Focal segmental glomerulonephritis
    (d) Rapidly progressive glomerulonephritis

60. Histological hallmark of rapidly progressive glomerulonephritis is *(Karnataka 2004)*
    (a) Crescents in most of the glomeruli
    (b) Loss of foot processes of epithelial cells
    (c) Subendothelial electron dense deposits
    (d) The thickening of glomerular capillary wall

61. ANCA is most specific and sensitive marker for *(UP 2000)*
    (a) Idiopathic cresenteric glomerulonephritis
    (b) Post streptococcal glomerulonephritis
    (c) Membranoproliferative glomerulonephritis
    (d) Focal segmental glomerulosclerosis

62. True about post streptococcal glomerulonephritis is: *(UP 2001)*
    (a) Linear deposition
    (b) Diffuse involvement
    (c) Tram track appearance
    (d) Global sclerosis

63. Most common in diabetic nephropathy is: *(UP 2002)*
    (a) Diffuse glomerulosclerosis
    (b) Diffuse cortical sclerosis
    (c) Nodular glomerulosclerosis
    (d) Renal atherosclerosis

64. Steroid responsive glomerulonephritis are all except: *(UP 2002)*
    (a) Post streptococcal glomerulonephritis
    (b) Minimal change disease
    (c) Membranoproliferative glomerulonephritis
    (d) Focal segmental glomerulosclerosis

65. All conditions lead to CRF except: *(UP 2002)*
    (a) Post streptococcal GN
    (b) Membranoproliferative GN
    (c) Minimal change GN
    (d) Focal glomerulosclerosis

66. Most characteristic finding in diabetic nephropathy is: *(UP-2002, 2004)*
    (a) Diffuse glomerulosclerosis
    (b) Nodular glomerulosclerosis
    (c) Diffuse cortical sclerosis
    (d) Renal atherosclerosis

67. All of the following are seen in Goodpasture's syndrome except: *(PGI-1999)(UP 2004)*
    (a) Cresenteric glomerulonephritis
    (b) Hemorrhage inflammation
    (c) Anti-GBM antibody
    (d) Diffuse alveolar involvement

68. All of the following are True about minimal change nephrotic disease except: *(PGI-1999)* *(UP 2004)*
    (a) Respond to steroids
    (b) Selective proteinuria
    (c) IgG deposition in mesangium
    (d) Common in the age group of 2-9 years

69. IgA depositions in mesangial cells are seen in
    (a) Goodpasture's syndrome *(UP 2005)*
    (b) Berger disease
    (c) Cresenteric glomerulonephritis
    (d) Alport syndrome

70. All are causes of rapidly progressive glomerulonephritis except: *(UP 2002, 2007)*
    (a) SLE
    (b) Polyarteritis nodosa
    (c) Post streptococcal GN
    (d) Rheumatoid arthritis

71. The cause of edema in nephritic syndrome is:
    (a) Decrease in plasma protein concentration *(UP 2007)*
    (b) Increase in plasma protein concentration
    (c) Reduced plasma osmotic pressure
    (d) Sodium and water retention

72. Hall mark of the IgA nephropathy is: *(UP 2007)*
    (a) Oedema
    (b) Hematuria
    (c) Hypertension
    (d) Proteinuria

73. Electron dense deposits in the region of hyalinosis and sclerosis, with diffuse loss of foot processes, seen in electron microscopy are features of: *(UP 2007)*
    (a) Minimal change disease
    (b) Membranous glomerulonephritis
    (c) Membranoproliferative GN
    (d) Focal segmental glomerulosclerosis

74. In hemolytic uremic syndrome there is:
    (a) Thrombocytopenia + Renal failure *(AP 2000)*
    (b) Normal coagulative profile
    (c) Microangiopathic hemolytic anemia
    (d) All of the above

75. Subepithelial deposits with 'M' spike is seen in:
    (a) Membranous glomerulonephritis *(AP 2001)*
    (b) Membranoproliferative glomerulonephritis
    (c) Minimal change disease
    (d) RPGN

76. Crescentic glomerulonephritis with pauci-immune glomerulonephritis is associated with: *(Mahe 2001, TN 1990, 1991) (AP 2002)*
    (a) Post infectious glomerulonephritis
    (b) Goodpasture's syndrome
    (c) Wegener's glomerulonephritis
    (d) Membranous glomerulonephritis

77. **Tram track appearance on histopathology of kidney is seen in:** *(AP 2005)*
    (a) Membranous nephropathy
    (b) Membranoproliferative glomerulonephritis
    (c) IgA nephropathy
    (d) Crescentic glomerulonephritis

78. **On electron microscopy, in most of the cases, characteristic splitting of GBM with sub-epithelial deposits in few cases is seen in:** *(AP 2008)*
    (a) RPGN
    (b) Membranous nephropathy
    (c) FSGS
    (d) Minimal change disease

79. **An old man from a village Ram Khilavan has progressively increasing back pain for last 6 months. He also had repeated bouts respiratory tract infections with Streptococcus pneumonia within past 10 months. He ignored these thinking they are associated with his age. However, he then notices the development of an edema on his lower limbs. He rushes to a physician in the city hospital. On examination, apart from pitting edema, his investigations reveal total serum protein 9.8 g/dL, albumin 3.6 g/dl, creatinine, 3.5 mg/dL; urea nitrogen, 30 mg/dL; and glucose is 80 mg/dL. There is absence of glucosouria and hematuria but presence of proteinuria (4.5 g/24 hr). Biopsy of the kidney followed by staining reveals the amorphous pink material deposited within glomeruli, interstitium, and arteries. What is the most probable diagnosis of the old man?**
    (a) Analgesic nephropathy
    (b) Goodpasture syndrome
    (c) Diabetes mellitus
    (d) Multiple myeloma

80. **A 6 year old child Devanand presented to the skin OPD with some honey-colored crusts on his face. Dr Priyanka sends a microbiological culture which comes out to be positive for group A β hemolytic streptococci. Antibiotics are initiated in the child. However, he returns to the hospital with his mother after 15 days with mild fever, malaise and a history of passage of smoky urine. His investigations reveal a serum antistreptolysin O titer of 1:1024. Which of the following is the most likely outcome in this child?**
    (a) Development of rheumatic heart disease
    (b) Chronic renal failure
    (c) Complete recovery without treatment
    (d) Progression to crescentic glomerulonephritis

81. **A 35-year-old woman Sumitra has had type 1 diabetes mellitus for 20 years. She is now developing advanced disease with visual complaints, foot ulcers, and renal disease. Which of the following features that might be seen on renal biopsy is most specific for diabetic glomerulosclerosis?**
    (a) Mesangial IgA deposits
    (b) Necrotic epithelial cells in tubules

(c) Nests of cells with abundant clear cytoplasm
(d) Ovoid, periodic acid-Schiff (PAS)-positive, hyaline masses

82. **A 60-year-old man develops oliguria and peripheral edema over a period of weeks. Urinalysis reveals hematuria and proteinuria; examination of the urinary sediment reveals red cell casts. Radiologic and ultrasound studies fail to demonstrate an obstructive lesion. Renal biopsy shows many glomerular crescents. This presentation is most suggestive of which of the following conditions?**
    (a) Anti-glomerular basement membrane disease
    (b) Diabetic nephropathy
    (c) Hypertensive nephropathy
    (d) Lupus nephritis

83. **An IV drug abuser Chulbul develops an aggressive form of nephrotic syndrome that does not respond to steroids. A renal biopsy is performed. Which of the following histological diagnoses will most likely be made from the biopsy tissue?**
    (a) Focal segmental glomerulosclerosis
    (b) IgA nephropathy
    (c) Membranous glomerulonephritis
    (d) Membranoproliferative glomerulonephritis

Most Recent Questions

83.1. **All of the following decrease in Nephrotic syndrome except:**
    (a) Thyroxin   (b) Transferrin
    (c) Fibrinogen   (d) Albumin

83.2. **Crescents are derived from which of the following?**
    (a) Epithelial cells + fibrin + macrophage
    (b) Mesangial cell + fibrin + macrophage
    (c) Tubular cell + mesangial cell + fibrin
    (d) Neutrophil + tubular cell + fibrin

83.3. **Flea bitten appearance of the kidney is seen in:**
    (a) Malignant hypertension
    (b) Benign hypertension
    (c) Chronic pyelonephritis
    (d) Diabetes mellitus

83.4. **Most common cause of nephritic syndrome in adults is:**
    (a) Rapidly progressive glomerulonephritis
    (b) Focal segmental glomerulosclerosis
    (c) Membranous glomerulonephritis
    (d) Minimal change disease

83.5. **Most common cause of nephrotic syndrome in adults is:**
    (a) Membranous glomerulonephritis
    (b) Minimal change disease
    (c) Acute GN
    (d) Focal segmental glomerulosclerosis

83.6. **The crescent forming glomerulonephritis is:**
    (a) Acute GN
    (b) Rapidly progressive glomerulonephritis

Kidney and Urinary Bladder

(c) Membranous GN

(d) Membranoproliferative GN

83.7. Microalbuminuria is defined as protein levels of:

(a) 100-150 mg/d   (b) 151-200 mg/d

(c) 30-300 mg/d   (d) 301-600 mg/d

83.8. Post streptococcal glomerulonephritis in children is diagnosed by:

(a) Heavy protienuria, high cholesterol, high ASO titre

(b) Heavy protienuria, hematuria, low ASO titre

(c) Mild protienuria, hematuria, high ASO titre

(d) Mild protienuria, high cholesterol, normal ASO titre

83.9. IgA nephropathy is characterized by all of the following except:

(a) Hypertension

(b) Hematuria

(c) Nephritic syndrome

(d) Renal biopsy having thin basement membrane

83.10. In which one of the primary glomerulonephritis the glomeruli are normal by light microscopy but shows loss of foot processes of the visceral epithelial cells and no deposits by electron microscopy

(a) Poststreptococcal glomerulonephritis

(b) Membrano-proliferative glomerulonephritis type I

(c) IgA nephropathy

(d) Minimal change disease

83.11. Type I membranoproliferative glomerulonephritis is commonly associated with all except:

(a) SLE

(b) Persistent hepatitis C infections

(c) Partial lipodystrophy

(d) Neoplastic diseases

83.12. RBC cast seen in:

(a) Minimal change disease

(b) Renal vein thrombosis

(c) Bladder schistomiasis

(d) Rapidly progressive glomerulonephritis

83.13. Most common glomerulonephritis associated with HIV is which of the following?

(a) Focal segmental glomerulonephritis

(b) Diffuse glomerulosclerosis

(c) Membrano-proliferative glomerulonephritis

(d) Crescentic glomerulonephritis

TUBULAR DISEASE AND RENAL CALCULI

84. A lady presents with complaints of abdominal pain. Contrast enhanced CT scan shows bilateral papillary necrosis. Which of the following test shall not be done to investigate the cause of her papillary necrosis?

(a) Culture for bacteria   *(AIIMS Nov 2011)*

(b) Sickling test

(c) Urine acidification

(d) Urine PCR for TB

85. Urine analysis of a patient with haematuria and hypercalciuria is most likely to reveal which of the following?   *(AIIMS Nov 2011)*

(a) Isomorphic RBCs

(b) RBC casts

(c) Nephrotic range proteinuria

(d) Eosinophiluria

86. All of the following about xanthogranulomatous pyelonephritis are true except: *(AI 2011, AIIMS May 2010)*

(a) On cut section yellowish nodules are seen

(b) Associated with tuberculosis.

(c) Foam cells are seen

(d) Giant cells are seen

87. In which of the following conditions bilateral contracted kidneys are characteristically seen?

(a) Amyloidosis   *(AI 2005)*

(b) Diabetes mellitus

(c) Rapidly progressive glomerulonephritis

(d) Benign nephrosclerosis

88. Necrotizing papillitis may be seen in all of the following conditions except: *(AI 2002)*

(a) Sickle cell disease

(b) Tuberculous pyelonephritis

(c) Diabetes mellitus

(d) Analgesic nephropathy

89. Mercury affects which part of the kidney?

(a) PCT   *(AIIMS May 2007)*

(b) DCT

(c) Collecting duct

(d) Loop of Henle

90. Nephrocalcinosis is seen in all except:

(a) Sarcoidosis   *(AIIMS May 2007)*

(b) Distal RTA

(c) Milk alkali syndrome

(d) Medullary cystic kidney

91. Pulmonary, renal syndrome is seen in:

(a) Goodpasture's syndrome.   *(PGI Dec 2003)*

(b) Leptospirosis.

(c) Legionella.

(d) Wegener's granulomatosis.

(e) Hanta virus infection

92. Renal papillary necrosis is seen in:

(a) Thalassemia   *(PGI June 2001)*

(b) DM

(c) Phenacetin abuse

(d) Alcoholism

(e) Cortical necrosis

93. Causes of Nephrocalcinosis are: *(PGI June 2001)*

(a) Hyperparathyroidism

(b) T.B. Kidney

(c) Hypercalcemia

(d) Glomerulonephritis

(e) MCD

94. **Bilaterally enlarged kidneys are seen in:**
    (a) Chronic glomerulonephritis   *(PGI Dec 2002)*
    (b) Chronic pyelonephritis
    (c) Benign nephrosclerosis
    (d) Polycystic Kidney disease
    (e) Amyloidosis

95. **Hereditary nephritis is seen in:**
    (a) Analgesic nephropathy   *(PGI Dec 2003)*
    (b) Balkan nephropathy
    (c) Alport syndrome.
    (d) Eosinophilic nephritis

96. **Nephrocalcinosis is seen in:**   *(PGI June 2004)*
    (a) Hypoparathyroidism
    (b) Medullary sponge kidney
    (c) DM
    (d) RTA

97. **Histology of acute rejection of renal transplant are:**
    (a) Arteriolar hyalinosis   *(PGI June 2005)*
    (b) Eosinophilic infiltration
    (c) Glomerular vasodilatation
    (d) Neutrophilic infiltration
    (e) Necrotizing vasculitis.

98. **Which of the following is seen in hemolytic uremic syndrome?**   *(Delhi PG-2007)*
    (a) Spherocytes   (b) Schistocytes
    (c) Target cells   (d) Heinz bodies

99. **All are true about nephronophthisis except:**
    (a) Interstitial fibrosis   *(Delhi PG-2006)*
    (b) Cortical tubular hypertrophy
    (c) Cysts in the medulla
    (d) 20% cases are non-familial

100. **Most common cause of papillary necrosis is:**
    (a) Diabetes Mellitus   *(Delhi PG-2005)*
    (b) Acute Pyelonephritis
    (c) Sickle cell disease
    (d) Analgesic Nephropathy

101. **Renal calculi are commonly made up of**
    (a) Calcium oxalate   *(Karnataka 2006)*
    (b) Magnesium ammonium phosphate
    (c) Uric acid
    (d) Cystine

102. **Salt losing nephritis is due to**   *(UP 2000)*
    (a) Lupus nephritis
    (b) Streptococcal infection
    (c) Interstitial nephritis
    (d) Goodpasture's syndrome

103. **Most common cause of renal papillary necrosis is:**
    (a) Analgesic nephropathy   *(UP 2000)*
    (b) Sickle cell disease
    (c) Diabetes mellitus
    (d) Chronic pyelonephritis

104. **Tubulo-interstitial disease are all except:**
    (a) Hypokalemic nephropathy   *(UP 2002)*
    (b) Lupus nephritis
    (c) Hypercalcemic nephropathy
    (d) Analgesic nephropathy

105. **Renal pathology in SLE includes all except:**
    (a) Focal glomerulonephritis   *(UP 2008)*
    (b) Diffuse glomerulonephritis
    (c) Diffuse membranous glomerulonephritis
    (d) Lipoid nephrosis

106. **Pathologic feature of malignant hypertension is:**
    (a) Fibrinoid necrosis   *(RJ 2004)*
    (b) Papillary necrosis
    (c) Hard exudate
    (d) All

107. **Contracted kidneys are seen in all of the following diseases except:**   *(RJ 2006)*
    (a) Chronic glomerulonephritis
    (b) Chronic renal failure
    (c) Amyloidosis
    (d) Analgesic nephropathy

108. **Hematuria with dysmorphic RBC are seen in:**
    (a) Acute glomerulonephritis   *(RJ 2006)*
    (b) Renal TB
    (c) Renal Calculi
    (d) Chronic renal failure

109. **Birefringent crystals in urine is seen with:**   *(Bihar 2004)*
    (a) Calcium oxalate stone (b) Uric acid stone
    (c) Struvite stones   (d) None

110. **Anti-GBM antibodies are seen in:**   *(Kolkata 2005)*
    (a) Goodpasture's syndrome
    (b) RPGN
    (c) Membranous GN
    (d) Minimal change disease

111. **A 30 year old company executive gets up at night with severe waxing and waning abdominal pain on right side radiating to the groin and rushes to his physician Dr. Shiv Narayan at RG Clinic. On examination, he is afebrile and has a blood pressure of 118/74 mm Hg. His blood and urine samples are sent for investigations. Reports show serum Na+, 140 mmol/L; K+, 4.2 mmol/L; glucose, 80 mg/dL: creatinine, 1.0 mg/dL; calcium, 8.9 mg/dL; and phosphorus, 2.4 mg/dL. Urine had pH of 7.1; specific gravity of 1.018 and absence of protein, glucose or ketones. He is advised to drink plenty of water but even after following this advice, he continues to have similar episodes. Which of the following is most likely substance to be increased in his urine?**
    (a) Mucoprotein
    (b) Calcium oxalate
    (c) Magnesium ammonium phosphate
    (d) Uric acid

112. **A 28 year young female Katrina present to your OPD with complaints of suprapubic pain, urinary frequency and dysuria. She also passed blood in last voided urine**

about 30 minutes ago. Her urinanalysis demonstrate the presence of pyuria but no white cell casts. On physical examination, she has suprapubic tenderness on palpation. Which of the following is the likely diagnosis in this patient?
(a) Acute pyelonephritis
(b) Chronic pyelonephritis
(c) Cystitis
(d) Fanconi syndrome

113. A 27 year old female Kareena presents to your office with urinary frequency, urgency, and burning during urination. She has also noticed a scant vaginal discharge. The symptoms started two days ago. Which of the following additional findings would be most suggestive of pyelonephritis in this patient?
(a) Fever
(b) Bacteriuria
(c) White blood cell casts
(d) Sterile pyuria

114. A female patient Nargis comes to your OPD with complaints of fever, malaise, increased frequency, urgency and painful micturition. Further investigations reveal that she is suffering from acute urinary tract infection. Which of the following is not a risk factor for the increased predisposition of females for development of UTI?
(a) Shorter urethra in females
(b) Absence of antibacterial properties in vaginal fluid
(c) Hormonal changes affecting adherence of bacteria to the mucosa
(d) Urethral trauma during sexual intercourse

115. At autopsy, a patient who had died with acute anuria and uremia is found to have ischemic necrosis of the cortex of both kidneys with relative sparing of the medulla. These pathological findings are most likely related to which of the following underlying conditions?
(a) Disseminated intravascular coagulation
(b) Multiple myeloma
(c) Sickle cell anemia
(d) Pyelonephritis

116. A 51-year-old man Sonu with a history of recurrent calcium-containing renal stones presents to the emergency room with excruciating flank pain and blood in the urine. This patient is likely to have which of the following underlying disorders?
(a) Anemia of chronic disease
(b) Chronic Proteus infection
(c) Hyperparathyroidism
(d) Hyperaldosteronism

117. A 54 old man Girish is admitted to the hospital because of shortness of breath. He has severe pedal edema and his blood pressure is 75/50 mm Hg. His serum urea nitrogen (BUN) 36 mg/dL and serum creatinine 1.0 mg/dL. A chest x-ray shows cardiac enlargement and perihilar infiltrates. Which of the following most likely accounts for his BUN and creatinine levels?
(a) Decreased renal perfusion
(b) Distal urinary tract obstruction
(c) Increased synthesis of urea
(d) Renal tubulointerstitial disease

Most Recent Questions

117.1. Alports syndrome is inherited by al the following inheritances except
(a) X linked
(b) Co-dominant
(c) AD
(d) AR

117.2. Renal papillary necrosis is almost always associated with one of the following conditions:
(a) Diabetes mellitus
(b) Analgesicnephropathy
(c) Chronic pyelonephritis
(d) Post streptococcal GN

117.3. All are causes of granular contracted kidneys except:
(a) Benign nephrosclerosis
(b) Diabetes mellitus
(c) Chronic Pyelonephritis
(d) Chronic glomerulonephritis

117.4. Periglomerular fibrosis is considered typical of:
(a) Chronic pyelonephritis
(b) Chronic glomerulonephritis
(c) Arterionephrosclerosis
(d) Malignant hypertension

117.5. Nephrocalcinosis is seen in which one of the following?
(a) Hyperparathyroidism
(b) Diabetes mellitus
(c) Amyloidosis kidney
(d) End stage kidney

117.6. Thimble bladder is typically seen in which one of the following?
(a) Acute bacterial cystitis
(b) Tuberculous cystitis
(c) Bilharziasis
(d) Transitional cell carcinoma

117.7. Marker of acute kidney injury includes all of the following except: *(AIIMS Nov 2013)*
(a) Cystatin C (b) N gal
(c) Kim 1 (d) Micro RNA -122

117.8. Which of the following increases tuberculosis?
(a) Asbestosis (b) Sarcoidosis
(c) Silicosis (d) Berylliosis

117.9. Which one of the following statements is incorrect regarding uric acid stones?
(a) They are radiolucent
(b) Crystals are hexagonal
(c) Formed in acidic urine
(d) Can be seen with normouricemia

117.10. **Characteristic histopathological feature of kidney in DM?**
   (a) Nodular glomerulosclerosis
   (b) Fibrin cap
   (c) Papillary necrosis
   (d) Diffuse glomerulosclerosis

RENAL TUMOURS: RCC, WILMS TUMOUR

118. **Which of the following is not associated with renal cell carcinoma?** *(AIIMS May 2011)*
   (a) Polycythemia
   (b) Amyloidosis
   (c) Cushing's syndrome
   (d) Hypertension

119. **Wilm's tumor is associated with all of the following except** *(AIIMS May 2010)*
   (a) Hemihypertrophy
   (b) Aniridia
   (c) Hypertension
   (d) Bilateral polycystic kidney

120. **The cytogenetics of chromophilic renal cell carcinoma is characterized by:** *(AI 2010)*
   (a) Mutant VHL gene
   (b) Loss of 3p
   (c) Trisomy 7/17
   (d) Loss of 5q 3

121. **The most common histological variant of renal cell carcinoma is** *(AIIMS Nov 2005)*
   (a) Clear cell type
   (b) Chromophobe type
   (c) Papillary type
   (d) Tubular type

122. **In which of the following conditions, Aniridia and Hemi-hypertrophy are most likely present**
   (a) Neuroblastoma *(AIIMS May 2004)*
   (b) Wilm's tumor
   (c) Non-Hodgkin's lymphoma
   (d) Germ cell tumor

123. **In Wilm's tumor the following leads to emergence of resistance to chemotherapy:** *(Delhi 2009 RP)*
   (a) Nephrogenic rests
   (b) Monophasic morphology
   (c) Anaplasia
   (d) Capsular infiltration

124. **True statement regarding Wilm's tumour is:**
   (a) Common in adult *(UP 2004)*
   (b) Associated with deletion of chromosome 11p13
   (c) Associated with MIC-2 genes
   (d) Commonest presentation is hematuria

125. **Most common histological type of renal cell carcinoma is:** *(AP 2003)*
   (a) Clear cell

   (b) Medullary
   (c) Papillary
   (d) Mixed type

126. **A 60 year old security guard Dharam Chaudhary presents to the his physician because he is having malaise, fever and weakness. On taking history, a positive history of multiple episodes of passage of altered colored urine is present. However, this is not associated with urinary frequency, dysuria, or nocturia. Physical examination is insignificant but his urine analysis reveals 4 + hematuria; 1 + proteinuria and absence of glucose or ketones by the dips stick method. Which of the following is the next most appropriate step for the management of this patient?**
   (a) Straining of urine for calculi
   (b) Abdominal CT scan for renal mass
   (c) Collection of a 24 hour urine specimen for protein
   (d) Percutaneous renal biopsy

127. **A pediatrician Dr. Jyoti Jain discovers a large mass in the abdomen of a 3-year-old child. Ultrasound examination demonstrates that the mass appears to arise from the right kidney. Which of the following tumors is most likely present?**
   (a) Cortical adenoma
   (b) Hemangioma
   (c) Nephroblastoma
   (d) Oncocytoma

128. **An anxious couple brings in a 18 month boy with gonadal dysgenesis to a pediatric clinic for a follow-up visit. The physician Dr. Mayank Dhamija notices a large abdominal mass during his physical examination. Which of the following disorders does the patient most likely have?**
   (a) Renal cell carcinoma
   (b) Renal hamartoma
   (c) Wilms' tumor
   (d) Transitional cell carcinoma of the bladder

Most Recent Questions

128.1. **Most important prognostic factor of wilms tumour:**
   (a) Histopathology and ploidy of cells
   (b) Tumour stage
   (c) Age of patient
   (d) Mutation of chromosome 1p

128.2. **Oncocytic carcinoma arises from:**
   (a) Perivascular tissue
   (b) Glomerulus
   (c) Loop of henle
   (d) Collecting duct

128.3. **Gene for Wilm's tumour is located on which of the following?**
   (a) Chromosome 1
   (b) Chromosome 10
   (c) Chromosome 11
   (d) Chromosome 12

128.4. Deletion of short arm of chromosome 11 is seen in:
- (a) Osteosarcoma
- (b) Meningioma
- (c) Wilm's tumor
- (d) Colon Carcinoma

URINARY BLADDER DISEASE

129. Michaelis Gutmann bodies are seen in

(AIIMS May 2007)
- (a) Xanthogranulomatous pyelonephritis
- (b) Malacoplakia
- (c) Nail patella syndrome
- (d) Tubercular cystitis

130. Chronic urethral obstruction due to benign prostatic hyperplasia can lead to the following change in kidney parenchyma *(Karnataka 2007)*
- (a) Hyperplasia
- (b) Hypertrophy
- (c) Atrophy
- (d) Dysplasia

131. Michaelis Guttmann bodies are present in:
- (a) Analgesic nephropathy *(RJ 2001,2003)*
- (b) Homman's ulcer
- (c) Malacoplakia
- (d) Erythroplasia

132. Bence Jones proteins are: *(RJ 2001)*
- (a) Light chain
- (b) Heavy chain
- (c) Medium chain
- (d) All

Most Recent Questions

132.1. Transitional cell carcinoma bladder is associated with which of the following?
- (a) Schistosomiasis
- (b) Ascariasis
- (c) Malaria
- (d) Any of the above

132.2. Metabolic complication in CRF include all of the following except
- (a) Hyperkalemia
- (b) Hypophosphatemia
- (c) Hypocalcemia
- (d) Hypokalemia

EXPLANATIONS

1. **Ans. (d) Alport's syndrome** *(Ref: Robbins 8th/931-2)*
Presentation of male patient with lenticonus and end stage renal disease with a family history of renal disease is highly suggestive of Alport syndrome.
   - AR polycystic kidney is ruled out because the age of presentation in ARPKD is childhood and most of the affected children do not survive beyond their childhood.
   - AD polycystic kidney is ruled out because there is no association of ADPKD with lenticonus as is mentioned in our question.
     - *Alport syndrome is manifest by hematuria with progression to chronic renal failure, accompanied by nerve deafness and various eye disorders, including lens dislocation, posterior cataracts, and corneal dystrophy.*
     - In about 85% cases, it is inherited as an **X-linked trait**. So, males express the full syndrome, and *females are carriers in whom manifestations of disease are typically limited to hematuria.*
     - Autosomal recessive and autosomal dominant forms also exist in which both the sexes are equally susceptible.
     - In Alport syndrome, **Hematuria is the earliest manifestation** and the *sensorineural deafness* is the *commonest extra renal abnormality.*

2. **Ans. (d) Tricuspid valve prolapse** *(Ref: Robbins 8th/959 9/e p947)*
Mitral valve prolapse (and not tricuspid valve prolapse) and other cardiac valvular anomalies occur in 20% to 25% of patients.
Adult polycystic kidney disease (APKD) is a hereditary disorder characterized by multiple expanding cysts of both kidneys that ultimately destroy the renal parenchyma and cause renal failure. It is an *autosomal dominant* condition caused by mutation in PKD1 gene encoding for *polycystin-1*. This protein is present on distal tubular epithelial cells. It is involved in cell-cell and cell-matrix interactions. The *PKD2* gene product *polycystin-2* is localized to all segments of the renal tubules and may act as a Ca^{2+}-permeable cation channel for regulatoring intracellular Ca^{2+} levels.

3. **Ans. (a) Berry Aneurysm in Circle of Willis** *(Ref: Robbins 7th/964 9/e p947)*

4. **Ans. (b) Hypertension is rare** *(Ref: Robbins 7th/964, 9/e p 947)*
Hypertension is common in patients with autosomal dominant polycystic kidney disease. It is present in 75% of adult patients and 25% of children.

5. **Ans. (e) Renal failure seen in middle life** *(Ref: Robbins 7th/963-64, 9/e p947, Harrison 17th/1797-1798)*
Salient points about Adult polycystic kidney disease

   - Due to mutation of *PKD 1 gene* (Chromosome 16) and *PKD 2 gene* (on chromosome 4).
   - PKD 1 and 2 genes encode for polycystin 1 and 2 proteins (and not genes) respectively.
   - Autosomal dominant
   - Kidneys are enlarged bilaterally.
   - Disease may present at any age but most frequently produces symptoms in the 3rd or 4th decade
   - Leads to CRF at 40-60 years of life.
   - Other than kidney, cysts are found in Liver (most commonly), Pancreas, Spleen Ovaries, and Lung.
   - Other associated lesions include berry aneurysm, mitral valve prolapsed and colonic diverticula
   - The goals of treatment are to slow the rate of progression of renal disease and to minimize the symptoms.
   - There is no contraindication to renal transplantation.

6. **Ans. (b) 4 and 16.** *(Ref: Robbins 8th/960; 9/e p946)*

7. **Ans. (b) Dialysis** *(Ref: Robbins 9/e p949, 8th/960; 7th/962, 966)*

8. **Ans. (d) Renin** *(Ref: Robbins 8th/957-958, 9/e p 946-47)*
The disease is adult polycystic kidney disease, which is an autosomal dominant condition that typically manifests in middle age. The kidneys appear very badly deformed but they function surprisingly well because the cystic spaces actually only affect 10% or less of the nephrons. Pressure exerted by the cysts can compromise blood flow to some glomeruli, increasing renin secretion followed by hypertension.

ACTH (choice A) can stimulate cortisol (choice B) secretion, and the cortisol (in high amounts) can have enough mineralocorticoid activity to cause hypertension. However, this is associated with a pituitary tumor, adrenal tumor, or with exogenous corticosteroid use.

8.1. **Ans. (d) Bowman's capsule** *(Ref: Robbins 8/e p910, 9/e p900)*
Podocytes (or **visceral epithelial cells**) are cells in the Bowman›s capsule in the kidneys that wrap around the capillaries of the glomerulus.

8.2. **Ans. (a) Autosomal dominant….. Too obvious at this stage friend…For details, read text.**

8.3. **Ans. (a) Cardiovascular disease** *(Ref: Cambell's Urology, 8/e p346,349)*
Principal causes of death in renal transplant patients (in decreasing order)
  • **Heart disease**[Q]   • *Infection*   • *Stroke*

8.4. **Ans. (b) Excretion of less than 500 ml in 24 hrs**
  • **Oliguria**[Q] refers to a **24-h urine output of <500 mL**[Q], and
  • **Anuria**[Q] is the complete absence of urine formation **(<50 mL)**[Q].

8.5 **Ans. (a) 3** *(Ref: Harrison 18/e p 339; CMDT 2014/e p879)*
The minimum number of red blood cells per microliter of urine required for diagnosis of hematuria is **>3 RBC/HPF of centrifuged specimen.**
Persistent or significant hematuria (>3 RBCs/ HPF on three urinalyses, a single urinalysis with >100 RBCs, or gross hematuria) is associated with significant renal or urologic lesions…Harrison

8.6. **Ans (d) Brain** *(Ref: Robbbins 9/e p947)*
About 40% have one to several cysts in the liver (polycystic liver disease) that are usually asymptomatic. Cysts occur much less frequently in the spleen, pancreas, and lungs.

9. **Ans. (b) Hyperplastic arteriosclerosis** *(Ref: Robbins 8th/950-951, 9/e p939)*
Histological alterations characterizing blood vessels in malignant hypertension
  • **Fibrinoid necrosis of arterioles:** This appears as an eosinophilic granular change in the blood vessel wall, which stains positively for fibrin by histochemical or immunofluorescence techniques.
  • In the interlobular arteries and arterioles, there is intimal thickening caused by a proliferation of elongated and concentrically arranged smooth muscle cells with deposition of collagen. This alteration has been referred to as **onion-skinning** because of its concentric appearance. The lesion, also called **hyperplastic arteriolitis**, *correlates well with renal failure in malignant hypertension.*
  • *Malignant nephrosclerosis is the form of renal disease associated with the malignant or accelerated phase of hypertension.* Small, pinpoint petechial hemorrhages may appear on the cortical surface from rupture of arterioles or glomerular capillaries, giving the kidney a peculiar **"flea-bitten" appearance.**
  • **Hyaline arteriolosclerosis** is narrowing of the lumens of arterioles and small arteries, caused by thickening and hyalinization of the walls. It is seen with *Benign nephrosclerosis.* Nephrosclerosis is associated with **increasing age,** more frequent in blacks than whites, and *may be seen in the absence of hypertension.* **Hypertension** and **diabetes mellitus,** however, *increase the incidence and severity of the lesions.*

10. **Ans. (a) Alport's syndrome** *(Ref: Robbins 8th/931-2, 9/e p924)*
COL4A5 chain represents the a5 chain of collagen type IV. It is associated with the development of Alport syndrome.

Genetic Mutation in Chain	Disease
Gene encoding α5 **chain** of collagen type IV	Alport syndrome
Gene encoding α4 **chain** of collagen type IV	**Benign familial hematuria/Thin membrane disease**
Gene encoding α3 **chain** of collagen type IV	Goodpasture syndrome

Alport syndrome

  • Nephritic disorder characterized by the involvement of the triad of **kidney, ear and eye**.
  • Fundamental *defect in the a5-chain of collagen type IV*
  • **Light microscopy** glomerular involvement in the form of the presence of *foam cells* in the interstitial cells.
  • **Electron microscopy (Diagnostic for this disorder**[Q]**)**
  • It shows the presence of irregular foci of thickening and *thinning in the GBM* with splitting and lamination of lamina densa called as *"basket weave appearance"*. *Absence of a5 staining is seen even on skin biopsy apart from glomerular and tubular basement membrane.*

11. **Ans. (b) NPHS 2** *(Ref: Robbins 8th/927, 9/e p918)*

Gene	Chromosome	Protein	Location	Disease
NPHS 1	19q13	Nephrin	Slit diaphragm	Steroid sensitive/Finnish type of nephrotic syndrome
NPHS 2	1q25	Podocin	Slit diaphragm	Steroid resistant nephrotic syndrome

12. **Ans. (a) Focal segmental glomerulosclerosis** *(Ref Robbins 8th/926, 9/e p918)*
Direct quote Robbins 8th/926.... '*Focal segmental glomerulosclerosis occurs as a component of the adaptive response to loss of renal tissue in advanced stage of other renal disorders such as **reflux nephropathy, hypertensive nephropathy** and **unilateral renal agenesis**.*'

13. **Ans. (c) No IgG deposits or C3 deposition on renal biopsy** *(Ref: Robbin's 8th/925-6, 9/e 910)*
The clinical symptoms and the findings in the stem of the question (child with generalised swelling because of reduced serum protein secondary to massive proteinuria with urinary lipid casts) are suggestive of nephrotic syndrome. The commonest cause in a child of nephrotic syndrome is lipoid nephrosis or minimal change disease. So option 'a' and 'd' are ruled out. Both cause hematuria as a finding.
Electron microscopic examination in minimal change disease show the presence of effacement of foot processes of podocytes[Q].
Summary of salient features of some diseases causing nephrotic syndrome

Glomerular microscopic findings				
Disease	Clinical presentation	Light Microscopy	Fluorescence	Electron Microscopy
Membranous glomerulopathy	Nephrotic syndrome	Diffuse capillary wall thickening	Granular IgG and C3; diffuse	Subepithelial deposits
Minimal change disease	Nephrotic syndrome	Normal; lipid in tubules	Negative	Loss of foot processes; no deposits
Focal segmental glomerulosclerosis	Nephrotic syndrome; non-nephrotic proteinuria	Focal and segmental sclerosis and hyalinosis	Focal; IgM and C3	Loss of foot processes; epithelial denudation
Membranoproliferative glomerulonephritis (MPGN) Type I	Nephrotic syndrome	Mesangial proliferation; basement membrane thickening; splitting	(I) IgG + C3; C1q + C4	(I) Subendothelial deposits

Note: MPGN Type II (Dense deposit disease) is associated with hematuria.

14. **Ans. (b) Focal necrotizing glomerulonephritis** *(Ref: Robbins 9/e p511-512, 8th/516-7, 7th/541, Harrison 17th/2121-3)*
   • Robbins .....'The renal lesions range from a mild/early disease, where glomeruli show acute focal necrosis with thrombosis of isolated glomerular capillary loops (focal and segmental necrotizing glomerulonephritis) whereas advanced glomerular lesions are characterized by diffuse necrosis and parietal cell proliferation to form crescents (crescentic glomerulonephritis)'.
   • Direct quote from Harrison........ "Necrotizing vasculitis of small arteries and veins *with granuloma formation* is seen in pulmonary tissue whereas granuloma formation is *rarely seen* on *renal biopsy*".

15. **Ans. (a) Autosomal recessive inheritance** *(Ref: Heptinstall's pathology of kidney vol 1/931)*
Fibronectin nephropathy is a disease with the following features:

   • Autosomal dominant[Q] mode of inheritance.
   • Presents with proteinuria and slowly progressive loss of renal function.
   • Proteinuria is the most common presentation with patients also having microscopic hematuria and mild hypertension.
   • The fibronectin levels in serum are normal.
   • The principal light microscopic change is glomerular enlargement and lobulation resulting from PAS and trichrome-positive mesangial deposits and mild mesangial proliferation
   • Special stains for amyloid are negative
   • By immunofluorescence microscopy, the glomeruli do not stain for immunoglobulin or complement components
   • The most consistent ultrastructural finding is large (giant), mesangial and subendothelial electron-dense deposits that mirror the location of the PAS-positive, fibronectin deposits.

16. **Ans. (d) Focal glomerular sclerosis** *(Ref: Robbins 9/e p1118-1119, 8th/1141-1142)*
Diabetes may cause nodular and diffuse glomerulosclerosis but not focal glomerular sclerosis.

17. **Ans. (a) Loss of antithrombin III (AT III)** *(Ref: Robbins 9/e p914, 8th/922, 7th/978 CMDT 2010)*
Thrombotic and thromboembolic complications are common in nephrotic syndrome due to loss of anticoagulant factor (e.g. antithrombin III, protein C and S) combined with increased platelet activation. Renal vein thrombosis is most often a **consequence** of this hypercoagulative state. There is also **increased synthesis of fibrinogen** in the liver.

18. **Ans. (a) Nephrin** *(Ref: Robbins 9/e p918, 8th/927)*
Direct quote Robbins..."*A mutation in the Nephrin (NPHS 1) gene causes a hereditary form of congenital Nephrotic syndrome (Finnish type) with minimal change glomerular morphology whereas mutations in NPHS2 coding for podocin results in steroid resistant nephrotic syndrome*".

Gene	Chromosome	Protein	Location	Disease
NPHS 1	19q13	Nephrin	Slit diaphragm	Steroid sensitive/Finnish type of nephrotic syndrome
NPHS 2	1q25	Podocin	Slit diaphragm	Steroid resistant nephrotic syndrome

19. Ans. (a) Microscopic polyangiitis *(Ref: Robbins 9/e p912, 8th/920)*

Crescentic Glomerulonephritis

Type I RPGN (Anti-GBM antibody)	Type II RPGN (Immune complex)	Type III RPGN (Pauci immune)
• Idiopathic • Goodpasture's syndrome.	• Idiopathic • Post infectious • SLE, Henoch Schonlein Purpura.	• Idiopathic. • ANCA associated. • Wegener's granulomatosis. • Microscopic polyangitis.
Immunofluorescence finding	*Immunofluorescence finding*	*Immunofluorescence finding*
• *Linear GBM deposits of IgG and C3*	• *"Lumpy bumpy" granular pattern of staining.*	• *No immunoglobulin or complement deposits in GBM.*

20. Ans. (A) Nephrin *(Ref: Robbins 9/e p912, 8th/918, Nelson 17th/1757)*
- Lipoid nephrosis or nephrotic syndrome is also called as minimal change disease. Congenital nephrotic syndrome occurs as a result of mutation in the **nephrin** gene. (Finnish type of nephrotic syndrome)

Also now

- Megalin in involved is the pathogenesis of membranous glomerulonephritis
- Podocin and α_4 actinin can also result in congenital nephrotic syndrome.

21. Ans. (b) Alport syndrome *(Ref: Robbins 9/e p912, 8th/920, 7th/523-4)*
As discussed earlier, crescentic glomerulonephritis is the alternative name of RPGN.

Alport syndrome is a hereditary nephritis characterized by associated nerve deafness and eye disorders like lens dislocation, posterior cataracts and corneal dystrophy. Histologically foam cells (interstitial cells having fats and mucopolysaccharides) are seen.

22. Ans. (b) Mesangiocapillary GN *(Ref: Anderson 10th/2076; Robbins 7th/979)*
Glomerular lesions with increased cells in the tufts are often known as proliferative glomerulonephritis.

Conditions with Proliferative Glomerulonephritis

- SLE (particularly class II, mesangial hypercellularity defined as >3 cells in mesangial regions)
- HIV
- Membranoproliferative/Mesangiocapillary glomerulonephritis
- Neoplasia (particularly CLL and MALT lymphoma)
- Post streptococcal glomerulonephritis

Rest all options are non proliferative glomerulonephritis.

23. Ans. (a) Thrombotic microangiopathy *(Ref: Robbins 9/e p941, 8th/952, 7th/1009, 612, Harrison 17th/1813-4)*
The term thrombotic microangiopathy encompasses a spectrum of clinical syndromes that include TTP and HUS. *DIC is not included because these disorders (TTP and HUS) are associated with normal coagulation times and normal fibrin degradation products.*

Microthrombi are demonstrated in renal arterioles and capillaries. In HUS, microthrombi mainly contain fibrin whereas in TTP, these are composed of platelet aggregates, fibrin and VWF. More than 90% patients with HUS have significant renal failure whereas < 10% cases of classic TTP have anuria.

24. Ans. (a) Post streptococcal glomerulonephritis *(Ref: Robbins 9/e p918, 8th/919, Harrison's 17th/1786)*
- Although all conditions mentioned in the question are associated with low complement levels. Persistently depressed levels' are not seen in post streptococcal glomerulonephritis.
- **In post streptococcal glomerulonephritis:** serum C_3 levels are depressed within 2 weeks, however, these usually return to normal levels within 6 to 8 weeks.
- **Persistently depressed levels after this period should suggest another cause such as presence of C3 nephritic factor (Membranoproliferative glomerulonephritis).**

25. Ans. (c) Diarrhea associated hemolytic uremic syndrome *(Ref: Harrison 17th/1813-1814, 9/e p942)*

Nephritic syndrome associated with low C3

Immune complex glomerulonephritis	
• Post streptococcal glomerulonephritis	• Crescenteric glomerulonephritis
• Lupus nephritis	• Idiopathic proliferative glomerulonephritis
• Cryoglobulinemia	• Atheroembolic renal disease
• Bacterial endocarditis	• Sepsis
• Shunt nephritis	• Acute Pancreatitis/advanced liver disease
• Membranoproliferative glomerulonephritis	

*Hemolytic uremic syndrome is associated with normal C_3 levels.

26. **Ans. (c) Goodpasture's disease** *(Ref: Harrison's 17th/1788)*

27. **Ans. (d) Absence of associated proteinuria is pathognomic** *(Ref: Robbin's 7th/986-988, 9/e p923)*
    Berger's disease (IgA nephropathy) is a frequent cause of gross or microscopic hematuria. Mild proteinuria is frequently present and occasionally nephrotic syndrome may develop.

    • Microscopically, mesangioproliferative glomerulonephritis is seen more commonly than focal proliferative and crescentic (least) glomerulonephritis.
    • Immunofluorescence shows deposition of IgA with C3 and properdin.
    • Electron dense deposits are seen in mesangium on electron microscopy.

28. **Ans. (b) Rapidly progressive glomerulonephritis** *(Ref: Robbins 9/e p912, 8/e p920-921)*
    • Rapidly progressive glomerulonephritis, also known as crescentic glomerulonephritis is characterized by the presence of crescents in most of the glomeruli.
    • Crescents are produced by proliferation of the *parietal epithelial cells of Bowman's capsule and by infiltration of monocytes and macrophages*.

29. **Ans. (c) Crescentic glomerulonephritis** *(Ref: Robbins 9/e p912, 8th/516-7, 7th/541, Harrison 17th/2121-3)*
    Discussed earlier.

30. **Ans. (c) Alport syndrome** *(Ref: Robbins 9/e p924, 8th/932, 7th/988, Rubin pathology/361)*
    Alport syndrome is the commmest type of Hereditary nephritis (refers to a group of heterogenous familial renal diseases associated primarily with glomerular injury). The other important intity is *thin basement membrane disease.*
    Rubins mentions 'The **most diagnostic morphologic lesion** is seen **only by electron microscopy** as an irregularly thickened GBM, with splitting of the lamina densa into interlacing lamellae that surround electron-lucent areas'
    Robbins 8th. 'The characteristic electron microscopic finding of Alport syndrome is that the glomerular basement membrane shows irregular foci of thickening alternating with attenuation (thinning), with pronounced splitting and lamination of the lamina densa, often with a distinctive **basket-weave appearance'.**
    Important info

    Thin basement membrane disease is the most common cause of benign familial hematuria.

31. **Ans. (b) Collapsing** *(Ref: Robbin's 8th/926, 9th/p 920, 7th/985)*
    • **Five mutually exclusive variants of focal segmental glomerulosclerosis (FSGS) may be distinguished by the pathological findings seen on renal biopsy**
        – Collapsing variant
        – Glomerular tip lesion variant
        – Cellular variant
        – Perihilar variant
        – Not otherwise specified variant (NOS)
    • The **NOS** variant is the *most common* subtype and collapsing FSGS has worst prognosis.

32. **Ans. (c) Podocin** *(Ref: Robbins 9/e p918, 8th/927, 7th/983-4)*
    • Mutations in NPHS1 gene that codes for nephrin results in congenital nephrotic syndrome of Finnish type.
    • NPHS2 gene coding for podocin mutation result in steroid resistant nephrotic syndrome.
    Mnemonic:

    • *NPHS1 contains 1, which suggest first letter (means N) that stands for Nephrin whereas NPHS2 contains 2, which suggest second letter (means P) that stands for Podocin.*
    • *1 comes first, so NPHS1 mutations cause congenital nephrotic syndrome whereas 2 comes later, so NPHS2 mutations cause acquired disease (steroid resistant nephrotic syndrome)*

33. **Ans. (d) Hypertrophy and necrosis of visceral epithelium** *(Ref. Robbin's 9/e p920, 8th/926, 7th/983-4)*

Collapsing Glomerulopathy is characterised by

- A characteristic feature is proliferation and hypertrophy of glomerular visceral epithelial cells.
- The minimum diagnostic criteria for defining a collapsing variant of FSGS is the presence by light microscopy of at least one glomerulus showing segmental or global obliteration of the glomerular capillary lumen by wrinkling and collapse of glomerular basement membrane in association with hypertrophy and hyperplasia of overlying visceral epithelial cells.

34. **Ans. (b) NPHS-2** *(Ref: Robbin 9/e p918, 8th/927, 7th/983-4)*

35. **Ans. (c) Collapsing glomerulopathy** *(Ref: Harrison 17th/1796, Robbins, 9/e p920, 8th/928,7th/982- 3)*

36. **Ans. (d) Amyloidosis** *(Ref: Robbins 9/e p926, 8th/252,610-1,927-8)*
    - Mesangial deposits of **monoclonal kappa/lambda** light chains suggest the diagnosis of **Amyloidosis.** In primary Amyloidosis **AL protein** is deposited in the organs, which is made of light chains (usually lambda type) of immuno-globulins. Renal amyloidosis is the **most common cause of death due to amyloidosis** (including both primary and secondary amyloidosis).

    Other options:

    - **Mesangioproliferative glomerulonephritis** shows mesangial deposits of IgG, IgA and C_3.
    - **Focal and segmental glomerulosclerosis** shows hyaline deposits of IgM, C_3 and IgA and fibrinogen in juxtamedullary capillaries.
    - In **Kimmelstiel-Wilson disease** (or nodular glomerulosclerosis), the hyaline masses are deposited in the mesangial core of the glomerular lobules consist of **lipids** and **fibrin.**

37. **Ans. (b) Has molecular weight slightly greater than the molecules normally getting filtered** *(Ref: Robbins 9/e p914, 8th/910, Harrison 18th/2334, Ganong 21st/709-10; Guyton 10th/373)*
    - There are **three main types of plasma proteins** which include Albumin, Globulin and Fibrinogen
    - Normally, the glomerular filtration layer **does not** allow **any plasma protein** to pass through it. However, in any renal disease, it allows protein molecules to pass through it and **albumin is the first protein** to appear in the urine.
    - The filtration of any substance through glomerular filtration layer depends on **two** factors as described below:

    Size of the substance

    The glomerular filtration layer is thick and porous membrane. *Any neutral substance ≤ 4A diameter freely filters through this layer. However, the filterability of any neutral substance with diameter between 4 nm and 8 nm is inversely proportional to its size. The filterability of substances of diameter more than 8 nm is zero.*

    Charge of the substance

    The **sialoproteins** contained in the glomerular filtration layer are **negatively charged** causing repulsion of *all negatively charged particles including proteins.* This explains the negligible filtration of **albumin anion** which has diameter of **7 nm**

    In some renal diseases, the **anionic charge of the filtration membrane is lost** and this allows negatively charged particles of diameter **8nm** to pass through it resulting in proteinuria. Albumin has a diameter of **7nm** and it *starts appearing in urine as soon as the negative charge of filtration layer disappears.*

38. **Ans. (a) Fusion of foot process of the glomerular epithelial cells** *(Ref: Robbins 9/e p917, 8th/925)*
    - The child is presenting with features likely of Nephrotic syndrome whose most frequent cause in children is minimal change disease or lipoid nephrosis.
    - Light microscopy there is no abnormality whereas on electron microscopy there is fusion of foot processes of the glomerular epithelial cells with normal glomeruli.

39. **Ans. (a) Number of crescents** *(Ref: Robbins 6th/453, Essential of nephrology by K visweswaran 2nd/102)*
    As discussed in text the prognosis in RPGN is related to the number of crescents. However, this point is not mentioned in the 7th, 8th and 9th editions of Robbins.

Poor prognostic factors	Good prognostic factors
• *Oliguria* and *azotemia* at presentation • *More than 80% circumferential crescents* have poor response to therapy • Glomerular tuft necrosis, global glomerular sclerosis, gaps in Bowman capsule and interstitial fibrosis	• *Pauci immune RPGN has best prognosis* • *Non- circumferential crescents in less than 50% glomeruli have indolent course.* • *Associated endocapillary proliferation is a good prognostic factor*

Essential of nephrology writes that '*oliguria is related to crescent formation*'.

40. **Ans. (d) No change seen** *(Ref: Robbins 9/e p917, 7th/981-982)*

41. **Ans. (d) Glomerular function is lost due to loss of polyanionic charge on both sites of glomerular foot process.** *(Ref: Harrison 17th/1790, Robbins 9/e p900)*

As discussed earlier, *Glomerular barrier function* depends on the molecular size (the larger, the less permeable) and charge (the more cationic, the more permeable) is done. The anionic moieties present within the capillary wall including the acidic proteoglycans of the GBM and the sialoglycoproteins of epithelial and endothelial cells are responsible for the virtually complete exclusion of albumin (also having anionic charge) from the filtrate. In addition, the *visceral epithelial cell* (or po-docyte) is important for the maintenance of glomerular barrier function. The slit diaphragm of the podocyte is composed of nephrin, actin and podocin, so, any defect in any of these is responsible for increased protein excretion from the kidney. In a patient of minimal change disease, there is presence of visceral epithelial injury leading to the loss of glomerular poly-anions resulting in low molecular weight proteinuria (selective proteinuria).

Clarifying Option c; Foot process of the podocyte is effaced. However, it **appears** to be normal on **light microscopy**.

42. **Ans. (a) Alport's syndrome** *(Ref: Robbins 9/e p924, 8th/931-2, 7th/988-9)*

Genetic Mutation in Chain	Disease
Mutation in the gene encoding α5 chain of collagen type IV	Alport syndrome
Mutation in the gene encoding α4 chain of collagen type IV	Benign familial hematuria
Mutation in the gene encoding α3 chain of collagen type IV	Goodpasture syndrome

Alport's syndrome is a hereditary nephritis, characterized by microscopic hematuria (first symptom) and deafness.

43. **Ans. (a) Post streptococcal glomerulonephritis** *(Ref: Robbins 9/e p910, Harrison 17th/1786-1787)*

44. **Ans. (a) PSGN; (b) MPGN; (e) Infective endocarditis:** *(Ref: Robbins 9/e p910, Harrison 17th/1788)*

45. **Ans. (a) MPGN-1; (c) PSGN; (d) Membranous GN; (e) RPGN** *(Ref: Robbins 9/e p910, 7th-975)*

Summary of Glomerular Deposits

Subepithelial	Subendothelial	Basement membrane	Mesangial
• Acute GN (like PSGN) • Membranous GN • Heyman GN • RPGN (some cases) • MPGN (Type I) rarely	• MPGN (Type I) • SLE • Acute GN	• MPGN (Type II) • Membranous • Glomerulopathy	• IgA nephropathy • HSP • Anti-GBM diseases like • RPGN and Goodpasture syndrome

46. **Ans. (a) Proteinuria; (b) Hyperlipidemia; (c) Oedema; (e) Lipiduria** *(Ref: Robbins 9/e p914, 8th/907, 7th/978)*

47. **Ans. (a) Albumin** *(Ref: Robbins 9/e p914, 7th/958, Vasudevan-Sreekumari 4th/224)*
Albuminuria is seen in nephrotic syndrome.

48. **Ans. (b) Massive proteinuria; (d) Edema; (e) Hyperlipidemia.** *(Ref: Robbins 7th/978, 9/e p914)*

49. **Ans. (a) Heymann antigen is called megalin; (d) Subepithelial aspect of basement membrane has deposit.**

(Ref: Robbins 7th/968 – 970, 9/e p903, 915)

* The Heyman model of rat glomerulonephritis is induced by immunizing rat with an **antigen containing preparation of proximal tubular brush border.**
* The rats develop antibodies to this antigen and a membranous glomerulopathy, resembling human membranous glomerulopathy. The **antigen is called megalin** and has homology to LDL receptor.
* On electron microscopy, the glomerulopathy is characterized by presence of numerous electron dense deposits along the **subepithelial** *aspect of basement membrane. Immunofluorescence microscopy shows granular deposits.*

50. **Ans. (b) Malignant nephrosclerosis.** *(Ref: Robbins 7th/1008, 9/e p939)*

51. **Ans. (a) Foamy cells in interstitium; (d) Thinning of GBM < 100 nm:** *(Ref: Robbins 7th/988, 9/e p924)*
Histological characteristics of Alport's syndrome:

• Diffuse basement membrane thinning • Foam cells in interstitium • In advanced stage there is focal or global glomerulosclerosis	• Vascular sclerosis • Tubular atrophy • Interstitial fibrosis

On electron microscopy (diagnostic of this disorder), GBM shows

• Irregular foci of thickening alternating with thinning • Pronounced splitting and lamination of lamina densa (**basket weave appearance**)[Q].

Info: Immunohistochemistry shows failure to stain α-3, 4, 5 collagen.

52. **Ans. (b) Wegener's granulomatosis (c) Goodpasture's syndrome (e) Microscopic polyangitis** *(Ref: Robbins 9/e p912, 7th/977)*

53. **Ans. (a) Subepithelial deposits; (b) Nephritis along with acute renal failure; (c) Low complement levels; (d) HTN and proteinuria:** *(Ref: Robbins 7th/974-5, 9/e p910-911)*

54. **Ans. (c) Microscopic polyangitis** *(Ref: Robbin 7th/540, 9/e p912, Harrison 17th/1789)*
   - In microscopic polyangitis, there is a paucity of immunoglobulin demonstrable by immunofluorescence microscopy **(pauci-immune injury)**. There are few or no immune deposits in this type of vasculitis.
   Pauci immune injury is also seen in Churg Strauss syndrome and Wegener granulomatosis.

55. **Ans. (a) Diabetic Nephropathy** *(Ref: Robbin 7th/991, 9/e p1118)*

56. **Ans. (a) Goodpasture's syndrome** *(Ref: Robbins 7th/745-746, 9/e p912)*

57. **Ans. (a) Diabetic glomerulosclerosis** *(Ref: Robbins 7th/991, 9/e p1118)*

58. **Ans. (a) Normal C3** *(Ref: Robbins 7th/974-5, 9/e p910-911)*

59. **Ans. (b) Mesangioproliferative glomerulonephritis** *(Ref: Robbins 7th/403-405 , 9/e p393)*

   - Visceral leishmaniasis is caused by *L. donovani*
   - Mucocutaneous leishmaniasis is caused by *L. braziliensis*.
   - Visceral leishmaniasis is characterized by the clinical features of hepatosplenomegaly, lymphadenopathy, pancytopenia, fever and weight loss. There is hyperpigmentation of the skin, so it is also called as "Kala azar".
   - In the renal involvement in this disease, there is presence of mesangioproliferative glomerulonephritis and in advanced cases, there is presence of amyloidosis.

60. **Ans. (a) Crescents in most of glomeruli** *(Ref: Robbins 975 7th/20-6, 9/e p910)*

61. **Ans. (a) Idiopathic cresenteric glomerulonephritis** *(Ref: Robbins 9/e p910-911, 8th/920; 7th/977)*

62. **Ans. (b) Diffuse involvement** *(Ref: Robbins 9/e p911, 8th/919; 7th/975)*

63. **Ans. (a) Diffuse glomerulosclerosis** *(Ref: Robbins 9/e p1118, 8th/934; 7th/990-992)*

64. **Ans. (c) Membranoproliferative glomerulonephritis** *(Ref: Robbins 8th/929; 7th/985)*

65. **Ans. (a) Post streptococcal GN** *(Ref: Robbins 8th/920; 7th/975)*

66. **Ans. (b) Nodular glomerulosclerosis** *(Ref: Robbins 9/e p1118, 8th/934; 7th/991)*

67. **Ans. (d) Diffuse alveolar involvement** *(Ref: Robbins 8th/709-710, 9/e p913)*

68. **Ans. (c) IgG deposition in mesangium** *(Ref: Robbins 9/e p923, 8th/925-926; 7th/981)*

69. **Ans. (b) Berger disease** *(Ref: Robbins 9/e p923, 8th/929-930; 7th/986)*

70. **Ans. (d) Rheumatoid arthritis** *(Ref: Robbins 9/e p912, 8th/920; 7th/977)*

71. **Ans. (d) Sodium and water retention** *(Ref: Robbins 9/e p922, 8th/407-408; 7th/522)*

72. **Ans. (b) Hematuria** *(Ref: Robbins 9/e p923, 8th/930, 7th/986)*

73. **Ans. (d) Focal segmental glomerulosclerosis** *(Ref: Robbins 9/e p919, 8th/926, 7th/983)*

74. **Ans. (d) All of the above** *(Ref: Robbins 9/e p942, 8th/669-670; 7th/1009-1010)*

75. **Ans. (a) Membranous glomerulonephritis** *(Ref: Robbins 9/e p915, 8th/918, 923; 7th/984,979-981)*

76. **Ans. (c) Wegener's glomerulonephritis** *(Ref: Robbins 9/e p903, 8th/920; 7th/993,997)*

77. **Ans. (b) Membranoproliferative glomerulonephritis** *(Ref: Robbins 9/e p920, 8th/929; 7th/984)*

78. **Ans. (b) Membranous nephropathy** *(Ref: Robbins 9/e p915, 8th/918,920; 7th/975, 979)*

79. **Ans. (d) Multiple myeloma** *(Ref: Robbins 9/e p937, 8th/948)*

   - Elevated total serum protein with normal albumin point towards the large amount of serum globulin. This is combination with other features like back pain (from lytic lesions), immunosuppression (manifesting as recurrent infections), and amyloid deposition enlarging the kidneys are all pointing towards the likely diagnosis of multiple myeloma.
   - Analgesic nephropathy can lead to tubulointerstitial nephritis and papillary necrosis.
   - Absence of both hemoptysis and history of anti glomerular basement antibodies rules out option 'b'
   - The serum glucose is normal so, diabetes mellitus is ruled out. Glomerulosclerosis is not the same as amyloid.

80. **Ans. (c) Complete recovery without treatment** *(Ref: Robbins 9/e p911, 8th/917-9)*

The findings in the stem of the question are characteristic of poststreptococcal glomerulonephritis. There are different strains of streptococci which cause glomerulonephritis and rheumatic fever. Majority of the children with post streptococcal glomerulonephritis recover without treatment. Rarely, few children develop a rapidly progressive glomerulonephritis. The progression to chronic renal failure is more common in affected adults.

81. **Ans. (d) Ovoid, periodic acid-Schiff (PAS)-positive, hyaline masses** *(Ref: Robbins 8th/142, 9/e p1118)*

The most specific lesion (pathognomonic) of diabetic glomerulosclerosis is the Kimmelstiel-Wilson nodule. These are ovoid, hyaline, PAS-positive structures found in the mesangial core at the edge of the glomerulus.
Mesangial IgA deposits (option A) are a feature of Berger disease (IgA nephropathy).
- Necrotic epithelial cells in tubules (option B) are a feature of acute tubular necrosis.
- Nests of cells with abundant clear cytoplasm (option C) are a feature of renal cell carcinoma.

82. **Ans. (a) Anti-glomerular basement membrane disease** *(Ref: Robbins 8th/920-921, 9/e p912)*

The two principal causes of rapidly progressive glomerulonephritis are anti-glomerular basement membrane (including both Goodpasture's syndrome and isolated anti-glomerular basement disease) and primary systemic vasculitis (including Wegener's granulomatosis, microscopic polyarteritis, idiopathic rapidly progressive glomerulonephritis, Churg-Strauss syndrome, polyarteritis nodosa, giant-cell arteritis, and Takayasu's arteritis).

> Diabetic nephropathy (choice B) typically begins with microalbuminuria and hypertension and progresses to renal failure. Hypertensive nephropathy (choice C) due to essential hypertension typically presents with slowly rising BUN and creatinine; hypertensive nephropathy due to malignant hypertension presents with more rapidly rising BUN and creatinine. Lupus nephritis (choice D) has the most typical presentation as proteinuria.

83. **Ans. (a) Focal segmental glomerulosclerosis** *(Ref: Robbins 8th/928, 9/e p920)*

There is a specific association between focal segmental glomerulosclerosis and both IV drug abuse and HIV nephropathy. This disorder usually presents as an aggressive form of nephrotic syndrome with poor prognosis and non responsive to steroid therapy (called as 'collapsing variant').

83.1. **Ans. (c) Fibrinogen** *(Ref: Robbins 8/e p922, Heptinstall's Pathology of the Kidney 6/e p131)*

Direct quote from Heptinstall's Pathology.. "Many factors increase in nephrotic syndrome usually due to lowering of serum albumin to which they are usually bound. These factors include **fibrinogen**, factors **V, VII, VIII and von Willebrand factor**. On the other hand, substances like factors XI and XII, plasminogen an anti-thrombin III."
Thrombotic and thromboembolic complications are common in nephrotic syndrome due to loss of anticoagulant factor (e.g. antithrombin III, protein C and S) combined with increased platelet activation. Renal vein thrombosis is most often a **consequence** of this hypercoagulative state. There is also **increased synthesis of fibrinogen** in the liver.

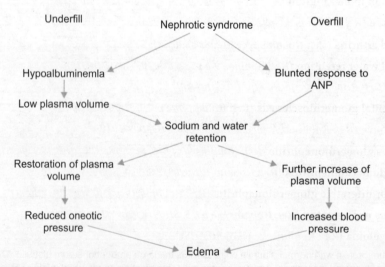

Figure: Mechanisms of edema formation in the nephrotic syndrome left. The classic view of edema formation, in which a low blood volume (underfill) serves as the signal for secondary renal sodium retention Right. The mechanism of edema formation in most patient with the nephrotic syndrome who have normal or slightly elevated blood volumes (overfill). The blunted response to atrial natriuretic peptide observed in patients with the nephrotic syndrome may be the stimulus for primary renal sodium retention that plays a central role in edema formation. ANP, atrial natriuretic peptide.

Edema in nephrotic syndrome is attributed to the following:
- **Underfill hypothesis/classical hypothesis**:
    - Seen in patients with low plasma volume
    - *Hypovolemia is the primary stimulus* leading to sodium and water retention leading to edema by alteration of Starling forces
- **Overfill hypothesis/classical hypothesis**:
    - Seen in patients with normal or increased plasma volume
    - *Sodium retention is the primary mechanism* leading to increased blood pressure and then alteration in Starling forces and edema formation.

83.2. Ans. (a) Epithelial cells + fibrin + macrophage *(Ref: Robbins 8/e p921, 9/e p913)*
Crescents are formed by proliferation of **parietal cells** and by **migration of monocytes and macrophages** into the urinary space. Neutrophils and lymphocytes may be present. **Fibrin strands** are frequently prominent **between the cellular layers in the crescents.** The escape of fibrinogen into Bowman space and its conversion to fibrin are an important contributor to crescent formation.
Rapidly progressive glomerulonephritis is characterized histologically by domination of distinctive **crescents**. It is also known as Crescentic glomerulonephritis. The crescents eventually obliterate Bowman space and compress the glomerular tuft. So, the prognosis is dependent on the number of crescents in the kidney biopsy.

83.3. Ans. (a) Malignant hypertension *(Ref: Robbins 8/e p950, 9/e p939)*

Mnemonic for differential diagnosis of flea bitten kidney: We HaTe PSM
We: Wegener's granulomatosis
HaTe – **H**enoch schonlein purpura; **H**US;**T**TP
P- **P**oststreptococcal glomerulonephritis (PSGN); **P**olyarteritis nodosa (PAN)
S-**S**ub acute bacterial endocarditis (SABE)
M- **M**alignant hypertension

83.4. Ans. (a) Rapidly progressive glomerulonephritis *(Ref: Robbins 8/e p920, 9/e p912-913)*
Easy question friends given the fact that all the other options "b", "c" and "d"' are associated with nephrotic syndrome.

Just brush up!
- *IgA nephropathy is a frequent cause of recurrent gross or microscopic hematuria and is probably the most common type of **primary glomerulonephritis** worldwide.*
- MC primary cause of nephritic syndrome in children: post streptococcal glomerulonephritis[Q]
- MC **primary** cause of **nephrotic** syndrome in **children: minimal change disease**[Q]
- MC **primary** cause of **nephrotic** syndrome in **adults: focal segmental glomerulosclerosis**[Q]
- MC **overall/ secondary** cause of **nephrotic** syndrome in **adults: diabetes mellitus**[Q]

83.5. Ans. (d) Focal segmental glomerulosclerosis *(Ref: Robbins 8/e p926, 9/e p 918)*
Focal segmental glomerulosclerosis is the **commonest cause** of **nephrotic syndrome** in the **adults** in the World. It is characterized by

NEET Points to be brushed up!
- Associated with loss of renal tissue as **unilateral renal agenesis**[Q]or advanced stages of reflux nephropathy or hypertensive nephropathy.
- Also seen with with conditions like **Sickle cell anemia**[Q], **HIV infection**[Q], Heroin abuse, Obesity
- Degeneration and focal *disruption of the visceral epithelial cells* is the hallmark feature of focal segmental glomerulosclerosis.
- Is chief renal lesion in **HIV associated nephropathy** (especially **collapsing**[Q]variant)

83.6. Ans. (b) Rapidly progressive glomerulonephritis… discussed earlier *(Ref: Robbins 7/e p976-977, 9/e p912)*

83.7. Ans. (c) 30-300 mg/d *(Ref: Robbins 8/e p1145, 9/e p1120)*
- The **earliest manifestation** of diabetic nephropathy is the appearance of low amounts of albumin in the urine (**>30 mg/day, but <300 mg/day**), that is, *microalbuminuria*.
- Microalbuminuria is also a *marker for greatly increased cardiovascular morbidity and mortality* for persons with either type 1 or type 2 diabetes

83.8. Ans. (c) Mild proteinuria, hematuria, high ASO titre *(Ref: Robbins 9/e p910-911)*
In post streptococcal glomerulonephritis, there elevated levels of antistreptolysin O or ASO and anti DNAase antibodies [Q] (indicative of streptococcal infection) and *reduced levels of serum C3*

Glomerular Syndromes

Acute nephritic syndrome	Hematuria, azotemia, variable proteinuria, oliguria, edema, and hypertension
Rapidly prog. glomerulonephritis	Acute nephritis, proteinuria, and acute renal failure
Nephrotic syndrome	• >3.5 gm proteinuria, hypoalbuminemia, hyperlipidemia, lipiduria
Chronic renal failure	• Azotemia uremia progressing for years

83.9 Ans. (d) Renal biopsy having thin basement membrane *(Ref: Robbins 9/e p925)*

Benign familial hematuria is common hereditary entity manifested clinically by familial asymptomatic hematuria—usually uncovered on routine urinalysis—and morphologically by diffuse thinning of the GBM to widths between 150 and 225 nm (compared with 300 to 400 nm in healthy adults).

83.10. Ans (d) Minimal change disease *(Ref: Robbins 9/e p 917)*

The glomeruli are **normal** by light microscopy. By electron microscopy the GBM appears normal, and no electrondense material is deposited. The principal lesion is in the visceral epithelial cells, which show a *uniform and diffuse effacement of foot processes.*

Foot process effacement is also present in other proteinuric states (e.g., membranous glomerulopathy, diabetic nephropathy); it is only when effacement is associated with normal glomeruli by light microscopy that the diagnosis of minimal-change disease can be made.

83.11. Ans (c) Partial lipodystrophy *(Ref: Robbins 9/e p 922)*

Secondary MPGN (invariably type I) is more common in adults and arises in the following:

- Chronic immune complex disorders, such as SLE; hepatitis B infection; hepatitis C infection, usually with cryoglobulinemia; endocarditis; infected ventriculoatrial shunts; chronic visceral abscesses; HIV infection; and schistosomiasis
- α1-Antitrypsin deficiency
- Malignant diseases particularly CLL which have formation of autoantibodies

Robbins 8th mentioned that partial lipodystrophy is associated with *C3 nephritic factor (C3NeF)*. It is associated with type II membranoproliferative glomerulonephritis.

83.12. Ans. (d) Rapidly progressive glomerulonephritis *(Ref: Robbins 9/e p912)*

RBC casts are a feature of glomerular damage. Normally < 3 RBC/HPF are going to leak. But in case of glomerular damage the number of RBC in the urine will exceed the limit mentioned above and these RBC get impinged on Tamm Horsfall protein. The resultant RBC casts can be seen under microscopic examination of urine.

83.13. Ans. (a) Focal segmental glomerulonephritis *(Ref: Robbins 9/e p919)*

A morphologic variant of FSGS is called collapsing glomerulopathy and is the most characteristic lesion of HIV-associated nephropathy.

84. Ans. (d) Urine PCR for TB *(Ref: Robbins 9/e p943, 8th/947, Harrisons 18th/2372)*

Major causes of Papillary necrosis are:
- Analgesic nephropathy
- Sickle cell nephropathy
- Diabetes with urinary tract infection

Option 'a' can detect urinary tract infection which may be associated with UTI.

Option 'b' is helpful for detecting sickle cell disease.

Option 'c' can detect renal tubular acidosis. Analgesic nephropathy is an important cause of distal tubular acidosis.

- Renal TB is least likely cause of papillary necrosis and therefore, urine PCR for B is the answer of exclusion. Please note that TB can cause focal papillary necrosis of the kidney rarely.

85. Ans. (a) Isomorphic RBC *(Ref: Paediatric Nephrology 5th/141, 190 by R.N. Srivastava, Arvind Bagga (senior faculty from AIIMS)*

Approach to patient with hematuria to determine source of bleeding

	Parenchymal Intrarenal	Collecting system Extrarenal
Appearance of urine	Tea colored	Bright red, blood clots
Pattern of hematuria	Total hematuria (throughout the stream)	Initial, terminal hematuria
Urinary symptoms	Painless	Dysuria, urgency, frequency
Associated features	Sore throat, HTN, edema	Fever, colicky pain
Family history	Deafness, renal failure	Renal stones, urinary infection
Proteinuria	High grade (urine protein: creatinine ratio >1)	Low grade
Other urinary findings	RBC casts (highly specific less sensitive)	Crystals
RBC morphology	Dysmorphic	Eumorphic

Page 141 mentions …Eosinophiluria (>1% WBCs) is observed in acute interstitial nephritis.

86. Ans. (b) Associated with tuberculosis *(Ref: Robbins 8th/943, 9/e p934)*

As discussed in text, Xanthogranulomatous pyelonephritis is associated with E. coli Proteus mirabilis, Pseudomonas, Streptococcus faecalis and Klebsiella.

87. Ans. (d) Benign Nephrosclerosis *(Ref: Robbins 9/e p938, 8th/949, 7th/992, 1006; Chandrasoma taylor 3rd/275)*

Direct quote Robbins.. *'In benign nephrosclerosis, kidneys are either normal or moderately reduced in size on gross appearance. The loss of mass is due mainly to cortical scarring and shrinking'.*

Causes of contracted kidneys

Symmetric	Asymmetric
• Chronic glomerulonephritis • Benign nephrosclerosis	• Chronic pyelonephritis

Causes of enlarged kidneys

• Amyloidosis • Rapidly progressive glomerulonephritis (RPGN) • Myeloma kidney	• Diabetic renal disease [Kimmelstiel Wilson nodules are pathognomic] • Polycystic kidney disease • Bilateral obstruction (hydronephrosis)

Important info

Contracted kidneys:Less than 8 cm length of kidney is taken as chronic contracted kidney. Normal size corresponds to 3 times the length of L1 vertebrae *or 2/3rd of additive length of T11, T12 and L1 vertebrae.*

Note: In some patients of diabetes (especially in late stages), kidney may be reduced in size.

88. Ans. (b) Tuberculous pyelonephritis *(Ref: Robbins 7th/1004, 9/e p936, Harrison 17th/1825 – 1826)*

Necrotizing papillitis is the other name of acute papillary necrosis. When infection of renal pyramids develop in association with vascular diseases of the kidney or with urinary tract obstruction, renal papillary necrosis is likely to result. In the given options, DM is the commonest and TB is the rarest cause of papillary necrosis

- Diabetes mellitus
- Sickle cell disease
- Chronic alcoholism
- Vascular disease
- Analgesic abuse nephropathy

89. Ans. (a) PCT *(Ref: Robbins 9/e p928, 8th/937-8, 7th/918)*

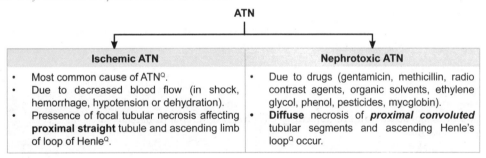

Clinical info:Harrison 18th

It is the most common cause of acute renal failure (ARF). ARF is defined as rapid and reversible deterioration of renal function leading to reduction of urine outflow to less than 400 ml per day within 24 hours.

90. Ans. (d) Medullary cystic kidney *(Ref: Harrison 18th/2383, 16th/1807, Robbin's 9/e p948, 8th/947, 7th/1005)*

Nephrocalcinosis is a diffuse deposition of calcium salts in the interstitium of the kidney.

Conditions associated with nephrocalcinosis are:

• Hyperoxaluria • Hyperparathyroidism • Prolonged immobilization • Hypervitaminosis D • Hypophosphatemic rickets • Excessive bone destruction in metastasis • Cortical necrosis malignancies (such as multiple myeloma) • Cushing syndrome	• Hyperthyroidism • Hyperuricosuria • Renal candidiasis • Excessive calcium intake (*milk alkali syndrome*) • *Sarcoidosis* • *Renal tubular acidosis (distal)* • *Medullary sponge kidney*

91. **Ans. (a) Goodpasture's syndrome; (b) Leptospirosis; (d) Wegener's granulomatosis; (e) Hantan virus infection;** *(Ref: Harrison 17th/1793)*
Pulmonary renal syndrome is seen in

- Goodpasture's syndrome: pulmonary hemorrhage and renal failure
- Leptospirosis: Renal and hepatic dysfunction, Hemorrhagic pneumonia, bleeding diathesis
- Hantan virus also cause pulmonary renal syndrome.
- Wegener's granulomatosis: Lung and kidney involvement common.
- Other causes of pulmonary renal syndrome include Henoch Schonlein purpura, Churg Strauss vasculitis, microscopic polyangiitis and cryoglobulinemia.

Please note that Legionella does not affect kidneys. It causes atypical pneumonia, diarrhea and hyponatremia.*

92. **Ans. (b) DM, (c) Phenacetin abuse, (d) Alcoholism** *(Ref: Harrison 17th/1826, Robbins 9/e p936, 8th/947, 7th-1004)*

Causes of papillary necrosis				
	Diabetes mellitus	**Analgesic nephropathy**	**Sickle cell disease**	**Obstruction**
M:F	1:3	1:5	1:1	9:1
Time course	10 years	7 years of abuse	Variable	Variable
Infection	80%	25%	+ or −	90%
Calcification	Rare	Frequent	Rare	Frequent
Number of papillae affected	Several; all of same stage	Almost all; all in different stages of necrosis	Few	Variable

93. **Ans. (a) Hyperparathyroidism; (b) T.B. Kidney; (c) Hypercalcemia** *(Ref: Harsh Mohan 6th/685, Robbins 9/e p937, 7th/1005)*
Causes of Nephrocalcinosis

• Distal RTA	• Hyperparathyroidism	• Multiple myeloma
• Severe hypercalcemia	• Hypercalcemia	• Vitamin D intoxication
• Medullary sponge kidney	• TB kidney	• Metastatic bone disease

94. **Ans. (d) Polycystic kidney disease; (e) Amyloidosis:** *(Ref: Robbins 7th/964, 992, 989, 9/e 947)*

Causes of bilaterally enlarged kidneys	Causes of small contracted kidney
• Polycystic kidney diseases	• Benign nephrosclerosis
• Amyloidosis of kidney	• Chronic glomerulonephritis
• DM	• Chronic Pyelonephritis

95. **Ans. (c) Alport's syndrome** *(Ref: Robbins 7th/988, 9/e p924, Harrison 17th/1794)*
Hereditary Nephritis refers to a group of heterogenous hereditary familial diseases associated primarily with glomerular injury. These are: **Alport's syndrome** and **Thin membrane disease.**

96. **Ans. (b) Medullary sponge kidney; (D) RTA** *(Ref: Robbins 7th/1005, 9/e p937,948)*

97. **Ans. (d) Neutrophilic infiltration; (e) Necrotizing vasculitis:** *(Ref: Robbins 7th/220)*
Acute rejection can be caused by either cellular or humoral mechanisms
The histologic features of **acute humoral rejection** (within days) in renal transplants are:
- Necrotizing vasculitis
- Endothelial cell necrosis
- Neutrophilic infiltration
- Deposition of immunoglobulins
- Complement and fibrin deposition and thrombosis.
- There is extensive necrosis of renal parenchyma.

In acute cellular rejection
- Extensive interstitial mononuclear cell infiltration
- Edema
- Interstitial hemorrhage is seen.

In hyper acute rejection (within minutes or hours)
- Fibrinoid reactions are seen

In chronic rejection (over period of 4-6 months)
- Vascular changes consisting of dense, obliterative intimal fibrosis, principally in the cortical arteries seen. It clinically presents with progressive rise in serum creatinine.

98. **Ans. (b) Schistocytes** *(Ref: Harrison 17th/723, Robbin 9/e p644)*

The presence of a severe hemolytic anemia with schistocytes or fragmented red blood cells in the peripheral blood smear is characteristic of microangiopathic hemolytic anemia such as in Hemolytic uremic syndrome and Thrombotic thrombocytopenic purpura.

99. **Ans. (b) Cortical tubular hypertrophy** *(Ref: Robbins 8th/959, 7th/966)*
   * Cortical tubulo-interstitial damage occurs in nephronophthisis.

   Nephronophthisis (Uremic Medullary Cystic Disease Complex)
   * It is a group of progressive renal disorders that usually have onset in childhood.
   * Common characteristic is the presence of a variable number of cysts in the medulla, usually concentrated at the cortico-medullary junction.
   * Cortical tubulo-interstitial damage occurs.
   * 4 variants of this disease are:
     – Sporadic/non familial (20%)
     – Familial juvenile nephronophthisis (40-50% autosomal recessive).
     – Renal-retinal dysplasia (15% autosomal recessive)
     – Adult-onset medullary cystic disease (15% autosomal dominant).
   * Affected children present first with polyuria and polydipsia which reflect a marked tubular defect in concentrating ability.
   * Sodium wasting and tubular acidosis are also prominent.
   * Renal failure occurs in a period of 5-10 years.
   * In gross appearance, the kidneys are small, have contracted granular surfaces and show cysts in the medulla, most prominently at the cortico-medullary junction.
   * Small cysts are also seen in the cortices and are lined by flattened or cuboidal epithelium.
   * In the cortex, there is widespread atrophy and thickening of the basement membranes of proximal and distal tubules together with interstitial fibrosis.
   * In general, glomerular structure is preserved.

100. **Ans. (a) Diabetes Mellitus** *(Ref. Robbins 7th/991, 1004, 9/e p936)*

101. **Ans. (a) Calcium oxalate** *(Ref: Robbins 7th/1014, 9/e p951)*

102. **Ans. (c) Interstitial nephritis** *(Ref: Robbins 9/e p930, 8th/938-939, 7th/1002-1003)*

103. **Ans. (c) Diabetes mellitus** *(Ref: Robbins 9/e p936, 8th/934; 7th/1003)*

104. **Ans. (b) Lupus nephritis** *(Ref: Robbins 8th/939, 9/e p929)*

105. **Ans. (d) Lipoid nephrosis** *(Ref: Robbins 9/e p222-223, 8th/218, 7th/231-232)*

106. **Ans. (a) Fibrinoid necrosis** *(Ref: Robbins 9/e p939, 8th/950, 7th/1007)*

107. **Ans. (c) Amyloidosis** *(Ref: Robbins 8th/254, 7th/263) Harsh Mohan*

108. **Ans. (a) Acute glomerulonephritis** *(Ref: Robbins 9/e p911, 8th/936)*

109. **Ans. (a) Calcium oxalate stone** *(Ref: Robbins 9/e p951, 8th/962, 7th/1014)*

110. **Ans. (a) Goodpasture's syndrome** *(Ref: Robbins 9/e p912, 8th/920, 7th/745)*

111. **Ans. (b) Calcium oxalate** *(Ref: Robbins 9/e p951, 8th/962)*
   The patient has typical features suggestive of a ureteric colic. Most of the renal stones are composed of calcium oxalate crystals. Patients with these stones tend to have hypercalciuria without hypercalcemia. Uric acid stones and cystine stone are radiolucent and tend to form in acidic urine. Triple phosphate (magnesium ammonium phosphate) stones occur more frequently with UTI caused by urease positive bacteria like Proteus sp. Mucoproteins may fuse together to form hyaline casts which are asymptomatic because they are very small.

112. **Ans. (c) Cystitis** *(Ref: Robbins 8th/974-5, 9/e p962)*
   The clinical presentation of the patient in the stem of the question is of cystitis, which is characterized by pyuria and hematuria but absence of white cell casts in the urine.
   Patients with acute pyelonephritis present with fever, leucocytosis, flank tenderness, urinary white cells, and white cell casts in the urine. Chronic pyelonephritis is almost always the result of chornic urinary tract obstruction and repeated bouts of acute inflammation in the kidneys.

113. **Ans. (c) White blood cell casts** *(Ref: Robbins 9/e p933, 8th/942)*

WBC casts are pathognomonic for pyelonephritis when UTI is present. They are **formed only in tubules**, where **leukocytes are precipitated by the Tamm Horsfall protein** secreted by tubular epithelial cells. Urethritis and cystitis are both characterized by the clinical features of dysuria, frequency, urgency, pyuria, and bacterium, but suprapubic pressure and tenderness is more specific to cystitis. If pathogens ascend via the ureter to penetrate kidney parenchyma, systemic signs of the disease become prominent. Symptoms of acute pyelonephritis include fever, chills, nausea, vomiting, flank/abdominal pain, and costovertebral angle (CVA) tenderness. Urine sediment microscopy reveals WBCs, WBC casts, and bacteria.

- (Choice A) Abdominal pain is a non-specific symptom. It can be seen in acute pyelonephritis and in a large number of other conditions, like pelvic inflammatory disease.
- (Choice B) Fever is a sign of any systemic infection. In acute pyelonephritis, it may also be accompanied by shaking chills, nausea, vomiting, diarrhea, muscle aches, and anorexia.
- (Choices C and D) Bacteriuria is found in both upper (acute pyelonephritis) and lower (cystitis, urethritis) UTIs.

114. **Ans. (b) Absence of antibacterial properties in vaginal fluid** *(Ref: Robbins 8th/939, 9/e p931)*
Females are more susceptible to UTIs due to having urethras that are both closer to the rectum and shorter than in males. Sexual intercourse is often a precipitating factor for UTI. The increased predisposition is also attributed to the absence of antibacterial substances which are present in prostatic fluid. Moreover, thinking logically, the anti infective substances in vaginal fluid will prevent vaginal infection. They cannot prevent UTI.

115. **Ans. (a) Disseminated intravascular coagulation** *(Ref: Robbins 8th/954, 9/e p944)*
Diffuse cortical necrosis is usually seen in the setting of disseminated intravascular coagulation, typically associated with overwhelming sepsis. It can also be seen following hypotension combined with vasoconstriction.
Multiple myeloma (option B) is associated with renal deposition of amyloid protein and damage to both glomeruli and tubules.
Pyelonephritis (option D) would produce inflammation, often most severe in the renal pelvis. Sickle cell anemia (option c) usually affects the medulla most severely, and can cause papillary necrosis.

116. **Ans. (c) Hyperparathyroidism** *(Ref: Robbins 8th/962, 9/e p951)*
The patient's history of recurrent urolithiasis with calcium-containing stones implies a disorder in the regulation of calcium concentration. Hyperparathyroidism is associated with increased parathormone (PTH) levels, which can produce hypercalcemia, hypercalciuria, and, ultimately, renal stones.

- Anemia of chronic disease (option A) does not produce calcium stones. The patient presents with a chronic condition and hematuria but the urinary blood loss is not usually significant enough to produce an anemic state.
- Hyperaldosteronism (option D) results in potassium depletion, sodium retention, and hypertension. Primary hyperaldosteronism (Conn's syndrome) is associated with adrenocortical adenomas in 90% of patients and is characterized by decreased renin. Secondary hyperaldosteronism results from excessive stimulation by angiotensin II that is caused by excess renin production (plasma renin-angiotensin levels are high). Neither condition is associated with renal stones.

117. **Ans. (a) Decreased renal perfusion** *(Ref: Robbins 8th/906, 9/e p898)*
The patient's ankle edema, shortness of breath, and relatively low blood pressure suggest the development of congestive heart failure (confirmed by the cardiac enlargement and perihilar infiltrates). This is an important prerenal cause for the azotemia resulting in elevated serum urea nitrogen with normal serum creatinine.
Postrenal causes of azotemia are typically due to urinary tract obstruction distal to the kidney (option B), and usually cause a rise in both urea and creatinine, with the rise in urea being larger than that in creatinine.
Increased synthesis of urea (option C) is seen in severe burns and prolonged high fever.
Renal tubulointerstitial disease (option D) severe enough to cause renal failure will cause both urea and creatinine to rise; the creatinine may rise out of proportion to the urea, particularly in acute tubular necrosis.

117.1. **Ans. (b) Co-dominant** *(Ref: Robbins 8/e p931-2, 9/e p924)*
Friends, read the following lines from Robbins carefully....
- *Alport syndrome* is manifested by *hematuria with progression to chronic renal failure, accompanied by nerve deafness and various eye disorders, including lens dislocation, posterior cataracts, and corneal dystrophy.*
- The disease is inherited as an **X-linked trait** in approximately **85%** of cases. In this X-linked form, *males express the full syndrome and females are carriers* in whom manifestations of disease are typically limited to hematuria.

- **Autosomal recessive** and **autosomal dominant** pedigrees also exist, in which males and females are equally susceptible to the full syndrome

117.2. Ans. (a) Diabetes mellitus *(Ref: Robbins 8/e p947, 9/e p 936, Top 3 Differentials in Radiology: A Case Review Thieme pg 121)*

The most common cause of papillary necrosis is **diabetes mellitus**[Q].....Top 3 Differentials in Radiology

Encyclopedia of Imaging, Vol 2; pg 1192.. *"diabetes mellitus is the most common condition associated with renal papillary necrosis accounting for >50% of all cases."*

Clinical Pathology Oxford press pg220.. **"acute papillary necrosis** is most often a complication of acute pyelonephritis in **diabetes**. Chronic papillary necrosis is seen most often in association with analgesic nephropathy".

Conditions with papillary necrosis: Mnemonic is POSTCARDS

• **P**yelonephritis
• **O**bstruction of the urinary tract
• **S**ickle cell hemoglobinopathies, including sickle cell trait
• **T**uberculosis
• **C**irrhosis of the liver, **C**hronic alcoholism
• **A**nalgesic abuse
• **R**enal transplant rejection, **R**adiation
• **D**iabetes mellitus
• **S**ystemic vasculitis

117.3. Ans. (b) Diabetes mellitus *(Ref: Robbins 8/e p934, 7/e p991-992)*

Causes of contracted kidneys

Symmetric	Asymmetric
• Chronic glomerulonephritis	• Chronic pyelonephritis
• Benign nephrosclerosis	
Causes of enlarged kidneys	
• Amyloidosis	• Diabetic renal disease [Kimmelstiel winos nodules are pathognomonic]
• Rapidly progressive glomerulonephritis (RPGN)	• Polycystic kidney disease
• Myeloma kidney	• Bilateral obstruction (hydronephrosis)

117.4. Ans. (a) Chronic pyelonephritis *(Ref: Robbins 9/e p934, 8/e p943, 7/e p989)*

In the morphology of chronic pyelonephritis, glomeruli may appear normal except for **periglomerular fibrosis.**

117.5. Ans. (a) Hyperparathyroidism *(Ref: Robbins 9/e p937)*

- Disorders *characterized by hypercalcemia*, such as *hyperparathyroidism, multiple myeloma, vitamin D intoxication, metastatic bone disease, or excess calcium intake (milk-alkali syndrome),* may induce the formation of calcium stones and deposition of calcium in the kidney (**nephrocalcinosis**).

117.6. Ans. (b) Tuberculous cystitis *(Ref: Bailey 25/e p1108)*

TB Urinary Bladder

• Bladder tuberculosis *is almost always secondary to renal tuberculosis*[Q].
• The disease **starts at the ureteric opening**, the earliest evidence being pallor of the mucosa due to submucosal edema.
• Subsequently tiny white transluscent tubercles develop all over. Gradually these tubercles enlarge and may ulcerate (but **do not cause bladder perforation**[Q]).
• These tubercles lend **'cobblestone' appearance**[Q] on cystoscopy.
• There is considerable suhmucous fibrosis which causes diminished capacity of bladder. *Scarred & ftbrosed, small capacity bladder* is known as **thimble bladder**[Q].
• The fibrosis which usually starts around the ureter, contracts to cause a pull at the ureters. This either leads to a stricture or displaced, dilated and rigid wide mouthed ureter called as **golf hole ureters**[Q] (this almost always leads to *ureteral reflux*.)

117.7. Ans. (d) Micro RNA -122 *(Ref: Harrison 18/e p2304-5)*

New question friends and highly likely to be repeated…..

Name of marker	Significance
Kidney injury molecule-1 (KIM-1) and Clusterin	* Type-1 cell membrane glycoprotein upregulated in de differentiated proximal tubule epithelial cells * ***Elevated urinary levels are highly sensitive and specific for A****KI*
Cystatin C	* Important extracellular inhibitor of cysteineproteases * Elevated urinary levels **reflect tubular dysfuncti**on; high levels may predict poorer outcome
NGAL	* Expression upregulated in kidney proximal tubule cells and urine following ***ischemic or cisplatin induced renal injury*** * Found to be an early indicator of AKI following cardiopulmonary bypass
IL-18	* Constitutively expressed in distal tubules; strong immunoreactivity in proximal tubules with transplant rejection * Elevated urinary levels found to be ***early marker*** of AKI and ***independent predictor of mortality*** in critically ill patients
Na⁺/H⁺ exchanger 3 (NHE 3)	* For ***discrimination between prerenal azotemia and AKI*** in ICU patients
L-FABP	Biomarker in **CKD and diabetic nephropathy**
Osteopontin	* Correlates with inflammation and tubulointerstitial fibrosis
β₂-Microglobulin	* Light chain of the MHC I molecule; * An ***early marker of tubular dysfunction***
α₁-Microglobulin	* Synthesized by the liver; tubular dysfunction marker
Microalbumin	Marker for monitoring progression of chronic kidney disease

NGAL is Neutrophil gelatinase associated lipocalin, Liver fatty acid–binding protein (L-FABP);

In addition, *N*-Acetyl--(D) glucosaminidase (NAG), Retinol-binding protein, Cysteine-rich protein CYR 61, Exosomal fetuin-A and enzymes like Alanine aminopeptidase (AAP), alkaline phosphatase (AP), Glutathione-*S*-transferase (α-GST) Glutamyl transpeptidase (γ-GT) are other markers of acute kidney injury (AKI).

117.8. Ans (c) Silicosis *(Ref: Robbins 9/e p690)*

117.9. Ans (b) Crystals are hexagonal *(Ref: Robbins 9/e p 952)*

Hexagonal stones are seen in cystine stones whereas uric acid stones are barrel or diamond shaped.

Uric acid stones are common in individuals with hyperuricemia, such as patients with gout, and diseases involving rapid cell turnover, such as the leukemias.

A tendency to excrete urine of pH below 5.5 may predispose to uric acid stones, because uric acid is insoluble in **acidic urine**. In contrast to the radiopaque calcium stones, *uric acid stones are radiolucent.*

117.10. Ans (a) Nodular glomerulosclerosis *(Ref: Harsh Mohan 6/e p678)*

Nodular lesions of diabetic glomerulosclerosis are also called as *Kimmelstiel-Wilson (KW) lesions or intercapillary glomerulosclerosis*. These lesions are specific for type 1 diabetes.

118. Ans. None or 'c' Cushing syndrome. *(Ref: Robbins 8th/966, Kidney Cancer: Principles and Practice (2012) pg 71, Springer, Harrison 17th/592: 618)*

Friends, ideal answer of this question would be none. Robbins 8th/966…. 'renal cell carcinomas produce a number of paraneoplastic syndromes, ascribed to abnormal hormone production, including polycythemia, hypercalcemia, hypertension, hepatic dysfunction, feminization or masculinization, Cushing syndrome, eosinophilia, leukemoid reactions, and amyloidosis.'

However, a table from Kidney Cancer: Principles and Practice is given underneath to help you decide the fact that if we have to compulsorily mark one option as the answer, then it has to be Cushing syndrome (option 'c') because it has the rarest incidence.

Paraneoplastic manifestations of renal cell cancer syndromes with their incidence

Paraneoplastic syndrome	Incidence
Endocrinological	
Hypercalcemia	13-20%
Hypertension	40%
Polycythemia	1-8%
Stauffer syndrome	3-20%
Elevated Alkaline phosphatase	10%
Cushing syndrome	2%
Thrombocytosis	-
Cachexia	30%
Non endocrine	
Amyloidosis	3-8%
Anemia	20%
Neuromyopathy	3%
Vasculopathy	-
Nephropathy	-
Fever	20%

Stauffer syndrome *is the name give to non metastatic hepatic dysfunction.*

119. **Ans. (d) Bilateral polycystic kidney** *(Ref: Robbins 8th/479-480, 9/e p479-480)*
Wilm's tumor (Nephroblastoma) is the **most common primary renal tumor of childhood** in USA. It is associated with the following:

> **WAGR syndrome**
> It is characterized by aniridia, genital anomalies, and mental retardation and increased choice of developing Wilms' tumor. Patients with WAGR syndrome carry constitutional (germline) deletions of two genes WT1 and PAX6 both located at chromosome **11p13**[Q].
>
> **Denys-Drash syndrome**
> It is characterized by gonadal dysgenesis (male pseudohermaphroditism) and early-onset nephropathy leading to renal failure.
>
> **Beckwith-Wiedemann syndrome**
> It characterized by enlargement of body organs (organomegaly), macroglossia, hemihypertrophy, omphalocele and abnormal large cells in adrenal cortex (adrenal cytomegaly).

Clinical features include presentation as a large abdominal mass extending across the midline[Q] and down into the pelvis. The patient may also present with fever and abdominal pain, with hematuria, intestinal obstruction or hypertension[Q] as a result of pressure from the tumor.

120. **Ans. (c) Trisomy 7/17** *(Ref: Robbins 8th/964-964, 9/e p953-954, Harrison 17th/592)*
Friends, answer to the question is very easy for us to understand provided we are aware of the fact that chromophilic renal cell cancer is the other name of papillary renal cell cancer because 80% of chromophilic renal cell cancers show a tubulopapillary architecture. (source….British Journal of Cancer 1996,74; 1605-1614.). As discussed in text, Papillary cancer is associated with trisomy 7, 16, 17.

121. **Ans. (a) Clear cell type** *(Ref: Robbins 7th/1016, 1017, 9/e p953)*

122. **Ans. (b) Wilm's tumor** *(Ref. Robbins 8th/479, 9/e p479)*
Wilm's tumor is increased in WAGR syndrome, Dennys-Drash syndrome and Beckwith-wiedemann syndrome.
The features mentioned in the question point to a diagnosis of WAGR syndrome. The components of this syndrome are

> W – Wilm's tumor
> A – Aniridia
> G – Genital anomalies
> R – Mental retardation

123. **Ans. (C) Anaplasia** *(Ref: Robbins 8th/481, 9/e p481)*
5% of tumors reveal **anaplasia**, defined as the presence of cells with large, hyperchromatic, pleomorphic nuclei and abnormal mitoses and the presence of anaplasia correlates with underlying *p53* mutations and the emergence of resistance to chemotherapy.

124. Ans. (b) Associated with deletion of chromosome 11p13 *(Ref: Robbins 9/e p479, 8th/479-481; 7th/504-506)*

125. Ans. (a) Clear cell *(Ref: Robbins 9/e p953, 8th/964; 7th/1016)*

126. Ans. (b) Abdominal CT scan for renal mass *(Ref: Robbins 9/e p955, 8th/964-6)*
Painless hematuria in an old patient is highly suggestive of a renal malignancy. Moreover, additional presence of constitutional symptoms, such as fever and weakness, increase the suspicion of a renal cell carcinoma.

> - Urinary tract calculi usually cause severe, colicky pain when they are passed.
> - Nephrotic syndrome, which manifests with proteinuria, typically is not associated with hematuria,
> - A renal biopsy has a less diagnostic yield in a condition without an acute onset renal disease, and it is not very effective for diagnosing neoplasms.

127. Ans. (c) Nephroblastoma *(Ref: Robbins 8th/481, 9/e p481)*
- Nephroblastoma (Wilms tumor) characteristically affects children between 2 and 4 years of age and can form large spherical masses composed of variegated tissues including primitive renal epithelial elements, a sarcomatous-appearing stroma, abortive glomeruli and tubules, and heterologous tissues such as muscle, cartilage, fat, and bone.

> - Cortical adenoma (option A) is a small (under 2 cm) benign tumor that is usually found incidentally at autopsy.
> - Hemangiomas (option B) can occur in the kidney, but would not usually produce a large mass.
> - Oncocytomas (option D) are benign tumors that can be large but do not usually affect young children.

128. Ans. (c) Wilms' tumor *(Ref: Robbins 8th/481, 9/e p479-481)*
The only childhood malignancy in the given options is Wilms' tumor, which commonly presents in a toddler as a large abdominal mass. There is now a 90% survival rate for this tumor with combined therapy with surgery, chemotherapy, and radiotherapy.

> Renal cell carcinoma (choice A) and transitional cell carcinoma of the bladder (choice D) are malignant tumors of adults. Renal hamartoma (fibroma; choice B) causes a small, gray, benign module in the renal pyramids and is usually only identified as an incidental finding.

128.1. Ans. (b) Tumour stage *(Ref: Robbins 8/e p, Rudolph Pediatrics; Robbins 9/e p481)*
Also revise that anaplsia is an adverse prognostic factor because it increases the resistance to chemotherapy and increased chances of recurrence.

Good prognostic factors	Poor prognostic factors
- Age < 2 years - Early stage disease (stage I,II) - Favourable histology - Tumour < 500 gms	- Age > 2 years - Late stage disease (stage III,IV) - Anaplasia (unfavourable histology) - Tumour > 500 gms - Loss of genetic material on 11q,16q - Gain of material on 1q - Renal vessel and capsule invasion

128.2. Ans. (d) Collecting duct *(Ref: Robbins 8/e p964, 9/e p953)*

Oncocytoma

> - Arises from the **intercalated cells of collecting ducts**[Q].
> - Epithelial tumor composed of large **eosinophilic cells** having small, round, benign-appearing nuclei that have large nucleoli.
> - *Ultrastructurally the eosinophilic cells have* **numerous mitochondria**[Q].

128.3. Ans. (c) Chromosome 11 *(Ref: Robbins 8/e p479-80, 9/e p479-480)*
Easiest way to remember that info..... count the number of letters in Wilms tumour..yea it is exactly 11...the location of both genes associated with Wilms tumour ☺
So, the two genes associated with Wilms tumour **WT1** gene (located on **chr 11p13**)and WT2 gene (located on **chr 11p15**).

128.4. Ans. (c) Wilm's tumor.... Discussed in a separate question *(Ref: Robbins 8/e p479-480, 9/e p479-480)*

129. Ans. (b) Malacoplakia *(Ref: Robbins, 9/e p963, 8th/975, 7th/1027-8)*
Michaelis-Gutmann bodies are laminated mineralized concretions typically present within the macrophages resulting from deposition of calcium in enlarged lysosomes. It is seen in malacoplakia. Similar lesions are also seen in the colon, lungs, bones, kidneys, prostate, and epididymis. In this conditions, there is presence of PAS+ macrophages.

130. **Ans. (c) Atrophy** *(Ref: Robbins 7th/9, 1012, 9/e p950)*

Chronic urethral obstruction because of urinary calculi, prostatic hypertrophy, tumors, normal pregnancy, uterine prolapse or functional disorders cause **hydronephrosis** which by definition is used to describe *dilatation of renal pelvis* and calyces associated with *progressive atrophy of the kidney* due to obstruction to the outflow of urine.

Concept

> Atrophy is shrinkage in size of the cell by loss of cell substance. *Atrophied cells are only decreased in size; they are not dead*

131. **Ans. (c) Malacoplakia** *(Ref: Robbins 9/e p963, 8th/975, 7th/1027)*

132. **Ans. (a) Light chain** *(Ref: Robbins 9/e p937-938, 8th/948, 7th/1005)*

132.1. **Ans. (a) Schistosomiasis** *(Ref: Robbins 8/e p979, 9/e p965)*

Direct lines from Robbins...

Schistosoma haematobium infections in endemic areas like Egypt and Sudan are an established risk. The ova are deposited in the bladder wall and incite a brisk chronic inflammatory response that induces progressive mucosal squamous metaplasia and dysplasia and, in some instances, neoplasia.

Most of these cancers are **squamous cell**[Q] carcinomas.

132.2. **Ans. (b) Hypophosphatemia** *(Ref: Harrison 18/e)*

- Hyponatremia
- Hyperkalemia
- **Hyperphosphatemia**

GOLDEN POINTS FOR QUICK REVISION / UPDATED INFORMATION FROM 9TH EDITION OF ROBBINS (KIDNEY AND URINARY BLADDER)

Robbins 9th/898....Chronic kidney disease is elaborated

> *Chronic kidney disease* (previously called chronic renal failure) is defined as the presence of a diminished GFR that is persistently **less than 60 mL/minute/1.73 m2 for at least 3 months,** from any cause, and/or persistent albuminuria.

Robbins 9th/915....Membranous Nephropathy with New Autoantigen

> **Primary** (also called idiopathic) **membranous nephropathy** is now considered to be an *autoimmune disease linked to certain HLA alleles such as* **HLA-DQA1** *and caused in most cases by antibodies to a* **renal autoantigen**. In many adult cases the autoantigen is the **phospholipase A2 receptor**. This antigen is the counterpart of the megalin antigen complex in the rats.

Robbins 9th/938............Bile Cast Nephropathy

> *Hepatorenal syndrome* refers to impairment of renal function in patients with acute or chronic liver disease with advanced liver failure. This can be associated with highly elevated bilirubin levels with *bile cast formation* (also known as **cholemic nephrosis**) in distal nephron segments. The casts can extend to proximal tubules, resulting in both direct toxic effects on tubular epithelial cells and obstruction of the involved nephron. The tubular bile casts can range from yellowish-green to pink. The reversibility of the renal injury depends upon the severity and duration of the liver dysfunction.

Robbins 9th/953....Additional Risk Factor of Renal Cell Cancer

> **Hereditary leiomyomatosis and renal cell cancer syndrome**: This autosomal dominant disease is caused by mutations of the *FH* gene, which expresses fumarate hydratase, and is characterized by *cutaneous and uterine leiomyomata and an aggressive type of papillary carcinoma* with increased propensity for metastatic spread.
>
> **Birt-Hogg-Dubé syndrome:** The autosomal dominant inheritance pattern of this disease is due to mutations involving the *BHD* gene, which expresses folliculin. The syndrome features a constellation of skin (fibrofolliculomas, trichodiscomas, and acrochordons), pulmonary (cysts or blebs), and renal tumors with varing histologies.

Additional variant of renal cell cancer (as if clear cell, papillary, chromophobe and collecting duct were not enough!!!)... **Robbins 9th/954**

> *Xp11 translocation carcinoma* is a genetically distinct subtype of renal cell carcinoma. It often occurs in young patients and is defined by translocations of the *TFE3* gene located at Xp11.2 with other genes resulting in over expression of TFE3. The neoplastic cells consist of clear cytoplasm with a papillary architecture.

NOTES

CHAPTER 12

Gastrointestinal Tract

The normal layers present in the gastrointestinal tract are:
1. *Mucosa* consisting of epithelial layer, lamina propria and muscularis mucosae
2. *Submucosa* having submucosal glands and Meissner's plexus
3. *Muscularis propria* consisting of inner circular layer, outer longitudinal layer and having Auerbach's plexus in between these two layers.
4. *Serosa*.

ESOPHAGUS

It is a muscular tube almost **25 cm in length in adults** (it is about 10 cm in a newborn) taking the food from the oral cavity into the stomach. The esophagus is having the following four constrictions in it:

- **Cricopharyngeus** constriction: present at 15 cm **(6 inches)** from the incisor teeth[Q].
- **Aortic arch constriction:** present at 22.5 cm **(9 inches)** from the incisor teeth[Q].
- **Left bronchus constriction:** present at 27.5 cm **(11 inches)** from the incisor teeth[Q].
- **Diaphragmatic** and **lower esophageal sphincter** constriction: present at 40 cm **(16 inches)** from the incisor teeth[Q].

There is presence of a functional sphincter at the lower end of the esophagus (LES) which prevents the reflux of the gastric contents back into the esophagus.

ACHALASIA CARDIA

It is a disease characterized by loss of ganglion cells in the Auerbach's plexus the cause of which may be unknown (**Primary achalasia**) or it may be due to secondary cause like **Chagas'** disease (caused by T. cruzi) or *Varicella zoster* infection. This result in the incomplete relaxation of the LES and its increased resting tone. There is selective loss of function of inhibitory neurons like those secreting vasoactive intestinal peptide and nitric oxide whereas *cholinergic innervation is intact*. It is characterized by the triad of *incomplete LES relaxation, increased LES tone and aperistalsis of the esophagus.*

Clinical features include *progressive dysphagia* (difficulty in swallowing increases with time as the disease progresses) for food though usually dysphagia is more for the liquid food as compared to solid food particles.

Screening test
***Cholecystokinin*[Q] (CCK) test:** CCK normally causes a fall in the sphincter pressure (because of the relaxant effect of inhibitory neurotransmitters like VIP and nitric oxide) but in achalasia cardia it causes paradoxical increase in LES tone (loss of inhibitory neurons).
Diagnosis
• Barium swallow shows **'bird beak'**[Q] **or 'rat tail'**[Q] **appearance** of the esophagus (due to normal upper esophagus with tapering in the lower part).   • *Manometry is the most confirmatory investigation.*[Q]
Treatment
It is medically managed with *botulinum toxin* but the treatment of choice is surgical excision of the muscle of the lower esophagus and cardia (*Heller myotomy*[Q]).

Serosa is absent in the esophagus *except* for intra-abdominal portion.

The **submucosa** is the **strongest** layer of the gut. Surgically, it provides strength to intestinal anastomosis

Calcifying epithelial odontogenic tumour is called as "Pindborg tumour".

CCK test causes paradoxical increase in LES tone in achalasia cardia

The **gastric bubble** is usually **absent** in chest X-ray.

HIATAL HERNIA

It is characterized by the separation of the diaphragmatic crura and increased space between the muscular crura and the esophageal wall. It can be of two types:

1. **Sliding hernia** (95%): Characterized by upward dislocation of cardioesophageal junction. Esophagitis resulting from the reflux is commonly seen.
2. **Paraesophageal/Rolling hernia** (5%): A part of the stomach enters the thorax without any displacement of the cardioesophageal junction. Dysphagia is common and chest pain may also be present (usually relieved by a loud belch).

Treatment is achieved only with surgical repair of the defect.

MALLORY-WEISS TEARS

Most of the cases (90%), the tear is present at the cardia

Mallory-Weiss tears are mucosal tears in the *esophagogastric junction or the gastric cardiac mucosa* caused *due to vigorous vomiting usually seen in alcoholics*. In most of the cases (**90%**), the tear is present immediately **below the squamocolumnar junction at the cardia** ^{Q} whereas in 10% cases, it is present in the esophagus. These tears **never involve the muscular layer** of the esophagus whereas, in contrast, in **Boerhaave syndrome**, *rupture of all the esophageal layers* is seen including the muscle layer. Most common location of the perforation in this syndrome is in *left posterolateral part* 3-5 cm above the gastroesophageal junction.

ESOPHAGITIS

Barrett's esophagus is the most important risk factor for the development of esophageal adenocarcinoma.

Inflammation of the esophageal mucosa is known as esophagitis and *reflux of the gastric contents into the lower esophagus* is its *most important cause. Gold standard* for the diagnosis of reflux esophagitis is *24 hours pH study* ^{Q}. The reflux is associated with obesity, alcohol intake, smoking, pregnancy and overeating.

BARRETT'S ESOPHAGUS

Concept

Intestinal goblet cells differ from normal mucus secreting foveolar cells of the stomach by the fact that in the former, there is presence of distinct mucous vacuoles (not present in gastric foveolar cells).

Barrett's esophagus is the **metaplastic change** in the esophageal lining in which the normal squamous epithelium is changed to columnar epithelium due to prolonged gastroesophageal reflux disease (GERD). It is classified as **long segment** (if **>3 cm** is involved) or **short segment** (if **<3 cm** is involved). Microscopically, esophageal squamous epithelium is replaced by columnar epithelium. *Definite diagnosis is made only when columnar mucosa contains the intestinal goblet cells.* ^{Q}

Note: Barrett's ulcer is the ulcer in the columnar lined portion of Barrett's esophagus.

CARCINOMA OF THE ESOPHAGUS

Triad of Plummer Vinson syndrome = *iron deficiency anemia + esophageal webs + glossitis*

It is a cancer affecting individuals of mid to late adulthood which is of two main types: **squamous cell cancer and adenocarcinoma.**

Risk factors for squamous cell cancer

- Tobacco and alcohol consumption
- Hot beverages or food
- Longstanding esophagitis
- Achalasia
- *Plummer Vinson syndrome* (also known as *Patterson Kelly syndrome*)
- Ingestion of nitrites in diet
- Nutritional deficiency of vitamins A, vitamin C, riboflavin, zinc, molybdenum
- *Tylosis et palmaris* (hyperkeratosis and pitting of palms and soles)
- Longstanding celiac disease
- Other conditions like ectodermal dysplasia and epidermolysis bullosa
- **Genetic alterations** include amplification of cyclin D1, c-MYC and Epithelial Growth Factor Receptor (EGFR)

The investigation of choice in esophageal cancer is **endoscopy and biopsy.**

Most of the cancers are well differentiated and the morphological patterns include:

   i.   Exophytic protruding lesion in the lumen (60%)
   ii.   Flat, diffuse infiltrative form spreading in the esophageal wall (15%)
   iii. Ulcerative lesion (25%)

Risk factors for Adenocarcinoma

- Barrett's esophagus[Q] (*Most important*)
- Tobacco exposure
- Obesity
- *Genetic alterations* include over expression of p53, amplification of c-ERB-B2 and nuclear translocation of β-catenin (biomarkers of disease progression).

Microscopically, most of the cancers are mucin producing glandular tumors exhibiting intestinal type features. Multiple foci of dysplastic epithelium are present adjacent to the mucosa.

Clinical features include progressive dysphagia (more for solids as compared to liquids), weight loss, chest pain and vomiting. The lymph node metastasis is dependent on the anatomic site of the primary tumor.

- Cancer in the upper 1/3rd of the esophagus: metastasis to cervical lymph nodes.
- Cancer in the middle 1/3rd of the esophagus: metastasis to paratracheal, mediastinal and tracheobronchial lymph nodes.
- Cancer in the lower 1/3rd of the esophagus: metastasis to gastric and celiac lymph nodes.

Treatment: It is mainly surgical with **partial or total esophagectomy**.

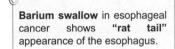

Barium swallow in esophageal cancer shows **"rat tail"** appearance of the esophagus.

- MC type of esophageal cancer in India: *Squamous cell cancer*[Q]
- MC type of esophageal cancer in upper 1/3rd of esophagus: *Squamous cell cancer*[Q]
- MC type of esophageal cancer in middle 1/3rd of esophagus: *Squamous cell cancer*[Q]
- MC type of esophageal cancer in lower 1/3rd of esophagus: *Adenocarcinoma*[Q].

STOMACH

CELLS AND THEIR SECRETIONS

Parietal (Oxyntic) cells	• **Secrete acid** (from the proton pump, H^+-K^+ ATPase) • **Secrete intrinsic factor** (required for vitamin B_{12} absorption)
Chief (Zymogenic) cells	• Secrete the **proenzymes pepsinogen I and II** (activated to pepsin)
Endocrine cells	• Secrete **gastrin in antrum** (by G cells), **histamine** in the body
Foveolar cells	• Secrete **mucin layer** over the mucosal cells

GASTRITIS

Gastritis is the inflammation of the gastric mucosa. It can either be acute gastritis or chronic gastritis.

Risk factors of acute gastritis

- Heavy smoking and alcohol consumption
- Excessive NSAID use (particularly aspirin)
- Uremia
- Ischemia and shock
- Stress (trauma, burns, surgery)
- Others (nasogastric intubation, distal gastrectomy, systemic infections)

Microscopically

Presence of neutrophils above the basement membrane in direct contact with the epithelial cells is indicative of active inflammation[Q].

Risk factors of chronic gastritis

- Chronic infection with *H. pylori*
- Autoimmune cause (pernicious anemia)
- Alcohol and smoking
- Radiation

Humans are the **only** known host of *H.pylori*.

H.pylori. gastritis causes involvement of the **antrum**

- Antrectomy with gastroenterostomy
- Others (amyloidosis, graft-versus-host disease, uremia, Crohn's disease).

MICROSCOPICALLY

> *Chronic gastritis has the presence of lymphocytes and plasma cells associated with intestinal metaplasia and mucosal atrophy.*

Chronic gastritis can be of the following **two types**:

1. **Associated with *H. pylori* (in 90% patients)**

   H. pylori is a gram-negative flagellated bacteria producing enzymes like phospholipase and urease, adhesion molecules like BabA (responsible for enhanced binding in people having **blood group O**) and toxins like CagA and VacA. It causes gastritis in *two patterns*:

   > a. ***Antral predominant gastritis:*** Seen in individuals having *lower IL-1β* production and associated with *high acid production* and increased risk of *duodenal ulcer*.
   >
   > b. ***Pangastritis followed by multifocal atrophic gastritis***—Seen in individuals having *higher IL-1β production* and *lower gastric acid production* and increased risk of *adenocarcinoma*.

   Intraepithelial neutrophils and *subepithelial plasma cells* (meaning plasma cells in the lamina propria) are *characteristic* of H. pylori gastritis. *H. pylori is also associated with peptic ulcer disease, gastric cancer and gastric mucosa associated lymphoma*[Q].

2. **Autoimmune gastritis (in 10% patients)**

   It is caused due to formation of autoantibodies against the proton pump, gastrin receptor and intrinsic factor and is associated with pernicious anemia, Hashimoto's thyroiditis, Addison's disease, type 1 diabetes, gastric cancer and carcinoid tumor. This is particularly associated with damage to the *mucosa of the body and fundus with less involvement of the antrum*. Hyperplasia of gastrin producing G cells in the antral mucosa may result in gastric carcinoid tumor formation.

The **histologic features** of chronic gastritis include regenerative change, intestinal metaplasia (columnar absorptive cells and goblet cells of intestinal type), atrophy and dysplasia. In autoimmune gastritis, there is presence of inflammatory infiltrate having lymphocytes, macrophages in the deeper layers. *Plasma cells in the superficial lamina propria* are characteristically *absent*.

Clinical features include nausea, vomiting and epigastric pain. Autoimmune gastritis maybe associated with symptoms seen in pernicious anemia (beefy tongue, paresthesia, numbness, sensory ataxia, loss of vibration and position sense).

PEPTIC ULCER DISEASE

Any breach in the mucosa of the GIT that involves the submucosa or deeper due to exposure to gastric acid is called peptic ulcer. It is usually a chronic and *solitary lesion less than 4 cm* caused due to imbalance between gastroduodenal protective and damaging factors:

Damaging factors	Protective factors
• Gastric acid	• Mucus and bicarbonate secretion
• Pepsin	• Mucosal blood flow
• Smoking, alcohol	• Prostaglandin production
• Drugs like NSAIDs	• Epithelial regenerative capacity
• H. pylori	
• Ischemia and shock	
• Delayed gastric emptying	
• Duodenal gastric reflux or gastric hyperacidity	

Autoimmune gastritis causes involvement of the **fundus** and **body**.

Histology remains the gold standard for detection of *H. pylori*. The special stains used for H. pylori include **non-silver stains** (like Giemsa, Diff-Quick, Gimenez, Acridine orange) and **silver stains** (like Warthin-Starry, Steiner etc.)

H. pylori is the most important cause of peptic ulcer.

The **location of the peptic ulcer** (in decreasing order of frequency) is:

- **Duodenum (first part)**[Q]
- Stomach **(lesser curvature near the junction of body and antrum**[Q]**)**
- Gastroesophageal junction in GERD or Barrett's esophagus
- Margins of jejunostomy
- Stomach, duodenum and/or jejunum of patients with Zollinger-Ellison syndrome
- In ileal Meckel's diverticulum containing ectopic gastric mucosa.

Males are more commonly affected than females

Duodenal ulcers are located near the pyloric ring and gastric ulcers are predominantly located near the lesser curvature and the antrum. More commonly, there is involvement of the *anterior wall of the duodenum* as compared to the posterior wall. Benign peptic ulcer is classically punched with margins of the ulcer usually at level with the surrounding mucosa whereas heaping up of the margins is more frequently associated with malignancy. Histologically the zones in peptic ulcer are:

i. Base and margins having necrotic fibrinoid debris
ii. Zone of neutrophil predominant infiltrate
iii. Base having active granulation tissue with mononuclear cells
iv. Zone of fibrous or collagenous scar

Clinical features include burning epigastric pain (usually getting worse at night), nausea, vomiting and bloating.

Complications of Peptic Ulcer

Bleeding	
• Most frequent complication[Q]. • More common in posterior wall duodenal ulcers[Q]	
Perforation	
• Most common cause of death in peptic ulcer[Q] • More common in anterior wall duodenal ulcers[Q]	
Gastric outlet obstruction (GOO)	
• Results in persistent vomiting leading to fluid and electrolyte imbalance (metabolic alkalosis due to loss of acid in vomitus)	
Malignancy	
• Associated with gastric ulcer but never with duodenal ulcer.	

> **Gastroduodenal artery** is the source of the bleeding in **duodenal ulcer** whereas *left gastric artery* bleeds in *gastric ulcer*

Duodenal and Gastric peptic ulcer

Features	Duodenal ulcer	Gastric ulcer
Site	1st part of duodenum	Along lesser curvature
Incidence	More common	Less common
Age	25 – 50 yrs, M>F	Beyond 6th decade, M>F
Etiology	Almost all patients have H. pylori infection	Less stronger association
Acid level	High	Usually normal; ↑ if hypergastrinemia
Pain after food intake	Relieved	Aggravated
Clinical features	Night pain and melena more common	No night pain, hematemesis more common
	No vomiting/no weight loss	Vomiting common/weight loss is present
Complications	No malignant change	Malignant change present (though rarely)

Investigations

- **Screening test:** Serum ELISA for antibodies against *H. pylori*
- Urea breath test (radiolabeled urea is broken down to radiolabeled CO_2 by urease enzyme which is detected by breath analyzer, thus suggesting presence of *H. pylori* infection)
- **Gold standard:** Staining of *H. pylori* with silver stain or Warthin starry stain[Q]
- **Most specific investigation:** Culture of bacteria[Q] (done on Skirrow's medium)

Treatment: with "triple drug therapy"[Q] (combination of lansoprazole, clarithromycin and metronidazole) for 2 weeks.

> **Concept**
> Urea breath test is used to ensure the efficacy of the treatment for peptic ulcer disease.

> **Menetrier disease:** It is characterized by diffuse foveolar cell hyperplasia due to **excessive secretion of TGF-α**. It is associated with *enlarged gastric rugae* and *protein losing enteropathy*.

> **Concept**
> Infection with *H. pylori* is associated with *distal intestinal type* and **not** with diffuse, proximal carcinoma.

> Diffuse involvement of the stomach in cancer is called **linitis plastica** or **"leather bottle"** appearance of the stomach. It is also seen in metastasis from cancers of breast and lung.

> **H. pylori** is a **Type 1 carcinogen** for **gastric cancer**.

> Metatasis to anterior left axillary lymph node is called as **Irish Nodes**

Vital Information

- **Cushing ulcer** is seen in esophagus, stomach or the duodenum and is associated with *intracranial disease or head injury*. It is caused by gastric acid hypersecretion due to vagal nuclei stimulation.
- **Curling ulcer** is seen in proximal duodenum and is associated with *burns or trauma*. It is caused due to reduced blood supply and systemic acidosis in burns or trauma.

GASTRIC CANCER

Gastric cancer is the *most common gastric malignancy*. The risk factors for this cancer are:

Environmental factors	Genetic factors	Host factors
• H. pylori infection • Nitrites in diet • Nutritional (vitamin C, E) deficiency • Smoking	• Family history of gastric cancer • Blood group A • Hereditary nonpolyosis colon cancer syndrome (HNPCC) • Familial gastric cancer syndrome (*due to E-cadherin mutation*)	• Chronic gastritis • Intestinal metaplasia • Partial gastrectomy • Gastric adenoma • Barrett's esophagus • Menetrier disease

Classification of gastric cancer
1. **Based on Lauren's histological classification**
   i. *Intestinal type*: This is localized type of cancer composed of the neoplastic intestinal glands which exhibit an expanding sheet pattern of spread due to cohesion of the cells.
   ii. *Diffuse type*: Poorly differentiated non-cohesive cells which do not form glands. The appearance of the cells is **"signet ring"** appearance[Q] (because mucin in the cell pushes the nucleus to the periphery). It is seen more frequently with *E-cadherin mutation*.
2. **Based on Depth of invasion**
   i. *Early gastric cancer*: Characterized by the involvement of *mucosa and the submucosa* irrespective of the involvement of perigastric lymph nodes and is associated with better prognosis.
   ii. *Late gastric cancer*: Characterized by the involvement of the *muscle layer*[Q] of the stomach and is associated with poor prognosis.
3. **Based on Macroscopic pattern**
   i. Protruding mass or *exophytic* (type I lesion)
   ii. *Flat* or depressed: No obvious mass in the mucosa (type II lesion)
   iii. *Excavated:* Erosion is present in stomach wall (type III lesion).

Clinical features

The most common location of the gastric cancer is the antrum of the stomach[Q]

Symptoms include postprandial heaviness in the abdomen (*earliest symptom*), weight loss (*most common symptom*), vomiting and anorexia.

Investigation of choice: Endoscopy with biopsy and brush cytology[Q].

Metastasis occurs to the liver (first organ to be affected) followed by lungs, bone, ovary (where it is known as **Krukenberg's tumor**), periumbilical lymph nodes (*Sister Mary Joseph nodule*), peritoneal cul-de-sac (Blumer's shelf palpable on rectal or vaginal examination) and left supraclavicular lymph node (*Virchow's lymph node*[Q]).

Treatment: Surgical resection is the only curative treatment in gastric cancer. Chemotherapy may be given in advanced cancers with ECF regime (**E**pirubacin, **C**isplatin and 5-**F**luorouracil).

GASTROINTESTINAL STROMAL TUMOR (GIST)

The cells controlling the gastrointestinal peristalsis are present in the muscularis propria and are called as *interstitial cells of Cajal*.[Q] Gastrointestinal stromal tumor (GIST) is the **most common mesenchymal tumor** of the abdomen and majority is present in the stomach. These tumors arise from *interstitial cells of Cajal*. Increased incidence of GIST is seen in NF-1. The most useful diagnostic marker is **c-kit (CD117)** detectable in 95% of the patients. Other markers like CD34 and vimentin can also be expressed by some tumor cells.

Microscopically the tumor may show either epithelioid cells, spindle cells or mixed (both the epithelioid cells and spindle cells).

Diagnosis: CT scan either alone or *with PET scan* (preferable) is the *investigation of choice*.

Treatment: The localized tumors are surgically resected and the metastatic or non-excisable tumors are managed with tyrosine kinase inhibitors called **imatinib mesylate** or sunitinib.

> **Interstitial cells of Cajal** are known as the *pacemaker* cells of the *GIT*.

> **Carney's triad** is gastric GIST + paraganglioma + pulmonary chondroma.

INTESTINE

Infectious Diseases

The important causes of infections in the intestine are as follows:

I. *Enteric fever (typhoid)*

   It is caused because of infection with Salmonella species usually affecting the ileum and the colon.
   – It is associated with ulceration of the Peyer's patches in the terminal ileum and presence of **longitudinal ulcers**[Q] (oval ulcers with long axis along the long axis of the ileum). Microscopic examination reveals the presence of macrophages having bacteria and red blood cells (*erythrophagocytosis*[Q])
   – In the liver, the hepatocytes are replaced by an aggregation of macrophages called as "typhoid nodule"[Q]. Involvement of gallbladder results in development of chronic carrier state. Healing in ulcer is *uncommonly associated with fibrosis or stricture formation*.
   – Clinically, the patient develops *step-ladder pyrexia, rose spots* (erythematous macular lesions on chest and abdomen), abdominal pain, vomiting and diarrhea. *Salmonella osteomyelitis* is particularly common in patients having *sickle cell disease*.
   – Complications include hemorrhage and perforation.
   – *Blood culture* is the mainstay of diagnosis and Widal test is use for measuring the antibody titer.
   – Drug of choice for the treatment is *ciprofloxacin/ceftriaxone* and for *carriers*, it is *ampicillin + probenecid*.

II. *Tuberculosis*: It can present itself in two of the following forms:

> **Erythrophagocytosis** is a characteristic feature of **enteric fever.**

> **Hemorrhage** occurs in **3rd week** of typhoid infection.

Primary infection
- Caused by infection due to *Mycobacterium bovis* (due to intake of infected/non pasteurised milk) and results in the development of hyperplastic tuberculosis. The infection is present in the lymphoid follicles of the intestine and associated with thickening and narrowing of the lumen of the intestine. It usually affects the *ileocecal region* and is associated with subacute intestinal obstruction. The mesenteric lymph nodes are enlarged; matted and caseous. This is known as **tabes mesenterica**.
- *Clinical features* of the patient include acute abdominal pain and intermittent diarrhea. Investigations show widening of the ileocecal angle (known as **"pulled up cecum"**) on barium radiography.

> *Unlike typhoid*, **stricture formation** is **common** in intestinal **tuberculosis**

> **Secondary infection**
>
> - Caused by *Mycobacterium tuberculosis* secondary to swallowing of infected sputum in a patient of pulmonary tuberculosis. It is characterized by presence of the **transverse ulcers** in the intestine particularly the ileum.
> - *Clinical features* of the patient include weight loss and intermittent diarrhea. Investigations show "*filling defect* in the ileum, cecum and ascending colon" on barium radiography. Complications include perforation of the intestine and fistula formation.

Treatment is by administration of antitubercular therapy (conservative management) or surgical resection of the affected part of the intestine (in case of obstruction or fistula formation).

III. *Amoebiasis*

It is caused by infection with an anaerobic protozoa *E. histolytica* and results in the development of **flask shaped ulcers**^{Q} (ulcer with a broad base but narrow neck). The disease affects the cecum and ascending colon followed by sigmoid colon, rectum and appendix. The ulcers usually involve the mucosa and the submucosa (not the muscle layer) and have the presence of liquefactive necrosis. Liver is another important organ affected by the disease resulting in the development of hepatic abscess having necrotic material and hemorrhage (called as "**anchovy sauce pus**" ^{Q}). The invasive disease is diagnosed with ELISA.

> The drug of choice for amoebiasis is metronidazole.

Microbiology link!

- Rotavirus is the most common cause of diarrhea in children of age 6-24 months.
- *Giardia lamblia* is the most common pathogenic parasitic infection in the humans.
- Cholera is caused by *Vibrio cholerae* resulting in the passage of "rice water" stools.

■ PSEUDOMEMBRANOUS COLITIS (ANTIBIOTIC ASSOCIATED COLITIS)

It is a condition most commonly caused by *Clostridium difficile* and is characterized by inflammation in the colon associated with the formation of a pseudomembrane (layer of inflammatory cells and necrotic material overlying the sites of mucosal injury). In normal individuals, the normal flora of the gut is responsible for the production of chemicals called bacteriocins in the intestine. On administration of broad spectrum antibiotics (*most commonly, IIIrd generation cephalosporins*), the normal bacteria are destroyed resulting in increased proliferation of the Clostridium bacteria which then produces large amounts of two toxins, toxin A and toxin B. These toxins induce cytokine production and host cell apoptosis resulting in diarrhea. The disease is diagnosed with the demonstration of *C. difficile* cytotoxin in stool.

> Treatment of Pseudomembranous colitis is done with either **metronidazole (drug of choice)** or vancomycin.

Malabsorption Syndromes

Defective absorption of fats, vitamins, proteins, carbohydrates and fats is called malabsorption. Its hallmark feature is steatorrhea and chronic diarrhea is the most common clinical presentation. The important causes are as follows:

1. *Celiac Disease (Celiac Sprue or Gluten Sensitive Enteropathy or Non-troical sprue)*

   It is a disease characterized by increased sensitivity to a protein called **gluten** or its alcohol soluble fraction **α-gliadin** ^{Q} present in the grains like wheat, oat, barley and rye resulting in a T-cell mediated chronic inflammatory reaction in the small intestine and impaired absorption. It is associated with **HLA-DQ2 or HLA-DQ8**. Clinical features include diarrhea, flatulence, weight loss and fatigue and a characteristic skin lesion called '*dermatitis herpetiformis*'.

   Biopsy of the intestine shows the diffuse enteritis (lymphocytes and plasma cells in lamina propria) with marked atrophy of the villi and elongated and hyperplastic crypts (**overall mucosal thickness is unaltered**^{Q}). The disease also demonstrates the presence of antigliadin, antiendomysial^Q (most useful) or antitransglutaminase antibodies^Q (useful for screening test) whereas definitive diagnosis is made by the following three features:

> Dapsone is the drug of choice for dermatitis herpetiformis.

- Clinical documentation of malabsorption
- Demonstration of small intestinal lesion by biopsy
- Improvement in clinical features and mucosal histology on gluten withdrawal from the diet.

Treatment is intake of the *gluten-free diet* and substitution by rice, millet, tapioca, potato and maize in the diet.

2. *Tropical Sprue (Post Infectious Sprue) is now called as Environmental Enteropathy*
It is a disease similar in features to celiac sprue but present in the tropical region. Though the exact cause is unknown, but bacterial overgrowth particularly *E. coli and Hemophilus* have been implicated. Biopsy of the intestine shows the diffuse enteritis with *atrophy of the villi*. Treatment is done with the help of antibiotics.

Concept

In tropical sprue, the features in the intestine **do not** reverse on gluten free diet

Note:
- There is characteristically involvement of the **proximal intestine in celiac sprue** resulting in iron deficiency anemia whereas *in tropical sprue, there is generalized involvement of the small intestine* (resulting in megaloblastic anemia because B12 and folic acid are absorbed from the terminal ileum).
- Another important difference between the two is that *tropical sprue is not associated with cancer development* whereas **celiac sprue is associated with cancers** like non Hodgkin's lymphoma, small intestine adenocarcinoma and esophageal squamous cell cancer.

3. *Whipple's Disease*
- It is a systemic infectious disease caused by an actinomycete, *Tropheryma whippelii* affecting the triad of *small intestine, CNS and joints*[Q]. The bacteria characteristically proliferate inside the macrophages without getting destroyed.
- The **hallmark feature** of the disease is *small intestinal mucosa having macrophages in the lamina propria* and these macrophages show the *presence of PAS positive, diastase resistant granules*[Q] *and rod shaped bacteria on electron microscopy*. There is mucosal edema, dilation of the lymphatics and involvement of mesenteric lymph nodes. The macrophages having the bacteria can also be found in the *joints, brain, cardiac valves etc with absence of inflammation* being a typical feature.
- Clinical features include arthropathy (initial presentation), diarrhea, weight loss, hyperpigmentation and dementia. *The diarrhea is due to impaired lymphatic transport.*
- Diagnosis is confirmed by identification of *T. whipplei* by polymerase chain reaction (PCR). Treatment is done with **cotrimoxazole** (*drug of choice*) for one year.

Concept

The presence of *T. whipplei* **outside of macrophages is more important** indicator of active disease than is their presence inside the macrophages.

Note:
- Hallmark of Whipple's disease had been presence of PAS positive macrophages containing the characteristic small bacilli. But, similar picture (PAS +ve macrophages with bacilli) can also be seen with M. avium complex (cause of diarrhea in AIDS). However, these organisms are acid fast whereas Tropheryma is not.
- The organs in which these foamy macrophages can be seen are Liver, Small intestine, Lymph nodes, Heart, Eyes, CNS and synovial membranes of joints.

Disorders Associated with Abnormalities in Small-Bowel Biopsy Specimens

Biopsy has diagnostic value (Diffuse Lesions)	
Whipple's disease:	Lamina propria infiltrated with macrophages containing PAS-positive glycoproteins
Abetalipoproteinemia:	Villus structure normal; epithelial cells vacuolated due to excess fat
Agammaglobulinemia:	Flattened or absent villi; increased lymphocytic infiltration; absence of plasma cells
Mycobacterium avium complex	

contd...

contd...

Biopsy may have diagnostic value (Patchy lesions)	
Intestinal lymphoma:	Infiltration of lamina propria and submucosa with malignant cells
Intestinal lymphangiectasia:	Dilated lacteals and lymphatics in lamina propria; clubbed villi
Eosinophilic enteritis:	Diffuse or patchy eosinophilic infiltration in lamina propria and mucosa
Amyloidosis:	Presence of amyloid confirmed by special stains
Regional enteritis:	Noncaseating granulomas
Parasitic infestations:	Parasitic invasion of mucosa; adherence of trophozoites to mucosal surface, as in Giardiasis
Systemic mastocytosis:	Mast cell infiltration of lamina propria

Biopsy is abnormal but not diagnostic		
Celiac sprue	Collagenous sprue	Tropical sprue
Folate deficiency	Vitamin B12 deficiency	Acute radiation enteritis
Systemic scleroderma	Bacterial overgrowth syndromes	

Inflammatory Bowel Disease (IBD)

It is a group of chronic inflammatory conditions as a result of unregulated and persistent activation of the immune system in genetically susceptible persons. It is primarily of two types: Crohn's disease and ulcerative colitis.

CROHN'S DISEASE

It is a chronic granulomatous disease which can affect any part of the gut from the esophagus to the large intestine but the *most commonly affected part is small intestine particularly the ileum*. So, it is also called as *"terminal ileitis" or "granulomatous colitis"*[Q]. It is associated with HLA-DR1/DQw5 and NOD2 genes and an abnormal T-cell response particularly, CD4+ T cells (T_H1 cells[Q]).

MORPHOLOGY:

- The *earliest lesion* in Crohn's disease is the **aphthous ulcer**. Many such ulcers may fuse together to from *serpentine ulcers* arranged longitudinally.
- Grossly, involved bowel segment typically has a rigid, strictured or **thickened wall with creeping fat**.[Q]
- Full thickness of the intestine is affected in the disease i.e. there is **transmural inflammation**[Q]. This causes weakness in the wall thereby leading to *fissure and fistula formation* in Crohn's disease. Fibrosis is also commoner in this type of IBD. *Perianal fistula is the most common fistula seen*.
- There is patchy involvement of the intestine which is known as presence of *"skip lesions"*. The intervening area between two affected portions is absolutely normal. So, the mucosa appears to be irregular which is known as *"cobblestone mucosa"*[Q]
- There is a presence of **non-caseating**[Q] granulomas.
- Clinical features are intermittent attacks of abdominal pain, blood in stools, fever, steatorrhea and megaloblastic anemia (the last two features result because there is impairment in the absorption of bile acids and vitamin B_{12} respectively from the ileum).
- **Screening test** is *presence of ASCA* (**Anti-Saccharomyces cerevisae Antibody**[Q]). Antibody formation is common against cell wall of yeast, *Saccharomyces cerevisae* in patients of Crohn's disease. The investigation done in these patients to confirm the diagnosis is endoscopy and colonoscopy so that direct visualization of the lesions can be done and even a biopsy can be taken if needed.

Gastrointestinal Tract (side margin)

"Skip lesions" and **non-caseating granulomas** are characteristic features of . Crohn's disease

Radiological appearance on barium meal follow-through is known as **"String Sign of Kantor"** because of the decreased lumen in the affected part of the intestine.

m
The mnemonic for important features of Crohn's disease is **SISTER**

Important features of Crohn's disease

S	–	**S**kip lesions
I	–	**I**leum (MC affected site)
S	–	**S**accharomyces cerevisae antibody present
T	–	**T**ransmural involvement
E	–	**E**xtra fibrosis and fistula formation (as compared to ulcerative colitis)
R	–	**R**adiological sign- *String sign of Kantor*, **R**ectum is *usually spared*.

ULCERATIVE COLITIS

It is a chronic inflammatory condition affecting the colon. It most commonly starts from the rectum and affects the superficial layers, the mucosa and the submucosa[Q] (*muscularis propria is rarely affected*). It is **associated with HLA-DR2,** polymorphism in IL-10 gene and an abnormal T-cell response particularly of CD4+ T cells (**TH2 cells**[Q]).

MORPHOLOGY:

- The disease involves the entire colon (**pancolitis**)[Q] starting from the rectum (retrograde involvement). There is presence of regenerating mucosa which projects in the lumen and is called "**pseudopolyps**"[Q]
- In extreme cases, there is involvement of the nerve plexus in the muscularis layer resulting in decrease in the motility of the colon and increase in its size over a period of time giving rise to "**toxic megacolon**"[Q]
- The characteristic feature of the disease is **mucosal damage continuously** from the rectum and extending proximally. This may also lead to "*backwash ileitis*". This type of IBD is more commonly associated with progression to the development of cancer.
- There is **absence of granulomas**[Q].
- Clinical features are intermittent attacks of abdominal pain, bloody mucoid stools and fever.
- There is presence of **p-ANCA**[Q] (perinuclear antineutrophil cytoplasmic antibodies).

Important features of ulcerative colitis

Ulcerative	–	**U**lcers in mucosa and submucosa (Muscle layer **not** effected)
C	-	**C**ontinuous retrograde involvement (No skip lesions)
O	-	**O**riginates in the rectum
L	-	**L**ead pipe appearance
I	-	**I**ncreased chances of cancer (More than that in Crohn's disease)
T	-	**T**oxic megacolon (Due to involvement of transverse colon)
I	-	**I**ncreased growth from the mucosa ("Pseudopolyps")
S	-	**S**ymptoms are severe (As compared to Crohn's disease)

- The extraintestinal manifestations in the IBD are *uveitis, iritis, ankylosing spondylitis, clubbing, migratory polyarthritis, sacroiliitis, primary sclerosing cholangitis, pyoderma gangrenosum, erythema nodosum* etc.

- The disease is treated with sulfasalazine (5-aminosalicylic acid is the principal therapeutic moiety), infliximab (TNF-α antagonist) and steroids.

- IBD is a *precancerous condition* and can increase the risk of development of cancer of the colon.

CARCINOID TUMOR

Carcinoid tumor arises from the endocrine cells called as argentaffin tissue (also called as **Kulchitzsky cells** of crypts of Lieberkuhn) with the GIT and the lungs as the main sites of origin of this cancer. The clinical features are due to release of peptide and non-peptide hormones from these cells. The gastrointestinal carcinoid tumors can be of the following types:

1. Foregut carcinoid tumors: Arise from the esophagus, stomach and the duodenum proximal to the ligament of Treitz, these are usually benign.

Radiological appearance on barium meal follow-through is known as **"lead pipe" appearance.**

m

The mnemonic for important features of Ulcerative colitis is Ulcerative **COLITIS**

Concept

Polymorphism of the **IL-23 receptor** is **protective** in both the types of inflammatory bowel disease.

Smoking is a strong exogenous risk factor for development of **CD** whereas smoking partly *relieves symptoms in UC*.

Concept

The cardiac changes are **largely right sided** due to inactivation of both serotonin and bradykinin in the blood during passage through the lungs by the monoamine oxidase present in the pulmonary vascular endothelium.

497

2. **Midgut carcinoid tumors:** Arise from the jejunum and ileum; these are aggressive and **m**etastasize frequently.

3. Hindgut carcinoid tumors: Arise from the appendix, colon and rectum; usually benign.

Morphology:

On section, the tumors show a characteristic solid, yellow tan appearance and on electron microscopy, the tumor cells show **dense core granules** in the cytoplasm which stain positively with *chromogranin A, neuron-specific enolase and synaptophysin* [Q] on immunocytochemistry.

Carcinoid syndrome is present in 1% patients of carcinoid tumor and it is due to excessive release of serotonin (5-HT)[Q] It is strongly associated with metastatic disease.

Cardiac lesions are present in 50% of the patients with the *carcinoid syndrome.* They consist of **fibrous intimal thickenings** on the inside surfaces of the cardiac chambers and valvular leaflets. And are located mainly in the **right ventricle, tricuspid and pulmonic valves**, and *occasionally in the major blood vessels.* The commonest cardiac manifestation is the *tricuspid regurgitation* (tricuspid stenosis is relatively uncommon) followed by pulmonary regurgitation.

Hepatic metastasis is usually present in this tumor. The **most sensitive screening test** for small intestine carcinoids is the **plasma level of chromogranin A**. The levels of 5-HT and its metabolite *5-hydroxyindoleacetic acid*[Q] (5-HIAA) is elevated in the urine.

POLYPS

Polyps are seen most commonly in colon but can also be seen in other parts of GIT.

Polyps

Non-Inflammantory	Neoplastic polyps
• Inflammatory polyp • Hyperplastic polyps • Hamartomatous polyps: they of 2 types – Juvenile polyp (MC in rectum) – Peutz jegher polyp (MC in jejunum)	• Adenomatous polyp – Tubular adenoma (most common) – Villous adenomas (maximum malignant potential) – Tubulovillous adenoma

Concept

• Dysplasia may be seen in a small number of juvenile polyps and the juvenile polyposis syndrome is associated with increased risk of colonic cancer.

• Peutz Jegher polyp is a benign polyp but Peutz Jegher's syndrome is characterized by multiple hamartomatous polyps scattered throughout the GIT and melanotic mucosal and cutaneous pigmentation around the lips, oral mucosa, face, genitalia and palmar surface of the hands.

Adenomatous polyps are usually asymptomatic.

Also Know

Hamartomatous polyps can occur sporadically or as a part of syndromes such as Juvenile polyposis, Peutz-Jegher syndrome, Cowden syndrome and Cronkhite-Canada syndrome. All these syndromes have autosomal dominant inheritance **except Cronkhite-Canada syndrome, which is a non-hereditary disorder.**

CARCINOMA OF THE COLON

The cancer of the colon is seen frequently in old age (peak age 60-79 years). It is an **adenocarcinoma** in almost all the patients. The risk factors for the colon cancer are:

A. GENETIC FACTORS

i. *Hereditary Non-polyposis Colon Cancer (HNPCC) syndrome* (also called as **Lynch syndrome**[Q])

It is an autosomal dominant condition characterized by the increased incidence of colon cancer and extraintestinal cancer particularly the ovarian and endometrial cancer. The hallmark is the *mutation in the DNA repair genes (MSH2 and MLH1) leading to microsatellite instability*. Colon cancers in these patients affect **right or ascending colon** and occurs at younger age (<50 years). The proximal colon tumors in HNPCC have a better prognosis than sporadic tumors from patients of similar age.

ii. *Familial Adenomatous Polyposis (FAP)*

It is caused by the mutation of adenomatous polyposis coli (APC) gene present on the long arm of chromosome 5^Q (5q21). Some FAP patients without APC mutation have a mutation in the nucleotide base excision repair gene called MUTYH. Colorectal carcinoma develop in 100% of untreated FAP patients often before age 30. As a result, prophylactic colectomy is the standard therapy in patients with APC mutations.

Subtypes of FAP

Classic FAP syndrome

- The patient has a large number of adenomatous polyps and retinal pigment epithelial hypertrophy. There should be a minimum of *100 polyps^Q* to make a diagnosis of this syndrome. Most of the adenomatous polyps are tubular polyps.

Attenuated FAP syndrome

- The patient has a lower number of adenomatous polyps (around 30) which are located in proximal colon.

Gardener syndrome^Q

- Intestinal polyps + epidermal cysts + fibromatosis + osteomas (of the mandible, long bones and skull).

Turcot syndrome^Q

- Adenomatous colon polyposis + CNS tumors (medulloblastoma in 2/3rd and gliomas in 1/3rd patients).

iii. *Mutations affecting p53 and K-RAS genes*

B. ENVIRONMENTAL FACTORS

Factors increasing risk	Factors decreasing risk
• Increased calorie intake and obesity^Q	• Increased intake of dietary fiber^Q
• Decreased intake of micronutrients	• Intake of ω-3 fatty acids (fish)^Q
• Smoking and alcohol^Q	• NSAID use (especially Aspirin)^Q
• Streptococcus bovis septicemia or endocarditis	• Intake of folic acid and calcium^Q
• Ureterosigmoidostomy^Q	• Hormone replacement therapy
• Inflammatory bowel disease^Q	
• Acromegaly	
• Pelvis irradiation	

Molecular pathogenesis

1. **APC/β-catenin pathway** (also called *adenoma-carcinoma sequence*): Loss of tumor suppressor APC gene is followed by increased β-catenin transcriptional activity (normal APC protein degrades β-catenin) leading to localized colon epithelial proliferation and formation of small adenoma. This is followed by dysplastic change due to activating mutation in K-ras and inhibition of tumor suppressor genes like SMAD2, SMAD4 and p53 leads ultimately to cancer.

2. **Microsatellite instability pathway**: Genetic lesions in 90% cases involve **MSH2 and MLH1 genes** which are *DNA mismatch repair genes*. These genes correct any genetic disruption which may arise whenever the colonic cells are multiplying rapidly. Any mutation in these genes causes activation of BRAF and inhibition of BAX protein

Concept

Prophylactic colectomy in FAP **does not** decrease risk for cancer due to adenomas at other sites specially ampulla of Vater and stomach.

and TGF-β type II gene thereby increasing the chances of development of colonic cancer. Kras and p53 are not typically mutated.

Colon cancer exemplifies the concept of Multi-step carcinogenesis

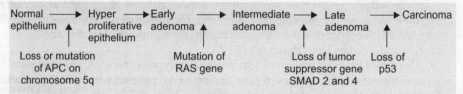

MORPHOLOGY

Most of the cancers arise from the **rectum**[Q] *followed by the sigmoid colon*. Microscopically, it is an adenocarcinoma and invasive cancers invoke a strong desmoplastic response. Cancers in the **anorectal region** are **squamous cell cancers**.

CLINICAL FEATURES OF COLORECTAL CARCINOMA

Features	Right sided/proximal	Left sided/distal
Sites in colon	Caecum and ascending colon	Descending colon and sigmoid colon
Gross appearance	Fungating/ulcerative type polypoid carcinoma Large cauliflower-like soft friable mass projecting into lumen	Obstructive type Carcinomatous ulcers have Napkin ring configuration
Infiltration	Absent	Present
Clinical features	Fatigue, weakness, Iron deficiency anemia, bleed readily	Occult bleeding change in bowel habits carmpy lower left quadrant discomfort, Melena, diarrhea, constipation
Diagnosis	Later	Early stage (theoretically) due to symptoms
Prognosis	Good	Poor

Metastasis occurs in order of preference, to regional lymph nodes, liver, lungs and bones.

Diagnosis

- **Tumor markers:** Colonic cancer is associated with the elevated levels of tumor markers CEA (carcinoembryonic antigen) and CA 19-9.

- **Colonoscopy** may also be done which helps in the direct visualization of the cancer and may also be used to take a biopsy. **Gross** appearance of the colon is called as **"napkin ring"**[Q] **appearance** (caused by annular and constricting lesions in distal colon).

Most important prognostic indicator of colon cancer is the **stage** which means the extent of tumor at the time of diagnosis. **Duke's staging** was used for colon cancer which has *now been replaced by the TNM staging*.

TREATMENT

- *Right colon cancer* is surgically treated with *resection and ileocolic anastomosis* whereas for *Left sided colon* cancer, *Hartman's procedure* (surgical resection of the affected lesion and proximal diversion with the help of colostomy) is done.

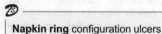

Napkin ring configuration ulcers have increased fibrous tissue forming annular ring and have central ulceration with slightly elevated margins

The **occult blood loss** in the stool can be detected with the help of **Guaiac test**.

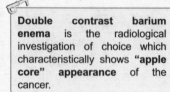

Double contrast barium enema is the radiological investigation of choice which characteristically shows **"apple core" appearance** of the cancer.

Gastrointestinal Tract

MULTIPLE CHOICE QUESTIONS

ESOPHAGUS

1. Barrett's esophagus shows   *(AIIMS May 2010)*
   (a) Intestinal dysplasia
   (b) Intestinal metaplasia
   (c) Columnar cell metaplasia
   (d) Columnar cell dysplasia

2. Predisposing factor for esophageal cancer is all except
   (a) Mediastinal fibrosis   *(AIIMS May 2009)*
   (b) Diverticula
   (c) Caustic alkali burn
   (d) HPV

3. Most common cause of esophagitis is
   (a) Smoking   *(AIIMS May 2009)*
   (b) Alcohol
   (c) Reflux disease
   (d) Increased intake of spices

4. Best site for taking biopsy for viral esophagitis is
   (a) Edge of ulcer   *(AIIMS Nov 2001)*
   (b) Base of ulcer
   (c) Adjacent indurated area around ulcer
   (d) Surrounding normal mucosa

5. Which of the following viruses does not produce viral esophagitis?   *(Delhi PG 2009)*
   (a) Herpes   (b) Adenovirus
   (c) Varicella   (d) Cytomegalovirus

6. Which of the following is true about Barret's esophagus?
   (a) Squamous to columnar metaplasia   *(Delhi PG-2007)*
   (b) Columnar to squamous metaplasia
   (c) Does not increase risk of malignancy
   (d) None of the above

7. Barrett esophagus can result from: *(UP 2004)*
   (a) *H. pylori* infection
   (b) *H. simplex* infection
   (c) Gastroesophageal reflux
   (d) Varices

8. Plummer-Vinson syndrome is characterized by all except: *(UP 2006)*
   (a) Glossitis
   (b) Esophageal webs
   (c) Megaloblastic anemia
   (d) Esophageal dysphagia

9. A 60- year-old man Jivan Kumar with a 4-year history of GERD presents with persistent pyrosis (hearburn) and acid regurgitation. He has had similar symptoms for the past 4years. Considering the long history of GERD, an upper GI endoscopy is performed to rule out Barrett esophagus. However, the results reveal that Barrett esophagus, is indeed present. Which of the following is true of Barrett esophagus?
   (a) A biopsy will show a histologic finding of columnar to squamous metaplasia.
   (b) It is a known precursor of carcinoma of the stomach.
   (c) The most common location is the proximal (upper) third of the esophagus.
   (d) It is a known precursor of adenocarcinoma of the esopohagus.

10. A 50 year old male Grisham who complains of nocturnal cough undergoes an esophageal biopsy which shows elongation of the lamina propriae, many eosinophils, and occasional neutrophils within the squamous epithelium. He takes metformin and enalapril for his diabetes and hypertension. He is started on omeprazole: after 2 weeks, his coughing symptoms resolve. Which of the following is the most likely cause of his symptoms?
    (a) Pill-induced esophageal mucosa damage
    (b) Gastroesophageal junction incompetence
    (c) Mucosal disruption from fungal infection
    (d) Absent esophageal peristaltic movements

11. A 80 year old man Baba complains of pain in the upper portion of his neck on swallowing. He occasionally regurgitates undigested food shortly after eating. Which of the following is the most likely etiology of his problems?
    (a) Mallory-Weiss tears
    (b) Zenker's diverticulum
    (c) Schatzki rings
    (d) Traction diverticula

12. A 43-year-old female Divya with chronic dysphagia undergoes an upper endoscopy that reveals massive dilation of the distal esophagus. The esophagus is kinked and tortuous and partly filled with undigested foods. What is the most likely diagnosis for this patient?
    (a) Achalasia
    (b) Barrett's esophagus
    (c) Hiatal hernia
    (d) Plummer-Vinson syndrome

13. Which of the following locations is most likely for the development of carcinoma in a 50-year-old mason who has chewed tobacco for 25 years?
    (a) Floor of the mouth
    (b) Lower lip
    (c) Tongue
    (d) Buccal mucosa

14. A middle aged man Nitesh complains of increasing difficulty in swallowing over the past 3 years. He reports a feeling of pressure in his chest occurring 2-3 seconds after swallowing a solid bolus. He also experiences regurgitation of undigested food eaten hours previously. Manometry shows the absence of esophageal peristalsis with swallowing and a lower esophageal sphincter that fails to relax. What is the most likely diagnosis?
   (a) Achalasia
   (b) Diffuse esophageal spasm
   (c) Incompetent lower esophageal sphincter
   (d) Oropharyngeal dysphagia

Most Recent Questions

14.1. Most common anatomical location of tongue cancer is:
   (a) Anterior third
   (b) Lateral margin
   (c) Dorsum
   (d) Posterior third

14.2. All are precancerous for carcinoma of esophagus except:
   (a) Achalasia
   (b) Peterson Kelly syndrome
   (c) Zenker diverticulum
   (d) Ectodermal dysplasia

STOMACH: GASTRITIS, PUD, GIST, GASTRIC CANCER

15. A 50 years old male presents with obstructive symptoms. Biopsy of stomach reveals the likely diagnosis to be gastrointestinal stromal tumour (GIST). The most appropriate marker for this tumor would be which of the following?   *(AIIMS May 2011)*
   (a) CD 34
   (b) CD 117
   (c) CD 30
   (d) CD 10

16. Sister Mary Joseph nodule is most commonly seen in with which of the following?   *(AIIMS May 2010)*
   (a) Ovarian cancer
   (b) Stomach cancer
   (c) Colon cancer
   (d) Pancreatic cancer

17. Most appropriate marker of GIST:
   (a) CD117   *(AI 2010, AIIMS Nov 09)*
   (b) CD 34
   (c) CK
   (d) Vimentin

18. Which of the following is a specific marker for GIST?
   (a) CD 117   *(AI 2009)*
   (b) CD34
   (c) CD23
   (d) S-100

19. Which one of the following is the most significant risk factor for development of gastric carcinoma?   *(AI 2006)*
   (a) Paneth cell metaplasia
   (b) Pyloric metaplasia
   (c) Intestinal metaplasia
   (d) Ciliated metaplasia

20. When carcinoma of stomach develops secondarily to pernicious anemia, it is usually situated in the:
   (a) Prepyloric region   *(AI 2006)*
   (b) Pylorus
   (c) Body
   (d) Fundus

21. Sister Mary Joseph nodules are found in:
   (a) Gastric carcinoma   *(AIIMS May 2009)*
   (b) Pancreatic carcinoma
   (c) Lung carcinoma
   (d) Ovary carcinoma

22. Gastrointestinal stromal malignancy arises from which of the following: *(AIIMS May 2002)*
   (a) Smooth muscle
   (b) Nerve cells
   (c) Interstitial cells of Cajal
   (d) Vascular endothelium

23. Histologic examination of the lesion in stomach reveal fat-laden cells, likely cause is:
   (a) Lymphoma   *(AIIMS Nov 2001)*
   (b) Postgastrectomy
   (c) Signet-cell carcinoma stomach
   (d) Atrophic gastritis

24. The following have strong causal association with *H. pylori* infection except   *(Karnataka 2008)*
   (a) Chronic gastritis
   (b) Peptic ulcer disease
   (c) Gastric carcinoma
   (d) Gastric adenoma

25. In early gastric carcinoma malignancy is confined to
   (a) Mucosa   *(Karnataka 2004)*
   (b) Mucosa and submucosa
   (c) Gastric wall without lymph node metastasis
   (d) Gastric glands

26. In pernicious anemia, antibody is formed against:
   (a) G-cell   *(Bihar 2006)*
   (b) Parietal cell
   (c) Stem cell
   (d) All

27. A 60 years old fashion photographer and smoker Alok Nath complaints of severe nausea, vomiting, early satiety, and a 10 kg weight loss over the past 5 months. His physical examination reveals the presence of mild muscle wasting. An upper GI endoscopy reveals the erosion of entire gastric mucosa. In addition, there is presence of erythematous cobblestone appearance of the mucosa. The stomach is also found to be shrunken and reduced in size. Upper gastrointestinal radiographs

show that the stomach is small and shrunken. Which of the following is the likely microscopic finding in this man?
(a) Early gastric carcinoma
(b) Gastrointestinal stromal tumor
(c) Signet ring cell adenocarcinoma
(d) Chronic atrophic gastritis

28. A 56-year-old man with a history of glomerulonephritis is diagnosed with renal failure. The man subsequently complains of heartburn and nausea, and gives a history that he has been vomiting each morning for the last few days. Which of the following forms of gastritis would most likely be found in this patient?
(a) Acute gastritis
(b) Chronic antral gastritis
(c) Lymphocytic gastritis
(d) Hypertrophic gastritis

29. Which of the following conditions would mostly likely be associated with chronic gastritis (Type A) resulting from autoimmune destruction of parietal cells?
(a) Decreased growth of luminal bacteria
(b) Decreased likelihood of developing gastric carcinoma
(c) Decreased plasma concentration of gastrin
(d) Increased production of macrocytic red blood cells

30. Which of the following sites contains striated muscle that is not under voluntary control?
(a) Bladder
(b) Colon
(c) Esophagus
(d) Gallbladder

31. An old man being evaluated for abdominal pain and weight loss undergoes endoscopy showing a broad region of the gastric wall in which the rugae are flattened. Biopsy of this area shows infiltration by numerous polygonal tumor cells with small, dark, round or ovoid nuclei pushed to the margin of the cell by large, clear, cytoplasmic structures. These cells might be expected to have which of the following properties?
(a) Keratohyalin granules observed by electron microscopy
(b) Melanosomes and premelanosomes by electron microscopy
(c) Positive staining for gastrin by light microscopy
(d) Positive staining for mucin by light microscopy

Most Recent Questions

31.1. Most common site of GIST is:
(a) Ileum   (b) Esophagus
(c) Colon   (d) Stomach

31.2. Which of the following is not true about GIST?
(a) Stomach is the most common site
(b) High propensity of malignant change
(c) Associated with c-KIT mutation
(d) Histology shows spindle shaped cells

31.3. One of the following can have malignant transformation:
(a) Gastric ulcer
(b) Duodenal ulcer
(c) Stomal ulcer
(d) Stress ulcer

31.4. Gastrointestinal stromal tumor originates in which of the following?
(a) Parietal cells
(b) Chief cells
(c) Neuroendocrine cells
(d) Interstitial cells of Cajal

31.5. Which of the following artery is responsible for duodenal ulcer hemorrhage?
(a) Superior pancreaticoduodenal artery
(b) Inferior pancreaticodudenal artery
(c) Gastroduodenal artery
(d) Left gastric artery

31.6. The best prognosis is gastric carcinoma is in type:
(a) Linitis plastic
(b) Polypoidal growth
(c) Ulcerative
(d) Superficial spreading

INTESTINE: INFECTIONS, MALABSORPTION DISEASES

32. Which of the following is a histological feature of Whipple's disease?   *(AI 2008)*
(a) Infiltration of histiocytes in the lamina propria
(b) Granuloma in the lamina
(c) Macrophages with PAS (+) material inside the lamina propria
(d) Eosinophils in the lamina propria

33. Gluten sensitive enteropathy is most strongly associated with: *(AI 2003)*
(a) HLA-DQ2   (b) HLA-DR4
(c) HLA-DQ3   (d) Blood group 'B'

34. In the intra-epithelial region of the mucosa of intestine the predominant cell population is that of   *(AI 2002)*
(a) B cell   (b) T-cells
(c) Plasma cells   (d) Basophils

35. Macrophages containing large quantities of undigested and partial digested bacteria in intestine are seen in
(a) Whipple's disease   *(AI 2002)*
(b) Amyloidosis
(c) Immunoproliferative small intestinal disease
(d) *Vibrio cholerae* infection

36. The histological features of celiac disease include all of the following, except: *(AI 2002)*
(a) Crypt hyperplasia
(b) Increase in thickness of the mucosa
(c) Increase in intraepithelial lymphocytes
(d) Increase in inflammatory cells in lamina propria

37. **Type of anemia caused by Ileocecal TB:**
    (a) Iron – deficiency   *(AIIMS Nov 2009)*
    (b) Megaloblastic
    (c) Sideroblastic
    (d) Normocytic Normochromic

38. **The following cereals should be avoided in patients with celiac diseases, except:** *(AIIMS Nov 2003)*
    (a) Wheat   (b) Barley
    (c) Maize   (d) Rye

39. **Which of the following organs is not involved in Whipple's disease?** *(Delhi PG 2009)*
    (a) Heart   (b) CNS
    (c) Lungs   (d) GI Tract

40. **Morphological features of celiac disease include all except:** *(Delhi PG 2009 RP)*
    (a) Increase in intraepithelial lymphocytes
    (b) Increase in crypt: villous ratio
    (c) Distended macrophages with PAS positive granules in lamina propria
    (d) Elongated hyperplastic and tortuous crypts

41. **All are true about amoebic ulcer except:** *(UP 2002)*
    (a) Commonest site is ascending colon and cecum
    (b) Flask shaped ulcer
    (c) Perforation is common
    (d) Paucity of inflammatory cells

42. **Intestinal biopsy in not diagnostic in** *(UP 2002)*
    (a) Abetalipoproteinemia
    (b) Tropical sprue
    (c) Agammaglobulinemia
    (d) Intestinal lymphangiectasis

43. **Transverse ulcers are seen in:** *(UP 2004)*
    (a) Typhoid   (b) Tuberculosis
    (c) Amoebiasis   (d) Ulcerative colitis

44. **Aphthous ulcers are also known as** *(UP 2007)*
    (a) Canker sores   (b) Marjolin's ulcer
    (c) Curling's ulcer (d) Cushing's ulcer

45. **All are complication of typhoid ulcers except:** *(UP 2008)*
    (a) Perforation   (b) Stricture formation
    (c) Hemorrhage   (d) Sepsis

46. **Which one of the following tumors is most commonly associated with pseudomyxoma peritonei?** *(AP 2006)*
    (a) Appendix   (b) Gall bladder
    (c) Stomach   (d) Pancreas

47. **All are true about typhoid ulcer except:**
    (a) Mainly affects ileum   *(Kolkata 2005)*
    (b) Multiple ulcer and transverse
    (c) Perforation occurs at 3rd week
    (d) Perforation treated by surgery

48. **A 28 year old lady Kulraj Kandhawa presents to the medicine OPD with complaints of diarrhea and fatigue. She also had weight loss of 4 kg over last 5 months. Her physical examination is non significant** and investigations do not reveal occult blood, ova, or parasites in the stool. An endoscopy is performed and after thorough microscopic examination, her diet is modified. She is started on a special diet with no wheat or barley grain products. The dietary substitution causes marked improvement in her symptoms. Which of the following is the most likely microscopic finding to be seen in the biopsy specimen?
    (a) Lymphatic obstruction
    (b) Noncaseating granulomas
    (c) Atrophy of the villi with blunting and flatterning
    (d) Foamy macrophages within the lamina propria

49. **A middle aged man Humesh was cooking in his kitchen when there was an accidental cooking gas cylinder bursting episode. He suffered extensive burns for which he is admitted to Burns Care Hospital. The patient was stabilized by the health care team but after 15 days, he passed altered colored (black) stools. His blood pressure also dropped and his hematocrit just is 20%. The patient worsened within a short time and eventually expired. If an autopsy is conducted, which of the following organs would show the presence of gastrointestinal ulcerations?**
    (a) Esophagus   (b) Stomach
    (c) Duodenum   (d) Ileum

50. **A complete endoscopic examination is performed on a middle aged female Bebo having abdominal pain and alteration in the bowel habits. She was reassured by her gastroenterologist Dr. S. Sarin that her lesions were non malignant in nature. Which of the following is most likely to have been picked up by her physician?**
    (a) Colorectal villous adenoma
    (b) Crohn disease
    (c) Duodenal peptic ulcer
    (d) Familial multiple polyposis

51. **A woman Mallika Sehrawat presents to the medicine OPD with complaint of low volume watery diarrhea associated with flatulence. The symptoms occur off and on and have been present since 10 months. She has no fever, nausea, vomiting or abdominal pain but has lost 3.5 kg weight during this period. Her stool test is negative for occult blood, ova, and parasites, and a stool culture. Endoscopy is performed and the biopsy from the duodenum shows villous atrophy with a chronic inflammatory infiltrate in the lamina propria. Which of the following antibodies is likely to be seen in this patient?**
    (a) Anticentromeric antibody
    (b) Anti-DNA topoisomerase I antibody
    (c) Antimitochondrial antibody
    (d) Antigliadin antibody

52. **Over the last 6 months, a 40 year old lady has noticed gradual yellowing of her skin. She visits her physician who observes that she is afebrile and has scleral icterus and generalized jaundice. Her blood investigations**

reveal total serum bilirubin of 9.2 mg.dL; direct bilirubin of 7.0 mg/dL, serum ALT of 120 U/L, and serum AST of 110 U/L. A liver biopsy is performed which on microscopic examination shows sclerosing cholangitis. Which of the following disease of the gastrointestinal tract may coexist in this lady?
(a) Chronic pancreatitis
(b) Diverticulosis
(c) Celiac sprue
(d) Ulcerative colitis

53. A patient who recently underwent a gastrectomy procedure complains of nausea, diarrhea, sweating, palpitations, and flushing soon after eating a meal. This patient should be instructed to
(a) eat less frequent, larger meals that are high in carbohydrates
(b) eat more frequent, smaller meals that are high in fat
(c) eat more frequent, larger meals that are high in protein
(d) eat more frequent, smaller meals that are high in carbohydrates

54. A female patient has severe arthritis involving the lower back. Before making a diagnosis of ankylosing spondylitis, the patient should be questioned by the physician about which of the following diseases?
(a) Carcinoid syndrome
(b) Celiac disease
(c) Crohn's disease
(d) Whipple's disease

55. A patient with intestinal malabsorption is found to markedly improve when flour products (bread, noodles, etc.) are removed from his diet. At the height of the patient's disease, marked histologic changes would be seen at which of the following sites?
(a) Distal large bowel
(b) Distal small bowel
(c) Proximal small bowel
(d) Entire small bowel

56. A 25-year-old man presents to a rheumatologist with complaints of joint pain involving the large joints of the legs which exacerbates frequently accompanied by diarrhea. Which of the following gastrointestinal diseases is most likely to be implicated as the cause of the patient's joint problems?
(a) Amebic colitis
(b) Chronic appendicitis
(c) Diverticulosis
(d) Ulcerative colitis

57. Based on epidemiological studies, which of the following has been found to be most protective against colon cancer? *(AIIMS May 2011)*
(a) High fiber diet   (b) Low fat diet
(c) Low selenium diet (d) Low protein diet

Most Recent Questions

57.1. Diverticulum most common site is:
(a) Sigmoid colon   (b) Ileum
(c) Ascending colon (d) Transverse colon

57.2. Which of the following is the commonest site of intestinal tuberculosis?
(a) Stomach   (b) Jejunum
(c) Ileum   (d) Colon

57.3. The most common site for amoebiasis:
(a) Sigmoid colon   (b) Transverse colon
(c) Cecum   (d) Liver

57.4. Anti-gliadin antibodies are detectable in:
(a) Tropical sprue
(b) Whipple's disease
(c) Celiac disease
(d) Intestinal lymphoma

57.5. Which of the following is not associated with celiac sprue?
(a) Turner syndrome
(b) Down syndrome
(c) Klinefleter syndrome
(d) Type 1 diabetes

57.6. Paneth cells contain:
(a) Zinc   (b) Copper
(c) Molybdenum   (d) Selenium

57.7. Which is incorrect of typhoid ulcers:
(a) Hemorrhage is common
(b) Occurs on lymphoid aggregation
(c) Horizontal ulcers
(d) Longitudinal ulcers

57.8. Perforation of typhoid ulcer usually occurs during which week?
(a) 1st   (b) 2nd
(c) 3rd   (d) 4th

57.9. Serum amylase level are raised in all of the following EXCEPT:
(a) Duodeneal ulcer perforation
(b) Pancreatitis
(c) Appendicitis
(d) Small Bowel Strangulation

57.10. Which of the following is not considered a premalignant lesion:
(a) Leukoplakia
(b) Erythroplakia
(c) Chronic hyperplastic candidiasis
(d) Oral lichen planus

57.11. Diagnosis of typhoid in first week is by:
(a) Widal test
(b) Stool culture
(c) Urine culture
(d) Blood culture

57.12. Purtscher's retinopathy is seen in:
(a) Meningitis
(b) Pancreatitis
(c) Uncontrolled hypertension
(d) Unilateral carotid artery occlusion

57.13. Usually, gall stones consists of these types, except:
(a) Oxalate
(b) Bile salts
(c) Bile pigments
(d) Cholesterol

INTESTINE: IBD, POLYP, TUMOURS

58. Most important prognostic factor for colorectal carcinoma is *(AIIMS May 2011)*
(a) Site of lesion
(b) Tumour size and characteristics
(c) Age of patient
(d) Lymph node status

59. Which of the following is NOT true about FAP?
(a) AR inheritance *(AIIMS May 2011)*
(b) Screening done by sigmoidoscopy
(c) Polyps develop in early adulthood
(d) Epidermal cysts and osteomas may occur

60. In Peutz-Jeghers syndrome, polyps are mainly seen in
(a) Rectum *(AIIMS May 2010)*
(b) Colon
(c) Esophagus
(d) Jejunum

61. Which of the following is not true about FAP?
(AIIMS May 2010, May 2011)
(a) Autosomal recessive inheritance
(b) Screening done by sigmoidoscopy
(c) Polyps develop in early adulthood
(d) Epidermal cysts and osteomas may occur

62. Colon carcinoma is associated with all except:
(a) Rb *(AI 2009)*
(b) Mismatch repair genes
(c) APC
(d) β-catenin

63. In ulcerative colitis, which of the following is seen?
(a) Cryptitis *(AIIMS May 2008)*
(b) Crypt loss
(c) Crypt branching
(d) Proliferating mucosa

64. Which of the following would be the best morphological feature to distinguish ulcerative colitis from Crohn's disease? *(AIIMS May 2004)*
(a) Diffuse distribution of pseudopolyps
(b) Mucosal edema
(c) Crypt abscesses
(d) Lymphoid aggregates in the mucosa

65. Which of the following statements about Crohn's disease is incorrect? *(Delhi PG 2009)*
(a) Granulomas present frequently
(b) It is separate and distinct from ulcerative colitis
(c) Cigarette smoking is a risk factor
(d) Rectum spared in 50% patients with large bowel involvement

66. Commonest endocrine tumour of pancreas artses from which of the following cells? *(Karnataka 2009)*
(a) α cells   (b) β cells
(c) Delta cells   (d) VIPoma

67. Skin lesions are seen in *(Karnataka 2006)*
(a) Ulcerative colitis   (b) Crohn's disease
(c) Both (a) and (b)   (d) None of the above

68. Polyps in Peutz-Jegher's syndrome are
(a) Adenomatous polyps *(Karnataka 2004, 2008)*
(b) Hyperplastic polyps
(c) Hamartomatous polyps
(d) Pseudopolyps

69. All are malignant in nature except *(UP 2000)*
(a) Juvenile polyp   (b) Familial polyp
(c) Carcinoid tumor (d) Villous adenoma

70. All are true about Crohn's disease except
(a) Rectal involvement is common *(UP 2001)*
(b) Granuloma formation
(c) Erythema nodosum
(d) Fistula formation

71. Most common tumor of appendix is *(UP 2005)*
(a) Carcinoid tumor
(b) Pseudomyxoma-peritonitis
(c) Adenocarcinoma
(d) Mucocele

72. Skip lesions are seen in *(UP 2005)*
(a) Ulcerative colitis
(b) Crohn's disease
(c) Carcinoid syndrome
(d) Whipple's disease

73. Fistula is most common in *(UP 2007)*
(a) Crohn's disease
(b) Ulcerative colitis
(c) Infective enterocolitis
(d) Celiac sprue

74. Most common site of carcinoid tumor is *(RJ 2000)*
(a) Stomach   (b) Jejunum
(c) Distal ileum   (d) Appendix

75. Most common site of carcinoma pancreas is *(RJ 2000)*
(a) Head   (b) Body
(c) Tail   (d) Equal incidence at all sites

76. Carcinoid tumor produces all except *(RJ 2003)*
(a) Flushing   (b) Diarrhea
(c) Bronchodilation (d) Raynaud's phenomenon

Gastrointestinal Tract

77. **Which organ is always involved in ulcerative colitis?**
    (a) Jejunum   *(RJ 2005)*
    (b) Ileum
    (c) Rectosigmoid
    (d) Duodenum

78. **Two identical specimen of the intestine obtained following colectomy shows on examination hemorrhagic cobblestone appearance; one of them however, shows longitudinal grooving. It is likely to be a specimen of:**
    (a) Ulcerative colitis   *(Kolkata 2002)*
    (b) Ischemic colitis
    (c) Multiple polyposis
    (d) Crohn's disease

79. **Carcinoma of colon is associated with all except:**
    (a) High fat diet   *(Kolkata 2005)*
    (b) High fiber diet
    (c) Streptococcus bovis infection
    (d) Ulcerative colitis

80. **Backwash ileitis is seen in:**   *(Bihar 2006)*
    (a) Crohn's disease
    (b) Ulcerative colitis
    (c) Colonic carcinoma
    (d) Ileal polyp

81. **Granulomatous inflammation is found in:** *(Bihar 2006)*
    (a) Crohn's disease   (b) Ulcerative colitis
    (c) Amoebiasis   (d) Giardiasis

82. **Continuous involvement of colonic mucosa is seen in:**
    (a) Ulcerative colitis   *(Bihar 2006)*
    (b) Crohn's disease
    (c) Carcinoma colon
    (d) Colonic polyp

83. **All are true about carcinoid syndrome except:**
    (a) Wheezing   *(Jharkhand 2006)*
    (b) Pulmonary stenosis
    (c) Flushing
    (d) Splenomegaly

84. **A 24 year old male Anil B. with a 4-year history of abdominal pain, periodic diarrhea, low-grade fever, and easy fatigability is found to have an enteroenteric fistula on contrast radiography. Colonoscopy shows "cobblestone" mucosa that has linear ulcerations with "skip areas" of normal bowel wall. Which of the following is the most likely explanation of fistula formation in this patient?**
    (a) Intramural granulomas
    (b) Transmural inflammation
    (c) Marked lymphoid reaction
    (d) Skip lesions of the intestinal wall

85. **A 51 year young man Firdaus had been receiving antibiotics for severe folliculitis. He develops fever, toxicity, and severe diarrhoea. Which of the following is the most likely diagnosis?**

    (a) CMV infection
    (b) Pseudomembranous colitis
    (c) Ulcerative colitis
    (d) Whipple disease

86. **A 50-year-old man Bhupi presents to his doctor with diarrhea, flushing and wheezing. Physical examination is significant for a grade II/VI diastolic murmur located at the right sternal border at the 4th intercostal space. Which of the following substances is most likely to be elevated in this patient's urine?**
    (a) 5-HIAA   (b) HVA
    (c) Phenylalanine   (d) Selegiline

87. **Biopsy of a small, rounded rectal polyp demonstrates glands and sawtooth crypts composed of a proliferation of goblet and columnar epithelial cells. No atypia is seen. This polyp is best classified as which of the following?**
    (a) Hyperplastic polyp
    (b) Peutz-Jeghers polyp
    (c) Tubular adenoma
    (d) Tubulovillous adenoma

Most Recent Questions

87.1. **Toxic megacolon is seen in:**
    (a) Chronic nonspecific ulcerative colitis
    (b) Crohn's disease
    (c) Colonic diverticulosis
    (d) Hamartomatous polyp

87.2. **Which of the following is inheritance of Gardner syndrome?**
    (a) Autosomal recessive
    (b) Autosomal dominant
    (c) X linked dominant
    (d) X linked recessive

87.3. **Osteomas, adenomatous polyps of intestine and periampullary carcinomas are seen in which oif the following conditions?**
    (a) Cowden syndrome
    (b) Peutz Jegers syndrome
    (c) FAP
    (d) Gardener syndrome

87.4. **True about ulcerative colitis, all except:**
    (a) Rectum involved
    (b) Pseudopolyps
    (c) Pancolitis
    (d) Noncaseating granuloma

87.5. **Which of the following is the most common location of carcinoid tumour?**
    (a) Pancreas
    (b) Lung
    (c) Gastrointestinal tract
    (d) Gonads

87.6. Carcinoid tumour develops from:
- (a) Hematopioetic cells
- (b) Kulschitsky cells
- (c) Neuroglial cells
- (d) Chromaffin cell

87.7. Pseudopolyps are seen in:
- (a) Crohn's disease
- (b) Ulcerative colitis
- (c) Juvenile polyposis
- (d) Tuberculosis

87.8. The highest malignant potential is seen in:
- (a) Crohn's disease
- (b) Ulcerative colitis
- (c) Familial polyposis
- (d) Infantile polyp

87.9. Commonest malignant small intestinal tumor
- (a) Adenocarcinoma
- (b) Lymphosarcoma
- (c) Leiomyosarcoma
- (d) Carcinoid tumor

87.10. Most common site of carcinoma pancreas is
- (a) Head
- (b) Body
- (c) Tail
- (d) None

87.11. Which of the following is a special stain for rhabdo-myosarcoma?
- (a) Cytokeratin
- (b) Synaptophysin
- (c) Desmin
- (d) Myeloperoxidase

87.12. Which of the following type of anemia would be associated with carcinoma of the colon?
- (a) Megaloblastic anemia
- (b) Iron deficiency anemia
- (c) Aplastic anemia
- (d) Hemolytic anemia

87.13. Following statements regarding ulcerative colitis is:
- (a) Smoking does not have a protective effect
- (b) Smoking has a protective effect
- (c) No relation with smoking
- (d) Smoking causing relapses

87.14. Zollinger Ellison syndrome is not caused by tumors from:
- (a) Pancreas
- (b) Ovary
- (c) Colon
- (d) Duodenum

87.15. Crohn disease is associated with:
- (a) NOD2/CARD15 gene
- (b) P53 gene
- (c) Philadelphia chromosome
- (d) BRCA1 gene

87.16. A highly sensitive and specific marker for detecting intestinal inflammation in ulcerative colitis is:
- (a) CRP
- (b) Fecal lactoferrin
- (c) Fecal calprotectin
- (d) Leukocytosis

87.17. The minimum number of polyps necessary for a diagnosis of Familial Adenomatous Polyposis (FAP) is:
- (a) 05
- (b) 10
- (c) 50
- (d) 100

87.18. Antibody suggestive of diagnosis of ulcerative colitis?
- (a) p-ANCA
- (b) c-ANCA
- (c) A.M.A
- (d) A.N.A

EXPLANATIONS

1. **Ans. (b) Intestinal metaplasia** *(Ref: Robbins 8th/770, 9/e 757)*
   Direct quote from Robbins …. 'Barrett esophagus is a complication of chronic GERD that is characterized by intestinal metaplasia within the esophageal squamous mucosa'.

2. **Ans. (a) Mediastinal fibrosis** *(Ref: Robbins 7th/607, 8th/773, 9/e p758-759)*
   - **External beam irradiation** but **not mediastinal fibrosis** is a risk factor for esophageal cancer.
   - **HPV DNA** is found frequently in esophageal squmaous cell carcinoma in high incidence regions..Robbins 7th/807
   - **Caustic ingestion, achalasia, bulimia, tylosis** (an inherited autosomal dominant trait), **Plummer-Vinson syndrome, external-beam radiation,** and **esophageal diverticula** all have known associations with squamous cell cancer......
     ...Sabiston textbook of surgery 18th edn

3. **Ans. (c) Reflux disease** *(Ref: Robbins 8th/769, 9/e p755)*
   Robbins clearly states that "*Reflux of gastric contents into the lower esophagus is the most important cause of esophagitis*".

4. **Ans. (a) Edge of the ulcer** *(Ref: Robbins 8th/768)*
   - *Herpes viruses* typically cause *punched-out ulcers*; the nuclear inclusions of herpes virus are found in a narrow rim of degenerating epithelial cells at the *margin of the ulcer.*
   - *CMV* causes linear ulceration of the esophageal mucosa; the histologic findings of CMV-associated change with both intranuclear and cytoplasmic inclusions are found in capillary endothelium and stromal cells in the *base of the ulcer.*

   > For diagnosis, the biopsy should be taken from edge of ulcer in HSV and base of ulcer in CMV.

   So, friends both a and b options are correct. But as we have to choose only one, we will go for option (a) because Herpes simplex is the most common virus causing esophagitis.

5. **Ans. (b) Adenovirus** *(Ref: Robbins 8th/768, 9/e p754, Harrison 17th/1853)*
   Viruses that can cause esophagitis are: HSV-1, HSV-2, Varicella zoster virus, Cytomegalovirus and HIV For diagnosis, the biopsy should be taken from **edge of ulcer in HSV and base of ulcer in CMV**.
   Findings in biopsy of edge of ulcer in HSV are:
   - Ballooning degeneration
   - Ground glass changes in nuclei
   - Cowdry type A intranuclear inclusion bodies.

6. **Ans. (a) Squamous to columnar metaplasia** *(Ref: Robbins 7th/804, 9/e p757)*

7. **Ans. (c) Gastroesophageal reflux** *(Ref: Robbins 9/e p757, 8th/770-1; 7th/804-805, 808-809)*

8. **Ans. (c) Megaloblastic anemia** *(Ref: Robbins 9/e p753, 8th/662; 7th/776)*

9. **Ans. (d) It is a known precursor of adenocarcinoma of the esopohagus.** *(Ref: Robbins 9/e p758, 8th/769-772)*
   Barrett esophagus is columnar metaplasia of the esophageal squamous epithelium (squamous–to–columnar). The columnar epithelium is often of the intestinal type with goblet cells. Barrett esophagus is a complication of long-standing gastroesophageal reflux disease and is a precursor of esophageal adenocarcinoma. The most common location is in the distal (lower) third of the esophagus.

10. **Ans. (b) Gastroesophageal junction incompetence** *(Ref: Robbins 9/e p755, 8th/769)*
    Gastrointestinal reflux disease (GERD) is a common condition manifesting as heartburn and regurgitation. However, some patients can have "silent GERD," which means they may have symptoms like dysphagia, nocturnal cough, and sore throat even though they don't feel heartburn.

    > Gastroesophageal junction incompetence is the primary pathophysiologic mechanism responsible for GERD. This incompetence is most commonly caused by transient lower esophageal sphincter relaxations and a hypotensive lower esophageal sphincter (LES). Acidic gastric contents reflux back into the esophagus and irritate the esophageal mucosaleading to an inflammatory reaction and epithelial repair.

    Basal zone hyperplasia, elongation of lamina propria papillae, and inflammatory cells (eosinophils, neutrophils and lymphocytes) are characteristic histologic findings.

(Choice A) Pill-induced esophagitis is commonly seen with tetracycline antibiotics, potassium chloride, and bisphosphates. Metformin and enalapril do not cause esophagitis.

(Choices C) Candida albicans is the most common cause of infectious esophagitis. White plaques on the erythematous mucosa are seen on endoscopy. Light microscopy shows Pseudo hyphae and budding spores embedded in necrotic debris. Candida is the most common cause of oropharyngeal dysphagia odynophagia in HIV and immunocompromised patients.

(Choice D) Absent esophageal peristaltic movements is seen in achalasia and scleroderma.

11. **Ans. (b) Zenker's diverticulum** *(Ref: Robbins 8th/767, 9/e p753)*

This is the classic presentation of *Zenker's diverticulum*, which is a *false diverticulum* formed by herniation of the mucosa at a point of weakness at the junction of the pharynx and esophagus in the posterior hypopharyngeal wall. It is also associated with halitosis, and if the diverticulum fills completely with food, it can cause dysphagia or obstruction of the esophagus.

> • Mallory-Weiss tears (option A) are mucosal tears at the gastroesophageal junction secondary to repeated, forceful vomiting. They are often seen in alcoholics.
> • Schatzki rings (option C) are mucosal rings found in the distal esophagus at the squamocolumnar junction.
> • In contrast to a Zenker's diverticulum, the usually asymptomatic traction diverticula (option D) are true diverticula involving all of the layers of the esophagus. They are typically caused by adherence of the esophagus to a scarred mediastinal structure.

12. **Ans. (a) Achalasia** *(Ref: Robbins 8th/768, 9/e p753)*

13. **Ans. (d) Buccal mucosa** *(Ref: Robbins 8th/811, 9/e p721-732)*

14. **Ans. (a) Achalasia** *Read explanation below (Ref: Robbins 9/e p753)*

> • Achalasia is an acquired insidiously developing esophageal motility disorder due to the loss of inhibitory enteric neurons of the esophageal body and lower esophageal sphincter. The primary complaint with diffuse esophageal spasm (choice B) is mid-sternal pain that can be misdiagnosed as cardiac pain. The pain is caused by prolonged contraction of the entire esophageal body. A manometric study may show poor peristalsis in the smooth muscle portion of the esophageal body, but **lower esophageal sphincter function is unaffected.**
> • The primary complaint with incompetent lower esophageal sphincter (choice C) is heart burn and regurgitation due to gastroesophageal reflux. A manometric study would show lower-than-normal resting tone in the lower esophageal sphincter, or a sphincter that relaxes inappropriately.
> • Since the patient's symptoms do not occur until 2-3 seconds after a swallow suggests that oropharyngeal dysphagia (choice D) is not the diagnosis. The presence of cough, hoarseness, or nasal regurgitation commonly occurs with this disorder. Oropharyngeal dysphagia is often due to neurological or muscle disorders like stroke, amyotrophic lateral sclerosis, muscular dystrophy, or myasthenia gravis.

14.1. **Ans. (b) Lateral margin**
 • **Oral Cancer: Diagnosis, Management, and Rehabilitation** pg 100 mentions that '*60-70% arise from the lateral surface of the middle third of the tongue*'.

14.2. **Ans (c) Zenker diverticulum** *(Ref: Robbins 9/e p 758-9)*

15. **Ans. (b) CD 117** *(Ref Robbins 8th/789-790, 9/e p776)*
Direct quote Robbins… 'The most useful diagnostic marker for GIDT is c-kit^Q (also known as CD117^Q)'.

16. **Ans. (b) Stomach Cancer** *(Ref: Robbins 8th/786, 9/e p776)*

17. **Ans. (a) CD117** *(Ref: Robbins 8th/789-790, 7th 826-827, Harrison 17th/573)*
The most useful diagnostic marker is **c-kit (CD117)** detectable in 95% of the patients. Other markers like CD34 and vimentin can also be expressed by some tumor cells. **CD34** is also present on **pluripotent hematopoetic stem cell**.

18. **Ans. (a) CD117** *(Ref: Robbins 8th/790, 9/e p776)*

19. **Ans. (c) Intestinal metaplasia** *see text for details (Ref: Harrison 17th/572)*

20. **Ans. (d) Fundus** *(Sleisenger & Fordtrans text book of Gastrointestinal disease 7th/813)*
Pernicious anemia is associated with autoimmune atrophic gastritis affecting the fundic glands. Intestinal metaplasia (premalignant for gastric carcinoma), is characteristically seen in this area of atrophic gastritis. Atrophic glands with extensive intestinal metaplasia are most characteristically confined to the fundus in patients with pernicious anemia.

21. **Ans. (a) Gastric carcinoma** *(Ref: Robbins 8th/786)*

Metastasis in gastric cancer

- *Liver (first organ to be affected)*
- Ovary (where it is known as Krukenberg's tumor)
- Periumbilical lymph nodes (*Sister Mary Joseph nodule*)
- Peritoneal cul-de-sac (Blumer's shelf palpable on rectal or vaginal examination)
- Left supraclavicular lymph node (*Virchow's lymph node*[Q]).

22. **Ans. (c) Interstitial cells of cajal** *(Ref: Robbins 7th/826, 9/e p775)*

23. **Ans. (d) Atrophic gastritis > (b) Postgastrectomy** *(Ref: Sternberg's diagnostic surgical pathology, Volume 2, page 1451, LWW, Biopsy interpretation of the gastrointestinal tract mucosa by EA Montgomery, Lippincott William Wilkins; 120, multiple journals)*

    Sternberg.. '*Multifocal atrophic gastritis with intestinal metaplasia is present commonly in postgastrectomy stomach*. It is not clear whether it is pre-existing (for which surgery was done) or develops after gastrectomy'.

    Biopsy interpretation of the gastrointestinal tract mucosa... '*some authors have associated gastric xanthoma with atrophic gastritis*'. *Digestive Diseases and Sciences, Vol. 31,1986,page 925-8* mentions... 'It says **xanthomatosis** is characterized by collections of lipid-laden macrophages, or foam cells , plaques or nodules in many tissues, most commonly the skin. Involvement can occur in all regions of the gastrointestinal tract, but is **most common in the stomach**. It is more common in patients with gastritis, gastric ulcer, and with duodeno-gastric reflux after gastric surgery and mucosal damage has been postulated to play an important role in its pathogenesis. There is *no documented relationship between degree of hyperlipidemia or hypercholesterolemia* and presence of gastric xanthomatosis. Rather, *it is associated with atrophic gastritis*.

    Turkish Journal of gastroenterology.. 'Lipid islands are found in the stomach only when there are pathological changes such as chronic gastritis, intestinal metaplasia, *atrophic gastritis*, gastric ulcer,and changes caused by bile reflux or **partial gastrectomy**'.

    ### Clinical importance of knowing about gastric xanthoma

    Atypical xanthoma cells can be easily confused with signet-ring adenocarcinoma cell. However, xanthoma cells are negative with periodic acid-Schiff (PAS) stain but show a positive reaction with Oil red 0 and weakly positive reaction with Masson trichrome. (Ref...Acta Cytol. 2006 Jan-Feb;50(1):74-9).

    Signet-ring adenocarcinoma cells showed a **strongly positive** reaction with **PAS stain, cytokeratin and mucicarmine.**

24. **Ans. (d) Gastric adenoma** *(Ref: Robbins 7th/817, 823, 826, 9/e p770)*
    - *H. pylori is also associated with peptic ulcer disease, gastric cancer and gastric mucosa associated lymphoma* (called MALToma or mucosa associated lymphoid tissue tumor)
    - Gastric adenoma are polypoid lesions of the stomach found in the antrum most commonly.

25. **Ans. (b) Mucosa and submucosa** *(Ref: Robbins 7th/824, 825; fig/17-25, 9/e p771-772)*

    GASTRIC CARCINOMA

    Classification – On the basis of

Depth of invasion	Macroscopic pattern	Histologic subtype
(a) **Early**-involving mucosa and submucosa (b) **Advanced**-extending into muscularis propria and beyond	1. Exophytic 2. Flat or depressed 3. Excavated	(a) Intestinal type (b) Diffuse type

26. **Ans. (b) Parietal cell** *(Ref: Robbins 8th/657; 7th/641, 9/e p765)*

27. **Ans. (c) Signet ring cell adenocarcinoma** *(Ref: Robbins 8th/772)*

    The description is indicative of the presence of leather bottle appearance (linitis plastica) of diffuse gastric carcinoma. Microscopic examination reveals that in this cancer, diffuse infiltration of the stomach wall by gastric type mucus cells is present. The tumor cells have a signet ring appearance because the cytoplasmic mucin pushes the nucleus to one side.

    - **Early gastric carcinoma** is confined to the **mucosa and submucosa**.
    - **Gastrointestinal stromal tumors** tend to be **bulky masses**.
    - In **chronic atrophic gastritis**, there is *no significant scarring or shrinkage* but **rugal folds are lost**.

    Info

    In the comparison of the whole GIT, granulomas are rarest in the stomach.

28. **Ans. (a) Acute gastritis** *(Ref: Robbins 8th/773, 9/e p763)*

    Acute gastritis, characterized by patches of erythematous mucosa, sometimes with petechiae and ulceration, can be seen as a complication of a variety of other conditions (alcohol use, aspirin and other NSAIDs use, smoking, shock, steroid use, and uremia), which usually have in common disruption of the mucosal barrier of the stomach.

- Chronic antral (type B) gastritis (option B) is associated with Helicobacter pylori.
- Lymphocytic gastritis (option C) is thought to be a gastric manifestation of celiac sprue.
- Hypertrophic gastritis (Menetrier's disease; option D) is an idiopathic condition characterized by markedly enlarged mucosal folds.

29. Ans. (d) Increased production of macrocytic red blood cells *(Ref: Robbins 8th/778-779, 9/e p765)*

Autoimmune destruction of parietal cells would lead to decreased secretion of gastric acid and intrinsic factor followed by poor absorption of dietary vitamin B12 and then pernicious anemia. It is characterized by increased production of macrocytes (megaloblasts) by the bone marrow.

The luminal bacteria (option A) would most likely exhibit increased (not decreased) growth due to sterilizing action of the acid.

A decrease in acid secretion leads to increased secretion of gastrin by antral G cells because low gastric pH (less than 3) inhibits gastrin secretion via paracrine release of somatostatin from cells in the gastric mucosa that can sense the acidity. With decreased parietal cells, the pH of the gastric lumen would rise and remove this inhibitory component.

Because less acid would be delivered to the duodenum with parietal cell destruction, less secretin would be released into the blood.

30. Ans. (c) Esophagus *(Read explanation below)*

Striated (skeletal) muscle not under voluntary control is an unusual feature of the upper third of the esophagus. The middle third of the esophagus contains roughly half striated and half smooth muscle; the lower third contains only smooth muscle. All the other structures listed in the answer choices contain smooth muscle.

31. Ans. (d) Positive staining for mucin by light microscopy *(Ref: Robbins 8th/785)*

31.1. Ans. (d) Stomach *(Ref: Robbins 8/e p789-90, 9/e p776)*

NEET Key points about Gastrointestinal stromal tumor GIST

• Arise from pacemakers of the GIT known as *interstitial cells of Cajal*[Q].
• GIST is the **most common mesenchymal tumor**[Q] of the abdomen
• The most common location of the GIST is the **stomach**[Q]
• This is associated with patients having **neurofibromatosis-1**[Q].
• **Microscopically** the tumor may show either epithelioid cells, spindle cells or mixed (both the epithelioid cells and spindle cells).
• The most useful diagnostic marker is **c-kit (CD117)**[Q] detectable in 95% of the patients.
• It is **best diagnosed with CT scan *with PET scan*[Q]** (preferable) or CT scan.
• **Treatment** is done with **surgical resection** (localized tumors) and non-excisable tumors are managed with tyrosine kinase inhibitors called **imatinib mesylate**[Q] or sunitinib.

31.2. Ans. (b) High propensity of malignant change *(Ref: Robbins 8/e p789-90, 9/e p775-776)*

High-yield Imaging: Gastrointestinal p213

Direct quote from **High yield**.. "90% of stomach GISTs are found to be **benign**". Do revise all features of GIST from earlier question.

31.3. Ans. (a) Gastric ulcer *(Ref: Bailey 25/e p1055, Robbin 9/e p767)*

Chronic duodenal ulcers are not associated with malignancy but, in contrast, gastric ulcers are.

- It is fundamental that any gastric ulcer should be regarded as being malignant, no matter how classically it resembles a benign gastric ulcer.
- *Stomal ulcers* occur *after a gastroenterostomy or a gastrectomy of the Billroth II type.* The ulcer is usually found on the jejunal side of the stoma.

31.4. Ans (d) Interstitial cells of Cajal *(Ref: Robbins 9/e p 775)*

31.5. Ans (c) Gastroduodenal artery *(Ref: Robbins 9/e p767; Bailey 25/e p1064)*

31.6. Ans (d) Superficial spreading *(Ref: Robbins 9/e p772-3)*

32. Ans. (c) Macrophages with PAS (+) material inside the lamina propria *(Ref: Harrison 18th/2474, Robbins 9/e p792)*

• Hallmark of Whipple's disease had been presence of PAS positive macrophages containing the characteristic small bacilli.
• Just revise friends that the presence of *T. Whipplei* **outside of macrophages is more important** indicator of active disease than is their presence inside the macrophages.

33. **Ans. (a) HLA – DQ2** *(Ref: Harrison's 17th/2051, Robbins 9/e p782)*
    Celiac sprue is associated with HLA DQ2. For other diseases associated with HLA; refer to the table in the chapter of Immunity (chap-6)

34. **Ans. (b) T-lymphocyte** *(Ref: Mucosal Immunology Elsevier, 3rd/565)*
    Direct quote.. 'IEL are a distinctive population of T cells dispersed among the luminal epithelial cells. Particularly in the small intestine, there is a predominance of CD 8+T cells.

    - Increase in IEL is defined as > 40 lymphocytes per 100 enterocytes.

35. **Ans. (a) Whipple's Disease** *(Ref: Robbins 7th/884 9/e p792, Harrison 17th/1884)*
    The hallmark of Whipple's disease is a small intestinal mucosa laden with distended macrophages in the lamia propria. The macrophages contain periodic acid– Schiff (PAS) positive granules and small rod shaped bacilli)

36. **Ans. (b) Increased in thickness of mucosa** *(Ref: Robbins 7th/843, 9/e p783, Harrison's 17th/1881)*
    - Characteristic **histological features** seen on duodenal/jejunal biopsy in celiac sprue are:

      1. Absence or reduced height of villi, resulting in '**flat**' appearance.
      2. Crypt cell hyperplasia compensate for villous atrophy and **mucosal thickness remain same**
      3. Cuboidal appearance and nucleus that are no longer basally oriented and increased intraepithelial lymphocytes.
      4. Increased lymphocytes and plasma cells in lamina propria.

    - These features are **characteristic of celiac sprue but not diagnostic** because similar features can be seen in:

      1. Tropical sprue, 2. Eosinophilic enteritis, 3. Milk-protein intolerance in children

    - So, for establishing the diagnosis of celiac sprue, the **characteristic histological picture on small intestinal biopsy should also revert back to normal on gluten free diet.** Gluten free diet also reverses the symptoms as well as serological markers (anti-endomysial antibodies).

37. **Ans. (b) Megaloblastic** *(Ref: Harsh Mohan 6th/569-571, Harrison 17th/649)*
    In intestinal tuberculosis the ileocecal junction is the commonest site of involvement. Ileum is the physiological site for absorption of vitamin B$_{12}$. Also, TB is mentioned to be a cause of folic acid deficiency which is therefore going to result in megaloblastic anemia.

38. **Ans. (c) Maize** *(Ref: Robbin's 8th/796, 9/e p782)*
    - It is a disease characterized by increased sensitivity to a protein called gliadin present in the grains like wheat; oat, barley and rye resulting in a T-cell mediated chronic inflammatory reaction in the small intestine and impaired absorption. It is associated with HLA-DQ2 or HLA-DQ8.

39. **Ans. (c) Lungs** *(Ref: Robbins 9/e p792, 8th/804, Harrison 17th/1884)*
    The organs in which these foamy macrophages can be seen are *Liver, Small intestine*, Lymph nodes, Heart, Eyes, *CNS* and *synovial membranes of joints.*

40. **Ans. (c) Distended macrophages with PAS positive granules in lamina propria** *(Ref: Robbins 9/e p792, 8th/795, 803)*
    It is feature of Whipple's disease.

41. **Ans. (c) Perforation is common** *(Ref: Robbins 9/e p795, 8th/806; 7th/839)*

42. **Ans. (b) Tropical sprue** *(Ref: Robbins 9/e p784, 8th/796, 7th/844)*

43. **Ans. (b) Tuberculosis** *(Ref: Robbins 8th/798, 9/e p376)*

44. **Ans. (a) Canker sores** *(Ref: Robbins 9/e p728, 8th/742, 7th/776)*

45. **Ans. (b) Stricture formation** *(Ref: Robbins 9/e p789, 8th/801-802)*

46. **Ans. (a) Appendix** *(Ref: Robbins 9/e p816, 8th/828; 7 th/871-872,1097)*

47. **Ans. (b) Multiple ulcer and transverse** *(Ref: Robbins 8th/801, 9/e p789)*

48. **Ans. (c) Atrophy of the villi with blunting and flatterning** *(Ref: Robbins 8th/796-7, 9/e p782-783)*
    - The description of a malabsorption disorder that responded to dietary treatment is suggestive of celiac disease (gluten sensitivity). The microscopic features are mucosal flattening, diffuse and severe villous atrophy and chronic inflammation of the lamina propria. Intraepithelial lymphocytes are also increased.
    - Lymphatic obstruction and foamy macrophages the lamina propria containing PAS-positive granules occurs in Whipple disease.
    - Noncaseating granulomas are present in the intestinal wall in Crohn's disease.

49. Ans. (b) Stomach *(Ref: Robbins 9/e p762, 8th/775-6)*

- The presentation of the patient is suggestive of stress ulcers called as Curling ulcers when they occur in patients with burn injuries. These small shallow ulcers never penetrate the muscular is propria, but may can bleed profusely. Esophageal varices occur in patients with portal hypertension usually associated with cirrhosis.
- **Duodenal ulcer** are typically peptic ulcers in individuals with **Helicobacter pylori** infection.
- Ileal ulcerations and colonic ulcerations can either be idiopathic or inflammatory bowel disease or infections.

50. Ans. (c) Duodenal peptic ulcer *(Ref: Robbins 8th/780-1, 9/e p767, Bailey and Love 25th/1055-6, Harsh Mohan 6th/553)*
Peptic ulcer of the duodenum is not a precursor lesion to carcinoma. This is in contrast to gastric peptic ulcer disease which are premalignant in nature (though rarely).

- Familial multiple polyposis has almost 100% chance of progression to a malignancy.
- Colorectal villous adenomas may also undergo malignant change. The same holds true of inflammatory bowel disease (ulcerative colitis has higher of progression to a malignancy than Crohn's disease).

Duodenal and Gastric peptic ulcer

Features	Duodenal ulcer	Gastric ulcer
Site	1st part of duodenum	Along lesser curvature
Incidence	More common	Less common
Age	25 – 50 yrs, M>F	Beyond 6th decade, M>F
Etiology	Almost all patients have H. pylori infection	Less stronger association
Acid level	High	Usually normal; ↑ if hypergastrinemia
Pain after food intake	Relieved	Aggravated
Clinical features	Night pain and melena more common	No night pain, hematemesis more common
	No vomiting/no weight loss	Vomiting common/weight loss is present
Complications	No malignant change	Malignant change present (though rarely)

51. Ans. (d) Antigliadin antibody *(Ref: Robbins 9/e p783, 8th/795)*
The features in the stem of the question suggest likely diagnosis of **celiac disease**. These patients have anti-transglutaminase, anti-gliadin and **anti-endomysial (most useful)** antibodies. Women are affected more than men. Celiac disease results from gluten sensitivity. Exposure to the **gliadin** protein in **wheat, oats, barley, and rye** (but not rice) results in intestinal inflammation. Gliadin sensitivity causes epithelial cells to produce IL – 15 which activates CD8+ T cells. These T cells damage the enterocyte. **Dermatitis herpetiformis**, and **enteropathy associated T-cell lymphoma**s may be seen in some individuals.

- **Anticentromeric antibody** is most specific for **limited scleroderma (CREST syndrome)**.
- **Anti- DNA topoisomerase I** antibody is most specific for **diffuse scleroderma** in which GIT may be affected and malabsorption may be present.
- **Antimitochondrial antibody** is more specific for **primary biliary cirrhosis**.

52. Ans. (d) Ulcerative colitis *(Ref: Robbins 8th/811, 9/e p800)*
Sclerosing cholangitis is an extraintestinal manifestation of inflammatory bowel disease, more commonly associated with ulcerative colitis and less often with, Crohn disease. Explaining other options,

- Pancreatitis has no association with sclerosing cholangitis. It may cause bilary tract lithiasis.
- Diverticulosis may be complicated by diverticulitis, but the liver is not involved.
- Celiac disease may be associated with dermatitis herpetiformis, but not with liver disease. Peptic ulcer disease does not lead to hepatic complications.

53. Ans. (b) Eat more frequent, smaller meals that are high in fat
Read explanation below
The postgastrectomy symptoms in the given question is called the **dumping syndrome**. Since all or part of the stomach is removed, an ingested meal will be delivered to the small intestine more quickly than normal. The large increase in tonicity in the small intestine causes an osmotic fluid shift from the extracellular fluid (plasma) into the lumen of the gut. The increased distention of the small intestine increases motility through reflex mechanisms and causes diarrhea. The blood volume contraction and concomitant release of vasoactive substances such as bradykinin and/or vasoactive intestinal peptide can create hypotension and reflex tachycardia.

These patients should be instructed to eat more frequent, smaller meals to reduce the osmotic and/or carbohydrate load that is delivered to the small intestine. Furthermore, since fats are the slowest to be absorbed, a diet that is higher in fat will also reduce the problem of rapid absorption.

54. Ans. (c) Crohn's disease *(Ref: Robbins 8th/811, 9/e p799-800)*

55. Ans. (c) Proximal small bowel *(Ref: Robbins 8th/795-796, 9/e p782-783)*

The patient has celiac disease, which is apparently an acquired hypersensitivity to the gluten (such as gliadin) in wheat. Unlike tropical sprue (which may be related to enterotoxigenic E. coli infection), which involves the entire small bowel, celiac sprue is usually limited to the proximal small bowel.

56. Ans. (d) Ulcerative colitis *(Ref: Robbins 8th/811, 9/e p800)*

The most frequent GIT disorder which can be associated with sacroiliitis (related to HLA-B27) or lower limb arthritis is the chronic inflammatory bowel diseases, ulcerative colitis and Crohn's disease. Other GI diseases associated with arthropathy include bypass surgery, Whipple's disease, Behcet's syndrome, and celiac disease.

Amebic colitis (choice A) is caused by ingestion of infectious cysts (typically from Entamoeba histolytica). Cecal amebiasis can resemble acute appendicitis.

Diverticulosis (choice C) is usually a disease of older adults. It is often asymptomatic unless inflammation supervenes.

57. Ans. (a) High fiber diet *(Ref Robbins 8th/822-3, 9/e p811)*

The dietary factors predisposing to a higher incidence of cancer are
- Excess dietary caloric intake relative to requirements,
- A low content of unabsorbable vegetable fiber,
- A corresponding high content of refined carbohydrates,
- Intake of red meat, and
- Decreased intake of protective micronutrients.

Concept

- **Reduced fiber content** leads to decreased stool bulk, increased fecal transit time in the bowel, and an altered bacterial flora of the intestine. Potentially toxic oxidative byproducts of carbohydrate degradation by bacteria are therefore present in higher concentrations in the stools and are held in contact with the colonic mucosa for longer periods of time.
- **High fat intake** (red meat) enhances the synthesis of cholesterol and bile acids by the liver, which may be converted into potential carcinogens by intestinal bacteria.
- Refined diets also contain less of vitamins A, C, and E, which may act as oxygen-radical scavengers.
- **NSAIDs** like aspirin are **protective in colon cancer** because they inhibit the COX-2 enzyme which is responsible for the proliferation of the colonic mucosa. The COX-2 expression is upregulated by TLR4 which recognizes lipopolyaccharides and is over-expressed in adenoma and carcinoma.

57.1. Ans. (a) sigmoid colon *(Ref: Robbins 8/e p814-5, 9/e p803, Bailey 25/e p1160)*
- The condition is found in the **sigmoid colon** in 90% of cases.
- Interestingly in South-east Asia, **right-sided diverticular disease**[Q] is twice as common as the left.
- The main morbidity of the disease is due to **sepsis**[Q].

57.2. Ans. (c) Ileum *(Ref: Robbins 8/e p372)*
Although any portion of the gastrointestinal tract may be affected, **the terminal ileum** and *the cecum* are the sites most commonly involved"... **Harrison 18th**

57.3. Ans. (c) Cecum *(Ref: Robbins 9/e p795, 8/e p806, 7/e p839)*
Amoebiasis is seen most frequently in the cecum and ascending colon.......Robbins

57.4. Ans. (c) Celiac disease *(Ref: Robbins 9/e p783, 8/e p795-796, 7/e p843)*
- The **most sensitive tests** are the presence of IgA antibodies to tissue transglutaminase or IgA or IgG antibodies to **deamidated gliadin.**
- **Anti-endomysial antibodies** are **highly specific** but less sensitive than other antibodies.

57.5. Ans. (c) Klinefelter syndrome *(Robbins 8/e p795, 9/e p782-783)*
Direct line... 'There is also an association of celiac disease with other immune diseases including *type 1 diabetes, thyroiditis, and Sjögren syndrome, as well as ataxia, autism, depression, some forms of epilepsy, IgA nephropathy, Down syndrome* and *Turner syndrome*'

57.6. Ans. (a) Zinc *(Ref: Robbins 8/e p804)*
Paneth cells contain zinc along with lysozyme. They are involved in gut defence.

57.7. Ans. (c) Horizontal ulcers *(Ref: Bailey 25/e p1174)*

Typhoid ulcer
- Perforation of a typhoid ulcer usually occurs **during the third week**[Q] and is occasionally the first sign of the disease.
- The ulcer is **parallel to the long axis of the gut**[Q] and
- Is usually situated in the **lower ileum**[Q].

57.8. Ans. (c) 3rd *(Ref: Bailey 25/e p1174)*

Perforation of a typhoid ulcer usually occurs **during the third week**[Q] and is occasionally the first sign of the disease.

57.9. Ans. (c) Appendicitis *(Ref: Bailey 25/e p1132)*

Causes of raised serum amylase level other than *acute pancreatitis*[Q]

- Upper gastrointestinal tract perforation[Q]
- Mesenteric infarction[Q]
- *Torsion of an intra-abdominal viscus*
- *Retroperitoneal haematoma*
- *Ectopic pregnancy*
- **Macroamylasaemia**
- **Renal failure**
- **Salivary gland inflammation**

57.10. Ans. (d) Oral lichen planus *(Ref: Bailey 25/e p735)*

Conditions associated with malignant transformation

High-risk lesions	Medium-risk lesions	Low-risk/equivocal-risk lesions
*Erythroplakia	*Oral submucous fibrosis	*Oral lichen planus
*Speckled erythroplakia	*Syphilitic glossitis	*Discoid lupus erythematosus
*Chronic hyperplastic candidiasis	*Sideropenic dysphagia	*Discoid keratosis congenita

- In the Indian subcontinent oral submucous fibrosis is very common. This condition is characterized by limited opening of mouth and burning sensation on eating of spicy food.

57.11. Ans. (d) Blood culture....remember the acronym *BASU* for <u>b</u>lood, <u>a</u>ntibody, <u>s</u>tool and <u>u</u>rine.

57.12. Ans (b) Pancreatitis

Purtscher's retinopathy is manifested by a sudden and severe loss of vision in a patient with acute pancreatitis. It is caused by occlusion of the posterior retinal artery with aggregated granulocytes. There are cotton-wool spots and hemorrhages confined to an area limited by the optic disc and macula.

57.13. Ans (a) Oxalate *(Ref: Robbins 9/e p876)*

There are two general classes of gallstones: cholesterol stones, containing more than 50% of crystalline cholesterol mono-hydrate, and pigment stones composed predominantly of bilirubin calcium salts.

58. Ans. (d) Lymph node status *(Ref: Robbins 8th/825, 9/e p813)*

Direct quote Robbins .. 'the two most important prognostic factors are depth of invasion and the presence or absence of lymph node metastasis.

59. Ans. (a) Autosomal recessive inheritance *(Ref Robbins 8th/820-821, 9/e p809)*

Prophylactic colectomy does not decrease risk for cancer due to adenomas at other sites specially ampulla of Vater and stomach.

60. Ans. (d) Jejunum *(Ref: Robbins 8th/817, 9/e p806)*

The polyps of Peutz-Jeghers syndrome are **most common in the small intestine**, although they may occur in the stomach and colon, and, with much lower frequency, in the bladder and lungs.

61. Ans. (a) Autosomal recessive inheritance *(Ref: Robbins 8th/820-821, , 9/e p809)*

Familial polyposis syndrome (FAP) is an **autosomal dominant**[Q] disorder. It is caused by mutation in the adenomatous polyposis coli or APC gene on chromosome 5q21. Atleast 100 polyps are necessary for a diagnosis of FAP.

Option 'c'..Robbins clearly writes that colorectal carcinoma develop in 100% of untreated FAP patients often before age 30. As a result, prophylactic colectomy is the standard therapy in patients with APC mutations.

62. Ans. (a) RB *(Ref: Robbins 8th/823-824, 9/e p811)*

Two distinct genetic pathways are described in adenocarcinoma of colon:

Adenoma-carcinoma sequence: It accounts for 80% of sporadic colon cancers. Mutation of APC gene occurs early or is inherited. Whenever second allele of APC is mutated or inactivated, β-catenin accumulates [APC protein degrades β-catenin]. Beta–catenin translocates to nucleus and activates genes like myc and cyclin D1.
Additional mutations occuring later are:
- Kras
- SMAD-2 and SMAD-4
- p53

Microsatellite instability pathway: Mutations in DNA mismatch repair genes (MSH2 and MLH1) results in expansion of microsatellites. This microsatellite instability may result in decreased functioning of TGF- β type II and bax proteins. Mutations in BRAF and epigenetic silencing of genes by hypermethylation may also occur. Kras and p53 are not typically mutated.

Some people were of the opinion that Rb was not the option but the option in the exam was K-RAS. In such a situation, we can understand that the answer would be none.

63. **Ans. (a) Cryptitis** *(Ref: Robbins 7th/849-850; 9/e 800, Harrison 17th/1888)*
The pathology in ulcerative colitis typically involves distortion of crypt architecture, inflammation of crypts (cryptitis), frank crypt abscess, and hemorrhage or inflammatory cells in the lamina propria.
The **mnemonic** for important features is Ulcerative **COLITIS** *(described in text)*.

64. **Ans. (a) Diffuse distribution of pseudopolyps** *(Ref: Harrison 17th/2077, Robbins 8th/807-13, 9/e p800)*
- Pseudopolyps (inflammatory polyps) can be seen in both Crohn's disease and ulcerative colitis.
- Even Mucosal edema, crypt abscess and mucosal lymphoid aggregates are features common to both the types of inflammatory bowel disease.
- However, diffuse distribution of these polyps is observed only in ulcerative colitis because in Crohn's disease, there is presence of skip lesions in which there is presence of normal area adjacent to diseased segments of the intestine. So, patchy distribution of polyps is observed in Crohn's disease.

65. **Ans. (d) Rectum spared in 50% patients with large bowel involvement.** *(Ref: Robbins 8th/810-2, 9/e p799, Harrison 17th/1888)*

66. **Ans. (b) B cells** *(Ref: Robbins 7th/1205)*

67. **Ans. (c) Both a and b** *(Ref: Robbins 7th/849-851, 9/e p800)*
Please don't confuse 'skin lesions' with 'skip lesions', the latter are seen only in *Crohn disease.*

68. **Ans. (c) Hamartomatous polyp** *(Ref: Robbins 7th/858, 9/e p806)*
- **Peutz-Jegher's polyps** are **hamartomatous polyps** that involve mucosal epithelium, lamina propria and muscularis mucosa. Peutz-Jegher's polyps are located usually in small intestine *most commonly in jejunum.*
- When they occur in multiple numbers, condition is called **Peutz-Jegher's syndrome.** It is rare autosomal dominant syndrome characterized by multiple hamartomatous polyps scattered throughout GIT, along with mucosal and cutaneous melanotic pigmentation along lips, face, genitalia and palms
Genetic basis of Peutz-Jegher's syndrome is mutation in gene STKII (LKB1) located on chromosome 19 which encodes protein with serine/threonine kinase activity.

69. **Ans. (a) Juvenile polyp** *(Ref: Robbins 9/e p805, 8th/817; 7th/857)*

70. **Ans. (a) Rectal involvement is common** *(Ref: Robbins 9/e p799, 8th/810-811; 7th/851)*

71. **Ans. (a) Carcinoid tumor** *(Ref: Robbins 9/e p816, 8th/828, 7th/871)*

72. **Ans. (b) Crohn's disease** *(Ref: Robbins 9/e p799, 8th/810; 7th/851)*

73. **Ans. (a) Crohn's disease** *(Ref: Robbins 9/e p800, 8th/810-811, 7th/849)*

74. **Ans. (c) Distal ileum** *(Ref: Robbins 9/e p774, 8th/788, 7th/866-867)*

75. **Ans. (a) Head** *(Ref: Robbins 9/e p893, 8th/900-903, 7th/950)*

76. **Ans. (c) Bronchodilation** *(Ref: Robbins 9/e p774, 8th/321-322, 7th/868)*

77. **Ans. (c) Rectosigmoid** *(Ref: Robbins 9/e p800, 8th/812, 7th/849)*

78. **Ans. (d) Crohn's disease** *(Ref: Robbins 9/e 799, 8th/810-811, 7th/847-848)*

79. **Ans. (b) High fiber diet** *(Ref: Robbins 8th/811, 7th/864)*

80. **Ans. (b) Ulcerative colitis** *(Ref: Robbins 9/e 800, 8th/810-811; 7th/848)*

81. **Ans. (a) Crohn's disease** *(Ref: Robbins 9/e p799, 8th/810-811; 7th/848)*

82. **Ans. (a) Ulcerative colitis** *(Ref: Robbins 9/e p800, 8th/811-812; 7th/849)*

83. **Ans. (d) Splenomegaly** *(Ref: Robbins 9/e p774, 8th/789; 7th/868)*

84. **Ans. (b) Transmural inflammation** *(Ref: Robbins 9/e p799-800, 8th/810)*
The typical presentation of Crohn's disease is abdominal pain and diarrhea in a 20-30 year old patient. Weight loss,

fatigability, low grade fever, and aphthous ulcers of the oral mucosa are also common.

Transmural inflammation explains the two most common complications of Crohn's disease: strictures, and fistulas. Chronic inflammation causes edema and fibrosis leading to narrowing of the intestinal lumen (strictures). Necrosis of the intestinal wall causes ulcer formation. Ulcers can penetrate the entire thickness of the affected intestinal wall, leading to the formation of a fistula.

> Please contrast with ulcerative colitis in which only the mucosa and submucosa are inflamed, so, strictures and fistulas are not common.

- **(Choices a and d)** Intramural granulomas and skip lesions are commonly found in Crohn's disease. They do not, however, predispose to fistula formation.
- **(Choice c)** A chronic inflammatory infiltration that consists predominantly of monocytes and lymphocytes is characteristic of Crohn's disease. However, it is not the composition of the inflammatory infiltrate, rather the fistula's depth that is responsible for fistula formation.

85. **Ans. (b) Pseudomembranous colitis** *(Ref: Robbins 9/e p791, 8th/803)*

Severe diarrhoea, fever, and toxicity following broad-spectrum antibiotic therapy is likely due to pseudomembranous colitis. This is associated with overgrowth of Clostridium difficile, a commensal microorganism indigenous to the bowel. The clostridia remain intraluminal, but secrete an enterotoxin that is responsible for the clinical and pathologic manifestations of the disorder.

- IIIrd generation cephalosporins[Q] are the most notorious antibiotics causing pseudomembranous colitis.

86. **Ans. (a) 5-HIAA** *(Ref: Robbins 9/e p774, 8th/788-789)*

5-HIAA is a metabolite of serotonin, a major secretory product of carcinoid tumors. The signs and symptoms of carcinoid syndrome include diarrhea, flushing, and wheezing. The cardiac abnormalities are commonly concentrated in the right heart because carcinoid secretory products are degraded or detoxified in the lung.

The correct answer is D

87. **Ans. (a) Hyperplastic polyp** *(Ref: Robbins 9/e p804, 8th/819)*

This is a hyperplastic polyp; these polyps comprise 90% of all colonic polyps and have no malignant potential.

Peutz-Jeghers polyps (choice 'b') also have no malignant potential, but tend to be larger and have a complex branching pattern.

Tubular adenomas and tubulovillous adenomas, (choices c and d) are all true neoplastic polyps containing dysplastic epithelium; the malignant potential of these polyps increases with size and the percentage of the polyp which has a villous configuration.

87.1. **Ans. (a) Chronic nonspecific ulcerative colitis** *(Ref: Robbins 9/e p800, 8/e p812)*

In **ulcerative colitis**, inflammation and inflammatory mediators can damage the muscularis propria and disturb neuro-muscular function leading to colonic dilation and **toxic megacolon**, which carries a significant risk of perforation

87.2. **Ans. (b) Autosomal dominant** *(Ref: Robbins 9/e p809, 8/e p820)*

Familial Adenomatous Polyposis is caused by the mutation of adenomatous polyposis coli (APC) gene present on the long arm of chromosome 5[Q] (5q21). It is inherited as an autosomal dominant disorder.

Subtypes of FAP

Classic FAP syndrome
• The patient has a large number of adenomatous polyps and retinal pigment epithelial hypertrophy. There should be a minimum of 100 polyps[Q] to make a diagnosis of this syndrome. Most of the adenomatous polyps are tubular polyps.
Attenuated FAP syndrome
• The patient has a lower number of adenomatous polyps (around 30) which are located in proximal colon.
Gardener syndrome[Q]
• Intestinal polyps + epidermal cysts + fibromatosis + osteomas (of the mandible, long bones and skull).
Turcot syndrome[Q]
• Adenomatous colon polyposis + CNS tumors (medulloblastoma in 2/3rd and gliomas in 1/3rd patients).

87.3. **Ans. (d) Gardener syndrome** *(Ref: Robbins 9/e p809, 8/e p816)*

Explained in the earlier question

87.4. **Ans. (d) Noncaseating granuloma** *(Ref: Robbins 9/e p799, 8/e p810-2)*

- Noncaseating granuloma is a feature of **Crohn disease** and **not ulcerative colitis.**

Key points about ulcerative colitis

Ulcerative – **U**lcers in mucosa and submucosa
C - Continuous retrograde involvement (No skip lesions)
O - Originates in the rectum
L - Lead pipe appearance
I - Increased chances of cancer (More than that in Crohn's disease)
T - Toxic megacolon (Due to involvement of transverse colon)
I - Increased growth from the mucosa ("Pseudopolyps")
S - Symptoms are severe (As compared to Crohn's disease)

87.5. Ans. (c) Gastrointestinal tract *(Ref: Robbins 9/e p774, 8/e p788 , Harrison 18/e p)*

Direct quote from Harrison.. "The **GI tract** is the **most common** site for these tumors, accounting for 64%, with the respiratory tract a distant second at 28%."

87.6. Ans. (b) Kulschitsky cells *(Ref: Robbins 9/e p774, 8/e p787)*

Carcinoid tumour arises from the neuroendocrine cells called **Kulschitsky cells**. These cells are also called as **Enterochromaffin (EC) cells** and are present in gastrointestinal tract and the respiratory tract.

87.7. Ans. (b) Ulcerative colitis *(Ref: Robbins 9/e p800, 8/e p811, 7/e p849)*

Though pseudopolyps may be seen in both Crohn disease and ulcerative colitis, it is more common in ulcerative colitis.

87.8. Ans. (c) Familial polyposis *(Ref: Robbins 9/e p809, 8/e p820-821, 7/e p862)*

Direct line.. *"Colorectal cancer develops in 100% of untreated FAP patients often before the age of 30".*

87.9. Ans. (a) Adenocarcinoma

- **Small intestinal adenocarcinomas**[Q] and carcinoids have roughly equal incidence, followed in order by lymphomas and sarcomas. However, other texts mention that adenocarcinomas are common. So, its he answer of consensus here.
- Most common **benign** small intestinal tumor is **adenoma**[Q]. It is located most commonly **near Ampulla of Vater**[Q].

87.10. Ans. (a) Head *(Ref: Robbins 9/e p893)*

Carcinoma of the pancreas

• More than 85% of pancreatic cancers are **ductal adenocarcinomas** [Q].
• Ductal adenocarcinomas arise most commonly in the **head of the gland**[Q].
• **Painless jaundice** [Q] secondary to obstruction of the distal bile duct is the most common symptom.
• The jaundice may be associated with nausea and epigastric discomfort.
• On examination, there may be evidence of jaundice, weight loss, a palpable liver and **a palpable gall bladder**[Q]
• If there is a genuine suspicion of a tumour in the head of the pancreas, the preferred test is a **contrast- enhanced CT scan**[Q]
• The standard resection for a tumour of the pancreatic head or the ampulla is a **pylorus-preserving pancreatoduodenectomy.**[Q] This is considered better than the earlier performed **Whipple procedure**.

87.11. Ans. (b) Juvenile polyp *(Ref: Robbin 8/e p 816-7)*

- *Juvenile polyps* are focal malformations of the mucosal epithelium and lamina propria.
- The vast majority of juvenile polyps occur in *children less than 5 years*[Q] of age.
- *The majority of juvenile polyps are located in the rectum*[Q] and **most present with rectal bleeding**[Q].

87.12. Ans (b) Iron deficiency anemia *(Ref: Robbins 9/e p 813)*

The underlying cause of iron deficiency anemia in an older man or postmenopausal woman is GI cancer until proven otherwise.

87.13. Ans. (b) Smoking has a protective effect *(Ref: Robbins 9/e p 800)*

87.14. Ans (c) Colon *(Ref: Robbins 9/e p 769; Harrison 18/e p 2455-6)*

- Zollinger-Ellison syndrome is caused by gastrin-secreting tumors. These gastrinomas are most commonly found in the small intestine or pancreas.
- The extrapancreatic sites of these tumors are *duodenum* (*most common extrapancreatic site*), stomach, bones, ovaries, heart, liver, and lymph nodes.

Also revise!

Gastrinoma triangle (confluence of the cystic and common bile ducts superiorly, junction of the second and third portions of the duodenum inferiorly, and junction of the neck and body of the pancreas medially).

87.15. Ans (a) NOD2/CARD15 gene *(Ref: Robbins 9/e p 797)*

One of genes *most strongly associated with Crohn disease is NOD2* (nucleotide oligomerization binding domain 2), which encodes an intracellular protein that binds to bacterial peptidoglycans and activates signaling events, including the NF-κB pathway.

87.16. Ans (b) Fecal lactoferrin *(Ref: Harrison 18/e)*

In ulcerative colitis, active disease can be associated with a rise in acute-phase reactants C-reactive protein (CRP), platelet count, erythrocyte sedimentation rate (ESR), and a decrease in hemoglobin.

Direct line... *"Fecal lactoferrin is a highly sensitive and specific marker for detecting intestinal inflammation"*.

- Fecal calprotectin levels correlate well with histologic inflammation, predict relapses, and detect pouchitis.
- Leukocytosis may be present but is not a specific indicator of disease activity.

Fecal lactoferrin is a marker of fecal leukocytes and is more sensitive and is available in latex agglutination and enzyme-linked immunosorbent assay formats.

87.17. Ans (d) 100 *(Ref: Robbins 9/e p809)*

At least 100 polyps are necessary for a diagnosis of classic FAP, but as many as several thousand may be present.

87.18. Ans. (a) p-ANCA *(Ref: Robbins 9/e p860)*

p-ANCA is also called now by the name of anti myeloperoxidase (MPO-ANCA). It is directed against a lysosomal granule constituent and is seen in the following conditions:

- Ulcerative colitis
- Churg-Strauss syndrome
- Primary sclerosing cholangitis
- Microscopic polyangiitis
- Focal necrotising and crescentic glomerulonephritis
- Rheumatoid arthritis

GOLDEN POINTS FOR QUICK REVISION
(GASTROINTESTINAL TRACT)

- **Allgrove (triple A) syndrome**, an autosomal recessive disorder characterized by *achalasia, alacrima,* and *adrenocorticotrophic hormone-resistant adrenal insufficiency.*
- The most common cause of gastroesophageal reflux is *transient lower esophageal sphincter relaxation.*
- *Reflux of gastric contents* into the lower esophagus is the most frequent cause of esophagitis.
- The malabsorptive diarrhea of Whipple disease is due to **impaired lymphatic transport**.
- *Gastritis* is a mucosal inflammatory process. When neutrophils are present, the lesion is referred to as acute gastritis. When inflammatory cells are rare or absent, it is termed as *gastropathy.*
- The *most common cause of chronic gastritis* is infection with the bacillus *H. pylori.*
- **Autoimmune gastritis** is the most common cause of **diffuse atrophic gastritis.** It is the most common form of *chronic gastritis in patients without H. pylori infection.*
- *Carney triad*, a nonhereditary syndrome of unknown etiology is seen primarily in young females and includes *gastric GIST, paraganglioma, and pulmonary chondroma.*
- *Carney-Stratakis syndrome* (different from Carney triad) is caused by loss of succinate dehydrogenase complex (SDH) function. It increases the risk of *GIST and paraganglioma*
- *Celiac disease* is associated with a higher incidence of other autoimmune diseases like including *type 1 diabetes, thyroiditis, and Sjögren syndrome, IgA nephropathy,* and neurologic disorders, such as *ataxia, autism, depression, epilepsy, Down syndrome, and Turner syndrome.*
- Individuals with celiac disease have a higher than normal rate of malignancy. The most common celiac disease-associated cancer is *enteropathy-associated T-cell lymphoma.* The patients also have increased risk of small intestinal adenocarcinoma.

CHAPTER 13

Liver

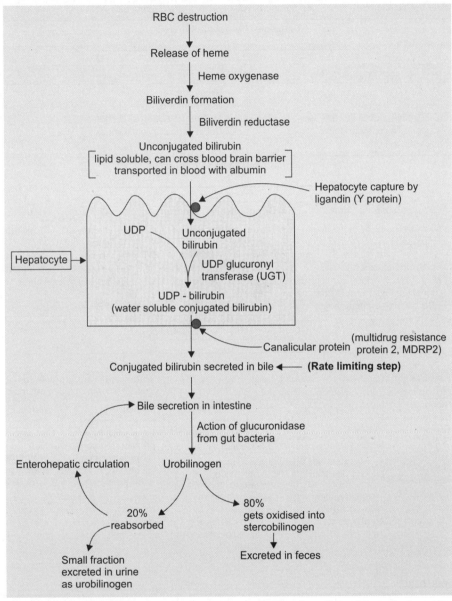

RBC destruction

↓

Release of heme

↓ Heme oxygenase

Biliverdin formation

↓ Biliverdin reductase

Unconjugated bilirubin
[lipid soluble, can cross blood brain barrier transported in blood with albumin]

Hepatocyte capture by ligandin (Y protein)

UDP → Unconjugated bilirubin

Hepatocyte

↓ UDP glucuronyl transferase (UGT)

UDP - bilirubin
(water soluble conjugated bilirubin)

Canalicular protein (multidrug resistance protein 2, MDRP2)

↓

Conjugated bilirubin secreted in bile ← **(Rate limiting step)**

↓

Bile secretion in intestine

↓ Action of glucuronidase from gut bacteria

Enterohepatic circulation   Urobilinogen

20% reabsorbed

80% gets oxidised into stercobilinogen

Small fraction excreted in urine as urobilinogen

Excreted in feces

The adult liver is an important organ of the body weighing around 1.5 kg and supplied by portal vein (60% of blood flow) and hepatic artery (40% of blood flow). It is responsible for plasma protein synthesis and metabolism of endogenous waste products and xenobiotics.

The functional unit of the liver is a hexagonal lobule having hepatic vein at its centre and portal tract (composed of hepatic artery, portal vein and bile duct) at its periphery.

The hepatic sinusoids are lined by fenestrated and discontinuous endothelial cells. There is presence of Kupffer cells and stellate cells in the extra sinusoidal space (called *space of Disse*).

The *stellate cells or Ito cells are required for vitamin A metabolism and get transformed into collagen producing myofibroblasts during hepatic inflammation.*

Jaundice is characterized by hyperbilirubinemia and yellowing of the skin and sclera (due to elastin fibers).

Indirect hyperbilirubinemia is called when unconjugated bilirubin is 85% or more of the total bilirubin whereas direct hyperbilirubinemia corresponds to conjugated bilirubin more than 15% of total.

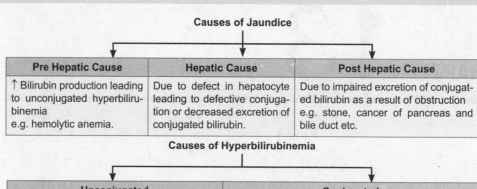

Causes of Jaundice

Pre Hepatic Cause	Hepatic Cause	Post Hepatic Cause
↑ Bilirubin production leading to unconjugated hyperbiliru-binemia e.g. hemolytic anemia.	Due to defect in hepatocyte leading to defective conjuga-tion or decreased excretion of conjugated bilirubin.	Due to impaired excretion of conjugat-ed bilirubin as a result of obstruction e.g. stone, cancer of pancreas and bile duct etc.

Causes of Hyperbilirubinemia

Unconjugated	Conjugated
• Physiological jaundice of newborn • Hemolytic anemia • Diffuse hepatocellular disease • Criggler Najjar syndrome • Gilbert syndrome	• Biliary tract obstruction • Biliary tract disease like primary biliary cirrhosis and primary sclerosing cholangitis • Dubin Johnson syndrome • Rotor syndrome

Unconjugated Hyperbilirubinemia

Physiological jaundice	Criggler Najjar Syndrome	Gilbert Syndrome
• Due to immaturity of the liver • Increased changes with prematurity and **erythroblastosis fetalis**[Q]. • May result in kernicterus (unconjugated bilirubin crosses BBB causing brain damage[Q])	• Due to decreased UGT activity • Type I → **Absence** of UGT enzyme; 100% fatal • Type II **Reduced** UGT activity.	• Decreased bilirubin glucuronidation • Jaundice associated with stress like **illness, fasting** or **exercise**[Q].

> **Type II Criggler Najjar Syndrome** is treated with **pheno-barbitone**.

Conjugated Hyperbilirubinemia

Biliary Tract Obstruction	Biliary Tract Disease		Dubin Johnson Syndrome	Rotor Syndrome
– Stones – Stricture – Cancers – Fluke (*Clonorchis sinensis*)	**Primary Biliary Cirrhosis** – Autoimmune liver disease having inflammation of **intrahepatic bile duct**[Q] – F > M; 30-65 years	**Primary Sclerosing Cholangitis** – Chronic liver disease having segmental inflammation of **extrahepatic**[Q] **bile ducts** – M > F; 20-40 years – Usually associated with ulcerative colitis[Q]	– Defective canalicular protein[Q] – Pigmented liver present (pigment is **epinephrine** not bilirubin[Q])	– Defect in bilirubin excretion – **Non pigmented liver**[Q]

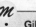

> • **G**ilbert and **C**riggler **N**ajjar: Glucuronide Conjugation Not present
> • **D**ubin Johnson and **R**otor: Defect in Removing conjugated bilirubin

CIRRHOSIS

It is the end stage liver disease characterized by disruption of the liver architecture by fibrotic bands that divide the liver into nodules of regenerating liver parenchyma. It can be *micronodular* (if nodule is <3mm) or *macronodular* (>3 mm) or mixed.

CAUSES

- **Alcoholic liver disease** (*most common cause*[Q])
- Viral hepatitis
- Biliary tract disease
- Hemochromatosis

> **Most common** cause of cirrhosis is **alcoholic liver disease**.
>
> **Non-alcoholic fatty liver disease** is the most common cause of *cryptogenic cirrhosis*.

- Cryptogenic/idiopathic (**non alcoholic fatty liver disease** is its *commonest cause*)
- Wilson disease
- α-1-antitrypsin deficiency

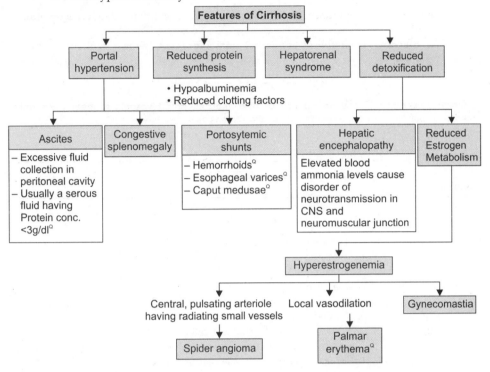

> The **fibrosis** is produced by the **hepatic stellate cell or Ito cell** and there is deposition of primarily **type I and type III collagen** in the lobule.

Non-Cirrhotic Portal Fibrosis (NCPF)/Idiopathic Portal Hypertension (IPH)

It is a condition characterized by portal hypertension and moderate portal fibrosis without cirrhosis. Though the exact etiology is unknown, it has been associated with the following:

- **Infections:** sepsis, diarrhea in children, bacterial infections
- **Immunological mechanisms:** associated with HLA DR-3
- **Chemical exposure:** *arsenic*, vinyl chloride, copper sulfate, hypervitaminosis A, drugs (steroid)

Histopathological Features

Intimal fibroelastosis of medium sized portal veins (Obliterative portovenopathy of liver): characteristic finding. Other findings include: *portal fibrosis* (intra portal but **not bridging fibrosis**), portal vein sclerosis, portal tract edema and *lymphocytic infilteration,* pseudolobulation, and atrophy of liver parenchyma with no regenerative capacity.

FIGURE EXPLAINING THE PATHOGENESIS OF NCPF

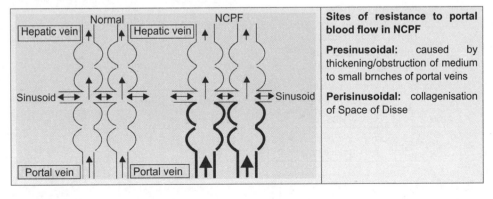

Sites of resistance to portal blood flow in NCPF

Presinusoidal: caused by thickening/obstruction of medium to small brnches of portal veins

Perisinusoidal: collagenisation of Space of Disse

Most common cause of Portal hypertension

Adults: Cirrhosis *followed by* NCPF

Children: Extra hepatic portal vein obstruction **(EHPVO).**

CLINICAL FEATURES

- Presentation in the *3rd-4th decade* of life
- Low socio economic strata
- Slight sex preponderance *M>F* (this may vary however depending on geographical areas)
- **GI bleeding** (*commonest symptom*), **massive splenomegaly** with **normal liver function tests**.

Clinical significance of NCPF

Massive splenomegaly and **emergence of new aberrant blood vessels** is **most commonly** associated with NCPF out of all causes of portal hypertension.

INFECTIOUS DISORDERS OF LIVER

Hepatitis

ACUTE HEPATITIS

1. Swelling of the hepatocytes called *"Ballooning"*.
2. Presence of apoptotic hepatocytes giving rise to *Councilman bodies*. Apoptosis of a single hepatocyte is called '**spotty necrosis**'.
3. Disruption of lobular architecture of the liver.
4. Necrosis connecting portal to portal, portal to central, central to central regions of adjacent lobules is called **bridging necrosis**
5. Infiltration of portal tract with inflammatory cells.
6. Spilling of inflammatory cells in the adjacent parenchyma causing necrosis of adjacent cells (**Interface hepatitis** or **piecemeal necrosis**).

CHRONIC HEPATITIS

Older classification of chronic hepatitic

Chronic persistant Hepatitis	Chronic active hepatitis	Chronic lobular hepatitis
• Inflammation limited to portal tracts • Lobular structure of liver is preserved	• Inflammation involving both parenchyma and portal tracts • Associated with *"piecemeal necrosis"* and *"bridging necrosis"* • Lobular structure not preserved.	• Inflammation limited to the lobules

Latest classification of hepatitis is based on

1. *Cause* (Viral hepatitis, autoimmune hepatitis, drug associated hepatitis etc.)
2. *Histological activity or grade*
   - Grading is based on necrosis and inflammation which include assessment of the following factors:
   - Periportal necrosis including piecemeal necrosis and bridging necrosis
   - Portal inflammation
   - Intralobular necrosis
   - Fibrosis
3. *Degree of progression or stage*

Staging is done based on the degree of fibrosis

Absent	Mild	Moderate	Severe	Cirrhosis
0	1 (Fibrosis confined to portal tracts with portal expansion)	2 (Portal and peri-portal fibrosis)	3 (Bridging fibrosis)	4 (Cirrhosis)

Liver

1. **Hepatitis A virus (Infectious Hepatitis)**
   - It is a benign and self-limiting disease.
   - Incubation period of HAV is 2-6 weeks.
   - It **does not** cause chronic hepatitis or carrier state in hepatitis.
   - HAV is an unenveloped, single stranded RNA virus belonging to Picornavirus family.
   - **Feco-oral route** is the predominant route of spread.
   - HAV is present in stools 2-3 weeks before and 1 week after onset of jaundice.
   - IgM antibody appearing in blood with onset of symptoms is a marker of acute infection whereas IgG antibody provides life long immunity.

2. **Hepatitis B virus (Serum Hepatitis)**
   - It can cause acute hepatitis, non-progressive chronic hepatitis, progressive chronic hepatitis leading to cirrhosis, fulminant hepatitis, carrier state and hepatocellular carcinoma.
   - Incubation Period of HBV is 30-180 days.
   - HBV is present in all physiologic and pathologic body fluids, *except in stools* (unlike HAV).

Mode of Infection

- Blood products, needle sticks etc. (30%)
- Sexual transmission
- Vertical transmission is responsible for development of carrier state
- The virus is a double stranded DNA belonging to Hepadnaviridae family.
- It is a spherical, double layered 'Dane particle' 42 mm in size.

Genome

The genome of the virus has several genes coding for different proteins or enzymes. These include:

'S' gene	'C' gene	'P' gene	'X' gene
• Codes for envelope protein, **HBs Ag**[Q] (surface antigen)	• Codes for 2 nucleocapsid proteins: • **HBc Ag:**[Q] Intracellular nucleocapsid core antigen • **HBe Ag:**[Q] Nucleocapsid protein with a core and precore region.	• Codes for **DNA polymerase** having **reverse transcriptase activity**[Q]	• Codes for **HBx protein**[Q] required for viral replication and transcriptional activator of viral and host genes. • Particularly important in the development of **hepatocellular carcinoma**[Q].

- The precore region directs the release of HBe Ag towards secretion in the blood. Uncommonly, mutated strains called *precore mutants* of HBV emerge that do not produce HBe Ag but are replication competent and express HBc Ag. In these patients, the HBe Ag may be undetectable despite the presence of HBV viral load. A **mutation in the core promoter region** can also lead to an HBeAg negative phenotype. Clinically both these conditions are characterized by the presence of elevated liver enzymes and active viral multiplication is indicated only by the high levels of DNA polymerase.

PHASE OF INFECTIONS

There is an *initial proliferative phase* in which the viral DNA is present in an episomal form leading to the formation of complete virion with associated antigens. This is followed by expression of viral antigens with MHC class I molecules resulting in CD8+ T cells activation and destruction of infected hepatocytes. There is presence of an *integrative phase* in which the viral DNA is incorporated into host DNA. This usually occurs in hepatocytes not destroyed by immune response.

Carrier state is defined by the presence of **HBs Ag** in the serum for **6 months or longer** after initial detection.

HBc Ag never appears in the blood.

Concept

An important mutation seen in HBV is **"escape mutants"** due to amino acid substitution causing a conformational change in HBsAg resulting in *loss of neutralizing activity by anti-HBs*. It is seen in association with active and passive immunization and in liver transplant patients. In both these conditions, there is increased concentration of anti HBs leading to mutation in the virus so that it can escape from the protective effect of anti-HBs.

Most useful indicator of **prior infection** with HBV is **Anti HBc Ag**

Microscopically, **HBs Ag** is responsible for **"ground glass" hepatocytes** whereas *'HBc Ag"* gives *"sanded nuclei"* appearance.

Focal macrovesicular fatty changes indicates **HCV** infection

Panlobular micro and macrovesicular steatosis indicates *Alcohol* as the etiology

Bile duct damage and lymphoid aggregates in portal tract are indicative of chronic HCV infection.

Sequential Appearance of Hepatitis B Markers and Significance

HBs Ag	• Present in *acute disease*[Q]
	• Continued presence indicates chronic disease or carrier state
HBe Ag **HBV DNA** **DNA polymerase**	• Seen with active viral replication and denotes *high infectivity*[Q]
IgM anti HBc	• Antibody detectable shortly before onset of symptoms
	• *Marker of window period*[Q]
	• IgM anti HBc is indicator of recent disease whereas IgG anti HBc is seen with chronic infection or prior infection
Anti HBe Ab	• Detected after HBe Ag disappears and denotes *low infectivity*[Q]
IgG anti HBs	• Appears after disappearance of HBs Ag
	• Provides protection against Hepatitis B and *indicates immunity*[Q]
	• Seen in prior infection and in vaccinated persons[Q]

NUTSHELL OF HEPATITIS B SEROLOGY

	HBs Ag	IgM anti HBc	IgG anti HBc	IgG anti HBs
Acute HBV infection	+	+	–	–
Window period	–	+	–	–
Chronic infection	+	+/-	+	–
Prior infection	–	–	+	+
Immunization	–	–	–	+

In addition: Remember that the presence of HBe Ag denotes high infectivity and its absence denotes low infectivity.

Immunology concept
Immunization for HBV is based on the fact that anti HBs Ab is protective in nature. So, vaccination with non- infectious HBs Ag still retaining its immunogenic potential is done.

3. **Hepatitis C virus (Transfusion Associated Hepatitis)**
   – HCV is a single stranded RNA virus belonging to Flaviviridae family.
   – Incubation Period is 2-26 weeks.
   – Acute HCV infection is generally undetectable clinically whereas chronic disease occurs in majority of infected individuals.
   – Spread of the virus is through inoculation and blood transfusion (more frequently) and less commonly through sexual and vertical transmission.
   – Acute illness is usually asymptomatic/mild.
   – Initially, there is IgM anti-HCV followed by the presence of IgG anti-HCV antibodies.
   – Chronic infection is associated with episodic elevations in serum transaminases with intervening normal period associated with persistence of HCV RNA in the blood.

Note: Antibody against HCV is IgG anti-HCV which does not provide effective immunity because the virus demonstrates genomic instability and antigenic variability.

4. **Hepatitis D virus (Delta Agent)**
   – It is a single stranded RNA virus.
   – Replication is defective and can cause infection only when encapsulated by HBs Ag.

Liver

- So, it can cause infection in 2 conditions:
  - **Acute co-infection**: In which there is simultaneous exposure to both HBV and HDV. However, HBV must establish first. This is associated with 90% chances of recovery and only rare chances of development of chronic hepatitis.
  - **Super infection**: In which chronic carriers of HBV get infected with HDV. This is associated with majority developing chronic hepatitis.

The serology shows the presence of *IgM Anti HDV* which is the *most reliable marker of recent infection*.

5. **Hepatitis E virus**

   - It is a single stranded RNA unenveloped **enterically transmitted** virus accounting for more than 50% of cases of acute hepatitis in India.
   - Incubation period is 2-8 weeks.
   - It causes sporadic infection in young to middle aged adults (rare in children).
   - The **disease is self limiting** (*not associated with chronic disease*).
   - The serology shows the HEV RNA and presence of virions in stool and the liver even before onset of clinical illness.
   - IgM anti-HEV IgG anti HEV followed by is seen in 2-4 weeks.

> HEV is associated with high mortality in pregnancy.

6. **Hepatitis G virus**

   It is a single stranded RNA virus transmitted by the parenteral route i.e. by the contaminated blood or blood products and possibly by the sexual route. In up to 75% of infections, HGV is cleared from the plasma and the infection becomes chronic in the remaining 25%. The site of HGV replication is *mononuclear cells*, so, it does not cause any rise in serum amino transferases and is **non pathogenic**. It co-infects patients with HIV and the dual infection is protective against HIV disease.

Clinicopathologic Syndromes

1. **Acute asymptomatic infection with recovery:**
   This is identified incidentally with the help of elevated serum transaminases or the presence of antiviral antibodies

2. **Acute viral hepatitis:** It has got 4 phases:

Incubation period
Peak infectivity during last days of incubation period and early days of acute symptoms.
Symptomatic pre-icteric phase
Nonspecific, constitutional symptoms, malaise, general fatigability, nausea, and loss of appetite.
Symptomatic icteric phase
Caused mainly by conjugated hyperbilirubinemia, dark urine and light stools
Convalescence
Recovery due to T cell activity against infected hepatocytes.

3. **Chronic viral hepatitis:** Symptomatic, biochemical or serologic evidence of continuing or relapsing disease for > *6 months* with histologic documentation of inflammation and necrosis. Chronic hepatitis constitutes a "Carrier State". Healthy carriers are individuals having the virus without adverse effects. Vertical transmission with HBV produces carrier in 90-95% cases. The most common symptom is fatigue; less common symptoms are malaise, loss of appetite, and occasionally mild jaundice.

4. **Fulminat hepatitis:** Progression of hepatic insufficiency *from onset* of symptoms *to hepatic encephalopathy* within *2-3 weeks*, is called *fulminant hepatic failure*. The progression in upto 3 months is called subfulminant failure.

ALCOHOLIC LIVER DISEASE

Alcoholic liver disease

Hepatic steatosis	Alcoholic hepatitis	Alcoholic cirrhosis
• Also called fatty liver • Characterized by the presence of small (microvesicular) or large (macrovesicular) lipid droplets inside the hepatocytes • Initial centrilobular involvement followed by entire lobule involved • Reversible if there is abstinence from alcohol.	• Having hepatocyte swelling and necrosis **(ballooning degeneration)** • Neutrophilic infiltration in lobule • Perivenular and periportal fibrosis (due to ito cell in space of sisse) • Some hepatocytes show the presence of eosinophilic, cytokeratin filaments called **'Mallory Hyaline bodies'**.	• Irreversible form of alcoholic liver disease • Initially, liver is enlarged and later there is presence of micronodules and macronodules • Later, the whole liver has tough, pale scar tissue **(Laennec Cirrhosis)**.

Conditions where Mallory Hyaline bodies are seen (Mnemonic: New Indian WATCH)

New - **N**on-alcoholic fatty liver disease (NAFLD)

Indian - **I**ndian childhood cirrhosis

W - **W**ilson's disease

A - α_1- **A**T deficiency; **A**lcoholic Liver Disease

T - **T**umor of liver (Hepatocellular carcinoma)

C - **C**hronic cholestatic conditions

H - **H**epatic or Primary Biliary cirrhosis (it is **not** seen in Secondary biliary cirrhosis)

Non Alcoholic Fatty Liver Disease (NAFLD)

• It is a condition that resembles alcohol-induced liver disease but occurs in patients who are not heavy drinkers. Men and women are equally affected.

Association

• Strong association with **obesity**[Q], **dyslipidemia**[Q], **hyperinsulinemia**[Q] and **insulin resistance**[Q].

Spectrum of disease

• NAFLD includes simple hepatic steatosis, steatosis with non specific inflammation and non-alcoholic steatohepatitis (NASH). Some patients may develop cirrhosis. Patients are largely asymptomatic, with abnormalities only in biochemical laboratory tests.

Clinical Significance

• NAFL is now the *most common cause of "cryptogenic" cirrhosis*[Q]. It also contributes to the progression of other liver diseases like hepatitis C viral infection.

Diagnosis

• NAFL is a diagnosis of exclusion (excessive alcohol intake has to be excluded).
• *Liver biopsy*[Q] is the most important diagnostic tool for NASH. It is also associated with AST/ALT ratio less than 1 (in alcoholic steatohepattis the same ratio is >2.0).

Clinically

• The patients are asymptomatic with elevated enzyme levels. **Cardiovascular disease**[Q] is a frequent cause of death.

NODULAR HYPERPLASIAS

These are represented by two conditions: **Focal nodular hyperplasia** and **Nodular regenerative hyperplasia**.

Focal nodular hyperplasia

• Presents as a spontaneous mass lesion

• Most frequently in **young** to middle-aged adults

• **Female** preponderance

• Associated with long term use of **anabolic hormones** or **contraceptives**

• Typically, there is a **central** grey-white, depressed **stellate scar** from which fibrous septa radiate to the periphery. The central scar contains large vessels, usually arterial, that typically exhibit fibromuscular hyperplasia with eccentric or concentric narrowing of the lumen.

Nodular regenerative hyperplasia

- Associated with the development of **portal hypertension** and its clinical manifestations.
- Occurs in conditions affecting intra hepatic blood flow like **rheumatoid arthritis (most commonly)**, Felty syndrome, myeloproliferative disorders, hyperviscosity syndromes, solid organ (particularly renal and liver) transplantation, bone marrow transplantation, **HIV infection** (Robbins), vasculitic conditions and **drugs (anabolic steroids and cytotoxics).**
- Characteristically, there is **absence of fibrosis** in this condition.

Hepatic Tumors

Hepatic tumors

Benign	Malignant

• Cavernous hemangioma
  – *Most common benign lesion of liver*
• Liver cell adenoma (hepatic adenoma)
  – Seen in young females
  – Associated with oral contraceptive intake
  – Microscopically, the cells have clear cytoplasm and the portal tracts are absent.
	• Hepatoblastoma
	  – *Most common liver tumor of young children*
	  – Activation of Wnt/β catein signaling pathway causes carcinogenesis
	• Angiosarcoma
	  – Associated with previous exposure to arsenic vinyl chloride or thorotrast
	• Hepatocellular carcinoma
	• Cholangiocarcinoma

▌ HEPATOCELLULAR CARCINOMA (HCC)

It is the *most common primary malignant tumor of the liver*. It usually affects old patients with a M:F ratio of 3:1.

Risk factors for development of HCC
- Chronic Hepatitis (Hepatitis B, Hepatitis C)
- Alcoholism
- Aflatoxins (due to *Aspergillus flavus* infection of peanuts, grains)
- Tyrosinemia
- Hereditary hemochromatosis

Pathogenesis: HBV has the presence of HBX protein which causes activation of host cell proto-oncogenes and disruption of cell cycle control. Aflatoxins cause mutations in proto-oncogenes or p53 (tumor suppressor gene).

Clinical features include malaise, upper abdominal pain, weight loss and fatigue. Laboratory investigations show elevation of serum α-fetoprotein (AFP). AFP elevation can also be seen in yolk sac tumors, cirrhosis, massive liver necrosis, chronic hepatitis, normal pregnancy, fetal distress or death, fetal neural tube defects (anencephaly and spina bifida).

Histologically, HCC can present as a unifocal mass, multifocal mass or diffuse infiltrative cancer involving the entire liver. All the three variants have a strong *tendency for vascular invasion* and intrahepatic metastasis. These can involve portal vein or inferior vena cava extending upto right side of the heart. There is presence of Mallory Hyaline bodies (eosinophilic intracytoplasmic inclusions of keratin filaments).

Distinguishing features of Fibrolamellar cancer (from hepatocellular cancer)

- Seen in **young adults** (20-40 years).
- **Equal incidence in males and females,** [In India, however, females > males]
- **No association** with HBV or cirrhosis risk factors.
- Has **better prognosis**.
- **No elevation of serum AFP** levels.
- Microscopic examination shows well differentiated cells separated by dense collagen bands.
- Fibrolamellar variant usually affects **left lobe** of the liver more commonly.
- It spreads by *lymphatic route*.

> **Hep–par 1 or hepatocyte paraffin 1** is specific for hepatocyte mitochondria and is considered the **most specific** and **sensitive marker** of normal and neoplastic hepatocytes. It has been used in diagnosing hepatocellular carcinomas.

> The staining for **Glypican-3** is used to distinguish early hepatocellular carcinoma from a dysplastic nodule. Other tests cannot be used because the levels of serum α-fetoprotein are inconclusive in this condition.

> The tumor marker of fibrolamellar variant of hepatocellular carcinoma is *Neurotensin*.

> The marker of choice for differentiating between hepatocellular cancer and its fibrolamellar variant is *AFP*.

Metastasis from HCC takes place to:

1. Contiguous spread through hepatic vessels – *"Satellite nodules"*
2. Lungs
3. Perihilar, peri-pancreatic and para-aortic lymph nodes.

CHOLANGIOCARCINOMA

Cholangiocarcinoma (CC)

CC typically refers to mucin-producing adenocarcinomas that arise from the bile ducts.
Classification
Extrahepatic- 90% • Perihilar-60% • Distal bile duct – 20 to 30% **Intra-hepatic** – 10%.
Risk factors (Mnemonic: All have alphabet '**C**')
• Primary sclerosing **C**holangitis • Liver flukes like **C**lonorchis sinensis and Opisthorchis viverrini • Cause of chronic biliary inflammation and injury (**C**holedocholithiasis) • **C**ontrat material: thorotrast • Chronic alcoholic liver disease • **C**ongenital fibropolycystic diease (**C**holedochal cysts, **C**aroli's disease)
Genetic predisposition
There is **over expression of IL-6** and **K-RAS and reduced expression of p53**.
Clinical features
Painless jaundice, often with pruritus or weight loss, and acholic stools.
Microscopically
It is an *adenocarcinoma associated with dense collagenous stroma* (desmoplastic reaction). The differentiated bile duct epithelial cells do not produce bile, so, this cancer is **rarely bile stained**.
Diagnosis
• Percutaneous biopsy for peripheral liver lesions. • Endoscopic retrograde cholangiopancreatography (ERCP) for central lesions.
Tumor markers
• Tumors stain **positively** for **cytokeratin 7, 8, and 19** and *negatively for cytokeratin 20*. • CEA, CA 19-9, and **CA-125** are non specific and are **useful for following response to therapy**.
Metastasis
Spread of the cancer takes place to lungs, vertebrae, adrenals, brain and regional lymph nodes.

▌ METASTATIC TUMORS

Secondary liver cancers are more common than primary liver cancers. The common primary sites include breast, colon and lung. The metastatic nodules have central necrosis and umbilication.

Klatskin tumors are located at *junction of right and left hepatic ducts*. They are the commonest sub type of **cholangiocarcinoma**.

All risk factors of **cholangio-carcinoma** start with **alphabet 'C'**)

Liver

MULTIPLE CHOICE QUESTIONS

BILIRUBIN METABOLISM, HYPERBILIRUBINEMIAS

1. **Which of the following condition is associated with unconjugated hyperbilirubinemia?** *(DPG 2011)*
   (a) Dubin-Johnson syndrome
   (b) Rotor syndrome
   (c) Gilbert syndrome
   (d) Gall stones

2. **A patient with unconjugated bilirubinemia has increased excretion of urobilinogen in his urine. This can be seen in all of the following conditions, except:**
   (a) G6 PD deficiency *(AI 2010)*
   (b) Hemolytic anemia
   (c) Hereditary spherocytosis
   (d) Biliary cirrhosis

3. **In post-hepatic jaundice, the concentration of conjugated bilirubin in the blood is higher than that of unconjugated bilirubin because:** *(AIIMS Nov 2002)*
   (a) There is an increased rate of destruction of red blood cells
   (b) The unconjugated bilirubin is trapped by the bile stone produced in the bile duct.
   (c) The conjugation process of bilirubin in liver remains operative without any interference.
   (d) The UDP glucuronyl transferase activity is increased manifold in obstructive jaundice

4. **Function of hepatic stellate cells is/are:**
   (a) Formation of sinusoids *(PGI June 2001)*
   (b) Vitamin A storage
   (c) Increases blood perfusion
   (d) Phagocytosis

5. **Which of the following diseases is not a cause of indirect hyperbilirubinemia?** *(Delhi PG 2009)*
   (a) Rotor's syndrome
   (b) Criggler Najjar syndrome
   (c) Gilbert syndrome
   (d) Hereditary spherocytosis

6. **In unconjugated hyperbilirubinemia, the fraction of unconjugated bilirubin to total bilirubin exceeds**
   (a) 0.65 *(UP 2002)*
   (b) 0.50
   (c) 0.35
   (d) 0.80

7. **A 40 years old woman Hema Thapar presents with generalized pruritus for last 4 months which is not relieved by various lotions available in the market. On physical examination is unremarkable but her blood sample is sent to the laboratory. Her reports are as follows:**

- Total serum bilirubin of 2.0 mg/dL
- Direct bilirubin of 1.4 mg/dL
- SGOT 58 U/L
- SGPT 52U/L
- Alkaline phosphate is 300U/L
- Total protein is 7.2 g/dL with serum albumin of 3.5 g/dL
- Total cholesterol of 350 mg/dL.

Which of the following serologic test findings is most likely to be positive in this patient?
   (a) Anti-parietal cell antibody
   (b) Antimitochondrial antibody
   (c) Anti-centromere antibody
   (d) Anti ribonucleoprotein antibody

Most Recent Questions

7.1. **Primary biliary cirrhosis is positive for:**
   (a) p-ANCA
   (b) Anti nuclear antibody
   (c) Anti-microsomal antibody
   (d) Anti-mitochondrial antibody

7.2. **Which of the following is not a function of liver:**
   (a) Production of vitamin K
   (b) Production of albumin
   (c) Detoxification of ammonia
   (d) Metabolism of drugs

CIRRHOSIS, NCPF

8. **A 30 years old man Surajmal visits his physician because he noticed the development of yellowish skin during last 5 days. His physical examination has absence of abdominal pain or tenderness. His blood reports are as follows: Haemoglobin 11.5 g/dL, MCV 94μm3, platelet count 1,80,000/mm3, WBC count 6930/mm3, albumin 3.7g/dL, total protein 5.6 g/dL, total bilirubin 8.2 mg/dL, direct bilirubin, 0.5 mg/dL, AST, 45 U/L, ALT 32 U/L, and alkaline phosphatase, 340U/L. What of the following is the most likely diagnosis?**
   (a) Cholelithiasis
   (b) HAV infection
   (c) Micronodular cirrhosis
   (d) Hemolytic anemia

9. **Which one of the following is not a feature of liver histology in *Non cirrhotic portal fibrosis*?**
   (AI 05, DPG '10)
   (a) Fibrosis in and around the portal tracts

(b) Thrombosis of the medium and small portal vein branches

(c) Non specific inflammatory cell infiltrates in the portal tracts

(d) Bridging fibrosis

10. 'Nutmeg liver' is seen in   *(Karnataka 2005)*
   (a) Portal cirrhosis
   (b) Biliary cirrhosis
   (c) Chronic venous congestion of liver
   (d) Fatty liver

11. Commonest site of varices in portal hypertension is
   (a) Esophagus   *(UP 2000)*
   (b) Anal canal
   (c) Periumbilical
   (d) Liver

12. In cirrhosis of liver collagen is laid down by
   (a) Hepatocytes   *(AP 2005)*
   (b) Hepatic stellate cells
   (c) Biliary epithelial cells
   (d) Kupffer cells

13. An old alcoholic Chivas R Signature presents to the medical emergency of GS Hospital with confusion and lethargy. The medical specialist on duty, Dr. Thamim carried out the physical examination in which Mr Signature was visibly jaundiced with ascites. His blood sample was taken and sent to the laboratory. The investigations reveled increased prothrombin time and prolonged activated partial thromboplastin time, as well as significantly increased serum ammonia levels. With the known finding of significantly increased serum ammonia, which of the following physical findings may be expected in this patient?
   (a) Capillary telangiectasias
   (b) Asterixis
   (c) Caput medusae
   (d) Gynecomastia

14. A 50-year-old chronic alcoholic with jaundice and ascites secondary to known cirrhosis becomes disoriented and confused. Asterixis (flapping tremor) can be demonstrated. Which of the following is not associated with the development of ascites?
   (a) Hypoalbuminemia
   (b) Increased hepatic lymph formation
   (c) Increased portal venous pressure
   (d) Portal-systemic venous shunting

15. A 42-year-old woman Kiran with polycythemia vera develops progressive severe ascites and tender hepatomegaly over a period of several months. Liver function tests are near normal. Which of the following tests would be most likely to establish the probable diagnosis?
   (a) Endoscopic retrograde cholangiopancreatography
   (b) Hepatic venography
   (c) Serum alpha fetoprotein
   (d) Serum iron

Most Recent Questions

15.1. Nutmeg liver is seen in which of the following conditions?
   (a) Right sided heart failure
   (b) Left sided heart failure
   (c) Increased pulmonary pressure
   (d) Decreased pulmonary pressure

15.2. Nutmeg liver is seen in:
   (a) Right sided heart failure
   (b) Left sided heart failure
   (c) Increased pulmonary pressure
   (d) Decreased pulmonary pressure

15.3. Micronodular cirrhosis is seen in all except:
   (a) Alcoholic cirrhosis
   (b) Viral hepatitis
   (c) Budd-Chiari syndrome
   (d) Indian childhood cirrhosis

HEPATITIS

16. A 20 yr old man with HBs Ag +ve, HbeAg –ve with SGOT and SGPT raised 5 times the normal value. The HBV DNA copies are 1,00,000/ml. Which is the likely diagnosis?   *(AI 2010)*
   (a) Wild type HBV   (b) Surface mutant HBV
   (c) PreCore mutant HBV   (d) Inactive HBV carrier

17. Which one of the following diseases characteristically causes fatty change in liver?   *(AI 2005)*
   (a) Hepatitis B virus infection
   (b) Wilson's disease
   (c) Hepatitis C infection
   (d) Chronic alcoholism

18. Councilman bodies are seen in: *(AIIMS Nov 2007)*
   (a) Wilson disease   (b) Alcoholic hepatitis
   (c) Acute viral hepatitis (d) Auto immune hepatitis

19. In Chronic Viral Hepatitis   *(AIIMS May 2004)*
   (a) Hepatitis A virus infection is a common cause in children
   (b) Morphological classification into Chronic Active Hepatitis and Chronic Persistent Hepatitis are important
   (c) Fatty change is pathognomic of Hepatitis C virus infection
   (d) Grading refers to the extent of necrosis and inflammation

20. The liver biopsy in acute hepatitis due to hepatitis B virus is likely to show all of the following, except
                    (AIIMS May 2004)
   (a) Ballooning change of hepatocytes
   (b) Ground glass hepatocytes
   (c) Focal or spotty necrosis
   (d) Acidophil bodies

21. **All are correctly matched except:** *(PGI June 2006)*
    (a) Hepatitis B - Ground glass hepatocytes
    (b) Reye's syndrome - Ground glass hepatocytes
    (c) Alcohol - Mallory bodies
    (d) Wilson disease - Mallory bodies
    (e) Acute hepatitis - councilman bodies

22. **Centrilobular necrosis of liver occurs in**
    (a) Phosphorus *(UP 2000)*
    (b) Phenol
    (c) Arsenic
    (d) Mercury

23. **Most common Pathological change seen in acute viral hepatitis is** *(UP 2002)*
    (a) Ballooning degeneration
    (b) Neutrophilic infiltration
    (c) Piece meal necrosis
    (d) Periportal fatty change

24. **Steatosis is NOT seen in** *(UP 2004)*
    (a) Hepatitis-B infection
    (b) Hepatitis-C infection
    (c) Alcoholic person
    (d) Protein malnutrition

25. **Piece meal necrosis is seen in** *(RJ 2001)*
    (a) Alcoholic hepatitis
    (b) Toxic hepatitis
    (c) Chronic active hepatitis
    (d) Malignancy

26. **In pregnancy, which viral infection has maximum mortality?** *(RJ 2003)*
    (a) Hepatitis A Virus
    (b) Hepatitis B Virus
    (c) Hepatitis C Virus
    (d) Hepatitis E Virus.

27. **Hepatitis B virus is not associated with** *(RJ 2004)*
    (a) Fulminant hepatitis
    (b) Chronic active hepatitis
    (c) Hepatocellular carcinoma
    (d) Cholangiocarcinoma

28. **Piece meal necrosis is pathognomic of** *(RJ 2006)*
    (a) Alcoholic Liver disease
    (b) Chronic active hepatitis
    (c) Toxic hepatitis
    (d) Wilson disease

29. **Hepatitis E is transmitted by** *(AP 2004)*
    (a) Blood
    (b) Feco-oral
    (c) Venereal
    (d) All of the above

30. **Incubation period of hepatitis B is** *(Bihar 2004)*
    (a) 6 weeks to 6 months
    (b) 6 days to 6 weeks
    (c) 6 months to 6 years
    (d) More than 6 years

31. **Indicator of active multiplication of hepatitis B virus is:** *(Bihar 2004)*
    (a) HBs Ag
    (b) HBc Ag
    (c) Hbe Ag
    (d) Anti-HBs Ab

32. **Chronic carrier stage is not found in** *(RJ 2003)*
    (a) Hepatitis B Virus
    (b) Hepatitis C Virus
    (c) Both a and b
    (d) Hepatitis A Virus

33. **A 30 year old woman Aishwarya goes to her gynecologist Dr. Harmeet for a pre-pregnancy examination. Routine prenatal laboratory testing demonstrates normal hematological profile with controlled sugar as well negative TORCH infections. She normal liver function tests with the following profile: HBsAg negative, anti-HBcAg (-), anti- HBeAg (-), HBV DNA polymerase (-) but anti- HBsAg is positive. Which of the following likely represents the status of the patient?**
    (a) Hepatitis B carrier
    (b) Recently infected with hepatitis B
    (c) Immunized against hepatitis B
    (d) Infected with hepatitis B and highly transmissible

34. **In a pioneering clinical study at Spartans Institute, patients having infection with infectious hepatitis, (as in hepatitis A, B, C, D, E, F, and G) are being followed for 40 months. During that time the subjects are required to undergo regular investigations like prothrombin time, serum AST, ALT, alkaline phosphatase, total bilirubin, and ammonia. Every 6months, a liver biopsy is performed microscopically examined. Which of the following is the best predictor of development of chronic disease progressing to cirrhosis?**
    (a) Presence of inflammatory cell in the sinusoids on a liver biopsy specimen
    (b) Degree to which hepatic transaminase enzymes are elevated.
    (c) Length of time that hepatic enzymes remain elevated
    (d) Specific form of hepatitis virus responsible of the infection

35. **An eminent hepatobiliary expert Dr. Sarin conducts a study in hepatitis B patients for which the patients are followed for almost a decade. Their detailed history regarding the mode of transmission of HBV is taken. A battery of tests including periodic serologic testing for HBs Ag, anti HBs and anti-HBc, and serum levels of bilirubin, SOT, SGPT, alkaline phosphatase, and prothrombin time is conducted. Dr. Sarin finds that a particular group of patients happen to be chronic carriers of HBV. This finding is most likely to be associated with which of the following modes of transmission of HBV?**
    (a) Blood transfusion
    (b) Heterosexual transmission
    (c) Vertical transmission during childbirth
    (d) Needle stick injury

36. A 34-year-old man Bholu presents to his physician with loss of appetite, nausea and vomiting, and fatigue. Laboratory examination confirms the diagnosis of hepatitis B, and the man becomes icteric 2 weeks later. This patient may also be particularly vulnerable to the development of which of the following disorders?
    (a) Berry aneurysm
    (b) Coronary artery aneurysm
    (c) Polyarteritis nodosa
    (d) Giant cell arteritis

37. After passing his physical exam, a young army recruit gives urine and blood samples for further testing. Serum analysis yields elevated ALT, HBsAg, Anti-HBc, HBeAg, and bilirubin. All other values are normal. Which of the following is the hepatitis B status of this recruit?
    (a) Asymptomatic carrier
    (b) Chronic active carrier
    (c) Fulminant hepatitis B
    (d) Recovered from acute self-limited HBV

ALCOHOLIC LIVER DISEASE, NODULAR HYPERPLASIA

38. In a chronic alcoholic all the following may be seen in the liver except   (AI 2002)
    (a) Fatty degeneration
    (b) Chronic hepatitis
    (c) Granuloma formation
    (d) Cholestatic hepatitis

39. Nodular regenerative changes in liver most commonly occur in: (AIIMS May 2009)
    (a) Drugs induced hepatitis
    (b) Alcoholic hepatitis
    (c) Hepatitis B
    (d) Autoimmune hepatitis

40. Mallory hyaline is seen in: (PGI Dec 2000)
    (a) Alcoholic liver disease
    (b) Hepatocellular carcinoma
    (c) Wilson's disease
    (d) I.C.C. (Indian childhood cirrhosis)
    (e) Biliary cirrhosis

41. All of the following are true except?
    (DPG &AIIMS Nov 10)
    (a) LKM 1 – Autoimmune hepatitis
    (b) LKM 2– Drug induced
    (c) LKM 1– Chronic hepatitis C
    (d) LKM 2– Chronic hepatitis D

42. A chronic alcoholic has an elevated serum alpha fetoprotein levels. Which of the following neoplasms is most likely seen?   (Delhi PG 09 RP)
    (a) Prostatic adenocarcinoma
    (b) Multiple myeloma
    (c) Hepatocellular carcinoma
    (d) Glioblastoma multiforme

43. Mallory's hyaline is seen in: (Delhi PG 2009 RP)
    (a) Hepatitis C infection
    (b) Amoebic liver abscess
    (c) Indian childhood cirrhosis
    (d) Autoimmune hepatitis

44. Mallory hyaline body is seen in all except:
    (a) Indian childhood cirrhosis   (Delhi PG-2007)
    (b) Alcoholism
    (c) Secondary biliary cirrhosis
    (d) α-1 antitrypsin deficiency

45. Mallory bodies are composed of:
    (a) Fat droplets   (Karnataka 2009)
    (b) Mitochondria
    (c) Lysosomal enzymes
    (d) Intermediate filaments

46. Alcoholic hyaline seen in alcoholic liver disease is composed of   (UP 2007)
    (a) Lipofuschin
    (b) Eosinophilic intracytoplasmic inclusions
    (c) Basophilic intracytoplasmic inclusions
    (d) Hemazoin

47. In Alcoholic liver disease, which of the following pigments is deposited in the hepatocytes?
    (a) Hemosiderin   (UP 2008)
    (b) Hemoglobin
    (c) Lipofuschin
    (d) Melanin

48. Mallory bodies are seen is   (RJ 2006)
    (a) Viral hepatitis
    (b) Toxic hepatitis
    (c) Alcoholic hepatitis
    (d) All

49. Mallory bodies are seen in all except   (AP 2004)
    (a) Alcoholic cirrhosis
    (b) Biliary cirrhosis
    (c) Cardiac cirrhosis
    (d) Wilson disease

50. A 46-year-old man, Sushil who has a long history of excessive drinking presents with signs of alcoholic hepatitis. Microscopic examination of a biopsy of this patient's liver reveals irregular eosinophilic hyaline inclusions within the cytoplasm of the hepatocytes. These eosinophilic inclusions are composed of which of the following substances?
    (a) Immunoglobulin
    (b) Excess plasma proteins
    (c) Prekeratin intermediate filaments
    (d) Basement membrane material
    (e) Lipofuscin

Most Recent Questions

50.1. Mallory bodies contain:
    (a) Vimentin   (b) Cytokeratin
    (c) Keratin   (d) Collagen

50.2. Which of the following is not associated with Mallory hyaline bodies?
(a) Alcoholic liver disease
(b) Primary biliary cirrhosis
(c) Secondary biliary cirrhosis
(d) Indian childhood cirrhosis

50.3. Which of the following may not cause microvesicular steatosis?
(a) Alcoholic fatty liver
(b) Tetracycline toxicity
(c) Acute fatty liver of pregnancy
(d) Reye's syndrome

50.4. The following are true attributes of hepatitis B infection except:
(a) Infants develop chronic infections
(b) HBc Ag in serum is indicative of active infection
(c) Can cause hepatocellular cancer
(d) Interferons are used for treatment

HEPATIC TUMOURS

51. Which of the following most significantly increases the risk of hepatocellular cancer?
(a) Hep A *(AIIMS May 2012)*
(b) Hep B
(c) CMV
(d) EBV

52. True about Fibrolamellar carcinoma of Liver is all, except: *(AIIMS Nov 2001)*
(a) Females do not increased incidence than males
(b) Has good prognosis
(c) Not associated with liver cirrhosis
(d) Serum AFP levels are usually > 1000 mg/litre

53. Which of the following is not correct about fibrolamellar variant of hepatocellular carcinoma? *(Delhi PG 2009 RP)*
(a) Occurs in young males and females
(b) Hepatitis B virus is an important risk factor
(c) Often has a better prognosis
(d) Is a hard scirrhous tumor

54. Most common primary malignant tumour of liver in adult is *(UP 2002)*
(a) Squamous cell carcinoma
(b) Hepatoblastoma
(c) Hepatocellular carcinoma
(d) Hepatoma

55. Which is not correct about hepatocellular carcinoma? *(Jharkhand 2004)*
(a) More in females
(b) Rise of AFP noted
(c) Has stronger propensity to invade vascular channels.
(d) Chronic HBV has high rate of hepatocellular carcinoma

56. A young woman Ms Shaano who is otherwise normal goes for an annual examination in a nursing home. Her blood investigations reveal hemoglobin is 15 gm/ dl, TLC is 7,000/mm3, ESR is 12mm/hr. Her kidney and liver function tests are also normal. She undergoes a radiological scanning too. Dr. Sethi, the radiologist describes her findings to be normal except a mass in the right lobe of the liver. A biopsy is taken which confirms the diagnosis of a liver adenoma. Which of the following is likely to be associated with this lesion?
(a) Polycythemia vera
(b) Hepatitis B
(c) Oral contraceptives
(d) Polyvinyl chloride

Most Recent Questions

56.1. Thorium induced tumor:
(a) Angiosarcoma of liver
(b) Renal cell carcinoma
(c) Lymphoma
(d) Astrocytoma

56.2. Commonest benign tumor of liver is:
(a) Hamartoma
(b) Hemangioma
(c) Adenoma
(d) Nodular focal hyperplasia

BILIARY TRACT DISORDER

57. Most common site of Cholangiocarcinoma is?
(a) Distal biliary tree *(AIIMS Nov 2008)*
(b) Hilum
(c) Intrahepatic biliary duct
(d) Multifocal

58. Cholangiocarcinoma of liver is caused by
(a) *Hepatitis B* infection *(UP 2008)*
(b) Cirrhosis of liver
(c) Antitrypsin deficiency
(d) *Clonorchis sinensis* infection

59. Most common bile duct tumor is *(RJ 2000)*
(a) Adenocarcinoma
(b) Squamous cell cancer
(c) Transitional cell carcinoma
(d) All

60. A 50-year-old male film actor Sallu Kahn looses weight rapidly for one of his forthcoming films. He experiences occasional abdominal discomfort few days after that and guided by his physician, he undergoes a radiological scan (HIDA scan) is shown to have slow and incomplete gallbladder emptying in response to cholecystokinin stimulation. This patient is likely to develop which of the following?
(a) Black pigment stones
(b) Brown pigment stones
(c) Biliary sludge
(d) Phospholipid stones

61. A middle aged woman comes to the emergency room complaining of severe, right-sided abdominal

pain, fever, and chills for the past several hours. She has a history of gallstones and her family doctor recommended a cholecystectomy after a similar episode several months ago. Upon examination, she has a temperature of 102.7°F (39.3°C), is tender in the right upper quadrant, and is visibly jaundiced. Her white blood count is 18,000/mm³. In which of the following locations is a gallstone most likely lodged in this patient?

(a) Common bile duct
(b) Cystic duct
(c) Fundus of gallbladder
(d) Proximal duodenum

Most Recent Questions

61.1. Which is risk factor for cholangiocarcinoma:
(a) Obesity
(b) Primary sclerosing cholangitis
(c) Salmonella carrier state
(d) HBV infection

61.2. Klatskin tumor is:
(a) Nodular type of cholangiocarcinoma
(b) Fibrolamellar hepatocellular carcinoma
(c) Gall bladder carcinoma
(d) Hepatocellular carcinoma

61.3. All of the following are risk factors for carcinoma gall bladder, except:
(a) Typhoid carriers
(b) Adenomatous gall bladder polyps
(c) Choledochal cysts
(d) Oral contraceptives

61.4. Focal diffuse gall bladder wall thickening with comet tail reverberation artifacts on USG are seen in:
(a) Adenomyomatosis of gall bladder
(b) Carcinoma gall bladder
(c) Adenomatous Polyps
(d) Xanthogranulomatous gall bladder

61.5. Onion skin fibrosis of the common bile duct is:
(a) Primary biliary cirrhosis
(b) Primary sclerosing cholangitis
(c) Extrahepatic biliary fibrosis
(d) Congenital hepatic fibrosis

■ MISCELLANEOUS

62. True about hemochromatosis is: *(AI 2009)*
(a) Complete penetrance
(b) Autosomal recessive
(c) Phlebotomy leads to cure
(d) More common in females

63. All are seen in hemochromatosis except:
(a) Hypogonadism *(AI 2008)*
(b) Arthropathy
(c) Bronze diabetes
(d) Desferrioxamine is the treatment of choice

64. Liver granulomas may be associated with all of the following except *(AI 2002)*
(a) Candida
(b) Halothane
(c) Sarcoidosis
(d) Hepatic metastasis

65. Histological finding in Reye's syndrome is
(a) Budding and branching of mitochondria
(b) Swelling of endoplasmic reticulum
(c) Para-nuclear micro-dense deposits
(d) Glycogen depletion

66. Finding on histopathological examination of liver in case of malaria is *(AIIMS May 2007)*
(a) Microabscess formation
(b) Kupffer's cell hyperplasia with macrophage infiltration around periportal area laden with pigments.
(c) Non caseating granuloma
(d) Non specific finding of neutrophilic infiltration

67. Pigmentation in the liver is caused by all except
(a) Lipofuscin *(PGI Dec 01)*
(b) Pseudomelanin
(c) Wilson's disease
(d) Malarial pigment
(e) Bile pigment

68. True statements about α-l antitrypsin deficiency is
(a) Autosomal dominant disease *(PGI June 2003)*
(b) Emphysema
(c) Fibrosis of portal tract
(d) Diastase resistant positive hepatocytes
(e) Orcein positive granules

69. "Kayser-Fleischer ring" is seen in *(UP 2007)*
(a) Wilson's disease
(b) α-1 antitrypsin deficiency
(c) Hemochromatosis
(d) Primary biliary cirrhosis

70. All are true about Wilson's disease except
(a) ↑Liver Cu *(RJ 2000,2004,2006)*
(b) ↑Urine Cu
(c) ↑Ceruloplasmin
(d) ↑Serum Cu

71. α-1 antitrypsin deficiency causes *(AP 2000)*
(a) Congenital cystic fibrosis
(b) Neonatal hepatitis
(c) Pulmonary fibrosis
(d) All of the above

72. Centrilobular necrosis is seen in *(Kolkata 2005)*
(a) CCl_4
(b) White phosphorus
(c) Yellow fever
(d) Eclampsia

73. A retired man Pradyuman R complains of vague abdominal pain since last 6 months. One fine day, he experienced acute chest pain with dyspnea. He was rushed to the emergency of Gangaram Hospital where his chest and abdomen CT scans demonstrate a

Liver

pulmonary embolus. The radiologist Dr. Sandeep Goel also notices a 7.5 cm mass in the body of the pancreas. His blood investigations reveal elevated levels of CEA and CA 19-9. Which of the following genetic mutations is likely to be associated with this pancreatic mass?
(a) BRCA -2
(b) K-RAS
(c) PRSS1
(d) SPINK1

Most Recent Questions

73.1. Liver in hemochromatosis is stained by which of the following stain?
(a) Perls iron stain
(b) Alcian blue
(c) Congo Red
(d) Masson trichome

73.2. Bronze diabetes is seen in:
(a) Wilson's disease
(b) Sarcoidosis
(c) Lead intoxication
(d) Hemochromatosis

73.3. Copper is mainly transported by:
(a) Albumin
(b) Haptoglobin
(c) Ceruloplasmin
(d) Globulin

73.4. Gene of Wilsons disease is:
(a) ATP 7A
(b) ATP 7B
(c) ADP 7A
(d) ADP 7B

EXPLANATIONS

1. **Ans. (c) Gilbert syndrome** *(Ref: Harrison 17th/1929, 9/e p854)*

2. **Ans. (d) Biliary cirrhosis** *(Ref: Robbins 8th/868, 9/e p853-854)*
   Biliary cirrhosis is characterized by conjugated hyperbilirubinemia. Rest all the mentioned options cause unconjugated hyperbilirubinemia.

3. **Ans. (c) The conjugation process of bilirubin in liver remains operative without any interference** *(Ref: Harrison 17th/262-3, Ganong 22nd/503, 9/e p853)*
   Post hepatic jaundice is due to impaired excretion of conjugated bilirubin as a result of obstruction. However, the process of conjugation is not interfered with.

4. **Ans. (b) Vitamin A storage:** *(Ref: Robbins' 7th/878, 9/e p436)*

   > The hepatic stellate cells (also called Ito cells) are of mesenchymal origin, found in space of Disse. The stellate cells play a role in the storage and metabolism of vitamin A and are transformed into collagen producing myofibroblasts when there is inflammation and cause fibrosis of liver.

5. **Ans. (a) Rotor's syndrome** *(Ref: Robbins 9/e p854, 8th/841, Harrison 17th/26)*

6. **Ans. (d) 0.80** *(Ref: Robbins 9/e p853, Harrison 17th/262)*
   Indirect hyperbilirubinemia is called when unconjugated bilirubin is 85% or more of the total bilirubin whereas direct hyperbilirubinemia corresponds to conjugated bilirubin more than 15% of total.

7. **Ans. (b) Anti mitochondrial antibody** *(Ref: Robbins 8th/867, 9th/858)*
   The findings in the stem of the question are suggestive of clinical condition of primary biliary cirrhosis. It is seen in middle aged women in which the jaundice may progress due to progressive intrahepatic destruction. In these patients, there is presence of anti mitochondrial antibodies.
   Other options

   > - Anti parietal antibodies are seen in pernicious anemia.
   > - Anti-centromere antibody is seen in systemic sclerosis.
   > - Anti-ribonucleoprotein antibody is seen in different connective tissue disorders.

   The following disorders present with insidious onset of features of obstructive jaundice like pruritus, jaundice, malaise dark urine, light stools and hepatosplenomegaly.

   Features of the Bile Duct Disorders

	Primary Biliary Cirrhosis	Secondary Biliary Cirrhosis	Primary Sclerosing Cholangitis
Cause	Possibly autoimmune	Biliary atresia, gallstones, stricture, cancer of pancreatic head	Autoimmune; usually associated with inflammatory bowel disease
Sex predilection	Female to male: 6:1	None	Female to male: 1:2
Distribution	Intrahepatic bile duct obstruction	Extrahepatic bile duct obstruction	Extra + intra hepatic duct affected
Lab. findings	Same as secondary biliary cirrhosis with elevated serum IgM antimitochondrial antibody	↑conjugated bilirubin, ↑serum alkaline phosphatase with increased cholesterol	Same as secondary biliary cirrhosis with hypergammaglobulinemia (↑IgM), atypical p-ANCA (+)
Histological findings	Dense lymphocytic infiltrate in portal tracts with granulomatous destruction of bile ducts	Bile stasis in bile ducts, bile ductules proliferation with surrounding neutrophils, portal tract edema	Periductal portal tract fibrosis (onion skin fibrosis), segmental stenosis of extra and intrahepatic bile ducts

   > An important feature is Atypical p-ANCA (+) is seen with primary sclerosing cholangitis but that this antibody is directed against a nuclear envelope protein and not myeloperoxidase seen with typical p-ANCA antibodies.

7.1. **Ans. (b) Anti-mitochondrial antibody** *(Ref: Robbins 8/e p867, 9/e p858)*
   Friends, please do not get confused between options "b" and "d".
   - **Antimicrosomal antibodies** are autoantibodies, directed against the microsomes (in particular peroxidase) of the thyroid cells leading to thyroiditis, tissue damage, and disruption of thyroid function. It is associated with autoimmune conditions like **Hashimoto's thyroiditis** and **Grave's disease**.

Liver

- Anti-mitochondrial antibody is seen in primary biliary cirrhosis.

Key points for primary biliary cirrhosis

- Non-suppurative, inflammatory destruction of medium-sized *intrahepatic[Q] bile ducts*.
- Female to male ratio 6 : 1
- Serum *alkaline phosphatase and cholesterol are almost always elevated[Q]*, even at onset; hyperbilirubinemia is a late development and usually signifies incipient hepatic decompensation.
- *Antimitochondrial* **antibodies[Q]** are present in 90% to 95% of patients.
- Associated with *increased risk to develop hepatocellular carcinomas[Q]*.
- The major cause of death is **liver failure[Q]**,

7.2. Ans. (a) Production of vitamin K *(Ref: Robbins 9/e p 822)*

- Vitamin K is produced by the bacteria of gut and is used by liver for gamma carboxylation of factor 2/7/9/10.
- Liver produces albumin which falls in liver cirrhosis producing ascites/edema
- Ammonia is combined with carbon dioxide to produce urea which in turn is excreted by the liver.
- The cytochrome p450 is responsible for metabolism of drugs.

8. Ans. (d) Hemolytic anemia *(Ref: Robbins 8th/840-1, 9/e p853)*

The patient has unconjugated hyperbilirubinemia which can result in the given options from hemolytic anemia. Option (a), Cholelithiasis results in conjugated hyperbilirubinemia.

Option (c) and (d), hepatitis and micronodular cirrhosis can present with both unconjugated and conjugated hyperbilirubinemia though conjugated bilirubin predominates.

9. Ans. (d) Bridging fibrosis *(Ref: Tropical Hepato-Gastroenterology by Tandon Elsevier 1st/391, Histopathology of the liver in non-cirrhotic portal hypertension of unknown etiology Histopathology 1996;28:195–204 by Nakanuma Y et al., Non-cirrhotic portalfibrosis: current concept and management by Sarin SK, Kapoor D in J Gastroenterol Hepatol 2002; 17:526-534)*

The Following is a Figure explaining the pathogenesis of NCPF along with Histologically findings in NCPF

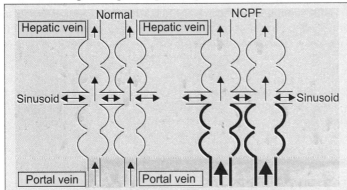

- **Portal fibrosis** (intra portal but not bridging fibrosis)
- Portal vein sclerosis
- Subcapsular scarring
- Pseudolobulation
- Portal tract edema and lymphocytic infilteration
- *Intimal fibroelastosis of medium sized portal veins;* **obliterative portal venopathy (characteristic lesion)**
- Sclerosis and obliteration of portal vein radicals
- Atrophy of liver parenchyma with no regenerative capacity
- Collagen deposition in the space of Disse

So, the answer is clear from the above mentioned features given collectively in all the references mentioned above. **Bridging fibrosis is not seen in NCPF.**

10. Ans. (c) Chronic venous congestion of liver *(Ref: Robbins 7th/122-3, 9/e p864)*

Congestion is a passive process resulting from impaired outflow from a tissue. In long standing or chronic venous congestion, the stasis results in chronic hypoxia resulting in parenchymal cell death. The central part of hepatic lobule is red brown and slightly depressed (due to loss of cells) and is accentuated against surrounding zone of uncongested tan liver. This is called **nutmeg liver**. Microscopically, there is presence of *hemosiderin laden macrophages*.

In severe cases (as with heart failure); there may be presence of hepatic fibrosis which is called *cardiac cirrhosis*.

11. Ans. (a) Esophagus *(Ref: Robbins 9/e p830,8th/839; 7th/885, 7th/885)*

12. Ans. (b) Hepatic stellate cells *(Ref: Robbins 9/e p822, 8th/837; 7th/883)*

13. Ans. (b) Asterixis *(Ref: Robbins 8th/836, 9/e p826)*

- Asterixis is a flapping tremor of the hands associated with hepatic encephalopathy. Failure of the liver to detoxify metabolites absorbed from the gastrointestinal tract results in accumulation of nitrogenous wastes that are neurotoxic.
- Disturbed mental status is also attributed to production of false neurotransmitters, increased CNS sensitivity to GABA, reduced activity of urea cycle enzymes due to zinc deficiency and swelling of astrocytes. Ref 2013 **(CMDT)**.

- Caput medusa results from dilation of the periumbilical venous collaterals as a result of portal hypertension and opening of portal-caval anastomoses. Other findings like palmar erythema, capillary telangiectasias, and gynecomastia results from the inability of the liver to metabolize estrogen leading to hyperestrinism.

14. **Ans. (d) Portal-systemic venous shunting** *(Ref: Robbins 8th/839, 9/e p830, Harrison 18th/2600)*
Portal-systemic venous shunting leads to encephalopathy in end-stage cirrhosis. It is also contributing to other features like esophageal varices, rectal haemorrhoids, and distention of periumbilical venous collaterals. Other factors like hypoalbuminemia, increased hepatic lymph formation and increased portal venous pressure mentioned as the options contribute to the development of ascites, but not to encephalopathy.

15. **Ans. (b) Hepatic venography** *(Ref: Robbins 8th/872-873, 9/e p863-864)*
The clinical presentation is most consistent with **Budd-Chiari syndrome** (hepatic vein obstruction), which may occur as a complication of thrombogenic and myeloproliferative disorders including polycythemia vera. The presentation in the question is the most common. **Hepatic venography is the best technique** of those listed to demonstrate the occlusion of the hepatic venous system.

- Endoscopic retrograde cholangiopancreatography (choice A) is most useful in demonstrating lesions of the biliary tree.
- Serum alpha fetoprotein (choice C) is a marker for hepatocellular carcinoma.
- Serum iron studies (choice D) are useful when considering hemochromatosis as a cause of cirrhosis.

15.1. **Ans. (a) Right sided heart failure** *(Ref: Robbins 8/e p872, 9/e p864)*
- *Right-sided cardiac decompensation leads to passive congestion of the liver.* In long standing or chronic venous congestion, the central part of hepatic lobule is red brown and slightly depressed (due to loss of cells) and is accentuated against surrounding zone of uncongested tan liver. This is called **nutmeg liver.**
- In severe cases this is called as *cardiac sclerosis or cardiac cirrhosis*.

15.2. **Ans. (a) Right sided heart failure explained earlier** *(Ref: Robbins 9/e p864)*

15.3. **Ans. (b) Viral hepatitis** *(Ref: Clinical Hepatology: Principles and Practice of Hepatobiliary Diseases: Volume 2 Springer publications p952)*
- Common causes of **micronodular cirrhosis** (nodules **<3mm in diameter**) Alcohol, Metabolic, Hemachromatosis, Wilson's Disease, Indian childhood cirrhosis, chronic venous outflow tract obstruction, bile duct obstruction
- Common causes of macronodular cirrhosis (nodules **>3mm in diameter**) Viruses, Toxins, Poisoning
Budd-Chiari syndrome is characterized by the obstruction of two or more major hepatic veins produce liver enlargement, pain, and ascites. So, it is a cause of hepatic venous outflow obstruction.

16. **Ans. (c) preCore mutant HBV** *(Ref: Robbins 8th/846, Harrison 17th/1935-6)*
The precore region directs the release of HBeAg towards secretion in the blood. Uncommonly, mutated strains called **precore mutants** of HBV emerge that do not produce HBeAg but are replication competent and express HBcAg. In these patients, the HBeAg may be undetectable despite the presence of HBV viral load. Another **mutation in the core promoter region** can also lead to an HBeAg negative phenotype. Clinically both these conditions are characterized by the presence of elevated liver enzymes and active viral multiplication is indicated only by the high levels of DNA polymerase.

Additional info

Another important mutation seen in HBV is **"escape mutants"** due to amino acid substitution causing a conformational change in HBs Ag resulting in **loss of neutralizing activity by anti-HBs.** It is seen in association with active and passive immunization and in liver transplant patients. In both these conditions, there is increased concentration of anti HBs leading to mutation in the virus so that it can escape from the protective effect of anti-HBs.

17. **Ans. (d) Chronic alcoholism** *(Ref: Robbins 7th/903-4, 9/e p 842, Harrisons 17th/1982)*
Alcoholic liver disease (ALD) is the most common cause of fatty liver. So, Fatty liver is characteristically seen in chronic alcoholism. However, now many other causes of fatty liver have also been elucidated known as Non-Alcoholic fatty liver disease (NAFLD) or Non-alcoholic steatohepatitis (NASH). These are explained in the chapter review.
- Sternberg 4th mentions "*although fatty change has been reported as a common feature of hepatits C, the degree of fatty changes is usually minimal and absence is not unusual.*"

18. **Ans. (c) Acute viral hepatitis** *(Ref: Robbin's 7th/899, 9/e p823; Harrison 17th/1929)*
Councilman bodies are feature of acute hepatitis. These are associated with the cellular phenomers of opposit.

19. **Ans. (d) Grading refers to the extent of necrosis and inflammation** *(Ref: Harrison 17th/1955), Sternberg's diagnostic surgical pathology 4th/1682*
The new classification system of **hepatitis** is based on **its etiology, grade or stage.** Grading refers to the assessment of necroinflammatory activity whereas the staging refers to degree of progression.

Concept

Regarding option 'c', Sternberg writes clearly 'although fatty change has been reported as a common feature of hepatits C, the degree of fatty changes is usually minimal and absence is not unusual. Fatty change due to virus is most likely associated with genotype 3. Biopsy in hepatitis B and C is done for purpose of staging and grading and not for diagnosis'.

20. **Ans. (b) Ground glass hepatocytes** *(Ref: Harrison 17th/1727; Robbins 7th/899, 8th/851, 9/e p837)*
Ground glass hepatocytes are large hepatocytes containing surface antigen. Their cytoplasm is ground glass in appearance. These cells are a feature of chronic hepatitis and not acute hepatitis.

21. **Ans. (b) Reye's syndrome—ground glass appearance of hepatocytes.** *(Ref: Robbins 7th 898, 9/e p841, H Mohan 6th-602)*
   • In *acute hepatitis B*, hepatocytes show *ground glass appearance.*
   • In Reye's syndrome, hepatocytes show microvesicular fatty change.
   • Mallory bodies are seen in alcoholic hepatitis, primary biliary cirrhosis, non-alcoholic fatty liver disease, Wilson's disease, chronic cholestatic jaundice and hepatocellular carcinoma.

22. **Ans. (b) Phenol** *(Ref: Robbins 7th/903)*

23. **Ans. (a) Ballooning degeneration** *(Ref: Robbins 9/e p838, 8th/851; 7th/897-9)*

24. **Ans. (a) Hepatitis-B infection** *(Ref: Robbins 9/e p841-842, 8th/846; 7th/907-8)*

25. **Ans. (c) Chronic active hepatitis** *(Ref: Robbins 8th/852-3, 7th/899)*

26. **Ans. (d) Hepatitis E Virus** *(Ref: Robbins 9/e p835, 8th/849, 7th/897)*

27. **Ans. (d) Cholangiocarcinoma** *(Ref: Robbins 9/e p833, 841-842, 8th/845-7, 7th/926)*

28. **Ans. (b) Chronic active hepatitis** *(Ref: Robbins 8th/851-2, 7th/899)*

29. **Ans. (b) Feco-oral** *(Ref: Robbins 9/e p835, 8th/849, 7th/896)*

30. **Ans. (a) 6 weeks to 6 months** *(Ref: Robbins 9/e p831-832, 8th/845; 7th/891)*

31. **Ans. (c) HBeAg** *(Ref: Robbins 9/e p832, 8th/846; 7th/893)*

32. **Ans. (d) Hepatitis A Virus** *(Ref: Robbins 9/e p831, 8th/844, 7th/891)*

33. **Ans. (c) Immunized against hepatitis B** *(Ref: Robbins 9/e 832-833, 8th/846, Harrison 18th/2550)*
Ms Aishwarya is positive only for the antibody to the hepatitis B antigen. This is suggestive of her being vaccinated for hepatitis B virus (HBV). The vaccine consists of recombinantly produced HBV surface antigen (HBsAg) alone and the antibodies to this protein provide immunity.
HBsAg would be seen in the serum within the first 3-4 months after initial infection. Antibodies to the core protein (anit-HBcAg) appear during acute illness and between the disappearance of HBsAg and the appearance of anti-HBsAg, the "window period." Anti-HBeAg appears during the window period as well. HBeAg and HBV DNA polymerase are the indices of infectivity.
Nutshell of Hepatitis B Serology

	HBs Ag	IgM anti HBc	IgG anti HBc	IgG anti HBs
Acute HBV infection	+	+	–	–
Window period	–	+	–	–
Chronic infection	+	+/-	+	–
Prior infection	–	–	+	+
Immunization	–	–	–	+

Also know: The presence of HBe Ag denotes high infectivity and its absence denotes low infectivity.

34. **Ans. (d) Specific form of hepatitis virus responsible of the infection** *(Ref: Robbins 9th/836)*
The best predictor for viral disease progressing to chronic liver disease and even cirrhosis is decided by the causative agent of the viral hepatitis. On comparing all viruses, hepatitis C is the commonest cause of chronic viral hepatitis.
Other viruses like hepatitis A, hepatitis E and hepatitis G never progress to chronic hepatitis. The histologic changes, degree and duration of transaminase elevation don't influence the progression to chronic hepatitis.

35. **Ans. (c) Vertical transmission during childbirth** *(Ref: Robbins 8th/845, 9/e p832)*
Hepatitis B infection is not commonly transmitted through blood transfusion now (due to mandatory screening of blood and its products), heterosexual transmission and needle stick injury (much more chances in comparison to HIV and HCV).

Important concept

- In adults, the viral hepatitis develops because they are immunocompetent, so, HBV induced T cells induce apoptosis of infected liver cells.
- Vertical transmission during childbirth is responsible for HBV chronic carrier stage. This is attributed to the fact that unlike the adults, the immune responses in the neonatal period are not fully developed thereby preventing the development of hepatitis.
- **Clinical significance** of high carrier rate is **increased risk of development of hepatocellular cancer.**

36. **Ans. (c) Polyarteritis nodosa** *(Ref: Robbins 8th/514, 9/e p509)*

Thirty percent of patients with polyarteritis nodosa have hepatitis B antigenemia. Polyarteritis is a systemic necrotizing vasculitis that can be difficult to diagnose, since the vascular involvement is typically widely scattered, and the specific symptoms depend on the specific vessels (small- to medium-sized arteries) involved. Patients typically present with low-grade fever, weakness, and weight loss. Abdominal pain, hematuria, renal failure, hypertension, and leukocytosis may occur. The disease is frequently fatal if untreated.

37. **Ans. (b) Chronic active carrier** *(Ref: Robbins 8th/846, 9/e 837)*

The presence of elevated ALT, HBsAg, anti-HBc, HBeAg, and bilirubin all point to active hepatitis B.
- An asymptomatic carrier (choice A) does not have elevated ALT and bilirubin.
- The absence of findings on physical examination rules out fulminant hepatitis B (choice C).
- Recovery from acute self-limited HBV (choice D) is associated with the presence of anti-HBs and the decrease in HBsAg and HBeAg.

38. **Ans. (c) Granuloma formation** *(Ref: Robbins 7th/94 - 905, 9/e 842 Harrison - 17th/1970)*

Spectrum of alcoholic liver disease includes:
- **Fatty Liver (Hepatic steatosis)**
- **Alcoholic hepatitis** - Hallmark of alcoholic hepatitis is hepatocyte injury characterized by ballooning degeneration, spotty necrosis, polymorphonuclear infiltrate and fibrosis in the perivenular and perisinusoidal space of Disse. Mallory bodies may also be present.
- **Alcoholic Cirrhosis**

Granuloma is **not** seen in alcoholic liver disease.

39. **Ans. (a) Drugs induced hepatitis** *(Ref: Robbins 8th/876, Diseases of the liver and biliary system by Sheila Sherlock, Sheila Sherlock (Dame.), James S. Dooley Blackwell Science 11th/530)*

Nodular regenerative hyperplasia: summary from Robbins and Sherlock

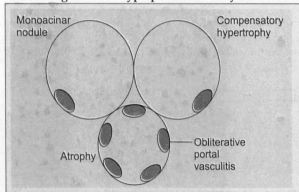

- Associated with the development of portal hypertension and its clinical manifestations.
- Occurs in conditions affecting intra hepatic blood flow like **rheumatoid arthritis (most commonly)**, Felty syndrome, myeloproliferative disorders, hyperviscosity syndromes, solid organ (particularly renal and liver) transplantation, bone marrow transplantation, **HIV infection** (Robbins), vasculitic conditions and **drugs (anabolic steroids and cytotoxics).**
- Characteristically, there is absence of fibrosis in this condition.

40. **Ans. (a) Alcoholic liver disease; (b) Hepatocellular carcinoma; (c) Wilson's disease; (d) ICC (Indian childhood cirrhosis); (e) Biliary cirrhosis** *(Ref: Robbins' 7th/905, 9/e p843)*

Mallory bodies- scattered hepatocytes accumulate tangled skeins of cytokeratin intermediate filaments and other proteins, visible as eosinophilic cytoplasmic inclusions in degenerating hepatocytes.

41. **Ans. d) LKM 2- Chronic hepatitis D** *(Ref: Harrison 17th/1956, 1968 CMDT/595-600, Robbin 839-840)*

LKM stand for liver kidney microsomal antibodies

Type of LKM antibody	Associated conditions
Anti LKM 1 antibodies	Chronic hepatitis C, Autoimmune hepatitis type 2
Anti LKM 2 antibodies	Drug induced hepatitis
Anti LKM 3 antibodies	Chronic hepatitis D, type 2 autoimmune hepatitis (rarely)

Liver

42. Ans. (c) Hepatocellular carcinoma *(Ref: Robbins 8th/879-880, 9/e p873)*
Elevated levels of serum α-fetoprotein are found in 50 to 75% of patients with HCC.
False-positive results are encountered with yolk-sac tumors and many non-neoplastic conditions, including cirrhosis, massive liver necrosis, chronic hepatitis, normal pregnancy, fetal distress or death, and fetal neural tube defects such as anencephaly and spina bifida.
Concept

> The staining for Glypican-3 is used to distinguish early hepatocellular carcinoma from a dysplastic nodule. Other tests cannot be used because the levels of serum α-fetoprotein are inconclusive in this condition.

43. Ans. (c) Indian childhood cirrhosis *(Ref: Harsh Mohan 6th/621-622)*

44. Ans. (c) Secondary biliary cirrhosis *(Ref: Robbin 7th/904, 9/e p843)*

45. Ans. (d) Intermediate filaments *(Ref: Robbins 7th/905, 9/e p843)*
Scattered hepatocytes accumulate tangled skeins of cytokeratin intermediate filaments and other proteins, visible as eosinophilic cytoplasmic inclusions in degenerating hepatocytes called as **Mallory bodies.** These inclusions are a characteristic but not specific feature of alcoholic liver disease.

46. Ans. (b) Eosinophilic intracytoplasmic inclusions *(Ref: Robbins 8th/858; 7th/612, 9/e p843)*

47. Ans. (a) Hemosiderin *(Ref: Robbins 8th/857; 7th/905)*

48. Ans. (c) Alcoholic hepatitis *(Ref: Robbins 9/e p843, 8th/858, 7th/905)*

49. Ans. (c) Cardiac cirrhosis *(Ref: Robbins 9/e p843, 8th/858; 7th/905,911)*

50. Ans. (c) Prekeratin intermediate filaments; *(Ref: Robbins 7th/34, 37- 41, 423, 905 9/e p843)*
- Hyaline is a nonspecific term that is used to describe any material, inside or outside the cell, that stains a red homogeneous color with the routine H&E stain.
- Alcoholic hyaline inclusions (Mallory bodies) are irregular eosinophilic hyaline inclusions that are found within the cytoplasm of hepatocytes. These are composed of pre-keratin intermediate filaments. They are a nonspecific finding and can be found in patients with several diseases other than alcoholic hepatitis, such as Wilson's disease, and in patients who have undergone bypass operations for morbid obesity.
Other options

> - **Immunoglobulins** may form intracytoplasmic or extracellular oval hyaline bodies called **Russell bodies**.
> - Excess plasma proteins may form hyaline droplets in proximal renal tubular epithelial cells or hyaline membranes in the alveoli of the lungs.
> - The hyaline found in the walls of arterioles of kidneys in patients with benign nephrosclerosis is composed of basement membranes and precipitated plasma proteins.

50.1. Ans. (b) Cytokeratin *(Ref: Robbins 8/e p858, 9/e p843)*
Mallory bodies are visible as eosinophilic cytoplasmic clumps in hepatocytes. They are composed of tangled skeins of **cytokeratin intermediate filaments**[Q] such as cytokeratin 8 and 18, in complex with other proteins such as ubiquitin.

50.2. Ans. (c) Secondary biliary cirrhosis *(Ref: Robbins 9/e 843, 8/e 858, 7/e p905)*
Mallory Hyaline bodies are seen in conditions memorized by Mnemonic: New Indian WATCH.

50.3. Ans. (a) Alcoholic fatty liver *(Ref: Robbins 9/e p830, 841, 8/e p857-8, Schiffs Diseases of the Liver)*
Steatosis is considered to be microvesiuclar when multiple small cytoplasmic vacuoles tend to leave the nucleus centrally placed. In contrast, macrovesicular steatosis has a single large fat vacuole which displaces the nucleus to the periphery.

Causes of Microvasicular steatosis
• Reye syndrome, acute fatty liver of pregnancy, drugs (tetracycline, valproate, aspirin, nucleoside analogs of anti HIV drugs)
Causes of Macrovasicular steatosis
• Malnutrition, diabetes, obesity, malabsorption, steroid therapy, some metabolic diseases

Alcohol intake can be associated with both microvesicular (initially) and macrovesicular steatosis (later on continued drinking).

50.4. Ans (b) HBc Ag in serum is indicative of active infection *(Ref: Robbins 9/e p833)*
HBe Ag and *not HBc Ag* in serum is *indicative of active infection*.

> • Persistence of HBeAg is an important indicator of continued viral replication, infectivity, and probable progression to chronic hepatitis.

51. **Ans. (b) Hep B** *(Ref: Robbins 8th/878-9, 9/e p870)*

    Risk factors for development of hepatocellular cancer (HCC)

    - Chronic Hepatitis (Hepatitis B, Hepatitis C)
    - Alcoholism
    - Aflatoxins (due to *Aspergillus flavus* infection of peanuts, grains)
    - Tyrosinemia
    - Hereditary hemochromatosis

52. **Ans. (d) Serum AFP levels are usually greater than 1000mg/liter** *(Ref: Robbins 7th/925, 9/e p873)*

    As discussed in text fibrolammelar cancer is not associated with elevated AFP levels.

53. **Ans. (b) Hepatitis B is an important risk factor** *(Ref: Robbins 8th/879, 9/e p873)*

54. **Ans. (c) Hepatocellular carcinoma** *(Ref: Robbins 8th/878; 7th/922-4, 9/e p869)*

55. **Ans. (a) More in females** *(Ref: Robbins 9/e p873, 8th/878; 7th/925)*

56. **Ans. (c) Oral contraceptives** *(Ref: Robbins 8th/877, 9/e p868)*

    Liver adenomas are benign liver tumors commonly associated with ***oral contraceptive*** use in young women (usually 3-4th decade of life). They may resemble hepatocellular carcinoma. If they are subscapular, they can rupture, causing intra-abdominal haemorrhage leading to acute abdominal pain.

    - **Hepatitis B** may lead to **hepatocellular carcinoma**.
    - **Polycythemia vera** is associated with **thrombosis of the hepatic veins**.
    - **Polyvinyl chloride, thorotrast** (a contrast material) and **arsenic** are the risk factors for development of **angiosarcoma of the liver**. Immunohistochemical staining of these *tumor cells is positive for* the **CD 31** cell marker.

56.1. **Ans. (a) Angiosarcoma of liver** *(Ref: Robbins 8/e p877, 9/e p875)*

    Angiosarcoma of the liver is a highly aggressive tumor which is associated with exposure to:

    - **Vinyl chloride**[Q],
    - **Arsenic**[Q], or
    - **Thorotrast**[Q],

    Thorotrast is a suspension containing particles of the radioactive compound thorium dioxide. It emits **alpha particles** due to which it has been found to be extremely carcinogenic.

56.2. **Ans. (b) Hemangioma** *(Ref: Robbins 9/e p867, 8/e p876, 7/e p922)*

    - Cavernous hemangiomas are the most common benign liver tumours.

57. **Ans. (b) Hilum** *(Ref: Robbins 9/e 874, 8th/880, Harrison 17th/585)*

    The commonest location of the cholangiocarcinoma is at the hilum. Klatskin tumors are located at the junction of the right and the left hepatic ducts.

58. **Ans. (d) *Clonorchis sinensis* infection** *(Ref: Robbins 9/e p874, 8th/880; 7th/671)*

59. **Ans. (a) Adenocarcinoma** *(Ref: Robbins 9/e p874, 8th/888, 7th/926-927)*

60. **Ans. (c) Biliary sludge** *(Ref: Robbins 9/e p876, 8th/882-4. Harrison 18th/2617-9)*

    The demonstration of slow or incomplete gallbladder emptying in response to cholecystokinin stimulation is called gall-bladder hypomotility. This is usually associated with *risk factors* like *pregnancy, rapid weight loss prolonged use of total parenteral nutrition or octreotide, and high spinal cord injuries*.

    Gallbladder hypomotility frequently results in the formation of biliary sludge, which results from bile precipitation. Biliary sludge typically contains cholesterol monohydrate crystals, calcium bilirubinate, and mucus and is a known precursor to stone formation. Complications such as acute cholecystitis occur in up to 20% of patients with biliary sludge.

    - (Choice b) **Brown pigment** stones are most likely to arise in cases of **biliary tract infection**.
    - (Choice a) **Black pigment stones** are most likely to arise in cases of **intravascular hemolysis**.
    - (Choice d) Gallstones **do not** typically *contain phospholipid* as a primary ingredient.

    ### Concept

    Gallbladder hypomotility often results in bile precipitation and the formation of biliary sludge.

61. **Ans. (a) Common bile duct** *(Ref: Robbins 9/e p877, 8th/887)*

    The patient is probably suffering from choledocholithiasis, a condition in which a gallstone becomes lodged in the common bile duct.

She is displaying "**Charcot's triad**" (**fever, jaundice, and right upper quadrant pain**), which is indicative of cholangitis (infection of the biliary tree proximal to an obstruction such as a gallstone or malignancy).

The important point in this case is the fact that the patient is jaundiced, eliminating all options other than a stone in the common bile duct. Stones within the cystic duct (option B) or gallbladder (option C) or small intestine (options D) do not cause jaundice.

61.1. Ans. (b) Primary sclerosing cholangitis *(Ref: Robbins 8/e p880)*

Risk factors (Mnemonic: All have alphabet 'C')

- Primary sclerosing **C**holangitis
- Liver flukes like **C**lonorchis sinensis and Opisthorchis viverrini
- **C**ause of chronic biliary inflammation and injury (**C**holedocholithiasis)
- **C**ontrat material: thorotrast
- **C**hronic alcoholic liver disease
- **C**ongenital fibropolycystic diease (**C**holedochal cysts, **C**aroli's disease)

61.2. Ans. (a) Nodular type of cholangiocarcinoma *(Ref: Robbins 9/e p874, 8/e p880)*

- *According to their localization,* cholangiocarcinomas (CCAs) *are classified into intrahepatic and extrahepatic forms.*
- Eighty to 90% of the tumors are **extrahepatic**[Q].
- The extrahepatic forms include perihilar tumors known as *Klatskin tumors*[Q], which are located at the **junction of the right and left hepatic ducts**[Q] forming the common hepatic duct, and distal bile duct tumors.
- Most extrahepatic CCAs appear as **firm, gray nodules**[Q] within the bile duct wall
- Klatskin tumors generally have slower growth than other CCAs, show *prominent fibrosis*, and *infrequently involve distal metastases.*

61.3. Ans. (d) Oral contraceptives *(Ref: Robbins 9/e p879, 8/e p888, Cancer Nursing: Principles and Practice 7/e p1317)*

Risk factors of gall bladder cancer
- Gallstones: most important risk factor associated with gallbladder carcinoma.
- Gholedochal cyst
- Carcinogens and chemicals including nitrosamines, rubber and textile industries
- Rubber plant workers
- Obesity
- Estrogen
- Typhoid carrier
- Porcelain gall bladder (calcification of the gallbladder wall)
- Gall bladder polyps
- Anomalous pancreatobiliary duct junction

Also know
- Only 0.5% of patients with gallstones develop gallbladder cancer after twenty or more years
- In Asia, where pyogenic and parasitic diseases of the biliary tree are common, the coexistence of gallstones in gallbladder cancer is much lower.

61.4. Ans. (a) Adenomyomatosis of gallbladder *(Ref: Learning Ultrasound Imaging p9, Harrison 17/e 1998)*

Focal diffuse gall bladder wall thickening with comet tail reverberation artifacts on USG is a diagnostic finding of Adenomyomatosis of gall bladder.

61.5. Ans. (b) Primary sclerosing cholangitis *(Ref: Robbins 9/e p860)*

62. Ans. (b) Autosomal recessive *(Ref: Robbins 9/e p847-849, 8th/861, Harrison 18th/3166)*

- Hemochromatosis is characterized by **excessive accumulation of iron** in the body.
- It **is an autosomal recessive** disorder most commonly caused by **mutations in HFE gene** located at **6p**21.3.
- It is more common in males characterized by the triad of
  *Micronodular cirrhosis   *Diabetes mellitus and   *Skin pigmentation
- Most of the cells of the body have increased amounts of hemosiderin in them but skin pigmentation is primarily due to increased intracellular melanin.
- **Inflammation** is characteristically **absent**
- Deposition of hemosiderin in the joint synovial lining can result in acute synovitis and pseudogout.
- Derangement of the hypothalamo-pituitary axis results in hypogonadism (loss of libido and impotence in male and amenorrhea in the female).
- Treatment is removal of excessive iron and it is accomplished by weekly or twice weekly phlebotomy.
- Chelating agents like desferrioxamine are indicated only when anemia or hypoproteinemia is severe enough to preclude phlebotomy.
- Cardiac failure and hepatocellular carcinoma are the most common causes of death.

63. Ans. (d) Desferrioxamine is the treatment of choice *(Ref: Harrison 18th/3166; Robbins 7th/615-7, 9/e p849)*
- *Desferrioxamine* is the drug of choice.
- The treatment of choice is phlebotomy at regular intervals.

64. Ans. (d) Hepatic Metastasis *(Ref: Harrison's 17th/1983; Oxford Texbook of Pathology by McGeel 1312t, Robbins 9/e p841)*

Causes of Hepatic Granulomas

Systemic disease	Infections	Drugs
• *Sarcoidosis* • Hodgkin's and Non-Hodgkin's lymphoma • Primary biliary cirrhosis • Berylliosis • Crohn's disease • Wegener's granulomatosis • Idiopathic	- Tuberculosis - MAC, Leprosy - Brucellosis - EBV, CMV, Chicken pox - Histoplasmosis, *Candidiasis* - Schistosomiasis - Q fever - Syphilis	• Sulfonamides • Isoniazid • Allopurinol • Methyldopa • Quinidine • Phenylbutazone • *Halothane*

65. Ans. (d) Glycogen depletion *(Ref: OP Ghai 6th/524; 7th/543, CPDT 18th/662-3)*

Reye's Syndrome/Jamshedpur Fever

- Described as a diffuse fatty infiltration of the liver, kidney and cerebral edema with diffuse mitochondrial injury.
- An acute self-limiting metabolic insult resulting in generalized mitochondrial dysfunction due to inhibition of fatty acid β-oxidation due to:
  - Salicylates
  - Inborn error of coenzyme A dehydrogenase
  - Varicella or Influenza B viral infections
  - Contamination of food with aflatoxin
  - Usually observed from 2 month - 15 years of age.

Clinical features
- Child presents with *vomiting, anorexia, listlessness followed by altered sensorium, irregular breathing, seizures* and coma.
- Hepatomegaly is present in 50% cases. Jaundice and focal neurological signs are absent.

Diagnosis
- Liver biopsy shows fatty change and glycogen depletion but no NECROSIS of liver cells.
- Liver is showing **fatty change,** so these lipids can be stained with *Oil Red – O.*

66. Ans. (b) Kupffer's cell hyperplasia with macrophage infiltration around periportal area laden with pigments
(Ref: Robbins 7th/402, 9/e p391-392)

- In severe infections with *Plasmodium falciparum,* the vital organs are *packed with erythrocytes* containing mature form of the parasite. There is abundant *intra and extraerythrocytic* pigment and organs such as *liver, spleen* and *placenta* may be grey black in color.

Liver and spleen in severe malaria

Liver
- Liver is generally enlarged and may be black from malarial pigment.
- There is congestion of the centrilobular capillaries with sinusoidal dilatation and Kupffer cell hyperplasia
- The Kupffer cells are heavily laden with malarial pigment, parasites and cellular debris.
- Sequestration of parasitized erythrocytes is associated with variable cloudy swelling of the hepatocytes and perivenous ischemic change and sometimes centrizonal necrosis.
- Hepatic glycogen is often present despite hypoglycemia.

Spleen
- The spleen is often dark or black from malarial pigment enlarged, soft and friable.
- It is full of erythrocytes containing mature and immature parasites.
- There is evidence of reticular hyperplasia and architectural reorganization.
- The soft and acutely enlarged spleen of acute lethal infections **contrasts** with the *hard fibrous enlargement* associated with **repeated malaria**.

Also know

Durck's granuloma is pathognomic of malignant cerebral malaria.

67. **Ans. None** *(Ref: Harsh Mohan 6th/628; Robbins' 39, 910, 914)*
    Pigmentation in liver is caused by:

> 1. Lipofuscin: It is an insoluble pigment known as lipochrome and 'wear and tear' pigment. It is seen in cells undergoing low, regressive changes and is particularly prominent in liver and heart of ageing patient or patients with severe malnutrition and cancer cachexia.
> 2. Pseudomelanin: After death, a dark greenish or blackish discoloration of the surface of the abdominal viscera results from the action of sulfated hydrogen upon the iron of disintegrated hemoglobin. Liver is also pigmented.

> 3. Wilson's disease: Copper is usually deposited in periportal hepatocytes in the form of reddish granules in cytoplasm or reddish cytoplasmic coloration stained by rubeanic acid or rhodamine stain for copper or orcein stain for copper associated protein. Copper also gets deposited in chronic obstructive cholestasis.
> 4. Malarial pigment: Liver colour varies from dark chocolate red to slate-grey even black depending upon the stage of congestion.
> 5. In biliary cirrhosis liver is enlarged and greenish-yellow in colour due to cholestasis. So liver is pigmented due to bile.

68. **Ans. (b) Emphysema; (c) Fibrosis of portal tact; (d) Diastase resistance positive hepatocytes** *(Ref: Robbins 7th/911-2, 9/e p850-851)*
    - This is **an autosomal recessive** disease characterized by deficiency of α_1-antitrypsin (important protease inhibitor).
    - There is **portal tract fibrosis**^{Q} in neonatal hepatitis. About 10% - 20% of newborn with α_1-antitrypsin deficiency develop neonatal hepatitis and cholestasis.
    - Hepatocellular carcinoma develops in 2-3 % α_1 - antitrypsin deficiency in adults.
    - The treatment and cure, for severe hepatic disease is *orthotopic liver transplantation.*
    - Most important treatment for pulmonary disease is to avoid cigarette smoking because it accelerates the development of **emphysema**.

69. **Ans. (a) Wilson's disease** *(Ref: Robbins 9/e p850, 8th/864, 7th/911)*

70. **Ans. (c) ↑Ceruloplasmin** *(Ref: Robbins 8th/863-4, 9/e p849-850, Harrison 17th/1492)*

71. **Ans. (b) Neonatal hepatitis** *(Ref: Robbins 9/e p851, 8th/865-6; 7th/492,719)*

72. **Ans. (a) CCl$_4$** *(Ref: Robbins 8th/872, 7th/882)*

73. **Ans. (b) K-RAS** *(Ref: Robbins 8th/900-2, 9/e p892)*
    Presence of pulmonary thromboembolism with a pancreatic mass in an old man suggests a diagnosis of pancreatic cancer with Trosseau syndrome. This is also supported with elevated serum levels of tumor markers like CEA and CA 19-9.
    The *K-RAS* gene (chromosome 12p^Q) is the **most frequently altered oncogene in pancreatic cancer.** This oncogene is activated by point mutation in 80% to 90% of pancreatic cancers.
    Other options

> - BRCA 2 mutation may be associated with some pancreatic cancers but usually there is a history of other cancers like breast cancer, prostate cancer (in males) and breast and ovarian cancers (in females).
> - **PRSS1** mutation is also associated with **pancreatic cancer** but this is usually a cancer starting early in life secondary hereditary pancreatitis.
> - **SPINK1** is only associated with **hereditary pancreatitis** but **not pancreatic cancer.**

73.1. **Ans. (a) Perls iron stain** *(Ref: Robbins 8/e p862, 9/e p849)*
    In the liver, iron becomes evident as golden yellow **hemosiderin granules** in the cytoplasm of periportal hepatocytes which stain blue with **Prussian blue stain**. The last mentioned stain is also called as Perls iron stain.

73.2. **Ans. (d) Hemochromatosis** *(Ref: Robbins 8/e p862, 9/e p849)*
    In hemochromatosis, there is iron deposited in different tissues in the form of hemosiderin. This deposition along with **increased epidermal melanin** production leads to a characteristic slate-gray color to the skin. The development of diabetes in these patients is therefore termed as **bronze diabetes**.

73.3. **Ans. (c) Ceruloplasmin** *(Ref: Robbins 8/e p863, 9/e p849-850)*
    Wilson disease is an autosomal recessive disorder caused by mutation of the *ATP7B gene*^{Q}, resulting in impaired copper excretion into bile and a failure to incorporate copper into *ceruloplasmin*^{Q}.

73.4. **Ans. (b) ATP 7B.. see above explanation.....**(Ref: Robbins 8/e p863, 9/e p849)*

GOLDEN POINTS / UPDATED INFORMATION FROM 9TH EDITION OF ROBBINS

(LIVER)

- The receptor for HAV is HAVcr-1, a 451–amino acid class I integral-membrane mucin-like glycoprotein.

Liver failure *(Robbins 9th/825)*

The most severe clinical consequence of liver disease is liver failure. It may be the result of sudden and massive hepatic destruction, *acute liver failure*, or, more often, *chronic liver failure,* which follows upon years or decades of insidious, progressive liver injury.

In some cases, individuals with chronic liver disease develop **acute on- chronic liver failure**, in which an unrelated acute injury supervenes on a well-compensated late-stage chronic disease or the chronic disease itself has a flare of activity that leads directly to liver failure.

Acute liver failure is defined as an acute liver illness associated with encephalopathy and coagulopathy that occurs **within 26 weeks** of the initial liver injury in the absence of pre-existing liver disease. It is most commonly caused by hepatitis B/C in Asia and by intake of paracetamol in USA.

The liver is small and shrunken.

Clinical features include nausea, vomiting, and jaundice, followed by life threatening encephalopathy, and coagulation defects. The serum liver transaminases are markedly elevated. Other manifestations of acute liver failure include progressively increasing jaundice and icterus, *hepatic encephalopathy* (alterations in the nervous system *including* disturbances in consciousness, confusion and stupor, to deep coma), *coagulopathy* (increased bleeding tendency), *portal hypertension, ascites, and hepatorenal syndrome* (a form of renal failure occurring in liver failure patients with no intrinsic morphologic or functional causes for kidney dysfunction).

Mnemonic for causes of acute liver failure (Robbins 9th/830)

- **A**: **A**cetaminophen, hepatitis **A**, **a**utoimmune hepatitis
- **B**: Hepatitis **B**
- **C**: Hepatitis **C**, **C**ryptogenic
- **D**: **D**rugs/toxins, hepatitis **D**
- **E**: Hepatitis **E**, **E**soteric causes (Wilson disease, Budd-Chiari)
- **F**: **F**atty change of the microvesicular type (fatty liver of pregnancy, valproate, tetracycline, Reye syndrome)

Chronic liver failure and cirrhosis

Liver failure in chronic liver disease is most often associated with cirrhosis, a condition marked by the diffuse transformation of the entire liver into regenerative parenchymal nodules surrounded by fibrous bands and variable degrees of vascular (often portosystemic) shunting.

The leading causes of chronic liver failure worldwide include chronic hepatitis B, chronic hepatitis C, nonalcoholic fatty liver disease, and alcoholic liver disease.

The Child-Pugh classification of cirrhosis distinguishes between **class A** (well compensated), **B** (partially decompensated), and **C** (decompensated), which correlate with different morphologic features histologically. *This classification helps to monitor the decline of patients on the path to chronic liver failure.*

Portopulmonary hypertension

Portopulmonary hypertension refers to pulmonary arterial hypertension arising in liver disease and portal hypertension. It is caused by excessive pulmonary vasoconstriction and vascular remodeling. The most common clinical manifestations are dyspnea on exertion and clubbing of the fingers.

Precursor Lesions of HCC... *Robbins 9th /871-2*

Several cellular and nodular precursor lesions apart from hepatocellular adenoma have been identified.

1. Cellular dysplasias

These changes serve as markers in biopsy specimens to indicate patients requiring more aggressive cancer surveillance.

a. **Large cell change**: it is a *marker of increased risk of HCC in the liver as a whole, but in hepatitis B they may also be directly premalignant.*

It has scattered hepatocytes that are larger than normal hepatocytes and with large and often multiple pleomorphic nuclei with the nuclear-cytoplasmic ratio being normal.

b. Small cell change: it is thought to be directly premalignant.

This has hepatocytes have high nuclear: cytoplasmic ratio and mild nuclear hyperchromasia and/or pleomorphism.

2. Dysplastic nodules

These are usually detected in cirrhosis, either radiologically or in resected specimens and have a different appearance (in size or vascular supply or appearance) from the surrounding cirrhotic nodules. They can be of the following types:

I. *Low-grade dysplastic nodules:* their presence indicates a higher risk for HCC in the liver as a whole. These nodules are devoid of cytologic or architectural atypia and are clonal.

II. *High-grade dysplastic nodules:* these are probably the most important primary pathway for emergence of HCC in **viral hepatitis** and **alcoholic liver disease**. These nodules have cytologic (e.g., small cell change) or architectural features (occasional pseudoglands, trabecular thickening) suggestive of, but still insufficient for diagnosis of overt HCC.

Precursor Lesions of Hepatocellular and Cholangiocarcinoma

	Hepatocellular Cancer					Cholangiocarcinoma		
	Hepatocellular Adenoma	Small Cell Change	Large Cell Change	Low Grade Dysplastic Nodule	High Grade Dysplastic Nodule	BilIN-3	Mucinous Cystic Neoplasm	Intraductal Papillary Biliary Neoplasia
Focality in liver	Single or multiple (adenomatosis)	Diffuse	Diffuse	Single or multiple	Single or multiple	Diffuse or multifocal	Single	Focal or diffuse
Premalignant	Yes	Yes	In some HBV*	Uncertain*	Yes	Yes	Yes	Yes
Association with cirrhosis	Rare	Common	Comon	Usual	Usual	Sometimes	No	No
Commonly associated diseases	NAFLD, Sex hormone exposures Glycogen storage diseases	HBV, HCV, Alcohol, NAFLD, A1AT, HH, PBC	HBV, HCV, Alcohol, NAFLD, A1AT, HH PBC	HBV, HCV, Alcohol, NAFLD, A1AT, HH PBC	HBV, HCV, Alcohol, NAFLD, A1AT, HH, PBC	PSC, Hepatolithiasis Liver flukes	None	None
Occurrence without identified predisposing condition	Occasional	No	No	No	No	Yes	Yes	Yes
Need for surveillance cancer screening	± depending on presence of predisposing condition	Yes	Yes	Yes	Yes	Yes	No	Yes

*While these are not certain to be directly premalignant, they are always at least an indication of increased risk for malignancy in the liver as a whole.
BilIN-3, Bliary intraepithelial neoplasia, high grade; NAFLD, nonalcoholic fatty liver disease; HBV, hepatitis B virus; hepatitis C virus; A1AT, α_1 −antitrypsin deficiency; HH, hereditary hemochromatosis PBC, primary biliary cirrhosis, PSC, primary sclerosis cholangitis.

Precursor Lesions of Cholangiocarcinoma ......Robbins 9th/874

Premalignant lesions for cholangiocarcinoma are also known, the most important of which are biliary intraepithelial neoplasias (low to high grade, BilIN-1, -2, or -3).

BilIN-3, the highest grade lesion, incurs the *highest risk of malignant transformation.*

Rarer are *mucinous cystic neoplasms* and intraductal *papillary biliary neoplasia.*

NOTES

MALE GENITAL TRACT

Penis

- Congenital malformations affecting the penis are *abnormal locations of urethral openings and phimosis*. These abnormal locations may produce obstruction of urinary tract infection or infertility.
- **Phimosis** occurs when the orifice of the prepuce (foreskin) is too small to permit normal retraction. It may be due to abnormal development or more commonly due to inflammatory scarring. It interferes with cleanliness and favors the development of secondary infections and possibly carcinoma.
- **Paraphimosis** is inability to roll back the prepuce after forcible retraction over glans penis. It is extremely painful and may cause obstruction of urinary tract (cause of acute urinary retention) or blood flow (may lead to necrosis of penis).
- **Balanoposthitis** is a non-specific infection of glans and prepuce. It is mostly caused by Candida, anerobic bacteria and Gardernella.

Tumors of penis may be benign [condyloma acuminata] or malignant [carcinoma in-situ and invasive carcinoma].

- **Condyloma acuminatum** is a benign tumor caused by human papilloma virus (HPV), most commonly type 6 and sometimes type 11. **Koilocytosis** is a characteristic of infection with HPV. It is seen in condyloma as well as carcinoma.

- **Carcinoma in-situ** refers to epithelial lesions in which cytological changes of malignancy are confined to epithelium, with no evidence of local invasion or metastasis. These are considered as **pre-cancerous lesions**. In about 80% of cases, these lesions are associated with HPV-16. **Bowen disease, Erythroplasia of Queyrat** (a variant of Bowen's disease) **and Bowenoid papulosis** are examples of carcinoma in-situ. Bowen disease may transform into invasive squamous cell carcinoma in 10% patients and is associated with occurrence of visceral cancers in about one thirds of patients. In contrast, *bowenoid papulosis never develops into invasive carcinoma* and many times, it spontaneously regresses.
- **Squamous cell carcinoma** is associated with cigarette smoking and infection with HPV-16 (more commonly) and HPV-18. Mostly, squamous cell carcinoma invades tissue as finger like projections (papillary) of atypical squamous epithelial cells. These show varying degree of differentiation. A variant of squamous cell carcinoma is **verrucous carcinoma** [also known as Giant condyloma or **Buschke-Lowenstein tumor**] which invades the underlying tissue along a broad front (in contrast, papillary carcinoma invades as finger like projections).

TESTIS AND EPIDIDYMIS

- **Cryptorchidism** (undescended testes) is found in 1% of 1-year-old boys and is mostly unilateral (Right > Left). Testicular descent has two phases; transabdominal and inguino-scrotal. Transabdominal phase is controlled by Mullerian-inhibiting substance whereas inguino-scrotal phase is androgen dependent (mediated by androgen induced release of CGRP from genitofemoral nerve). Grossly, testis is small, brown and atrophic. Microscopically, tubules are atrophic with thickened basement membranes. **Leydig cells are spared and appear to be prominent**. Occasionally, proliferation of Sertoli cells may also be seen. Smaller but definite

Hypospadias

Urethral opening located on *ventral (inferior) surface* of the penis.

Results from failure of urethral folds to close.

Epispadias

Urethral opening located on *ventral (inferior) surface* of the penis.

Results from faulty position of genital tubercle.

It is **associated with exstrophy of urinary bladder and undescended testes**.

Koilocytosis is clear vacuolization of superficial, prickle cell layers of epithelial cells associated with **HPV infection**.

Squamous cell carcinoma's risk is **reduced by circumcision**; therefore it is rare in Jews and Muslims.

Buschke-Lowenstein tumor is a **well differentiated** variant of squamous cell carcinoma.

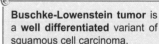

Increased risk of malignancy *(most commonly seminoma)* occurs with undescended testes (more for abdominal than for inguinal).

Concept

The **risk of malignancy** is **NOT REDUCED** by orchiopexy.

Superficial inguinal pouch is the *most common site* of **ectopic testis**.

Gonorrhea and tuberculosis almost invariably arise in epididymis whereas **syphilis affects the testis first**.

Prehan sign: Manually lifting of scrotal sac causes:
↑ pain in torsion:
↓ pain in orchitis.

Concept

Transillumination is helpful in differentiation of cysts (which transilluminate) and tumors (which do not).

Inguino-scrotal ultrasound is used to confirm the diagnosis.

Sertoli cell only syndrome:
Absence of germ cells
Results in infertility due to absence of spermatogenesis.

Seminomas are the most common type of *germ cell tumors* (50%).

Yolk sac tumor is the commonest testicular tumor in **infants and children** up to 3 years of age.

Seminoma is commonest testicular tumor in **young adults**.

Lymphoma is commonest testicular tumor in **elderly**.

risk of malignancy is present for contra-lateral, correctly placed testis. Persistently undescended testes require orchiopexy (placement in scrotal sac) preferably before 2 years before histological deterioration sets in. Orchiopexy does not guarantee fertility.

> **Note:** Cryptorchidism is *associated with trisomy 13* and genitourinary malformations like *hypospadias* or in-utero *exposure of DES*.

- **Ectopic testes** is the deviation of testes from normal path of descent. Gubernaculum testis has five tails (namely scrotal, pubic, perineal, inguinal and femoral). Normally scrotal tail is strongest, so testes descend to scrotum. If other accessory tails become strong, testis may drain toward that tail. Difference of ectopic testis from undescended testis is that former is fully developed and hence has **normal spermatogenesis** whereas latter lacks spermatogenesis.
- **Scrotal swelling** may occur due to inflammation, abnormality of blood vessels, cysts or tumors of testes or epididymis.
- Non-specific inflammations in a sexually active young patient **(< 35 years)** is mostly caused by *Chlamydia trachomatis* and *Neisseria gonorrhea* whereas most common culprit in men **older than 35 years** *are E. coli and pseudomonas*.
- Twisting of spermatic cord resulting in cut-off of the venous drainage and arterial supply to testis may result in **TORSION**. Neonatal torsion lacks any associated anatomical defect whereas adult torsion results from a bilateral anatomical defect in which testes have increased mobility [**bell-clapper abnormality**]. If untwisted within 6 hours, testes may remain viable. To prevent subsequent torsion, contralateral normal testis is fixed to scrotum [orchiopexy].

> **Note:** Doppler flow studies and testicular scintigraphy are useful if testicular torsion is expected clinically.

- **Benign scrotal cysts** may form from abnormalities of tunica vaginalis. Processus vaginalis is an outpouching of the peritoneum that enters into the scrotum. When testis reaches the scrotum, proximal portion of processus vaginalis obliterates whereas distal portion persists and forms tunica vaginalis. Cysts involving tunica vaginalis can be **hydrocele** [contain clear fluid], **hematocele** [results from hemorrhage into a hydrocele], **chylocele** [accumulation of lymph in tunica due to elephantiasis) or **spermatocele** (cystic enlargement of efferent ducts or rete testis with numerous spermatocytes present]. **Varicocele** results from dilatation of testicular veins in pampiniform plexus. It is associated with oligospermia (< 20 million spermatozoa/ml of semen) and is most common cause of infertility. Left side is affected more commonly.
- **Sertoli cell only syndrome** also known as **Del-Castillo's syndrome** is a condition in which seminiferous tubules are lined by only Sertoli cells.

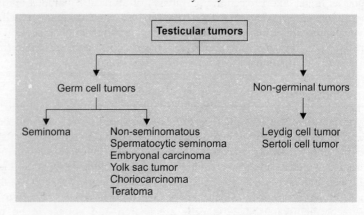

Testicular Germ Cell Tumors

Most of these arise from *intra tubular germ cell neoplasia* (ITGCN) except **spermatocytic seminoma** and **teratoma.**

Predisposing factors for germ cell tumors are:

- Cryptorchidism [abdominal > inguinal]
- Testicular dysgenesis [feminization and Klinefelter]
- Siblings of affected person (have tenfold higher risk)
- Isochromosome of short arm of chromosome 12, **i (12p) is seen in all germ cell tumors [both testicular as well as ovarian]**

Clinically germ cell tumors of testes can be divided into seminoma and non-seminomatous germ cell tumors (NSGCT).

SEMINOMATOUS GERM CELL TUMORS

- **Seminomas** are characterized by *large cells with distinct cell membranes and clear cytoplasm, large central nucleus with prominent one or two nucleoli. Cytoplasm contains glycogen.* Classical seminomas **do not contain alpha fetoprotein (AFP)**. Human chorionic gonadotropin (hCG) is present in 15% of seminomas that contain syncytiotrophoblasts. **Spermatocytic seminoma** is a distinctive tumor characterized by being found in *old age and having excellent prognosis* [do not metastasize]. Histologically, it is characterized by maturation of tumor cells, some of which resemble secondary spermatocytes. **Spermatocytic seminoma** is seen only in testis. There is **no ovarian counterpart**.

NON-SEMINOMATOUS GERM CELL TUMORS

These may be embryonal carcinoma, yolk sac tumors, choriocarcinoma or teratoma.

- **Choriocarcinomas** have a mixture of malignant cytotrophoblasts and syncytiotrophoblasts. These are most aggressive variants. **Malignant teratomas** have tissue derived from all three germ layers with scattered immature neural elements. In children, differentiated mature teratomas are considered benign whereas in post-pubertal males, all teratomas are regarded as malignant.
- **Embryonal cell carcinomas** present as sheets of undifferentiated cells. Focal glandular differentiation may be present. Elevated AFP and hCG is seen in this tumor.
- **Yolk sac tumor or infantile embryonal carcinoma or endodermal sinus tumor** are the *most common testicular tumor in infants and children up to 3 years of age*. These have very good prognosis. Half of tumors show **Schiller-Duval bodies or glomeruloid structures** [structures resembling endodermal sinuses]. Presence of **AFP** is highly characteristic of **yolk sac tumors.**

Seminoma	NSGCT
1. *Radiosensitive*	Radio resistant
2. *Localized to testes for long duration (70% present in stage 1)*	Early dissemination (60% present in stage II & III)
3. *Metastasis first to lymph nodes*	Early hematogenous metastasis
4. *Tunica albuginea spared*	Tunica breached mostly

Important points about germ cell tumors

- Painless enlargement of testis is a characteristic feature.
- Lymphatic spread is common to all testicular tumors. Retroperitoneal nodes are first involved.
- Hematogenous spread is primarily to lungs.

Testicular Germ Cell Tumors
Most of these arise from intra tubular germ cell neoplasia (ITGCN) except spermatocytic seminoma and teratoma.

Seminomas almost never occur in infants.

Counterpart of seminoma in ovary is dysgerminoma.

Pure choriocarcinoma is most aggressive testicular tumor.

Yolk sac tumor are characterized by **elevated AFP** and *choriocarcinoma* by *elevated hCG*. AFP is never elevated in seminoma.

Concept

Biopsy of testicular neoplasm is associated with risk of tumor spillage, therefore radical orchiectomy should be done on presumption of malignancy.

Extragonadal site of germ cell tumors include **mediastinum (commonest),** retroperitoneum and pineal gland.

Rod shaped **crystalloids of Reinke** are seen in about 25% of **Leydig cell tumors.**

Non-Germinal Tumors

- **Leydig cell tumors** are derived from stroma and Sertoli cell tumors from sex cords. *Sertoli cell tumors* are also known as *Androblastoma*. Both these tumors are benign.
- **Gonadoblastoma** contains a **mixture** of germ cells and gonadal stromal elements.

Lymphomas are most common testicular neoplasms in men over the age of 60 years. The prognosis is extremely poor. These are most common cause of bilateral testicular tumors.

PROSTATE

In a normal adult prostate weighs about 20g. It is divided into peripheral, central, transitional zones and the region of anterior fibromuscular stroma. Prostate is a **combined tubuloalveolar organ**. Characteristically, the glands are lined by *two layer of cells*, basal layer of cuboidal cells covered by a layer of columnar secretory cells. Three important conditions of prostate are inflammations, hyperplasia and tumors.

Inflammation of prostate (prostatitis)

It is characterized by finding at least **15 leukocytes per high power field** in prostatic secretions.
- Acute prostatitis present with sudden onset of fever, chills and dysuria. It is mostly caused by E. coli
- Chronic bacterial prostatitis is associated with recurrent UTI.
- Chronic abacterial prostatitis is associated with infections with Chlamydia or Ureaplasma.
- Granulomatous prostatitis is mostly caused by intravesical administration of BCG (used for treatment of superficial bladder carcinoma).

Malacoplakia is a granulomatous disease with defective intracellular lysosomal digestion of bacteria. It is mostly caused by E. coli. Sharply demarcated spherical structures with concentric owl eye (known as *Michaelis-Guttmann bodies*) are seen histologically.

Nodular hyperplasia

It is also known as *benign prostatic hyperplasia* (BPH). Clinical symptoms are urinary frequency, nocturia, difficulty in starting or stopping urination, dribbling and dysuria. Histologically, nodules are composed of hyperplastic stromal cells and hyperplastic glands. **Glands consist of two layer of cells; cuboidal and columnar [in carcinoma single layers of cells are present in glands]** with intervening stroma. Histological signs of malignancy are absent. Development of BHP is associated with advanced age and high testosterone levels. Di-hydrotestosterone (DHT) is produced from testosterone with the help of an enzyme, 5α-reductase type 2. DHT is the main substance responsible for prostatic growth. In addition to mechanical effects of enlarged prostate, clinical symptoms are also due to smooth muscle mediated contraction of prostate by α_{1A} receptors.

Note: In some cases, nodular enlargement may project up into the floor of urethra as a hemispherical mass, which is termed as "median lobe hypertrophy".

Tumors

Adenocarcinoma of prostate is most common form of cancer in men. Advancing age, race (more in American blacks, least in Asians), dietary factors (increases with more fat consumption, decreases with lycopene, vitamin A, vitamin E, selenium and soy products), androgens and genetic factors are implicated in pathogenesis of prostate cancer. *Genetic factors include germ line mutations of BRCA2 tumor suppressor gene, chromosomal re-arrangements that juxtapose ERG or ETV1 next to androgen regulated TMPRSS2 promoter and epigenetic alterations like hypermethylation of glutathione 5-transferase (GSTP1) gene causing down regulation of GSTP1 expression.* Local extension most commonly involves seminal vesicles and later base of bladder; **Fascia of Denonvilliers prevents the backward extension of the tumor.** Hematogenous spread occur chiefly to bones (**osteoblastic secondaries**) *most commonly to lumbar spine.* Lymphatic

BPH mostly originates from *transitional zone* of prostate whereas **carcinoma** mostly arises from **peripheral zone**.

Concept

BHP is NOT a pre-malignant condition.

5-α-reductase inhibitors (e.g. **finasteride**) and α_{1A} receptor antagonists (e.g. **tamsulosin**) can be used for treatment of BPH.

Most of the prostatic carcinomas are acinar adenocarcinoma and arise in peripheral zone, classically in a posterior location.

Concept

Feature that differentiate benign and malignant prostate gland is that benign glands contain basal cells [two layered; basal cells and columnar cells] that are absent in cancer [single layered cells].

Genital System and Breast

spread occurs initially to obturator nodes. Histologically, most lesions are adenocarcinomas characterized by small **glands that appear "back to back" without intervening stroma** or that appear to be infiltrating beyond the normal prostate lobules.

Most *prostate cancers* arise peripherally, away from urethra; therefore *urinary symptoms occur late.* Osteoblastic secondaries in bone are virtually diagnostic of prostate cancer.

Grading of prostate cancer

Grade 1 is well differentiated and Grade 5 shows no glandular differentiation. Grade 2, 3 and 4 are in-between. Most tumors contain more than one pattern, so primary grade is assigned to dominant pattern and secondary grade to sub-dominant pattern. Combined Gleason score is derived by addition of these two grades. Tumors with only one pattern are assumed to have both primary and secondary grade as same. Thus Gleason score for these is double the grade. Score of 2-4 are considered well-differentiated, 5-6 as moderately differentiated, 7 moderate to poorly differentiated and 8-10 high grade cancers. Grading is of particular importance in prostatic cancer, as it is the best marker, along with stage, for predicting prognosis.

> **Gleason score** is used for **Grading** of prostate cancer.

> **Minimum Gleason score is 2** (1 + 1) and is most differentiated whereas **maximum score is 10** (5 + 5), least differentiated.

Major role of transrectal ultrasonography (TRUS) in prostate cancer is in guiding the placement of needle biopsies to thoroughly sample the gland. Transperineal or transrectal biopsy is required for diagnosis.

Prostate specific antigen (PSA): 20-40% patients with prostate cancer have PSA value of 4 ng/ml or less and so, four different refinements in PSA value can be utilized.

a. *PSA density:* It is the ratio of serum PSA value and volume of prostate. It reflects PSA produced per gram of prostate tissue. Upper normal limit is 0.15.

b. *Age specific reference range*

> PSA is organ specific but not cancer specific because it may be elevated in BHP, prostatitis, infarct, ejaculation etc. apart from prostatic cancer.

Age	Upper normal value
40-49 years	2.5 ng/ml
50-59 years	3.5 ng/ml
60-69 years	3.5 ng/ml
70-79 years	6.5 ng/ml

c. *PSA velocity:* It is rate of change of PSA with time. At least 3 PSA measurements should be taken over a period of 1.5 to 2 years.

d. *Percentage of free PSA:* It is calculated as

> **PSA velocity** of *0.75 ng/ml/ year best distinguishes* between cancer and benign lesions.

$$\text{Free PSA/Total PSA} \times 100$$

It is more valuable, when total PSA is in 'gray zone' of 4 to 10 ng/ml. Free PSA less than 10% indicates high risk of carcinoma whereas value > 25% indicates lower risk.

FEMALE GENITAL TRACT

Embryology

The paired genital ducts consist of the mesonephric (Wolffian) duct, which extends from the mesonephros to the cloaca, and the paramesonephric (Mullerian) duct, which runs parallel and lateral to the Wolffian duct.

- The **mesonephric ducts in males**, if stimulated by testosterone (secreted by the Leydig cells), develop into the *vas deferens, epididymis, and seminal vesicles.* In contrast, because normal females do not secrete testosterone, the Wolffian ducts regress and form vestigial structures. They may, however, form mesonephric cysts in the cervix or vulva, or they may form Gartner duct cysts in the vagina. The cranial group of mesonephric tubules (the epoophoron) remains as vestigial structures in the broad ligament above the ovary, while the caudal group of mesonephric tubules (the paroophoron) forms vestigial structures in the broad ligament beside the ovary.

> **Mesonephric ducts in males**: develop into the *vas deferens, epididymis, and seminal vesicles.*
>
> **Mesonephric ducts in females:** Gartner duct cysts *in the vagina.*

- The **paramesonephric ducts in the female** form the *fallopian tubes, the uterus, the uppermost vaginal wall, and the hydatid of Morgagni.* The lower portion of the vagina and the vestibule develop from the urogenital sinus. Males secrete Mullerian-inhibiting factor (MIF) from the Sertoli cells of the testes, which causes regression of the Mullerian ducts. This results in the formation of the vestigial appendix testis.
- Several **abnormalities** result from abnormal embryonic development of the Mullerian ducts.
  - **Uterine agenesis** may result from abnormal development or fusion of these paired paramesonephric ducts. Developmental failure of the inferior portions of the Mullerian ducts results in a **double uterus**, while failure of the superior portions to fuse (incomplete fusion) may form a **bicornuate uterus**.
  - Retarded growth of one of the paramesonephric ducts along with incomplete fusion to the other paramesonephric ducts results in the formation of a **bicornuate uterus with a rudimentary horn**.

GENITAL CYSTS

Obstruction of the ducts of any of the glands found within the female genitalia may cause the formation of a genital cyst.

- **Bartholin's cyst:** The paired Bartholin's glands, which are analogous to the bulbourethral glands of the male, are located in the lateral wall of the vestibule. If these are obstructed, a cyst may form that is usually lined with transitional epithelium.
- **Gartner's duct cysts:** These are derived from Wolffian (mesonephric) duct remnants and are located in the lateral walls of the vagina.
- **Mesonephric cysts:** Cysts derived from the same Wolffian duct may also be found on the lateral aspect of the vulva and are called mesonephric cysts.
- **Nabothian cysts:** Obstruction of the ducts of the mucous glands in the endocervix may result in small mucous (Nabothian) cysts.
- **Epithelial inclusion cysts:** Cysts may also be found within the skin of the vulva. These cysts, which contain white, cheesy material, are called keratinous (epithelial inclusion) cysts. Clinically they are referred to as sebaceous cysts, which is a misnomer.
- **Follicular cysts:** These are benign cysts of the ovary.

DISEASES OF VULVA

1. Leukoplakia

Several pathologic conditions are associated with the formation of white plaques on the vulva, which are clinically referred to as leukoplakia.

- **Lichen sclerosis** is seen histologically as atrophy of the epidermis with underlying dermal fibrosis.

The **four cardinal histologic features** are:

- Atrophy (thinning) of the epidermis, with disappearance of the rete pegs
- Hydropic degeneration of the basal cells
- Replacement of the underlying dermis by dense collagenous fibrous tissue
- A monoclonal bandlike lymphocytic infiltrate

- Loss of pigment in the epidermis (**vitiligo**) can also produce leukoplakia.
- Inflammatory skin diseases, squamous hyperplasia and vulvar intraepithelial neoplasia can also present with leukoplakia.

2. Benign Tumors

a. Papillary Hidradenoma

Hidradenomas consist of tubular ducts lined by a single or double layer of nonciliated columnar cells, with a layer of flattened "myoepithelial cells" underlying the epithelium. These myoepithelial elements are characteristic of sweat glands and sweat gland tumors. It is identical in appearance to intraductal papillomas of the breast.

b. Condyloma Acuminatum

Condylomata acuminata are sexually transmitted, benign tumors that have a distinctly verrucous gross appearance. Condylomata are caused by HPV, principally types 6 and 11. It is not considered to be precancerous lesions.

> Koilocytotic atypia (nuclear atypia and perinuclear vacuolization) caused by HPV is considered a viral "cytopathic" effect.

3. Premalignant and Malignant Neoplasms

i. **Squamous cell carcinoma**

It may be *associated with high-risk HPV or with squamous cell hyperplasia and lichen sclerosus.*

- Rare variants of squamous cell carcinoma include *verrucous carcinomas*, which are fungating tumors resembling condyloma acuminatum, and *basal cell carcinomas*, which are identical to their counterparts on the skin. Neither tumor is associated with papillomaviruses.

> Most (85%) of the malignant tumors of vulva are squamous cell carcinomas.

ii. **Paget's disease**

- It manifests grossly as pruritic, red, crusted, sharply demarcated map-like areas.
- Histologically, it reveals single anaplastic tumor cells infiltrating the epidermis. These cells are characterized by having **clear spaces ("halos")** between them and the adjacent epithelial cells. These malignant cells stain positively with PAS or mucicarmine stains.

iii. **Malignant melanoma**

Malignant melanoma of the vulva may resemble Paget's disease, however, these malignant cells **stain positively with a melanin stain or S100** immunoperoxidase stain.

> *Concept*
>
> Paget's disease of the vulva (extramammary Paget's disease) is similar to Paget's disease of the nipple except that *100% of cases of Paget's disease of the nipple are associated with an underlying ductal carcinoma* of the breast, while **vulvar lesions are most commonly confined to the skin.**

DISEASES OF VAGINA

1. Adenocarcinoma

- The tumors are most often located on the anterior wall of the vagina, usually in the upper third.
- These are often composed of vacuolated, glycogen-containing cells, hence the term clear cell carcinoma. These cancers can also arise in the cervix.
- A probable precursor of the tumor is **vaginal adenosis**, a condition in which glandular columnar epithelium of Müllerian type either appears beneath the squamous epithelium or replaces it.

> Clear cell adenocarcinomas are seen in young *women whose mothers* had been treated with **diethylstilbestrol (DES) during pregnancy**

2. Embryonal rhabdomyosarcoma or sarcoma botryoides

- It is an uncommon vaginal tumor most frequently found in infants and in children **younger than 5 years** of age.
- The tumor consists predominantly of malignant embryonal rhabdomyoblasts and is thus a type of rhabdomyosarcoma.
- These tumors have the appearance and consistency of **grapelike clusters** (hence the designation botryoides, meaning grapelike).

> **Sarcoma botryoides or Embryonal rhabdomyosarcoma**
>
> Tumor cells have **"tennis racket" appearance.**

DISEASES OF CERVIX

1. Cervicitis

- **Acute cervicitis** is characterized by acute inflammatory cells, erosion, and reactive or reparative epithelial change.
- **Chronic cervicitis** includes inflammation, usually mononuclear, with lymphocytes, macrophages, and plasma cells.

Risk factors for cervical neoplasia

- Early age at first intercourse
- Multiple sexual partners
- Increased parity
- A male partner with multiple previous sexual partners
- Presence of a cancer-associated HPV
- Exposure to oral contraceptives and nicotine
- Genital infections (chlamydia)
- Persistent detection of a high viral load of high-risk HPV.
- Certain HLA and viral subtypes

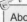

About 95% of squamous carcinomas are composed of relatively large cells, either keratinizing (well-differentiated) or nonkeratinizing (moderately differentiated) patterns.

- HSV is most strongly associated with epithelial ulcers (often with intranuclear inclusions in epithelial cells) and a lymphocytic infiltrate, and *C. trachomatis* with lymphoid germinal centers and a prominent plasmacytic infiltrate. Epithelial spongiosis is associated with *T. vaginalis* infection.

2. Intraepithelial and Invasive Squamous Neoplasia

a. *Cervical Intraepithelial Neoplasia (CIN)*

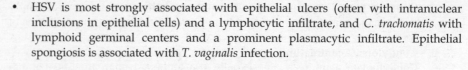

CIN can be divided into three grades; CIN I, CIN II and CIN III

- **CIN I:** These lesions are on the extreme low end of the spectrum and are often indistinguishable histologically from condylomata acuminata . These have a low rate of progression to cancer.
- **CIN II:** These consist of the appearance of atypical cells in the lower layers of the squamous epithelium but nonetheless with persistent (but abnormal) differentiation toward the prickle and keratinizing cell layers.
- **CIN III:** As the lesion evolves, there is progressive loss of differentiation accompanied by greater atypia in more layers of the epithelium, until it is totally replaced by immature atypical cells, exhibiting no surface differentiation (CIN III).

b. *Squamous Cell Carcinoma*
   – Invasive cervical carcinoma manifests in three somewhat distinctive patterns: fungating (or exophytic), ulcerating, and infiltrative cancers. The most common variant is the fungating tumor, which produces an obviously neoplastic mass that projects above the surrounding mucosa.
   – On histologic examination, a small subset of tumors (less than 5%) are poorly differentiated small cell squamous or, more rarely, small cell undifferentiated carcinomas (neuroendocrine or oat cell carcinomas). The latter closely resemble oat cell carcinomas of the lung and have an unusually poor prognosis owing to early spread by lymphatics and systemic spread. These tumors are also frequently associated with a specific high-risk HPV, type 18.

Clear cell adenocarcinomas of the cervix in DES-exposed women are similar to those occurring in the vagina.

DISEASES OF UTERUS

1. Endometeritis

- The endometrium and myometrium are relatively resistant to infections. Therefore, inflammation of the endometrium (endometritis) is rare.
- **Acute endometritis** is usually caused by bacterial infection following delivery or miscarriage and is characterized by the presence of **neutrophils** in non-menstrual endometrium.
- The histologic diagnosis of **chronic endometritis** depends on finding **plasma cells** within the endometrium. All it takes is one plasma cell to make the diagnosis.
- Chronic endometritis may be seen in patients with intrauterine devices (IUDs), pelvic inflammatory disease (PID), retained products of conception (postpartum), or tuberculosis.

2. Endometriosis and Adenomyosis

- Adenomyosis is thought to result from the abnormal down growth of the endometrium into the myometrium. Symptoms produced by adenomyosis include *menorrhagia, colicky dysmenorrhea, dyspareunia, and pelvic pain.*
- Endometriosis is thought to possibly arise from metaplasia of celomic epithelium into endometrial tissue or implantation of normal fragments of menstrual endometrium either via the fallopian tubes or via the blood vessels. Histologically, it reveals endometrial glands, stroma, and hemosiderin pigment (from the cyclic bleeding).

Presence of *benign endometrial glands* surrounded by endometrial stroma **within the myometrium** (conventionally atleast 2.5 mm below the endomyometrial junction), is called **adenomyosis.**

Ectopic endometrial tissue outside of the uterus is called **endometriosis**

Cysts containing blood clots in **endometriosis** are called as **"chocolate cysts.**

Repeated cyclic bleeding in patients with endometriosis can lead to the formation of cysts (3-5 cm diameter) that contain areas of new and old hemorrhages. "

- Sites of endometriosis include the ovary, uterine ligaments (associated with dyspareunia), the rectovaginal pouch (associated with pain on defecation and low back pain), the fallopian tubes (associated with peritubular adhesions, infertility, and ectopic pregnancies), the urinary bladder (associated with hematuria), the GI tract (associated with pain, adhesions, bleeding and obstruction), and the vagina (associated with bleeding).

> Most common site of endo-metriois is **ovary.**

3. Menstrual abnormalities

With normal menstruation about 30 to 40 ml of blood is lost. Amount greater than 80 ml lost on a continued basis are considered to be abnormal.

- **Menorrhagia** refers to excessive bleeding at the time of menstruation, either in the number of days or the amount of blood. A submucosal leiomyoma could produce menorrhagia.
- **Metrorrhagia** refers to bleeding that occurs at *irregular intervals.*
- **Menometrorrhagia** refers to *excessive* bleeding that occurs at *irregular intervals*. Causes of metro or menometrorrhagia include cervical polyps, cervical carcinoma, endometrial carcinoma, or exogenous estrogens.
- **Oligomenorrhea** refers to infrequent bleeding that occurs at *intervals greater than 35 days.* Causes include polycystic ovarian syndrome and too low a total body weight.
- **Polymenorrhea** refers to *frequent, regular* menses that are *less than 22 days* apart. It is commonly associated with anovulatory cycles, which can occur at menarche.

> **Postmenopausal bleeding** occurs **more than 1 year** *after the normal cessation of menses at menopause.*

> **Dysmenorrhea** refers to **painful menses**. It is associated with increased levels of **prostaglandin F** in the menstrual fluid.

4. Dysfunctional uterine bleeding (DUB)

DUB is defined as abnormal uterine bleeding that is due to a **functional abnormality** rather than an organic lesion of the uterus.

The three main categories of DUB are:
- Anovulatory cycles (the most common form),
- Inadequate luteal phase
- Irregular shedding.

> **DUB:** *Abnormal uterine bleeding* due to a **functional abnormality; NO organic lesion** of the uterus.

Anovulatory cycles consist of *persistence of the Graffian follicle without ovulation.* This results in continous and excess estrogen production without the normal postovulatory rise in progesterone levels. With no progesterone production, no secretory endometrium is formed. Instead, biopsies reveal proliferative endometrium with mild hyperplasia. The mucosa becomes too thick and is sloughed off, resulting in the abnormal bleeding.

> **Avovulatory cycles** characteristically occur at **menarche and menopause;** are also associated with **polycystic ovary (Stein-Leventhal) syndrome.**

If there is ovulation but the functioning of the corpus luteum is inadequate, then the levels of progesterone are decreased, resulting in asynchrony between the chronologic dates and the histologic appearance of the secretory endometrium. This is referred to as an inadequate luteal phase (luteal phase defect).

The luteal phase defect is an important cause of infertility. Biopsies are usually performed several days after the predicted time of ovulation. If the histologic dating of the endometrium lags 4 or more days behind the chronologic date predicted by menstrual history, the diagnosis of luteal phase defect can be made. Clinically, these patients exhibit low serum progesterone, FSH, and LH levels.

Prolonged functioning of the corpus luteum (**persistent luteal phase** with continued progesterone production) results in prolonged heavy bleeding at the time of menses. Histologically, there is a combination of secretory glands mixed with proliferative glands (irregular shedding). Clinically, these patients have regular periods, but the menstrual bleeding is excessive and prolonged (lasting 10 to 14 days).

5. Endometrial hyperplasia (Endometrial Intraepithelial Neoplasia)

It is related to excess estrogens and is important clinically because of its relation to the development of endometrial adenocarcinoma. The types of endometrial hyperplasia include simple hyperplasia and complex hyperplasias.

Note: The shift in gland morphology from benign to precancerous is often highlighted by a loss of PTEN gene expression.

6. Endometrial carcinoma

- Endometrial carcinomas that are associated with hyperplasia tend either to be well-differentiated, mimicking normal endometrial glands (*endometrioid*) in histologic appearance, or to display altered differentiation (mucinous, tubal, squamous differentiation).
- Endometrial cancer not associated with pre-existing hyperplasia are generally more poorly differentiated, including tumors that resemble subtypes of ovarian carcinomas (papillary *serous carcinomas*). Overall, these tumors have a **poorer prognosis** than estrogen-related cancers do. In contrast to endometrioid tumors, serous subtypes infrequently display microsatellite instability and are linked to **mutation of** p53.

- *Histologically most of the endometrial carcinomas are adenocarcinomas.*
- If there are areas of *squamous differentiation* within these tumors, they are called *adenoacanthomas*.
- If there are areas of ***malignant squamous differentiation***, they are called ***adenosquamous carcinomas***.

7. Tumors of the Endometrium with Stromal Differentiation

a. *Carcinosarcomas or malignant mixed Müllerian tumors*
   Carcinosarcomas consist of endometrial adenocarcinomas in which malignant stromal differentiation takes place. The stroma tends to differentiate into a variety of malignant mesodermal components, including muscle, cartilage, and even osteoid. On histology, the tumors consist of adenocarcinoma mixed with the stromal (sarcoma) elements Sarcomatous components may mimic extrauterine tissues (i.e., striated muscle cells, cartilage, adipose tissue, and bone).

b. *Adenosarcomas*
   It consists of malignant appearing stroma, which coexists with benign but abnormally shaped endometrial glands.

c. *Stromal Tumors*
   The endometrial stroma occasionally gives rise to neoplasms that may resemble normal stromal cells. Stromal neoplasms may be benign stromal nodules or endometrial stromal sarcomas.

8. Tumors of Myometrium

- **Fibroids (Leiomyoma)** of the uterus arise in the myometrium, submucosally, subserosally, and mid-wall, both singly and several at a time. They are benign smooth-muscle tumors that are sharply circumscribed, firm, gray-white, and **whorled** on cut section.
- Their malignant counterpart, **leiomyosarcoma** of the uterus, is quite rare in the *de novo* state and arises even more rarely from an antecedent leiomyoma.

DISEASES OF OVARIES

1. Stein-Leventhal syndrome/Polycystic ovarian disease (PCOD)

- The symptoms of patients with this syndrome are related to *increased androgen production*, which causes hirsutism, and decreased ovarian follicle maturation, which can lead to amenorrhea.
- The cause of this syndrome is thought to be the abnormal secretion of gonadotropins by the pituitary. *Increased secretion of LH* stimulates the thecal cells to secrete excess amounts of androgens, which are converted to estrone by the peripheral aromatization of androgens by the adrenal gland. Excess estrogens in turn increase the levels of gonadotropin-releasing hormone (GnRH) but decrease the levels of

---

M

Endometrial cancer risk factors (Mnemonic: **ENDOME**Trial)

E	**E**lderly
N	**N**ulliparity
D	**D**iabetes
O	**O**besity
M	**M**enstrual irregularity
E	**E**strogen therapy
T	**T**ension (hypertension)

Concept

Mitoses are the most important criteria in assessing malignancy in smooth-muscle tumors of the uterus.

PCOD patients typically have **excess androgens** (androstenedione), **increased estrogen** levels, **increased LH levels,** *increased GnRH* levels, and ***decreased FSH*** levels (with a **high LH/FSH ratio**).

FSH. The GnRH increases the levels of LH, which then stimulate the thecal cells of the ovary to secrete more androgens, and the hormonal cycle begins again.

The ovaries in these patients are enlarged and show thick capsules, hyperplastic ovarian stroma, and numerous follicular cysts, which are lined by a hyperplastic theca interna. Because these patients do not ovulate, there is a markedly decreased number of corpora lutea, which, in turn, results in decreased progesterone levels.

Concept

PCOD is associated with *increased risk of developing endometrial hyperplasia and endometrial carcinoma* because of the excess estrogen production.

2. Ovarian tumors

Ovarian neoplasms may be divided into four main categories; epithelial tumors, sex cord-stromal tumors, Germ cell tumors and metastases.

Mnemonic:

WHO classification of ovarian tumors

1. Surface Epithelial Tumors		2. Germ Cell Tumors	
My	Mucinous	Doctor	Dysgerminoma
Servant	Serous	Examined	Endodermal Sinus tumor
Began	Brenner	The	Teratoma
Experiencing	Endometrioid	Ovaries	Ovarian choriocarcinoma
Cancer	Clear		
3. Sex cord Stromal Tumors		4. Metastatic	
She	Sertoli-Leydig	Killed:	Krukenberg
Felt	Fibroma-thecoma		
Grim	Granulosa theca		

A. Surface Epithelial Tumors

These are derived from the surface celomic epithelium, which embryonically gives rise to the Mullerian epithelium. Therefore, these ovarian epithelial tumors may recapitulate the histology of organs derived from the Mullerian epithelium.

a. **Serous ovarian tumors**

These are composed to ciliated columnar serous epithelial cells, which are similar to the *lining cells of the fallopian tubes.*
   - They commonly involve the *surface of ovary*.
   - Bilaterality is common, occurring in 20% of benign cystadenomas, 30% of borderline tumors, and approximately 66% of cystadenocarcinomas.
   - Concentric calcifications (psammoma bodies) characterize serous tumors, although they are not specific for neoplasia when they are found alone.

b. **Mucinous ovarian tumors**

Benign mucinous tumors are characterized by a lining of tall columnar epithelial cells with apical mucin and the absence of cilia, akin to *benign cervical or intestinal epithelia.* In gross appearance, the mucinous tumors differ from the serous variety in several ways:

   - They are characterized by more cysts of variable size and a rarity of surface involvement.
   - They are less frequently bilateral.
   - Mucinous tumors tend to produce larger cystic masses, and some have been recorded with weights of more than 25 kg.

   - One group of typically benign or borderline mucinous tumors arises in endometriosis and is termed "Müllerian mucinous" cystadenoma, resembling endometrial or cervical epithelium. These tumors are uncommonly malignant.
   - The second, more common group includes tumors exhibiting abundant gland-like or papillary growth with nuclear atypia and stratification and is strikingly similar to tubular adenomas or villous adenomas of the intestine. These tumors

Surface epithelial tumors are the **most common tumors of ovary**.

Serous cystadenocarcinomas account for approximately 40% of all cancers of the ovary and are the **most common malignant ovarian tumors.**

Serous tumors are also the **most common bilateral tumors of the ovaries**.

are presumed precursors to most cystadenocarcinomas. Cystadenocarcinomas contain more solid growth with conspicuous epithelial cell atypia and stratification, loss of gland architecture, and necrosis, and are similar to colonic cancer in appearance.

– Pseudomyxoma peritonei refers to the formation of multiple mucinous masses within the peritoneum. This condition results from the spread of mucinous tumors, either from metastasis or rupture of an ovarian mucinous cyst.

c. **Endometrioid ovarian tumors**

These are composed of nonciliated columnar cells, which are *similar to the epithelial cells of the endocervical glands.*

d. **Clear cell carcinoma of the ovary**

It is similar histologically to clear cell carcinoma of the kidney, or more accurately, the clear cell variant of endometrial adenocarcinoma or the glycogen-rich cells associated with pregnancy.

e. **Brenner tumor**

It is similar to the *transitional lining of the renal pelvis or bladder*. This ovarian tumor is associated with benign mucinous cystadenomas of the ovary. Most Brenner tumors are benign, but borderline (proliferative Brenner tumor) and malignant counterparts have been reported.

f. **Cystadenofibromas**

These are variants in which there is more pronounced proliferation of the fibrous stroma that underlies the columnar lining epithelium. They may be composed of mucinous, serous, endometrioid, and transitional (Brenner tumors) epithelium.

B. Sex-Cord Stromal Tumors

Examples of ovarian stromal tumors include thecomas, fibromas, granulosa cell tumors, and Sertoli-Leydig cell tumors.

- **Thecomas** are composed of *spindle-shaped cells with vacuolated cytoplasm*. They are vacuolated because of *steroid hormone (estrogen) production*, which can be stained with an Oil Red O stain.
- **Fibromas** are also composed of *spindle-shaped cells, but they do not produce steroid hormones* and are Oil Red O-negative.
- **Granulosa cell tumor**: These are the most common type of ovarian tumor that is composed of cells that *stain positively with inhibin*. Histologically, the cells may form Call-Exner bodies, which are gland-like structures formed by the tumor cells aligning themselves around a central space that is filled with acidophilic material. The tumor cells may secrete estrogens and cause precocious sexual development in girls or increase the risk for endometrial hyperplasia and carcinoma in women. Less commonly granulosa cell tumors can secrete androgens and produce masculinization.
- **Sertoli-Leydig tumors (Androblastomas)**: These also may secrete androgens and produce virilization in women. The tumor cells may *stain positively with inhibin, but Call-Exner bodies are not present*. Granulosa cell tumors vary in their clinical behavior, but they are considered to be potentially malignant.
- **Hilus cell tumors (Pure Leydig cell tumor)**: The ovarian hilum normally contains clusters of polygonal cells arranged around vessels (hilar cells). *Hilus cell tumors* are rare tumors derived from these cells and are *mostly unilateral*. These are characterized histologically by large lipid-laden cells with distinct borders. Typically, patients with hilus cell tumors present with evidence of masculinization, hirsutism, voice changes, and clitoral enlargement. True hilus cell tumors are almost always benign.
- **Small cell carcinoma** of the ovary is the another tumor of possible stromal origin. These malignant tumors occur predominantly in young women and may be associated with hypercalcemia.

Most cases of **Pseudomyxoma peritonei** result from spread of a mucinous tumor located in the appendix (mucocele).

Meig's syndrome = *ovarian fibroma + ascites + hydrothorax.* (usually right sided).

Concept

Granulosa cell tumor: *Stain positively with inhibin;* **Call-Exner bodies are present**.

Sertoli-Leydig tumors: May *stain positively with inhibin*, but **Call-Exner bodies are NOT present.**

Reinke crystalloids is a typical cytoplasmic structure characteristic of **Leydig cells** is usually present.

Genital System and Breast

C. Germ Cell Tumors

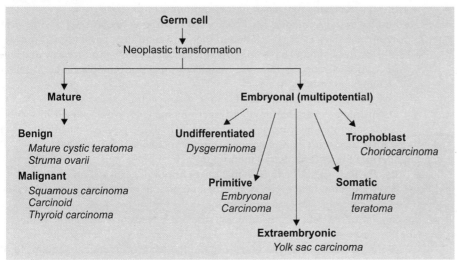

Concept

Most consistent lab finding in Hilus cell tumors is *an elevated 17-ketosteroid excretion level unresponsive to cortisone suppression.*

a. **Teratomas:** These are divided into three categories: mature (benign), immature (malignant), monodermal or highly specialized.

    Mature (Benign) Teratomas:

    –   Cystic teratomas are usually found in young women during the active reproductive years.

        •   Characteristically, they are unilocular cysts containing hair and cheesy sebaceous material.
        •   Within the wall, it is common to find tooth structures and areas of calcification.

    –   On histologic examination, the cyst wall is composed of stratified squamous epithelium with underlying sebaceous glands, hair shafts, and other skin adnexal structures.

    –   In most cases, structures from other germ layers can be identified, such as cartilage, bone, thyroid tissue, and other organoid formations.

    –   About 1% of the dermoids undergo malignant transformation of any one of the component elements (e.g., thyroid carcinoma, melanoma, but most commonly, squamous cell carcinoma).

    –   These tumors arise from an ovum after the first meiotic division.

    Monodermal or Specialized Teratomas:

    –   The most common of the specialized teratoma are struma ovarii and carcinoid. They are always unilateral.

        •   Struma ovarii is composed entirely of mature thyroid tissue. Interestingly, these thyroidal neoplasms may hyperfunction, causing hyperthyroidism.

    –   The **ovarian carcinoid** presumably arises from intestinal epithelium in a teratoma and may result in carcinoid syndrome. Primary ovarian carcinoid can be distinguished from metastatic intestinal carcinoid, the latter virtually always bilateral.

    –   Even more rare is the **strumal carcinoid**, a combination of struma ovarii and carcinoid in the same ovary.

    Immature Malignant Teratomas:

    –   These are rare tumors that differ from benign teratomas in that the component tissue resembles that observed in the fetus or embryo rather than in the adult.

    –   The tumor is found chiefly in prepubertal adolescents and young women, the mean age being 18 years.

    –   On microscopic examination, there are varying amounts of immature tissue differentiating toward cartilage, glands, bone, muscle, nerve, and others.

Most **benign teratomas** are cystic and are known as **dermoid cysts; they arise from** the ectodermal differentiation of **totipotential cells.**

The karyotype of all benign ovarian teratomas is 46, XX.

All **dysgerminomas** are **malignant.**

These neoplasms are **extremely radiosensitive.**

Characteristic histologic feature of **yolk sac tumor** is a glomerulus-like structure composed of a central blood vessel enveloped by germ cells within a space lined by germ cells (**Schiller-Duval body**).

Concept

In contrast to choriocarcinomas arising in placental tissue, those arising in the ovary are generally unresponsive to chemotherapy and are often fatal.

Krukenberg tumors are often found in **both ovaries.**

Stomach is the primary site in most of the cases of Krukenberg tumor.

b. **Dysgerminoma**
   - It is the **ovarian counterpart of the seminoma** of the testis.
   - Similar to the seminoma, it is composed of large vesicular cells having a clear cytoplasm, well-defined cell boundaries, and centrally placed regular nuclei.
   - Most of these tumors have no endocrine function. A few produce elevated levels of chorionic gonadotropin and may have syncytiotrophoblastic giant cells on histologic examination.
   - These are **usually unilateral** (80% to 90%) and solid.
   - On histologic examination, the dysgerminoma cells are dispersed in sheets or cords separated by scant fibrous stroma. As in the seminoma, the fibrous stroma is infiltrated with mature lymphocytes and occasional granulomas.

c. **Endodermal Sinus (Yolk Sac) Tumor**
   - It is the second most common malignant tumor of germ cell origin.
   - It is thought to be derived from differentiation of malignant germ cells toward extraembryonic yolk sac structure.
   - Similar to the yolk sac, the tumor is rich in *a-fetoprotein and a1-antitrypsin*.

d. **Choriocarcinoma**
   - More commonly of placental origin, the choriocarcinoma, similar to the endodermal sinus tumor, is an example of extraembryonic differentiation of malignant germ cells.
   - Most ovarian choriocarcinomas exist in combination with other germ cell tumors, and pure choriocarcinomas are extremely rare.
   - Like all choriocarcinomas, they elaborate high levels of chorionic gonadotropins that are sometimes helpful in establishing the diagnosis or detecting recurrences.

e. **Other Germ Cell Tumors**
   - These include **embryonal carcinoma** (another highly malignant tumor of primitive embryonal elements, histologically similar to tumors arising in the testes), **polyembryoma** (a malignant tumor containing so-called embryoid bodies) and **mixed germ cell tumors** (containing various combinations of dysgerminoma, teratoma, endodermal sinus tumor, and choriocarcinoma).

Gonadoblastoma is an uncommon tumor thought to be composed of germ cells and sex cord-stroma derivatives. It occurs in individuals with abnormal sexual development and in gonads of indeterminate nature. Eighty per cent of patients are phenotypic females, and 20% are phenotypic males with undescended testicles and female internal secondary organs. On microscopic examination, the tumor consists of nests of a mixture of germ cells and sex cord derivatives resembling immature Sertoli and granulosa cells. A coexistent dysgerminoma occurs in 50% of the cases. The prognosis is excellent.

D. Metastatic tumors of ovary

- The most common "metastatic" tumors of the ovary are probably derived from tumors of Mullerian origin: the uterus, fallopian tube, contralateral ovary, or pelvic peritoneum.
- The most common extramullerian primaries are the breast and gastrointestinal tract, including colon, stomach, biliary tract, and pancreas.
- Also included in this group are the rare cases of pseudomyxoma peritonei, derived from appendiceal tumors.
- **Krukenberg tumor** classically refers to a metastatic ovarian malignancy whose primary site arose in the gastrointestinal tract or breast. Microscopically, they are characterized by appearance of **mucin-secreting signet-ring cells** in the tissue of the ovary; when the primary tumor is discovered, the same signet-ring cells are typically found. Carcinomas of colon, appendix, and breast (mainly invasive lobular carcinoma) are the next most common primary sites. Rare cases of Krukenberg tumor originating from carcinomas of the gallbladder, biliary tract, pancreas, small intestine, ampulla of Vater, cervix, and urinary bladder/urachus have been reported

SECONDARY AMENORRHEA

Secondary amenorrhea refers to absent menses for 3 months in a woman who had previously had menses. Causes of secondary amenorrhea include pregnancy (the most common cause), hypothalamic/pituitary abnormalities, ovarian disorders, and end organ (uterine) disease.

The remainder of the disorders causing secondary amenorrhea can be differentiated by examining gonadotropin (FSH and LH) levels along with the results of a progesterone challenge test.

- Withdrawal bleeding following progesterone administration indicates that the endometrial mucosa had been primed with estrogen, which, in turn, indicates that the hypothalamus/pituitary axis and ovaries are normal.
- **Hypothalamic/pituitary disorders**, which are characterized by decreased FSH and LH levels, include functional gonadotropin deficiencies, such as can be seen in patients with a weight loss syndrome. In these patients, markedly decreased body weight (> 15% below ideal weight) causes decreased secretion of GnRH from the hypothalamus. Decreased gonadotropin levels decrease estrogen levels, which results in amenorrhea and an increased risk for osteoporosis. Because of the decreased estrogen levels, progesterone challenge does not result in withdrawal bleeding.
- **Ovarian conditions**, such as surgical removal of the ovaries, would most likely produce elevated gonadotropin levels due to the lack of negative feedback from estrogen and progesterone. Because of the decreased estrogen levels, a progesterone challenge would not result in withdrawal bleeding.
- **Uterine (end organ) disorders** are characterized by normal FSH and LH levels. An example is Asherman's syndrome. (Describe alongside) A patient with Asherman's syndrome would have no response to progesterone.

GESTATIONAL TROPHOBLASTIC DISEASES

The diseases in this category include; benign hydatidiform mole (partial and complete), invasive mole, placental site trophoblastic tumor and choriocarcinoma.

1. **Hydatidiform mole**: Both partial and complete, are composed of *avascular, grape-like structures* that do not invade the myometrium. .

Differentiating features between partial and complete mole

- In complete (classic) moles, all the chorionic villi are abnormal and fetal parts are not found. In partial moles, only some of the villi are abnormal and fetal parts may be seen.
- Complete moles have a 46, XX diploid pattern and arise from the paternal chromosomes of a single sperm by a process called androgenesis. In contrast, partial moles have a triploid or a tetraploid karyotype and arise from the fertilization of a single egg by two sperm.
- Another way to differentiate these two disorders is to use immunostaining for p57, which is a gene that is paternally imprinted (inactivated). Because the complete mole arises only from paternal chromosomes, immunostaining for p57 will be negative.

2. **Invasive moles**: This is defined as a mole that penetrates and may even perforate the uterine wall. There is invasion of the myometrium by hydropic chorionic villi, accompanied by proliferation of both cytotrophoblast and syncytiotrophoblast. Hydropic villi may embolize to distant sites, such as lungs and brain, but do not grow in these organs as true metastases.

3. **Placental site trophoblastic tumor**: In contrast to syncytial cytotrophoblast, which is present on the chorionic villi, intermediate trophoblast is found in the implantation site and placental membranes. Intermediate trophoblasts may give rise to *placental site trophoblastic tumors* (PSTTs). PSTTs comprise less than 2% of gestational trophoblastic neoplasms and present as neoplastic polygonal cells infiltrating the endomyometrium. PSTTs may be preceded by a normal pregnancy (one-half),

Concept

Pregnancy can be **diagnosed** by obtaining a clinical history along with a pregnancy test that determines serum or urine beta-human chorionic gonadotropin **(beta-hCG) levels**.

Asherman's syndrome is a clinical condition caused by numerous aggressive dilatation and curettage of the endometrium for menorrhagia leading to removal of the stratum basalis. It is also associated with absence of the glandular epithelium.

Concept

It is important to differentiate between partial and complete mole these two disorders because about **2% of complete moles may develop into chriocarcinoma**, but *partial moles are rarely followed by malignancy*

spontaneous abortion (one-sixth), or hydatidiform mole (one-fifth). Distinction of PSTTs from normal exaggerated placental implantation site trophoblast may be difficult and can be achieved by using biomarkers (Mel-Cam and Ki-67) that detect increased proliferation in the trophoblastic cells.

4. **Gestational choriocarcinomas:** These are composed of malignant proliferations of both cytotrophoblasts and syncytiotrophoblasts without the formation of villi, can arise from either normal or abnormal pregnancies: 50% arise in hydatidiform moles, 25% in cases of previous abortion, 22% in normal pregnancies, and the rest in ectopic pregnancies or teratomas. Both hydatidiform moles and choriocarcinomas have high levels of human chorionic gonadotropin (hCG); the levels are extremely high in choriocarcinoma unless considerable tumor necrosis is present.

BREAST

Pain (mastalgia or mastodynia) is the most common breast symptom.

Discrete *palpable masses* are the second most common breast symptom. A breast mass usually does not become palpable until it is about 2 cm in diameter. Approximately 50% of carcinomas arise in the upper outer quadrant, 10% in each of the remaining quadrants, and about 20% in the central or subareolar region.

Nipple discharge is a less common presenting symptom but is of concern when it is spontaneous and unilateral. Bloody or serous discharges are most commonly associated with benign lesions but, rarely, can be due to a malignancy. The most common etiologies for discharge are a solitary large duct papilloma, cysts, or carcinoma.

The principal mammographic signs of breast carcinoma are densities and calcifications:

> **DCIS** is the most common malignancy associated with calcifications

- Densities. Most neoplasms grow as solid masses and are radiologically denser than the intermingled connective and adipose tissue of the normal breast. Mammography can detect masses before they become palpable. The most common lesions that are detected as densities are invasive carcinomas, fibroadenomas, and cysts. Ductal carcinoma in situ (DCIS, or carcinoma limited to the ductal system) rarely presents as a density.
- Calcifications. Calcifications are associated with secretory material, necrotic debris, and hyalinized stroma. Calcifications associated with malignancy are commonly small, irregular, numerous, and clustered or linear and branching.

INFLAMMATIONS

Acute Mastitis

> **Acute mastitis** occuring during lactation is usually caused by *Staphylococcus aureus*.

Almost all cases of acute mastitis occur during lactation usually caused by *Staphylococcus aureus*.

Periductal Mastitis/Zuska disease

This condition is also known by the names of recurrent subareolar abscess or squamous metaplasia of lactiferous ducts. Both women, as well as men, present with a painful erythematous subareolar mass. The main histologic feature is keratinizing squamous epithelium extending to an abnormal depth into the orifices of the nipple ducts.

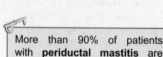

> More than 90% of patients with **periductal mastitis** are smokers.

Mammary Duct Ectasia

This disorder tends to occur in the fifth or sixth decade of life, usually in multiparous women, and, unlike periductal mastitis, is not associated with cigarette smoking.

Patients present with a poorly defined palpable periareolar mass, sometimes with skin retraction, often accompanied by thick, white nipple secretions. This lesion is characterized chiefly by dilation of ducts, inspissation of breast secretions, and a marked periductal and interstitial chronic granulomatous inflammatory reaction.

Fat Necrosis

Fat necrosis can present as a painless palpable mass, skin thickening or retraction, a mammographic density, or mammographic calcifications.

BENIGN EPITHELIAL LESIONS

Nonproliferative Breast Changes (Fibrocystic Changes)

Three principal patterns of morphologic change:
1. Cyst formation, often with apocrine metaplasia;
2. Fibrosis; and
3. Adenosis

Cysts: Small cysts form by the dilation and unfolding of lobules. When cystic lobules coalesce, larger cysts are formed. Unopened cysts are brown to blue (blue-dome cysts) owing to the contained semitranslucent, turbid fluid. Cysts are lined either by a flattened atrophic epithelium or by cells altered by apocrine metaplasia. Metaplastic cells have an abundant granular, eosinophilic cytoplasm, with round nuclei, resembling the apocrine epithelium of sweat glands.

Fibrosis: Cysts frequently rupture, with release of secretory material into the adjacent stroma. The resulting chronic inflammation and fibrous scarring contribute to the palpable firmness of the breast.

Adenosis: Adenosis is defined as an increase in the number of acini per lobule.

The acini are often enlarged (blunt duct adenosis) and are not distorted as is seen in sclerosing adenosis.

Concept

"Milk of calcium" is a term radiologists use to describe calcifications in large cysts that look as if they are lining the bottom of a rounded cyst on mammography.

Proliferative Breast Disease without Atypia

This group of disorders is characterized by proliferation of ductal epithelium and/or stroma without cellular abnormalities suggestive of malignancy. The following entities are included in this category: **(1)** moderate or florid epithelial hyperplasia, **(2)** sclerosing adenosis, **(3)** complex sclerosing lesions, **(4)** papillomas, and **(5)** fibroadenoma with complex features.

Epithelial Hyperplasia
- In the normal breast, only myoepithelial cells and a single layer of luminal cells are present above the basement membrane. Epithelial hyperplasia is defined by the presence of more than two cell layers.

Sclerosing Adenosis
- The number of acini per terminal duct is increased to at least twice the number found in uninvolved lobules. The normal lobular arrangement is maintained. The acini are compressed and distorted in the central portions of the lesion but characteristically dilated at the periphery. Myoepithelial cells are usually prominent.

Complex Sclerosing Lesion (Radial Scar)
- Radial scars are stellate lesions characterized by a central nidus of entrapped glands in a hyalinized stroma.

Papillomas
- Papillomas are composed of multiple branching fibrovascular cores, each having a connective tissue axis lined by luminal and myoepithelial cells. Growth occurs within a dilated duct.
- Small duct papillomas have been shown to be a component of proliferative breast disease and increase the risk of subsequent carcinoma.

Proliferative Breast Disease with Atypia

Proliferative disease with atypia *includes atypical ductal hyperplasia (ADH) and atypical lobular hyperplasia (ALH).*

- **ADH** is recognized by its histologic resemblance to ductal carcinoma in situ, including a monomorphic cell population, regular cell placement, and round lumina. However, the lesions are characteristically limited in extent, and the cells are not completely monomorphic in type or they fail to completely fill ductal spaces.
- **ALH** refers to a proliferation of cells identical to those of LCIS (described later), but the cells do not fill or distend more than 50% of the acini within a lobule.

Concept

Atypical hyperplasia is a cellular proliferation resembling ductal carcinoma in situ (DCIS) or lobular carcinoma in situ (LCIS) but lacking sufficient qualitative or quantitative features for a diagnosis of carcinoma in situ.

Non-proliferative changes do not increase the risk of cancer. Proliferative disease is associated with a mild increase in risk. Proliferative disease with atypia (ADH and ALH) confers a moderate increase in risk.

CARCINOMA OF THE BREAST

Carcinoma is the most common malignancy of the breast, and breast cancer is the most common non-skin malignancy in women.

PROGNOSTIC FACTORS

Major

- Invasive carcinoma has worse prognosis than in-situ carcinoma
- Distant metastasis indicates bad prognosis.
- Axillary lymph node involvement is associated with worse prognosis.
- Tumor Size: Less than 1 cm good prognosis, more than 2 cm bad prognosis.
- Local invasion into skeletal muscle carries poor prognosis.
- Inflammatory carcinoma has poor prognosis.

Minor

- **Histological type:** Invasive ductal carcinoma (no special type; NST) carries poor prognosis. Special types have good prognosis except medullary.
- **Nottingham histological score (Scarff-Bloom-Richardson grade):** Grade 1 good prognosis, grade 3 poor
- **Estrogen and Progesterone receptor** positivity indicates good response to anti-estrogen therapy.
- **HER2/neu overexpression:** Poor prognosis
- **Lymphovascular invasion:** poor prognosis
- High proliferative rate indicates worse prognosis
- **Aneuploidy** indicates bad prognosis
- *The major risk factors for the development of breast cancer are hormonal and genetic (family history).* Breast carcinomas can, therefore, be divided into sporadic cases, possibly related to hormonal exposure, and hereditary cases, associated with family history or germ-line mutations.

Hereditary Breast Cancer

Mutated *BRCA1* also markedly increases the risk of developing ovarian carcinoma, which is as high as 20 to 40%. *BRCA2* confers a smaller risk for ovarian carcinoma (10 to 20%) but is associated more frequently with male breast cancer. *BRCA1* and *BRCA2* carriers are also susceptible to other cancers, such as colon, prostate, and pancreas, but to a lesser extent. BRCA1-associated breast cancers are commonly poorly differentiated, have medullary features and do not express hormone receptors or HER2/neu (so called, *triple negative phenotype*). Their gene profile signature is similar to basal-like breast cancers. These are frequently associated with loss of inactive X-chromosome and reduplication of active X, resulting in absence of Barr body. BRCA2 are also poorly differentiated but are more commonly estrogen receptor positive.

Sporadic Breast Cancer

The major risk factors for sporadic breast cancer are related to hormone exposure: gender, age at menarche and menopause, reproductive history, breast-feeding, and exogenous estrogens. The majority of these cancers occur in postmenopausal women and overexpress estrogen receptors (ER).

CLASSIFICATION OF BREAST CARCINOMA

Almost all breast malignancies are adenocarcinomas, all other types (i.e., squamous cell carcinomas, phyllodes tumors, sarcomas, and lymphomas) making up fewer than 5% of the total.

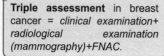

Breast cancer is the *most common* malignancy in women in **India**

Axillary lymph node status is the *most important prognostic factor for invasive carcinoma* in the absence of distant metastases.

Triple assessment in breast cancer = *clinical examination+ radiological examination (mammography)+FNAC.*

In comparison to BRCA1, **BRCA2** is associated more frequently with **male breast cancer**.

Carcinomas are divided into in situ carcinomas and invasive carcinomas.

Noninvasive carcinomas (carinoma in situ) may be located within the ducts (intraductal carcinoma) or within the lobules (lobular carcinoma in situ). There are several variants of intraductal carcinoma, including comedocarcinoma, cribriform carcinoma, and intraductal papillary carcinoma. Comedocarcinoma grows as a solid intraductal sheet of cells with a central area of necrosis, that commonly undergoes calcification. It is frequently associated with the erb B2/neu oncogene and a poor prognosis. Cribriform carcinoma is characterized by round, ductlike structures within the solid intraductal sheet of epithelial cells, while intraductal papillary carcinoma has a predominant papillary pattern.

Infiltration of the nipple by large cells with clear cytoplasm is diagnostic of Paget's disease. These cells are usually found both singly and in small clusters in the epidermis. Paget's disease is always associated with (in fact, it begins with) an underlying intraductal carcinoma that extends to infiltrate the skin of nipple and areola. **Paget cells** may resemble the cells of superficial spreading melanoma, but they are *PAS-positive and diastase-resistant (mucopolysaccharide-or mucin-positive)*, unlike melanoma cells.

INVASIVE (INFILTRATING) CARCINOMA

Invasive breast carcinoma is divided into two main types:
- No- special type carcinoma **[Intraductal]**
- **Special carcinoma**
  - Lobular
  - Cribriform
  - Colloid
  - Medullary
  - Papillary
  - Metaplastic

Invasive carcinomas of no special type include the majority of carcinomas (70 to 80%) that cannot be classified as any other subtype.

Invasive Carcinoma, No Special Type (NST; Invasive Ductal Carcinoma)

On gross examination, most carcinomas are firm to hard and have an irregular border. Within the center of the carcinoma, there are small pinpoint foci or streaks of chalky white elastotic stroma and occasionally small foci of calcification. There is a characteristic grating sound (similar to cutting a water chestnut) when cut or scraped. Five major patterns of gene expression in the NST group are noted:

- **Luminal A (40-55%):** ER positive and HER2/neu negative. These are generally slow growing and respond to hormonal treatments.
- **Luminal B (15-20%):** Triple positive cancers i.e. ER, PR and HER2/neu positive. These are of higher grade and more likely to have lymph node metastasis.
- **Normal breast-like (6-10%):** Well-differentiated ER positive and HER2/neu negative.
- **Basal-like (13-25%):** Triple negative cancers i.e. ER, PR and HER2/neu negative. Express markers of typical myoepithelial cells (e.g. basal keratins, P-cadherin, p63 or laminin), progenitor cells or putative stem cells (cytokeratin 5 and 6). Members of this group include medullary carcinoma, metaplastic carcinoma (e.g. spindle cell carcinoma or matrix producing carcinoma) and carcinomas with a central fibrotic focus. Many cancers in women with BRCA-1 mutations are of this type.
- **HER2 positive (7-12%):** ER negative but overexpress HER2/neu. In more than 90%, it is due to amplification of the segment of DNA on chromosome 17q21.

Lobular Carcinoma

Lobular carcinoma (invasive) of breast is one of the very few carcinomas which are **seen bilaterally**. Histologic hallmark is the presence of dyscohesive infiltrating tumor cells, often arranged in *single file* or in loose clusters or sheets. *Tubule formation is absent.* Signet ring cells containing intracytoplasmic mucin droplets are common. It metastasizes frequently to peritoneum, retroperitoneum, leptomeninges, GIT and ovaries. The incidence of this

Concept

Paget cells may resemble the cells of superficial spreading melanoma, but they are *PAS-positive and diastase-resistant (mucopolysaccharide-or mucin-positive)*, unlike melanoma cells.

Intraductal carcinoma is most common carcinoma of breast and carries poor prognosis.

Special type carcinomas carry good prognosis but inflammatory carcinoma has poor prognosis.

Lobular carcinoma (invasive) of breast occurs **bilaterally**.

Concept

Both lobular carcinoma of breast and signet ring carcinoma of GIT are characterized by the loss of E-cadherin.

carcinoma is increasing among postmenopausal females presumably because of increasing use of HRT.

Medullary Carcinoma

The tumor has a soft, fleshy consistency (*medulla* is Latin for "marrow") and is well-circumscribed. The carcinoma is characterized by

- Solid, syncytium-like sheets (occupying more than 75% of the tumor) of large cells with vesicular, pleomorphic nuclei, containing prominent nucleoli
- Frequent mitotic figures
- A moderate to marked lymphoplasmacytic infiltrate surrounding and within the tumor
- A pushing (non-infiltrative) border.

Medullary carcinomas have slightly better prognosis than do NST carcinomas, despite the almost universal presence of poor prognostic factors. These show overexpression of E-cadherin and basal like gene expression.

Mucinous (Colloid) Carcinoma

The tumor cells are seen as clusters and small islands of cells within large lakes of mucin that push into the adjacent stroma.

Tubular Carcinoma

These tumors consist exclusively of well-formed tubules. However, a myoepithelial cell layer is absent, and tumor cells are in direct contact with stroma.

Invasive Papillary Carcinoma

Invasive carcinomas with a papillary architecture are rare and represent 1% or fewer of all invasive cancers. Papillary architecture is more commonly seen in DCIS.

Metaplastic Carcinoma

"Metaplastic carcinoma" includes a wide variety of rare types of breast cancer (<1% of all cases), including conventional adenocarcinomas with a chondroid stroma, squamous cell carcinomas, and carcinomas with a prominent spindle cell component that might be difficult to distinguish from sarcomas. Some of these carcinomas express genes in common with myoepithelial cells and likely to arise from this cell type.

MULTIPLE CHOICE QUESTIONS

MALE GENITAL TRACT

1. Alpha fetoprotein is *Not* raised in which testicular tumors?   *(AI 2010)*
   (a) Choriocarcinoma
   (b) Teratocarcinoma
   (c) Yolk sac tumor
   (d) Embryonal cell carcinoma

2. Which one of the following is not used as a tumor marker in testicular tumors?   *(AI 2005) (DNB 2007)*
   (a) AFP   (b) LDH   *(Kolkata 2008)*
   (c) hCG   (d) CEA

3. All of the following statements about Gleason grading system are true except: *(AIIMS Nov 2008)*
   (a) Score range from 1 to 10
   (b) High score is associated with bad prognosis
   (c) Helps in grading of tumor
   (d) Helps decide treatment modality

4. Infertility is a common feature in "Sertoli cell only" syndrome because: *(AIIMS May 2003)*
   (a) Too many Sertoli cells inhibit spermatogenesis via inhibin
   (b) Proper blood testis barrier is not established
   (c) There is no germ cell in this condition
   (d) Sufficient numbers of spermatozoa are not produced

5. Predisposing factors for germ cell tumor are:
   (a) Cryptorchidism   *(PGI Dec 2002)*
   (b) Testicular feminizing syndrome
   (c) Klinefelter's syndrome
   (d) Smoking
   (e) Right side more common than left side.

6. In the testis intratubular germ cell neoplasia is seen in all, except: *(Delhi 2009 RP)*
   (a) Seminomas
   (b) Spermatocytic seminoma
   (c) Yolk sac tumor of testis
   (d) Embryonal carcinoma

7. Condyloma are mostly caused by HPV types:
   (a) 11 and 13   *(Delhi PG-2006)*
   (b) 6 and 11
   (c) 6 and 13
   (d) 30 and 33

8. Which one of the following is not used as a tumor marker in testicular tumors?   *(DNB- 2007)*
   (a) AFP   (b) LDH
   (c) HCG   (d) CEA

9. Gleason's classification is used for: *(UP 2008)*
   (a) Carcinoma breast
   (b) Carcinoma prostate
   (c) Carcinoma pancreas
   (d) Carcinoma rectum

10. Which of the following is not a malignant tumor of germ cell origin?   *(AP 2002)*
    (a) Mature teratoma
    (b) Choriocarcinoma
    (c) Dysgerminoma
    (d) Embryonal carcinoma

11. Metastasis is least common with: *(AP 2007)*
    (a) Embryonal cell carcinoma
    (b) Endodermal sinus tumor
    (c) Teratocarcinoma
    (d) Spermatocytic seminoma

12. A 25-year-old man, Ramesh presents with a testicular mass and is found to have high serum levels of α-fetoprotein (AFP). Microscopic examination of a biopsy from this mass reveals sheets of undifferentiated cells along with focal primitive glandular differentiation. The tumor cells have large and hyperchromatic nuclei. Further workup fails to reveal the presence of any metastatic disease as the tumor is confined within the testis. Based on all of these findings, which of the following best characterizes this tumor?

Tumor Aggressiveness	Grade	Stage
(a) Benign	Low	Low
(b) Benign	Low	High
(c) Malignant	Low	Low
(d) Malignant	High	Low
(e) Malignant	High	High

13. In which of the following respects do a seminoma involving the testis and a dysgerminoma involving the ovary differ most significantly?
    (a) Most common age of presentation
    (b) Number of mitoses
    (c) Potential to contain foci of more aggressive tumors
    (d) Ultrastructural appearance

14. A 10-year-old child develops a testicular mass and undergoes orchiectomy. On cut section, the mass shows a variety of appearances and colors. Histologically, many different tissues are seen, including cartilage, thyroid, and neural tissue. A small focus of clear-cut squamous cell carcinoma is seen. Which of the following is the most appropriate classification for this tumor?

(a) Dermoid cyst
(b) Teratoma with malignant transformation
(c) Immature teratoma
(d) Solid mature teratoma

Most Recent Questions

14.1. Which one of the following is not used as a tumor marker in testicular tumors?
(a) AFP
(b) LDH
(c) HCG
(d) CEA

14.2. Benign hyperplasia of prostate first develops in:
(a) Central zone
(b) Peripharal zone
(c) Periurethral transition zone
(d) Any of the above

14.3. The commonest site for extragonadal germ cell tumour is:
(a) Pineal gland
(b) Mediastinum
(c) Retroperitoneum
(d) Sacrococyygeal region

FEMALE GENITAL TRACT

15. The cytogenicity of solid tumors is not easily assessed especially in carcinoma cervix because
(a) Metaphase is distinct   (AIIMS Nov 2010)
(b) Due to contamination with infectious agents
(c) High mitotic rate
(d) Deficient tissue sample

16. With regard to the malignant behavior of leiomyosarcoma, the most important criterion is:
(a) Blood vessel penetration by tumor cells   (AI 2006)
(b) Tumor cells in lymphatic channels
(c) Lymphocyte infiltration
(d) The number of mitoses per high power field

17. All are true about polycystic ovarian disease except:
(a) Persistently elevated LH   (AIIMS Nov 2008)
(b) Increased LH/FSH ratio
(c) Increased DHEAS
(d) Increased prolactin

18. Sections from a solid-cystic unilateral ovarian tumor in a 30-year old female show a tumor composed of diffuse sheets of small cells with doubtful nuclear grooving and scanty cytoplasm. No Call-Exner bodies are seen. The ideal immunohistochemistry panel would include:
                                    (AIIMS May 2006)
(a) Vimentin, epithelial membrane antigen, inhibin, CD99
(b) Desmin, S-100 protein, smooth muscle antigen, cytokeratin
(c) Chromogranin, CD45, CD99, CD20
(d) CD3, Chromogranin, CD 45, Synaptophysin

19. An ovarian neoplasm in a 14-year old girl is most likely to be: (Delhi 2009)
(a) Germ cell tumor
(b) Epithelial tumor
(c) Sertoli-Leydig cell tumor
(d) Granulosa cell tumor

20. The incidence of bilaterality in a dermoid cyst is approximately: (Delhi 2009)
(a) 10%   (b) 30%
(c) 50%   (d) 70%

21. The risk of sarcoma developing in a fibroid uterus is approximately: (Delhi 2009)
(a) < 1%   (b) 10%
(c) 30%   (d) 50%

22. Uterine leiomyoma is least likely to undergo:
(a) Malignant change   (Delhi PG-2005)
(b) Hyaline change
(c) Calcification
(d) Red degeneration

23. Carcino-sarcoma occurs in: (UP 2003)
(a) Uterus   (b) Liver
(c) Breast   (d) Lungs

24. Schiller – Duval bodies are seen in: (UP 2005, 2007)
(a) Teratoma
(b) Seminoma
(c) Yolk-Sac tumor
(d) Choriocarcinoma

25. Call-Exner bodies are seen in: (UP 2007)
(a) Mature teratoma
(b) Endodermal sinus tumor
(c) Granulosa cell tumor
(d) Sertoli Leydig cell tumor

26. Hormone produced by endodermal sinus tumor is
(a) AFP   (RJ 2002)
(b) Alpha1 antitrypsin
(c) Both
(d) hCG

27. Choriocarcinoma is characterized by all except:
(a) Primarily trophoblastic tumor   (AP 2004)
(b) It can occur following hydatidiform mole
(c) Villi present
(d) It can metastasize to lungs

28. Call-Exner bodies are characteristic feature of (AP 2005)
(a) Granulosa theca cell tumor
(b) Brenner tumor
(c) Dysgerminoma
(d) Endodermal sinus tumor

29. Tennis Racquet cells are seen in :   (AP 2007)
(a) Rhabdomyoma
(b) Rhabdomyosarcoma
(c) Histiocytoma
(d) Eosinophilic granuloma

Genital System and Breast

30. A 30-year-old woman Shagun visits her gynecologist for a surgery. After laparotomy, a mass is removed which on microscopic examination demonstrates a cystic cavity filled with hair and keratin debris, and the wall contains skin, adnexal tissue, thyroid tissue, and neural tissue. All of the tissues are similar to those normally found, and no malignant changes are seen. Which of the following is the most likely diagnosis?
    (a) Immature teratoma
    (b) Leiomyoma
    (c) Leiomyosarcoma
    (d) Mature teratoma

31. Bilateral ovarian masses are identified on pelvic examination of a 40-year-old woman for which she undergoes total abdominal hysterectomy. Pathologic examination demonstrates papillary carcinoma producing serous fluid. Which of the following tumor markers would be most useful in monitoring for recurrence?
    (a) Alpha-fetoprotein
    (b) Bombesin
    (c) CA-125
    (d) PSA

32. A patient with chronic pelvic pain undergoes a hysterectomy. The resected uterus is filled with nodules composed of benign smooth muscle cells. Which of the following terms best describes these nodules?
    (a) Angiosarcoma   (b) Leiomyoma
    (c) Leiomyosarcoma (d) Rhabdomyoma

Most Recent Questions

32.1. An adenofibroma of the ovary in which the epithelial component consists of the nests of transitional cells is called:
    (a) Thecoma
    (b) Brenner tumour
    (c) Serous cystadenoma
    (d) Granulose cell tumor

32.2. Endodermal sinus tumor is characterized by:
    (a) Call Exner body
    (b) Psammoma body
    (c) Schiller duval body
    (d) Homer wright body

BREAST TISSUE

33. Lesions affecting the teminal duct lobulat unit (TDLU) in breast are all except   (DPG 2011)
    (a) Nipple adenoma
    (b) Blunt duct adenosis
    (c) Intraductal papilloma
    (d) Fibroadenoma

34. The type of mammary ductal carcinoma in situ (DCIS) most likely to result in a palpable abnormality in the breast is: (AI 2006)

    (a) Apocrine DCIS
    (b) Neuroendocrine DCIS
    (c) Will-differentiated DCIS
    (d) Comedo DCIS

35. BRCA 1 gene is located on: (AIIMS Nov 2008)
    (a) Chromosome 13   (b) Chromosome 11
    (c) Chromosome 17   (d) Chromosome 22

36. Increased susceptibility to breast cancer is likely to be associated with a mutation in the following gene:
    (a) p53   (b) BRCA-1 (AIIMS Nov 2004)
    (c) Retinoblastoma (Rb) (d) H-Ras

37. A female patient presented with a firm mass of 2 × 2 cms in the upper outer quadrant of the breast. She gives a family history of ovarian carcinoma. The investigation that needs to be done to assess for mutations is:
    (a) p53   (b) BRCA-2 (AIIMS May 2002)
    (c) Her 2/Neu gene   (d) C-myc gene

38. Bilateral breast carcinoma is: (PGI June 2002)
    (a) Scirrhous carcinoma (b) Medullary carcinoma
    (c) Lobular carcinoma   (d) Ductal carcinoma
    (e) Paget's carcinoma

39. Rare histological variants of carcinoma breast with better prognosis include all except: (Delhi 2009)
    (a) Colloid carcinoma
    (b) Medullary carcinoma
    (c) Inflammatory carcinoma
    (d) Tubular carcinoma

40. Tumor marker useful in the diagnosis of the cancer of the breast is: (Karnataka 2005)
    (a) CEA   (b) AFP
    (c) CA-125   (d) CA-15-3

41. Histologic hallmark of Paget's disease of nipple is:
    (a) Caseous necrosis   (Karnataka 2004)
    (b) Infiltration of the epidermis by malignant cells
    (c) Atypical lobular hyperplasia
    (d) Desmoplasia

42. BRCA-1 gene lies on chromosome: (DNB- 2008)
    (a) 17   (b) 18
    (c) 20   (d) 21

43. Commonest carcinoma of the breast with multifocal origin is: (UP 2001)
    (a) Scirrhous carcinoma (b) Adenocystic carcinoma
    (c) Lobular carcinoma   (d) Ductal carcinoma

44. Which of the following breast tumors is bilateral?
    (a) Colloid carcinoma   (UP 2003)
    (b) Invasive ductal carcinoma
    (c) Invasive lobular carcinoma
    (d) Medullary carcinoma

45. Indian file pattern is seen in histopathological examination of: (RJ 2006)
    (a) Infiltrating duct carcinoma
    (b) Fibroadenoma
    (c) Fibro carcinoma
    (d) Lobular carcinoma

46. Fleshy, soft lymphatic infiltration of skin in breast cancer appears as: *(TN 1996) (AP 2001)*
    (a) Puckering
    (b) Peau 'd orange
    (c) Cancer encurasse
    (d) All of the above

Most Recent Questions

46.1. BRCA-1 gene lies on chromosome:
    (a) 17
    (b) 18
    (c) 20
    (d) 21

46.2. A 54-year-old female Shanti presents for an annual exam. Her right breast is swollen, red, and tender. The physician palpates a firm area in the breast and suspects inflammatory breast cancer. Which of the following best describes the histological changes observed in this disorder?
    (a) Acute inflammation in breast carcinoma
    (b) Chronic inflammation in breast carcinoma
    (c) Dermal lymphatic invasion by cancer cells
    (d) Epidermal invasion by cancer cells

46.3. Paget's disease of the nipple is:
    (a) Infection
    (b) Dermatisis
    (c) Neoplasia
    (d) Hypopigmentation

CONCEPTUAL QUESTIONS

1-3. **Will have two statements, assertion and reason. Read both of them carefully and answer according to these options.**
    (a) Both assertion and reason are true and reason is correct explanation of assertion.
    (b) Both assertion and reason are true and reason is not the correct explanation of assertion.
    (c) Assertion is true and reason is false.
    (d) Both assertion and reason are false.

1. **Assertion:** Stromal cells are responsible for androgen dependent prostatic growth
   Reason: Stromal cells have 5α reductase activity which produces testosterone in prostate.

2. **Assertion:** Struma ovarii is mature teratoma
   Reason: It is responsible for production of the gonadotropins

3. **Assertion:** Seminoma is germ cell tumor with good prognosis.
   Reason: The tumor cells rarely have areas of necrosis and hemorrhage

EXPLANATIONS

1. **Ans. (a) Choriocarcinoma** *(Ref: Robbins 9/e p978, 8th/327, 989-991, 7th/339)*
   AFP is a marker of hepatocellular cancer and non-seminomatous germ cell tumors of testes.
   Non-seminomatous germ cell tumors may be embryonal carcinoma, yolk sac tumors, choriocarcinoma or teratoma.
   - **Embryonal cell carcinomas** and Yolk **sac tumor** have elevated AFP levels.
   - **Dorland's** dictionary 27th edition writes that **Teratocarcinoma** refers to a germ cell tumor that is a mixture of teratoma with embryonal carcinoma, or with choriocarcinoma, or with both. So, it may be having elevated levels of AFP.
   - **Choriocarcinomas** have elevated levels of HCG which can be readily demonstrated in the cytoplasm of syncytiotrophoblastic cells.

2. **Ans. (d) CEA** *(Ref: Robbins 7th/1045, 9/e p979, Harrison 17th/602)*
   - Biological markers of germ cell testicular tumors include AFP, hCG, placental alkaline phosphatase, placental lactogen and LDH. AFP, hCG and LDH are widely used clinically and have proved to be valuable in the diagnosis and management of testicular cancer.
   - CEA is an onco-fetal antigen and may be used as a tumor marker in adenocarcinoma of colon, pancreas, lung, breast and ovary. It is however not used as marker for Germ cell tumors.
   - About 70% patients with non-seminomatous germ cell tumors (NSGCT) show increased concentration of AFP or hCG. Latter may also be elevated in 10% of seminomas. **But AFP is never increased in seminoma.**
   "The presence of increased AFP level in a patient whose tumor shows only seminoma indicates that an occult NSGCT component exists".
   - LDH levels are not as specific as AFP or hCG but are increased in 50-60% patient with NSGCT and up to 80% patients with advanced seminoma.
   - AFP, hCG and LDH levels should be determined before and after orchiectomy. Reappearance of these markers or failure to decline according to predicted half life is an indication of persistent or recurrent tumor.

3. **Ans. (a) Score range from 1 to 10** *(Ref: Schwartz 8th/1216, Robbins 9/e 987)*
   - A **Gleason score** is given to prostate cancer based upon its microscopic appearance. Cancers with a higher Gleason score are more aggressive and have a worse prognosis. Most tumors contain more than 1 pattern.
   - The pathologist assigns a *grade* to the most common tumor, and a second *grade* to the next most common tumor. The two *grades* are added together to get a Gleason *score*. For example, if the most common tumor was grade 3, and the next most common tumor was grade 4, the Gleason *score* would be 3 + 4 = 7.
   - The Gleason *grade* ranges from 1 to 5, with 5 having the worst prognosis. The Gleason *score* ranges from 2 to 10, with 10 having the worst prognosis.
   - It should be noted that for Gleason score 7, a Gleason 4+3 is a more aggressive cancer than a Gleason 3+4. Also, there is not really any difference between the aggressiveness of a Gleason score 9 or 10 tumour.
   - **Gleason scores are associated with the following features:**

     - **Grade 1**: The cancerous prostate closely resembles normal prostate tissue. The glands are small, well-formed, and closely packed
     - **Grade 2**: The tissue still has well-formed glands, but they are larger and have more tissue between them.
     - **Grade 3**: The tissue still has recognizable glands, but the cells are darker. At high magnification, some of these cells have left the glands and are beginning to invade the surrounding tissue.
     - **Grade 4**: The tissue has few recognizable glands. Many cells are invading the surrounding tissue.
     - **Grade 5**: The tissue does not have recognizable glands. There are often just sheets of cells throughout the surrounding tissue

   The Gleason score is used to help evaluate the prognosis of men with prostate cancer. Together with other parameters, the Gleason score is incorporated into a strategy of prostate cancer staging which predicts prognosis and helps guide therapy.

4. **Ans. (c) There is no germ cells in this condition** *(Ref: Anderson 10th 2177)*
   'Sertoli cell only' syndrome also called as Germ cell aplasia has small seminiferous tubules. In this condition seminiferous tubules are smaller than normal and are lined by a single layer of Sertoli cells and no germ cells. Without germ cell, spermatogenesis does not take place resulting in infertility.

5. **Ans. (a) Cryptorchidism ; (b) Testicular feminising syndrome; (c) Klinefelter syndrome; (e) Rt. side has more common flow than Lt. side** *(Ref: Robbins' 7th/1041, 9/e p975, Harrison' 16th/550)*

   The predisposing factors of germ cell tumors of testes are:
   - Cryptorchidism
   - Testicular feminization syndrome
   - Klinefelter syndrome
   - Excess 12P copy number either in the term of i(l2P) or increased 12P an aberrantly banded marker chromosome.
   - Prior germ cell tumor
   - Strong family history of germ cell tumor
     - In most large testicular tumour approximately 10% associated with cryptorchidism.
     - Abdominal cryptorchid testes are at higher risk than inguinal cryptorchid testes.
     - Klinefelter's syndrome is associated with mediastinal GCT.
     - An isochromosome of short arm of chromosome 12[i(l2P)] is pathognomic of GCT in all histological types.
     - Blacks have very low incidence of germ cell neoplasms.
     - Seminoma is most common GCT.

6. **Ans. (b) Spermatocytic seminoma** *(Ref: Robbins 8th/988, 9/e p975,)*

   Most testicular germ cell tumors originate from intratubular germ cell neoplasia (ITGCN).

   ITGCN is seen adjacent to all germ cell tumors in adults except for spermatocytic seminoma and epidermoid and dermoid cysts. With rare exceptions, it is also not seen in pediatric tumors (teratomas, yolk sac tumors... Robbins 7th edition page 1096)

   So, obviously friends, if we have to choose between options b and c, we would prefer option b as the answer. ITCGN is seen with a high frequency in the following conditions:
   - Cryptorchidism
   - Prior germ cell tumors
   - Strong family history of germ cell tumor
   - Androgen insensitivity syndrome
   - Gonadal dysgenesis syndrome.

   Untreated ITGCN progresses to invasive germ cell tumor in approximately 50% of cases over 5 years of follow-up.

7. **Ans. (b) 6 and 11** *(Ref: Robbins 7th/1035, 9/e p970)*
   - Condyloma are most commonly caused by HPV types 6 and 11.
   - Condyloma acuminatum is a benign tumor caused by human papilloma virus (HPV).
   - It is related to the common wart (verruca vulgaris) and may occur on any moist mucocutaneous surface of the external genitalia in either sex.
   - Also, HPV and associated diseases are sexually transmitted.
   - On the penis, these lesions occur most often about the coronal sulcus and inner surface of the prepuce.
   - They consist of single or multiple sessile or pedunculated, red papillary excrescences that vary from 1 mm to several mm in diameter.
   - Histologically a branching, villous, papillary connective tissue stroma is covered by a thickened hyperplastic
   - Epithelium that may have considerable superficial hyperkeratosis and thickening of the underlying epidermis (acanthosis).
     - The normal orderly maturation of the epithelial cells is preserved.
     - Clear vacuolization of the prickle cells (Koilocytosis), characteristic of HPV infection, is noted in these lesions.
     - The basement membrane is intact, and there is no evidence of invasion of the underlying stroma.
     - Condyloma acuminata tend to recur but do not evolve into invasive cancers.

8. **Ans. (d) CEA** *(Ref: Robbins 8th/327, 9/e p979)*

9. **Ans. (b) Carcinoma prostate** *(Ref: Robbins 8th/999-1000, 9/e p987)*

10. **Ans. (a) Mature teratoma (Mature teratoma is a benign tumour)** *(Ref: Robbins 9/e p979, 8th/1047; 7th/1093,1096)*

11. **Ans. (b) Endodermal sinus tumor** *(Ref: Robbins 8th/1049, 9/e p977)*

12. **Ans. (d)** *(Ref: Robbins 7th/335, 1043, 9/e p977, Chandrasoma/307-308)*
    - An embryonal carcinoma is testicular malignancy that secretes alpha-fetoprotein (α-AFP) and is composed of undifferentiated cells along with primitive glandular differentiation. Once the diagnosis of malignancy is established, prognosis for the patient is estimated through the process of grading and staging.
    - It is important to understand the difference between these two terms. First of all, note that these terms are applied only to malignant neoplasms. Basically, **grading is done histologically, while staging is done clinically**.
    - Lower grades, such as grades I and II, are more differentiated, less aggressive and have a better prognosis, while

higher grades, such as grades III and IV, are less differentiated, more aggressive and have a worse prognosis. Tumors composed of malignant cells that appear primitive or undifferentiated are classified as high grade tumors.

- In contrast to grading, the staging of cancers is based on the size of the primary lesion, the presence of lymph node metastases, and the presence of blood-borne metastases. Two main staging systems are Union International Centre le Cancer (UICC) and American Joint Committee (AJC), UICC classification is called the TNM classification. AJC staging system generally divides cancers into stages 0 through IV. Lower stage tumors are smaller, localized, and have a better prognosis, while higher stage tumors are larger, widespread, and have worse prognosis.

13. **Ans. (a) Most common age of presentation** *(Ref: Robbins 8th/988, 1049, 9/e p976, 1030)*
    - Seminomas and dysgerminomas are very similar tumors but differ in two significant respects: the most common age of presentation in men is in the fourth decade, while in women, it is in the third decade. Also, seminomas are relatively common in men (30% of testicular germ cell tumors), while dysgerminomas are rare in women (1% of ovarian tumors).
    - Both of these tumors are composed of sheets of uniform polyhedral cells with intervening fibrous septa of connective tissue, lymphocytes, and multinucleated giant cells. The number of mitoses (choice B) per high-power field and ultrastructural appearance (choice D) do not differ greatly between the two tumors.
    - These tumors in pure form are very radiosensitive but can be much more aggressive (choice C) if foci of other germ cell tumors (notably embryonal carcinoma, choriocarcinoma, and yolk sac tumors) are present.

14. **Ans. (b) Teratoma with malignant transformation** *(Ref: Robbins 8th/991, 9/e p978)*
    - This is teratoma with malignant transformation. The possibility of malignant transformation is the reason why mature teratomas with very well differentiated tissues should be completely excised. Malignant transformation is more common in teratomas in adults than in children or babies.
    - Dermoid cyst (choice A) is a cystic form of mature teratoma, usually found in the ovaries.
    - Immature teratoma (choice C), while clinically malignant, shows embryonal tissues and often displays no clear-cut cytological evidence of malignancy.
    - Solid mature teratoma (choice D) without the added descriptor "with malignant transformation" is by definition a benign tumor. Careful extensive sampling is required to exclude minute foci of cancerous transformation.

14.1. **Ans. (d) CEA** *(Ref: Robbins 8/e 327, 9/e p979)*
    Carcino embryonic antigen is increased in cancers of the pancreas and colon.

14.2. **Ans. (c) Periurethral transition zone** *(Ref: Robbins 9/e p982)*

14.3. **Ans. (b) Mediastinum** *(Ref: Robbins 9/e p475; Harsh Mohan 6/e p703)*

15. **Ans. (b) Due to contamination with infectious agents** *(Ref: Enzinger and Weiss Soft Tissue Tumors, 5th/73, Wintrobes Hematology, 12th/50-60)*
    - Cytogenetics is the study of chromosome structure which can be done with techniques like karyotyping or molecular techniques (FISH, spectral karyotyping/multicolor FISH, comparative genomic hybridization). These techniques needs metaphase (more commonly) but can be applied to interphase also. Cytogenetics is easy if the metaphase is distinct. So, culture is often done in solid tumors to get the cells in metaphase.
    - Cytogenetics is also easier if mitotic rate is high.

    The problems with cytogenetics are:

    - Unpredictable growth of the neoplastic cells in tissue culture
    - Overgrowth of neoplastic cells by reactive non-neoplastic cells
    - Contamination of tumor cultures by bacteria or fungi
    - Predominance of nonviable tumor (necrotic sample)

    Deficient tissue sampling like sampling from nonrepresentative areas or the necrotic areas will impair the results in most of the solid tumors but the commonest problem with cancer of the cervix is the high contamination rate. So, option 'B' is better than option 'D'.

16. **Ans. (d) The number of mitoses per high power field** *(Ref: Robbins 7th/1090, 9/e p1021)*
    - The most important criterion for distinction of leiomyosarcoma from leiomyoma (malignant transformation) is the number of mitoses present.
    - Ten high power fields (hpf) are examined. If > 10 mitoses are seen, it signifies malignancy. If cellular atypia is also present, ≥ 5 mitoses are enough to make a diagnosis of leiomyosarcoma.

17. **Ans. (d) Increased Prolactin** *(Ref: Shaw 13th/353, 9/e p1022)*

The diagnosis of polycystic ovarian syndrome (PCOS) is straightforward using the **Rotterdam criteria**, even when the syndrome is associated with a wide range of symptoms.

Standard diagnostic assessments

- History-taking, specifically for menstrual pattern, obesity, hirsutism, and the absence of breast discharge. A clinical prediction rule found that these four questions can diagnose PCOS with a sensitivity of 77.1% (95% CI 62.7-88.0%) and a specificity of 93.8% (95% CI 82.8-98.7%).
- Gynecologic ultrasonography, specifically looking for small ovarian follicles. These are believed to be the result of disturbed ovarian function with failed ovulation, reflected by the infrequent or absent menstruation that is typical of the condition. In normal menstrual cycle, one egg is released from a dominant follicle - essentially a cyst that bursts to release the egg. After ovulation the follicle remnant is transformed into a progesterone producing corpus luteum, which shrinks and disappears after approximately 12-14 days. In PCOS, there is a so called "follicular arrest", i.e. several follicles develop to a size of 5-7 mm, but not further. No single follicle reach the preovulatory size (16 mm or more). According to the Rotterdam criteria, **12 or more small follicles** should be seen in an ovary on ultrasound examination. The follicles may be oriented in the periphery, giving the appearance of a 'string of pearls'. The numerous follicles contribute to the increased size of the ovaries, that is, 1.5 to 3 times larger than normal.
- Laparoscopic examination may reveal a thickened, smooth, pearl-white outer surface of the ovary.
- Serum (blood) levels of androgens (male hormones), including androstenedione, testosterone and dehydroepian-drosterone sulfate may be elevated: free testosterone is more sensitive than total. Free testosterone is reflected as the ratio of testosterone to sex hormone-binding globulin (SHBG).
- Some other blood tests are suggestive but not diagnostic. The ratio of LH (Luteinizing hormone) to FSH (Follicle stimulating hormone) is greater than 1:1, as tested on Day 3 of the menstrual cycle. The pattern is not very specific and was present in less than 50% in one study. There are often low levels of sex hormone binding globulin, particularly among obese women.

18. **Ans. (a) Vimentin, epithelial membrane antigen, inhibin, CD99** *(Ref. Sternberg Pathology/2581, 2583, 2543, 2579, 2652 Ackerman's Pathology/1694, 1675, 1681, 687)*

The specimen in the given question is most likely to be of granulosa cell tumor of ovary:

The features pointing toward this diagnosis are:
- Unilateral tumor
- Small cells arranged in sheets
- Scant cytoplasm
- Solid and cystic areas
- Nuclear grooving

The only point against this diagnosis is absence of Call-Exner bodies, but note that these structures if found are diagnostic of Granulosa cell tumors but these are not prerequisite for diagnosis.

Vimentin, EMA, inhibin and CD99 all are the markers of granulosa cell tumors.

19. **Ans. (A) Germ cell tumor** *(Ref: Robbins 8th/1047-1049, 9/e p1029, Harrison 17th/606, 604)*
- Epithelial tumors of ovary usually occur in old age
- Germ cell tumors of ovary generally occur in younger women. About 75% of these occur in women <30 years old
- Stromal tumors (like Sertoli Leydig tumors and granulosa cell tumors) occur in all ages.
- *Granulosa- theca cell tumors are mostly seen in post- menopausal women.*   *- Robbins/1050*
- Sertoli-Leydig cell tumors occur in women of all ages, although the peak incidence is in second and third decade
                                                                                                                        -Robbins/1051

Thus, we are left with two options: Germ cell tumors and Sertoli Leydig cell tumors. But, if we see the frequency of tumors; germ cell tumors have 15-20% whereas all sex-cord stromal tumors (Sertoli Leydig is one of them) together constitute only 5-10% of ovarian neoplasms

Thus, a 14-year-old girl is most likely to have germ cell tumor.

Important Points About Ovarian Neoplasms

- These may develop from epithelial cells (like serous, mucinous, Brenner tumor etc), germ cells (like granulose cell tumor, Sertoli-Leydig cell tumors etc).
- *Most common* ovarian neoplasms are *epithelial tumors*
- *Most common* malignant *ovarian neoplasms are epithelial tumors*.
- Two types of autosomal dominant familial cancers have been identified:
    - *Breast/ovarian cancer syndrome:* Due to mutations in BRCA1 or BRCA2 genes.
    - *Lynch type II syndrome:* Results due to mutations in mismatch repair genes. This is associated with Non-polyposis colorectal cancer, endometrial and ovarian cancer.
- CA-125 is marker of epithelial ovarian cancers
- Dysgerminoma is ovarian counterpart of seminoma and is highly sensitive to radiation therapy

20. **Ans. (a) 10%** *(Ref: Robbins 8th/1047, 9/e p1029)*
    - Germ cell tumors constitutes 15-20% of all ovarian tumors
    - Most are benign cystic teratoma, also known as dermoid cyst.
    - *Benign teratomas are bilateral in 0-15% of cases --- Robbins 1047*

21. **Ans. (a) < 1%** *(Ref: Robbins 8th/1037, 9/e p1020)*
    - Fibroid is the term used for uterine leiomyoma. *Malignant transformation (leiomyosarcoma) within a leiomyoma is extremely rare* -- Robbins/1037
    - Fibroids are most common tumor in women
    - They have characteristic whorled pattern of smooth muscle bundles on cut section as well as histologically
    - Differences between leiomyoma and leiomyosarcoma is mainly based on number of mitoses
    - If ≥10 mitoses per high power field are present or ≥ 5 mitoses with nuclear atypia are present, it indicates malignancy

22. **Ans. (a) Malignant change** *(Ref: Shaw's 13th/341, Robbins 9/e p1020)*
    Secondary changes (degenerations) in uterine leiomyoma:
    - **Atrophy:** It can be:
      - After menopause
      - After delivery
      Tumour becomes firmer and more fibrotic. It is due to diminished blood supply.
    - **Calcareous degeneration:** Phosphates and carbonates of lime are deposited in the periphery along the course of the vessels.
      - *'Womb-stones' in graveyard:* In old patients with long-standing myomas.
    - **Red (Carneous) degeneration:** It is more common during pregnancy. The myoma becomes tense and tender and causes severe abdominal pain with constitutional upset and fever. The tumour itself assumes a peculiar purple-red color and develops a fishy odour.
      - Although the patient is febrile with moderate leucocytosis and raised ESR, the condition is an aseptic one.
      - It needs to be differentiated from–
        - Appendicitis
        - Twisted ovarian cyst
        - Pyelitis
        - Accidental hemorrhage
    - **Sarcomatous change:** It is extremely rare. Incidence is no more than 0.5% of all myomas.
      - Intramural and submucous tumors have a higher potential than sub-serous.
      - It is rare for malignant change to develop in a women under the age of 40.
      - It is highly malignant and spreads through blood.
    - **Other complications:**
      - Torsion
      - Inversion
      - Capsular hemorrhage
      - Infection
      - Associated endometrial carcinoma

23. **Ans. (a) Uterus** *(Ref: Robbins 9/e p1018, 8th/1035; 7th/1088)*

24. **Ans. (c) Yolk-Sac tumour** *(Ref: Robbins 8th/1049, 9/e p1031)*

25. **Ans. (c) Granulosa cell tumour** *(Ref: Robbins 8th/1050, 9/e p1032)*

26. **Ans. (c) Both** *(Ref: Robbins 8th/1049, 9/e p1031)*

27. **Ans. (c) Villi present** *(Ref: Robbins 7th/1113, 9/e p1041)*

28. **Ans. (a) Granulosa theca cell tumor** *(Ref: Robbins 9/e p1032, 8th/1050; 7th/1102)*

29. **Ans. (b) Rhabdomyosarcoma** *(Ref: Robbins 9/e p1001, 8th/1017)*

30. **Ans. (d) Mature teratoma** *(Ref: Robbins 9/e p1029, 8th/1047-1048)*
    The lesion is a mature teratoma. Teratomas located in the ovary and containing a hair and keratin filled cyst are sometimes called dermoid cysts. They contain cells of a variety of types, often including skin, skin adnexal structures (hair follicles, sweat glands, sebaceous glands), connective tissues, neural tissue, muscle, and thyroid tissue. If immature tissues such as primitive neuroepithelial cells or developing skeletal muscle cells are seen, the lesion is considered potentially malignant and classified as an immature teratoma (option A).

31. **Ans. (c) CA-125** *(Ref: Robbins 9/e p1029, 8th/327)*
    - The tumors are serous papillary cystadenocarcinomas of the ovaries. These tumors express CA-125 and are apparently derived from the surface epithelium of the ovaries.
    - Bombesin (choice B) is a marker for neuroblastoma, small cell carcinoma, gastric carcinoma, and pancreatic carcinoma.

32. **Ans. (b) Leiomyoma** *(Ref: Robbins 8th/327, 9/e p1020)*

32.1. **Ans. (b) Brenner tumour** *(Ref: Robbins 9/e p1028)*
Transitional cell tumors contain neoplastic epithelial cells resembling urothelium and are usually benign. They comprise roughly 10% of ovarian epithelial tumors and are also referred to as Brenner tumors

32.2. **Ans. (c) Schiller duval body** *(Ref: Robbins 9/e p977)*

33. **Ans. (c) Intraductal papilloma** *(Ref: Pathology and Genetics of tumours of breast and female genital organs/81, Robbin 9/e p1044)*
Successive branching of the large ducts eventually leads to the terminal duct lobular unit (TDLU).
    - All breast cancers whether ductal or lobular originate from terminal duct lobular unit (TDLU).
    - Most of the benign breast diseases also originate from TDLU except intraductal papilloma, 90% of which occurs in large ducts in the central portion of breast.

34. **Ans. (d) Comedo DCIS** *(Ref: Robbins 7th/1139, 9/e p1057)*
    - **DCIS most frequently presents as mammographic calcifications. Less typically DCIS may present as a vaguely palpable mass. This is most likely with Comedocarcinomas.**
    - **Most of the breast malignancies are adenocarcinomas. These can be** *divided into insitu carcinomas and invasive carcinomas.*
    - **Carcinoma in situ** refers to a neoplastic population of cells limited to ducts and lobules by the basement membrane. It does not invade into lymphatics and blood vessels and cannot metastasize.
    - **Invasive carcinoma** (synonymous with "infiltrating" carcinoma) has invaded beyond the basement membrane into stroma. Here, the cells might also invade into the vasculature and thereby reach regional lymph nodes and distant sites. Even the smallest invasive breast carcinomas have some capacity to metastasize.
    - All carcinomas are thought to arise from the terminal duct lobular unit, and the terms "ductal" and "lobular" do not imply a site or cell type of origin.

CARCINOMA IN SITU

Ductal Carcinoma in Situ (DCIS; Intraductal Carcinoma)
- DCIS most frequently presents as mammographic calcifications. DCIS consists of a malignant population of cells limited to ducts and lobules by the basement membrane. The myoepithelial cells are preserved, although they may be diminished in number. DCIS is a clonal proliferation and usually involves only a single ductal system. The majority of cases of DCIS cannot be detected by either palpation or visual inspection of the involved tissue.
- **Occasional cases of comedocarcinoma are associated with sufficient periductal fibrosis to produce a thickening of the tissue, and punctate areas of necrosis ("comedone"-like) can be seen grossly.**

DCIS can be divided into
- **Comedocarcinoma:** It is characterized by **solid sheets of pleomorphic cells with high-grade nuclei and central necrosis**. The necrotic cell membranes commonly calcify and are detected on mammography as clusters or linear and branching microcalcifications. Periductal concentric fibrosis and chronic inflammation are common, and extensive lesions are sometimes palpable as an area of vague nodularity. Microinvasion (defined by foci of tumor cells less than 0.1 cm in diameter invading the stroma) is most commonly seen in association with comedocarcinoma.
- **Non-comedo DCIS** consists of a monomorphic population of cells with nuclear grades ranging from low to high. These may be cribriform (cookie cutter-like intraepithelial spaces), Solid (completely fills the involved spaces), Papillary (grows into spaces and lines fibrovascular cores typically lacking the normal myoepithelial cell layer) and Micropapillary (bulbous protrusions without a fibrovascular core).
- **Paget's disease** of the nipple is a rare manifestation of breast cancer and presents as a unilateral erythematous eruption with a scale crust. Pruritus is common, and the lesion might be mistaken for eczema. Malignant cells, referred to as Paget cells, extend from DCIS within the ductal system into nipple skin without crossing the basement membrane. The Paget cells are easily detected by nipple biopsy or cytological preparations of the exudate. The carcinomas are usually poorly differentiated and overexpress *HER2/neu.*

Lobular Carcinoma in Situ (LCIS)
LCIS is not associated with calcifications and is bilateral in 20-40% of women compared to 10-20% of cases of DCIS. LCIS is more common in young women.
- **Cells of LCIS and invasive lobular carcinoma are identical in appearance, and both lack expression of E-cadherin.** The loss of expression correlates with the histologic appearance of lobular carcinomas as single detached cells.

- Older studies indicated that both breasts were at equal risk of developing invasive carcinoma, but **a recent report suggests that the ipsilateral breast may be at greater risk** in women with lobular neoplasia.
- The abnormal cells consist of small cells that have oval or round nuclei with small nucleoli that do not adhere to one another. **Signet-ring cells containing mucin are present commonly. LCIS almost always expresses estrogen and progesterone receptors, and overexpression of** HER2/neu **is not observed.**

35. **Ans. (c) Chromosome 17** *(Ref: Harrison 17th/563, Robbin 9/e p1054)*
    - Tumor-suppressor gene, *BRCA-1*, has been identified at the chromosomal locus 17q21; this gene encodes a zinc finger protein, and the product therefore may function as a transcription factor. The gene appears to be involved in gene repair. Women who inherit a mutated allele of this gene from either parent have at least a 60–80% lifetime chance of developing breast cancer and about a 33% chance of developing ovarian cancer. The risk is higher among women born after 1940, presumably due to promotional effects of hormonal factors. Men who carry a mutant allele of the gene have an increased incidence of prostate cancer and breast cancer.
    - *BRCA-2*, which has been localized to chromosome 13q12, is also associated with an increased incidence of breast cancer in men and women.

36. **Ans. (a) p53** *(Ref: Robbins 7th/286, 300, 302, 8th/290-291, 9/e p1054, Harrison 16th/516, 517; 17th/563)*
    Breast cancer can be either familial (associated with germline mutation) or sporadic (associated with somatic mutation). The **familial breast cancer** is caused due to mutation in the following 4 genes:
    - **p53** tumor suppressor gene (called Li Fraumeni syndrome having multiple malignancies like breast cancer, osteo-genic sarcoma etc.)
    - **PTEN gene**: Gene on chromosome 10q associated with epithelial cancers of breast, endometrium and thyroid.
    - **BRCA1 gene**: Located on 17q: females having mutant gene have increased incidence of breast and ovarian cancer whereas males having mutant gene have high incidence of breast and prostate cancer.
    - **BRCA2 gene**: Located on chromosome 13q is associated with increased incidence of breast cancer in men and women.
    Sporadic breast cancer is associated with mutation in *p53 gene* (p53 defect is present in 40% of human breast cancer as an acquired defect) and *PTEN gene*.
    Since, incidence of sporadic cancer is much more than familial cancer, so the most important gene mutation increasing susceptibility to breast cancer should be answered as p53.

37. **Ans. (b) BRCA2** *(Ref: Harrison 17th/604, 9/e p1054)*
    In women with hereditary breast/ovarian cancer, there can be two susceptibility loci:
    - *BRCA1* located on chromosome 17q12-21, and
    - *BRCA2* located on 13q12-13.
    Both these are tumor-suppressor genes which produce nuclear proteins that interact with RAD 51 affecting genomic integrity.
    The cumulative risk of ovarian cancer with critical mutations of *BRCA1* or - *BRCA2* is 25%. Men in such families have an increased risk of prostate cancer.

38. **Ans. (c) Lobular Ca** *(Ref: Robbins 7th/1144/1141, 9/e p1065)*
    - Lobular carcinoma (invasive) of breast is one of the very few carcinomas which are seen bilaterally.
    - Lobular carcinoma in situ in 20-40% cases is bilateral.
    - Histologic hallmark is pattern of single infiltrating tumor cells often only one cell in width or in loose clusters or sheets.
    - Signet ring cells common.
    - Metastasize frequently to peritoneum, retroperitoneum, leptomeninges, GIT and ovaries.
    - The incidence of this carcinoma is increasing among postmenopausal females presumably because of increasing use of HRT.

39. **Ans. (c) Inflammatory carcinoma** *(Ref: Robbins 8th/1083)*

40. **Ans. (d) CA 15-3** *(Ref: Robbins 7th/339, 9/e p337, Anderson pathology 144-152)*

41. **Ans. (b) Infiltration of the epidermis by malignant cells** *(Ref: Robbins 7th/1140, 9/e p1057)*

42. **Ans. (a) 17** *(Ref: Robbins 8th/275-276, 9/e p1054)*

43. **Ans. (d) Ductal carcinoma** *(Ref: Robbins 8th/1080,1083, 9/e p1057)*

44. **Ans. (c) Invasive lobular carcinoma** *(Ref: Robbins 8th/1082; 7th/1142, 9/e p1059)*

45. **Ans. (d) Lobular carcinoma** *(Ref: Harsh Mohan 6th/762-763)*

46. **Ans. (b) Peau 'd orange** *(Ref: Robbins 9/e p1067, 8th/1083; 7th/122,1140,1142)*

46.1. **Ans. (a) 17** *(Ref: Robbins 8/e p275-276, 9/e p1054)*
   - BRCA 1 gene: chromosome 17
   - BRCA2 gene: chromosome 13

46.2. **Ans. (c) Dermal lymphatic invasion by cancer cells** *(Ref: Robbins 8th/1089, 9/e p1067)*
   - Inflammatory breast cancer is a pattern of invasive breast cancer in which the neoplastic cells infiltrate widely through the breast tissue. The cancer involves dermal lymphatics and therefore has a high incidence of systemic metastasis and a poor prognosis. If the lymphatics become blocked, then the area of skin may develop lymphedema and "peau d'orange," or orange peel appearance. The overlying skin in inflammatory breast cancer is usually swollen, red, and tender.
   - Acute inflammation (option A) is associated with secondary infection or abscess whereas chronic inflammation in breast cancer (option B) is a non-specific finding. In medullary breast cancer, a type of invasive ductal carcinoma, there are a large number of lymphocytes around the tumor and a desmoplastic reaction is often absent in the surrounding tissue.
   - Epidermal invasion by cancer cells (option D) is a poor prognostic indicator. Intraepidermal malignant cells are called Paget cells. Paget's disease of the nipple is a type of ductal carcinoma that arises in large ducts and spreads intraepidermally to the skin of the nipple and areola. There is usually an underlying ductal carcinoma.

46.3. **Ans. (c) Neoplasia** *(Ref: Robbins 9/e p1057)*
   Paget disease of the nipple is a rare manifestation of breast cancer (1% to 4% of cases) that presents as a unilateral erythematous eruption with a scale crust. Pruritus is common, and the lesion may be mistaken for eczema.

EXPLANATIONS TO CONCEPTUAL QUESTIONS

Explanations(1-3): *While solving assertion reason type of questions, we can use a particular method.*
1. First of all, read both assertion (A) and reason (R) carefully and independently analyse whether they are true or false.
2. If A is false, the answere will directly be (d) i.e. both A and R are false. You can note that all other options (i.e. a, b or c) consider A to be true.
3. If A is true, answer can be (a), (b) or (c), Now look at R. If R is false, answer will be (c)
4. If both A and R are ture, then we have to know whether R is correctly explaining A [answer is (a)] or it is not the explanation of assertion [answer is (b)]

1. **Ans. (c) Assertion is true and reason is false.** *(Ref: Robbins 8th/995, 9/e p983)*
   Stromal cells are responsible for androgen dependent prostatic growth. The main hormone responsible for androgen dependent prostatic growth is **dihydrotestosterone** (and not testosterone) because stromal cells have type 2 5α reductase enzyme which converts testosterone into dihydrotestosterone. DHT is more potent than testosterone because it binds more strongly to the androgen receptor.

   - **FGF-7**[Q] (fibroblast growth factor-7) is the most important factor mediating **paracrine** regulation of androgen dependent growth.
   - **Type 1**[Q] 5α **reductase** enzyme is minimally present in prostate and is mainly located mainly in **liver and skin**[Q].

2. **Ans. (c) Assertion is true and reason is false.** *(Ref: Robbins 8th/1048, 9/e p1030)*
   Struma ovarii is mature teratoma which is composed of **functioning thyroid tissue**. It is therefore responsible for production of the **thyroid hormones** (and not gonadotropins).

3. **Ans. (b) Both assertion and reason are true and reason is not the correct explanation of assertion.** *(Ref: Robbins 8th/988-9, 9/e p976)*
   Seminoma is a germ cell tumor with a good prognosis because it is an extremely radiosensitive and chemosensitive tumor. These tumors histologically have necrosis and hemorrhage only rarely.

Features	Seminoma	Non –seminoma
Localization	Localized to testes for long time	Metastasize early
Stage	70% patients present in stage I	60% in stage II and III
Metastasis	Mainly lymph node: hematogenous spread later	Hematogenous spread more frequent
Necrosis and hemorrhage	Rare	Common
Radiation sensitivity	Radiosensitive	Radio-resistant
General behavior	Less aggressive	More aggressive
Prognosis	Good	Bad

CEREBRAL HERNIATION

The cranial cavity is separated into compartments by infoldings of the dura. The two cerebral hemispheres are separated by the falx, and the anterior and posterior fossae by the tentorium. Herniation refers to displacement of brain tissue into a compartment that it normally does not occupy. These are of three main types: transtentorial, transfalcine (subfalcine) and tonsillar (foraminal).

> The **most common** herniations are **Transtentorial herniation**.

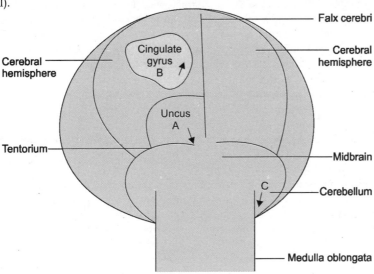

Transtentorial Herniation

The most common herniations are from the supratentorial to the infratentorial compartments through the tentorial opening, hence *transtentorial*. These may be divided into temporal (Uncal) or central herniations.

> **Uncal transtentorial herniation:** *compression of IIIrd cranial nerve; eye deviated down and out; mydriasis.*

- **Uncal transtentorial herniation** refers to impaction of the anterior medial temporal gyrus (the uncus) into the tentorial opening just anterior to and adjacent to the midbrain. The displaced brain tissue compresses the third nerve and results in *mydriasis and ophthalmoplegia (pupil point down and out) of the ipsilateral pupil.*
- **Central transtentorial herniation** denotes a symmetric downward movement of the thalamic medial structures through the tentorial opening with compression of the upper midbrain. Miotic pupils and drowsiness are the heralding signs.

Transfalcine Herniations

These are caused by herniation of the medial aspect of the cerebral hemisphere (cingulate gyrus) under the falx, which may compress the anterior cerebral artery.

Tonsillar Herniation

Masses in the cerebellum may cause tonsillar herniation, in which the cerebellar tonsils are herniated into the foramen magnum. This may compress the medulla and respiratory centers, causing death.

> *Concept*
>
> Tonsillar herniation may also occur if a lumbar puncture is performed in a patient with increased intracranial pressure. Therefore, **before** *performing a lumbar puncture*, the patient should be *checked for the presence of* **papilledema**.

DEVELOPMENTAL ABNORMALITIES OF THE BRAIN

Developmental abnormalities of the brain include the **Arnold-Chiari malformation**, the **Dandy-Walker malformation**, and the **Phakomatoses**, which include tuberous sclerosis, neurofibromatosis, von Hippel-Lindau disease, and Sturge-Weber syndrome.

- **Dandy-Walker malformation** has severe hypoplasia or absence of the cerebellar vermis. There is cystic distention of the roof of the fourth ventricle, hydrocephalus, and possibly agenesis of the corpus callosum.

- **Arnold-Chiari malformation** consists of herniation of the cerebellum and fourth ventricle into the foramen magnum, flattening of the base of the skull, and spina bifida with meningomyelocele. Newborns with this disorder are at risk of developing hydrocephalus within the first few days of delivery secondary to stenosis of the cerebral aqueduct.

- **Tuberous sclerosis** may show characteristic firm, white nodules (tubers) in the cortex and subependymal nodules of gliosis protruding into the ventricles (**"candle drippings"**) Facial angiofibromas (*adenoma sebaceum*) may also occur.
- **von Hippel-Lindau** disease shows multiple benign and malignant neoplasms including hemangioblastomas of the retina, cerebellum, and medulla oblongata; angiomas of the kidney and liver; and renal cell carcinomas.
- **Sturge-Weber syndrome** is a non-familial congenital disorder, display angiomas of the brain, leptomeninges, and ipsilateral face, which are called port-wine stains (nevus flammeus).
- **Syringomyelia**: Bilateral loss of pain and temperature sensations in both arms is most likely to be caused by syringomyelia, which is a chronic myelopathy that results from formation of a cavity (syrinx) involving the central gray matter of the spinal cord. This is the location where pain fibers cross to join the contralateral spinothalamic tract. Interruption of the lateral spinothalamic tracts results in segmental sensory dissociation with loss of pain and temperature sense, but preservation of the sense of touch and pressure or vibration, usually over the neck, shoulders, and arms. Other features of syringomyelia include wasting of the small intrinsic hand muscles (claw hand) and thoracic scoliosis. The cause of syringomyelia is unknown, although one type is associated with a Chiari malformation with obstruction at the foramen magnum.

NEURAL TUBE DEFECTS

These are caused by defective closure of the neural tube. These defects may occur anywhere along the extent of the neural tube and are classified as either caudal or cranial defects. Failure of development of the cranial end of the neural tube results in anencephaly, while failure of development of the caudal end of the neural tube results in spina bifida.

- Anencephaly, which is not compatible with life, is characterized by the absence of the forebrain. Instead, there is a mass of disorganized glial tissue with vessels in this area called a cerebrovasculosa. Ultrasound examination will reveal an abnormal shape to the head of the fetus with an absence of the skull.

- Spina bifida can be spina bifida occulta which results due to failure of closure of vertebral arches posteriorly. It is a mild disorder with normal meninges and spinal cord. If meninges also herniate out, it is known as meningocele whereas protruding out of both meninges as well as spinal cord is called meningomyelocele.

- Neural tube defects are associated with maternal obesity and decreased folate during pregnancy (folate supplementation in diet decreases the incidence of these development defects).

CEREBRAL HEMORRHAGE

It can be epidural, subarachnoid, subdural and intraparenchymal.

Central Nervous System

M

Dandy	**D**ilated 4th ventricle
Walker	**W**ater on the brain (hydrocephalus)
Syndrome	**S**mall or absent vermis

Triad of tuberous sclerosis: Seizures+mental retardation+ congenital white spots or macules (leukoderma).

The most common location of a syrinx is the **cervical region** and so, the loss of pain and temperature sensation **affects both arms**.

The diagnosis of syringomyelia is best made with **MRI of the cervical spine**.

Concept

Neural tube defects are associated with **increased** maternal serum levels of α-**fetoprotein (AFP)**, which is a glycoprotein synthesized by the yolk sac and the fetal liver. Increased serum levels are also associated with yolk sac tumors of the testes and liver cell carcinomas (note that **decreased AFP is associated with Down syndrome**).

Maternal folate level must be adequate **BEFORE** pregancy to decrease the risk of neural tube defects.

- **Epidural hemorrhage**: It results from hemorrhages into the potential space between the dura and the bone of the skull. These hemorrhages result from severe trauma that typically causes a skull fracture. The hemorrhage results from rupture of one of the meningeal arteries, as these arteries supply the dura and run between the dura and the skull. Since the bleeding is of arterial origin (high pressure), it is rapid and the symptoms are rapid in onset, although the patient may be normal for several hours (lucid interval). Bleeding causes increased intracranial pressure and can lead to tentorial herniation and death.

- **Subarachnoid hemorrhage**: It is much less common than hypertensive intracerebral hemorrhage. It most often results from the rupture of a berry aneurysm. These aneurysms are Saccular aneurysms that result from congenital defects in the media of arteries. They are typically located at the bifurcations of arteries. They are not the result of atherosclerosis. Instead, berry aneurysms are called congenital, although the aneurysm itself is not present at birth. The chance of rupture of berry aneurysms increases with age (rupture is rare in childhood). Rupture causes marked bleeding into the subarachnoid space and produces severe headaches, typically described as the "worst headache ever". Additional symptoms include vomiting, pain and stiffness of the neck (due to meningeal irritation caused by the blood), and papilledema. Death may follow rapidly.

- **Subdural Hemorrhage**: The space beneath the inner surface of the dura mater and the outer arachnoid layer of the leptomeninges is also a potential space.

CEREBRAL ISCHEMIA

Decreased brain perfusion may be generalized (global) or localized.

Global ischemia results from generalized decreased blood flow, such as with shock, cardiac arrest, or hypoxic episodes (e.g. near drowning or carbon monoxide poisoning).

- The gross changes produced by global hypoxia include watershed (border zone) infarcts, which typically occur at the border of areas supplied by the anterior and middle cerebral arteries, and laminar necrosis, which is related to the short, penetrating vessels originating from pial arteries.

- The microscopic changes produced by global hypoxia are grouped into three categories. The earliest histologic changes, occurring in the first 24 h, include the formation of *red neurons (acute neuronal injury)*, characterized by eosinophilia of the cytoplasm of the neurons, and followed in time by pyknosis and karyorrhexis. Subacute changes occur at 24 h to 2 weeks. These include tissue necrosis, vascular proliferation, and reactive gliosis.

INTRACRANIAL ANEURYSMS

- **Charcot-Bouchard aneurysms**: It results from weakening of the wall of cerebral artery by lipohyalinosis (deposition of lipids and hyaline material) caused by hypertension. Hypertensive hemorrhage shows a *predilection for the distribution of the lenticulostriate arteries (branch of middle cerebral artery)* with small (lacunar) hemorrhages, or large hemorrhages obliterating the corpus striatum, including the putamen and internal capsule. Hypertensive hemorrhages also commonly occur in cerebellum and pons and are often fatal.

- **Berry aneurysms** (small saccular aneurysms) are the result of congenital defects in the **media of blood vessels** and are located at the bifurcations of arteries.

- **Atherosclerotic aneurysms** are fusiform (spindle-shaped) aneurysms usually located in the major cerebral vessels. They rarely rupture, but may become thrombosed.

- **Mycotic (septic) aneurysms** result from septic emboli, most commonly from subacute bacterial endocarditis.

The artery involved in **epidural hemorrhage** is usually the **middle meningeal artery**, which is a branch of the maxillary artery, as the skull fracture is usually in the **temporal area**.

Excluding trauma, *Berry aneurysm is the commonest cause of subarachnoid hemorrhage.*

Berry aneurysms are most commonly found in the **circle of Willis**, typically either at the junction of the anterior communicating artery with the anterior cerebral artery or at the junction of the middle cerebral artery and the posterior communicating artery.

Subdural hemorrhage most commonly occurs due to **rupture of bridging veins.**

The **Purkinje cells of the cerebellum** and the **pyramidal neurons of Sommer's sector in the hippocampus** are particularly sensitive to ischemic damage.

CNS INFECTIONS

- Meningoencephalitis caused by HIV (human immunodeficiency virus) is characterized by microglial nodules within the brain that are composed of mononuclear cells, microglia, and scattered multinucleated giant cells.

- Herpes simplex virus produces characteristic Cowdry type A intranuclear inclusions in neurons and glial cells.

- Rabies form characteristic inclusions within neurons called Negri bodies. Rabies, caused by a single-stranded RNA rhabdovirus, is transmitted by the bite of a rabid animal, usually a dog, and travels to the brain via peripheral nerves. Symptoms caused by destruction of neurons in the brainstem include irritability, difficulty in swallowing and spasms of the throat (these two resulting in "hydrophobia"), seizures, and delirium. The illness is almost uniformly fatal.

- Enlarged cells (cytomegaly) with intranuclear and intracytoplasmic inclusions are seen with cytomegalovirus infection.

The pathognomonic feature of **PML** is the **oligodendrocytes** in areas of demyelination, which have a **"ground-glass"** appearance of their nuclei due to infection with the viral particles.

DORSALIS
D **D**orsal column degeneration
O **O**rthopedic pain (Charcot joints)
R **R**eflexes decreased (deep tendon)
S **S**hooting pain
A **A**rgyll-Robertson pupils
L **L**ocomotor ataxia
I **I**mpaired proprioception
S **S**yphilis

Progressive multifocal leukoencephalopathy (PML): It is a demyelinating disease of the central nervous system that results from infection of oligodendrocytes by the **JC polyomavirus**. Signs and symptoms of PML are varied but include dementia and ataxia along with abnormal vision and speech. PML occurs as a terminal complication in immunosuppressed individuals, especially individuals with AIDS.

Neurosyphilis: Neurosyphilis, a tertiary stage of syphilis, includes syphilitic meningitis, paretic neurosyphilis, and tabes dorsalis.

- Syphilitic meningitis is characterized by perivascular infiltrates of lymphocytes and plasma cells that cause obliterative endarteritis and meningeal fibrosis.

- *Tabes dorsalis* is the result of degeneration of the posterior columns of the spinal cord. This is caused by compression atrophy of the posterior spinal sensory nerves, which produces impaired joint position sensation, ataxia, loss of pain sensation (leading to joint damage, i.e. *Charcot joints*), and *Argyll Robertson pupils* (pupils that react to accommodation but not to light).

Prion diseases: The spongiform encephalopathies include Creutzfeldt-Jakob disease (CJD), Gerstmann-Straussler-Scheinker syndrome (GSS), fatal familial insomnia, and kuru. Microscopically, there is characteristic spongiform change in the gray matter ("cluster of grapes" vacuolation) without inflammation.

All of the spongiform encephalopathies are associated with abnormal forms of a prion protein (PrP). Disease results from alternate folding of the normal α-helix (called PrP^C) to an abnormal β-pleated sheet form (called PrP^{SC}). This conformational change can occur spontaneously at a very slow rate. Once formed, however, PrP^{SC} can combine with PrP^C to much more quickly form many more PrP^{SC} particles, which can "crystallize" and form plaques. PrP^C can also form PrP^{SC} at much higher rates if mutations are present in PrP^C, which can result from mutations in the gene that codes for PrP^C called PRNP. Mutations in this gene have been identified in patients with the familial forms of CJD, GSS, and fatal familial insomnia.

Note: *SOD1 mutations are seen with amyotrophic lateral sclerosis (ALS), FGFR3 mutations with achondroplasia, UBE3A mutations with Angelman's syndrome, and PTEN mutations with endometrial and prostate cancers.*

CSF Findings in CNS Infections

Parameters	Normal values	Bacterial Meningitis	Tuberculous Meningitis	Viral Meningitis
Pressure	50-180 mm water	Raised	Raised	Raised
Gross appearance	Clear and colorless	Turbid	Clear (may clot)	Clear
Protein	20 – 50 mg/dL	High	Very High	Slightly high
Glucose	40-70 mg/dL	Very low	Low	Normal
Chloride	116 – 122 µg/dL	Low	Very low	Normal
Cells	< 5/microlitre	Neutrophils	Pleocytosis	Lymphocytosis

Central Nervous System

Meningitis [inflammation of the arachnoid and the cerebrospinal fluid (CSF)] may be classified as acute pyogenic, aseptic, or chronic. The etiology and CSF findings vary in these three groups.

- The CSF in acute pyogenic meningitis, which is usually caused by bacteria, is grossly cloudy (not bloody, which is suggestive of a subarachnoid hemorrhage) and displays increased pressure, increased neurophils, increased protein, and decreased glucose.
- With chronic meningitis, such as that caused by *Mycobacterium tuberculosis*, the CSF is clear grossly, with only a slight increase in leukocytes (either mononuclear cells or a mixed infiltrate), a markedly increased protein level, increased pressure, and moderately decreased or normal amounts of sugar.
- **Brain abscesses and subdural empyemas,** which are parameningeal infections rather than direct meningeal infections, cause increased CSF pressure (more marked with abscess because of mass effect) along with increased inflammatory cells (lymphocytes and polymorphonuclear cells) and increased protein but a normal glucose level. The *CSF is clear.*
- Encephalitis, also not a direct infection of the meninges, results in clear CSF, increased pressure, increased protein, normal glucose, and possibly increased lymphocytes.

> In **bacterial meningitis**, majority of organisms originate in **nasopharynx** whereas
>
> **Viral meningitis** is most often transmitted by **fecal-oral route**.

> **Meningitis**
> ↑ CSF protein (viral, bacterial, fungal)
> ↓ CSF glucose (bacterial, fungal)

DEMYELINATING DISORDERS

Multiple Sclerosis

In primary CNS demyelination there is loss of myelin sheaths with relative preservation of axons. Primary demyelination is seen predominately in multiple sclerosis, in the perivenous encephalomyelopathies, and in progressive multifocal leukoencephalopathy (PML). Multiple sclerosis (MS), a disease of unknown etiology, causes disseminated but focal plaques of primary demyelination anywhere in the CNS, but often in the white matter near the angles of the lateral ventricles. It primarily affects young adults between 20 and 40 years of age, with the onset of symptoms such as abnormalities of vision, tremors, paresthesias, and incoordination. The course is typically remitting and relapsing. Early findings include weakness of the lower extremities and visual abnormalities with retrobulbar pain.

> Multiple sclerosis is the most common demyelinating disease.

Apart from the Charcot triad, another pathognomonic feature in MS is **internuclear ophthalmoplegia** (INO), also known as the **MLF syndrome**, which results from demyelination of the *medial longitudinal fasciculus*. It results in medial rectus palsy in attempted lateral gaze and monocular nystagmus in abducting eye with convergence.

Examination of the CSF in patients with MS reveals increased T lymphocytes, increased protein, and normal glucose. *Protein electrophoresis of the CSF reveals oligoclonal bands* (individual monoclonal spikes), although this latter finding is not specific for MS.

> The **classic (Charcot) triad** in patients with MS consists of **scanning speech, intension tremor,** and Nystagmus (*mnemonic is SIN*).

Neuromyelitis Optica (also known as Devic disease)

It is characterized by the development of synchronous bilateral optic neuritis and spinal cord demyelination.

DEGENERATIVE DISORDERS

The degenerative diseases of the CNS are diseases that affect the gray matter and are characterized by the progressive loss of neurons in specific areas of the brain.

Alzheimer's Disease

Alzheimer's disease (AD) is the **most common cause** of dementia in elderly (followed by vascular multi-infact dementia and diffuse Lewy body disease). AD often begins insidiously with impairment of memory and progresses to dementia. Histologically, AD is characterized by numerous neurofibrillary tangles and senile plaques with a central core of amyloid alpha-

AD: ↑ density of **NF tangles** and senile (neuritic) plaques in the brain.

NF tangles: hyperphosphorylated **tau protein** in neuron.

Age is the main risk factor for AD

Concept

The gene for beta-amyloid (A-beta) is located on chromosome 21 and so, the high incidence of Alzheimer's disease is seen in individuals with **trisomy 21 (Down Syndrome).**

Idiopathic Parkinson's disease is the *most common cause of parkinsonism.*

Lewy bodies (eosinophilic intracytoplasmic inclusions) are found in the surviving neurons of the **substantia nigra** in PD.

Concept

Unlike Parkinson's disease, however, no mutations in the gene that codes for alpha-synuclein have been found with the Shy-Drager syndrome.

HD involves the extrapyramidal system and atrophy of the **caudate nuclei and putamen.**

protein. Both tangles and plaques are found to a lesser extent in other conditions, for example, neurofibrillary tangles in Down syndrome. Silver stains demonstrate tangles and plaques and Congo red shows amyloid deposition in plaques and vascular walls (**amyloid angiopathy**). In AD there are also numerous **Hirano bodies,** and granulovacuolar degeneration is found in more than 10% of the neurons of the hippocampus. Grossly, brain atrophy (narrowed gyri and widened sulci) is predominant in the frontal and superior temporal lobes.

The etiology of AD is not well understood, but it is clear that there are multiple etiologic pathways to this disease state. Alzheimer's disease has been linked to abnormalities involving four specific genes. Cleavage of the beta-amyloid precursor protein (beta-APP) by alpha-secretase precludes beta-A formation; but cleavage of beta-APP by beta-secretase (BACE-1) or gamma-secretase produces fragments that tend to aggregate into the pathogenic amyloid fibrils. Beta-amyloid deposition is necessary but not sufficient for the development of Alzheimer's disease. Early-onset familial Alzheimer's is also related to **mutations in presenilins**. The presenilin 1 (PS1) gene is located on *chromosome 14*, while the presenilin 2 **(PS2) gene** is located on *chromosome 1*.

Parkinson's Disease

It is characterized by a mask-like facial expression, coarse tremors, slowness of voluntary movements, and muscular rigidity, there is degeneration and loss of pigmented cells in the substantia nigra, resulting in a decrease in dopamine synthesis. The decreased synthesis of dopamine by neurons originating in the substantia nigra leads to decreased amounts and functioning of dopamine in the striatum. This results in decreased dopamine inhibition and a relative increase in acetylcholine function, which is excitatory in the striatum. The effect of this excitation, however, is to increase the functioning of GABA neurons, which are inhibitory. The result, therefore, is increased inhibition or decreased movement. The severity of the motor syndrome correlates with the degree of dopamine deficiency.

Lewy Body Disorders

Lewy bodies are intracytoplasmic eosinophilic inclusions that are composed of fine filaments, which are densely packed in the core but loose at their rim. These filaments are composed of neurofilament antigens, parkin, and ubiquitin, but the major component of the Lewy body is alpha-synuclein. The histologic presence of Lewy bodies can be seen in several disorders (Lewy body disorders) that differ in the location where the Lewy bodies are found.

- In **classic Parkinson's disease**, Lewy bodies are found in the *nigrostriatal system* (producing extrapyramidal movement disorder).
- In **Lewy body dementia**, Lewy bodies are found in the *cerebral cortex* (producing dementia; this is the third most common cause of dementia).
- In **Shy-Dragger syndrome**, Lewy bodies are found in *sympathetic neurons in the spinal cord* (causing *autonomic dysfunction*, including orthostatic hypotension, impotence, abnormal sweat and salivary gland secretion, and pupillary abnormalities).

Huntington's Disease: (HD)

It is characterized by choreiform movements and progressive dementia that appear after the age of 30. It is an **autosomal dominant** disorder that results from an abnormal gene (showing CAG repeats) on **chromosome-4**. Choreiform movements and progressive dementia appear after the age of 30. There is degeneration of *GABA neurons* in the striatum, which leads to decreased function (decreased inhibition) and increased movement.

Note: Huntington's disease is one of four diseases that are characterized by long repeating sequences of three nucleotides (the other diseases being fragile X syndrome, myotonic dystrophy, and spinal and bulbar muscular atrophy).

Amyotrophic Lateral Sclerosis (ALS)

Amyotrophic lateral sclerosis (ALS), also known as **Lou Gehrig's disease**, is a degenerative disorder of motor neurons, principally the anterior horn cells of the spinal cord, the motor nuclei of the brainstem, and the upper motor neurons of the cerebral cortex. Clinically, this disease is a combination of lower motor neuron (LMN) disease with weakness and fasciculations and upper motor neuron (UMN) disease with spasticity and hyperreflexia. Early symptoms include weakness and cramping and then muscle atrophy and fasciculations. Reflexes are hyperactive in upper and lower extremities, and a positive extensor plantar (Babinski) reflex develops because of the loss of upper motor neurons. The clinical course is rapid, and death may result from respiratory complications.

> The **triad** of *atrophic weakness of hands and forearms, slight spasticity of the legs, and generalized hyperreflexia*—**in the absence of sensory changes** suggests the diagnosis of ALS.
>
> **Riluzole** *(NMDA antagonist)* and **baclofen** are used for the treatment of ALS.

▍TUMORS

CNS tumors can be gliomas, neuronal tumors, poorly differentiated neoplasms, meningiomas and metastatic tumors.

1. Gliomas: These are most common group of primary brain tumors. These include astrocytoma, oligodendroglioma and ependymoma.

> **Metastatic tumors** are most common intra—cranial tumors.

   a. **Astrocytoma**

   It is the **most common primary brain tumors in adults** and range from low grade to very high grade (glioblastoma multiforme). These grades of astrocytomas include:

   > **Astrocytoma** is the *most common* **primary** *brain tumors* in **adults**

   Grade I The least aggressive and histologically difficult to differentiate from reactive astrocytosis.
   Grade II Some plemorphism microscopically.
   Grade III Anaplastic astrocytoma, characterized histologically by increased pleomorphism and prominent mitoses.
   Grade IV Glioblastoma multiforme. A highly malignant tumor characterized histologically by endothelial proliferation and serpentine areas of necrosis surrounded by peripheral palisading of tumor cells. It frequently crosses the midline (**"butterfly tumor"**).

   > **Glioblastoma multiforme**: *high grade astrocytoma with* **worst prognosis.**

   Progression of low grade astrocytoma to a higher grade (secondary glioblastoma multiforme) is associated with several genetic abnormalities, such as disruption of the p16/CDKNZA gene or overexpression of PDGF-A and its receptor.

   b. **Oligodendroglioma**

   These most commonly involve the cerebrum (hemispheres) in adults, are slow-growing tumors that have a high recurrence rate. Some oligodendrogliomas do proliferate in a rapid and aggressive fashion and may be associated with a malignant astrocytoma component. Histologically, oligodendrogliomas consist of sheets of cells with clear halos (**"fried-egg" appearance**) and various amounts of calcification (which can be seen on x-ray). Cytogenetic abnormalities have therapeutic significance for this type of tumor, as only tumors with deletion involving 19q or 1p respond to chemotherapy.

   c. **Ependymoma**

   These most often arise next to the ependyma-lined ventricular system, including central canal of spinal cord. Spinal cord ependymoma frequently occur in setting of neurofibromatosis type 2.

   > **MC Site of Ependymoma**
   >
   > In *children*: typically near *fourth ventricle* whereas
   >
   > In *adults*: *spinal cord*.

2. **Neuronal tumors**

   The most common CNS tumor containing mature appearing neurons (ganglion cells) is ganglioglioma. These are most commonly found in temporal lobe and frequently contain ganglion cells with binucleated forms.

3. **Poorly differentiated neoplasms**

   Most common among these is medulloblastoma. Others include atypical tetroid/rhabdoid tumor.

   a. **Medulloblastoma**

   Primitive neuroectodermal tumors (PNETs) are a type of malignant embryonal tumor that can be found at sites within or outside of the central nervous system.

Medulloblastoma is the most common tumor located in the posterior fossa of a child.

Meningioma contain calcified bodies called **psammoma bodies.**

Lung cancer is the most common cancer causing metastasis to the brain.

Choriocarcinoma has high likelihood of metastasizing to brain whereas *prostatic carcinoma almost never grow in the brain.*

An example of a PNET located outside of the CNS is Ewing's sarcoma of bone. PNETs of the CNS can be divided into supratentorial tumors (sPNET) and infratentorial tumors (iPNET). The latter are also called as medulloblastoma and they usually arise in the midline of the cerebellum (the vermis) but in adults, where the incidence is much less than in children, they are more apt to arise in the cerebellar hemispheres in a lateral position. In about one-third of cases, these show rosette formation centered by neurofibrillary material. Medulloblastomas grow by local invasive growth and may block cerebrospinal fluid circulation (CSF block) via compression of the fourth ventricle.

4. **Meningioma**

    A tumor that is attached to the dura is most likely to be a meningioma. This type of tumor arises from the arachnoid villi of the brain or spinal cord. Although they usually occur during middle or later life, a small number occur in persons 20 to 40 years of age. They commonly arise along the venous sinuses (parasagittal, sphenoid wings, and olfactory groove).

> **Note:** Both oligodendroglioma and craniopharyngioma show calcification fairly frequently, oligodendroglioma is often located in the frontal lobe, whereas **craniopharyngioma** occurs around the third ventricle and demonstrates *suprasellar calcification*.

5. **Metastatic tumors**

    These are *most common intra – cranial tumors.* Five most common sites are

    Lung
    Breast
    Skin (melanoma)
    Kidney
    GIT.

> **Note:**
> *   Deletion of region 12 on chromosome 22 is the most common cytogenetic abnormality of meningiomas.
> *   Duplication of the long arm of chromosome 17 is the most common genetic abnormality seen in medulloblastomas.

CNS Tumors and Age

The location of a tumor and the age of the patient are both very important in the differential diagnosis of tumors of the central nervous system. Astrocytomas occur predominantly in the cerebral hemispheres in adult life and old age, in the cerebellum and pons in childhood, and in the spinal cord in young adult. The pilocytic astrocytoma is a subtype that is the most common brain tumor in children, and therefore it is also called a juvenile pilocytic astrocytoma. It is characterized by its location in the cerebellum and better prognosis. Meningiomas, found within the meninges, have their peak incidence in the fourth and fifth decades. The highly malignant glioblastoma multiforme is also found primarily in adults. Oligodendrogliomas also involve the cerebrum in adults. Ependymomas are found most frequently in the fourth ventricle, while the choroid plexus papilloma, a variant of the ependymoma, is found most commonly in the lateral ventricles of young boys. The medulloblastoma is a tumor that arises exclusively in the cerebellum and has its highest incidence toward the end of the first decade. In children medulloblastomas are located in the midline, while in adults they are found in more lateral locations.

PERIPHERAL NERVE SHEATH TUMOR

Schwannomas

These are benign tumors that generally appear as extremely cellular spindle cell neoplasms, sometimes with metaplastic elements of bone, cartilage, and skeletal muscle. Schwannomas (neurilemomas) are single, encapsulated tumors of nerve sheaths, usually benign, occurring on peripheral, spinal, or cranial nerves.

Acoustic neuromas typically located at the cerebellopontine angle or in the internal acoustic meatus. Initially, when they are small, these tumors produce symptoms by compressing CN VIII and CN VII (facial). CN VIII symptoms include unilateral tinnitus (ringing in the ear), unilateral hearing loss, and vertigo (dizziness). Involvement of the facial nerve produces facial weakness and loss of corneal reflex. Histologically, an acoustic neuroma consists of cellular areas **(Antoni A)** and loose edematous areas **(Antoni B)**. **Verocay bodies** (foci of palisaded nuclei) may be found in the more cellular areas.

Familial Tumor Syndromes

a. **Tuberous sclerosis**

Tuberous sclerosis is an autosomal dominant syndrome characterized by the **clinical triad of angiofibromas ("adenoma sebaceum"), seizures, and mental retardation**. Patients develop hamartomas in the central nervous system including "tubers", which are film areas with haphazardly arranged neurons and glia with stout processes. The syndrome is associated with the development of several different types of tumors, including subepedymal giant cell tumor, rhabdomyoma of the heart, and angiomyolipoma of the kidney. Mutations at several loci have been associated with tuberous sclerosis including the TSC1 locus, which codes for hamartin, and the TSC2 locus, which codes for tuberin. These two proteins inhibit mTOR, which is the mammalian target of rapamycin. mTOR plays a central role in the regulation of cell growth.

> **Note:** Dysregulation of mTOR activity is associated with several hamartoma syndromes, including the tuberous sclerosis, von Hippel-Lindau syndrome, Peutz-Jegher's syndrome, and the PTEN-related hamartoma syndromes.

b. **von Hippel-Lindau disease**

In this rare autosomal dominant disorder, multiple benign, and malignant neoplasms occur. These include hemangioblastomas of retina and brain (cerebellum and medulla oblongata), angiomas of kidney and liver, and renal cell carcinomas (multiple and bilateral) in 25 to 50% of cases.

c. **Neurofibromatosis type 1**

Classic neurofibromatosis (NF-1) is an autosomal dominant disorder. It is characterized by **cafe-au-lait skin macules, axillary freckling, multiple neurofibromas, plexiform neurofibromas, and Lisch nodules** (pigmented iris hamartomas). Lisch nodules are found in 95% of patients after age 6. There is increased risk of developing meningiomas or even pheochromocytoma. A major complication of NF-1 is the malignant transformation of a neurofibroma to a neurofibrosarcoma. The gene for the classic form (NF-1) is lcoated on chromosome 17. It encodes for neurofibromin, a protein that regulates the function of p21 oncoprotein.

d. **Neurofibromatosis type 2**

Central neurofibromatosis (NF-2) is an autosomal-dominant disorder in which patients develop a range of tumors, most commonly **bilateral VIII nerve schwannomas and multiple meningiomas**. Gliomas, typically ependymomas of the spinal cord, also occur in these patients. Many individuals with NF2 also have non-neoplastic lesions, which include nodular ingrowth of Schwann cells into the spinal cord (schwannosis), meningioangiomatosis (a proliferation of meningeal cells and blood vessels that grows into the brain), and glial hamartia (microscopic nodular collections of glial cells at abnormal locations, often in the superficial and deep layers of cerebral cortex). The *NF2 gene is located on chromosome 22 and encodes for merlin.*

The **acoustic neuroma** is an example of a Schwannoma that arises from the **vestibulocochlear nerve (CN VIII)**.

Clinical triad of tuberous sclerosis is angiofibromas ("adenoma sebaceum"), seizures, and mental retardation.

Rhabdomyoma of the heart is highly predicitve of tuberous sclerosis.

Hamartomas of the iris are not present in central or acoustic neurofibromatosis (NF-2), though both types of neurofibromatosis produce cafe-au-lait macules and neurofibromas.

Only the central, or acoustic, form produces bilateral acoustic neuromas; the classic form may produce unilateral acoustic neuroma.

MULTIPLE CHOICE QUESTIONS

DEVELOPMENTAL DEFECTS, CEREBRAL HEMORRHAGE, ANEURYSM

1. Cervical syringomyelia all are seen except
   (a) Burning sensation in hands   *(AIIMS Nov 2012)*
   (b) Hypertrophy of abductor pollicis brevis
   (c) Extensor plantar response is present
   (d) Absent biceps reflex.

2. The best described etiology for Berry aneurysm is which of the following?   *(AIIMS May 2011)*
   (a) Degeneration of internal elastic lamina
   (b) Degeneration of tunica media
   (c) Defect in muscular layer
   (d) Low grade inflammation in the vessel wall

3. The defect in Berry aneurysm is   *(AIIMS May 2010)*
   (a) Degeneration of internal elastic lamina
   (b) Degeneration of media
   (c) Deposition of mucoid material in media
   (d) Low grade inflammation of vessel wall

4. Which of the following would distinguish hydrocephalus due to aqueductal stenosis when compared to that due to Dandy walker malformation?
   (a) Third ventricle size   *(AIIMS Nov 2002)*
   (b) Posterior fossa volume
   (c) Lateral ventricular size
   (d) Head circumference

5. Most common site for berry aneurysm is: *(UP 2002)*
   (a) Basilar artery
   (b) Anterior communicating artery
   (c) Posterior communicating artery
   (d) Posterior cerebral artery

Most Recent Questions

5.1. Middle meningeal vessel damage results in:
   (a) Subdural hemorrhage
   (b) Extradural hemorrhage
   (c) Subarachnoid hemorrhage
   (d) Intracerebral hemorrhage

CNS INFECTIONS, DEMYELINATING DISEASE

6. Enzymes found in CSF: *(AIIMS Nov 2012)*
   (a) GGT+ALP
   (b) ALP+CK-MB
   (c) CK+LDH
   (d) Deaminase and Peroxidase

7. A 17 year old female presents with a history of fever and headache and now develops altered sensorium. CT scan shows basal exudates with meningeal enhancement. The CSF is most likely to show   *(AIIMS Nov 2011)*
   (a) Lymphocytic pleocytosis, low sugar, low protein
   (b) Polymorphonuclear pleocytosis, normal sugar, high protein
   (c) Lymphocytic pleocytosis, low sugar, high protein
   (d) Lymphocytic pleocytosis, normal sugar, high protein

8. Inclusion body in oligodendroglia is a feature of which of the following?   *(AIIMS Nov 2010)*
   (a) Progressive Multifocal Leucoencephalopathy
   (b) Japanese Encephalitis
   (c) Polio
   (d) CJD

9. Which of the following is not a Prion disease?
   (a) Creutzfeldt- Jakob disease   *(DPG 2011)*
   (b) Fatal familial insomnia
   (c) Gerstmann-Straussler-Scheinker syndrome
   (d) Parkinson's disease

10. All of the following diseases show abnormal folding of proteins except: *(AIIMS Nov 2008)*
    (a) Creutzfeldt-Jakob disease
    (b) Prion disease
    (c) Multiple sclerosis
    (d) Amyloidosis

11. Prion includes: *(AIIMS Nov 2007)*
    (a) DNA and RNA   (b) Only RNA
    (c) Proteins   (d) Only DNA

12. Pathologic features of brain in AIDS are all, except:
    (a) Perivascular giant cell invasion   *(AIIMS Nov 2001)*
    (b) Microglial nodules
    (c) Vasculitis
    (d) Temporal lobe infarction

13. Febrile response in CNS is mediated by: *(PGI Dec 2003)*
    (a) Bacterial toxin   (b) IL-l
    (c) IL-6   (d) Interferon
    (e) Tumor Necrosis Factor

14. Cerebral infarction is caused by: *(PGI June 01)*
    (a) Toxoplasma   (b) Cryptococcus
    (c) Aspergillus   (d) Mucor
    (e) Histoplasma

15. Complications of tubercular meningitis are:
    (a) Endarteritis   *(PGI Dec 2000)*
    (b) Hydrocephalus
    (c) Deafness
    (d) Venous sinus infarct

16. The pathogenesis of cerebral malaria includes:
    (a) Cytoadhesion   *(PGI Dec 2000)*
    (b) Sequestration of cerebral vessels by RBCs
    (c) Reticulocytopenia
    (d) Also caused by P. vivax
    (e) Sporozoites are sequestrated in blood

17. Brain infarct is seen in: *(PGI Dec 2003)*
    (a) TB
    (b) Cryptococcosis
    (c) Aspergillosis
    (d) Toxoplasmosis
    (e) Rabies

18. Commonest cause of cerebral infarction is: *(DNB- 2000)*
    (a) Arterial thrombosis
    (b) Arteritis
    (c) Venous thrombosis
    (d) Embolism

19. Albumino-cytologic dissociation occurs in cases of:
    (a) Guillain Barre syndrome   *(DNB- 2004)*
    (b) TB meningitis
    (c) Motor neuron disease
    (d) Demyelinating disorder

20. Most common type of pathological changes seen in Rabies are: *(UP 2000)*
    (a) Meningitis   (b) Cranial arteritis
    (c) Ventriculitis   (d) Brain stem encephalitis

Most Recent Questions

20.1. All of the following are seen in thymoma except
    (a) Hypogamma globulinemia
    (b) Hyperalbuminemia
    (c) Red cell aplasia
    (d) Myasthenia Gravis

20.2. Spongiform degeneration of cerebral cortex occurs in which of the following?
    (a) Subacute sclerosing panencephalitis
    (b) Fatal familial insomnia
    (c) Creutzfeldt-Jakob disease
    (d) Cerebral toxoplasmosis

20.3. What is the histological appearance of brain in Creutzfeldt-Jakob disease?
    (a) Neuronophagia
    (b) Spongiform change in brain
    (c) Microabscesses
    (d) Demyelination

20.4. Perivascular lymphocytes and microglial nodules are seen in:
    (a) Multiple sclerosis
    (b) CMV meningitis
    (c) Bacterial meningitis
    (d) HIV encephalitis

20.5. Albumino-cytologic dissociation occurs in cases of:
    (a) Guillain Barre syndrome
    (b) TB meningitis
    (c) Motor neuron disease
    (d) Demyelinating disorder

20.6. Dissociated sensory loss is seen in:
    (a) Syringomyelia
    (b) Vitamin B12 deficiency
    (c) Transverse myelitis
    (d) Pellagra

20.7. Locomotor ataxia, a late manifestation of syphilis due to parenchymatous involvement of the spinal cord is called:
    (a) General paralysis of insane
    (b) Tabes dorsalis
    (c) Meningovascular syphilis
    (d) Syphilitic amyotrophy

ALZHEIMER DISEASE, PARKINSON DISEASE AND OTHER DEGENERATIVE DISEASE

21. Disease or infarction of neurological tissue causes it to be replaced by: *(AI 2002)*
    (a) Fluid
    (b) Neuroglia
    (c) Proliferation of adjacent nerve cells
    (d) Blood vessel

22. Nucleus involved in Alzheimer's disease is:
    (a) Nucleus Basalis of Meynert   *(Delhi PG-2005)*
    (b) Superior salivary nucleus
    (c) Ventromedial nucleus of thalamus
    (d) All of the above

23. Damage to nervous tissue is repaired by:
    (a) Neuroglia   *(DNB- 2001,2005)*
    (b) Fibroblasts
    (c) Axons
    (d) Microglia

24. The following is not a feature of Alzheimer's disease:
    (a) Neurofibrillary tangles   *(DNB- 2007)*
    (b) Senile (neuritic) plaques
    (c) Amyloid angiopathy
    (d) Lewy bodies

25. Neurofibrillary tangles are seen in: *(UP 2007)*
    (a) Parkinsonism
    (b) Alzheimer's disease
    (c) Multiple sclerosis
    (d) Perivenous encephalomyelitis

26. Dementia in an old man with senile plaques is usually associated with: *(AP 2004)*
    (a) Alzheimer's disease
    (b) Picks disease
    (c) Parkinson's disease
    (d) All of the above

Most Recent Questions

26.1. Most common site for medulloblastoma is:
- (a) Medulla
- (b) Cerebellum
- (c) Cerebrum
- (d) Pineal gland

26.2. Medulloblastoma most common metastasis is to:
- (a) Lung
- (b) Liver
- (c) Spleen
- (d) CNS

26.3. Rosenthal fibres are seen in which of the following tumours?
- (a) Pilocytic astrocytoma
- (b) Glioblastoma
- (c) Medulloblastoma
- (d) Ependymoma

26.4. Most common cerebellar tumor in children?
- (a) Medulloblastoma
- (b) Ependymoma
- (c) Astrocytoma
- (d) PNET

26.5. Commonest type of intracranial tumor is:
- (a) Astrocytoma
- (b) Medulloblastoma
- (c) Meningioma
- (d) Secondaries

26.6. Which of the following is affected in patients with Alzheimer's disease?
- (a) Parietal and frontal lobe
- (b) Parietal and temporal lobe
- (c) Temporal and occipital lobe
- (d) Parietal and occipital lobe

26.7. Lewy bodies are found in the substantia nigra neurons in
- (a) Alzheimer disease
- (b) Parkinson disease
- (c) Huntington disease
- (d) Pick disease

26.8. Tuberous sclerosis is associated with all EXCEPT:
- (a) Ash leaf macule
- (b) Shagreen patch
- (c) Schwannoma
- (d) Adenoma sebaceum

CNS TUMOURS

27. Which of the following receptor on neuronal membrane that induces development of glioma? *(AIIMS Nov 2012)*
- (a) CD45
- (b) CD133
- (c) CD33
- (d) CD24

28. Pituitary adenomas are regarded as macroadenomas when their size is *(AI 2012)*
- (a) > 1 cm
- (b) > 1.5 cm
- (c) > 2 cm
- (d) > 2.5 cm

29. Which is not a neuronal tumor? *(AI 2011)*
- (a) Ependymoma
- (b) Neuroblastoma
- (c) Gangliocytoma
- (d) Ganglioglioma

30. Which of the following brain tumors does not spread via CSF? *(DPG 2011)*
- (a) Germ cell tumors
- (b) Medulloblastoma
- (c) CNS Lymphoma
- (d) Craniopharyngioma

31. A metastatic carcinoma in the brain of an adult, most often comes from a primary in the: *(AIIMS Nov 2005)*
- (a) Stomach
- (b) Ovary
- (c) Oral cavity
- (d) Lung

32. Which of the following is true about Medulloblastoma? *(PGI Dec 2005)*
- (a) Radiosensitive tumor
- (b) Spreads through CSF
- (c) Surgical treatment not done
- (d) Occurs in young age group

33. Commonest type of intracranial tumor is: *(DNB- 2000, 2004, 2007)*
- (a) Astrocytoma
- (b) Medulloblastoma
- (c) Meningioma
- (d) Neurofibroma
- (e) Secondaries

34. Most common CNS tumor is: *(RJ 2000)*
- (a) Astrocytoma
- (b) Meduloblastoma
- (c) Meningioma
- (d) Oligodendroma

35. Glial fibrillary proteins are present in: *(RJ 2002, 2006)*
- (a) Astrocytoma
- (b) Meduloblastoma
- (c) Ependymoma
- (d) All

36. Enamel like superstructure is seen in which CNS lesion? *(AP 1998, TN 1 (AP 2001)*
- (a) Craniopharyngioma
- (b) Pituitary tumour
- (c) Astrocytoma
- (d) Glioma

37. Pseudorosettes are seen in all except: *(AP 2002)*
- (a) Neuroblastoma
- (b) Retinoblastoma
- (c) Medulloblastoma
- (d) Thecoma

38. Most common intracranial malignancy is:
- (a) Glioblastoma multiforme *(Jharkhand 2003)*
- (b) Ependymoma
- (c) Choroid angioma
- (d) Pinealoma

39. Worst prognosis meningioma is: *(Jharkhand 2005)*
- (a) Syncytial
- (b) Fibroblastic
- (c) Anaplastic
- (d) Atypical

Most Recent Questions

39.1. Commonest cause of cerebral infarction is:
- (a) Arterial thrombosis
- (b) Arteritis
- (c) Venous thrombosis
- (d) Embolism

39.2. Damage to nervous tissue is repaired by:
- (a) Neuroglia
- (b) Fibroblasts
- (c) Axons
- (d) Microglia

39.3. The following is not a feature of Alzheimer's disease:
   (a) Neurofibrillary tangles
   (b) Senile (neuritic) plaques
   (c) Amyloid angiopathy
   (d) Lewy bodies

39.4. Which of the following is incorrect about neuro-blastoma?
   (a) Most common abdominal tumor in infants
   (b) X-ray abdomen shows calcification
   (c) Can show spontaneous regression
   (d) Urine contains 5H.I.A.A

ASSERTION AND REASON QUESTIONS

1-5. Will have two statements, assertion and reason. Read both of them carefully and answer according to these options.
   (a) Both assertion and reason are true and reason is correct explanation of assertion.
   (b) Both assertion and reason are true and reason is not the correct explanation of assertion.
   (c) Assertion is true and reason is false.
   (d) Both assertion and reason are false.

1. **Assertion:** Berry aneurysm is the commonest cause of subarachnoid hemorrhage
   Reason: Rupture of the aneurysm occurs commonly in childhood

2. **Assertion:** B12 deficiency causes subacute combined degeneration of the spinal cord
   Reason: B12 deficiency causes degeneration of both the ascending and descending tracts of the spinal cord

3. **Assertion:** Alzheimer's disease is associated with Down syndrome
   Reason: Beta amyloid gene is located on chromosome 21

4. **Assertion:** Shy-Dragger syndrome is characterized by autonomic dysfunction
   Reason: Lewy bodies are found in nigrostriatal neurons

5. **Assertion:** Huntington's disease is characterized by chorea and dementia
   Reason: Degeneration of GABA neurons in the striatum leads to decreased function (decreased inhibition) and increased movement.

EXPLANATIONS

1. **Ans. (b) Hypertrophy of abductor pollicis brevis** *(Ref: Robbins 8th/1286, 9/e p1258)*
Atrophy and *not hypertrophy* of the abductor pollicis brevis is a feature of syringomyelia.
Syringomyelia

- It is a chronic myelopathy that results from formation of a cavity (syrinx) involving the central gray matter of the spinal cord. The cause of syringomyelia is unknown, although one type is associated with a Chiari malformation with obstruction at the foramen magnum.
- Since the gray matter is the location where pain fibers cross to join the contralateral spinothalamic tract, the interruption of the lateral spinothalamic tracts results in *segmental sensory dissociation with loss of pain and temperature sense*, but *preservation of the sense of touch and pressure or vibration*, usually over the neck, shoulders, and arms.
- The most common location of a syrinx is the cervicothoracic region and therefore, **the loss of pain and temperature sensation affects both arms**.
- Other features of syringomyelia include **wasting of the small intrinsic hand muscles (claw hand) and thoracic scoliosis**. This is accompanied by areflexic weakness in the upper limbs. As the cavity enlarges, spasticity and weakness of the legs, bladder and bowel dysfunction as well as Horner syndrome appear due to compression of the long tracts.
- ***The diagnosis of syringomyelia is best made with MRI of the spine (cervical region should be examined first)***

2. **Ans. (b) Degeneration of tunica media** *(Ref: Robbins 8th/1297-8, 9/e p1270)*
Direct quote from Robbins... 'the berry aneurysms develop over time *because of an underlying defect in the media of the vessel"*.
Concept

It is different from other causes of aneurysm (atherosclerosis, trauma, infections) which cause **only cerebral infarction** and not subarachnoid hemorrhage.

Salient points about Berry aneurysm (saccular aneurysm)

Saccular aneurysm is the most common type of **intracranial aneurysm**.
Risk factors
Smoking and **hypertension** are the important risk factors for Berry aneurysm. They are **not the result of atherosclerosis** (which is a disease of intima).   Berry aneurysms are called congenital, although the aneurysm itself is not present at birth.
Location
Commonest location is in the circle of Willis, typically at the junction of the anterior communicating artery with the anterior cerebral artery[Q].   It is also present at the junction of the middle cerebral artery and the posterior communicating artery.
Clinically
It is responsible for a clinically significant *subarachnoid hemorrhage*. In fact, excluding trauma, berry aneurysm is the commonest cause of subarachnoid hemorrhage.   The chance of rupture of berry aneurysms increases with age (rupture is rare in childhood). Rupture causes marked bleeding into the subarachnoid space and produces severe headaches, typically described as the "worst headache ever".

3. **Ans. (b) Degeneration of media** *(Ref: Robbins 8th/1297-8, 9/e p1270)*
Direct quote from Robbins... 'the berry aneurysms develop over time because of an underlying defect in the media of the vessel".
Concept

It is different from other causes of aneurysm (atherosclerosis, trauma, infections) which cause **only cerebral infarction** and not subarachnoid hemorrhage.

4. **Ans. (b) Posterior fossa volume** *(Ref: Robbin's illustrated 6th/27691, 9/e p1255)*
   The basics of CSF production and drainage

> CSF production (Occurs by choroid plexus of lateral and IIIrd ventricle)
> ↓
> Foramen of Monro
> ↓
> Third ventricle
> ↓
> Aqueduct of Sylvius
> ↓
> Fourth ventricle
> ↓
> Foramen of Magendie and Lushka
> ↓
> Subarachnoid space (It is absorbed here, by arachnoid villi)

Both Aqueductal stenosis and Dandy Walker syndrome cause non-communicating hydrocephalus but the site of obstruction is different.
- Let us see the causes of hydrocephalus in aqueductal stenosis and Dandy-Walker malformation.

Aqueductal stenosis
- In aqueductal stenosis the aqueduct connecting the 3rd and 4th ventricle is stenosed which leads to hydrocephalus with the dilatation of ventricular system prior to the aqueduct, i.e. lateral ventricles and third ventricle.

Dandy Walker Malformation
- In Dandy Walker malformation there is cystic dilatation of the fourth ventricle in the posterior fossa with obstruction at the formation of Lushka and Magendie.
- So the ventricular system in this condition will also be dilated as in aqueductal stenosis but here the posterior fossa is also enlarged (in contrast to normal posterior fossa size in aqueductal stenosis). i.e.

5. **Ans. (b) Anterior communicating artery** *(Ref: Robbins 9/e p1270, 8th/1297; 7th/1367)*

5.1. **Ans. (b) Extradural hemorrhage** *(Ref: Robbins 9th/1261)*

6. **Ans. (c) CK and LDH** *(Ref: Chatterjee Shinde 8th/730)*
   The following enzymes are present in the CSF:

   Aspartate transaminase (AST): 5-12 units/ml. Its value increases in abscess, cerebral hemorrhage and infarction and in primary or metastatic malignant disease. It may increase in some patients with multiple sclerosis.

   Lactate dehydrogenase (LDH): normal value is 5-40IU/l. Its value increases in abscess, cerebral hemorrhage and infarction and in metastatic malignant disease.
   Increase in LDH4 isoenzyme of CSF is seen in tuberculous meningitis.

   Creatine kinase (CK): CK-BB is present in the brain. Its value increases in associated with meningitis, cerebral hemorrhage and infarction.
   >30 units/ml is suggestive of tubercular meningitis and <30 units/ml is suggestive of pyogenic meningitis.

   In MI, lDH1 increases but in heart failure, LDH 5 increases because right sided heart failure causing hepatic congestion and release of LDH5 from them. ....Dinesh Puri 3rd/122-3

7. **Ans. (c) Lymphocytic pleocytosis, low sugar, high protein** *(Ref: Harrison 18th/3426, Harsh Mohan 6th/appendix)*
   CT scan shows *basal exudates with meningeal enhancement* is highly suggestive of *tuberculous meningitis*. For CSF changes in CNS infection see text.

8. **Ans. (a) Progressive multifocal leukoencephalopathy (PML)** *(Ref: Robbins 8th/1305, 9/e p1278)*
   Progressive multifocal leukoencephalopathy (PML) is a demyelinating disease of the central nervous system that results from infection of oligodendrocytes by the JC polyomavirus. It occurs almost exclusively in immunocompromised individuals as in HIV due to reactivation of the virus.
   Microscopic examination shows lesions in the white matter which is an area of demyelination, in the center of which are scattered lipid-laden macrophages and a reduced number of axons. At the edge of the lesion are greatly **enlarged oligodendrocyte nuclei whose chromatin is replaced by glassy amphophilic viral inclusion**.....Robbins
   Significance of microscopic findings in PML

   In PML, the virus also **infects astrocytes**, leading to **bizarre giant forms** with irregular, hyperchromatic, sometimes multiple nuclei **that can be mistaken for tumor.**

OTHER OPTIONS

- In acute cases of **Polio**, there is mononuclear cell perivascular cuffs and neuronophagia of the **anterior horn motor neurons of the spinal cord**.
- In **CJD**, microscopically, there is characteristic **spongiform change in the gray matter** ("cluster of grapes" vacuolation) **without inflammation**.

9. **Ans. (d) Parkinson's Disease** *(Ref: Harrison 17th/2647, Robbins 8th/1308, 9/e p1281)*
Prion's disease of humans include:
- Iatrogenic Creutzfeldt-Jakob disease
- Sporadic Creutzfeldt-Jakob disease
- Variant Creutzfeldt-Jakob disease
- Fatal Familial Insomnia
- Gerstmann-Straussler-Scheinker syndrome
- Sporadic Fatal Insomnia
- Kuru

10. **Ans. (c) Multiple sclerosis** *(Ref: Harrison 17th/2647; Robbins 9/e p57, 1283-1284)*
Disorders caused by misfolding of proteins are
- Amyloidosis
- Alzheimer's disease and other neurodegenerative diseases
- Transmissible prion diseases like CJD
- Some genetic diseases caused by mutations that lead to misfolding of protein and loss of function, such as certain of the cystic fibrosis mutations.

Prions are infectious proteins that cause degeneration of the central nervous system (CNS). Prion diseases are disorders of protein conformation, the most common of which in humans is called Creutzfeldt-Jakob disease (CJD). CJD typically presents with dementia and myoclonus, is relentlessly progressive, and generally causes death within a year of onset.
Four new concepts have emerged from studies of prions:

- Prions are the only known infectious pathogens that are devoid of nucleic acid; all other infectious agents possess genomes composed of either RNA or DNA that direct the synthesis of their progeny.
- Prion diseases may manifest as infectious, genetic, and sporadic disorders; no other group of illnesses with a single etiology presents with such a wide spectrum of clinical manifestations.
- Prion diseases result from the accumulation of PrP^{Sc}, the conformation of which differs substantially from that of its precursor, PrP^C.
- PrP^{Sc} can exist in a variety of different conformations, each of which seems to specify a particular disease phenotype. How a specific conformation of a PrP^{Sc} molecule is imparted to PrP^C during Prion replication to produce nascent PrP^{Sc} with the same conformation is unknown. Additionally, it is unclear what factors determine where in the CNS a particular PrP^{Sc} molecule will be deposited.

11. **Ans. (c) i.e. Proteins** *(Ref: Harrison 17th/2646; 16th/2495, 9/e p1281)*
- *Prions* are infectious proteins that cause degeneration of the central nervous system (CNS). Prion diseases are disorders of protein conformation, the most common of which in humans is called Creutzfeldt-Jakob disease (CJD).
- In mammals, prions reproduce by binding to the normal, cellular isoform of the *prion* protein (PrP^C) and stimulating conversion of PrP^C into the disease-causing isoform (PrP^{Sc}). PrP^C is rich in alpha-helix and has little beta-structure, while PrP^{Sc} has less alpha-helix and a high amount of beta-structure. This **alpha-to-beta structural transition** in the prion protein (PrP) is the fundamental event underlying prion diseases.
- Prions are the only known infectious pathogens that are devoid of nucleic acid; all other infectious agents possess genomes composed of either RNA or DNA that direct the synthesis of their progeny.
Prion diseases may be manifest as infectious, genetic, and sporadic disorders
- *The sporadic form of CJD is the most common prion disorder in humans.* Familial CJD (fCJD), Gerstmann-Straussler-Scheinker (GSS) disease, and fatal familial insomnia (FFI) are all dominantly inherited prion diseases that are caused by mutations in the PrP gene.
- Although infectious prion diseases account for <1% of all cases and infection does not seem to play an important role in the natural history of these illnesses, the transmissibility of prions is an important biologic feature. *Kuru is an infectious prion disease* thought to have resulted from the consumption of brains from dead relatives during ritualistic cannibalism in New Guinea.
- A major feature that distinguishes prions from viruses is the finding that both PrP isoforms are encoded by a chromosomal gene. In humans, the PrP gene is designated *PRNP* and is located on the short arm of chromosome 20.
- Accidental transmission of CJD to humans appears to have occurred with corneal transplantation, contaminated electroencephalogram (EEG) electrode implantation, surgical procedures, implantation of dura mater grafts and from contaminated human growth hormone preparations.
- On light microscopy, the pathologic hallmarks of CJD are spongiform degeneration and astrocytic gliosis. The lack of an inflammatory response in CJD and other prion diseases is an important pathologic feature of these degenerative

disorders. Spongiform degeneration is characterized by many 1- to 5-micrometers vacuoles in the neuropil between nerve cell bodies. Amyloid plaques have been found in ~10% of CJD cases.
- In variant CJD, a characteristic feature is the presence of "florid plaques." These are composed of a central core of PrP amyloid, surrounded by vacuoles in a pattern suggesting petals on a flower.
- The constellation of dementia, myoclonus, and periodic electrical bursts in an afebrile 60-year-old patient generally indicates CJD.

12. **Ans. (c) Vasculitis** *(Ref: Anderson10th/2728, Robbins 9/e p1278)*
Anderson clearly mentioned that "Unlike most other encephalitides, HIV does not seem to infect neurons and perivasculitis is conspicuously absent"
"Characteristic multinuclear Giant Cells of Macrophage origin are seen in white matter of frontal and temporal lobes particularly in perivascular location"
Feature of CNS involvement in AIDS

- Diffuse and focal spongiform changes
- Vacuolar myelopathy of posterior column of spinal cord
- Major cells affected are macrophages and monocytes
- Most characteristics finding is chronic inflammatory reaction with widely distributed infiltrates of microglial nodules

13. **Correct answer: (a) Bacterial toxin; (b) IL-l; (d) Interferon; (e) Tumor necrosis factor (TNF).** *(Ref: Robbins 7th/84, Harrison 16th/106)*
Fever is produced in response to substances called pyrogens that act by stimulating prostaglandin synthesis in the vascular and perivascular cells of hypothalamus.
They can be classified as
- Exogenous pyrogens→Lipopolysaccharides (bacterial toxin) stimulate WBCs to release endogenous pyrogens.
- Endogenous pyrogens→ IL-1 (α, β) and TNF-α, IL-6, Ciliary neurotropic factor and interferons that increase the enzyme (cyclooxygenase) that converts arachidonic acid into prostaglandins.
NSAIDs reduce fever by inhibiting cyclooxygenase.

14. **Ans. (a) Toxoplasma; (c) Aspergillus; (d) Mucor** *(Ref: Robbins 7th/1363, 1378)*
Arteritis of small and large vessels causes cerebral infarcts.
Causes of cerebral infarction:
- Syphilis
- Tuberculosis
- Infectious vasculitis in setting of immunosuppression
- Toxoplasmosis
- Aspergillosis
- CMV encephalitis
- Mucormycosis

15. **Ans. (a) Endarteritis; (b) Hydrocephalus** *(Ref: Robbins 9/e p1274, 7th/1371, OPG' 6th/520-22)*
Most serious complication of chronic tubercular meningitis

- Arachnoid fibrosis→ Hydrocephalous
- Obliterative endarteritis→ Arterial occlusion and infarction of underlying brain.
- Spinal roots may also be affected.
- Calcification
- Tuberculomas

16. **Ans. (a) Cytoadhesin ; (b) Sequestration of cerebral vessels by RBCs** *(Ref: Harrison 16th/1222, Robbins 9/e p391)*
Cerebral malaria is caused by *P. falciparum.*
Pathophysiology of cerebral malaria

Cytoadhesion: On the surface of infected RBC appears an antigen called $PfEMP_1$ (*P. falciparum* erythrocyte membrane protein-I). Due to this antigen infected RBCs adheres in the blood vessels.
Sequestration: It is the key events of falciparum pathology. Brain capillaries especially capillaries of white matter of brain are plugged with parasitized RBCs which terminally leads to thrombosis. Three receptors for parasitized RBC have been identified (ICAM - 1, CD_{36}, thrombospondin). These cause focal cerebral damage.
Rosetting occurs in middle of a sexual life cycle. It is seen in cerebral malaria in brain capillaries.

17. **Ans. (a) T.B.; (c) Aspergillosis; (d) Toxoplasmosis.** *(Ref: Robbins' 7th/1363, 1378)*

18. **Ans. (a) Arterial thrombosis** *(Ref: Robbins 8th/1291-1292, 9/e p1263)*

19. **Ans. (a) Guillain Barre syndrome** *(Ref: Harrison 17th/2667, Robbin 9/e p1231)*

20. **Ans. (d) Brain stem encephalitis** *(Ref: Robbins 9/e p1277, 8th/1304-1305; 7th/1375)*

20.1. **Ans. (b) Hyperalbuminemia** *(Ref: Robbins 8/e p636-7, 9/e p627)*
   Direct lines…"In addition to myasthenia gravis, other associated autoimmune disorders with thymoma include *hypogammaglobulinemia, pure red cell aplasia, Graves' disease, pernicious anemia, dermatomyositis-polymyositis, and Cushing syndrome*".

20.2. **Ans. (c) Creutzfeldt-Jakob disease (CJD)** *(Ref: Robbins 9/e p1282)*
   - In CJD, on microscopic examination, the pathognomonic finding is a **spongiform** *transformation of the cerebral cortex* and, often, deep gray-matter structures (caudate, putamen).
   - This multifocal process results in the uneven formation of small, apparently empty, microscopic vacuoles of varying sizes within the neuropil and sometimes in the perikaryon of neurons.
   - In advanced cases there is severe neuronal loss, reactive gliosis, and sometimes expansion of the vacuolated areas into cystlike spaces ("status spongiosus").
   - *No inflammatory infiltrate is present.*

20.3. **Ans. (b) Spongiform change in brain….see earlier explanation.** *(Ref: Robbins 9/e p1282)*

20.4. **Ans. (d) HIV encephalitis** *(Ref: Robbins 8/e p1375, 9/e p1278)*
   - HIV encephalitis is *best characterized* microscopically as a chronic inflammatory reaction with widely distributed infiltrates of **microglial nodules.**
   - The microglial nodules are also found in the vicinity of small blood vessels, which show abnormally prominent endothelial cells and *perivascular foamy or pigment-laden macrophages*. These changes occur especially in the subcortical white matter, diencephalon, and brainstem.
   - An important component of the microglial nodule is the macrophage-derived **multinucleated giant cell**.

20.5. **Ans. (a) Guillain Barre Syndrome** *(Ref: Robbins 8/e p1262, 9/e p1231, Harrison 17/e p2667)*
   In patients with Guillanin Barre syndrome, there is elevation of the CSF protein due to inflammation and altered permeability of the microcirculation within the spinal roots as they traverse the subarachnoid space. Inflammatory cells are contained within the roots, however, and there is little to no CSF pleocytosis. This is termed as albumin-cytological dissociation.

20.6. **Ans. (b) Syringomyelia** *(Ref: Robbins 9th/1258)*

20.7. **Ans. (b) Tabes dorsalis** *(Ref: Robbins 9th/1275)*
   - Tabes dorsalis is the result of damage to the sensory axons in the dorsal roots. This causes impaired joint position sense and ataxia (locomotor ataxia); loss of pain sensation, leading to skin and joint damage (Charcot joints); other sensory disturbances like the characteristic "lightning pains"; and absence of deep tendon reflexes.
   - Meningovascular neurosyphilis is chronic meningitis involving the base of the brain. It may be associated with obliterative endarteritis (Heubner arteritis) accompanied by a distinctive perivascular inflammatory reaction. Cerebral gummas (plasma cell-rich mass lesions) may also be present.
   - General paresis of the insane is caused by the invasion of the brain by T. pallidum. It manifests as progressive cognitive impairment associated with mood alterations (including delusions of grandeur) terminating in severe dementia.
   - Syphilitic amyotrophy presents with painless and progressive weakness.

21. **Ans. (b) Neuroglia** *(Ref: Robbins 7th/1349, 9/e p1252)*
   - **Neuroglia** (astrocytes) are the principal cells in the central nervous system responsible for reaction to injury repair and scar formation in the brain. They perform **function similar to fibroblasts** in the CNS.
   - **Gliosis** is the most important histopathological indicator of CNS injury. Astrocytes participate in this process by undergoing both hypertrophy and hyperplasia.
   - *Neuroglial cells can be ectodermal in origin (e.g. astrocytes and oligodendrocytes) or derived from mesoderm (microglia).*
   - Microglia resemble macrophages and act as scavenger cells whereas oligodendrocytes help in myelin formation [similar to Schwann cells in PNS]

22. **Ans. (a) Nucleus basalis of Meynert** *(Ref: Harrison 16th/2395, Robbins 9/e p1290)*
   - The brain of Alzheimer's disease patients shows severe neuronal loss in the *nucleus basalis of Meynert*, the major source of cholinergic input to cerebral cortex.
   - The major microscopic abnormalities of Alzheimer's disease are:
     - Neurofibrillary tangles, neuropil threads
     - Senile (Neuritic) plaques
     - Amyloid angiopathy
     - Granulovacuolar degeneration

- A dominant component of the plaque core is Aβ, a peptide of approximately 40-43 amino acid residues derived from a larger molecule, amyloid precursor protein (APP).
- Although neurofibrillary tangles are characteristic of Alzheimer's disease, they are not specific to this condition.
- **Hirano bodies:** Found especially in Alzheimer's disease, are elongated, glassy, eosinophilic bodies consisting of paracrystalline arrays of beaded filaments with actin as their major component.

23. **Ans. (d) Neuroglia** *(Ref: Robbins 8th/1282, 9/e p1252)*

24. **Ans. (d) Lewy bodies** *(Ref: Robbins 8th/1313-1317, 9/e p1290)*

25. **Ans. (b) Alzheimer's disease** *(Ref: Robbins 8th/1314)*

26. **Ans. (a) Alzheimer's disease** *(Ref: Robbins, 9/e p1290, 8th/1113-1117; 7th/1386)*

26.1. **Ans. (b) Cerebellum** *(Ref: Robbins 8/e p1336, 9/e p1312)*
Medulloblastoma

• In **children**, the location is in the **midline of the cerebellum**, but *lateral locations are more often found in adults.*
• Medulloblastomas are the *most common malignant brain tumor of childhood*
• 5% of children have it in association with **Gorlin syndrome**[Q] (the *most common of the inherited disorders* due to mutations in the patched-1; PTCH-1 gene.
• Histologically, there is presence of **Homer-Wright rosettes**[Q].

- *Dissemination through the CSF is a common complication*[Q], presenting as nodular masses elsewhere in the CNS, including metastases to the cauda equina that are termed **drop metastases**[Q].

26.2. **Ans. (d) CNS...............explained earlier** *(Ref: Robbins 9/e p1312)*

26.3. **Ans. (a) Pilocytic astrocytoma** *(Ref: Robbins 8/e p1333, 9/e p1309)*
On microscopic examination of *pilocytic astrocytoma*, the tumor is composed of bipolar cells with long, thin *"hairlike" processes* that are **GFAP-positive** and form dense fibrillary meshworks; **Rosenthal fibers** and *eosinophilic granular bodies*, are often present.

26.4. **Ans. (c) Astrocytoma** *(Ref: Robbins 8/e)*

26.5. **Ans. (d) Secondaries** *(Ref: Robbins 8/e p1339, 9/e p1315)*
- Metastatic lesions, mostly carcinomas, account for approximately a quarter to half of intra-cranial tumors in hospitalized patients.
- The meninges are also a frequent site of involvement by metastatic disease.

26.6. **Ans. (b) Parietal and temporal lobe** *(Ref: Robbin 8/e p1314)*
Grossly, the brain shows a variable degree of **cortical atrophy** marked by widening of the cerebral sulci that is most pronounced in the *frontal, temporal, and parietal lobes.. (Ref: Robbind 8/e p 1314*
- *Hippocampus and other medial temporal lobe* structures are the *earliest* and *most severely* affected in Alzheimer's disease.
- Bradley's Neurology mentions that.. "*cortical atrophy is most pronounced in the temporal and parietal lobe* with the *frontal lobe involvement being later* in the disease".

26.7. **Ans. (b) Parkinson disease** *(Ref: Robbins 9th/1294)*

26.8. **Ans. (c) Schwannoma** *(Ref: Robbins 9th/1316-7)*
- Tuberous sclerosis is an autosomal dominant syndrome characterized by the development of hamartomas and benign neoplasms involving the brain and other tissues. Elsewhere in the body, renal angiomyolipomas, retinal glial hamartomas, pulmonary lymphangioleiomyomatosis and cardiac rhabdomyomas develop over childhood and adolescence. Cysts may be found at various sites, including the liver, kidneys, and pancreas.
- Cutaneous lesions include angiofibromas, localized leathery thickenings (shagreen patches), hypopigmented areas (ash-leaf patches), sebaceous adenomas and subungual fibromas.

27. **Ans. (b) CD133** *(Ref: Wintrobe's 12th/2559)*
- CD 133 is used as a marker for leukemia and glioblastoma stem cell. It is also used for identifying immature leukemic stem cell in AML and pro B leukemia.
- CD 45 is required for lymphocyte activation. Its deficiency causes Severe Combined Immunodeficiency disease (SCID).

28. **Ans. (a) > 1cm** *(Ref: Robbins 8th/1100, 9/e p1075)*

Pituitary adenomas are designated as the following:
- *Microadenomas* if they are less than 1 cm in diameter and
- *Macroadenomas* if they exceed 1 cm in diameter

The **most common** cause of *hyperpituitarism* is an *adenoma arising in the anterior lobe.*

29. **Ans. (a) Ependymoma** *(Ref: Robbins 8th/1330, 9/e p1306)*
The four major classes of brain tumors are:

1. Gliomas
Astrocytoma
• Pleomorphic xanthoastrocytoma • Brainstem glioma • Pilocytic astrocytoma • Fibrillary (diffuse) astrocytomas • Glioblastoma
Oligodendroglioma
Ependymoma
2. Neuronal tumors
Ganglion cell tumors *Gangliocytoma* *Ganglioglioma* *Dysembryoplastic neuroepithelial tumor* *Cerebral neuroblastomas*
3. Poorly differentiated neoplasms
4. Meningiomas

30. **Ans. (d) Craniopharyngioma** *(Ref: Robbins 8th/1106, 9/e p1082)*
Brain tumors spreading via CSF are
- Ependymoma
- Medulloblastoma
- Choroid plexus carcinoma
- Astrocytoma
- Germinoma
- Pineoblastoma
- CNS Lymphoma

31. **Ans. (d) Lung** *(Ref: Robbins 8th/1339, 9/e p1315)*

32. **Ans. (a) Radiosensitive tumor; (B) Spreads through CSF; (D) Occurs in young age group.** *(Ref: Robbins 7th/1407; 9/e p1312 Harrison 16th/2455)*
Medulloblastoma:

- The tumor occurs predominantly in children and exclusively in cerebellum (infratentorial tumor).
- Histopathological hallmark is Homer-Wright rosettes.
- Dissemination of tumor occurs through CSF.
- The tumor is highly malignant.
- It is a radiosensitive tumor. Radiotherapy improves the survival in children.
- Cranio-spinal irradiation (CSI) reduces the recurrence from CSF dissemination.

33. **Ans. (e) Secondaries** *(Ref: Robbins 8th/1339, 9/e p1315)*
34. **Ans. (a) Astrocytoma** *(Ref: Robbins 8th/1330, 9/e p1306)*
35. **Ans. (a) Astrocytoma** *(Ref: Robbins 8th/1330, 9/e p1253)*
36. **Ans. (a) Craniopharyngioma** *(Ref: Robbins 9/e p1082, 8th/1106; 7th/1129)*
37. **Ans. (d). Thecoma** *(Ref: Robbins 8th/1051; 7th/1442)*
38. **Ans. (a) Glioblastoma multiforme** *(Ref: Robbins 8th/1330-1331, 9/e p1308)*
39. **Ans. (c) Anaplastic** *(Ref: Robbins 9/e p1315, 8th/1339; 7th/1409)*
39.1. **Ans. (a) Arterial thrombosis** *(Ref: Robbins 8/e p1291-1292)*
The majority of thrombotic occlusions are due to atherosclerosis. The most common sites of primary thrombosis causing cerebral infarction are the carotid bifurcation, the origin of the middle cerebral artery, and either end of the basilar artery…. Robbins

Central Nervous System

39.2. Ans. (d) Neuroglia *(Ref: Robbins 8/e p1282, 9/e p1252)*
"Gliosis is the most important histopathological indicator of CNS injury regardless of its etiology and is characterized by both hypertrophy and hyperplasia." The chief cell involved in this reaction is an astrocyte. Please remember that the oligodendrocytes and the ependyma do not participate in active response to injury.
In contrast, microglia are the fixed macrophage system in the CNS.

39.3. Ans. (d) Lewy bodies *(Ref: Robbins 8/e p1313-1317, 9/e p1290)*
The following are the histopathological features of Alzheimer's disease:
- Neuritic plaques : diagnostic feature
- Neurofibrillary tangles : diagnostic feature
- Cerebral amyloid angiopathy (CAA)
- Hirano bodies

39.4. Ans. (d) Urine contains 5H.I.A.A *(Ref: Robbins 9th/478)*
- Neuroblastoma is the most common extracranial solid cancer in childhood and the most common cancer in infancy.
- About 90% of neuroblastomas, regardless of location, produce catecholamines, which are an important diagnostic feature (i.e., elevated blood levels of catecholamines and elevated urine levels of the metabolites vanillylmandelic acid and homovanillic acid.
- Increased urinary 5HIAA is a feature of carcinoid tumour and not neuroblastoma.

EXPLANATIONS TO ASSERTION AND REASON QUESTIONS

Explanations (1-5): While solving assertion reason type of questions, we can use a particular method.
- First of all, read both assertion (A) and reason (R) carefully and independently analyse whether they are true or false.
- If A is false, the answer will directly be (d) i.e. both A and R are false. You can note that all other options (i.e. a, b or c) consider A to be true.
- If A is true, answer can be (a), (b) or (c), Now look at R. If R is false, answer will be (c)
- If both A and R are ture, then we have to know whether R is correctly explaining A [answer is (a)] or it is not the explanation of assertion [answer is (b)]

1. **Ans. (d) Both assertion and reason are false.** *(Ref: Robbins 8th/1297, 9/e p1270)*
   Already explained in text and answer 3.

2. **Ans. (a) Both assertion and reason are true and reason is correct explanation of assertion.** *(Ref: Robbins 8th/1321, 9/e p1304)*
   Vitamin B_{12} deficiency leads to a swelling of myelin layers, producing vacuoles that begin segmentally at the mid-thoracic level of the spinal cord in the early stages. With time, axons in both the ascending tracts of the posterior columns and the descending pyramidal tracts degenerate. This is called as *subacute combined degeneration of the spinal cord.*

   Concept

   > Though isolated involvement of descending or ascending tracts may be a feature of many spinal cord diseases, the combined degeneration of both ascending and descending tracts of the spinal cord is characteristic of vitamin B_{12} deficiency.

3. **Ans. (a) Both assertion and reason are true and reason is correct explanation of assertion.** *(Ref: Robbins 8th/1314, 9/e p1288)*
   The gene for **amyloid precursor protein** (APP) is located on **chromosome 21**. APP gene mutation causes increased generation of Aβ. Alzheimer disease is associated with trisomy 21. This is related to a gene dosage effect with increased production of APP and subsequently Aβ.
   Other genes linked to early-onset familial Alzheimer disease are:

   > Chromosomes **14ᵠ** and **1ᵠ** as these two chromosomes encode highly related intracellular proteins, **presenilin-1 (PS1)** and **presenilin-2 (PS2)**.

4. **Ans. (b) Both assertion and reason are true and reason is not the correct explanation of assertion.** *(Ref:Robbins 8th/1319-1321)*
   Shy-Dragger syndrome is characterized by autonomic dysfunction including orthostatic hypotension, impotence, abnormal sweat and salivary gland secretion, and pupillary abnormalities. The Lewy bodies are found in sympathetic neurons in the spinal cord.
   - Lewy bodies in the nigrostriatal neurons produce extrapyramidal symptoms and are a feature of **classic Parkinson's disease.**
   - Lewy bodies in the *cerebral cortex* produce dementia and are a feature of **Lewy body dementia.**

   Concept

   > Unlike Parkinson's disease, however, no mutations in the gene coding for alpha-synuclein has been found with the Shy-Drager syndrome.

5. **Ans. (a) Both assertion and reason are true and reason is correct explanation of assertion.** *(Ref: Robbins 8th/1322, 9/e p1297)*
   Huntington's disease has already been explained in the text.

NOTES

CHAPTER 16

Endocrine System

PANCREAS

The endocrine pancreas consists of the islets of Langerhans, which contain four major cell types-β, α, δ, and PP (pancreatic polypeptide) cells.

Cell	Hormone secreted
β cell	Insulin, Amylin
α cell	Glucagon
δ cells	Somatostatin
PP cells	*Pancreatic polypeptide* (vasoactive intestinal peptide, VIP)

Amylin reduces food intake and weight gain by acting on central neurons in the hypothalamus.

Diabetes Mellitus

Diabetes mellitus is a *group of metabolic disorders having the feature of hyperglycemia* which results from either defect in insulin secretion, insulin action, or both. The diagnosis of diabetes is established by elevation of plasma glucose by any one of three criteria:

Glysosylated hemoglobin A1C (HbA1C) is formed due to non enzymatic attachment of glucose with globin component of hemoglobin. It is used for diagnosis as well as a marker of glucose control in diabetics.

Its *target level during the treatment* of DM is **<7%.**

- A *random plasma glucose* concentration of *200 mg/dL or higher*, with classical signs and symptoms
- A *fasting glucose* concentration of *126 mg/dL or higher* on more than one occasion, or
- An abnormal oral glucose tolerance test (OGTT), in which the glucose concentration is 200 mg/dL or higher 2 hours after a standard carbohydrate load (75 gm of glucose).
- A level of glycated hemoglobin *(HbA1c) > 6.5 g/dL* (accepted as an additional criteria for the diagnosis of DM by American Diabetic Association.

Apart from over diabetics, the following types of individuals are there:
- *Euglycemic* individuals: serum fasting glucose values less than 110 mg/dL, or less than 140 mg/dL following an OGTT
- *Impaired glucose tolerance*: serum fasting glucose greater than 110 but less than 126 mg/dL, or OGTT values of greater than 140 but less than 200 mg/dL. It is associated with increased risk of progressing to diabetes.

The insulin gene is expressed in the β cells of the pancreatic islets. Preproinsulin synthesized in the rough endoplasmic reticulum is delivered to the Golgi apparatus where it is converted to insulin and a cleavage peptide, C-peptide.

The vast majority of cases of diabetes fall into one of two broad classes:

The **most important stimulus** that triggers **insulin synthesis** and release is **glucose it**self.

- **Type 1 diabetes**: it is characterized by an **absolute deficiency of insulin** secretion caused by pancreatic β-cell destruction, usually resulting from an autoimmune attack.
- **Type 2 diabetes**: it is caused by a "**relative insulin deficiency**" due to combination of peripheral resistance to insulin action and an inadequate compensatory response of insulin secretion by the pancreatic β cells.

Concept

Since both insulin and C-peptide are secreted in equal amounts equimolar quantities after physiologic stimulation, **C-peptide levels** are used a *marker for endogenous insulin secretion.*

PATHOGENESIS OF TYPE 1 DIABETES MELLITUS

The following are the risk factors for the development of type 1 DM:
1. **Genetic factors**: these could affect
   HLA genes (**commonest locus** being affected is on **chromosome 6p21(HLA D)** like HLA DR3/DR4 with DQ8 haplotype
   The non HLA genes like that for insulin or polymorphism in CD25 (normally regulated the function of T cells)

The presence of **islet cell antibodies** is used as a **predictive marker for type 1 DM**. There is characteristically presence of **insulitis** in these patients.

2. **Environmental factors**: viral infections like coxsackie B, mumps, rubella or cytomegalovirus.

The *failure of self tolerance in T cells* is the main defect in type 1 DM. The autoreactive Tcells (TH1 cells and CD8+ cytotoxic T cells) get activated and cause β cell injury resulting in the reduction of β cell mass. *Autoantibodies* against a variety of β-cell antigens, including insulin, islet cell autoantigen 512 and glutamic acid decarboxylase are also found in the patients.

PATHOGENESIS OF TYPE 2 DIABETES MELLITUS

The disease is characterized by the following metabolic defects:

- **Insulin resistance:** it is defined as resistance to the effects of insulin on glucose uptake, metabolism, or storage. It is a characteristic feature of most individuals with type 2 diabetes.
- **β-cell dysfunction:** inadequate insulin secretion in the presence of insulin resistance and hyperglycemia

There is *no autoimmune basis* of type 2 DM. The insulin resistance is being contributed maximally by the *loss of sensitivity in the hepatocytes.*

> The genetic factors are much more important in type 2 DM than in type 1 DM.

> The presence of **islet amyloid protein (amylin)** is a characteristic feature of long standing **type 2 DM.** There is **no insulitis in type 2 DM** (which is characteristically seen in type 1 DM).

> **Obesity** is the most important risk factor **insulin resistance.**

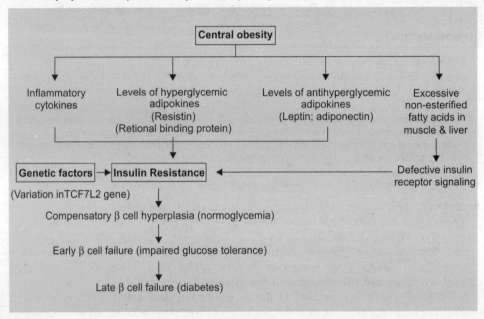

*An increase in the number of and size of islets is characteristic of non diabetic infants of diabetic mothers.

> 50% of carriers of **Glucokinase mutations** develop **Gestational diabetes mellitus.**
>
> Patients with lipoatrophic diabetes have hyperglycemia with loss of adipose tissue.

MONOGENIC FORMS OF DIABETES

The monogenic forms of diabetes can be due to the following causes:

Primary defect in β-cell function	Defect in insulin-insulin receptor signaling
• Autosomal-dominant inheritance with high penetrance • Early onset (usually before age 25) • Absence of obesity • Lack of islet cell autoantibodies	• Type A insulin resistance (severe insulin resistance + hyperinsulinemia + DM) • Lipoatrophic diabetes (insulin resistance + hypertriglyceridemia + DM + acanthosis nigricans + hepatic steatosis)

Pathogenesis of Complications of DM

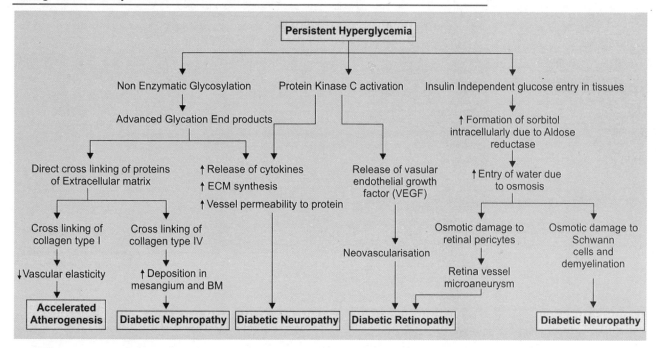

CLINICAL FEATURES OF DM

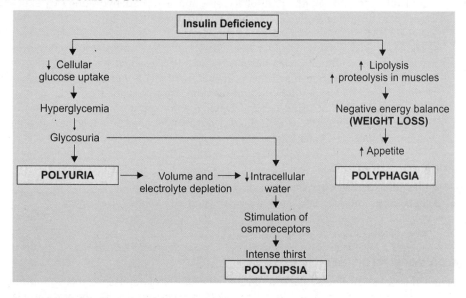

Concept

'**Honeymoon period**' is the *symptom free interval period* in a patient of DM in which the individual is asymptomatic. It is *due to the β reserve cell mass* in the pancreatic islets

The **paradoxical combination** of **weight loss and polyphagia** should make the physician suspicious of **DM**

Recent information

A family of proteins called *sirtuins*, identified to be involved in aging are now implicated in diabetes. Sirt-1 improves glucose tolerance, enhance β cell insulin secretion, and increase production of adiponectin.

Acute Complications of DM

1. **Type 1 DM**

    Diabetic ketoacidosis is an important complication seen in type 1 diabetics. It is usually precipitated by inadequate insulin therapy, intercurrent infection, emotional stress and excessive alcohol intake.

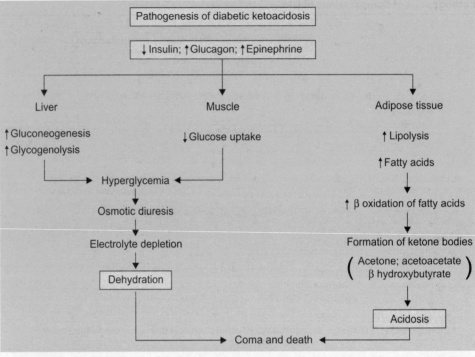

The clinical feature of these patients would be nausea, vomiting, respiratory difficulties, 'fruity' breath odour of acetone, and signs of dehydration (dry skin and poor skin turgor) and altered consciousness to coma.

2. **Type 2 DM**

These patients are usually older (>40 years) and frequently obese. It may present with polyuria and polydipsia but mostly it is diagnosed *after routine blood or urine testing*. A complication that is seen in these patients is *hyperosmolar nonketotic coma* due to the severe dehydration resulting from sustained osmotic diuresis in patients who do not drink enough water to compensate for urinary losses from chronic hyperglycemia. It is usually seen in elderly person who are unable to maintain adequate water intake.

CHRONIC COMPLICATIONS OF DM

The long-standing diabetes may involve:
- Both large- and medium-sized muscular arteries (*macrovascular disease*)
- Capillary dysfunction in target organs (*microvascular disease*): *diabetic retinopathy*, *nephropathy*, and *neuropathy*.

MACROVASCULAR DISEASE

It includes increased cardiovascular complications like MI, stroke and gangrene. The *hallmark* of diabetic macrovascular disease is *accelerated atherosclerosis* affecting the aorta and large and medium-sized arteries. It is having earlier onset and greater severity. Advanced vascular disease can lead to gangrene of the lower extremities. The LDL cholesterol is kept under 100mg/dL in these patients usually with statins. The vascular lesion in diabetics is **Hyaline arteriolosclerosis** (amorphous, hyaline thickening of the wall of the arterioles causing narrowing of the lumen).

Renal atherosclerosis and arteriolosclerosis is due to macrovascular disease in diabetics.

A characteristic feature of renal involvement in diabetics is **Hyaline arteriolosclerosis affecting both the afferent as well as the efferent arterioles**.

Concept

Type 2 DM patients **don't develop ketoacidosis** and its symptoms (nausea, vomiting, respiratory difficulties) because of elevated portal insulin levels. The **'fat sparing' effect of insulin** prevents the formation of ketone bodies by inhibiting the fatty acid oxidation in the liver.

Metformin is the *only oral agent* which *reduces macrovascular events* in type 2 DM.

MI is the *most common cause of death* in diabetics.

Endocrine System

608

MICROVASCULAR DISEASE

The most consistent morphologic feature of diabetic microangiopathy is **diffuse thickening of basement membranes.** However, the affected vessels (diabetic capillaries) are having increased permeability to plasma proteins. The microangiopathy is responsible for the development of diabetic nephropathy, retinopathy, and some forms of neuropathy.

1. *Diabetic nephropathy*

   The most important glomerular lesions are *capillary basement membrane thickening; diffuse increase in mesangial matrix,* and nodular glomerulosclerosis (PAS positive nodules called *Kimmelsteil Wilson* lesion). These patients also have increased risk of papillary necrosis. Clinical features include **microalbuminuria** (urinary excretion of 30-300 mg/day^Q of albumin). In uncontrolled diabetes, there is presence of glucosuria resulting in glycogen accumulation in PCT cells (called as **Armani Ebstein cells**). Patients with microalbuminuria are managed with ACE inhibitors. (See diabetic nephropathy for details in the chapter on kidney).

2. *Diabetic retinopathy*

   The ocular involvement may present as retinopathy, cataract formation, or glaucoma. Retinopathy is the most common pattern and can be of the following types: *nonproliferative (background) retinopathy* and *proliferative retinopathy.*

   Nonproliferative retinopathy includes intraretinal or pre-retinal hemorrhages, retinal exudates, microaneurysms (saccular dilations of retinal choroidal capillaries), venous dilations, edema, and, most importantly, thickening of the retinal capillaries (microangiopathy). The retinal exudates can be either "soft" (microinfarcts) or "hard" (deposits of plasma proteins and lipids).

   Proliferative retinopathy includes the process of neovascularization and fibrosis. Macular involvement can cause blindness whereas vitreous hemorrhages can result from retinal detachment. It is managed with laser photocoagulation.

3. *Diabetic Neuropathy*

   DM can affect both the central and peripheral nervous systems. The *most frequent* pattern of involvement is a *peripheral, symmetric neuropathy* of the lower extremities that affects both motor and sensory function. It can also manifest as *autonomic neuropathy* (can produce disturbances in bowel and bladder function) and *diabetic mononeuropathy* (can manifest as sudden foot drop, wrist drop, or isolated cranial nerve palsies). The neurological changes may be due to microangiopathy, increased permeability of the capillaries supplying the nerves and direct axonal damage due to alterations in sorbitol metabolism. The delayed gastric emptying is called diabetic gastroparesis and is managed with metoclopramide or erythromycin.

> Treatment of DM is done with insulin and/or anti-hyperglycemic agents. The latter include Sulfonylureas; (Glipizide, Glibenclamide), Biguanides (metformin), Meglitinides (Repaglinide), Glucosidase inhibitor (Acarbose) and DPP-4 inhibitors (Vildagliptin).

> **Diabetic nephropathy**
>
> *Most characteristic lesion: Nodular Glomerulosclerosis or Kimmelsteil Wilson lesion*
>
> *Most common lesion: Diffuse Glomerulosclerosis*

> **Peripheral, symmetric neuropathy** of the *lower extremities* is the commonest pattern in **diabetic neuropathy.**

> *Concept*
>
> **Dawn phenomenon** is an early morning rise in plasma glucose *requiring increased amounts of insulin* to maintain euglycemia.
>
> **Somogyi effect** is *rebound hyperglycemia* in the morning because of counter-regulatory hormone release *after an episode of hypoglycemia in the middle of the night.*

INSULINOMA

β-cell tumors (insulinomas) are the most common of pancreatic endocrine neoplasms. These benign tumors may be responsible for the elaboration of sufficient insulin to induce clinically significant hypoglycemia.

There is a characteristic **clinical triad** resulting from these pancreatic lesions:

1. *Attacks of hypoglycemia* occur with *blood glucose levels below 50 mg/dl*
2. The attacks consist principally of such central nervous system manifestations as confusion, stupor, and loss of consciousness
3. The attacks are precipitated by fasting or exercise and are promptly *relieved by feeding or parenteral administration of glucose.*

Hyperinsulinism may also be caused by *diffuse hyperplasia of the islets* which is usually seen in neonates and infants.

> **Insulinomas** are the *most common pancreatic endocrine neoplasms;* characterized by.the presence of **Whipple's triad.**

The critical laboratory findings in insulinomas are high circulating levels of insulin and a high insulin-glucose ratio. Surgical removal of the tumor is usually followed by prompt reversal of the hypoglycemia.

THYROID GLAND

It is a gland (weighing 15-20 g) responsible for the secretion of the thyroid hormones (T_3 and T_4) and calcitonin. Thyroid hormones are required for the development of brain and maintenance of basal metabolic rate whereas calcitonin is involved in calcium homeostasis. The two types of disorders associated with this gland are hyperthyroidism and hypothyroidism.

HYPERTHYROIDISM

It is a state of *hyperfunctioning of the thyroid gland* characterized by elevated levels of free T_3 and T_4 and associated with increased sympathetic activity. It should be differentiated from thyrotoxicosis which is a *hypermetabolic state due to elevated levels of free T_3 and T_4* (so, thyrotoxicosis includes hyperthyroidism as well as other causes). The causes for this condition include

1. Diffuse toxic hyperplasia (Graves' disease) (Accounts for 85% of cases)
2. Toxic multinodular goiter
3. Toxic adenoma
4. Uncommon causes:
   - Acute or subacute thyroiditis
   - Hyperfunctioning thyroid carcinoma
   - TSH secreting pituitary adenoma
   - Struma ovarii
   - Iatrogenic hyperthyroidism
   - Thyrotoxicosis factitia

Clinical features: The salient features include tachycardia, palpitations, diaphoresis (increased sweating), heat intolerance, tremors, diarrhea and weight loss despite a good appetite.

The diagnosis is made using serum TSH. It is the most useful screening test as its level may be altered in patients with even subclinical hyperthyroidism. **In primary hyperthyroidism**, serum *TSH is low* and free T_4 is increased whereas in **secondary** (due to increased TSH secretion from the pituitary) and **tertiary** (due to increased thyrotropin releasing hormone or TRH secretion from the hypothalamus) **hyperthyroidism**, serum *TSH is high*.

HYPOTHYROIDISM

It is caused due to decreased secretion of the thyroid hormones either due to a **primary** defect in the thyroid (*most common*[Q]) or a **secondary** (TSH deficiency) or rarely a **tertiary** (TRH deficiency) cause. This can result in *cretinism in children and myxedema (or Gull disease) in adults*. The clinical features of the disease include lethargy, sensitivity to cold, reduced cardiac output, constipation, *myxedema* [due to accumulation of glycoaminoglycans, proteoglycans and water resulting in deep voice, macroglossia (enlarged tongue) and non- pitting edema of hands and feet] and menorrhagia (increased menstrual blood loss).

The diagnosis is made using *serum TSH. It is the most useful screening test. Serum TSH is elevated in primary hypothyroidism and it is reduced in secondary and tertiary hypothyroidism.*

THYROIDITIS

It is defined as the inflammation of the thyroid gland which may be associated with illness and severe thyroid pain (as in infectious thyroiditis or subacute granulomatous thyroiditis) or can be painless (subacute lymphocytic thyroiditis or Reidel thyroiditis). The important types of thyroiditis include:

Nesidioblastosis is diffuse islet hyperplasia and is seen with maternal diabetes and Beckwith-Wiedemann syndrome.

Graves' disease is the commonest cause of thyrotoxicosis

Thyrotoxicosis factitia is Exogenous thyroid hormone induced hyperthyroidism

The **cardiac manifestations** are *the earliest and most consistent* feature of hyperthyroidism.

Serum TSH is best screening test for thyroid dysfunction.

Autoimmune hypothyroidism is the commonest cause of hypothyroidism in iodine sufficient areas of the world.

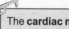

Primary hypothyroidism: ↓ serum T_4; ↑ **serum TSH.**

Secondary hypothyroidism: ↓ serum T_4; ↓ **serum TSH.**

Endocrine System

Hashimoto Thyroiditis (Chronic Lymphocytic Thyroiditis)

It is a chronic inflammation with lymphocytic infiltration of the thyroid gland (the latter responsible for the term '*struma lymphomatosa*'). It is more commonly seen in **females** (F: M ratio is 10:1) of the age group of 45-65 years. This condition is associated with HLA-DR5, HLA-DR3 and chromosomal defects like Turner and Down syndrome. Increased susceptibility to Hashimoto's thyroiditis has been associated with polymorphisms of cytotoxic T lymphocyte associated antigen-4 (CTLA4) and protein tyrosine phosphatase-22 (PTPN 22).

Pathogenesis: There is replacement of the thyroid cells with lymphocytic infiltration and fibrosis. There is presence of antithyroid antibodies (anti-TSH receptor antibodies, anti-thyroglobulin and anti-thyroid peroxidase antibodies) in the serum of the affected patients.

Morphology: The thyroid gland is diffusely enlarged with *intact capsule*. There is presence of *well developed germinal centers* and extensive infiltration of parenchyma by mononuclear inflammatory cells like lymphocytes and plasma cells. The thyroid follicles are atrophic and lined by epithelial cells having abundant eosinophilic and granular cytoplasm called **Hurthle cells**.[Q]

Clinical features: It is characterized by the presence of *painless enlargement* of the thyroid gland and a gradual loss of thyroid function (though initially, thyroid follicular disruption may cause transient hyperthyroidism). The disorder is *associated with autoimmune diseases* (like SLE, Sjögren syndrome, myasthenia gravis) and there is *increased risk of* development of *B-cell non-Hodgkin lymphoma*.

Subacute Lymphocytic Thyroiditis (or Silent/Painless Thyroiditis or Postpartum Thyroiditis)

It is a *self limiting*[Q] episode of thyrotoxicosis seen commonly in middle aged females especially in postpartum period. It is associated with HLA DR-3 and HLA DR-5 and is autoimmune in etiology. Painless and post-partum thyroiditis are variants of Hashimoto's thyroiditis.

Morphology: The thyroid gland has lymphocytic infiltration with hyperplastic germinal centers and patchy collapse of thyroid follicles.

Clinical features are *painless enlargement of the thyroid* and *transient hyperthyroidism* (lasting about 2-8 weeks). Investigations reveal elevated levels of T_3 and T_4 and reduced TSH.

Subacute Thyroiditis (Granulomatous Thyroiditis or De Quervain Thyroiditis)

It is a disorder seen commonly in females (Female: Male ratio is 3 to 5:1) of the age group 30-50 years. It is more commonly seen in summer, is *preceded by a viral infection* (caused by coxsackie virus, mumps, measles, adenovirus etc.) and is **associated with HLA-B5**.

Pathogenesis: It results due to virus induced host tissue damage or direct viral damage.

Morphology: The thyroid gland is diffusely enlarged with *intact capsule*. There is presence of patchy changes. In the initial stages, there is active inflammation characterized by disruption of follicles by neutrophils (forming micro abscess), lymphocytes, histiocytes, plasma cells and multi-nucleated giant cells which is followed by fibrosis.

Clinical features are *pain in neck, sore throat*, fever, fatigue, anorexia, myalgia, enlarged thyroid and the presence of **transient hyperthyroidism** which usually diminishes in 2-6 weeks. It may be followed by asymptomatic hypothyroidism but recovery is seen in most of the patients. Almost all patients have high T_3 and T_4 and low TSH initially which recovers in 6-8 weeks after the disease completes the course.

Reidel's Thyroiditis (or Fibrous Thyroiditis/Invasive Thyroiditis)

It is an idiopathic rare disorder characterised by the *destruction of the thyroid gland by dense fibrosis*. Fibrosis *of the surrounding structures like trachea and esophagus can also occur*. It is more commonly seen in females of middle age and is associated with retroperitoneal and mediastinal fibrosis.

GRAVES' DISEASE

It is the *commonest cause*[Q] of endogenous hyperthyroidism characterized by the **triad** of *hyperthyroidism* due to hyperfunctional diffuse enlargement of gland, *infiltrative ophthalmopathy* and localized, infiltrative *dermopathy* (also called as *pretibial myxedema*). The disorder is more

Thyroid acropachy is digital swelling and clubbing of fingers in Graves disease.

Concept

In Graves disease, there is crowding of cells with **papillae formation without fibrovascular core** (presence of the latter is the differentiating feature of papillary thyroid cancer).

In Toxic multinodular goiter: one or more nodules becom TSH independent.

***Exophthalmos and pretibial myxedema* are NOT seen in toxic multinodular goiter**

Presence of a hyper functioning nodule developing in MNG called as **Plummer Syndrome**.

Factors ↑ risk of neoplasia in STN (MY SR is Cool)
Male patients
Young patients
Solitary as compared to multiple nodules
Radiation exposure to head and neck is present
Cold nodule on radioactive scan (nodules taking less amount of radioactive iodine in imaging studies)

common in females of the age group of 20-40 years. It is associated with polymorphisms in HLA B8, HLA DR3, CTLA4 and PTPN-22.

Pathogenesis: It is an autoimmune disease most commonly due to formation of **antibodies to TSH receptors** (called TSI or LATS meaning *Thyroid Stimulating Immunoglobulin* and *Long Acting Thyroid Stimulator* respectively). The other antibodies found in this condition include **TGI** (Thyroid Growth stimulating Immunoglobulin) and **TBII** (TSH Binding Inhibitor Immunoglobulin), the latter sometimes responsible for *paradoxical hypothyroidism* seen in some of these patients. The anti-TSH antibodies stimulate the TSH receptor in this condition in contrast to Hashimoto's thyroiditis in which the antibodies inhibit the receptor.

Morphology: The thyroid gland is symmetrically enlarged with diffuse hypertrophy and hyperplasia. The capsule is intact.

Clinical features as described above include **hyperthyroidism**, **ophthalmopathy** (due to increased volume of extraocular muscle and retro-orbital connective tissue *as a result of expression of TSH receptor by orbital fibroblasts*) and localized, **infiltrative dermopathy** (most commonly in skin overlying shin). Investigations reveal increased levels of T_3 and T_4 with reduced TSH levels. There is a diffuse increase in the uptake of radioactive iodine.

DIFFUSE AND MULTINODULAR GOITER

Goiter is enlargement of the thyroid gland. Both diffuse and multinodular goiter are caused due to impaired synthesis of thyroid hormones most commonly due to dietary iodine deficiency. This results in increased secretion of TSH leading to hypertrophy and hyperplasia of the thyroid gland. The degree of enlargement is proportional to the level and duration of thyroid hormone deficiency. Usually, the enlargement takes place to maintain a euthyroid state but may also be associated with hyperthyroid state.

Diffuse Non-toxic Goiter (Colloid Goiter or Simple Goiter)

In this condition, the thyroid shows no nodules and there are colloid filled follicles (so, the other name is colloid goiter). It can be **endemic** (when >10% of population is affected usually due to low dietary iodine intake) or **sporadic** (seen more commonly in females during puberty; usually due to enzyme defects affecting thyroid hormone synthesis or ingestion of *Goitrogens* which are substances interfering with thyroid hormone synthesis like calcium, cabbage, cauliflower, turnip, cassava, etc.)

Histologically, there can be two stages: *initial hyperplastic stage* having diffuse, symmetrically enlarged gland with thyroid follicular hyperplasia and *later, the stage of colloid involution*.

MULTINODULAR GOITER (MNG)

This is a condition resulting from recurrent episodes of hyperplasia and involution resulting in *irregular enlargement* of thyroid gland. *The differential sensitivity of follicular cells for TSH results in multinodular goiter.* Grossly, there is presence of enlarged multinodular thyroid with presence of hemorrhage, fibrosis, calcification and cystic change.

Clinical features are due to mass effect (enlarged thyroid causing compression of esophagus, trachea, etc.) or cosmetic effect.

SOLITARY THYROID NODULE (STN)

It is a clinical entity seen more commonly in females. STN is *more likely to be neoplastic in* the presence of certain risk factor (mentioned alongside).

THYROID ADENOMA

These are solitary masses of the thyroid tissue composed of follicular epithelium and are therefore, called as follicular adenomas. They are formed due to chronic overactivation of

Endocrine System

cAMP pathway (due to somatic mutation of the TSH receptor or the α subunit of Gs receptor). They are usually asymptomatic and present as 'cold' nodules on radio imaging scans.

Morphologically, these are solitary, spherical lesions having an *intact capsule* Usually, the cells form uniform appearing follicles containing colloid but they can have the following subtypes:

- Follicular or simple colloid
- Microfollicular: Seen in fetal life
- Hurthle cell (oxyphil, oncocytic) adenoma: Cells have eosinophilic, granular cytoplasm
- Atypical adenoma: Increased variation in cellular and nuclear morphology
- Clear cell follicular adenoma: Cells have clear cytoplasm.

Concept

(Presence of **intact capsule** distinguishes a **benign follicular adenoma** from *follicular carcinoma* because in the latter the *capsule is **NOT** intact*).

THYROID CARCINOMAS

It is a cancer seen more commonly in females in early and middle adult life. The four histological types of thyroid cancers are:

1. Papillary cancer
2. Follicular cancer
3. Medullary cancer
4. Anaplastic cancer

Risk Factors for Thyroid Cancers

- **Papillary cancer**: It is associated with mutation in either tyrosine kinase receptors **RET** or **NTRK1** (Neurotrophic Tyrosine Kinase Receptor 1) or **BRAF oncogene**. RET is located on chromosome10 and translocation with chromosome 17 causes formation of a fusion gene ret/PTC (ret/papillary thyroid cancer) which is responsible for increased tyrosine kinase activity of cells resulting in papillary thyroid cancer. This cancer is also seen after exposure to **ionizing radiation** during first two decades of life.

- **Follicular cancer**: It is associated with mutation in RAS oncogenes particularly **N-RAS**. A specific translocation associated with follicular cancer is **t(2;3)** resulting in PAX8-PPARγ1fusion. PPAR is peroxisome proliferator-activated receptor required for terminal differentiation of the cell whereas PAX8 is a homeobox gene required for thyroid development.

- **Medullary cancer**: It is the only thyroid cancer to **arise from parafollicular 'C' cells**. It is associated with **mutation in RET proto-oncogene** resulting in constitutional activation of the receptor.

- Remember that ret/PPTC is NOT seen in medullary carcinoma of thyroid.

- **Anaplastic cancer**: It is associated with mutation in the **p53** tumor suppressor gene.

*All thyroid cancers arise from follicular epithelium **except** medullary cancer (arises from "C" cells)*

SALIENT FEATURES OF THYROID CANCERS

PAPILLARY CARCINOMA

- It is the *commonest type* of thyroid cancer[Q]
- Seen in 20-40 years old age group
- Spread is by *lymphatic route*[Q]
- *Carries excellent prognosis*[Q]
- **Microscopically** there is presence of **papillae with fibrovascular stalk**, calcified structures called **Psammoma bodies**[Q] and cancer cells have diagnostic nuclear features like presence of fine chromatin leading to 'ground glass' or '**Orphan Annie eye' nuclei**[Q], intranuclear inclusions (called '**pseudoinclusions**') or intranuclear longitudinal grooves.
- The variants include encapsulated variant (good prognosis), follicular variant (poor prognosis) and tall cell variant (poorest Prognosis).

M

Papillary Thyroid tumor (6Ps)

Popular (Most common)
Palpable Lymph nodes (Spreads by lymphatics)
Positive I (131) uptake
Positive Prognosis (Excellent prognosis)
Post radiation in head and neck (cause)
Psammoma bodies

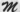

Follicular carcinoma (4Fs)

Female
Faraway metastasis
Favorable prognosis
Flow in blood (vascular invasions are common)

Medullary carcinoma (3Ms)

MEN association (associated with MEN IIa and MEN IIb)
Median node dissection
aMyloid (associated with amyloidosis)

FOLLICULAR CARCINOMA

- It is the 2nd most common form of thyroid cancer
- Seen in women of older age (40-50 yrs.)
- *Vascular invasion is common* (less lymphatic spread) to bone, lung, liver etc.
- **Microscopically**, there is presence of cells forming small follicles having colloid with *NO* Psammoma bodies. Uncommonly, cells have abundant, eosinophilic cytoplasm called as *Hurthle cells*[Q]
- Differentiation from follicular adenoma is based on the *presence of capsular invasion preferably* and vascular invasion[Q] (capsular vessel invasion).

MEDULLARY CARCINOMA

- Arises from *parafollicular cells/C cells and secretes calcitonin*[Q]
- *Sporadic in 80% of cases*
- *Associated with multiple endocrine neoplasia II (MEN) syndromes*[Q]
- **Only** thyroid cancer *associated with amyloidosis*[Q]
- *Unilateral in sporadic* cases and bilateral and multicentric in familial cases
- **Microscopically**, there is presence of polygonal, **spindle cells** in amyloid stroma. Familial cancers characteristically show the presence of multicentric C-cell hyperplasia.

ANAPLASTIC CARCINOMA

- Undifferentiated thyroid cancer
- Have the *worst prognosis*[Q]
- Seen mostly in elderly female patients
- 50% patients give a history of presence of multinodular goiter[Q]
- **Microscopically**, there is presence of highly anaplastic cells which can either be giant cells, spindle cells, mixed giant and spindle cells or small cells.

Quick revision of frequently asked MCQ's from thyroid cancers:

- Most common thyroid carcinoma -Papillary[Q]
- Least common thyroid carcinoma -Anaplastic[Q]
- Least malignant -Papillary[Q]
- Most malignant -Anaplastic[Q]
- Most common cancer after radiation -Papillary[Q]
- Cancer developing in Hashimoto's thyroiditis -Lymphoma[Q]
- Thyroid cancer developing in long standing multinodular goiter -Follicular, Anaplastic (rare)
- Type of thyroid cancer in MEN syndrome -Medullary[Q]
- Thyroid cancer associated with amyloidosis -Medullary[Q]
- Psammoma bodies seen in -Papillary[Q]
- Orphan-Annie Eyed Nuclei seen in -Papillary[Q]
- Thyroid Ca associated with dystrophic calcification -Papillary[Q]
- Carcinoma derived from 'C' cell of thyroid -Medullary[Q]
- Carcinoma developing in thyroglossal tract -Papillary[Q]

PARATHYROID GLAND

These are four glands situated near the thyroid gland and are composed of **chief cells** (containing PTH granules) and **oxyphil cells** (containing glycogen).

PTH secretion is responsible for elevating serum calcium level and increasing phosphate excretion in the urine. *Malignancy is the most common cause of clinically apparent hypercalcemia,* while primary hyperparathyroidism is the commonest cause of asymptomatic hypercalcemia. Increased calcium levels associated with malignancies can be because of osteolytic metastasis and secretion of a PTH related peptide (PTHrP).

The parathyroid gland activity is controlled by the concentration of **free calcium** in the body.

HYPERPARATHYROIDISM

Hyperparathyroidism can be primary (due to autonomous, spontaneous overproduction of PTH) or secondary. Rarely it can be tertiary.

Primary Hyperparathyroidism; 1° HPTH

It is the most important cause of asymptomatic hypercalcemia and can be due to a parathyroid adenoma, primary hyperplasia or parathyroid malignancy. Hyperparathyroidism can be familial or sporadic. The important *molecular defects associated with sporadic hyperparathyroidism include*

1. *PRAD 1 proto-oncogene on chromosome 11 causes over-expression of cyclin D1 resulting in proliferation of the parathyroid cells.*
2. *MEN I suppressor gene on 11 q 13.*

The **genetic syndromes associated with familial hyperparathyroidism** include
1. Multiple endocrine neoplasia I and II (**MEN-I and II**), the genes for which are located on chromosome 11q and 10 q respectively.
2. Familial hypocalciuric hypercalcemia (**FHH**) gene results in reduced sensitivity to extracellular calcium and is responsible for increased secretion of PTH.

Morphology

Adenoma: There is presence of solitary nodule with shrunken glands outside the adenoma.
Primary hyperplasia: There is asymmetric involvement of all four glands with the presence of chief cells.
Parathyroid carcinoma: Involvement of a single gland.

Clinical features: Usually asymptomatic, the only indicator for diagnosis is increased serum calcium and PTH. Symptomatic patients may have nephrolithiasis (urinary tract stones) or nephrocalcinosis (calcification of renal interstitium and tubules), osteoporosis, *osteitis fibrosa cystica* (bone marrow having foci of fibrosis, hemorrhage and cyst formation), metastatic calcification (in blood vessels, stomach and myocardium) and neurological changes like depression, lethargy, etc.

SECONDARY HYPERPARATHYROIDISM

It is seen in renal failure (most common cause), vitamin D insufficiency, steatorrhea and nutritional deficiency. The hypocalcemia due to any of these causes stimulates the secretion of PTH.

Morphology shows the presence of hyperplastic parathyroid glands.

Clinical features are similar to primary hyperparathyroidism. There is also presence of **calciphylaxis** (*vascular calcification causing organ ischemia*). Investigations reveal reduced serum calcium and increased PTH levels.

TERTIARY HYPERPARATHYROIDISM

Autonomous *excessive parathyroid activity even when serum calcium is increased* is called as tertiary hyperparathyroidism which is usually managed by parathyroidectomy.

HYPOPARATHYROIDISM

It is seen due to surgical removal (*commonest cause[Q]*), congenital absence (as in DiGeorge syndrome; failure of development of 3rd and 4th pharyngeal pouch leading to absence of thyroid and parathyroid glands) or is idiopathic.

Clinical features are due to hypocalcemia and the hallmark is tetany characterised by neuromuscular hyperexcitability, cataract, hypotension, QT prolongation on ECG, tingling in circumoral region and hands and feet. Investigations demonstrate the presence of *Chvostek sign* (percussion of facial nerve over ear causes contraction of facial muscles and upper lip) and *Trousseau sign* (inflation of blood pressure cuff more than the systolic blood pressure for around 3 minutes causes flexion at metacarpophalangeal joint with extension at interphalangeal joint). Diagnosis is made by low serum calcium levels.

Parathyroid adenoma is the *commonest cause* of **Primary HPTH**

Best intial screening test for Primary Hyperparathyroidism: intact serum PTH levels.

Concept
Invasion of surrounding tissue or metastasis is the only reliable criteria for diagnosis of malignancy.

Clinical features of Primary Hyperparathyroidism; 1° HPTH: "Stones, bones, abdominal groans, and psychic moans"

Renal failure is most common cause of **Secondary HPTH**

Surgical removal of the parathyroid gland is the commonest cause of **hypoparathyroidism.**

Concept
Hyperventilation worsens the symptoms because the alkalosis decreases free calcium levels.

Endocrine System

PITUITARY GLAND

It is a gland weighing 0.5g, present in sella turcica. It has two distinct lobes; anterior lobe and posterior lobe (stores oxytocin and antidiuretic hormone or vasopressin).

HYPERPITUITARISM

Depending on the size, adenoma can be **macrodenoma (> 1cm)** or *microadenoma (< 1 cm)*.

Concept

The absence of reticulin network and presence of cellular monomorphism differentiates pituitary adenoma from non-neoplastic anterior pituitary parenchyma.

It can be caused due to **adenoma** arising from the anterior lobe (*commonest cause*), hyperplasia and carcinoma. The majority of the adenomas are monoclonal in origin or can be associated with MEN I. Histologically; the adenomas are composed of polygonal cells with little reticulin or connective tissue. The common pituitary tumors include the following:

- **Prolactinoma**: It is the *most common pituitary tumor*. Small microadenomas secrete large amount of prolactin responsible for the clinical features of *amenorrhea, galactorrhea and infertility*. Since men will obviously not have amenorrhea and females are detected early due to menstrual problems, so, microadenomas are commoner in females.

  > Any mass in suprasellar compartment may disturb the normal inhibitory influence of the hypothalamus on prolactin secretion resulting in hyperprolactinemia. This is called **stalk effect.**

The best **initial** investigation is measurement of **serum IGF-I levels** (which would be elevated) and the *confirmatory test is failure to suppress GH production in response to an oral load of glucose.*

- **Growth hormone adenoma**: It is the second most common type of pituitary adenoma. Almost 40% of the patients have persistent GH activity resulting in hypersecretion of insulin like growth factor I (or IGF-I or somatomedin C) causing *gigantism in children and acromegaly in adults*. Gigantism is characterized by features of tall stature and long extremities whereas acromegaly has features of prominent jaw (prognathism), flat, broad forehead, enlarged hands and feet and enlargement of internal organs like heart, spleen, kidney etc.
- Other pituitary tumors include corticotroph cell adenoma producing ACTH (causing Cushing disease), thyrotrope adenoma secreting TSH (causing hyperthyroidism), gonadotrope adenoma secreting FSH and LH.

HYPOPITUITARISM

Pituitary adenoma is the commonest cause of **panhypopituitarism**

It is usually seen when *more than 75% of* parenchyma is lost. GH and gonadotropins (FSH, LH) are typically lost early as compared to other hormones. The causes of hypopituitarism include:

- Compression of the normal pituitary tissue by tumors or cysts
- Pituitary surgery or radiation exposure
- Pituitary apoplexy (acute hemorrhagic infarction of a pre-existing pituitary adenoma)
- Ischemic necrosis
- Sheehan syndrome (postpartum pituitary necrosis due to obstetric hemorrhage or shock)
- Empty sella syndrome.

Sheehan syndrome is *postpartum* pituitary necrosis due to obstetric hemorrhage or shock

Clinical features depend upon the hormone whose function is lost for example, there can be growth failure (due to GH deficiency), loss of libido, amenorrhea, infertility (due to gonadotropin deficiency), hypothyroidism and hypoadrenalism. Loss of melanocyte stimulating hormone (MSH) may cause pallor of the skin.

Concept

In **Primary empty sella syndrome,** the herniation of the arachnoid mater and CSF from the defect in diaphragmatic sella causes pituitary compression whereas in **secondary empty sella**, surgical removal of adenoma results in hypopituitarism

POSTERIOR PITUITARY SYNDROMES

- **Diabetes insipidus**: It is caused due to deficiency of ADH or vasopressin resulting in polyuria, polydipsia, hypernatremia and hyperosmolality (due to excessive renal loss of free water) and dehydration.
- **Syndrome of inappropriate ADH secretion (SIADH)**: Excessive production of ADH can cause oliguria, retention of water, hyponatremia and cerebral edema. The causes of SIADH include *ectopic ADH secretion by small cell lung cancer (commonest)*, injury to hypothalamus or pituitary or both by head trauma and drugs (like vincristine).

ADRENAL CORTEX

Adrenal gland is divided into adrenal cortex and adrenal medulla. The cortex is further subdivided into the following three parts from outside to inside responsible for the secretion of the hormones mentioned in front of them.

- Zona **g**lomerulosa - Mineralocorticoids
- Zona **f**asciculata - Glucocorticoids
- Zona **r**eticularis – Sex steroids

So, Hyperadrenalism can have 3 distinctive patterns:

1. Cushing syndrome:Excess of glucocorticoids
2. Hyperaldosteronism: Excess of mineralocorticoids
3. Adrenogenital syndrome: Excess of sex steroids (androgens)

CUSHING SYNDROME

It has four important causes

1. *Primary hypersecretion* due to increased ACTH (also called **Cushing disease**), seen in women of 20-30 years due to an ACTH producing microadenoma.
2. *Adrenal over-secretion* due to adenomas or carcinomas (adrenal Cushing syndrome): There is no effect of ACTH, so, also known as ACTH independent Cushing syndrome.
3. Secretion of *Ectopic ACTH*: Small cell cancer of the lung, carcinoid tumors.
4. Administration of *exogenous corticosteroids*

Morphology:

In **adrenal gland**, there can be presence of:

1. Cortical atrophy- Seen with exogenous glucocorticoids which cause feedback inhibition of ACTH leading to cortical atrophy except in *zona glomerulosa* (it *functions independent of ACTH*).
2. Diffuse hyperplasia
3. Nodular hyperplasia

Diagnosis

There is an increased 24 hour free cortisol level in the urine with loss of normal diurnal pattern of cortisol secretion. For differentiating between the causes of Cushing syndrome, we use *dexamethasone suppression test.* (See *Review of Pharmacology* Chapter-6 *by the same authors* for details)

ADRENOGENITAL SYNDROME

It is an adrenal disorder due to excessive production of androgens resulting in virilization. It can be caused either by an adrenocortical carcinoma or more commonly congenital adrenal hyperplasia (CAH). CAH represents a group of autosomal-recessive inherited metabolic errors in which there is deficiency of the enzyme/s necessary for synthesis of cortisol. Steroidogenesis channeled into other pathways lead to increased production of androgens, which accounts for virilization. Cortisol deficiency induced increased secretion of ACTH results in adrenal hyperplasia. CAH can manifest as the following three syndromes:

1. *Salt wasting syndrome* – Total absence of 21-α hydroxylase.
2. *Simple virilising adrenogenitalism* – Presents as genital ambiguity due to partial deficiency of 21 α hydroxylase.
3. *Non classic adrenogenitalism* – Asymptomatic or may manifest as hirsutism.

Morphology

Adrenals are hyperplastic bilaterally with nodular cortex that is brown (as there is absence of lipid).

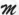

GFR

Layers of adrenal cortex from outside to inside: **G**lomerulosa, **F**asciculata and **R**eticularis

Administration of **exogenous corticosteroids** is the commonest cause of **Cushing syndrome.**

Concept

Pituitary Cushing: ↑ ACTH, ↑ Cortisol

Adrenal Cushing: ↓ ACTH, ↑ Cortisol

Ectopic Cushing: ↑↑ ACTH, ↑ Cortisol

In **Cushing Syndrome**, there is presence of light basophilic material due to accumulation of *intermediate keratin* filaments in the cytoplasm called as **Crooke hyaline change** in the **pituitary**.

Almost 90% of cases of CAH are due to **21 α hydroxylase deficiency** leading to defective conversion of progesterone to 11-deoxycorticosterone.

CLINICAL FEATURES

In 21-α hydroxylase deficiency, excessive androgenic activity causes signs of **masculinization** in females which may range from clitoral hypertrophy and pseudohermaphroditism in infants, to oligomenorrhea, hirsutism, and acne in post pubertal females. In males, androgen excess is associated with enlargement of the external genitalia and precocious puberty in prepubertal patients and oligospermia in older males.

HYPERALDOSTERONISM

The condition is characterized by elevated aldosterone levels leading to retention of sodium and excretion of potassium and hydrogen ions.

> **Primary aldosteronism:** *Diastolic hypertension* is **present** and there is ↓ **renin** secretion

> **Secondary aldosteronism:** *Diastolic hypertension* is **absent** and there is ↑ **renin** secretion

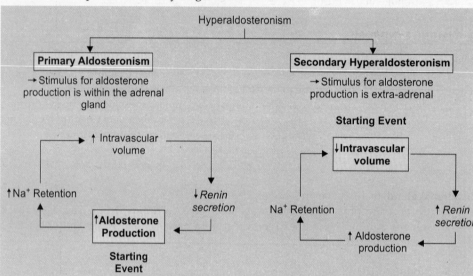

Causes	Causes
• Adrenocortical adenoma (Conn syndrome): - Commonest cause^Q • Primary adrenocortical hyperplasia → Due to overactivity of aldosterone synthase gene, CYP11B2 • Glucocorticoid remediable hyper aldosteronism due to fusion between CYP11B1 (11β hydroxylase) and CYP11B2 (Aldosterone synthetase) genes	• Decreased renal perfusion • Hypovolemia and edema (CHF and cirrhosis) • Pregnancy

> **Concept**
>
> The **adjacent adrenal cortex in adenoma producing aldosterone is not atrophic** *(it is atrophic in adenoma causing Cushing syndrome).*

Morphology: Adrenal adenomas are usually *unilateral (more common on the left as compared to right).* The aldosterone producing adenoma has the presence of eosinophilic laminated cytoplasmic inclusions called as *'spironolactone bodies'* seen after treatment with spironolactone.

Clinical features include hypokalemia induced polyuria, polydipsia and muscle weakness. There may be associated metabolic alkalosis because of excessive aldosterone secretion. Edema is uncommon in primary hyperaldosteronism because of *'escape effect'*.

ADRENAL INSUFFICIENCY

It can be due to **primary** adrenocortical insufficiency (primary hypoadrenalism) or ACTH deficiency induced reduced adrenal stimulation (**secondary** hypoadrenalism).

> **Abrupt withdrawal of corticosteriods** is the most common cause of **acute adrenocortical insufficiency.**

1. **Primary acute adrenocortical insufficiency**: It can be seen after stress, sudden withdrawal of steroids or massive adrenal hemorrhage. If the acute adrenal insufficiency is associated with *bilateral hemorrhagic infarction* of the adrenal glands associated with a *Neisseria infection* (septicemia) in a child, it can result in disseminated intravascular coagulation and rapidly developing hypotension and shock in the patient which is called **Waterhouse-Friedrichsen Syndrome**. The hemorrhage in this condition usually begins in the medulla and then involves the cortex.

> **TB** is the most common cause of **Addison's disease in India**

2. **Primary chronic adrenocortical insufficiency (Addison disease):** It is a slow and progressive disease resulting from adrenocortical hypofunction. Idiopathic atrophy (by autoimmune mechanism) is the commonest cause of adrenal destruction. Autoimmune adrenalitis is associated with Autoimmune Polyendocrine Syndrome (APS) 1 and 2. The loss of adrenal cortex can also be due to tuberculosis, sarcoidosis, AIDS, hemorrhage, trauma and metastatic involvement.

   Clinical features include initial manifestations of *progressive weakness and easy fatigability*, g*astrointestinal* disturbances like anorexia, nausea, vomiting, weight loss and diarrhea. In patients with primary adrenal disease, increased circulating levels of ACTH precursor hormone stimulate melanocytes, with resultant *hyperpigmentation* of the skin particularly of sun-exposed areas and at pressure points, such as neck, elbows, knees, and knuckles.

3. **Secondary adrenocortical insufficiency**: It occurs secondary to any disorder of the hypothalamus and pituitary, such as metastatic cancer, infection, infarction, or irradiation. Further, in adrenal insufficiency secondary to pituitary malfunction, marked hyponatremia and hyperkalemia are not seen.

ADRENAL MEDULLA

The adrenal medulla is composed of neuroendocrine cells called chromaffin cells and their supporting cells called sustentacular cells. The organ is responsible for the secretion of epinephrine and nor-epinephrine and is controlled by the autonomic nervous system.

PHEOCHROMOCYTOMA

It is a tumor of the adrenal medulla which produces catecholamines. The patients usually have severe headache, anxiety, increased sweating, tachycardia, palpitations and hypertensive episodes. The tumor is associated with a **'rule of 10's'** consisting of

- 10% are *bilateral*[Q]
- 10% are *extra-adrenal*[Q]
- 10% are *malignant*[Q]
- 10% occur in *children*[Q]
- 10% are not associated with hypertension[Q]

The tumor morphology shows the presence of small or large tumors that have yellow tan color that turns brown on incubation. There is presence of nests of chief or chromaffin cells with sustentacular cells (called **zellballen**[Q]) with abundant cytoplasm which contains catecholamine granules. The nuclei of the cells have **'salt and pepper'** appearance of the chromatin. The *immunomarkers* for this tumor include *chromogranin and synaptophysin in chief cells and S-100 for sustentacular cells.*

The definitive diagnosis of malignancy is based *exclusively on the presence of metastasis.*[Q]

The investigations reveal the presence of elevated urinary excretion of free catecholamines and their metabolites such as vanillylmandelic acid (VMA) and metanephrines.

Concept
In **secondary adrenocortical insufficiency disease**, the *hyperpigmentation* of primary Addison disease **is lacking** because melanotropic hormone levels are low.

Zellballen pattern is a feature of the **carotid body tumor** which is a prototype of **parasympathetic paraganglioma**.

Pheochromocytoma is 'rule of 10's' tumor.

Concept
Earlier, it was mentioned that 10% are familial but latest Robbins says "25% of the individuals with pheochromocytoma and paraganglioma have a germline mutation".

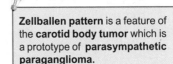

MEN III has three M
Medullary thyroid carcinoma
Medulla of adrenal (pheochromocytoma)
Mucosal neuroma

MEN II has two M (and one P)
Medullary thyroid carcinoma
Medulla of adrenal (pheochromocytoma)
Parathyroid hyperplasia

MEN I has three P
Pituiatry tumors
Pancreas tumors (insulinoma, gastrinoma)
Parathyroid tumors (hyperplasia)

Familial syndrome associated with pheochromocytoma

MEN IIA[Q]	MEN IIB/ MEN III[Q]	Sturge Weber syndrome[o]	Von Hippel Lindau syndrome[o]	Von Recklinghausen syndrome[o]
– Medullary thyroid cancer – Pheochromocytoma – Parathyroid hyperplasia	– Medullary thyroid cancer – Pheochromocytoma – Mucosal neuromas Marfanoid features	– Pheochromocytoma – Cavernous hemangioma of Vth cranial nerve distribution	– Pheochromocytoma – Renal cell cancer – Cerebellar hemangioblastoma – Angiomatosis – Renal, hepatic, pancreatic and epididymal cysts	– Pheochromocytoma – Neurofibromatosis – Cafe au lait skin spots[o] – Schwannoma, glioma; meningiomas

MULTIPLE CHOICE QUESTIONS

PANCREAS

1. Amylin is secreted by which group of cells of pancreas? *(All India 2012)*
   - (a) Alpha cells
   - (b) Beta cells
   - (c) D cells
   - (d) PP cells (Pancreatic polypeptide)

2. Diabetes is diagnosed by which of the following criteria? *(AIIMS Nov 2011)*
   - (a) The level of fasting glucose is ≥ 100 mg/dL and that of postprandial glucose is ≥ 140 mg/dL
   - (b) The level of fasting glucose is > 125 mg/dL and that of post prandial glucose is > 199 mg/dL
   - (c) The level of plasma insulin is ≥ 6 IU/dL
   - (d) The HbA1c level is ≥ 5.5%

3. All statements are true about Nesidioblastosis except?
   - (a) Hypoglycemic episodes are seen *(AI 2011)*
   - (b) Occurs more commonly in adults than in children
   - (c) Histopathology shows hyperplasia of Islet cells
   - (d) Diazoxide is used in treatment

4. Insulin increases glucose entry into skeletal muscle, adipose tissues and liver cells by: *(DPG 2011)*
   - (a) Increasing the number of glucose transporter GLUT2 in all these tissues
   - (b) Increasing the number of GLUT4 in muscle and adipose tissue and glucokinase in liver cells
   - (c) Increasing the number of GLUT3 in skeletal muscle and adipose tissues and GLUT4 in liver cells
   - (d) Increasing the number of GLUT1 in muscle, GLUT3 in adipose tissues and GLUT4 in liver cells

5. The term fetal adenoma is used for: *(UP 2003)*
   - (a) Hepatoma liver
   - (b) Fibroadenoma breast
   - (c) Follicular adenoma of thyroid
   - (d) Craniopharyngioma

6. Which of the following is used to measure control of blood sugar in diabetes mellitus? *(UP 2005)*
   - (a) HbA
   - (b) HbS
   - (c) HbA2
   - (d) HbA 1C

7. Two diabetic patients are seen by an endocrinologist, Dr. Saket. The first patient is a 16-year-old boy Raju who 2 years previously had presented with polyuria and polydipsia. The second patient is a 65-year-old woman Antara whose diabetes was identified by the presence of hyperglycemia on a routine blood glucose screen 10 years previously. Compared to Antara, Raju is more likely to
   - (a) Not have the HLA-DR3 or HLA-DR4 allele
   - (b) Become euglycemic with oral hypoglycemic agents
   - (c) Develop ketoacidosis
   - (d) Have relatively high endogenous insulin levels

8. A 62 year-old woman Omvati with advanced, metastatic lung cancer develops profound fatigue and weakness and alternating diarrhea and constipation. Physical examination demonstrates hyperpigmentation of skin, even in areas protected from the sun. Tumor involvement of which endocrine organ is most strongly suggested by this patient's presentation?
   - (a) Adrenal gland
   - (b) Endocrine pancreas
   - (c) Ovaries
   - (d) Pituitary gland

Most Recent Questions

8.1. Insulin resistance in liver disease is due to:
   - (a) Decreased insulin release
   - (b) Steatosis
   - (c) Hepatocyte dysfunction
   - (d) Decreased 'C' peptide level

8.2. According to ADA guidelines, the diagnosis of diabetes is made when the fasting blood glucose is more than
   - (a) 126 mg/dl
   - (b) 100 mg/dl
   - (c) 140 mg/dl
   - (d) 200 mg/dl

8.3. Mauriac's syndrome is characterized by all except
   - (a) Diabetes
   - (b) Obesity
   - (c) Dwarfism
   - (d) Cardiomegaly

8.4. Necrobiosis lipoidica is seen in
   - (a) Diabetes insipidus
   - (b) Lyme disease
   - (c) Diabetes mellitus
   - (d) Symmonds disease

THYROID, PARATHYROID

9. Which of the following term describes hyperthyroidism following intake of iodine in patients suffering from endemic goiter? *(All India 2012)*
   - (a) Wolff-Chaikoff effect
   - (b) Jod-Basedow effect
   - (c) Graves disease
   - (d) Hashimoto's thyroiditis

10. A 17 year old girl who was evaluated for short height was found to have an enlarged pituitary gland. Her T₄ was low and TSH was increased. Which of the following is the most likely diagnosis? *(AIIMS Nov 2011)*
    (a) Pituitary adenoma
    (b) TSH-secreting pituitary tumor
    (c) Thyroid target receptor insensitivity
    (d) Primary hypothyroidism

11. All are true about Hashimoto's thyroiditis except:
    (a) Follicular destruction   *(AIIMS Nov 2011)*
    (b) Lymphocytic infiltration
    (c) Oncocytic metaplasia
    (d) Orphan Annie eye nuclei

12. Hypothyroidism is seen in: *(AI 2011)*
    (a) Hashimoto's Thyroiditis
    (b) Graves' disease
    (c) Toxic Multinodular Goitre
    (d) Struma ovarii

13. All are true about Hashimoto's thyroiditis except:
    (a) Follicular destruction   *(AIIMS May 2010)*
    (b) Lymphocytic infiltration
    (c) Oncocytic metaplasia
    (d) Orphan Annie eye nuclei

14. MC thyroid cancer is: *(AI 2008)*
    (a) Papillary carcinoma
    (b) Follicular carcinoma
    (c) Medullary carcinoma
    (d) Anaplastic carcinoma

15. Which of the following gene defect is associated with development of medullary carcinoma of thyroid?
    (a) RET Proto-oncogene   *(AI 2004)*
    (b) FAP gene
    (c) Rb gene
    (d) BRCA 1 gene

16. Medullary carcinoma of the thyroid is associated with which of the following syndrome: `   *(AI 2003)*
    (a) MEN I
    (b) MEN II
    (c) Li-Fraumeni syndrome
    (d) Hashimoto's thyroiditis

17. The expression of the following oncogene is associated with a high incidence of medullary carcinoma of thyroid: *(AIIMS Nov 2005)*
    (a) p 53
    (b) Her 2 neu
    (c) RET proto oncogene
    (d) Rb gene

18. DeQuervain's thyroiditis is also known as:
    (a) Granulomatous thyroiditis   *(Delhi PG-2006)*
    (b) Struma lymphomatosa
    (c) Acute thyroiditis
    (d) Hashimoto thyroiditis

19. Hurthle cells are seen in: *(Delhi PG-2005)*
    (a) Granulomatous thyroid disease
    (b) Hashimoto's thyroiditis
    (c) Papillary carcinoma of thyroid
    (d) Thyroglossal cyst

20. Which of the following histological type of carcinoma thyroid most commonly metastasizes to lymph nodes?
    (a) Medullary   *(Delhi PG-2005)*
    (b) Anaplastic
    (c) Papillary
    (d) Follicular

21. Struma ovarii is composed entirely of
    (a) Mature thyroid tissue   *(Karnataka 2006)*
    (b) Immature-thyroid tissue
    (c) Primary ovarian carcinoid tissue
    (d) None of the above

22. Oncocytes are found in all of the following except:
    (a) Thyroid   *(DNB-2000, 2003, 2006, 2007)*
    (b) Pancreas
    (c) Pituitary
    (d) Pineal body
    (e) None of the above

23. Hurthle cells are seen in: *(DNB- 2000, 2005)*
    (a) Hashimoto's thyroiditis
    (b) Granulomatous thyroiditis
    (c) Carcinoma of thyroid
    (d) Acute thyroiditis

24. Calcitonin is a marker of thyroid: *(UP 2001)*
    (a) Papillary carcinoma
    (b) Medullary carcinoma
    (c) Anaplastic carcinoma
    (d) Adenocarcinoma

25. In Hashimoto's thyroiditis, there is infiltration of:
    (a) Macrophages   *(UP 2003)*
    (b) Neutrophils
    (c) Leukocytes
    (d) Eosinophils

26. Myasthenia gravis is associated with: *(UP 2006)*
    (a) Hypergammaglobulinemia
    (b) Thymoma
    (c) Squamous cell carcinoma
    (d) Hepatic adenoma

27. In MEN II B syndrome includes all except:
    (a) Hyperparathyroidism   *(UP 99, 2007)*
    (b) Marfanoid features
    (c) Medullary thyroid carcinoma
    (d) Pheochromocytoma

28. Plunging goiter is   *(RJ 2000)*
    (a) Solitary nodule
    (b) Colloid goiter
    (c) Retro-sternal goiter
    (d) Medullary ca

29. **All are parts of MEN-I except:** *(RJ 2006)*
    (a) Pituitary tumor
    (b) Parathyroid tumor
    (c) Pancreatic tumor
    (d) Medullary carcinoma of thyroid

30. **Psammoma bodies are seen in all except:**
    (a) Papillary carcinoma of thyroid *(AP 2002)*
    (b) Papillary adenoma of colon
    (c) Meningioma
    (d) Papillary cancer of the ovary

31. **Papillary carcinoma associated with aggressiveness are all except:** *(AP 2006)*
    (a) Follicular variant
    (b) Unencapsulated
    (c) Tall cell variant
    (d) Oxyphilic (Hurthle) cell type

32. **Which thyroid carcinoma is of C-Cell origin:**
    (a) Medullary carcinoma *(Kolkata 2003)*
    (b) Follicular carcinoma
    (c) Papillary carcinoma
    (d) Anaplastic carcinoma

33. **All of the following regarding thyroid carcinoma are true except:** *(Kolkata 2003)*
    (a) Prognosis of follicular carcinoma is worse than papillary carcinoma
    (b) Medullary carcinoma is autosomal recessive
    (c) Anaplastic carcinoma causes local invasion early
    (d) Medullary and papillary carcinoma both spread by lymphatic route

34. **Hurthle cell tumor is:** *(Kolkata 2005)*
    (a) Papillary carcinoma
    (b) Follicular carcinoma
    (c) Medullary carcinoma
    (d) Colloid carcinoma
    (e) Ionizing radiation in early decades is a major risk factor

35. **About papillary carcinoma of thyroid, all are true except:** *(Kolkata 2005)*
    (a) Prognosis better
    (b) Psammoma body present in 50% cases
    (c) Early metastasis with poor prognosis
    (d) Spreads by the lymphatic route

36. **A 51-year-old man Sonu with a history of recurrent calcium-containing renal stones presents to the emergency room with excruciating flank pain and blood in the urine. This patient is likely to have which of the following underlying disorders?**
    (a) Anemia of chronic disease
    (b) Chronic Proteus infection
    (c) Hyperparathyroidism
    (d) Hyperaldosteronism

Most Recent Questions

36.1. **Most common thyroid cancer after radiation exposure is:**
    (a) Papillary cancer
    (b) Medullary cancer
    (c) Follicular cancer
    (d) Anaplastic cancer

36.2. **Medullary carcinoma of the thyroid is associated with which of the following syndrome:**
    (a) MEN I
    (b) MEN II
    (c) Fraumeni syndrome
    (d) Hashimoto's thyroiditis

36.3. **Which thyroid carcinoma has amyloid?**
    (a) Papillary   (b) Follicular
    (c) Medullary   (d) Anaplastic

36.4. **Which is not seen in MEN I:**
    (a) Parathyroid adenoma
    (b) Pancreatic cancer
    (c) Prolactinoma
    (d) Medullary carcinoma thyroid

36.5. **Werner syndrome is:**
    (a) MEN I   (b) MEN IIA
    (c) MEN IIB   (d) AIP

36.6. **Orphan Annie eye nuclei appearance is characteristic of:**
    (a) Papillary carcinoma thyroid
    (b) Carcinoma pituitary
    (c) Paraganglioma
    (d) Meningioma

36.7. **The laboratory screening test which suggests normal thyroid function is**
    (a) TSH   (b) Free T4
    (c) T3   (d) Free T3

36.8. **Psammoma bodies are seen in?**
    (a) Papillary carcinoma thyroid
    (b) Medullary carcinoma thyroid
    (c) Follicular carcinoma thyroid
    (d) Anaplastic carcinoma

▎ PITUITARY

37. **Which of the following is true about pituitary tumor?**
    (a) It present in 10% of brain tumors. *(PGI Dec 2005)*
    (b) Erodes the sella and extends into surrounding area
    (c) Prolactinoma is least common
    (d) It is differentiated by reticulin stain

▎ ADRENAL GLAND

38. **Addison's disease was first reported by Thomas Addison. It is still being widely reported from various**

parts of the world/throughout the world. Which of the following is the most common cause of Addison's disease in India? *(AIIMS Nov 2011)*
- (a) Post-partum pituitary insufficiency
- (b) Tuberculous adrenalitis
- (c) HIV
- (d) Autoimmune adrenal insufficiency

39. All are true statements about pheochromocytoma except? *(AI 2011)*
- (a) 90% are malignant
- (b) 95% occur in the abdomen
- (c) They secrete catecholamines
- (d) They arise from sympathetic ganglia

40. All the following familial syndromes are associated with development of pheochromocytomas except:
- (a) Sturge-Weber syndrome *(AIIMS Nov 2002)*
- (b) Von Recklinghausen disease
- (c) MEN type II
- (d) Prader-Willi syndrome

41. The most common cause of Addison's disease is:
- (a) Autoimmune adrenalitis *(AIIMS May 2002)*
- (b) Meningococcal septicemia
- (c) Malignancy
- (d) Tuberculosis

42. Most important histopathological indicator of malignancy in Pheochromocytoma is:
- (a) Pleomorphism *(Delhi PG-2005)*
- (b) High mitotic activity
- (c) Vascular invasion
- (d) None

43. Which of the following is most often involved in multiple endocrine neoplasia I: *(DNB- 2007)*
- (a) Pituitary
- (b) Pancreas
- (c) Parathyroid
- (d) Thyroid

44. All are true about pheochromocytoma except:
- (a) 25% are malignant *(UP 2002)*
- (b) Variety of APUDOMA
- (c) Histological type is chromaffin cells
- (d) Most common neuroendocrine hormone secreting tumor

45. In Cushing syndrome, the tumor is associated with
- (a) Increased level of epinephrine *(UP 2004)*
- (b) Decreased level of epinephrine
- (c) Elevated levels of cortisol
- (d) Increased level of norepinephrine

46. Vanillylmandelic acid (VMA) is increased in
- (a) Hyperparathyroidism *(UP 2008)*
- (b) Pheochromocytoma
- (c) MEN-I
- (d) Addison's disease

47. Most common cause of Cushing's syndrome is
- (a) Exogenous corticosteroids *(RJ 2002)*
- (b) Pituitary tumor
- (c) Adrenal adenoma
- (d) Adrenal carcinoma

48. Submucosal neuroma is associated with: *(AP 2004)*
- (a) MEN I
- (b) MEN II A
- (c) MEN II B
- (d) None of the above

49. Most common site of pheochromocytoma after adrenal gland is: *(AP 2005)*
- (a) Hilum of kidney
- (b) Organs of Zuckerkandl
- (c) Neck
- (d) Urinary bladder

50. True about adrenal pheochromocytoma is: *(AP 2006)*
- (a) Chromaffin negative
- (b) Mostly malignant
- (c) Bilateral in 10% of cases
- (d) Unilateral in 10% of cases

51. Most common cause of Cushing's syndrome is:
- (a) Pituitary adenoma *(AP 2006)*
- (b) Adrenal adenoma
- (c) Exogenous steroids
- (d) Ectopic ACTH

52. Which of the following is not estrogen dependant carcinoma: *(Kolkata 2003)*
- (a) Lobular carcinoma breast
- (b) Follicular thyroid carcinoma
- (c) Endometrial leiomyosarcoma
- (d) Carcinoma prostate

53. A 40-year old man with central obesity, "buffalo hump" and vertical purple striae on the abdomen has fasting blood glucose is in the high normal range. Plasma levels of ACTH and cortisol are both increased compared to normal. An overnight high-dose dexamethasone test produces 75% suppression of cortisol levels. This patient most likely has
- (a) Addison's disease
- (b) an ectopic ACTH-secreting tumor
- (c) Conn's syndrome
- (d) Cushing's disease

Most Recent Questions

53.1. Tumor that follows rule of 10 is:
- (a) Pheochromocytoma
- (b) Oncocytoma
- (c) Lymphoma
- (d) Renal cell carcinoma

53.2. Ectopic pheochromocytoma may originate from which of the following?
- (a) Organ of Zuckerkandl
- (b) Bladder
- (c) Filum terminale
- (d) Meckel diveticulum

53.3. Which one of the following is not seen in pheochromocytoma?
- (a) Hypertension
- (b) Episodic palpitations
- (c) Weight loss
- (d) Diarrhea

53.4. In Conn's syndrome, all the following are seen, except
 (a) Hypokalemia (b) Hypernatremia
 (c) Hypertension (d) Edema

53.5. Dilutional hyponatremia is seen in:
 (a) Addison's disease
 (b) Diabetes insipidus
 (c) Diuretic therapy
 (d) None

ASSERTION AND REASON QUESTIONS

1–10. Will have two statements, assertion and reason. Read both of them carefully and answer according to these options.
 (a) Both assertion and reason are true and reason is correct explanation of assertion.
 (b) Both assertion and reason are true and reason is not the correct explanation of assertion.
 (c) Assertion is true and reason is false.
 (d) Both assertion and reason are false.

1. **Assertion:** C peptide levels are used as a surrogate marker for insulin secretion
 Reason: C peptide and insulin are secreted in equal amounts after β cell stimulation

2. **Assertion:** Pheochromocytoma is also referred to as 'rule of 10 tumor'
 Reason: Pheochromocytoma is seen in 10% familial cases

3. **Assertion:** FNAC is not useful for diagnosing follicular thyroid cancer
 Reason: Capsular invasion is the definitive feature differentiating follicular adenoma from follicular carcinoma

4. **Assertion:** Postpartum thyroiditis presents as a painful enlarged thyroid gland
 Reason: Postpartum thyroiditis is preceded by a viral infection (measles, mumps etc)

5. **Assertion:** Graves disease is most common cause of endogenous hyperthyroidism.
 Reason: Autoantibodies like TBIG may lead to reduced thyroid function

6. **Assertion:** Myocardial infarction is the commonest cause of death in diabetes
 Reason: Uncontrolled blood glucose leads to capillary dysfunction in target organs

7. **Assertion:** Skin hyperpigmentation is a feature of Addison's disease
 Reason: ACTH precursor has amino acid sequence similar to melanocyte stimulating hormone.

8. **Assertion:** Non ketotic hyperosmolar is a commoner complication than diabetic ketoacidosis in type 2 diabetes.
 Reason: Insulin has a 'fat sparing effect' preventing fatty acid oxidation.

9. **Assertion:** MEN 2A (Sipple syndrome) is characterized by pheochromocytoma, medullary carcinoma of thyroid and parathyroid hyperplasia.
 Reason: MEN 2A is associated with a loss of function mutation in RET proto-oncogene

10. **Assertion:** Amyloid deposition is associated with medullary variant of thyroid cancer
 Reason–T he altered cacitonin secreted by parafollicular cells gets deposited in the thyroid stroma

Endocrine System

EXPLANATIONS

1. **Ans. (b) Beta cells** *(Ref: Robbins 9/e p446, 8th/442, 1130)*
   - *Amylin is secreted by β cells of the pancreas. It reduces food intake and weight gain* by acting on central neurons in the hypothalamus.

2. **Ans. (b) The level of fasting glucose is > 125 mg/dL and that of post prandial glucose is > 199 mg/dL** *(Ref: Harrison 18th/2970, Robbin 9/e p1106)*

3. **Ans. (b) More common in adults than in children** *(Ref: Nelson Pediatrics 18th/660-662; Robbins, 9/e p1121)*
   - **Congenital hyperinsulinism** was formerly termed as Nesidioblastosis.
   - It is also known as *diffuse Islet cell hyperplasia*.
   - It can occur in adults also but **more commonly seen in neonates and children**.
   - Hypoglycemic episodes occur due hyperinsulinemia.
   - Medical management includes *Frequent feedings, Diazoxide and Somatostatin*.

4. **Ans. (b) Increasing the number of GLUT4 in muscle and adipose tissue and glucokinase in liver cells** *(Ref: Harrison 17th/2278-9, 2282 Robbins 8th/1134, 9/e p1112)*
   Insulin acts by binding to its receptor and stimulating intrinsic tyrosine kinase activity, leading to receptor autophosphorylation and the recruitment of intracellular signaling molecules, such as insulin receptor substrates (IRS). Activation of the phosphatidylinositol-3'-kinase (PI-3-kinase) pathway stimulates translocation of glucose transporters (e.g., **GLUT4**) to the cell surface, an event that is **crucial for glucose uptake by skeletal muscle and fat.** Activation of other insulin receptor signaling pathways induces glycogen synthesis, protein synthesis, lipogenesis, and regulation of various genes in insulin-responsive cells.

   Glucokinase catalyzes the formation of glucose-6-phosphate from glucose, a reaction that is **important for** glucose sensing by the beta cells and for **glucose utilization by the liver.** As a result of glucokinase mutations, higher glucose levels are required to elicit insulin secretory responses, thus altering the set point for insulin secretion, responsible for Maturity Onset Diabetes of Young-1 (MODY-1).

5. **Ans. (c) Follicular adenoma of thyroid** *(Ref: Robbins 9/e p1093, 8th/1118; 7th/1175, Harsh Mohan 6th/810)*

6. **Ans. (d) HbA 1C** *(Ref: Robbins 8th/1138, 9/e p1115)*

7. **Ans. (c) Develop ketoacidosis** *(Ref: Robbins 8th/1145, 9/e p1113-1114)*
   Raju probably has type 1 (juvenile onset) diabetes mellitus, while Antara probably has type 2 (maturity onset) diabetes mellitus. These two types of diabetes differ in many respects. Ketoacidosis is more likely to develop in type 1 diabetes.
   Type 1 diabetes has a strong association with HLA-DR3 and HLA-DR4 (option A), while type 2 does not have any strong HLA associations.
   Type 1 is usually apparently due to viral or immune destruction of beta cells, while type 2 is apparently usually due to increased resistance to insulin; consequently the 65-year-old, rather than the 16-year-old, is more likely to have relatively high endogenous levels of insulin (option D).
   Type 2 diabetes can often be controlled with oral hypoglycemic agents (option B), while type 1 diabetics generally require insulin. Note that some type 2 diabetics also may require insulin as the disease evolves.

8. **Ans. (a) Adrenal gland** *(Ref: Robbins 8th/1156-1157, 9/e p1130-11131)*
   This is Addison disease, in which severe adrenal disease produces adrenocortical insufficiency. Causes include autoimmune destruction, congenital adrenal hyperplasia, hemorrhagic necrosis, and replacement of the glands by either tumor (usually metastatic) or granulomatous disease (usually tuberculosis). The symptoms can be subtle and nonspecific (such as those illustrated), so a high clinical index of suspicion is warranted. Skin hyperpigmentation is a specific clue that may be present on physical examination, suggesting excess pituitary ACTH secretion. (The ACTH precursor has an amino acid sequence similar to MSH, melanocyte stimulating hormone.) Most patients have symptoms (fatigue, gastrointestinal distress) related principally to glucocorticoid deficiency. In some cases, however, mineralocorticoid replacement may also be needed for symptoms of salt wasting with lower circulating volume.

   - Except in the case of primary pancreatic cancer, complete tumor replacement of the endocrine pancreas (option B) would be uncommon. In any event, pancreatic involvement would be associated with diabetes mellitus.
   - Involvement of the ovaries (option C) by metastatic tumor (classically gastric adenocarcinoma) would produce failure of menstruation.
   - Involvement of the pituitary gland (option D) could produce Addisonian symptoms, but the pigmented skin suggests a primary adrenal problem rather than pituitary involvement.

8.1. Ans. (b) Steatosis *(Ref: Robbin 8/e p1136, Joslin's Diabetes Mellitus 14/e p436)*

Insulin resistance is defined as the failure of target tissues to respond normally to insulin. It leads to decreased uptake of glucose in muscle, reduced glycolysis and fatty acid oxidation in the liver, and an inability to suppress hepatic gluconeogenesis.

- The *loss of insulin sensitivity in the hepatocytes is likely to be the largest contributor to the pathogenesis of insulin resistance in vivo.*
- *Obesity* is the most important factor in the *development of insulin resistance.*

"*In type 2 diabetes patients, the presence of hepatic steatosis is associated with reduced insulin stimulated glucose uptake. Increased hepatic fat accumulation results in impaired peripheral insulin action*"....Joslin pg 436

8.2. Ans. (a) 126 mg/dl *(Ref: Robbins 9th/1106)*

8.3. Ans. (a) Diabetes *(Ref: internet)*

Mauriac syndrome is a rare complication of type 1 diabetes mellitus in children associated with hepatomegaly, growth impairment and cushingoid features.

8.4. Ans. (c) Diabetes mellitus *(Ref: Harrison 18th/chapter 53)*

Lesions of *necrobiosis lipoidica* are found primarily on the shins (90%), and patients can have *diabetes mellitus* or develop it subsequently. Characteristic findings include a central yellow color, atrophy (transparency), telangiectasias, and a red to red-brown border. Ulcerations can also develop within the plaques. Biopsy specimens show necrobiosis of collagen and granulomatous inflammation.

9. Ans. (b) Jod-Basedow effect *(Ref: Harrison 18th/2930, 2932)*

- **Jod Basedow effect** is characterized by **excessive thyroid hormone synthesis** caused by increased iodine exposure.
- **Wolff Chaikoff effect** is **iodide dependent suppression** of the thyroid.

10. Ans. (d) Primary hypothyroidism *(Ref: Robbins 8th/1109-1110, 9/e p1083-5)*

Analyzing all options,

- In pituitary adenoma/TSH secreting pituitary tumor increased TSH with increased T3/4 would be seen. (excludes 'a' and 'b')
- In thyroid hormone resistance *increased T_4 as well as T_3* with *low TSH* will be seen. (option 'c' excluded)
- **Primary hypothyroidism** is due to defect in the thyroid gland itself. This is associated with *high TSH with low T_4* will be seen.

11. Ans. (d) Orphan Annie eye nuclei *(Ref: Robbins 8th/1111, 9th/1087)*

Robbins writes…'The nuclei of **papillary carcinoma** cells contain finely dispersed chromatin, which imparts an optically clear or empty appearance, giving rise to the designation ground-glass or *Orphan Annie eye nuclei*'.

Salient features of Hashimoto Thyroiditis (Chronic Lymphocytic Thyroiditis)

Most common type of thyroiditis[Q] *Most common cause of hypothyroidism in areas having sufficient iodine levels.*
Genetic association
Associated with HLA-DR5, HLA-DR3 and chromosomal defects like Turner and Down syndrome.
Gland morphology
Diffusely enlarged gland with *intact capsule*.
Microscopic finding
Presence of *well developed germinal centers* and extensive lymphocytic infiltration
Atrophied[Q] thyroid follicles lined by epithelial cells having abundant eosinophilic and granular cytoplasm called **Hurthle cells**.[Q] (this is a metaplastic response of epithelium to the ongoing injury)
Chronic inflammation with lymphocytic infiltration[Q] of the thyroid gland (the latter responsible for the term '*struma lymphomatosa*').
Clinical findings
Painless enlargement of thyroid gland in a middle aged female. Associated with type 1 diabetes, SLE, Sjogren syndrome, myasthenia gravis, increased risk of B cell lymphoma

Endocrine System

12. **Ans. (a) Hashimoto's thyroiditis** *(Ref: Harrison 17th/2230, Robbins 9th/1087)*
Hashimoto's thyroiditis is a cause of hypothyroidism whereas other diseases mentioned like Graves' disease, toxic Multinodular goiter and struma ovarii result in hyperthyroidism.

Causes of Hypothyroidism
• Autoimmune hypothyroidism: **Hashimoto's thyroiditis**, atrophic thyroiditis
• Iatrogenic: ^{131}I treatment, subtotal or total thyroidectomy, external irradiation of neck for lymphoma or cancer
• Drugs: iodine excess (including iodine-containing contrast media and amiodarone), lithium, antithyroid drugs, *p*-aminosalicyclic acid, interferon-alpha and other cytokines, aminoglutethimide
• Congenital hypothyroidism: absent or ectopic thyroid gland, dyshormonogenesis, TSH-R mutation
• Iodine deficiency
• Infiltrative disorders: amyloidosis, sarcoidosis, hemochromatosis, scleroderma, cystinosis, Riedel's thyroiditis

Causes of hyperthyroidism
• Graves' disease
• Toxic multinodular goiter
• Toxic adenoma
• Functioning thyroid carcinoma metastases
• Activating mutation of the TSH receptor
• Activating mutation of G_{sa} (McCune-Albright syndrome)
• Struma ovarii
• Drugs: iodine excess (Jod-Basedow phenomenon)

13. **Ans. (d) Orphan Annie eye nuclei** *(Ref: Robbins 8th/1111, 9/e p1096)*
Robbins writes…'The nuclei of **papillary carcinoma** cells contain finely dispersed chromatin, which imparts an optically clear or empty appearance, giving rise to the designation ground-glass or *Orphan Annie eye nuclei'*.

14. **Ans. (a) Papillary carcinoma** *(Ref: Robbins 7th/735-736, 9/e p1095)*

15. **Ans. (a) RET proto-oncogene** *(Ref: Harrison's 17th/2361, Robbins 7th/1182, 9/e p1095)*
    - Medullary carcinoma of thyroid (MCT) pheochromocytoma and hyperparathyroidism are present in MEN-2A whereas the association of MCT, pheochromocytoma, mucosal neuroma and Marfanoid habitus is designated MEN-2B.
    - Most patients of MEN-2 have mutations of RET-proto-oncogene.
    - This gene is located on chromosome 10q11.2.
    - Most common germline mutation of RET is at codon 634 and is associated mostly with MEN 2A.
    - Most common somatic mutation of RET is at codon 918 and is mostly associated with MEN 2B.
    - Other genes given in the question can be remembered from their name only:
        – FAP: Familial adenomatous polyposis
        – Rb: Retinoblastoma
        – BRCA1: Breast cancer

16. **Ans. (b) MEN II** *(Ref: Robbins 7th/1222, 9/e p1099)*
Multiple endocrine neoplasia (MEN) syndromes are a group of genetically inherited diseases resulting in proliferative lesions (hyperplasia, adenoma and carcinoma) of multiple endocrine glands.

MEN I (Wermer's Syndrome)	MEN II A (Sipple's syndrome)	MEN II B
• Parathyroid hyperplasia/adenoma	• Parathyroid hyperplasia/adenoma	• Medullary carcinoma of thyroid
• Pancreatic islet cell hyperplasia/adenoma/ carcinoma	• Medullary carcinoma of thyroid	• Pheochromocytoma
• Pituitary hyperplasia/adenoma	• Pheochromocytoma	• Mucosal and gastrointestinal neuromas
• *Mutant gene is MEN 1*	• *Mutant gene is RET*	• Marfanoid features
		• *Mutant gene is RET*

17. **Ans. (c) RET proto-oncogene** *(Ref: Robbins 7th/294, 295, 9/e 1099)*
RET proto-oncogene is mutated in MEN-2A and MEN-2B syndromes. These are associated with medullary carcinoma of thyroid.

18. **Ans. (a) Granulomatous thyroiditis** *(Ref: Robbins 7th/1170, 9/e p1088)*
    - DeQuervain's thyroiditis is also referred to as granulomatous thyroiditis or subacute thyroiditis. *(For details, see text)*

19. **Ans. (b) Hashimoto's thyroiditis** *(Ref: Robbins 7th/1169, 76, 81, 9/e p1087)*
    - Hurthle cells (Oncocytes) are epithelial cells with abundant eosinophilic, granular cytoplasm.
    - Hurthle cells are seen in following conditions:

        – Hashimoto's thyroiditis
        – Hurthle cell adenoma of thyroid
        – Hurthle cell carcinoma of thyroid

- Hurthle cells are eosinophilic due to abundance of mitochondria.
- Hurthle cells are also called *Ashkanazy* cells or *oxyphil cells.*

20. **Ans. (c) Papillary** *(Ref: Robbins 7th/1180, 9/e p1097)*
    - Most papillary carcinoma present as asymptomatic thyroid nodules, but the first manifestation may be a mass in cervical nodes.
    - Follicular carcinoma has little propensity for lymphatics but high for vascular invasion and spreads to bones, lungs and CNS.
    - In anaplastic Ca direct spread (extensive local invasion) is more common than vascular.

21. **Ans. (a) Mature thyroid tissue** *(Ref: Robbins 7th/1100, 9/e p1030)*
    Struma ovarii is a specialized teratoma which is always unilateral and is composed of mature thyroid tissue. It may manifest itself with the features of hyperthyroidism.

22. **Ans. (d) Pineal body** *(Ref: Internet)*
    Oncocytes are large cells with small irregular nuclei and dense acidophilic granules due to the presence of abundant mitochondria. These are found in oncocytomas of the kidney, salivary glands, and endocrine glands (thyroid, parathyroid, pituitary, adrenal cortex and pancreatic islets).

23. **Ans. (a) Hashimoto's thyroiditis** *(Ref: Robbins 8th/1112, 9/e p1087)*

24. **Ans. (b) Medullary carcinoma** *(Ref: Robbins 9/e p1099, 8th/1125; 7th/1178)*

25. **Ans. (c) Leucocytes** *(Ref: Robbins 9/e p1087, 8th/1112; 7th/1169-1170)*

26. **Ans. (b) Thymoma** *(Ref: Robbins 8th/636-637, 9/e p1236)*

27. **Ans. (a) Hyperparathyroidism** *(Ref: Robbins 9/e p1136-1137, 8th/1162; 7th/1222)*

28. **Ans. (c) Retro-sternal goiter** *(Ref: Robbins 8th/1117, 9/e p1092)*

29. **Ans. (d) Medullary carcinoma of thyroid** *(Ref: Robbins 8th/1162, 9/e p1136)*

30. **Ans. (b) Papillary adenoma of colon** *(Ref: Robbins 9/e p1096, 1314, 1025, 8th/38,1122; 7th/859)*

31. **Ans. (a) Follicular variant** *(Ref: Robbins 9/e p1096-1097, 8th/1120-1122; 7th/1179)*

32. **Ans. (a) Medullary carcinoma** *(Ref. Robbins 8th/1121, 9/e p1099)*

33. **Ans. (b) Medullary carcinoma is autosomal recessive** *(Ref. Robbins 8th/1124-1126, 9/e p1095)*

34. **Ans. (b) Follicular carcinoma** *(Ref: Robbins 8th/1123, 9/e p1098)*

35. **Ans. (c) Early metastasis with poor prognosis** *(Ref: Robbins 8th/1121-1122, 9/e 1097)*

36. **Ans. (c) Hyperparathyroidism** *(Ref: Robbins 8th/962, 9/e p1103)*
    The patient's history of recurrent urolithiasis with calcium-containing stones implies a disorder in the regulation of calcium concentration. Hyperparathyroidism is associated with increased parathormone (PTH) levels, which can produce hypercalcemia, hypercalciuria, and, ultimately, renal stones.
    Anemia of chronic disease (option A) does not produce calcium stones. The patient presents with a chronic condition and hematuria but the urinary blood loss is not usually significant enough to produce an anemic state.
    Hyperaldosteronism (option D) results in potassium depletion, sodium retention, and hypertension. *Primary hyperaldosteronism (Conn's syndrome)* is associated with adrenocortical adenomas in 90% of patients and is characterized by *decreased renin.* **Secondary hyperaldosteronism** results from excessive stimulation by angiotensin II that is caused by **excess renin production** (plasma renin-angiotensin levels are high). Neither condition is associated with renal stones.

36.1. **Ans. (a) Papillary cancer** *(Ref: Robbins 8/e p1121, 9/e p1095)*
    - There is a marked increase in the incidence of **papillary carcinomas** among children exposed to **ionizing radiation** (particularly during the first 2 decades of life).
    - *Deficiency of dietary iodine* (and so, goiter) is linked with a higher frequency of **follicular carcinomas.**

36.2. **Ans. (b) MEN II** *(Ref: Robbins 8/e p1162, 9/e p1137)*
    - *MEN-2A,* or *Sipple syndrome,* is characterized by *pheochromocytoma, medullary carcinoma,* and *parathyroid hyperplasia.*
    - *MEN-2B* has significant clinical overlap with MEN-2A. Patients develop medullary thyroid carcinomas, which are usually multifocal and more aggressive than in MEN-2A, and pheochromocytomas. However, unlike in MEN-2A, *primary hyperparathyroidism is not present*

Endocrine System

36.3. **Ans. (c) Medullary** *(Ref: Robbins 8/e p1125, 9/e p1099)*
Acellular **amyloid deposits**, derived from altered calcitonin polypeptides, are present in the adjacent stroma in many cases of medullary thyroid cancer.

36.4. **Ans. (d) Medullary carcinoma thyroid** *(Ref: Robbins 8/e p1162, 9/e p1136)*
MEN-1, or *Wermer syndrome*, is characterized by abnormalities involving the *parathyroid, pancreas*, and *pituitary glands*; thus the mnemonic device, the *3Ps*

- *Parathyroid: Primary hyperparathyroidism* is the most common manifestation of MEN-1
- *Pancreas: Endocrine tumors of the pancreas* like gastrinomas associated with Zollinger-Ellison syndrome and insulinomas
- *Pituitary:* The most frequent anterior pituitary tumor encountered in MEN-1 is a *prolactinoma.*

36.5. **Ans. (a) MEN I....see earlier explanation......** *(Ref: Robbins 8/e p1162, 9/e p1136)*

36.6. **Ans. (a) Papillary carcinoma thyroid** *(Ref: Robbins 8/e p1122, 9/e p1096)*
- The nuclei of papillary carcinoma cells contain finely dispersed chromatin, which imparts an **optically clear** or **empty** appearance, giving rise to the designation **ground-glass** or **Orphan Annie eye nuclei.**

36.7. **Ans. (a) TSH** *(Ref: Robbins 9th /1083)*

36.8. **Ans.(a) Papillary carcinoma thyroid** *(Ref: Robbins 9th /1096)*

37. **Ans. (a) It is present in 10% of brain tumors; (b) Erodes the sella and extends into surrounding area (c) It is differentiated by reticulin stain;** *(Ref: Harrison 16th/208I; Robbins 7th/1159; 9/e p1075, Brains Neurology 11th/558)*
- 10% of all intracranial neoplasms are pituitary tumors.
- Benign adenomas are most common.
- The most common pituitary adenoma is microadenoma and about 70% microadenomas are prolactinoma.
- The tumor can erode the sella and extends into surrounding area and gives rise to local mass effect.
- Cellular monomorphism and absence of significant reticulin network distinguishes pituitary adenomas from non-neoplastic anterior pituitary parenchyma.

38. **Ans. (b) Tuberculous adrenalitis** *(Ref: Robbins 9/e p1130, 8th/1155-6, API 7th/1073, Harrison 18th/2955)*
The commonest cause of Addison's disease is as follows:
- In **developing** countries – **Tuberculosis**^{Q}
- In *developed countries – Autoimmune (Idiopathic atrophy)*^{Q}

39. **Ans. (a) 90% are malignant** *(Ref: Robbins 8th/1159, 9/e p1134)*
Pheochromocytoma is a tumor of the adrenal medulla which produces catecholamines. The patients usually have severe headache, anxiety, increased sweating, tachycardia, palpitations and hypertensive episodes.
Features of 'rule of 10's'in pheochromocytoma

- 10% are *bilateral*^{Q}
- 10% are *extra-adrenal*^{Q}
- 10% are *malignant* ^{Q}
- 10% occur in *children* ^{Q}
- 10% are not associated with hypertension ^{Q}

Please note

Earlier, it was mentioned that 10% are pheochromocytoma *are familial*^{Q} but latest Robbins says "**25% of the individuals with pheochromocytoma and paraganglioma have a germline mutation**"

40. **Ans. (d) Prader Willi syndrome** *(Ref: Robbins's illustrated 7th/1219, 9/e p1134)*
Pheochromocytoma is associated with the following familial syndromes.
- MEN syndromes type II and type III
- Von Hippel Lindau syndrome
- Von Recklinghausen disease
- Sturge Weber syndrome Famibial paraganglioma 1/3/4

41. **Ans. (a) Autoimmune adrenalitis** *(Ref: Harrison, 17th/2263, Robbins 9/e p1134)*
Addison's disease must involve >90% of the glands before adrenal insufficiency develops.
Idiopathic atrophy due to autoimmune adrenalitis is the most common cause of Addison's disease in the worldwhereas tuberculosis is the most common cause of the same in India.

42. **Ans. (d) None** *(Ref: Robbins 7th/1221, 9th/1135)*
- The histological pattern in pheochromocytoma is quite variable. The tumors are composed of polygonal to spindle-shaped chromaffin cells, clustered with their supporting cells into small nests or alveoli (*Zellballen*), by a rich vascular network.

- Cellular and nuclear pleomorphism is often present, especially in the alveolar group of lesions and giant and bizarre cells are commonly seen.
  Mitotic figures are rare and do not imply malignancy.
  Both capsular and vascular invasion may be encountered in benign lesions. Therefore the diagnosis of malignancy in pheochromocytoma is based exclusively on the presence of metastases. These may involve regional lymph nodes as well as more distant sites, including liver, lung and bone.

43. Ans. (c) Parathyroid *(Ref: Robbins 8th/1161-1162, 9/e p1136)*

44. Ans. (a) 25% are malignant *(Ref: Robbins 9/e p1134, 8th/1159-1160; 7th/1219)*

45. Ans. (c) Elevated levels of cortisol *(Ref: Robbins 9/e p1125, 8th/1150; 7th/1207)*

46. Ans. (b) Pheochromocytoma *(Ref: Robbins 8th/1161, 9/e p1136)*

47. Ans. (a) Exogenous corticosteroids *(Ref: Robbins 8th/1148, 9/e p1125)*

48. Ans. (c) MEN II B *(Ref: Robbins 9/e p1137, 8th/1163; 7th/1222)*

49. Ans. (b) Organs of Zuckerkandl *(Ref: Robbins 9/e p1134, 8th/1159-1161; 7th/1221)*

50. Ans. (c) Bilateral in 10% of cases *(Ref: Robbins 9/e p1134, 8th/1159-1161; 7th/1219)*

51. Ans. (c) Exogenous steroids *(Ref: Robbins 9/e p1125, 8th/1148; 7th/1207)*

52. Ans. (b) Follicular thyroid carcinoma *(Ref: Robbins 8th/1120-1121, 9/e p1095)*

53. Ans. (d) Cushing's disease *(Ref: Robbins 8th/1148-1150, 9/e p1125)*
This patient presents with "Cushingoid" signs and symptoms due to hypercortisolism. While the acute effect of cortisol is to produce lipolysis, patients with chronically increased cortisol levels develop a characteristic central obesity and buffalo hump. The mechanism for the redistribution of body fat is an interaction between cortisol and insulin. The weight gain with hypercortisolism usually results from increased appetite. Cortisol excess causes protein catabolism, which leads to poor wound healing, decreased connective tissue, and fragile blood vessels. The combination of thin skin and fragile blood vessels leads to abdominal stretch marks (striae) the are characteristically purple in color. Increased gluconeogenesis and decreased peripheral insulin sensitivity lead to elevated blood glucose. The hypercortisolism due to a functional tumor in the adrenal cortex (primary hypercortisolism) has low plasma ACTH level.

> - The patient in the question has increased cortisol and increased ACTH. This could result from either a functional ACTH-secreting tumor in the pituitary (Cushing's disease) or an ectopic tumor (such as a small cell carcinoma of the lung, choice B). To distinguish between these two, we administer high doses of the potent synthetic glucocorticoid, dexamethasone. High-dose dexamethasone should suppress ACTH secretion from the pituitary by at least 50%; secretion from an ectopic tumor typically is not suppressed by dexamethasone.
> - Addison's disease (choice A) is primary adrenal insufficiency, with increased plasma ACTH (producing hyperpigmentation) and decreased plasma cortisol and aldosterone compared to normal.
> - Conn's syndrome (choice C) results from hypersecretion of aldosterone by the adrenal cortex. In Cushing's disease, it is due in part to the mineralocorticoid-like effects of high plasma cortisol.

53.1. Ans. (a) Pheochromocytoma...discussed earlier in detail. *(Ref: Robbins 9/e p1134, 8/e p524-5)*

53.2. Ans. (a) Organ of Zuckerkandl *(Ref: Robbins 9th/1134)*
Ten percent of pheochromocytomas are extra-adrenal, occurring in sites such as the organs of Zuckerkandl and the carotid body.

53.3. Ans. (d) Diarrhea *(Ref: Robbins 9th/1135, Harrison 18th/2963)*
The dominant clinical manifestation of pheochromocytoma is hypertension, observed in 90% of patients. Approximately two thirds of patients with hypertension demonstrate paroxysmal episodes, which are described as an abrupt, precipitous elevation in blood pressure, associated with tachycardia, palpitations, headache, sweating, tremor, and a sense of apprehension.

53.4. Ans. (c) Hypernatremia > (d) Edema *(Ref: Sircar pg 532, Harrison 18th/2950)*
Harrison mentions that.... "The clinical hallmark of mineralocorticoid excess is hypokalemic hypertension; serum sodium tends to be normal due to the concurrent fluid retention, which in some cases can lead to peripheral edema".
Sircar Physiology writes.... Edema is not seen because of the escape mechanism: escape from the sodium retaining effects of hyperaldosteronism.

53.5. Ans. (b) Diabetes insipidus
Please don't get confused with the diuretic therapy because it can lead to increased ADH release and thus, may lead to hyponatremia.

EXPLANATIONS TO ASSERTION AND REASON QUESTIONS

Explanations(1-10): *While solving assertion reason type of questions, we can use a particular method.*

1. First of all, read both assertion (A) and reason (R) carefully and independently analyse whether they are true or false.
2. If A is false, the answere will directly be (d) i.e. both A and R are false. You can note that all other options (i.e. a, b or c) consider A to be true.
3. If A is true, answer can be (a), (b) or (c), Now look at R. If R is false, answer will be (c)
4. If both A and R are ture, then we have to know whether R is correctly explaining A [answer is (a)] or it is not the explanation of assertion [answer is (b)]

1. **Ans. (a) Both assertion and reason are true and reason is correct explanation of assertion.** *(Ref: Robbins 8th/1133, 9/e p1108)*
   Preproinsulin produced in rough endoplasmic reticulum is delivered to the Golgi apparatus where it is cleaed to generate mature insulin and C peptide. Both are stored in secretory granules and equimolar quantities are secreted after β cell simulation.
   • Most important stimulus for insulin synthesis and release is glucose itself.

2. **Ans. (c) Assertion is true and reason is false.** *(Ref: Robbins 8th/1159, 9/e p1134)*
   Pheochromocytoma is also referred to as 'rule of 10 tumor'. It is associated with the following:

• 10% are *bilateral*[Q]
• 10% are *extra-adrenal*[Q]
• 10% are *malignant* [Q]
• 10% occur in *children* [Q]
• 10% are not associated with hypertension [Q]

   Most of the earlier texts mention that 10% of these tumors are *familial*[Q] but Robbins 8th/1159 clearly says that it has been modified.
   "As many as 25% of the individuals with pheochromocytoma and paraganglioma have a germline mutation".

3. **Ans. (c) Assertion is true and reason is false.** *(Ref: Robbins 8th/1119, 9/e p1098)*
   FNAC is not useful for diagnosing follicular thyroid cancer because it can not distinguish between follicular adenoma from follicular carcinoma. The most reliable feature of follicular cancer is demonstration of capsular invasion or vascular invasion. This is best done with careful histologic examination after specimen resection.
   Intact capsule encircling the tumor is the hallmark of the benign tumor. …Robbins 8th/1119

4. **Ans. (d) Both assertion and reason are false.** *(Ref: Robbins 8th/1113, 9/e p1088)*
   Postpartum thyroiditis/subacute lymphocytic thyroiditis is a variant of Hashimoto's thyroiditis. It presents as a *painless enlargement of the thyroid* and *transient hyperthyroidism* (lasting about 2-8 weeks). Investigations reveal elevated levels of T_3 and T_4 and reduced TSH.
   How to differentiate between Hashimoto and subacute lymphocytic thyroiditis?
   • Hurthle cell metaplasia and fibrosis are not prominent as in Hashimoto's thyroiditis.
   (Granulomatous Thyroiditis (De Quervain Thyroiditis) is more commonly seen in females *preceded by a viral infection* (caused by coxsackie virus, mumps, measles). The thyroid gland is diffusely enlarged with *intact capsule*.
   Clinical features are *pain in neck, sore throat,* fever, fatigue, anorexia, myalgia, enlarged thyroid and the presence of transient hyperthyroidism lasting for 2-6 weeks. It may be followed by asymptomatic hypothyroidism but recovery is seen in most of the patients.

5. **Ans. (b) Both assertion and reason are true and reason is not the correct explanation of assertion.** *(Ref: Robbins 9/e p1089, 8th/1114-5)*
   Graves disease is most common cause of endogenous hyperthyroidism. This disease is characterized by breakdown in self tolerance to thyroid auto-antigens (most importantly TSH receptor). The antibodies seen in these patients are as follows:
   • **Thyroid stimulating immunoglobulin**: lead to hyperthyroidism
   • **Thyroid growth stimulating immunoglobulin**: lead to hyperthyroidism
   • **TSH binding inhibitor immunoglobulin (TBIG)**: lead to **episodes of hypothyroidism** in some patients.

6. **Ans. (b) Both assertion and reason are true and reason is not the correct explanation of assertion.** *(Ref: Robbins 8th/1138-9, 9/e p1117)*
   Myocardial infarction is the commonest cause of death in diabetes. It is caused by atherosclerosis of the coronary arteries. Large and medium sized vessel involvement is responsible for macrovascular disease (MI, stroke and lower extremity gangrene).
   Capillary dysfunction in target organs leads to microvascular disease (not macrovascular disease) leading to diabetic retinopathy, neuropathy and nephropathy.

7. **Ans. (a) Both assertion and reason are true and reason is correct explanation of assertion.** *(Ref: Robbins 8th/1157, 9/e p1130)*
Hyperpigmentation is quite characteristic of primary adrenal disease (Addison's disease) especially at pressure points and sun exposed areas. This is caused by elevated levels of pro-opiomelanocortin (POMC), which is derived from anterior pituitary and is a precursor of ACTH and melanocyte stimulating hormone (MSH).

8. **Ans. (a) Both assertion and reason are true and reason is correct explanation of assertion.** *(Ref: Robbins 9/e p1115, 8th/1143)*
Hyperosmolar nonketotic coma is due to the severe dehydration resulting from sustained osmotic diuresis in patients (commoner in elderly) who do not drink enough water to compensate for urinary losses from chronic hyperglycemia. These patients don't develop ketoacidosis and its symptoms (nausea, vomiting, respiratory difficulties) because of elevated portal insulin levels. The 'fat sparing' effect of insulin prevents the formation of ketone bodies by inhibiting the fatty acid oxidation in the liver.

9. **Ans. (c) Assertion is true and reason is false.** *(Ref: Robbins 8th/1162, 9/e p1137)*
MEN 2A (**Sipple syndrome**) is characterized by pheochromocytoma, medullary thyroid carcinoma and parathyroid hyperplasia. It is associated with a gain of function (not loss of function mutation) in RET proto-oncogene.

> **'Loss of function'** mutations in RET cause intestinal aganglionosis and Hirschprung disease[Q].

10. **Ans. (a) Both assertion and reason are true and reason is correct explanation of assertion.** *(Ref: Robbins 8th/1125, 9/e p1099)*
Amyloid deposition is associated with medullary thyroid cancer. The chemical nature of the amyloid in this condition is ACal. It is because of the deposition of the altered form of calcitonin which gets deposited in the thyroid stroma.

The **bone** is a type of connective tissue which is **composed of cells** (osteoclasts and osteoblasts) **and the extracellular matrix**. The extracellular components of bone consist of a solid mineral phase (consisting of calcium and phosphate) and an organic matrix consisting of type I collagen (90–95%), serum proteins such as albumin, cell attachment/signaling proteins such as thrombospondin, osteopontin and fibronectin, calcium-binding proteins such as matrix glial protein and osteocalcin and proteoglycans such as biglycan and decorin.

The mineral phase of bone is deposited initially in intimate relation to the collagen fibrils and is found in specific locations in the "holes" between the collagen fibrils. This architectural arrangement of mineral and matrix results in a two-phase material well suited to withstand mechanical stresses.

CELLS OF BONE

Osteoblasts synthesize and secrete the organic matrix. They are derived from cells of mesenchymal origin. As an osteoblast secretes matrix, which is then mineralized, the cell becomes an *osteocyte*. Mineralization is a carefully regulated process dependent on the activity of osteoblast-derived alkaline phosphatase, which probably works by hydrolyzing inhibitors of mineralization. Core-binding factor A1 (*CBFA1*, also called *Runx2*) regulates the expression of several important osteoblast proteins including osterix, osteopontin, bone sialoprotein, type I collagen, osteocalcin, and receptor-activator of NFκB (RANK) ligand. *Runx2* expression is regulated, in part, by bone morphogenic proteins (BMPs).

Osteoclasts carry out resorption of bone. **Macrophage colony-stimulating factor (M-CSF) plays a critical role** during several steps in the pathway and ultimately leads to fusion of osteoclast progenitor cells to form multinucleated, active osteoclasts. **RANK** ligand, expressed on the surface of osteoblast progenitors and stromal fibroblasts binds to the RANK receptor on osteoclast progenitors and stimulates osteoclast differentiation and activation. Alternatively, a soluble decoy receptor, referred to as osteoprotegerin, can bind RANK ligand and inhibit osteoclast differentiation. Several growth factors and cytokines (including interleukins 1, 6, and 11; TNF; and interferon-gamma modulate osteoclast differentiation and function.

Remodeling of bone

The cycle of bone remodeling is carried out by the basic multicellular unit (BMU), comprising a group of osteoclasts and osteoblasts. In cortical bone, the BMUs tunnel through the tissue, whereas in cancellous bone, they move across the trabecular surface. The process of bone remodeling is initiated by contraction of the lining cells and the recruitment of osteoclast precursors. These precursors fuse to form multinucleated, active osteoclasts that mediate bone resorption. Osteoclasts adhere to bone and subsequently remove it by acidification (protons secreted by type II carbonic anhydrase) and proteolytic digestion (by cathepsin K). As the BMU advances, osteoclasts leave the resorption site and osteoblasts move in to cover the excavated area and begin the process of new bone formation by secreting osteoid, which is eventually mineralized into new bone. After osteoid mineralization, osteoblasts flatten and form a layer of lining cells over new bone.

Remodeling of bone occurs along lines of force generated by mechanical stress.

Biochemical markers of bone resorption

a. Amino and carboxy terminal crosslinking telopeptide of bone collagen
b. Pyridinoline

Cleidocranial dysplasia is caused by heterozygous inactivating mutations in Runx2.

PTH and 1, 25-dihydroxyvitamin D activate receptors expressed by osteoblasts to assure mineral homeostasis.

Concept

Most hormones that influence osteoclast function do not directly target this cell but instead influence M-CSF and RANK ligand signaling by osteoblasts.

Both PTH and $1,25(OH)_2D$ increase osteoclast number and activity, whereas estrogen decreases osteoclast number and activity by this indirect mechanism.

Calcitonin, in contrast, binds to its receptor on the basal surface of osteoclasts and **directly inhibits osteoclast function.**

c. Free lysyl-pyridinoline
d. Tartarate-resistant acid phosphatase (TRAP)
e. Hydroxyproline (not very specific)

Biochemical markers of bone formation

a. Bone specific alkaline phosphatase
b. Procollagen type IC and IN propeptide
c. Osteocalcin
d. Alkaline phosphatase (not very specific)

PAGET'S DISEASE (OSTEITIS DEFORMANS)

Paget's disease (osteitis deformans) can be characterized as a *collage of matrix madness.* It is marked by regions of *furious osteoclastic bone resorption,* which is *followed by a period of hectic bone formation.* The net effect is a gain in bone mass. It has the following three stages:
i. Initial osteolytic stage
ii. Mixed osteoclastic-osteoblastic stage
iii. Burnt-out quiescent osteosclerotic stage.

Paget's disease usually begins after the age of 40 years and is more common in whites. It has been **linked to slow virus infection by paramyxovirus.** It can be involving one bone or monostotic (tibia, ilium, femur, skull, vertebra, humerus) in about 15% of cases and affecting multiple bones or polyostotic (pelvis, spine, skull) in the remainder. The *axial skeleton or proximal femur is involved in upto 80% of cases.*

On radiography, the Pagetic bone is typically enlarged with thick, coarsened cortices and cancellous bone. There is **increased serum alkaline phosphatase and increased urinary excretion of hydroxyproline.** The most common symptom is pain. Bone overgrowth in the craniofacial skeleton may produce *leontiasis ossea* and the weakened Pagetic bone may lead to invagination of base of skull (*platybasia*).

The **histologic hallmark** is the **mosaic pattern** of **lamellar bone** which is produced by prominent cement lines that anneal haphazardly oriented units of lamellar bone. The involved bones are weak and fracture easily.

The **complications** of the disease include arteriovenous shunts within the marrow resulting in *high output cardiac failure* and *increased risk of development of sarcomas* like osteosarcoma, chondrosarcoma, etc. *Secondary osteoarthritis* and *chalk-stick type fractures* are the other complications in Paget's disease.

BENIGN TUMORS OF THE BONE

Osteoma

Subperiosteal osteomas are benign tumors affecting most often the skull and facial bones. They are usually solitary and are detected in middle-aged adults. Multiple osteomas are seen in the setting of *Gardner's syndrome.*

Osteoid osteoma and osteoblastoma

Osteoid osteoma and *osteoblastoma* are terms used to describe benign bone tumors that have identical histologic features but that differ in size, sites of origin, and symptoms. **Osteoid osteoma** is *less than 2 cm* in size and usually affects patients in their teens and twenties. They *usually involve the femur or tibia,* where they commonly *arise in the cortex* and less frequently within the medullary cavity. Osteoid osteomas are painful lesions. The pain is characteristically *nocturnal,* and is dramatically relieved by aspirin.

Microscopically, there is a central nidus of osteoid surrounded by dense sclerotic rim of reactive cortical bone. X-ray shows the presence of central radiolucency surrounded by a sclerotic rim.

Osteochondroma (Exostosis)

It is a benign bony *metaphyseal* growth capped with cartilage originating from the epiphyseal growth plate. It is seen in adolescent males as a firm, solitary growth at the end of long bones. It may be asymptomatic or may cause pain and deformity. Rarely, it may undergo malignant transformation.

Multiple osteochondromas occur in *multiple hereditary exostosis,* which is an autosomal dominant hereditary disease.

There is inactivation of both copies of the *EXT* gene in growth plate chondrocytes in the pathogenesis of osteochondromas. Multiple osteochondromas become apparent during childhood.

Chondroma

Chondromas are benign tumors of hyaline cartilage that usually occurs in bones of endochondral origin. These can be

- *Enchondroma:* When origin is intramedullary
- *Subperiosteal or juxtacortical:* Originate from the surface of bone

Enchondromas are most common intraosseous cartilage tumors. Their *favored sites are short tubular bones of hand and feet.*

Enchondromas are composed of well-circumscribed nodules of cytologically benign hyaline cartilage. The center of the nodule can calcify whereas peripheral portion may undergo enchondral ossification. The unmineralized nodules of cartilage produce well-circumscribed oval lucencies that are surrounded by a thin rim of radiodense bone (**O ring sign**).

Patients with **Ollier's disease** may undergo malignant transformation to *chondrosarcoma* whereas those with **Maffuci's syndrome** have *increased risk of ovarian cancer and brain gliomas.*

Ollier's disease is a syndrome of multiple enchondromas (or enchondromatosis)

Maffuci's syndrome is association of soft tissue hemangiomas with enchondromatosis.

▌ MALIGNANT TUMORS OF THE BONE

Osteosarcoma

It is the **most common primary malignant tumor of the bone**. It has a *bimodal age distribution* with almost 75% occurring in patients younger than age 20. The second peak occurs in the elderly with conditions like Paget disease, bone infarcts, and prior irradiation. It is more commonly seen in the males with *increased risk of the development in patients with familial retinoblastoma.*

The patients usually have localized pain and swelling. It arises from the *metaphysis* of the long bones with the **knee** being the *most commonly affected site.* The tumor is a large, firm white-tan mass with necrosis and hemorrhage. Microscopically, there is presence of anaplastic cells producing osteoid and bone.

The tumor frequently breaks through the cortex and lifts the periosteum, resulting in reactive periosteal bone formation. The triangular shadow between the cortex and raised ends of periosteum is known radiographically as *Codman's triangle.*

The formation of bone by the tumor cells is characteristic of osteosarcoma.

Chondrosarcoma

These are group of tumors that produce neoplastic cartilage.
- Similar to chondroma, chondrosarcoma can be:
  - Intramedullary
  - Juxtacortical
- **Chondrosarcomas** are *second most common malignant matrix-producing tumor of bone* (*Most common is osteosarcoma*)
- **Histologically,** Chondrosarcomas are composed of malignant hyaline and myxoid cartilage. Spotty calcifications may be present and central necrosis may create cystic

The classic **X-ray** findings include bone destruction, **sunray pattern** due to radiating opacities in the tumor like sunrays and **Codman's triangle**.

spaces. Tumors vary in cellularity and cytological atypia. *Malignant cartilage infiltrates the marrow space and surrounds pre-existing bony trabeculae.*

- Chondrosarcomas commonly *arise in central portions of skeleton* (including pelvis, shoulder and ribs). In contrast to chondroma, chondrosarcoma rarely involve the distal extremities. The *clear cell variant* of chondrosarcoma characteristically *originates from Epiphysis of tubular long bones.*

Osteoclatoma or Giant cell tumor of bone

It is a malignant tumor containing multinucleated giant cells mixed with stromal cells. It is more commonly seen in the females and the most commonly affected age group is 20-40 years. The tumor involves the *epiphysis* of the long bones usually *around the knee* (distal femur and proximal tibia). Microscopically, there is presence of *osteoclast like giant* cells (having 100 or more nuclei) distributed in a background of mononuclear stromal cells. Most of the tumors are solitary.

Radiographically, giant cell tumors are large, *purely lytic, and eccentric*, and erode into the subchondral bone plate. The overlying cortex is frequently destroyed, producing a bulging soft tissue mass delineated by a thin shell of reactive bone. This gives rise to the **soap bubble appearance**. The tumor has high rate of recurrence after excision.

Ewing's sarcoma and primitive neuroectodermal tumor (PNET)

Ewing sarcoma and PNET are primary malignant *small round cell tumors* of bone and soft tissue. Both Ewing's sarcoma and PNET are the same tumor, differing only in their degree of neural differentiation. *Tumors that demonstrate neural differentiation by any analysis are called PNETs, and those that are undifferentiated are known as Ewing's sarcoma.*

> Of all bone sarcomas, Ewing's sarcoma has the youngest average age at presentation and approximately 80% patients are younger than age 20 years. Boys are affected slightly more frequently than girls. The classic translocation is t(11;22)(q24;q12) and the most common fusion gene (EWS-FLI1) generated acts as a dominant oncogenes to stimulate cell proliferation. The presence of p30/32, a product of mic-2 gene, is a cell surface marker form Ewing's sarcoma.

Ewing's sarcoma and PNET usually **arise in the diaphysis** of long tubular bones, especially the femur and the flat bones of the pelvis.

The tumor is composed of sheets of *uniform small, round cells that are slightly larger than lymphocytes having scant cytoplasm, which may appear clear because it is rich in glycogen.* There is presence of **Homer-Wright rosettes** (where the tumor cells are arranged in a circle about a central fibrillary space) which are *indicative of neural differentiation.*

They present as painful enlarging masses, and the affected site is frequently tender, warm, and swollen with the patients having systemic findings like fever, increased ESR, anemia and leukocytosis (all of which results in the tumor resembling infection). **X-ray** shows the characteristic periosteal reaction producing layers of reactive bone deposited in an '**onion-skin**' pattern.

> Note: *Metastatic tumors are the most common form of skeletal malignancy.*

SOFT TISSUE TUMORS

SYNOVIAL SARCOMA

These tumors forms about 10% of all soft tissue sarcomas. Less than 10% of them are intra-articular. 60-70% involve the lower extremities especially around knee and thigh. The **histologic hallmark** of biphasic synovial sarcoma is the **dual lining of differentiation of the tumor cells** (e.g. **epithelial-like and spindle cells**). The calcified concretions can be present which help in the diagnosis radiologically.

Immunohistochemically, these tumor cells yield **positive reactions for keratin and epithelial membrane antigen** (differentiating from most other sarcomas). Most synovial

---

Other giant cell lesions include:

- Brown tumor seen in hyperparathyroidism
- Giant cell reparative granuloma
- Chondroblastoma
- Pigmented villonodular synovitis

The presence of p30/32, the product of the *mic-2 gene* (which maps to the pseudo-autosomal region of the X and Y chromosomes) is a cell-surface marker for **Ewing's sarcoma** (and other members of a family of tumors called PNETs).

sarcomas show a characteristic chromosomal translocation **t(X ; 18)** producing SYT-SSX1 or -SSX2 fusion genes. This specific translocation is associated with poor prognosis.

Architectural Patterns in Soft Tissue Tumors

Pattern	Tumor Type
Fascicles of eosinophilic spindle cells **intersecting at right angles**	Smooth muscle
Short fascicles of spindle cells radiating from a central point (like **spokes on a wheel**)—storiform	Fibrohistiocytic
Nuclei arranged in columns—palisading	Schwann cell
Herringbone	Fibrosarcoma
Mixture of fascicles of spindle cells and groups of epithelioid cells—biphasic	Synovial sarcoma

INFLAMMATORY MYOPATHIES

The inflammatory myopathies represent the largest group of acquired and potentially treatable causes of skeletal muscle weakness. They are classified into **three major groups**: polymyositis (PM), dermatomyositis (DM), and inclusion body myositis (IBM).

Criteria for Diagnosis of Inflammatory Myopathies

Criterion	Polymyositis	Dermatomyositis	Inclusion body myositis
Myopathic muscle weakness	Yes	Yes	Yes; slow onset, early involvement of distal muscles, frequent falls
Electromyographic findings	Myopathic	Myopathic	Myopathic with mixed potentials
Muscle enzymes	Elevated (up to 50-fold) or normal	Elevated (up to 50-fold) or normal	Elevated (up to 10-fold) or normal
Muscle biopsy findings	"Primary" inflammation with the CD8/MHC-I complex and **no vacuoles**	Perifascicular, perimysial, or perivascular infiltrates, perifascicular atrophy	Primary inflammation with CD8/MHC-I complex; vacuolated fibers with amyloid deposits; **cytochrome oxygenase–negative** fibers; signs of chronic myopathy
Rash or calcinosis	Absent	**Present**	Absent

MUSCULAR DYSTROPHIES

The muscular dystrophies are a heterogeneous group of inherited disorders, often beginning in childhood, that are characterized clinically by *progressive muscle weakness and wasting*. The two most common forms of muscular dystrophy are **X-linked**: Duchenne muscular dystrophy (DMD) and Becker muscular dystrophy (BMD). **BMD is less common and much less severe than DMD.**

DMD and BMD are caused by abnormalities in a gene encoding a protein termed dystrophin.

Dystrophin and the dystrophin-associated protein complex form an interface between the intracellular contractile apparatus and the extracellular connective tissue matrix. The role of this complex of proteins is transferring the force of contraction to connective tissue, so, myocyte degeneration occurs in the absence of dystrophin.

Muscle biopsy specimens from patients with **DMD** show minimal evidence of dystrophin by both staining and Western blot analysis. **BMD** patients have a mutation causing a *reduced amount of altered dystrophin*.

Duchenne Muscular Dystrophy (DMD)
Doesn't **M**ake **D**ystrophin (no formation)

Panfascicular atrophy: characterized by the muscle fiber atrophy often involves an entire fascicle and is seen with **spinal muscular atrophy.**

Perifascicular atrophy: seen with **dermatomyositis**.

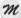

Becker Muscular Dystrophy (BMD)
Badly **M**ade **D**ystrophin (reduced formation of an altered protein)

Histopathologic abnormalities common to DMD and BMD include

- Variation in fiber size due to the presence of both small and enlarged fibers
- Increased numbers of internalized nuclei
- Degeneration, necrosis, and phagocytosis of muscle fibers
- Regeneration of muscle fibers
- Proliferation of endomysial connective tissue
  - **DMD** cases also often show *enlarged, rounded, hyaline fibers that have lost their normal cross-striations*, believed to be hypercontracted fibers, this finding is rare in BMD. In later stages, **the muscles eventually become almost totally replaced by fat and connective tissue**. Cardiac involvement consists of interstitial fibrosis, more prominent in the subendocardial layers.
- Boys with DMD are normal at birth, and early motor milestones are met on time. Walking is often delayed and weakness begins in the pelvic girdle muscles and then extends to the shoulder girdle giving rise to **Gower's sign** (child uses his hands to climb upon himself on getting up from the floor). Enlargement of the calf muscles associated with weakness, a phenomenon termed *pseudohypertrophy* caused initially by an increase in the size of the muscle fibers later by an increase in fat and connective tissue. **Cognitive impairment** is a component of the disease. Serum creatine kinase is elevated during the first decade of life but returns to normal in the later stages of the disease, as muscle mass decreases. *Death results from respiratory insufficiency, pulmonary infection, and cardiac decompensation.*
- Boys with **BMD** develop symptoms at a **later age** than those with DMD. The onset occurs in later childhood or in adolescence, and it is accompanied by a **slower and variable rate of progression**. Cardiac disease is frequently seen in these patients.

MULTIPLE CHOICE QUESTIONS

1. A 10 year old girl presents with a tibial mass. Histopathological examination reveals a small round cell tumor. Which of the following molecular findings is most likely to be present? *(All India 2012)*
   (a) 22q translocation
   (b) 11q deletion
   (c) 7p translocation
   (d) n-myc amplification

2. Which of the following is the most specific test for rheumatoid arthritis? *(All India 2012)*
   (a) Anti Ig M antibody
   (b) Anti CCP antibody
   (c) Anti Ig A antibody
   (d) Anti IgG antibody

3. Onion bulb appearance of nerve ending on biopsy is seen in *(AIIMS Nov. 2010)*
   (a) Diabetic neuropathy
   (b) Amyloid neuropathy
   (c) Leprous neuritis
   (d) Chronic inflammatory demyelinating polyneuropathy (CIDP)

4. The rate of newly synthesized osteoid mineralization is best estimated by *(AIIMS Nov. 2010)*
   (a) Tetracycline labeling
   (b) Alizarine red staining
   (c) Calceine stain
   (d) Von Kossa stain

5. Which of the following is false in relation to Osteosarcoma? *(DPG 2011)*
   (a) Paget's disease and prior irradiation are pre-disposing factors
   (b) Rb gene mutation is associated with hereditary variant
   (c) C-myc gene implicated in the genesis
   (d) Codman's triangle is the characteristic X-ray finding

6. Cytogenetics for synovial cell sarcoma is: *(AI 2008)*
   (a) t (X: 18)
   (b) t (17, 9)
   (c) t (9, 22)
   (d) t (11, 14)

7. MIC-2 mutation associated with: *(AIIMS Nov 2009)*
   (a) Osteosarcoma
   (b) Ewing sarcoma
   (c) Alveolar soft tissue sarcoma
   (d) Dermatofibrosarcoma protuberance

8. A 9-year-old girl has difficulty in combing hairs and climbing upstairs since 6 months. She has Gower's sign positive and maculopapular rash over metacarpophalangeal joints. What should be the next appropriate investigation to be done? *(AIIMS Nov 2008)*
   (a) ESR
   (b) RA factor
   (c) Creatine kinase
   (d) Electromyography

9. Antibody found in myositis is? *(AIIMS Nov 2008)*
   (a) Anti-Jo 1
   (b) Anti scl 70
   (c) Anti Sm
   (d) Anti Ku

10. CD-99 is for: *(AIIMS May 2008)*
    (a) Ewing's sarcoma
    (b) SLL
    (c) Dermatofibroma protruberans
    (d) Malignant histiocytic fibroma

11. Bone resorption markers are all except: *(AIIMS May 2008)*
    (a) Tartarate resistant alkaline phosphatase (TRAP)
    (b) Osteocalcin
    (c) Crosslinked-N-telopeptides
    (d) Urine total free deoxypyridinoline

12. A 50-year-old lady presented with a 3-month history of pain in the lower third of the right thigh. There was no local swelling; tenderness was present on deep pressure. Plain X-rays showed an ill-defined intramedullary lesion with blotchy calcification at the lower end of the right femoral diaphysis, possibly enchondroma or chondrosarcoma. Sections showed a cartilaginous tumor. Which of the following histological features (if seen) would be most helpful to differentiate the two tumors? *(AIIMS May 2006)*
    (a) Focal necrosis and lobulation
    (b) Tumor permeation between bone trabeculae at periphery
    (c) Extensive myxoid change
    (d) High cellularity

13. Dystrophic gene mutation leads to: *(AIIMS May 2003)*
    (a) Myasthenia gravis
    (b) Motor neuron disease
    (c) Poliomyelitis
    (d) Duchenne's muscular dystrophy

14. Giant cells are seen in: *(PGI Dec 2006)*
    (a) Osteoclastoma
    (b) Chondroblastoma
    (c) Chordoma
    (d) Osteitis fibrosa cystica

15. "Biphasic pattern" on histology is seen in which tumor?
    (a) Rhabdomyosarcoma *(Delhi 2010)*
    (b) Synovial cell sarcoma
    (c) Osteosarcoma
    (d) Neurofibroma

16. An epiphyseal bone lesion is: *(Delhi 2009 RP)*
    (a) Osteogenic sarcoma
    (b) Chondroblastoma
    (c) Ewing's sarcoma
    (d) Chondromyxoid fibroma

17. Mosaic pattern of lamellar bone histology is found in:
    (a) Osteopetrosis *(Delhi PG-2006)*
    (b) Osteoid osteoma
    (c) Osteitis deformans
    (d) Osteomalacia

18. Which one of the following inflammatory markers of muscle biopsy is diagnostic of polymyositis?
    (a) CD8/MHC-I complex *(Karnataka 2006)*
    (b) Vascular cell adhesion molecules
    (c) Intracellular adhesion molecules
    (d) Membrane attack complex

19. Bone tumor arising from epiphysis is: *(DNB 2001)*
    (a) Osteogenic sarcoma
    (b) Ewing's sarcoma
    (c) Chondromyxoid fibroma
    (d) Giant cell tumor

20. The commonest malignant bone tumor is: *(DNB 2001)*
    (a) Multiple myeloma
    (b) Osteosarcoma
    (c) Ewing's sarcoma
    (d) Giant cell tumor

21. Characteristics microscopic features of osteogenic sarcoma is: *(UP 2000)*
    (a) Osteoid formation
    (b) Osteoid formation by mesenchymal cells with pleomorphism
    (c) Codman's triangle
    (d) Predominant osteoclast

22. Ground glass appearance is found in: *(UP 2001)*
    (a) Inverted papilloma
    (b) Fibro calcification
    (c) Fibrous dysplasia of bones
    (d) Chronic osteomyelitis

23. Paget's disease increases the risk of: *(RJ 2003)*
    (a) Osteoma
    (b) Osteosarcoma
    (c) Fibrosarcoma
    (d) All

24. Osteoclast are stimulated by: *(RJ 2005)*
    (a) Thyroxine
    (b) PTH
    (c) Calcitonin
    (d) Estrogen

25. Large intracytoplasmic glycogen storage is seen in which malignancy? *(AP 2006)*
    (a) osteosarcoma
    (b) Mesenchymal chondrosarcoma
    (c) Ewing's sarcoma
    (d) Leiomyosarcoma

26. Osteoblastoma resembles histologically:
    (a) Osteosarcoma *(Kolkata 2002,2003)*
    (b) Osteoid osteoma
    (c) Chondroblastoma
    (d) Chondrosarcoma

27. Syncytial osteoclastic giant cells are seen in All Except:
    (a) Osteosarcoma *(Kolkata 2002,2003)*
    (b) Ewing's sarcoma
    (c) Chondroblastoma
    (d) Aneurysmal bone cyst

28. Hyaline cartilage contains which type of collagen:
    (a) Type I *(Kolkata 2008)*
    (b) Type II
    (c) Type III
    (d) Type IV

29. Tophi in gout are found in all regions, except:
    (a) Bone *(Bihar 2004)*
    (b) Skin
    (c) Muscle
    (d) Synovial membrane

30. Which of the following is true about psoriatic arthritis?
    (a) Involves distal joints of hand and foot
    (b) Pencil in cup deformity *(Bihar 2004)*
    (c) Sacroiliitis
    (d) All of the above

Most Recent Questions

30.1. Dystrophin is lacking in:
    (a) Polio
    (b) Duchenne's muscular dystrophy
    (c) Peroneal muscular atrophy
    (d) Spinal muscular atrophy

30.2. Ewings sarcoma arises from:
    (a) G cells
    (b) Totipotent cells
    (c) Neuroectodermal cells
    (d) Neurons

30.3. Most common malignant bone tumor –
    (a) Osteogenic sarcoma
    (b) Secondaries
    (c) Osteoma
    (d) Enchondroma

30.4. A 42 year-old woman Paro presents with slowly progressive syndrome comprising of features like pain and tenderness in multiple joints, with joint stuffiness on rising in the morning. Joint involvement is symmetric, with the proximal interphalangeal and metacarpophalangeal joints especially involved. The physician finds presence of tenderness in all the inflamed joints. Which of the following laboratory abnormalities is most likely associated in this patient?
(a) Antibodies to double-stranded DNA
(b) IgM anti-IgG antibodies
(c) HLA-B27 antigen
(d) Urate crystals and neutrophils in synovial fluid

30.5. In the giant cell tumor of the bone, the cell of origin is:
(a) Fibroblast cells
(b) Osteoclast and precursors
(c) Osteoblast and precursors
(d) Sinusoidal cells

30.6. Paget disease of the bone is also called:
(a) Osteitis fibrosa
(b) Brittle bone disease
(c) Fibrous dysplasia
(d) Osteomalacia

30.7. Polyarticular rheumatoid arthritis is diagnosed when more than _ joints are involved?
(a) Two
(b) Three
(c) Four
(d) Five

30.8. Which of these is characteristic of Gout?
(a) Podagra
(b) Anasarca
(c) Cheiroarthropathy
(d) Calcinosis cutis

ASSERTION AND REASON QUESTIONS

1–4. Will have two statements, assertion and reason. Read both of them carefully and answer according to these options.
(a) Both assertion and reason are true and reason is correct explanation of assertion.
(b) Both assertion and reason are true and reason is not the correct explanation of assertion.
(c) Assertion is true and reason is false.
(d) Both assertion and reason are false.

1. **Assertion:** Patients with Duchene's muscular dystrophy have difficulty in walking.
Reason: Altered dystrophin is responsible for muscular weakness in muscular dystrophy.
2. **Assertion:** Osteosarcoma is associated with the radiological appearance of Codman's triangle.
Reason: The tumor results in reactive periosteal bone formation.
3. **Assertion:** Great toe is the most commonly affected joint in gout.
Reason: Uric acid is deposited in less temperature
4. **Assertion:** Reiter syndrome is a n example of seronegative spondyloarthropathy
Reason: Reiter syndrome is associated with HLA B-27

EXPLANATIONS

1. **Ans. (b) 22q translocation** *(Ref: Robbins 8th/1232)*

Ewing sarcoma and primitive neuroectodermal tumor are primary malignant small round-cell tumors of bone and soft tissue. Both differ in their degree of differentiation. PNETs demonstrate neural differentiation whereas Ewing sarcomas are undifferentiated. Analyzing some features of Ewing sarcoma with the data in stem of the question:

- Arises in *diaphysis and metaphysis* (mass in the tibia in question)
- Most patients are *10 to 15 years old* (10 year old girl)
- Approximately 95% of patients with Ewing tumor have **t(11;22)**[Q] (q24;q12) or **t(21;22)**[Q] (q22;q12)
- Microscopically there are *sheets of small round cells* that contain *glycogen*.

Please note that the option 'b' (11q deletion) given in the question should not be confused with the answer because in Ewing sarcoma we find 11q translocation and not deletion ☺

Other features of Ewing sarcoma

- *Second most common pediatric bone sarcomas* after osteosarcomas.
- Boys are affected slightly more frequently than girls.
- The common chromosomal abnormality is a translocation that causes fusion of the EWS gene on 22q12 with a member of the ETS family of transcription factors usually the FL1 gene on 11q24, and the ERG gene on 21q22.
- The presence of **Homer-Wright** rosettes (tumor cells circled about a central fibrillary space) indicates neural differentiation. Please see the answer section of chapter 4 for an informative summary on rosettes.
- Periosteal reaction produces layers of reactive bone in **'onion skin'** fashion.
- Treatment includes chemotherapy and surgical excision

2. **Ans. (b) Anti-CCP antibody** *(Ref: Robbins 8th/1237-1240, Harrison 17th/2088)*

- Rheumatoid factor is an IgM antibody reactive with the Fc portions of the patients' own IgG. However, it is not specific for rheumatoid arthritis as it can also be seen in a wide range of autoimmune disorders, inflammatory disease and chronic infection.
- **Anti cyclic citrullinated peptide antibody** (anti CCP antibody) test is more specific than rheumatoid factor for diagnosis of rheumatoid arthritis. It is more commonly seen in the aggressive disease.

Key points about rheumatoid arthritis

- It is a type **III**[Q] **hypersensitivity reaction** (immune complex disease).
- Clinical features include **symmetrical arthritis** affecting the **small joints** of the hands and feet (though **typically sparing the distal interphalageal joint**[Q])
- **Rheumatoid nodules**[Q] are the most common cutaneouHs lesions in RA.
- Presence of **pannus**[Q] (synovial mass with inflammatory cells, granulation tissue and fibroblasts).
- **Felty syndrome**[Q] is RA+ spenomegaly+neutropenia
- **Caplan syndrome**[Q] is RA + pneumoconiosis
- Radiographic hallmarks are **juxta-articular osteopenia**[Q] and bone erosions with narrowing of the joint space from loss of articular cartilage.

3. **Ans. (d) Chronic inflammatory demyelinating polyneuropathy (CIDP)** *(Ref: Robbins 8th/1259)*

Segmental demyelination occurs in the absence of primary axonal abnormality when there is dysfunction or death of the Schwann cell (in hereditary motor and sensory neuropathy) or damage to the myelin sheath (in Guillain Barre syndrome). The process affects some Schwann cells while sparing others. The disintegrating myelin is engulfed initially by Schwann cells and later by macrophages. The denuded axon provides a stimulus for remyelination, with cells within the endoneurium differentiating to replace injured Schwann cells. These cells proliferate and encircle the axon and, in time, remyelinate the denuded portion. Remyelinated internodes, however, are shorter than normal and have thinner myelin in proportion to the diameter of the axon than normal internodes.

On transverse section, repetitive cycles of demyelination and remyelination cause an accumulation of tiers of Schwann cell processes that appear as concentric layers of Schwann cell cytoplasm and redundant basement membrane that surround a thinly myelinated axon (**onion bulbs**).

CIDP

- CIDP can result from altered triggering of T cells by antigen-presenting cells.
- Most cases occur in **adults**, and **males** are affected slightly more often than females.
- **Onset is usually gradual,** sometimes subacute; in a few, the initial attack is indistinguishable from that of GBS. An acute-onset form of CIDP should be considered when GBS deteriorates >9 weeks after onset or relapses at least three times.
- Symptoms are both motor and sensory in most cases. **Weakness of the limbs** is usually symmetric but can be strikingly asymmetric.
- **Death** from CIDP is **uncommon.**
- Biopsy typically reveals little inflammation and **onion-bulb changes** (imbricated layers of attenuated Schwann cell processes surrounding an axon) that result from recurrent demyelination and remyelination
- The diagnosis rests on characteristic clinical, CSF, and electrophysiologic findings. The CSF is usually acellular **with an elevated protein level.** Electrodiagnostically, variable degrees of conduction slowing, prolonged distal latencies, temporal dispersion of compound action potentials, and conduction block are the principal features.
- Treatment: If the disorder is mild, management can be awaiting spontaneous remission otherwise high-dose **IVIg, PE, and glucocorticoids** are all effective.

4. **Ans. (a) Tetracycline labeling** *(Ref: Bancroft 6th/358)*

Tetracycline is absorbed into bone and so, it is used as a marker of bone growth for biopsies in humans. Tetracycline binds to newly formed bone at the bone/osteoid (unmineralized bone) interface where it shows as a linear fluorescence. Tetracycline labeling is used to determine the amount of bone growth within a certain period of time, usually a period of approximately 21 days. Tetracycline is incorporated into mineralizing bone and can be detected by its fluorescence. In double tetracycline labeling, a second dose is given 11–14 days after the first dose, and the amount of bone formed during that interval can be calculated by measuring the distance between the two fluorescent labels.

5. **Ans. (c) C-myc gene implicated in the genesis** *(Ref: Robbins 8th/1225)*

- Osteosarcoma is defined as a malignant mesenchymal tumor in which the cancerous cells produce bone matrix. It is the most common primary malignant tumor of bone, exclusive of myeloma and lymphoma.
- It has a bimodal age distribution; 75% occur in patients younger than age 20. The smaller second peak occurs in the elderly, who frequently suffer from conditions like Paget disease, bone infarcts, and prior irradiation.
- The tumors usually arise in the metaphyseal region of the long bones of the extremities, and almost 60% occur about the knee
- Genetic mutations seen with osteosarcoma are that of RB gene, p53, CDK4, p16, INK4A, CYCLIN D1, and MDM2.
- **The formation of bone by the tumor cells is characteristic of Osteosarcoma**
- Osteosarcoma typically present as painful and progressively enlarging masses.
- Radiographs of the primary tumor usually show a large, destructive, mixed lytic and blastic mass that has permeative margins. The tumor frequently breaks through the cortex and lifts the periosteum, resulting in reactive periosteal bone formation.
- The triangular shadow between the cortex and raised ends of periosteum is known radiographically as **Codman triangle**

6. **Ans. (a) t (X: 18)** *(Ref: Robbins 7th/1323)*

7. **Ans. (b) Ewing's sarcoma** *(Ref: Harrison 17th/613)*

8. **Ans. (c) Creatine kinase** *(Ref: Harrison 17th/2699)*
- The diagnosis of the patient is most likely to be dermatomyositis (DM) as suggested by proximal muscle weakness (Gower's sign positive) and skin rash.
- The clinical picture of the typical skin rash and proximal or diffuse muscle weakness has few causes other than DM. However, proximal muscle weakness without skin involvement can be due to many conditions other than PM or IBM.
- Gowers sign is a medical sign that indicates weakness of the proximal muscles, namely those of the lower limb. The sign describes a patient that has to use his or her hands and arms to "walk" up his or her own body from a squatting position due to lack of hip and thigh muscle strength.
- Inflammatory myopathies
- The inflammatory myopathies are classified into three major groups: Polymyositis (PM), dermatomyositis (DM), and inclusion body myositis (IBM).
- DM affects both children and adults and women more often than men.

Features Associated with Inflammatory Myopathies

Characteristic	Polymyositis	Dermatomyositis	Inclusion Body Myositis
Age at onset	>18 yr	Adulthood and childhood	>50 yr
Familial association	No	No	Yes, in some cases
Extramuscular manifestations	Yes	Yes	Yes
Associated conditions			
Connective tissue diseases	Yes	Scleroderma and mixed connective tissue disease (overlap syndromes)	Yes, in up to 20% of cases
Systemic autoimmune diseases	Frequent	Infrequent	Infrequent
Malignancy	No	Yes, in up to 15% of cases	No
Viruses	Yes	Unproven	Yes
Drugs	Yes	Yes, rarely	No
Parasites and bacteria	Yes	No	No

Dermatomyositis

DM is a distinctive entity identified by a characteristic rash accompanying, or more often preceding, muscle weakness. The rash may consist of

- A blue-purple discoloration on the upper eyelids with edema (*heliotrope rash*),
- A flat red rash on the face and upper trunk, and erythema of the knuckles with a raised violaceous scaly eruption (*Gottron's sign*).
- The erythematous rash can also occur on other body surfaces, including the knees, elbows, malleoli, neck and anterior chest (often in a *V sign*), or back and shoulders (*shawl sign*), and may worsen after sun exposure.

Dilated capillary loops at the base of the fingernails are also characteristic. The cuticles may be irregular, thickened, and distorted, and the lateral and palmar areas of the fingers may become rough and cracked, with irregular, "dirty" horizontal lines, resembling *mechanic's hands*. The weakness can be mild, moderate, or severe enough to lead to quadriparesis.

At times, the muscle strength appears normal, hence the term *dermatomyositis sine myositis*. When muscle biopsy is performed in such cases, however, significant perivascular and perimysial inflammation is often seen.

DM usually occurs alone but may overlap with scleroderma and mixed connective tissue disease. Fasciitis and thickening of the skin, similar to that seen in chronic cases of DM, have occurred in patients with the eosinophilia-myalgia syndrome associated with the ingestion of contaminated L-tryptophan.

The CK level usually parallels disease activity, it can be normal in some patients with active IBM or DM, especially when associated with a connective tissue disease. The CK is always elevated in patients with active PM. Along with the CK, the serum glutamic-oxaloacetic and glutamate pyruvate transaminases, lactate dehydrogenase, and aldolase may be elevated. Muscle biopsy is the definitive test for establishing the diagnosis of inflammatory myopathy and for excluding other neuromuscular diseases. Inflammation is the histologic hallmark for these diseases; however, additional features are characteristic of each subtype.

As biopsy is not given in the options, we will mark CK as the answer.

9. **Ans. (a) Anti-Jo 1** (*Ref: Harrison 17th/2038*)

Some medically important autoantibodies:

Anti-actin antibodies	coeliac disease, autoimmune hepatitis, gastric cancer
Anti-ganglioside antibodies	
Anti-GD3	Guillain-Barré syndrome
Anti-GM1	Traveler's diarrhea
Anti-GQ1b	Miller-Fisher syndrome
Anti-glomerular basement membrane antibody (Anti-GBM antibody)	Good pasture syndrome
Anti-Hu antibody	Small cell lung carcinoma
Anti-Jo 1 antibody (anti-histidyl-tRNA synthetase)	Polymyositis
Anti-liver/kidney microsomal 1 antibody (anti-LKM 1 antibodies)	Autoimmune hepatitis

contd...

contd...

Anti-mitochondrial antibody	Primary biliary cirrhosis
Anti-neutrophil cytoplasmic antibody (ANCA)	Ulcerative colitis
Antinuclear antibody (ANA)	
Anti-p62 antibodies in Anti-sp100 antibodies in Anti-glycoprotein210 antibodies in Anti-ds DNA antibody	Primary biliary cirrhosis Primary biliary cirrhosis Primary biliary cirrhosis SLE
Anti-extractable nuclear antigen antibodies (Anti-ENA antibodies)-	
Anti-Ro antibody	Sjögren syndrome
Anti-La antibody	Sjögren syndrome
Anti-PM/Scl (anti-exosome) antibody	scleroderma + polymyositis/dermatomyositis.
Anti-Scl 70 antibody	Sclerosis and scleroderma
Anti-topoisomerase antibodies	
Anti-transglutaminase antibodies	
Anti-centromere antibodies	
Anti-tTG	Coeliac disease
Anti-eTG	Dermatitis herpetiformis

10. **Ans. (a) Ewing's sarcoma** *(Ref: Harrison 17th/614, 615)*
    - *CD 99 is a marker associated with the diagnosis of Ewing's sarcoma.*
    - *Granulosa cell tumour* is also often found to be associated with CD 99.

IMMUNOHISTOLOGICAL MARKERS FOR SOME CANCERS

CD-99	Ewing's/PNET, ovarian granulose cell tumors
LCA [CD-45]	Lymphoma
CD15	Hodgkin's lymphoma
	Adenocarcinoma
Desmin	Sarcoma
Vimentin	Sarcoma
CD-31	Kaposi's sarcoma
	Angiosarcoma
Thyroid transcription factor-1	Thyroid carcinoma, lung adenocarcinoma
CD-68 and HAM 56	Malignant fibrous histiocytoma
CD117	Gastrointestinal stromal tumors (GIST)
HMB-45	Melanoma
CD-103	Hairy cell leukemia

11. **Ans. (b) Osteocalcin** *(Ref: Harrison 17th/2368)*
    Osteocalcin is a protein secreted by **osteoblasts.** It is made virtually only by osteoblasts. Thus, it is a **bone formation marker,** i.e. *osteoblastic marker.*

Biochemical markers of bone resorption		Biochemical markers of bone resorption	
a.	Amino and carboxy terminal crosslinking telopeptide of bone collagen	a.	Amino and carboxy terminal crosslinking telopeptide of bone collagen
b.	Pyridinoline	b.	Pyridinoline
c.	Free Lysyl-pyridinoline	c.	Free Lysyl-pyridinoline
d.	Tartarate-resistant acid phosphatase (TRAP)	d.	Tartarate-resistant acid phosphatase (TRAP)
e.	Hydroxyproline (not very specific)	e.	Hydroxyproline (not very specific)

12. **Ans. (b) Tumour permeation between bony trabeculae at periphery** *(Ref: Robbins 8th/1227-1230; Sternberg's pathology 4th/276, 281)*
    - Chondromas are benign tumors of hyaline cartilage that usually occurs in bones of endochondral origin. These can be:
    - *Enchondroma:* when origin is intramedullary
    - *Subperiosteal or juxtacortical*: Origin from the surface of bone
    - **Ollier disease** is a syndrome of multiple enchondromas (or enchondromatosis)
    - **Maffucis syndrome** is associated of soft-tissue hemangiomas with enchondromatosis.
    - Enchondromas are composed of well-circumscribed nodules of cytologically benign hyaline cartilage. Centre of the nodule can calcify whereas peripheral portion may undergo enchondral ossification.
    - **Chondrosarcoma** – These are group of tumors that produce neoplastic cartilage
    - Similar to chondroma, chondrosarcoma can be:
        - Intramedullary
        - Juxtacortical
    - Chondrosarcomas are second most common malignant matrix-producing tumor of bone. (Most common is osteosarcoma).
    - Histologically, chondrosarcomas are composed of malignant hyaline and myxoid cartilage. Spotty calcifications may be present and central necrosis may create cystic spaces. Tumors vary in cellularity and cytological atypia.
    - Malignant cartilage infiltrates the marrow space and surrounds pre-existing bony trabeculae.
    - Chondrosarcomas commonly arise in central portions of skeleton (including pelvis, shoulder and ribs). In contrast to chondroma, chondrosarcoma rarely involve the distal extremities.
    - Clear cell variant of chondrosarcoma characteristically originate from epiphysis of tubular long bones.

13. **Ans. (d) Duchennes musculars Dystrophy** *(Ref: Robbins 8th/1268-1269)*
    Mutation in Dystrophin gene leads to Duchene muscular dystrophy.

    Important points about DMD

    - It is an **X-linked recessive disease**.
    - Weakness begins in the pelvic girdle muscles and then extends to the shoulder girdle giving rise to **Gower's sign** (child uses his hands to climb upon himself on getting up from the floor).
    - Enlargement of the calf muscles associated with weakness, a phenomenon termed *pseudohypertrophy* **caused** initially by an increase in the size of the muscle fibers later by an increase in fat and connective tissue.
    - Serum creatine kinase is elevated during the first decade of life but returns to normal in the later stages of the disease, as muscle mass decreases.
    - Death results from respiratory insufficiency, pulmonary infection, and cardiac decompensation.
    - Histologically, there is degeneration, necrosis, and phagocytosis of muscle fibers and proliferation of endomysial connective tissue.

14. **Ans. (a) Osteoclastoma.** *(Ref: Robbins 7th/1302)*
    Osteoclastoma (giant cell tumor) is so named because it contains a profusion of multinucleated osteoclast-type giant cells. This tumor is supposed to have a monocyte lineage and the giant cells are believed to form via fusion of the mononuclear cells.

    Other giant cell lesions include:

    - Brown tumor seen in hyperparathyroidism
    - Giant cell reparative granuloma
    - Chondroblastoma
    - Pigmented villonodular synovitis.

15. **Ans. (b) Synovial cell sarcoma** *(Ref: Harrison 17th/2184; Robbins 7th/1317)*
    Synovial cell sarcoma arise from primitive mesenchymal tissue that differentiate into epithelial and spindle cells.

16. **Ans. (b) Chondroblastoma** *(Ref: Robbins 8th/1228)*
    - Chondroblastoma is a rare benign tumor occurring in young patients in their teens with a *male-to-female ratio of 2:1*.
    - Most arise near the *knee*.
    - Chondroblastoma has a striking predilection for *epiphyses and apophyses* (epiphyseal equivalents, i.e., iliac crest). Chondroblastomas are usually *painful*.
    - Radiographically, they produce a *well-defined geographic lucency* that commonly has *spotty calcifications*.
    - The tumor cells are surrounded by *scant amounts of hyaline matrix* that is deposited in a lacelike configuration; nodules of well-formed hyaline cartilage are distinctly uncommon.
    - When the matrix calcifies, it produces a characteristic *chicken-wire pattern of mineralization*.

Osteogenic sarcoma and chondromyxoid fibroma arises from metaphysis whereas Ewing sarcoma arises from medullary cavity.

17. **Ans. (c) Osteitis deformans** *(Ref: Robbins 7th/1285)*
    - The histologic hallmark in *osteitis deformans (Paget's disease) is mosaic pattern of lamellar bone.*
    - This pattern which is likened to a jig saw puzzle, is produced by prominent cement lines that anneal haphazardly oriented units of lamellar bone.

18. **Ans. (a) CD8/MHC I complex** *(Ref: Robbins 7th/1343)*
    Polymyositis is an example of inflammatory myopathy which is characterized by the presence of symmetrical proximal muscle weakness and elevated muscle enzymes. It is diagnosed with the help of T cell infiltrates within the muscle fascicles (endomysial involvement). The presence of CD8/MHC I complex is required for the diagnosis of this condition.

    > **Note:** It differs from dermatomyositis by the absence of rash (no cutaneous involvement) and its occurrence mainly in the elderly. In DM, there is presence of perifascicular atrophy (defined by the presence of groups of atrophic fibers at the periphery of the fascicles).

    In another inflammatory myopathy called inclusion body myositis, there is presence of endomysial inflammation, basophilic granular deposits around the edge of slit-like vacuoles (rimmed vacuoles) and loss of fibers (being replaced with fat cells and connective tissue). There is characteristically presence of β amyloid deposits and cytochrome oxygenase negative fibers are seen.

19. **Ans. (d) Giant cell tumor** *(Ref: Robbins 8th/1233)*

20. **Ans. (a) Multiple myeloma** *(Ref: Robbins 8th/609-611)*

21. **Ans. (b) Osteoid formation by mesenchymal cells with pleomorphism** *(Ref: Robbins 8th/1226; 7th/1294-1296)*

22. **Ans. (c) Fibrous dysplasia of bones** *(Ref: Robbins 8th/1231; 7th/1300-1301)*

23. **Ans. (b) Osteosarcoma** *(Ref: Robbins 8th/1216)*

24. **Ans. (b) PTH** *(Ref: Robbins 8th/1207-1208)*

25. **Ans. (c) Ewing's sarcoma** *(Ref: Robbins 8th/1232 ; 7th/1295,1298,1301)*

26. **Ans. (b) Osteoid Osteoma** *(Ref: Robbins 8th/1224)*

27. **Ans. (a) Osteosarcoma** *(Ref: Robbins 8th/1226,1228,1234)*

28. **Ans. (b) Type II** *(Ref: Robbins 8th/1235)*

29. **Ans. (a) Bone** *(Ref: Robbins 8th/1243-1244 ; 7th/1312)*

30. **Ans. (d) All of the above** *(Ref: Robbins 8th/1241; 7th/1310)*

30.1. **Ans. (b) Duchenne's muscular dystrophy** *(Ref: Robbins 8/e p1268)*
    Mnemonic: **DMD**
    - Duchenne's muscular dystrophy: **D**oes not **M**ake **D**ystrophin
    Mnemonic: **BMD**
    - Becker's muscular dystrophy: **B**adly **M**ade **D**ystrophin

30.2. **Ans. (c) Neuroectodermal cells....see text for details ....**(*Ref: Robbins 8/e p1232*)

30.3. **Ans. (b)Secondaries..........**(*Ref: Robbins 8/e p1235*)
    Metastatic tumours are the most common form of skeletal malignancy..(Ref: Robbins)

30.4. **Ans. (b) IgM anti-IgG antibodies** *(Ref: Robbins 8th/1238-9)*
    Symmetric polyarthritis with involvement of the proximal interphalangeal and metacarpophalangeal joints in a female patient are characteristics of rheumatoid arthritis. Rheumatoid factor, an IgM antibody directed against the Fc portion of IgG, is found in about 80% of affected individuals.
    The most specific antibody for rheumatoid arthritis is anti-CCP (cyclic citrullinated peptide) antibody.

30.5. **Ans. (c) Osteoblast and precursors** *(Ref: Robbins 9/e p1203)*
    The neoplastic cells of giant cell tumor are *primitive osteoblast precursors* but they represent only a minority of the tumor cells. The bulk of the tumor consists of non-neoplastic osteoclasts and their precursors.

30.6. **Ans. (a) Osteitis fibrosa** *(Ref: Robbins 9/e p1189)*
    Paget disease is a disorder of increased, but disordered and structurally unsound, bone mass.

30.7. **Ans. (d) Five joints or more** *(Ref: Robbins 9/e p1209; Harrison 18/e p)*

- Rheumatoid arthritis is characterized by is a chronic inflammatory disorder of autoimmune origin that may affect many tissues and organs but principally attacks the joints, producing a non suppurative proliferative and inflammatory synovitis. The earliest involved joints are typically the small joints of the hands and feet.
- The initial pattern of joint involvement may be monoarticular, *oligoarticular (less than 4 joints)*, or **poly-articular (>5 joints)**, usually in a symmetric distribution.

30.8. Ans. (a) Podagra *(Ref: Robbins 9/e p1216)*

Podagra is the involvement of the great toe in a patient with gout. As the book mentions; most first attacks are monoarticular; 50% occur in the **first metatarsophalangeal joint.**

EXPLANATIONS TO ASSERTION AND REASON QUESTIONS

Explanations (1-4): While solving assertion reason type of questions, we can use a particular method.

1. First of all, read both assertion (A) and reason (R) carefully and independently analyse whether they are true or false.
2. If A is false, the answere will directly be (d) i.e. both A and R are false. You can note that all other options (i.e. a, b or c) consider A to be true.
3. If A is true, answer can be (a), (b) or (c), Now look at R. If R is false, answer will be (c)
4. If both A and R are ture, then we have to know whether R is correctly explaining A [answer is (a)] or it is not the explanation of assertion [answer is (b)]

1. **Ans. (b) Both assertion and reason are true and reason is not the correct explanation of assertion.** *(Ref: Robbins 8th/1268-9)*
Patients with Duchene's muscular dystrophy have difficulty in walking. This is attributed to the absence of the skeletal muscle contractile protein dystrophin in these patients.

Altered dystrophin is responsible for muscular weakness in patients of Becker's muscular dystrophy.

Mnemonic:
Duchenne Muscular Dystrophy (DMD)   Doesn't Make Dystrophin (no formation)
Becker Muscular Dystrophy (BMD)   Badly Made Dystrophin (reduced formation of an altered protein)

2. **Ans. (a) Both assertion and reason are true and reason is correct explanation of assertion.** *(Ref: Robbins 8th/1226)*
Osteosarcoma is associated with the radiological appearance of Codman's triangle because the the tumor frequently breaks through the cortex and lifts the periosteum, resulting in reactive periosteal bone formation.

The formation of bone by the tumor cells is characteristic of osteosarcoma.

3. **Ans. (a) Both assertion and reason are true and reason is correct explanation of assertion.** *(Ref: Robbins 8th/1243)*
- Great toe is the most commonly affected joint in gout because uric acid gets supersaturated in the peripheral joints (ankle and toes) especially so in the lower temperatures.

4. **Ans. (b Both assertion and reason are true and reason is not the correct explanation of assertion.** *(Ref: Robbins 8th/1241)*
The seronegative spondyloarthropathies include the following: Mnemonic: PAIR

P: Psoriatic arthritis
A: Ankylosing spondylitis
I: Inflammatory bowel disease (Crohn' disease and ulcerative colitis) associated arthritis
R: Reiter syndrome

These are called seronegative because they are not associated with specific autoantibodies although they are associated with HLA B-27 as well as a triggering infection.

Musculoskeletal System

1. SALIVARY GLAND TUMORS

About 65 to 80% of the salivary gland tumors arise within the parotid, 10% in the submandibular gland, and the remainder in the minor salivary glands, including the sublingual glands. *The likelihood of a salivary gland tumor being malignant is inversely proportional to the size of the gland* which means the tumors in minor salivary glands are more likely to be malignant and those in parotid are mostly benign.

These tumors usually occur in adults, with a slight female predominance except Warthin tumor which occur more often in males than in females.

Pleomorphic Adenoma or Mixed Tumors

- They are the *most common benign tumors* that are derived from a mixture of ductal (epithelial) and myoepithelial cells, and therefore they show both epithelial and mesenchymal differentiation. About 60% of tumors in the parotid are mixed tumors.
- *Radiation exposure* increases the risk. Most pleomorphic adenomas present as rounded, well-demarcated masses rarely exceeding 6 cm.
- The epithelial elements resemble ductal cells or myoepithelial cells and are typically dispersed within a mesenchyme-like background of loose myxoid tissue containing islands of chondroid and, rarely, foci of bone.
- Tumors present as painless, slow-growing, mobile discrete masses.
- A carcinoma arising in a pleomorphic adenoma is referred to as a *carcinoma ex pleomorphic adenoma* or a *malignant mixed tumor*. The incidence of malignant transformation increases with the duration of the tumor.

Warthins Tumor (Papillary Cystadenoma Lymphomatosum)

- It is the second most common benign salivary gland neoplasm. It arises almost always in the parotid gland and occurs more commonly in males than in females, usually in the fifth to seventh decades of life. About 10% are multifocal and 10% bilateral. It is more common in smokers.
- Most Warthin's tumors are round to oval, encapsulated masses, 2 to 5 cm in diameter.
- On microscopic examination, the cystic spaces are lined by a double layer of neoplastic epithelial cells resting on a dense lymphoid stroma. The **double layer of lining cells is distinctive**, with a surface palisade of columnar cells having an abundant, finely granular, eosinophilic cytoplasm, imparting an oncocytic appearance, resting on a layer of cuboidal to polygonal cells.

Mucoepidermoid Carcinoma

They occur mainly (60 to 70%) in the parotids. They are the **most common form of primary** *malignant* **tumor of the salivary glands**. Mucoepidermoid carcinomas can grow up to 8 cm in diameter, lack well-defined capsules and are often infiltrative at the margins. It is associated with a balanced translocation, **t(11;19)** producing a fusion gene made-up of MECT1 and MAML2.

The basic histologic pattern is that of cords, sheets, or cystic configurations of squamous, mucous, or intermediate cells. The hybrid cell types often have squamous features, with small to large mucus-filled vacuoles, best seen with mucin stains.

Two other salivary gland tumors include: Adenoid cystic carcinoma and acinic cell tumor.

Adenoid cystic carcinoma is a relatively uncommon tumor. In 50% of cases, it is found in the minor salivary glands (in particular; the palate). These tumors have a **tendency to invade perineural spaces.** They have high chances of recurrence and eventually, 50% or more disseminate widely to distant sites such as bone, liver, and brain.

The **acinic cell tumor** is composed of cells resembling the normal serous acinar cells of salivary glands. **Most arise in the parotids** and the small remainder arises in the submandibular glands. They *rarely involve the minor glands*. Most characteristically, the cells have apparently *clear cytoplasm*, but the cells are sometimes solid or at other times vacuolated. The cells are disposed in sheets or microcystic, glandular, follicular, or papillary patterns. There is usually little anaplasia and few mitoses. On histologic evaluation, they are composed of small cells having dark, compact nuclei and scant cytoplasm. These cells tend to be disposed in tubular, solid, or cribriform patterns. The spaces between the tumor cells are often *filled with a hyaline material* thought to represent **excess basement membrane.**

2. OTHER IMPORTANT TUMORS

a. Neuroblastoma

It is the **most common extracranial solid tumor of childhood** and the most frequently diagnosed tumor of infancy.

- Most cases are sporadic. *Familial* cases (1-2%) result *from germline mutation in anaplastic lymphoma kinase (ALK) gene.*
- *Most common site of origin is adrenal medulla (40%) followed by para-vertebral sympathetic chain in abdomen (25%) and posterior mediastinum (15%).*
- Adrenal neuroblastomas are malignant neoplasms arising from the sympathetic neuroblasts in the medulla of the adrenal gland. There are two clinical types, based on the differences in distribution of metastasis. First (**Pepper type**) occurs in the stillborn and in young infants and metastasizes to the liver and regional lymph nodes, then the lungs, and late in the course, the calvarium and other flat bones. The second (**Hutchinson**) type is characterized clinically by secondary growth in the orbit, meninges, skull and long bones and occurs in children up to 15 years of age.
- Histologically, it is one of the **small round blue cell tumor**. It shows central space filled with eosinophilic fibrillary material called *neuropil* surrounded by concentrically arranged tumor cells **(Homer-Wright pseudorosettes).**

Note: Other small round cell tumors can be remembered as (Sofia LOREN)

Sophia	**S**mall round cell tumors
L	Lymphoma
O	Oat cell carcinoma
R	Rhabdomyosarcoma
E	Ewing's Sarcoma
N	Neuroblastoma

- Tumor cells are *positive for neuron specific enolase and contain dense core granules.*
- Maturation of some of the cells (to form ganglion cells) along with presence of primitive neuroblasts is called **ganglioneuroblastoma.** Even better differentiation with few neuroblasts is designated **ganglioneuroma.**
- Only presence of ganglion cells is not enough for designation of maturation. **Presence of Schwannian stroma, mature Schwann cells and fibroblasts is a histologic prerequisite for the designation of ganglioneuroblastoma and ganglioneuroma.**
- Metastasis develops early and widely. Hematogenous spread may occur to liver, lungs, bone marrow and bones.
- About 60-80% children present with stage 3 or 4 tumors.
- Apart from stage 1, 2, 3 and 4, stage 4S (special stage) is present in neuroblastoma. It signifies localized primary tumor with dissemination limited to skin, liver and/or bone marrow. **Stage 4S is limited to infants < 1 year.**

Prognostic Factors

Factor	Favorable	Unfavorable
1. Stage	1, 2A, 2B, 4S	3, 4
2. Age	<18 months	>18 months
3. Histology Schwannian stroma Gangliocytic differentiation Mitotic rate Mitotic karyorrhexis index Intramural calcification	 Present Present Low <200/5000 cells (≤ 4%) Present	 Absent Absent High >200/5000 (> 4%) Absent
4. DNA Ploidy	Hyperdiploid or near triploid	Near diploid
5. N-Myc	Not amplified	Amplified
6. Genetics 17q gain 1p loss 11q loss TRKA expression TRKB expression MRP expression CD44 expression Telomerase expression	 Absent Absent Absent Present Absent Absent Present Absent	 Present Present Present Absent Present Present Absent Highly expressed

Note:
- Age for prognosis in 7th edition of Robbins was 1 year, in 8th edition, this has been changed to 18 months.
- Chromosome 11q loss, TRKB expression are included in prognostic factors in 8th edition of Robbins.

b. Retinoblastoma

- Retinoblastoma is the *most common malignant eye tumor of childhood.*
- 90% cases are diagnosed before 7 years. Hereditary retinoblastoma when affecting both eyes is called bilateral retinoblastoma.
- Bilateral retinoblastoma + pineal gland tumor in suprasellar or parasellar region is called **Trilateral retinoblastoma**
- These tumors *arise from neuroepithelium of the retina*
  - A characteristic feature is **Flexner Wintersteiner rosettes** consisting of clusters of cuboidal or short columnar cells arranged around a central lumen. The nuclei are displaced away from the lumen and photoreceptor like elements are produced from it. Retinoblastoma also shows **Homer Wright rosettes** which are radial arrangement of cells around a central tangle of fibrils.
- **Fleurettes** representing photoreceptor differentiation of tumor cells is also seen.

c. Wilms' Tumor

Wilms' tumor is the **most common primary renal tumor of childhood** in USA. The risk of Wilms's tumor is increased in association with at least three recognizable groups of congenital malformations:

1. *WAGR syndrome,* characterized by aniridia, genital anomalies, and mental retardation and a 33% chance of developing Wilms' tumor. Patients with WAGR syndrome carry constitutional (germline) deletions of two genes *WT1* and *PAX6,* both located at chromosome 11p13.
2. *Denys-Drash syndrome,* which is characterized by *gonadal dysgenesis* (male pseudo-hermaphroditism) and *early-onset nephropathy* leading to renal failure. The characteristic glomerular lesion in these patients is a *diffuse mesangial sclerosis.* These patients also have germline abnormalities in *WT1.* In addition to Wilms' tumors,

these individuals are also at increased risk for developing germ-cell tumors called *gonadoblastomas*.

3. *Beckwith-Wiedemann syndrome*, characterized by enlargement of body organs (organomegaly), macroglossia, hemihypertrophy, omphalocele, and abnormal large cells in adrenal cortex (adrenal cytomegaly). The genetic locus involved in these patients is in band p15.5 of chromosome 11 called "*WT2*". In addition to Wilms' tumors, patients with Beckwith-Wiedemann syndrome are also *at increased risk for developing hepatoblastoma, adrenocortical tumors, rhabdomyosarcomas, and pancreatic tumors*.

Morphology

Grossly, Wilms's tumor tends to present as a large, solitary, well-circumscribed mass and on cut section, the tumor is soft, homogeneous, and tan to grey with occasional foci of hemorrhage, cyst formation, and necrosis. **Microscopically,** Wilms's tumors are characterized by the *classic triphasic combination of blastemal, stromal, and epithelial cell types* observed in the vast majority of lesions.

d. Histiocytosis

Langerhans cell histiocytosis (LCH) has the following entities:
1. *Letterer-Siwe syndrome* (multifocal multisystem LCH)
2. *Pulmonary Langerhans' cell histiocytosis:* most often seen in adult smokers and can regress spontaneously on cessation of smoking.
3. *Eosinophilic granuloma.*
   - *Hand-Schuller-Christian triad* is composed of *calavrial bone defects, diabetes insipidus and exophthalmos.*
   - The tumor cells express **HLA-DR, S-100, and CD1a.**
   *The presence of **Birbeck's granules** in the cytoplasm is characteristic* which have a **tennis-racket appearance** under the electron microscope.

e. Mediastinal Tumors

The mediastinum is the region between the pleural sacs. It is separated into three compartments.
1. The *anterior mediastinum* extends from the sternum anteriorly to the pericardium and brachiocephalic vessels posteriorly. It contains the thymus gland, the anterior mediastinal lymph nodes, and the internal mammary arteries and veins.
2. The *middle mediastinum* lies between the anterior and posterior mediastinum and contains the heart; the ascending and transverse arches of the aorta; the venae cavae; the brachiocephalic arteries and veins; the phrenic nerves; the trachea, main bronchi, and their contiguous lymph nodes; and the pulmonary arteries and veins.
3. The *posterior mediastinum* is bounded by the pericardium and trachea anteriorly and the vertebral column posteriorly. It contains the descending thoracic aorta, esophagus, thoracic duct, azygos and hemiazygos veins, and the posterior group of mediastinal lymph nodes.

The most common lesions in the **anterior mediastinum** are *thymomas, lymphomas, teratomatous neoplasms, and thyroid masses.* The most common masses in the **middle mediastinum** are *vascular masses, lymph node enlargement from metastases or granulomatous disease, and pleuropericardial and bronchogenic cysts.* In the **posterior mediastinum**, *neurogenic tumors, meningoceles, meningomyeloceles, gastroenteric cysts, and esophageal diverticula* are commonly found.

THYMOMA

- The **thymus** is *derived from the third and fourth pharyngeal pouches* and is located in the anterior mediastinum. The thymus is composed of epithelial and stromal cells and lymphoid precursors.

- If a lymphoid cell within the thymus becomes neoplastic, the disease that develops is a lymphoma which is a **T cell lymphoblastic lymphomas** in most of the cases. **If the epithelial cells of the thymus become neoplastic, the tumor that develops is a thymoma.**
- **Thymoma is the most common cause of an anterior mediastinal mass in adults.** Thymomas are most common in the fifth and sixth decade. Majority (90%) of thymomas are in the anterior mediastinum. *Thymomas are epithelial tumors and all of them have malignant potential.* They may have a *variable percentage of lymphocytes within the tumor.* The epithelial component of the tumor may consist primarily of round or oval cells derived mainly from the cortex or spindle-shaped cells derived mainly from the medulla or combinations thereof.
- These tumors present clinically in 40% patients as causing symptoms due to compression on the mediastinal structures or due to their association with myasthenia gravis. In addition to myasthenia gravis, other paraneoplastic syndromes, such as acquired hypogammaglobulinemia, pure red cell aplasia, Graves disease, pernicious anemia, dermatomyositis-polymyositis, and Cushing syndrome, can be seen.
- *Epstein-Barr virus may be associated with thymomas.*

WHO Histologic Classification of Thymus Tumors

Type	Histologic Description
A	Medullary thymoma
AB	Mixed thymoma
B1	Predominantly cortical thymoma
B2	Cortical thymoma
B3	Well-differentiated thymic carcinoma
C	Thymic carcinoma

The genetic lesions in thymomas are not well characterized. Some data suggest that *Epstein-Barr virus may be associated with thymomas.*

3. SCLERODERMA

There are three major forms of scleroderma: diffuse, limited (CREST syndrome) and morphea/linear. Diffuse and limited scleroderma are both a systemic disease, whereas the linear/morphea form is localized to the skin.

Diffuse Scleroderma

Diffuse scleroderma (progressive systemic sclerosis) is the **most severe form**. It has a rapid onset, involves more widespread skin hardening, will generally cause much internal organ damage (especifically the lungs and gastrointestinal tract), and is generally more life-threatening.

Limited Scleroderma/CREST Syndrome

The limited form is much milder. It has a slow onset and progression. Skin hardening is usually confined to the hands and face, internal organ involvement is less severe, and a much better prognosis is expected. In typical cases of limited scleroderma, *Raynaud's phenomenon may precede scleroderma by several years.* The scleroderma may be limited to the fingers—known as **sclerodactyly.**

The limited form is often referred to as **CREST syndrome** characterized by:

- Calcinosis
- Raynaud's syndrome
- Esophageal dysmotility
- Sclerodactyly
- Telangiectasia

CREST is a limited form associated with **antibodies against centromeres** and usually spares the lungs and kidneys.

Morphea/Linear Scleroderma

Morphea/linear scleroderma involves isolated patches of hardened skin. There generally is no internal organ involvement.

Diagnosis is by clinical suspicion, presence of autoantibodies (especifically anti-centromere and anti-scl70/anti-topoisomerase antibodies) and occasionally by biopsy. Of the antibodies, 90% have a detectable anti-nuclear antibody. *Anti-centromere antibody is more common in the limited form (80-90%) than in the systemic form (10%), and anti-scl70 is more common in the diffuse form (30-40%).*

4. DEFICIENCIES AND TOXICITIES OF METALS

Element	Deficiency	Toxicity
Boron	No biologic function determined	Developmental defects, male sterility, testicular atrophy
Calcium	Reduced bone mass, osteoporosis	Renal insufficiency (milk-alkali syndrome), nephrolithiasis, impaired iron absorption
Copper	Anemia, growth retardation, defective keratinization and pigmentation of hair, hypothermia, degenerative changes in aortic elastin, osteopenia, mental deterioration	Nausea, vomiting, diarrhea, hepatic failure, tremor, mental deterioration, hemolytic anemia, renal dysfunction
Chromium	Impaired glucose tolerance	Occupational: renal failure, dermatitis, pulmonary cancer
Fluoride	Dental caries	Dental and skeletal fluorosis, osteosclerosis
Iodine	Thyroid enlargement, cretinism	Thyroid dysfunction, acne-like eruptions
Iron	Muscle abnormalities, koilonychia, pica, anemia, reduced work performance, impaired cognitive development, premature labor, increased perinatal and maternal mortality	Gastrointestinal effects (nausea, vomiting, diarrhea, constipation), iron overload with organ damage, acute systemic toxicity
Manganese	Impaired growth and skeletal development, reproduction, lipid and carbohydrate metabolism; upper body rash	*General:* Neurotoxicity, Parkinson-like symptoms *Occupational:* Encephalitis-like syndrome, Parkinson-like syndrome, psychosis, pneumoconiosis
Molybdenum	Severe neurologic abnormalities	Reproductive and fetal abnormalities
Selenium	Cardiomyopathy, heart failure, striated muscle degeneration	*General:* Alopecia, nausea, vomiting, abnormal nails, emotional lability, peripheral neuropathy, lassitude, garlic odor to breath, dermatitis *Occupational:* Lung and nasal carcinomas, liver necrosis, pulmonary inflammation
Phosphorous	Rickets (osteomalacia), proximal muscle weakness, rhabdomyolysis, paresthesia, ataxia, seizure, confusion, heart failure, hemolysis, acidosis	Hyperphosphatemia
Zinc	Growth retardation, altered taste and smell, alopecia, dermatitis, diarrhea, immune dysfunction, failure to thrive, gonadal atrophy, congenital malformations	*General:* Reduced copper absorption, gastritis, sweating, fever, nausea, vomiting *Occupational:* Respiratory distress, pulmonary fibrosis

Miscellaneous

MULTIPLE CHOICE QUESTIONS

1. The immune-cytochemical feature of Langerhans cell histiocytosis is positivity for which of the following?
   (a) CD1a *(AI 2012)*
   (b) CD99 (mic-2)
   (c) HMB-45
   (d) CD117

2. In the congenital dystrophic variety of epidermolysis bullosa, mutation is seen in the gene coding for
   (a) Laminin 4 *(AI 2012)*
   (b) Collagen type 7
   (c) Alpha 6 integerin
   (d) Keratin 14

3. The marker for Langerhans cell histiocytosis is:
   (a) CD 1a *(AI 2010)*
   (b) CD 20
   (c) CD 3
   (d) CD 30

4. For examination of fungus from a sample, uniformly stain by: *(AI 2010)*
   (a) Alizarin
   (b) PAS
   (c) MassonTrichome
   (d) Giemsa

5. All are components of photoreceptor matrix, except:
   (a) MMP *(AI 2008)*
   (b) TIMP
   (c) SPARC
   (d) MIMECAN

6. Acinic cell carcinomas of the salivary gland arise most often in the: *(AI 2006)*
   (a) Parotid salivary gland
   (b) Minor salivary glands
   (c) Submandibular salivary gland
   (d) Sublingual salivary gland

7. In familial Mediterranean fever, the gene encoding the following protein undergoes mutation *(AI 2005)*
   (a) Pyrin
   (b) Perforin
   (c) Atrial natriuretic factor
   (d) Immunoglobulin light chain

8. To which of the following events is 'good' outcome in Neuroblastoma associated *(AI 2004)*
   (a) Diploidy
   (b) N-myc amplification
   (c) Chromosome/p depletion
   (d) Trk A expression

9. Splenic macrophages in Gaucher's disease differ from those in ceroid histiocytosis by staining positive for:
   (a) Lipids *(AI 2004)*
   (b) Phospholipids
   (c) Acid-fast stain
   (d) Iron

10. A 70 years old male who has been chewing tobacco for the past 50 years presents with a six months history of a large, fungating, soft papillary lesions in the oral cavity. The lesion has penetrated into the mandible. Lymph nodes are not palpable. Two biopsies take from the lesion proper show benign appearing papillomatosis with hyperkeratosis and acanthosis infiltrating the subjacent tissues. The most likely diagnosis is: *(AI 2004)*
    (a) Squamous cell papilloma
    (b) Squamous cell carcinoma
    (c) Verrucous carcinoma
    (d) Malignant mixed tumour

11. Hereditary retinoblastoma develop the following chromosomal deletion: *(AI 2003)*
    (a) 13q14
    (b) 11p13
    (c) 14q13
    (d) 22q11

12. All the statement about lactoferin are true, except:
    (a) It is present in secondary granules of neutrophil
    (b) It is present in exocrine secretions of body *(AI 2003)*
    (c) It has great affinity for iron
    (d) It transports iron for erythropoiesis

13. Protein involved in intercellular connections is:
    (a) Connexins *(AI 2001)*
    (b) Integrins
    (c) Adhesins
    (d) None of the above

14. Which of the following stains is used to detect lipid in frozen section biopsy in histopathology laboratory?
    (a) PAS *(AIIMS Nov 2009)*
    (b) Oil Red O
    (c) NSE
    (d) Silver Methanamine

15. Young boy presented with multiple flaccid bullae and oral lesions. Diagnostic finding in skin biopsy immunofluorescence test would be: *(AIIMS Nov 2009)*
    (a) Fish net IgG in dermoepidermal junction
    (b) Linear IgG in dermoepidermal junction
    (c) Linear IgG in dermal papillae
    (d) Granular IgA in reticular dermis

16. **A 14 years old girl on exposure to cold develop pallor of extremities followed by pain and cyanosis. In later ages of life she is prone to develop?** *(AIIMS Nov 2008)*
    (a) Systemic lupus erythematosus
    (b) Scleroderma
    (c) Rheumatoid arthritis
    (d) Histiocytosis

17. **Which is false about acrodermatitis? enteropathica?** *(AIIMS Nov 2008)*
    (a) Triad of diarrhea, dementia and dermatitis
    (b) Low serum zinc levels
    (c) Symptoms improve with zinc supplementation
    (d) Autosomal recessive

18. **Which of the following statement is incorrect?** *(AIIMS Nov 2008)*
    (a) Selenium deficiency causes cardiomyopathy
    (b) Zinc deficiency causes pulmonary fibrosis
    (c) Increased calcium intake cause iron deficiency
    (d) Vitamin A deficiency occurs after 6 months to 1year of low vitamin A diet

19. **A patient presents with mediastinal mass with sheets of epithelial cells giving arborizing pattern of keratin reactivity along with interspersed lymphoid cells. The apt diagnosis would be:** *(AIIMS May 2008)*
    (a) Thymoma
    (b) Thymic carcinoid
    (c) Primary mediastinal lymphoma
    (d) Non-Hodgkin lymphoma

20. **Ultrastructural finding in case of Paraganglioma:**
    (a) Deposition of glycogen *(AIIMS May 2008)*
    (b) Enlarged mitochondria
    (c) Shrunken mitochondria
    (d) Dense core granules

21. **Brain natriuretic peptide is degraded by:**
    (a) Neutral endopeptidase *(AIIMS May 2007)*
    (b) Elastase
    (c) Collagenase
    (d) Ompatrilat

22. **Why fetal cells continue to divide but terminally differentiated adult cells do not divide:** *(AIIMS Nov 2006)*
    (a) There are many cyclin inhibitors which prevent cell to enter into S phase in adult
    (b) Phosphatase absent in fetal cells
    (c) Proteinase is absent in fetus
    (d) Absence of CD kinase

23. **All of the following are examples of a round cell tumor, except:** *(AIIMS Nov 2005)*
    (a) Neuroblastoma
    (b) Ewing's sarcoma
    (c) Non-Hodgkin's lymphoma
    (d) Osteosarcoma

24. **The tissue of origin of the Kaposi's sarcoma is:**
    (a) Lymphoid *(AIIMS May 2005)*
    (b) Vascular

(c) Neural
(d) Muscular

25. **"Tophus" is the pathognomic lesion of which of the following condition:** *(AIIMS May 2003)*
    (a) Multiple myeloma
    (b) Cystinosis
    (c) Gout
    (d) Eale's disease

26. **Which of the following diseases have an underlying mitochondrial abnormality?** *(PGI Dec 01)*
    (a) Krabbe's disease
    (b) Fabry's disease
    (c) Mitochondrial myopathy
    (d) Oncocytoma
    (e) Fanconi's syndrome

27. **Foam cells seen in:** *(PGI Dec 2005)*
    (a) Alport's syndrome
    (b) Niemann-Pick disease
    (c) Atherosclerosis
    (d) Pneumonia

28. **Which among the following is the best tissue fixative?**
    (a) Formalin *(Delhi PG-2007)*
    (b) Alcohol
    (c) Normal saline
    (d) Methylene blue

29. **All of the following are forms of panniculitis except:** *(Delhi PG-2006)*
    (a) Weber-Christian disease
    (b) Erythema induratum
    (c) Erythema nodosum
    (d) All of the above

30. **Warthin-Finkeldey cells are seen in:**
    (a) Measles
    (b) Rubella
    (c) Influenza
    (d) Rickettsial pox

31. **Pathogenesis is sequence of events in response to:** *(Delhi PG-2004)*
    (a) Expression of disease upto clinical manifestation
    (b) Expression of disease upto non-clinical manifestation
    (c) The etiological agent for the initial stimulus to the ultimate expression of disease
    (d) None

32. **All of the following characteristics are true of liposarcoma except that it:** *(Karnataka 2009)*
    (a) Is commonly found in the retroperitoneum
    (b) Frequently gives rise to embolization in lymphatics
    (c) Is the most common soft tissue sarcoma
    (d) Arises very rarely in subcutaneous tissue

33. **All of the following are correctly matched except:** *(Karnataka 2008)*
    (a) Russell bodies—Multiple myeloma

(b) Russell bodies – Alcoholic liver disease
(c) Michaelis Gutmann bodies – Langerhan's histio-cytosis
(d) Civatte bodies – Lichen planus

34. Most common second malignancy in patients with familial retinoblastoma is: *(Karnataka 2004)*
(a) Teratoma
(b) Medullary carcinoma
(c) Osteosarcoma
(d) Malignant melanoma

35. Hutchison's secondaries in skull are due to tumors in:
(a) Lung *(DNB-2000, 2003)*
(b) Breast
(c) Liver
(d) Adrenals
(e) Testes

36. Rosette shaped arrangement of cells are seen in:
(a) Thecoma of ovary *(DNB- 2000, 2006, 2007)*
(b) Ependymoma
(c) Neurofibroma
(d) Lymphoma

37. Spontaneous regression though rare is seen in:
(a) Burkitt's lymphoma *(DNB- 2000)*
(b) Wilms' tumor
(c) Neuroblastoma
(d) Melanoma

38. Peri-oral pallor and Dennie's lines are seen in:
(a) Atopic dermatitis *(DNB- 2008)*
(b) Chronic actinic dermatitis
(c) Blood dyscrasias
(d) Perioral contact dermatitis

39. Most common tumor of parotid gland is:
(a) Pleomorphic adenoma *(UP 2001)*
(b) Warthin's adenoma
(c) Mucoepidermoid carcinoma
(d) Mixed tumor

40. MC malignant tumor of parotid glands is:
(a) Pleomorphic adenoma *(UP 2001)*
(b) Mucoepidermoid carcinoma
(c) Warthin's tumor
(d) Mixed tumor of salivary gland

41. Punctate basophilia is found in: *(UP 2001)*
(a) DDT poisoning
(b) Mercury vapors inhalation
(c) Cyanide poisoning
(d) Lead poisoning

42. Epulis is *(UP-98, 2004)*
(a) Tumor of gingiva
(b) Tumor of enamel of tooth
(c) Disarrangement of tooth
(d) Dysplastic leukoplakia

43. Most common tumor of infancy is *(UP 2005)*
(a) Lymphangioma

(b) Rhabdomyoma
(c) Hemangioma
(d) Lipoma

44. Triad of biotin deficiency is *(UP 2005)*
(a) Dermatitis, glossitis, steatorrhea
(b) Dermatitis, glossitis, alopecia
(c) Mental changes, diarrhea, alopecia
(d) Dermatitis, dementia, diarrhea

45. Basophilic stippling is seen in: *(UP 2006)*
(a) Cadmium poisoning
(b) Lead poisoning
(c) Chromium poisoning
(d) Iron poisoning

46. Most common tumor of infancy is *(UP 2005, 2007)*
(a) Lymphangioma
(b) Rhabdomyoma
(c) Hemangioma
(d) Lipoma

47. Pleomorphic adenoma usually arises from
(a) Parotid gland *(UP 2007)*
(b) Submandibular gland
(c) Minor salivary gland
(d) Superficial lobe

48. Direct Coomb's test detects: *(UP 2008)*
(a) Antigen in serum
(b) Antibodies on RBC surface
(c) Antigen on RBC surface
(d) Antibodies in serum

49. In vitamin deficiencies, patient is vulnerable to infection with: *(RJ 2000)*
(a) Measles
(b) Mumps
(c) Rubella
(d) Whooping cough

50. Paralytic food poisoning is caused by: *(RJ 2000)*
(a) *Staphylococci*
(b) *E. coli*
(c) *B. cereus*
(d) *Clostridia*

51. Which is not present in anterior mediastinum?
(a) Lymphoma *(RJ 2000)*
(b) Thymoma
(c) Teratoma
(d) Neurofibroma

52. Nonbacterial verrucous endocarditis is associated with
(a) Rheumatic carditis *(RJ 2001)*
(b) Rheumatoid arthritis
(c) SLE
(d) Infective endocarditis

53. Frozen section biopsy in not used for: *(Bihar 2005)*
(a) Enzyme
(b) Amyloid
(c) Fat
(d) Proteins

54. Rodent ulcer is due to: *(RJ 2002)*
(a) Syphilis
(b) Burns
(c) Basal cell carcinoma
(d) TB

55. Most common salivary gland tumor in adult is:
(a) Mucoepidermoid carcinoma *(RJ 2003)*
(b) Lymphoma
(c) Pleomorphic adenoma
(d) None

56. Soft chancre is caused by: *(RJ 2003)*
(a) Syphilis
(b) TB
(c) Chancroid
(d) *L. donovani*

57. Kobner's phenomena is seen in: *(RJ 2003)*
(a) Psoriasis
(b) Lichen planus
(c) Toxic epidermal necrolysis
(d) All

58. Pellagra is characterized by all except: *(RJ 2003)*
(a) Diarrhea   (b) Dementia
(c) Dermatitis   (d) Diplopia

59. Smoking causes all cancers except: *(AP 2002)*
(a) Liver   (b) Pancreas
(c) Bladder   (d) Lung

60. Endothelial cells have: *(Bihar 2003)*
(a) Weibel Palade bodies
(b) Gamma Gandy bodies
(c) Both
(d) None

Most Recent Questions

60.1. Which one of the following conditions is NOT associated with occurrence of pellagra?
(a) People eating mainly corn-based diet
(b) Carcinoid syndrome
(c) Phototherapy
(d) Hartnup disease

EXPLANATIONS

1. **Ans. (a) CD1a** *(Ref: Robbins 8th/631-2)*

Entities in Langerhans cell histiocytosis

- Letterer-Siwe syndrome (multifocal multisystem LCH)
- Pulmonary Langerhans' cell histiocytosis: seen in adult smokers and can regress on cessation of smoking.
- Eosinophilic granuloma.

The tumor cells in Langerhans cell histiocytosis express HLA-DR, S-100^Q, and CD1a^Q.

2. **Ans. (b) Collagen type 7** *(Ref: Robbins 8th/1196)*

Epidermolysis bullosa are a group of non inflammatory disorders caused by defects in structural proteins which lend stability to the skin. It can be of the following types:
- **Simplex type**: defect in **basal layer of epidermis** due to mutation in gene for keratin 14 or 5
- **Junctional type**: blisters occur at the level of **lamina lucida**
- **Dystrophic type**: blisters beneath the **lamina densa** due to defect in COL7A1 gene for **collagen type VII^Q**

Clinical importance

Squamous cell cancers^Q can arise in these chronic blisters.
Non-Herlitz junctional epidermolysis bullosa is caused by defect in LAMB3 gene encoding *laminin Vβ3.*

3. **Ans. (a) CD 1a** *(Ref: Robbins 8th/631-632)*

Langerhans cell histiocytosis (LCH) has the following entities:
- *Letterer-Siwe syndrome* (multifocal multisystem LCH)
- *Pulmonary Langerhans' cell histiocytosis:* most often seen in adult smokers and can regress spontaneously on cessation of smoking.
- *Eosinophilic granuloma.*
- *Hand-Schuller-Christian triad* is composed of *calavrial bone defects, diabetes insipidus and exophthalmos.*
- The tumor cells express **HLA-DR, S-100, and CD1a.**
- *The presence of **Birbeck's granules** in the cytoplasm is characteristic* which have a **tennis-racket appearance** under the electron microscope.

4. **Ans. (b) PAS** *(Ref: Robbins 8th/336, Harsh Mohan 6th/12-13)*
- PAS (Periodic Acid Schiff) stain is used for Carbohydrates particularly glycogen and all mucins, amoebae and fungi

Other frequently asked stains:

Stains	Substance
Congo red with polarizing light	Amyloid
Ziehl Neilson stain	Tubercle bacilli
Masson's Trichrome	Extracellular collagen
Perl's stain	Hemosiderin, iron
Masson-Fontana	Melanin, argentaffin cells
Alizarin	calcium
Feulgen reaction	DNA
Giemsa	Campylobacter, leishmaniae, malaria parasites

- Silver methanamine is a better stain for fungi and stains *Pneumocystis* and the fungi black in color.
- Mucicarmine is for staining cryptococci

5. **Ans. (d) MIMECAN** *(Ref: Robbins 7th/105, 109-111; Retina; Stephen J.Ryan 4th/140)*
- Ryan says the retinal pigment epithelial (RPE) cells actively synthesize and degrade extracellular matrix (ECM) components. Deposition of ECM molecules is polarized with different components secreted apically and basally. The apical domain of the RPE cells is embedded in the interphotoreceptor matrix which is produced by RPE and inner segments of the photoreceptors. Degradation of ECM is regulated by the equilibrium between matrix metalloproteinases [(MMP) and their tissue inhibitors (TIMPs)].

- The normal RPE expresses membrane bound type I (MT_1-MMP) and type 2 (MT_2 MMP) metalloproteinase as well as the metalloproteinase inhibitors TIMP-1 and TIMP-3. TIMP-3 accumulates in Brusch membrane and is seen in age related macular degeneration (ARMD).
- Patients with SPARC (ostionectin) (Secreted Protein Acidic and Rich in Cysteine) contributes to tissue remodeling in response to injury and functions as an angiogenesis inhibitor. SPACR (sialyprotein associated with cones and rodes) is a glycoprotein identified in human interphotoreceptor matrix.
- MIMECAN is a member of small leucine rich proteoglycans (SLRP) gene family. They are essential for normal collagen fibrillogenesis in various connective tissues like cornea. It is not present in photorceptor matrix. It is also known as osteoglycin.

6. **Ans. (a) Parotid salivary gland***(Ref: Robbins 7th/794)*
- Acinic cell tumors of salivary glands are uncommon tumors representing 2 to 3% of salivary gland tumors.
- These are composed of cells resembling the normal serous acinar cells of salivary glands.
- Most of these arise in the parotids. The remainder arises in submandibular glands.
- Most parotid tumors are benign but half of submandibular and sublingual and most minor salivary gland tumors are malignant.

7. **Ans. (a) Pyrin***(Ref: Robbins 7th/261, Harrison 17th/2144)*
- **Familial Mediterranean fever (FMF)** is a group of inherited diseases characterized by recurrent episodes of fever with serosal, synovial or cutaneous inflammation and in some individuals, the eventual development of systemic AA amyloidosis.
- The FMF gene is located at **16p13.3** and encodes a protein denoted **PYRIN** (marenostrin) that is expressed in granulocytes, eosinophils, monocytes, dendritic cells and fibroblasts.
- Most of the gene mutations responsible for disease occurs in **exon 10** of the gene with a smaller group in exon 2 FMF follows **autosomal recessive** inheritance.
- **Treatment** of choice for FMF is daily oral **colchicine**, which decreases the frequency and intensity of attacks and prevents the development of systemic AA amyloidosis.

8. **Ans. (d) Trk A expression***(Ref: Robbins 7th/503)*
- Neuroblastoma has good prognosis in infants (< 1 year old) regardless of the stage. These tumors are hyperdiploid or near triploid.

Prognostic factors in Neuroblastoma
- **Age and stage:** Good prognosis in infants regardless of stage. In children > 1 year, stage III and IV poor prognosis as compared to stage I or II.
- **Genetics:** Hyperdiploid or near triploid and high expression of Trk-A have good prognosis whereas near-diploidly, deletion of chromosome 1p or 14, gain of chromosome 17q and N-myc amplification is associated with unfavorable outcome.
- 3. **Tumor markers:** Telomerase and MRP expression has poor prognosis whereas CD 44 expression associated with good prognosis.
- **Histology:** Differentiation (into Schwann cells and gangliocytes), low mitotic rate and intramural calcification has good prognosis.

Note: Most characteristic cytogenetic abnormality in neuroblastoma is 1p deletion.

9. **Ans. (a) Lipids***(Ref: Harrison 17th/2548, 2455)*
- Ceroid histiocytosis also known as neuronal cerebrolipofuschinosis is a group of diseases where lipofuschin, a yellow brown cytoplasmic pigment is deposited in the neurons. Lipofuschin is a lipid.
- In Gaucher's disease, all patients have a nonuniform infiltration of bone marrow by lipid laden macrophages termed Gaucher cells's.
Thus both these disorders have 'lipids' in the macrophages.

GAUCHER'S DISEASE
- It is autosomal recessive lysosomal storage disorder due to deficiency of enzyme α-glucosidase resulting in accumulation of glucosylceramide.
- Decreased activity (0-20%) of α-glucosidase in nucleated cells is required for diagnosis.
- Type 1 disease do not involve CNS and present as hepatosplenomegaly with skeletal dysplasia whereas Type 2 Gaucher's disease is a severe CNS disease leading to death by 2 year of age. Type 3 disease has highly variable manifestations in CNS and viscera.

10. **Ans. (c) Verrucous carcinoma** *(Ref: Robbins 7th/1037; Ackerman's surgical pathology 8th/235)*
Verrucous carcinomas also referred to as giant condyloma accuminatum or **Buschke-Lowenstein tumour** is considered an intermediate lesion between condyloma acuminata and invasive squamous cell carcinoma. It is important to distinguish verrucuous carcinomas from squamous cell carcinoma as these tend to remain localized and are cured by wide excision, however they may undergo malignant transformation to invasive squamous cell carcinomas.

Features of verrucuous carcinomas
- Predilection for **males** > 50 years
- Predisposed in **tobacco** users, poor oral hygiene
- **Grossly**, it is a soft, large, wart like (papillomatous) lesion which may show fungation
- **Microscopically:**
  - Cytological features of malignancy are absent or minimal and rare
  - Epithelium is thickened and thrown into papillary folds
  - The folds project both above and below the level of surrounding mucosa and crypt like surface grooves exhibit marked, pre-keratin plugging.
  - The deep border of epithelial projections is 'pushing' and not infiltrative.

11. **Ans. (a) 13q 14** *(Ref: Harrison's 17th/413)*
The term contiguous gene syndrome refers to genetic disorders that mimic single gene disorders. They result from deletion of a small number of tightly clustered genes. Because some are too small to be detected cytogenetically, they are termed as **microdeletion syndromes**
The important **microdeletion syndromes are:**

1. Wilms' tumor – Aniridia complex (WAGR syndrome)	11p 13
2. Retinoblastoma	13q 14.11
3. Prader-Willi syndrome	15q11-13
4. Angelman's syndrome	15q11-13
5. DiGeorge's syndrome/Velo-cardiofacial syndrome	22q 11
6. Miller-Dieker syndrome	17p 13

Deletions involving the long arm of chromosome 22 (22q 11) are the most common microdeletions identified to date.

Note: Important microduplication syndromes include Beckwith-Wiedemann syndrome (11p 15) and Charcot- Marie-Tooth syndrome type IA (17 p 11.2)

12. **Ans. (d) It transports iron for erythropoiesis** *(Ref: Harper 25th/775, Harrison 17th/378,815,847)*
- Transport of iron for erythropoiesis is done by transferin and not by lactoferin.
- Lactoferin is found in specific/secondary granules in neutrophils and in many exocrine secretions and exudates (milk, tears, mucus, saliva, bile, etc.)

13. **Ans. (a) Connexins** *(Ref: Harrison 17th/2479)*
- **Connexins** are complex protein assemblies that traverse the lipid bilayer of the plasma membrane and form a continuous channel. A pair of connexins from adjacent cells joins to form a gap junction that bridges the 2-4 mm gap between the cells. These are important for communications in neurons and glial cells.
- **Adhesions** are microbial surface antigens that frequently exist in the form of filamentous projection (pili or fimbria) and bind to specific receptors on epithelial cell membranes.
- **Integrins** are a family of cell membrane glycoproteins. These are involved in cell adhesion.

14. **Ans. (b) Oil Red O** *(Ref: Harsh Mohan 6th/12-13)*
Lipids are detected in histopathology by the use of the following stains:
- *Oil red O*: Mineral oils stain red and unsaturated fats stain pink
- *Sudan Black B*: Unsaturated fats stain blue black
- *Osmium tetroxide*: Unsaturated fats stain brown-black whereas saturated fats are unstained.

Regarding other options:
- PAS (Periodic Acid Schiff) stain is for carbohydrates particularly glycogen and all mucins
- Silver Methanamine is for fungi
- Non-specific esterase (NSE) is for staining myeloblast in patients of Acute myeloid leukemia (AML)

15. **Ans. (a) Fish net IgG in dermoepidermal junction** *(Ref: Robbins 8th/1192-1193, Harrison 17th/336-339)*
   - The inflammatory bullous lesions may be Pemphigus vulgaris, Bullous pemphigoid and dermatitis herpetiformis. The presentation of multiple flaccid bullae and oral lesions in a young boy is suggestive of *Pemphigus vulgaris*. An important histological finding in pemphigus is **acantholysis** which is dissolution, or lysis, of the intercellular adhesion sites within a squamous epithelial surface. The **suprabasal acantholytic blister** that forms is *characteristic of pemphigus vulgaris*. The antibody in pemphigus vulgaris reacts with *desmoglein 1 and 3*, a component of the desmosomes that appear to bind keratinocytes together. By direct immunofluorescence, lesional sites show a characteristic **netlike pattern** of intercellular IgG deposits.

   About other options:
   - Bullous pemphigoid generally affects *elderly* individuals. The *bullae are tense* and oral lesions are present in 10-15% of affected individuals. The **subepithelial acantholytic blister** is *characteristic of bullous pemphigoid*. The antibody in bullous pemphigoid reacts with bullous pemphigoid antigens 1 and 2 (BPAG 1 and 2) present in *dermoepidermal junction*. Linear IgG in dermoepidermal junction are seen by direct immunofluorescence. (option 'B').
   - Dermatitis herpetiformis is characterized by *urticaria and grouped vesicles*. The disease results from formation of antibodies against gliadin and is associated with *celiac disease*. By direct immunofluorescence, dermatitis herpetiformis shows granular deposits of **IgA** selectively localized in the *tips of dermal papillae*. (option 'D').
   - Pemphigus foliaceous is having the antibody reacting with *desmoglein 1 alone*. There is selective involvement of superficial epidermis at the level of the stratum granulosum. It usually affects the scalp, face, chest, and back, and the mucous membranes are only rarely affected. Linear IgG in dermal papillae is a feature of Pemphigus foliaceous. (option 'C').

16. **Ans. (b) Scleroderma** *(Ref: Harrison 17th/2096)*
   - The girl in this case is showing Raynaud's phenomenon and is likely to suffer later from systemic sclerosis.
   - **Raynaud's phenomenon** is characterized by episodic digital ischemia, manifested clinically by the sequential development of digital blanching, cyanosis, and rubor of the fingers or toes following cold exposure and subsequent rewarming. The blanching, or pallor, represents the ischemic phase of the phenomenon and results from vasospasm of digital arteries. During the ischemic phase, capillaries and venules dilate, and cyanosis results from the deoxygenated blood that is present in these vessels. A sensation of cold or numbness or paresthesia of the digits often accompanies the phases of pallor and cyanosis.
   - Raynaud's phenomenon is broadly separated into two categories: The **idiopathic** variety, termed *Raynaud's disease*, and the **secondary** variety, which is associated with other disease states or known causes of vasospasm
   - Raynaud's phenomenon occurs in **80–90% of patients with systemic sclerosis (scleroderma)** and is the presenting symptom in 30% of patients. It may be the only symptom of scleroderma for many years. Abnormalities of the digital vessels may contribute to the development of Raynaud's phenomenon in this disorder. Ischemic fingertip ulcers may develop and progress to gangrene and autoamputation. About 20% of patients with systemic lupus erythematosus (SLE) have Raynaud's phenomenon. Occasionally, persistent digital ischemia develops and may result in ulcers or gangrene. In most severe cases, the small vessels are occluded by a proliferative endarteritis. Raynaud's phenomenon occurs in about 30% of patients with dermatomyositis or polymyositis. It frequently develops in patients with rheumatoid arthritis and may be related to the intimal proliferation that occurs in the digital arteries.
   - Atherosclerosis of the extremities is a frequent cause of Raynaud's phenomenon in men >50 years. Thromboangiitis obliterans is an uncommon cause of Raynaud's phenomenon but should be considered in young men, particularly those who are cigarette smokers. The development of cold-induced pallor in these disorders may be confined to one or two digits of the involved extremity. Occasionally, Raynaud's phenomenon may follow acute occlusion of large and medium-sized arteries by a thrombus or embolus. Embolization of atheroembolic debris may cause digital ischemia. The latter situation often involves one or two digits and should not be confused with Raynaud's phenomenon. In patients with thoracic outlet compression syndrome, Raynaud's phenomenon may result from diminished intravascular pressure, stimulation of sympathetic fibers in the brachial plexus, or a combination of both. Raynaud's phenomenon occurs in patients with primary pulmonary hypertension; this is more than coincidental and may reflect a neurohumoral abnormality that affects both the pulmonary and digital circulations.

17. **Ans. (a) Triad of diarrhea, dementia and dermatitis** *(Ref: Harrison 17th/449)*
   - **Acrodermatitis enteropathica** also known as **Brandt Syndrome or Danbolt-Cross syndrome** is an autosomal recessive metabolic disorder affecting the uptake of zinc, characterized by periorificial and acral *dermatitis, alopecia and diarrhea*.
   - This disease is apparently caused by an inborn error of metabolism resulting in malabsorption of dietary zinc and can be treated effectively by parenteral or large oral doses of zinc. Zinc deficiency might in part account for the immunodeficiency that accompanies severe malnutrition.

- Features of acrodermatitis enteropathica start appearing in the first few months of life, as the infant discontinues breast milk. There are erythematous patches and plaques of dry, scaly skin. The lesions may appear eczematous, or may evolve further into crusted vesicles, bullas or pustules. The lesions are frequent around the mouth and anus, and also in hands, feet and scalp. There may be suppurative inflammation of the nail fold surrounding the nail plate-known as paronychia. Alopecia-loss of hair from scalp, eyebrows and eyelashes may occur. The skin lesions may be secondarily infected by bacteria such as *Staphylococcus aureus* or fungi like *Candida albicans*. These skin lesions are accompanied by diarrhea.
- Without treatment, the disease is fatal and affected individuals may die within a few years. There is no cure for the condition. Treatment includes lifelong dietary zinc supplementation in the range of greater than 1-2 mg/kg of body-weight per day.

18. Ans. (b) Zinc Deficiency Causes Pulmonary Fibrosis *(Ref: Harrison 17th/449)*

Element	Deficiency	Toxicity
Calcium	Reduced bone mass, osteoporosis	Renal insufficiency (milk-alkali syndrome), nephrolithiasis, impaired iron absorption
Selenium	Cardiomyopathy, heart failure, striated muscle degeneration	*General:* Alopecia, nausea, vomiting, abnormal nails, emotional lability, peripheral neuropathy, lassitude, garlic odor to breath, dermatitis *Occupational:* Lung and nasal carcinomas, liver necrosis, pulmonary inflammation
Zinc	Growth retardation, altered taste and smell, alopecia, dermatitis, diarrhea, immune dysfunction, failure to thrive, gonadal atrophy, congenital malformations	*General:* Reduced copper absorption, gastritis, sweating, fever, nausea, vomiting *Occupational:* Respiratory distress, pulmonary fibrosis

19. Ans. (a) Thymoma *(Ref: Harrison 17th/89, Devita 6th/1023)*
- Tumors made up of **two different lineage of cells,** i.e. lymphocytes and epithelial cells suggests the diagnosis of thymoma.
- Thymoma is the *most common cause of an anterior mediastinal mass in adults*, accounting for ~40% of all mediastinal masses. Thymomas are most common in the fifth and sixth decade. Some 90% of thymomas are in the anterior mediastinum. Thymomas are epithelial tumors and all of them have malignant potential. They may have a variable percentage of lymphocytes within the tumor, but genetic studies suggest that the lymphocytes are benign polyclonal cells. The epithelial component of the tumor may consist primarily of round or oval cells derived mainly from the cortex or spindle-shaped cells derived mainly from the medulla or combinations thereof.

20. Ans. (d) Dense core granules *(Ref: Robbin's 7th/769; Devita 6th/900)*
- Paraganglioma is a neuroendocrine tumor and **like other neuroendocrine tumors, the ultrastructure shows dense core granules** *(neurosecretory granules)*
- The tumor cells are separated by *fibrovascular stroma* and surrounded by *sustentacular cells.*
- *Chief cells are neuroendocrine cells and are positive for regular neuroendocrine markers, e.g.*
  - Chromogranin
  - Synaptophysin
  - euron specific enolase
  - Serotonin
  - Neurofilament
- The chief cells are **S-100 protein negative** but the **sustentacular cells are S-100 positive and are focally positive for glial fibrillary acid protein.**
- *Paraganglioma cells are never positive for cytokeratin like other neuroendocrine tumors.*

21. Ans. (a) Neutral endopeptidase *(Ref: Ganong 22nd/462, , Harrison's 17th/233,2146,2103)*
- **Brain natriuretic peptide (BND) or B type natriuretic peptide** is a hormone produced by the ventricles of the heart. It has been shown to increase in response to ventricular volume expansion and pressure overload.
- BNP is a marker of *ventricular systolic* and *diastolic function.*
  - BNP also has a prognostic significance in systemic sclerosis (with pulmonary artery hypertension) and in amyloidosis involving the heart.
- **Atrial natriuretic peptide** (ANP) is a hormone released by atrial walls of the heart when they become stretched. Because in heart failure, there is almost always excessive increase in both the right and left atrial pressures that stretch the atrial walls the circulating levels of ANP in the blood increase fivefold to tenfold in severe heart failure. The ANF in turn has a direct effect on the kidneys to increase greatly their excretion of salt and water. Therefore ANP plays a natural role to prevent the extreme congestive symptoms of cardiac failure.

- Both ANP as well as BNP are metabolized by neutral endopeptidases and the inhibitors of this enzyme (omapatrilat and sampatrilat) are used for the management of CHF.

22. **Ans. (a) There are many cyclin inhibitors which prevent cell to enter into S phase in adult** *(Ref: Robbins. 7th/42, 43, 308, 309)*
    - After a fixed number of divisions, normal cells become arrested in a *terminally non dividing state* known as replicative senescence. It occurs due to shortening of telomeres.
    - **Telomeres** are *short repeated sequences of DNA* present at the linear ends of chromosomes that are important for *ensuring the complete replication* of chromosomal ends and *protecting* chromosomal terminals from fusion and degradation. When somatic cells replicate a *small section* of the telomere is *not duplicated* and telomeres become *progressively shortened.* The loss of telomere function leads to *activation of p53 dependent cell cycle checkpoints causing proliferative arrest or apoptosis.*
    - *Germ cells, some stem cells and cancer cells continue to divide* because in these cells telomere *shortening is prevented by sustained function of the enzyme* **telomerase that maintains the length of the telomere** by nucleotide addition.

23. **Ans. (d) Osteosarcoma** *(Ref: Robbin's 7th/500, 8th/475)*
    - Most of the malignant pediatric neoplasms are unique in many respects:
      - They tend to have a more primitive *(embryonal)* rather than pleomorphic-anaplastic microscopic appearance, are often characterized by sheets of cells with small, round nuclei, and frequently exhibit features of organogenesis specific to the site of tumor origin. Because of this latter characteristic, these tumors are frequently designated by the suffix -*blastoma,* for example, nephroblastoma (Wilms' tumor), hepatoblastoma, and neuroblastoma.
      - Owing to their primitive histologic appearance, many childhood tumors have been collectively referred to as **small round blue cell tumors**.
      - The differential diagnosis of such tumors includes
        - Neuroblastoma
        - Wilms' tumor
        - Lymphoma
        - Rhabdomyosarcoma
        - Ewing sarcoma/Primitive neuroectodermal tumor.

24. **Ans (b) Vascular** *(Ref: Harrison 17th/1186-1187, Robbins 7th/548, 550)*
    - *Kaposi's sarcoma (KS)* is a multicentric neoplasm consisting of multiple vascular nodules appearing in the skin, mucous membranes, and viscera.
    - HHV-8 or KSHV has been strongly implicated as a viral cofactor in the pathogenesis of KS.
    - Lesions often appear in sun-exposed areas, particularly the tip of the nose, and have a propensity to occur in areas of trauma (Koebner phenomenon).
    - Because of the vascular nature of the tumors and the presence of extravasated red blood cells in the lesions, their colors range from reddish to purple to brown and often take the appearance of a bruise, with yellowish discoloration and tattooing.
    - KS lesions most commonly appear as raised macules.
    - Apart from skin, lymph nodes, gastrointestinal tract, and lung are the organ systems most commonly affected by KS.
    - Lesions have been reported in virtually every organ, including the heart and the CNS.
    - In contrast to most malignancies, in which lymph node involvement implies metastatic spread and a poor prognosis, lymph node involvement may be seen very early in KS and is of no special clinical significance.
    - A diagnosis of KS is based upon biopsy of a suspicious lesion. Histologically one sees a proliferation of spindle cells and endothelial cells, extravasation of red blood cells, hemosiderin-laden macrophages, and, in early cases, an inflammatory cell infiltrate.

25. **Ans. (c) Gout** *(Ref: Robbins 8th/1243-1246)*
    Tophi are formed by large aggregations of urate crystals. They are surrounded by macrophages, lymphocytes and foreign body giant cells. They are characteristic of gout.
    They are seen in the
    - Articular cartilage of joints*
    - Periarticular ligaments*
    - Tendons and soft tissues*
    - Achilles tendon*
    - Ear lobes*
    Other important points
    - Most common joint involved in Gout is Big Toe (First metatarsophalangeal joint)

- The diagnosis is made by presence of monosodium urate crystal in polarized light which are needle shaped and strongly negative birefringent crystal.

26. **Ans. (c) Mitochondrial myopathy** *(Ref: Robbins 7th/33, 1342, Harrison' 16th/2534, 374)*
Mutations in mitochondrial genes cause mitochondrial myopathies causing neurological and systemic involvements like:

- Mitochondrial Myopathy
- MELAS
- Leber's Hereditary Optic Neuropathy
- Myoclonic Epilepsy with Ragged Red Fibers syndrome (MERRF)
- Chronic progressive external ophthalmoplegia.
- Kearns-Sayre syndrome.

27. **Ans. (a) Alport's syndrome; (b) Niemann-Pick disease; (c) Atherosclerosis;** *(Ref: Robbin's 7th/523, 988 ,163)*
- Foam cells are lipid laden phagocytes. In Niemann-Pick disease, they are widely distributed in spleen, liver, lymph nodes, bone marrow, and tonsils.
- During atherosclerosis, oxidized LDL is ingested by macrophages forming foam cells.
- In Alport's syndrome, interstitial cells of kidney may acquire a foamy appearance owing to accumulation of neutral fats and mucopolysaccharides forming foam cells.

28. **Ans. (b) Alcohol** *(Ref: Harsh Mohan 6th/276)*
Formalin is the best tissue fixative.

29. **Ans. (d) All of the above** *(Ref: Robbins 7th/1265, 8th/1199)*
- Panniculitis is an inflammatory reaction in the subcutaneous fat that may affect principally the connective tissue septa separating lobules of fat or predominantly the lobules of fat themselves.
- The various forms of panniculitis are:
  - **Erythema nodosum: Most common form of panniculitis** and usually has an acute presentation. Its occurrence is often associated with infections (β-hemolytic streptococci, TB and less commonly, coccidiodomycosis, histoplasmosis and leprosy), drug administration (sulfonamides, oral contraceptives), sarcoidosis, inflammatory bowel disease, and certain malignant neoplasms.
  - **Erythema induratum:** Uncommon type of panniculitis that affects primarily adolescents and menopausal women. It is a primary vasculitis affecting deep vessels with subsequent necrosis and inflammation within the fat. There is no associated underlying disease.
  - **Weber-Christian disease** *(relapsing febrile nodular panniculitis)*: It is a rare form of lobular, nonvascular panniculitis seen in children and adults.
  - Factitial panniculitis: It is a result of self-inflicted trauma or injection of foreign or toxic substances, is a form of secondary panniculitis.
  - Lupus erythematosus may occasionally have deep inflammatory components with associated panniculitis.

30. **Ans. (a) Measles** *(Ref: Robbins 7th/364)*
In measles, the lymphoid organs typically have marked follicular hyperplasia, large germinal centers and randomly distributed multinucleate giant cells, called *Warthin-Finkeldey* cells, which have eosinophilic nuclear and cytoplasmic inclusion bodies.

Giant cells		Giant cells	
1.	Langhans giant cells	1.	TB
		2.	Sarcoidosis
2.	Touton giant cells	1.	Xanthoma
3.	Tumour giant cells	1.	Ca liver
		2.	Soft tissue sarcomas
4.	Foreign body giant cells	1.	Leprosy

31. **Ans. (c) The etiological agent for the initial stimulus to the ultimate expression of disease** *(Ref: Robbins 7th/4)*
Pathogenesis refers to the sequence of events in the response of cells or tissues to the etiological agent, from the initial stimulus to the ultimate expression of the disease".

32. **Ans. (b) Frequently gives rise to embolization in the lymphatics** *(Ref: Robbins 7th/1318)*
Liposarcomas are *one of the most common sarcomas* of adulthood and are uncommon in children. They usually *arise in the deep soft tissues* of the *proximal extremities and retroperitoneum* and are notorious for developing into large tumors. Histologically, liposarcomas can be divided into well-differentiated, myxoid, round cell, and pleomorphic variants. The cells in

well-differentiated liposarcomas are readily recognized as lipocytes. In the other variants, some cells indicative of fatty differentiation called **lipoblasts** are almost always present. The myxoid and round cell variant of liposarcoma has a **t(12;16)** chromosomal abnormality.

33. **Ans. (c) Michaelis Gutmann bodies—Langerhan's histiocytosis** *(Ref: Robbins 7th/1258, 680-681, 905, 1027-1028, 701-702)*

Russell bodies
Inclusions containing immunoglobulins present in the cytoplasm of patients of multiple myeloma; similar inclusions in the nucleus are called Dutcher bodies.

Mallory bodies
Eosinophilic cytokeratin inclusions seen in alcoholic liver disease (can also be seen in Wilson's disease, Indian childhood cirrhosis, chronic cholestatic conditions, hepatocellular cancer and primary biliary cirrhosis)

Civatte bodies
Lichen planus is a disease characterized by "purple, pruritic, polygonal papules" and characterized histologically by dense lymphocytic infiltrates along dermoepidermal junction. The lymphocytes are intimately associated with basal keratinocytes which show degeneration and necrosis contributing to *saw-toothing* of dermo-epidermal junction. Anucleate, necrotic basal cells may get incorporated into the inflamed papillary epidermis where they are called colloid or Civatte bodies.

Michaelis Gutmann bodies
Seen in Malacoplakia (vesicle inflammatory reaction associated with *E. coli* infection characterized by raised mucosal plaques and histologically by infiltration with large, foamy macrophages having laminated mineralized concretions of calcium inside lysosomes called Michaelis Gutmann bodies).

Langerhan's histiocytosis
It is a term used for proliferative disorders of dendritic cells which has three disorders namely Letterer-Siwe syndrome, Hand-Schuller-Christian disease and eosinophilic granuloma. The presence of *Birbeck's granules* in the cytoplasm is a characteristic feature. These granules have a rod-like structure and terminal dilated ends (**Tennis racket appearance**)

34. **Ans. (c) Osteosarcoma** *(Ref: Robbins 7th/299)*
    - Patients with familial retinoblastoma are also at greatly increased risk of developing osteosarcoma and some other soft tissue sarcomas *(Robbins pg 299)*
    - Alterations in 'RB pathway' involving INK 4a proteins, cyclin D-dependent kinases and RB family proteins which are present in normal cells lead on to inactivation of tumor suppressor gene (CRB gene) and associated somatic/inherited mutations cause the increased risk of other tumors.

35. **Ans. (d) Adrenals** *(Ref: Arch Ophthal. 1939; 22(4):575-580)*
    Adrenal neuroblastomas are malignant neoplasms arising from the sympathetic neuroblasts in the medulla of the adrenal gland. There are two clinical types, based on the differences in distribution of metastasis. First (**Pepper type**) occurs in the stillborn and in young infants and metastasizes to the liver and regional lymph nodes, then the lungs, and late in the course, the calvarium and other flat bones. The second (**Hutchinson**) type is characterized clinically by secondary growth in the orbit, meninges, skull and long bones and occurs in children up to 15 years of age.

36. **Ans. (b) Ependymoma** *(Ref: Robbins 8th/1334)*

37. **Ans. (c) Neuroblastoma** *(Ref: Robbins 8th/477)*

38. **Ans. (a) Atopic dermatitis** *(Ref: Robbins 8th/1187-1189)*

39. **Ans. (a) Pleomorphic adenoma** *(Ref: Robbins 8th/757; 7th/791)*

40. **Ans. (b) Mucoepidermoid carcinoma** *(Ref: Robbins 8th/759; 7th/791)*

41. **Ans. (d) Lead poisoning** *(Ref: Robbins 8th/407; 7th/432-433)*

42. **Ans. (a) Tumor of gingiva** *(Ref: Robbins 8th/748; 7th/776)*

43. **Ans. (b) Rhabdomyoma** *(Ref: Robbins 8th/584; 7th/614)*

44. **Ans. (b) Dermatitis, glossitis, Alopecia** *(Ref: Harsh Mohan 6th/254)*

45. **Ans. (b) Lead poisoning** *(Ref: Robbins 8th/406-407; 7th/433)*

46. **Ans. (b) Rhabdomyoma** *(Ref: Robbins 8th/584; 7th/614)*

47. **Ans. (a) Parotid gland** *(Ref: Robbins 8th/757)*

48. **Ans. (d) Antibodies in serum** *(Ref: Robbins 8th/653; 7th/736-737)*

49. **Ans. (a) Measles** *(Ref: Robbins 8th/432-433)*

50. **Ans. (d) Clostridia** *(Ref: Robbins 8th/378-379)*

51. **Ans. (d) Neurofibroma** *(Ref: Robbins 8th/730)*

52. **Ans. (c) SLE** *(Ref: Robbins 8th/220)*

53. **Ans. (b) Amyloid** *(Ref: Robbins 8th/253)*

54. **Ans. (c) Basal cell carcinoma** *(Ref: Robbins 8th/1180)*

55. **Ans. (c) Pleomorphic adenoma** *(Ref: Robbins 8th/261)*

56. **Ans. (c) Chancroid** *(Ref: Robbins 8th/366)*

57. **Ans. (d) All** *(Ref: Robbins 8th/1191-1192)*

58. **Ans. (d) Diplopia** *(Ref: Robbins 8th/438)*

59. **Ans. (a) Liver** *(Ref: Robbins 8th/273; 7th/923)*

60. **Ans. (a) Weibel Palade bodies** *(Ref: Robbins 8th/990; 7th/513)*

60.1. **Ans. (c) Phototherapy** *(Ref: Harrison, Chapter 74. Vitamin and Trace Mineral Deficiency and Excess)*

Niacin deficiency causes pellagra which can be due to the following reasons:
- People eating corn-based diets
- In alcoholics
- In congenital defects of intestinal and kidney absorption of tryptophan like Hartnup disease
- In patients with carcinoid syndrome

NOTES

AIIMS NOVEMBER 2014

1. Which of the following is the most common site of mucosa associated lymphoid tissue?
   (a) Duodenum
   (b) Jejunum
   (c) Ileum
   (d) Stomach

2. Which of the following is seen in schawannnoma?
   (a) Spindle cells
   (b) Storiform pattern
   (c) Target cells
   (d) Antoni A and B pattern

3. A young female presented with a right side thyroid nodule and was operated. A 2*2 cm thyroid nodule was resected and the following histology is seen. Which of the following is the most likely diagnosis?
   (a) Follicular goiter
   (b) Papillary thyroid cancer
   (c) Graves disease
   (d) Follicular carcinoma

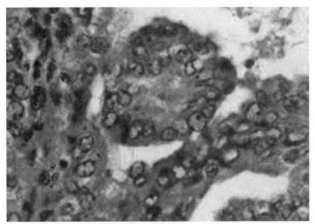

(For color version see plate 19)

4. A 45 year old patient has a history of recurrent ureteric stones and presents with off and on fever. The patient had to be operated and the appeared of the kidney is given alongside. Which of the following is the most likely diagnosis?
   (a) Renal cell cancer
   (b) Adult polycystic kidney
   (c) Hydronephrosis with chronic pyelonephritis
   (d) Cystic dysplastic kidney

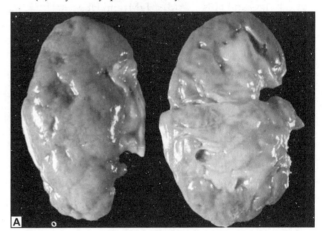

(For color version see plate 20)

5. Apoptosis is induced by which of the following
   (a) Iso-protenoids
   (b) Glucocorticoids
   (c) Mysteric acid
   (d) Oleic acid

6. Molecular classification of breast cancer is based on which of the following?
   (a) Gene expression profiling
   (b) Expression of hormone receptors like ER,PR, and HER-2 neu
   (c) Histology
   (d) Response to chemotherapy

7. Immuno-histopathological markers wrongly matched
   (a) Desmin-Carcinomas
   (b) Vimentin – Sarcomas
   (c) Leukocyte specific antigen-Lymphoma
   (d) S100-melanoma

8. Patient has been given penicillin 48 hours ago, with no history of drug allergy. Now he develops wheeze and hemolysis. Antibody for penicillin is positive. Type of hypersensitivity is which of the following:
   (a) Type I
   (b) Type II
   (c) Type III
   (d) Type IV

9. Which of the following is true regarding Non-specific interstitial pneumonia?
   (a) Honey combing on CT
   (b) Predominant in males
   (c) Affects elderly age group
   (d) Good prognosis

10. Nurse got a needle prick injury. Which of the following suggests active phase of hepatitis?
    (a) IgM anti HBc   (b) IgG anti HBc
    (c) IgG anti HBs   (d) IgM anti Hbe

11. Which of the following is the function of MHC I and II?
    (a) Signal transduction in T cells
    (b) Antibody class switching
    (c) Antigen presentation to T cells
    (d) Increase the secretion of cytokines

12. High calcium intake can lead to
    (a) Osteoporosis
    (b) Osteopetrosis
    (c) Milk alkali syndrome
    (d) Renal failure

13. Which of the following is rarely seen in rheumatic heart disease?
    (a) Mitral stenosis
    (b) Aortic stenosis
    (c) Pulmonary stenosis
    (d) Tricuspid stenosis

14. Which of the following is having a 90% association with HLA B27?
    (a) Ankylosing spondylitis
    (b) Rheumatoid arthritis
    (c) Psoriasis
    (d) Reiter syndrome

15. Angina, dyspnea and syncope is seen in:
    (a) Pulmonary stenosis
    (b) Atrial septal defect
    (c) Ventricular septal defect
    (d) Aortic stenosis

16. All of the following are premalignant except:
    (a) Ulcerative colitis
    (b) Peutz Jegher syndrome
    (c) Crohn disease
    (d) Familial adenomatous polyposis

17. Fine needle aspiration cytology is not able to detect which of the following?
    (a) Papillary carcinoma
    (b) Hashimoto thyroiditis
    (c) Follicular cancer
    (d) Medullary cancer

EXPLANATIONS

1. **Ans. (c) Ileum** *(Ref: Robbins 9th/772)*

Direct quote… "Although extranodal lymphomas can arise in virtually any tissue, they do so most commonly in the GI tract, particularly the stomach".

However, the question is regarding the most common site for MALT (and not MALToma) for which the answer is **ileum.**

Also know!

- In the stomach, MALT is induced *typically as a result of chronic gastritis.*
- *H. pylori* infection is the most common inducer in the stomach.

2. **Ans. (d) Antoni A and B pattern** *(Ref: Robbins 9th/1247)*
These are benign tumors that exhibit Schwann cell differentiation and often arise directly from peripheral nerves. They are a component of neurofibromatosis -2 (NF2). Microscopically, they are comprised of an admixture of dense and loose areas referred to as **Antoni A** and **Antoni B** areas, respectively.
The dense eosinophilic Antoni A areas often contain spindle cells arranged into cellular intersecting fascicles. Palisading of nuclei is common and "nuclear-free zones" that lie between the regions of nuclear palisading are termed **Verocay bodies.**

Also know!

- The Schwann cell tumors have a uniform immunoreactivity for S-100.
- Schwannomas may recur locally if incompletely resected, but *malignant transformation is extremely rare.*

Storiform pattern is seen in *dermatofibrosarcoma protuberans.* This is composed of closely packed fibroblasts arranged radially.

3. **Ans. (b) Papillary thyroid cancer** *(Ref: Robbins 9th/1095-6)*

Papillary carcinomas are the most common form of thyroid cancer. They occur most often between the ages of 25 and 50. It is associated with a previous exposure to ionizing radiation.

Histologically, papillary thyroid cancer is associated with **ground glass** or **Orphan Annie eye nuclei** (as shown in the figure). In this, the nuclei of papillary carcinoma cells contain finely dispersed chromatin. In addition, invaginations of the cytoplasm may give the appearance of intranuclear inclusions ("pseudo-inclusions") or intranuclear grooves. **The diagnosis of papillary carcinoma can be made based on these nuclear features**, even in the absence of papillary architecture. Concentrically calcified structures termed **psammoma bodies** are often present, usually within the cores of papillae. This structure is almost never found in follicular and medullary carcinomas, and so, is a strong indication that the lesion is a papillary carcinoma.

4. **Ans. (c) Hydronephrosis with chronic pyelonephritis** *(Ref: Robbins 9th/934)*
The characteristic changes of chronic pyelonephritis:
The kidneys usually are irregularly scarred; if bilateral, the involvement is asymmetric.
Hallmark feature: **coarse, discrete, corticomedullary scars overlying dilated, blunted, or deformed calyces, and flattening of the papillae.** The scars mostly are in the upper and lower poles, consistent with the frequency of reflux in these sites.

Microscopically, the tubules show atrophy in some areas and hypertrophy or dilation in others. Dilated tubules with flattened epithelium may be filled with casts resembling thyroid colloid **(thyroidization)**. There are varying degrees of chronic interstitial inflammation and fibrosis in the cortex and medulla.

Other options

- Renal cell cancer would be having a mass on the upper or lower pole. There is absence of thyroidisation in this condition.
- Adult polycystic kidney would have been The external surface appears to be composed solely of a mass of cysts with no intervening parenchyma.

5. **Ans. (b) Glucocorticoids..repeat question..see chapter 1 for details.**

6. **Ans. (a) Gene expression profiling** *(Ref: Robbins 9th/1061)*
Invasive carcinomas can be divided based on molecular and morphologic characteristics into several clinically important subgroups. Breast carcinomas have a wide variety of morphologic appearances. One third can be classified morphologically

into special histologic types, some of which are strongly associated with clinically relevant biologic characteristics. The remainder are grouped together and called "ductal" or no special type (NST).

Recent detailed description of *genomic alterations and gene and protein expression* in large cohorts of breast cancers has provided a framework for a **molecular classification** for this group of breast cancers.....Robbins 9th/ 1060

Gene expression profiling measures relative levels of mRNA expression...figure 23.20 Robbins

7. **Ans. (a) Desmin-Carcinomas** *(Ref: Robbins 9/e p11)*

Desmin is a marker of myogenic tumours and not carcinomas (keratin is marker in this cancer).

- *Lamin A, B, and C:* nuclear lamina of all cells
- *Vimentin:* mesenchymal cells (fibroblasts, endothelium)
- *Desmin:* muscle cells, forming the scaffold on which actin and myosin contract
- *Neurofilaments:* axons of neurons, imparting strength and rigidity
- *Glial fibrillary acidic protein:* glial cells around neurons
- *Cytokeratins:* 30 distinct varieties which are present in different cells, hence can be used as cell markers

8. **Ans. (b) Type II** *(Ref: Robbins 9th/205)*

Administration of penicillin causing no symptoms in 48 hours with no previous history of allergy rules out type I hypersensitivity reaction.

The patient presented with hemolysis which can be because of antibody formation against red cells. The formation of autoantibody is a feature associated with type II hypersensitivity reaction. Thus, it becomes the answer over here.

Clinically, antibody-mediated cell destruction and phagocytosis occur in multiple situations:

- *Transfusion reactions*, in which cells from an incompatible donor react with and are opsonized by preformed antibody in the host
- *Hemolytic disease of the newborn*: antigenic difference between the mother and fetus
- *Autoimmune hemolytic anemia*, agranulocytosis, and thrombocytopenia, in which individuals produce antibodies to their own blood cells, which are then destroyed.
- Certain drug reactions, in which *a drug acts as a "hapten" by attaching to plasma membrane proteins of red cells and antibodies are produced against the drug-protein complex.*

9. **Ans. (d) Good prognosis** *(Ref: Robbins 9th/686)*

Nonspecific interstitial pneumonia

- Nonspecific interstitial pneumonia may be idiopathic or associated with connective tissue disease.
- **Clinical features**
- Patients present with dyspnea and cough of several months' duration.
- More likely to be **female nonsmokers** in their sixth decade of life.
- High-resolution computed tomography scan: B/L, symmetric, predominantly lower lobe reticular opacities *(honeycomb pattern is absent)*.
- Patients have a *much better prognosis* than those with usual interstitial pneumonia.
- Having 2 patterns: cellular and fibrosing patterns. Those having the cellular pattern are somewhat younger than those with the fibrosing pattern and have a better prognosis
- In cellular pattern, there is mild to moderate chronic interstitial inflammation, in a uniform or patchy distribution.
- In fibrosing pattern, there is diffuse or patchy interstitial fibrotic lesions of roughly the same stage of development *(an important distinction from usual interstitial pneumonia)*
- Fibroblastic foci, **honeycombing, hyaline membranes** and **granulomas** are **absent.**

10. **Ans. (a) IgM anti HBc** *(Ref: Robbins 9th/833)*

IgM anti-HBc antibody becomes detectable in serum *shortly before* the onset of symptoms, concurrent with the *onset of elevated serum aminotransferase levels* (indicative of hepatocyte destruction).

11. **Ans. (c) Antigen presentation to T cells** *(Ref: Robbins 9th/194)*

The **function of MHC molecules** is to *display peptide fragments of protein antigens for recognition by antigen specific T cells.*

12. **Ans. (c) Milk alkali syndrome** *(Ref: Robbins 9th/65)*

Milk -alkali syndrome is due to excessive ingestion of calcium and absorbable antacids such as milk or calcium carbonate. This is associated with the development of metastatic calcification.

13. **Ans. (c) Pulmonary stenosis** *(Ref: Robbins 9th/558-559)*

In chronic disease the mitral valve is virtually always involved. The mitral valve is affected in isolation in roughly two thirds of RHD, and along with the aortic valve in another 25% of cases. Tricuspid valve involvement is infrequent, and the *pulmonary valve* is *only rarely affected.*

14. **Ans. (a) Ankylosing spondylitis** *(Ref: Robbins 9th/205)*

Direct quote… *"Approximately **90% of patients are HLA-B27 positive;** associations have also been found with the IL-23 receptor gene".*

Ankylosing spondylitis (also **rheumatoid spondylitis** and **Marie- Strümpell disease**)

It causes destruction of articular cartilage and bony ankylosis, especially of the *sacroiliac and apophyseal joints* (between tuberosities and processes).

It becomes symptomatic in the *2nd and 3rd decades* of life as lower back pain and spinal immobility.

15. **Ans. (d) Aortic stenosis** *(Ref: Robbins 9th/555)*

The valve area is approximately 0.5 to 1 cm2 in severe aortic stenosis whereas it is normally approximately 4 cm2. Left ventricular pressures rises leading to concentric left ventricular (pressure overload) hypertrophy. The hypertrophied myocardium tends to be ischemic (as a result of diminished microcirculatory perfusion, often complicated by coronary atherosclerosis), and angina pectoris may occur. Both systolic and diastolic myocardial function may be impaired; eventually, cardiac decompensation and CHF can ensue. The onset of symptoms (angina, CHF, or syncope) in aortic stenosis heralds cardiac decompensation and carries an extremely poor prognosis. If untreated, most patients with aortic stenosis *will die within 5 years of developing angina, within 3 years of developing syncope, and within 2 years of CHF onset.*

16. **Ans .(c) Crohn disease** *(Ref: Robbins 9th/800-1,806,809)*

Robbins pg 806……*Peutz-Jeghers syndrome* is associated with a markedly *increased risk of several malignancies*. Lifetime risk is approximately **40%** for these, and regular surveillance is recommended.

Pg 809…Colorectal adenocarcinoma develops in **100%** of *untreated FAP patients*, often before age 30 and nearly always by age 50.

> The risk of colonic adenocarcinoma is increased in patients with long-standing IBD affecting the colon. Please understand that *increased risk of cancer is seen in colonic variant of Crohn disease and not otherwise.* Ulcerative colitis is a premalignant condition.

17. **Ans. (c) Follicular cancer** *(Ref: Robbins 9th/1094)*

Direct quote… *"Because of the need for evaluating capsular integrity, the definitive diagnosis of adenomas can be made only after careful histologic examination of the resected specimen. Suspected adenomas of the thyroid are therefore removed surgically to exclude malignancy".*

AIIMS MAY 2014

1. In the entire human genome, coding DNA constitutes:
   (a) 2%
   (b) 1%
   (c) 0.1%
   (d) 4%

2. Methylation of cytosine leads to:
   (a) Increased expression of gene
   (b) Decreased expression of gene
   (c) No effect on gene expression
   (d) Mutation

3. The cells of the human body most sensitive to ischemia are:
   (a) Neurons
   (b) Nephrons
   (c) Cardiac myocyte
   (d) Hepatocytes

4. Which of the following regarding cellular events in acute inflammation is not correct?
   (a) PECAM/CD31 is responsible for neutrophil activation
   (b) Components of complement can assist in chemotaxis
   (c) Neutrophil margination is assisted by selectins
   (d) ICAM-1/VCAM-1 is responsible for neutrophil adhesion

5. Which of the following factors is morphogenic as well as mitogenic?
   (a) Fibroblast growth factor
   (b) Platelet derived growth factor
   (c) Bone morphogenetic protein
   (d) Insulin-like growth factor

6. ARDS is due to a defect/damage in:
   (a) Type 1 pneumocytes
   (b) Type 2 pneumocytes
   (c) Clara cells
   (d) Endothelial cells

7. Verocay bodies are seen in:
   (a) Meningioma
   (b) Hemangioma
   (c) Glioma
   (d) Schwannoma

8. Which of the following is not true regarding IgE antibodies?
   (a) It mediates release of histamine and other chemical mediators
   (b) It is the primary antibody involved in allergic reactions
   (c) It is involved in anti-parasitic immune responses
   (d) May cross the placenta and fix complement

9. Which of the following is not a characteristic feature of multiple myeloma?
   (a) Increased Ig levels in serum
   (b) Positive ANA
   (c) Plasmacytosis
   (d) M spike on electrophoresis

10. Anti-neutrophil cytoplasmic antibodies (ANCA) is seen in:
    (a) Wegener's Granulomatosis
    (b) Diabetes mellitus
    (c) Rheumatoid arthritis
    (d) Churg-Strauss syndrome

11. Which of the following is not an etiological factor for pancreatitis?
    (a) Abdominal trauma
    (b) Hyperlipidemia
    (c) Islet cell hyperplasia
    (d) Germline mutations in the cationic trypsinogen gene

12. Which of the following is not a part of HELLP syndrome?
    (a) Hemolysis
    (b) Elevated liver enzymes
    (c) Thrombocytopenia
    (d) Retroplacental hemorrhage

13. A 10-year old child presents with edema, oliguria and frothy urine. He has no past history of similar complaints. On examination, his urine was positive for 3+ proteinuria, no RBCs/WBCs and no casts. His serum albumin was 2.5 g/L and serum creatinine was 0.5 mg/dL. The most likely diagnosis is:
    (a) IgA nephropathy
    (b) Minimal change disease
    (c) Acute interstitial nephritis
    (d) Membranous nephropathy

14. A 6-year old girl presents with fever for the past 5 days, generalized erythematous rash, strawberry tongue and cervical lymphadenopathy. The most likely diagnosis is:
    (a) Kimura disease
    (b) Kawasaki disease
    (c) Scarlet fever
    (d) Rosie-Dorfman syndrome

15. Which of the following is NOT an example of a syndrome caused by uniparental disomy?
    (a) Prader-Willi syndrome
    (b) Angelman syndrome
    (c) Russell-Silver syndrome
    (d) Bloom syndrome

16. A 27-year old male presents with low backache, that occurs early in the morning, associated with stiffness, and persists for more than 30 minutes. On examination, his chest expansion is also restricted. The most probable diagnosis is:
    (a) Rheumatoid arthritis
    (b) Oteoarthritis
    (c) Gouty arthritis
    (d) Ankylosing spondylitis

17. Histopathologically, rosettes are not seen in:
    (a) Retinoblastoma
    (b) Neurocysticercosis
    (c) PNET
    (d) Medulloblastoma

EXPLANATIONS

1. **Ans. (a) 2%** *(Robbins 9th/2)*
   '98.5% of the human genome that does not encode proteins'..... direct quote from Robbins. So, it means that about 1.5% of the genome is used for coding proteins. The best answer therefore is option "a".

2. **Ans. (b) Decreased expression of gene** *(Robbins 9th/4)*
   High levels of *DNA methylation* in gene regulatory elements typically result in *transcriptional silencing*.

3. **Ans. (a) Neurons** *(Robbins 9th/ 130,1264)*
   Neurons undergo irreversible damage when deprived of their blood supply for **only 3 to 4 minutes**. Myocardial cells, although hardier than neurons, are also quite sensitive and die after only 20 to 30 minutes of ischemia...Robbins

Potential future questions!

> The most sensitive neurons in the brain are in the **pyramidal cell layer of the hippocampus** (especially area CA1, also referred to as *Sommer sector*), **cerebellar Purkinje cells** and **pyramidal neurons in cerebral cortex.**

4. **Ans. (a) PECAM/CD31 is responsible for neutrophil activation** *(Robbins 9th/ 76-7)*
   PECAM-1 (platelet endothelial cell adhesion molecule) is associated with transmigration (diapedesis) and not neutrophil activation.

   Other options

   > - **Chemotaxis** is assisted by **bacterial products, complement protein C5a, leukotriene B4** and interleukin (**IL-8**).
   > - **Selectins** are associated with rolling which also contributes to margination.
   > - *Integrins* are associated with **firm adhesion** of the white blood cells. They interact with vascular cell adhesion molecule 1 (*VCAM-1*) and intercellular adhesion molecule-1 (*ICAM-1*).

5. **Ans. (a) Fibroblast growth factor** *(Robbins 9th/ 19-20; 8th/87-88, Fetal and Neonatal Physiology 4th/867-8)*
   Fibroblast growth factor (FGF) contributes to wound healing responses, hematopoiesis, and development. They can be belonging to
   - Acidic FGF (aFGF, or FGF-1)
   - Basic FGF (bFGF, or FGF-2): necessary for angiogenesis
   - FGF-7 is also referred to as keratinocyte growth factor (KGF)

Growth Factor	Source	Functions
Epidermal growth factor (EGF)	Activated marcophages, selivary glands, keratinocytes, and many other cells	Mitogenic for keratinocytes and fibroblasts; stimulates karatinocytes migration; stimulates formation of granulation tissue
Transforming growth factor-α (TGF-α)	Activated marcophages, keratinocytes, many other cells types	Stimulates proliferation of hepatocytes and many other epithelial cells
Hepatocyte growth factor (HGF) scater factor	Fibroblasts, stromal cells in the liver, endothelial cells	Enhances proliferation of hepatocytes and other epithelial cells; increases cell motility.
Vascular endothelial growth factor (VEGF)	Messenchymal cells	Stimulates proliferation of endothelial cells; increases vascular parmeability
PLatelet-derived growth factor (PDGF)	Platelets, macrophages, endothelial cells, smooth muscle cells, keratino-cytes	Chemotactic for neutrophils, macrophages, fibroblasts, and smooth muscle cells, activates and stimulates proleferation of fibroblasts, endothelial, and other cells, stimulates ECM protein synthesis
Fibroblast growth factor (FGFs), including acidic (FGF-1) and basic (FGF-2)	Macrophages, mast cells, endothelial cells, many other cell types	Chemotactic and mitogenic for fibroblasts; stimulates anglogenesis and ECM protein synthesis.
Transforming growth factor β-(TGF-β)	Platelets, T lymphovcytes, macrophages, endothelial cells, keratinocytes, smooth muscle cells, fibroblasts	Chemotactic for leukocytes and fibroblasts; stimulates ECM protein synthesis; suppresses acute inflammation

Contd...

Contd...

Growth Factor	Source	Functions
Keratinocyte growth factor (KGF) (i.e., FGF-7)	Fibroblast	Stimulates keratinocyte migration, proliferation, and differentiation.
ECM, EXtracellular membrane		

6. **Ans. (d) Endothelial cells** *(Robbins 9th/672)*
   ALI/ARDS is initiated by injury of pneumocytes and pulmonary endothelium, setting in motion a viscous cycle of increasing inflammation and pulmonary damage.
   Endothelial activation is an important early event......Robbins 9th/672

Also revise

> The histologic manifestation of this disease is *diffuse alveolar damage* (DAD).

7. **Ans. (d) Schwannoma** *(Robbins 9th/ 1247)*
   Schwannomas are well-circumscribed, encapsulated masses that abut the associated nerve without invading it. Microscopically, they are comprised of an admixture of dense and loose areas referred to as **Antoni A** and **Antoni B** areas, respectively.

> - *The dense eosinophilic Antoni A* areas often contain spindle cells arranged into cellular intersecting fascicles. Palisading of nuclei is common and "nuclear-free zones" that lie between the regions of nuclear palisading are termed **Verocay bodies.**
> - In the loose, hypocellular **Antoni B** areas the spindle cells are spread apart by a prominent myxoid extracellular matrix that may be associated with microcyst formation.

8. **Ans. (d) May cross the placenta and fix complement (Harrison 18th/)**
   IgG (and *not IgE*) is the antibody which may cross the placental barrier and fix complement.

Also revise

> - **Heat labile antibody**
> - Has **homocytotropism** (affinity for cells of the same species)
> - Is increased in **allergic conditions** and **parasitic infections**.

9. **Ans. (b) Positive ANA** *(Robbins 9th/598-601)*
   Increased serum levels if immunoglobulins, plasmacytosis and M spike on electrophoresis are all seen in multiple myeloma. For details, see text of chapter 8.

10. **Ans. (a) Wegener's granulomatosis** *(Robbins 9th/511-2)*
    PR3-ANCAs are also present in up to 95% of cases; they are a useful marker of disease activity and may participate in Wegener's granulomatosis.

11. **Ans. (c) Islet cell hyperplasia** *(Robbins 9th/884)*

Etiological factors in acute pancreatitis

Metabolic
Alcoholism Hyperlipoprotelnemia Hypercalcemia Drugs (e.g., azathioprine)
Genetics
Mutations in genes encoding trypsin, trypsin regulators, or proteins that regulate calium metabolism
Mechanical
Gallstones Trauma Iatrogenic injury • Operative injury • Endoscopic procedures with dye injection

Contd...

Contd...

Vasular
Shock
Atheroembolism
Vasculitis

Infections
Mumps

12. Ans. (d) Retroplacental hemorrhage *(Robbins 9th/ 866)*

The subclinical hepatic disease may be the primary manifestation of preeclampsia, as part of a syndrome of **h**emolysis, **e**levated **l**iver enzymes, and **l**ow **p**latelets, dubbed the ***HELLP syndrome.***

13. Ans. (b) Minimal change disease *(Robbins 9th / 917)*
- Presence of edema, proteinuria *(frothy urine in stem of question)*, hypoalbuminemia etc. is suggestive of nephritic syndrome.
- *Minimal change disease* is the *most frequent cause* of **nephrotic syndrome in children**. There is commonly no hypertension or hematuria. The proteinuria usually is highly selective, most of the protein being albumin.
- No RBC casts in the urine is suggestive of absence of glomerulonephritis. So, options 'a' and 'c' are ruled out. Membranous nephropathy causes nephritic syndrome in adults. The best answer therefore is option 'b'

14. Ans. (b) Kawasaki disease *(Robbins 9th/510)*
- Kawasaki disease typically presents with *conjunctival and oral erythema* and blistering, *fever*, edema of the hands and feet, erythema of the palms and soles, *a desquamative rash*, and *cervical lymph node enlargement*. Hence, it is also called as *mucocutaneous lymph node syndrome*.
- It affects *infants or children*. 80% of patients are 4 years old or younger.

15. Ans. (a) Bloom syndrome *(Robbins 9th/314-5)*

Bloom syndrome is characterized by a defect in DNA repair genes as well as developmental defects. It is associated with increased risk of development of malignancies.

Prader-Willi Syndrome

- Characterized by diminished fetal activity, obesity, hypotonia, mental retardation, short stature, and hypogonadotropic hypogonadism.
- **Deletions of the paternal copy of** chromosome **15**

Angelman Syndrome

- Characterized by mental retardation, seizures, ataxia, and hypotonia,
- **Deletions involving the maternal copy** of chromosome **15**.

16. Ans. (d) Ankylosing spondylitis *(Robbins 9th/1213)*

Ankylosing spondylitis causes destruction of **articular cartilage and bony ankylosis, especially of the sacroiliac and apophyseal joints** (between tuberosities and processes). It is also known as *rheumatoid spondylitis* and *Marie- Strümpell disease*. Disease involving the sacroiliac joints and vertebrae becomes symptomatic in the **second and third decades of life** as **lower back pain and spinal immobility**. Involvement of peripheral joints, such as the hips, knees, and shoulders, occurs in at least one third of affected individuals. Approximately 90% of patients are *HLA-B27 positive*; associations have also been found with the IL-23 receptor gene.

17. Ans. (b) Neurocysticercosis *(Robbins 9th/ 1203,1312, 1339)*
- Retinoblastoma has the presence of Flexner-Wintersteiner rosette's and fleurettes reflecting photoreceptor differentiation. ....*(Robbins 9th/1339)*
- PNET (Primitive Neuro-Ectodermal Tumour): It is composed of sheets of uniform small, round cells that are slightly larger than lymphocytes. ....*(Robbins 9th/1203)*
- Medulloblastoma: The tumor may express neuronal (neurosecretory) granules, form Homer- Wright rosettes.... *(Robbins 9th/1312)*
- For details see the answer of a question in chapter of 'Neoplasia'

CHAPTER 20

Important Stains and Bodies

HEMATOXYLIN AND EOSIN (H & E)

This is the **most commonly used stain in routine pathology**. Hematoxylin, a basic dye stains acidic structures a purplish blue. Nuclei (DNA), ribosomes and rough endoplasmic reticulum (with their RNA) are therefore stained blue with H&E. Eosin, in contrast is an acidic dye which stains basic structures red or pink. Most cytoplasmic proteins are basic and therefore stained pink or pinkish red. In summary, H&E stains nuclei blue and cytoplasm pink or red.

PERIODIC ACID-SCHIFF (PAS)

This stain is versatile and has been used to stain many structures including glycogen, mucin, mucoprotein, glycoprotein, as well as fungi. PAS is useful for outlining tissue structures—basement membranes, glomeruli, blood vessels and glycogen—in the liver.

ROMANOWSKY STAINS

These histology stains are used for blood and bone marrow. Examples of Romanowsky histology stains include Wright's stain, Giemsa stain and Jenner's stain. These histology stains are based on a combination of eosin and methylene blue.

SILVER STAINS

These histology stains use silver. Argyrphilic tissue has an affinity for silver salts. The silver salts will be seen in argyrphilic tissues. Silver histology stains are used *to show melanin and reticular fibers*.

SUDAN STAINS

Sudan histology stains are used for staining of lipids and phospholipids. Examples of such histology stains are Sudan black, Sudan IV, and oil red O.

TYPE OF STAIN	Used for staining
Acid Fast Stain	Mycobacterial Organisms and other Acid Fast Organisms
Aldehyde Fuchsin	Pancreatic Islet Beta Cell Granules
Alician Blue	Mucins and Muco-substances
Alizarin Red S	Calcium
Bielschowsky Stain (Uses Silver)	Reticular Fibers, Neurofibrillary Tangles and Senile Plaques
Cajal Stain	Nervous Tissue
Congo Red	Amyloid
Cresyl Violet (Nissl Stain)	Neurons and Glia
Fontana Masson's	Melanin and Argentaffin Cells
Giemsa	Bone Marrow
Golgi Stain	Neurons
Gomori Methenamine Silver (GMS)	Fungi
Gram Stain (Taylor's)	Bacteria
Hematoxylin & Eosin (H&E)	General Stain Used in Routine Pathology

contd...

contd...

Luna Stain	Elastin and Mast Cells
Luxol Fast Blue (LFB)	Myelin
Masson's Trichrome	Connective Tissue, Collagen
Mucicarmine	Epithelial Mucin
Oil-Red-O (On Frozen Sections)	Lipid
Orcien Stain	Elastin fibers
Osmium Tetroxide	Lipids
Periodic Acid-Schiff (PAS)	Glycogen, Fungi
Phosphotungstic Acid-Haematoxylin	Fibrin, Cross Striations of Skeletal Muscle Fibres
Picrosirius Red (polarized)	Collagen
Reticulum Silver	Reticulum Fibres
Safranin O	Mucin, Cartilage and Mast cells
Toluidine Blue	Mast Cell Granules
Verhoeff Vangieson (VVG)	Elastic Fibres
Von Kossa	Calcium Salts

Inclusion Bodies

A. INTRA-CYTOPLASMIC

Rabies	Negri bodies
Small pox	Guarnieri bodies
Molluscum Contagiosum	Henderson Peterson bodies
Fowl pox	Bollinger bodies
Trachoma	Halberstaedter- Prowazeki bodies

B. INTRA-NUCLEAR

Cowdrey Type A	
Herpes Virus	Lipschutz Inclusions
Yellow fever	Torres Bodies

Cowdrey Type B
Adenovirus (Basophilic)
Poliovirus (acidophilic)

C. BOTH INTRANUCLEAR AND INTRACYTOPLASMIC

Measles Virus

Other Important Bodies

Asteroid body	Sarcoidosis and Sporotrichosis
Ferruginous body	Asbestosis
Torres body	Yellow fever
Lafora body	Myoclonic epilepsy
Michaelis Gutmann body	Malacoplakia

contd...

contd...

Mallory bodies	Primary biliary cirrhosis
	Alcoholic hepatitis
	Wilson's disease
	Chronic cholestasis
	Hepatocellular carcinoma
Miyagawa's Corpuscles	Buboes from LGV
Leishman Donovan Bodies	Kala –Azar
Babes- Ernst Granules	Corynebacterium diphtheriae
Donovan Bodies	Granuloma Inguinale
Lewis Bodies	Parkinsonism
Russell Bodies	Multiple Myeloma
Warthin- Finkedely Giant Cells	Measles
Owl-Eye Inclusions	CMV and Herpes
Keratin Pearls	Squamous Cell Carcinoma
Pick Body	Pick's Disease
Aschoff Bodies	Rheumatic Fever
Bodies of Arantius	Aortic Valve Nodules
Body of Highmore	Mediastinum Testis
Bollinger Bodies	Fowlpox
Brassy Body	Dark Shrunken Blood Corpuscle in Malaria
Call Exner Bodies	Granulosa Theca Cell Tumor
Chromatid Bodies	Entamoeba histolytica Pre-cyst
Citron Bodies	Clostridium septicum
Civatte Bodies	Lichen Planus
Councilman Bodies	Hepatitis
Coccoid X Bodies	Psittacosis
Creola Bodies	Asthma
Gamma Gandy Bodies	Congestive Splenomegaly
Guarnieri Bodies	Vaccinia
Henderson Peterson Bodies	Molluscum contagiosum
Heinz Bodies	G 6 PD Deficiency
Hirano Bodies	Alzheimer's Disease
Levinthal Coles Lille Bodies	Psittacosis
Mooser Bodies	Endemic Typhus
Moot Bodies	Multiple Myeloma
Psammoma Bodies	Papillary Carcinoma of Thyroid, Ovary and Salivary Glands,
	Meningioma, Mesothelioma
Reilly Bodies	Hurler's Syndrome
Rokitansky Bodies	Teratoma
Ross's Bodies	Syphilis
Rushton Bodies	Odontogenic Cyst
Sclerotic Bodies	Chromoblastomycosis
Sandstorm Bodies	Parathyroid Glands
Schiller Duval Bodies	Yolk Sac Tumor
Schaumann Bodies	Sarcoidosis
Verocay Bodies	Schwannoma
Winkler Bodies	Syphilis
Zebra Bodies	Metachromatic Leukodystrophy

NOTES

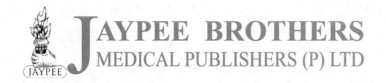

JAYPEE BROTHERS
MEDICAL PUBLISHERS (P) LTD

B-3, EMCA House, 23/23B, Ansari Road
Daryaganj, NEW DELHI - 110 002
Ph.: 011-23272143, 23282021, 23272703
+91-8860518516   Fax: +91-11-43574314

STUDENT FEEDBACK FORM

Name of the Student _____

Prof_____   College Name

City _____   Mobile No.

e-mail _____

ABOUT THE BOOK

Name of the Book_____

Author _____   Edn._____

_____

Feedback:

_____

_____

_____

_____

Suggestion (if any):

_____

_____

_____

_____

Post your feedback at the above mentioned address or mail at
jppgmee@gmail.com   _____

                                                              Signature

IMAGE BASED QUESTIONS

Image Based Questions

PLATE 1

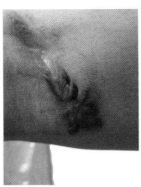

Q1. A 25 year old man of African American descent suffered from an injury and came back to your clinic with the complaint shown in the figure. What is the most likely diagnosis?
(a) Hypertrophic scar
(b) Normal scar
(c) Keloid
(d) Wound contraction

PLATE 2

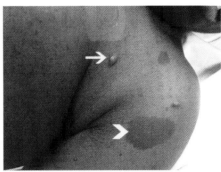

Q2. A 34-year-old man presents with the manifestation shown in the figure. He has a number of family members suffering from the same condition though the severity is different in different members. What is the likely diagnosis?
(a) Squamous cell cancer
(b) Basal cell cancer
(c) Neurofibromatosis 1
(d) Tuberous sclerosis

PLATE 3

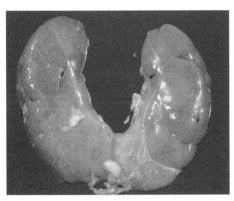

Q3. A patient having Turner syndrome was having the following lesion in the kidney. What is the lesion depicted?
(a) Polycystic kidney
(b) Horseshoe kidney
(c) Medullary cystic disease
(d) Hepatomegaly

PLATE 4

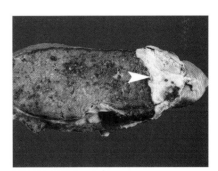

Q4. A patient presented with acute abdominal pain. He was operated and the appearance of the spleen is given in the figure. Which of the following organs can have the same appearance in the presence of ischemia?
(a) Intestine
(b) Heart
(c) Liver
(d) Lungs

Ans. 1. (c) Keloid

Ans. 2. (c) Neuro fibromatosis 1

Ans. 3. (b) Horseshoe kidney

Ans. 4. (bw) Heart

PLATE 5

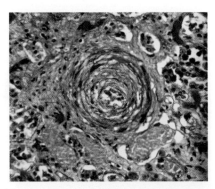

Q5. An old man presented in the medical emergency with complaints of severe headache and dizziness. His blood pressure was recorded to be 200/146 mmHg. A figure of the vascular changes is shown. Which of the following is the most expected change likely to be seen in his blood vessels?
(a) Hyaline arteriolosclerosis
(b) Hyperplastic arteriolosclerosis
(c) Neutrophilic infiltration
(d) Accumulation of plasma proteins in the vessel wall

PLATE 6

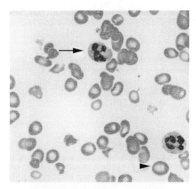

Q6. A strict vegetarian presented with complaints of numbness and tingling in her feet. She also had dyspnea, reduced ability of exertion and diarrhea. She had inflammation of tongue also. Her blood sample was taken and a peripheral smear was made. What is the most likely diagnosis for this lady?
(a) Iron deficiency anemia
(b) Immune thrombocytopenic purpura
(c) Megaloblastic anemia
(d) Aplastic anemia

PLATE 7

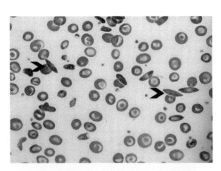

Q7. A young man presented with a chronic non-healing ulcer. He has episodes of severe pain the digits of hands and feet as well three episodes of priapism earlier. He was immunised earlier because the physician told him that he has greater chance of infection caused by capsulated organisms. His peripheral smear is shown in the figure. What is the likely diagnosis?
(a) Nutritional anemia
(b) Immune hemolytic anemia
(c) Hereditary spherocytosis
(d) Sickle cell anemia

PLATE 8

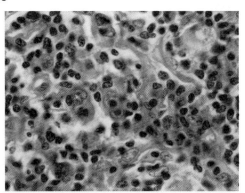

Q8. A 50-year-old female has complaints of painless cervical lymphadenopathy with fever, malaise and weight loss. A lymph node biopsy was taken and the finding is shown in the figure alongside which has cells with "owl eye appearance". What is the most likely diagnosis?
(a) Non-Hodgkin lymphoma
(b) Acute lymphadenitis
(c) Hodgkin disease
(d) Acute lymophoblastic leukemia

Ans. 5. (b) Hyperplastic arteriolosclerosis

Ans. 6. (c) Megaloblastic anemia

Ans. 7. (d) Sickle cell anemia

Ans. 8. (c) Hodgkin disease

PLATE 9

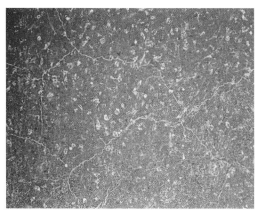

Q9. A child presented with a maxillary mass which on further investigation showed the presence of "starry sky appearance" in the biopsy. The likely diagnosis of this condition is:
(a) Mantle cell lymphoma
(b) Marginal zone lymphoma
(c) Burkitt lymphoma
(d) Hodgkin lymphoma

PLATE 10

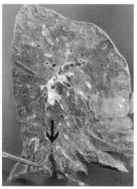

Q10. An old man with 20 years history of smoking presented with foul smelling sputum, fever and recurrent pulmonary infections. He died after few days. On autopsy his lung specimen showed the presence of the airways which were traced to the pleural surface. This man most probably was suffering from:
(a) Bronchogenic cancer
(b) Chronic bronchitis
(c) Bronchiectasis
(d) Emphysema

PLATE 11

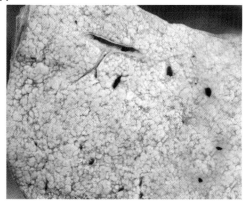

Q11. A chronic alcoholic had the complaints of yellowing of the skin and sclera, abdominal distension, hematemesis and alteration of sleep pattern. He could not be saved. The appearance of his liver is shown in the figure. The most likely diagnosis is:
(a) Gall bladder cancer with secondaries to the liver
(b) Alcholic fatty liver
(c) Cirrhosis
(d) Primary liver cell cancer

PLATE 12

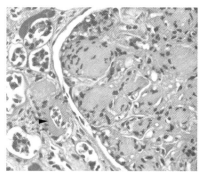

Q12. A 60-year man having uncontrolled diabetes presents with hypertension and frothiness in the urine. The urinary dipstick test showed the presence of proteinuria. A renal biopsy was taken which demonstrated the characteristic lesions of diabetic nephropathy. Which of the following is the finding observed in the photograph?
(a) Diffuse glomerulosclerosis
(b) Nodular glomerulosclerosis
(c) Basement membrane thickening
(d) Crescentic glomerulonephritis

Ans. 9. (c) Burkitt lymphoma

Ans. 10. (c) Bronchiectasis

Ans. 11. (c) Cirrhosis

Ans. 12. (b) Nodular glomerulosclerosis

PLATE 13

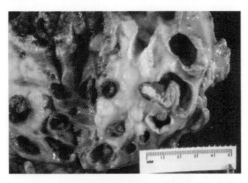

Q13. A patient was incidentally found to have the presence of renal stone which surprisingly cause massive destruction of the renal parenchyma. The history revealed that he had suffered from multiple episodes of urinary tract infection with Proteus organism earlier. A photograph of his kidney is revealed alongside. The most likely stone is:

(a) Calcium oxalate stone
(b) Triple stone
(c) Uric acid stone
(d) Cystine stone

PLATE 14

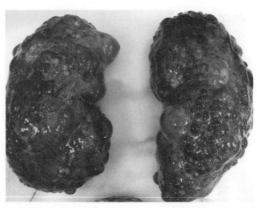

Q14. The kidneys shown in this image are from a 24-year-old man. What would have been the most likely cause of his death?

(a) A subarachnoid hemorrhage due to ruptured berry aneurysm
(b) A hypertensive crisis
(c) Chronic renal failure
(d) Metastatic renal cell carcinoma

PLATE 15

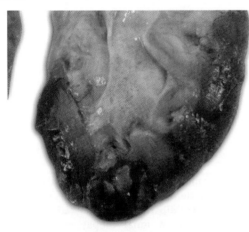

Q15. The kidney shown in the image was resected from a 63-year-old man with a history of smoking two packages of cigarettes a day for 40 years, who presented with hematuria. What is the most likely diagnosis?

(a) Papillary necrosis
(b) Renal cell carcinoma
(c) Angiomyolipoma
(d) Hemangioma

PLATE 16

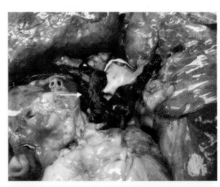

Q16. An old lady suffered from pelvic fracture because of which she was admitted in the ward and was immobile for 3 months. One night she complained of sudden onset of dyspnea and chest pain. On examination she had increased pulse rate. She expired after 20 minutes. Her autopsy showed the picture of the lung as is shown in the figure. What is the most likely diagnosis for this lady?

(a) Lung cancer
(b) Pulmonary thromboembolism
(c) Varicosities of the vein
(d) Deep vein thrombosis

Ans. 13. (b) Triple stone   Ans. 14. (c) Chronic renal failure

Ans. 15. (b) Renal cell carcinoma   Ans. 16. (b) Pulmonary thromboembolism

PLATE 17

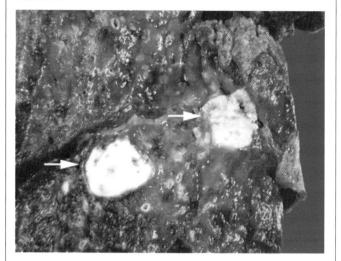

Q17. A labourer presented with the complained of night sweats, evening rise of fever, weight loss and two episodes of blood in the sputum. His lung demonstrated the lesion seen in the figure. The most probable diagnosis is:
(a) Pulmonary thromboembolism
(b) Pulmonary tuberculosis
(c) Bronchiectasis
(d) Bronchogenic cancer

PLATE 18

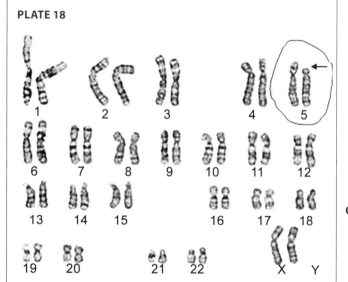

Q18. The most likely diagnosis in the picture is:
(a) Prader Willi syndrome
(b) Cri du chat syndrome
(c) Down syndrome
(d) Bloom syndrome

Ans. 17. (b) Pulmonary tuberculosis

Ans. 18. (b) Cri du chat syndrome

PLATE 19

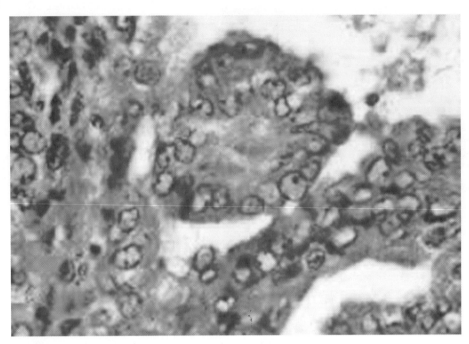

PLATE 20

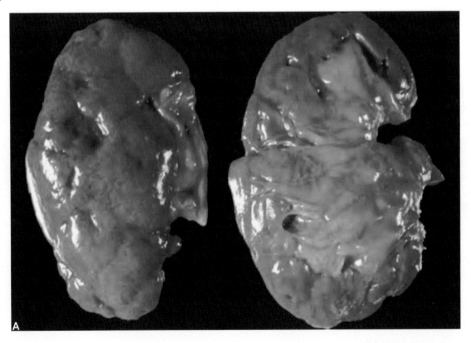

Aspiring to Serve Humanity
For All Those Who Want To Make A Difference
Lets Together Make A Difference............

ORTHO DHOOM DHADAKA 2015

Complete Discussion of Orthopedics with Visual Based Teaching to Prepare for
AIIMS/ AIPG NEET/ PGI/ DNB/ State PG Entrance Exams

will be held at

Ahmedabad	Bangalore	Chennai	Delhi
Hyderabad	Kolkata	Mumbai	Nagpur

by
Dr. Apurv Mehra

Leading Faculty, Motivator & Author of International Best Sellers
'Orthopedics Quick Review & MOM'S – Mehra's Orthopedics For MCI'

To Receive Registration Related Information
Interested Students Should Message Their Name/ Contact No./ College / E-mail Id
@ 8800222008 / 8800222009
or mail queries at: orthopedicsquickreview@gmail.com

A Glimpse of Grand Success of Ortho Dhoom Dhadaka 2014

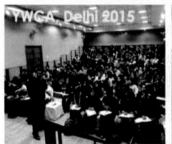

YWCA, Delhi 2015

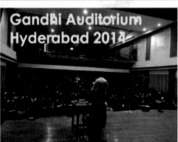

Gandhi Auditorium Hyderabad 2014

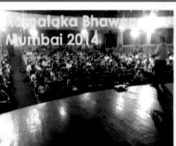

Karnataka Bhawan Mumbai 2014

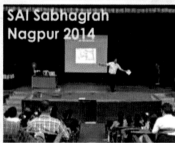

SAI Sabhagrah Nagpur 2014

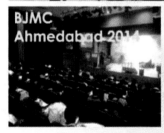

BJMC Ahmedabad 2014

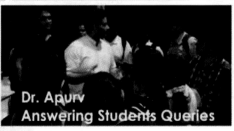

Dr. Apurv Answering Students Queries

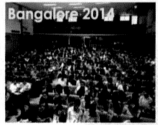

Bangalore 2014

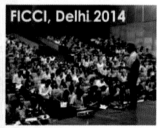

FICCI, Delhi 2014

What Toppers have to say.......

Dr.Apurv Mehra, his motivational classes, books & notes have been of great help to me.   - Dr.Siddharth Jain, Rank 1, AIIMS Nov. 2014

OPQR is the only book I read for Orthopedics, the chapter on Complete Summary Of Orthopedics is just awesome.   - Dr. Ravi Sharma, Rank 2, AIIMS Nov. 2014

Dr. Apurv Mehra's classes, the motivation he provided was of immense help in achieving Rank 4th, AIIMS May 2014. - Dr. Achintya Singh, Rank 4, AIIMS May 2014

'Attend To Be Benefitted Or Miss It Only To Repent'